Grayson's
Diseases of the Cornea

Grayson's Diseases of the Cornea

Robert C. Arffa, M.D.

Adjunct Associate Professor of
Ophthalmology
Medical College of Pennsylvania
Clinical Assistant Professor of
Ophthalmology
University of Pittsburgh School of
Medicine and
The Eye and Ear Institute of Pittsburgh
Pittsburgh, Pennsylvania

Fourth Edition

with 598 illustrations
including 215 in color

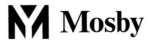 Mosby

St. Louis Baltimore Boston Carlsbad Chicago Naples New York Philadelphia Portland
London Madrid Mexico City Singapore Sydney Tokyo Toronto Wiesbaden

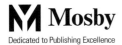

Mosby
Dedicated to Publishing Excellence

A Times Mirror Company

Publisher: Anne S. Patterson
Senior Editor: Laurel Craven
Developmental Editor: Kimberley J. Cox
Project Manager: Chris Baumle
Senior Production Editor: Stacy M. Loonstyn
Design Manager: Nancy J. McDonald
Manufacturing Manager: William A. Winneberger, Jr.
Cover Photo: Robert C. Arffa

FOURTH EDITION

Printed in the United States of America
Composition by Graphic Composition, Inc.
Printing/binding by Walsworth

Mosby–Year Book, Inc.
11830 Westline Industrial Drive
St. Louis, Missouri 63146

Library of Congress Cataloging-in-Publication Data

Arffa, Robert C.
  Grayson's diseases of the cornea. — 4th ed. / Robert C. Arffa.
     p.   cm.
  Includes bibliographical references and index.
  ISBN 0-8151-3654-4
  1. Cornea—Diseases.   I. Grayson, Merrill, 1919–   . II. Title.   III. Title: Diseases of
the cornea.
  [DNLM: 1. Corneal Diseases.   WW 220 A685d 1997]
  RE336.G76   1997
  617.7′19—DC21
DNLM/DLC   97-18628
for Library of Congress   CIP

97 98 99 00 01 / 9 8 7 6 5 4 3 2 1

Dedication

*To Sharon, Rachel, Lauren, and Matthew,
without whose understanding and support
this would not have been possible.*

Preface to the Fourth Edition

The reception to the third edition of *Diseases of the Cornea* was gratifying. In this edition, I have improved the clinical usefulness by adding two chapters on the differential diagnosis of conjunctivitis and corneal disease. These chapters are intended to provide an algorithm to narrow diagnostic possibilities in difficult cases, based on history and appearance.

I also added a new chapter on scleritis and episcleritis, including the diagnosis and treatment of infectious scleritis. The coverage of trauma has been expanded. The use of corneal topography analysis using videokeratography has been added to this edition, with references throughout the book. Many new references and figures have been added.

Diane Curtin has been instrumental with the new photographs. She took many of these slit lamp photographs, helped sort through the University of Pittsburgh archives, and produced many of the images. I am very grateful for her assistance.

Robert C. Arffa

Preface to the First Edition

Resident teaching has always been one of the major aims of my academic career. My desire has been to contribute to this dream by preparing and organizing the material of my major interest in ophthalmology so that it can more easily be assimilated by the student. I hope I have done this with *Diseases of the Cornea*.

Because of the close relationship between the conjunctiva and cornea, some diseases affecting both are discussed in the text. Primary corneal diseases and corneal manifestations of systemic diseases are stressed. Throughout the text, tables provide convenient and rapid association for study. *Diseases of the Cornea* is not to be considered an encyclopedia of corneal disease but a thorough aid to help one correlate and organize the large amount of material concerned. Discussion of therapy is included where it is considered necessary and helpful.

Many colleagues in the field have generously given permission to use their illustrations. Dr. Fred M. Wilson II and I took the color photographs of patients who attended the Cornea Service of the Department of Ophthalmology at Indiana University Medical Center. Kenneth Julian and Gene Louden are to be thanked for their generous aid in preparing many of the illustrations.

I greatly appreciate the work of my associate, Dr. Fred M. Wilson II, whose time, help, suggestions regarding the text, and close association in clinical consultation with numerous problems noted in this book were invaluable.

Merrill Grayson

Contents

Contents

Grayson's
Diseases of the Cornea

One

Anatomy

CONJUNCTIVA

Gross Anatomy

The *conjunctiva* is a mucous membrane that covers the inner surface of the lids and the outer surface of the globe. It allows independent movement of the lids and the globe, provides mucus for lubrication, and contains lymphoid tissue for immunologic protection. The conjunctival epithelium is derived from surface ectoderm.

The conjunctiva begins at the mucocutaneous junction on the lid margin, posterior to the orifices of the meibomian glands. It is firmly adherent to the lids over the tarsi and loosely attached in the fornices and over the globe, except at the limbus. Approximately 2 mm from the tarsal margin is a shallow groove, the subtarsal groove, which marks the transition from the nonkeratinized, stratified squamous epithelium of the lid margin to cuboidal epithelium.

In the primary position, the distance between the limbus and fornix is approximately 10 mm both superiorly and inferiorly (Figs. 1-1 and 1-2). The fornices are maintained by muscle fibers from the levator palpebra superioris and inferior rectus, respectively. The total surface area of the conjunctiva averages 16 cm² per eye.

Two specialized conjunctival structures are present medially, the plica semilunaris and the caruncle. The *plica semilunaris* is a fold of conjunctiva that extends from the superior to inferior fornices. It serves as a source of additional conjunctiva to permit lateral rotation of the globe. The *caruncle,* which lies medial to the plica and measures approximately 4 × 5 mm, is essentially modified skin tissue. Like skin, the caruncle contains hairs, sebaceous glands, and sweat glands. Unlike skin, it also contains lacrimal tissue (Krause's glands), and the surface epithelium is not keratinized.

Microscopic Anatomy

Like all mucous membranes, the conjunctiva has an epithelial layer and a submucosal lamina propria. The structure of the epithelial layer varies greatly in different regions. Stratified squamous epithelium is present on the lid margin, over the most peripheral 2 to 3 mm of the tarsi, and for 2 to 3 mm surrounding the lim-

1

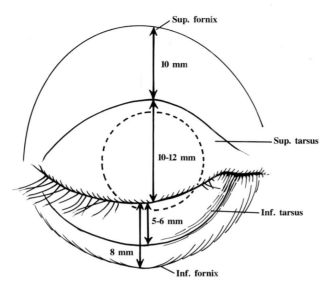

Figure 1-1
Frontal view of the lids and conjunctiva.

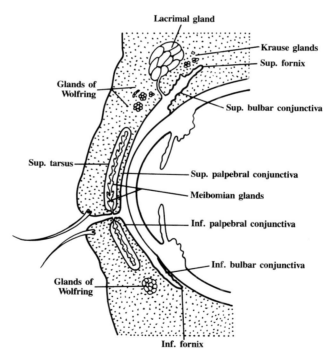

Figure 1-2
Sagittal view of the lids and conjunctiva.

bus. The remainder of the tarsal conjunctiva and the forniceal conjunctiva has from two to five epithelial cell layers, with cuboidal basal cells, cylindric superficial cells, and up to three layers of polyhedral cells between them (Fig. 1-3). The number of cell layers gradually increases over the bulbar conjunctiva, with the superficial cells becoming flatter and the basal cells taller, and increasing the number of polyhedral layers.

Goblet cells, which are mucus-secreting apocrine cells, can be found in all regions of the conjunctiva. They are most numerous over the tarsi and on the plica and least numerous in

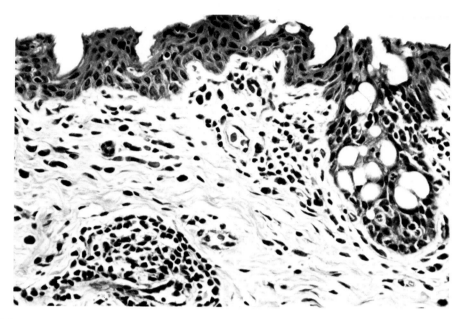

Figure 1-3
Forniceal conjunctiva. The epithelium contains goblet cells, and nests of lymphoid cells are present in the substantia propria. (Hematoxylin-eosin stain, ×500.) (Courtesy of Bruce L. Johnson, Pittsburgh.)

the interpalpebral bulbar conjunctiva. Goblet cells are oval or round, with a flattened nucleus near the base of the cell and a large intracellular collection of mucin (Fig. 1-3). The number of goblet cells can increase in some conjunctival inflammations and decrease in destructive conjunctival processes, such as Stevens-Johnson syndrome or cicatricial pemphigoid.[1]

The surfaces of the conjunctival epithelial cells are covered with microvilli and microplicae as well as a thin coating of glycocalyx and mucin.[2] This coating increases the surface area and aids in attachment of the tear film. The basal epithelial cells are attached to a typical basement membrane by hemidesmosomes. Melanocytes may be found among the basal epithelium.

The conjunctival stroma consists of two layers, a superficial lymphoid layer and a deeper fibrous layer. The lymphoid layer is made up of a connective tissue matrix containing a homogeneous-appearing population of lymphocytes (Fig. 1-3). Normally no germinal follicles are present. The lymphoid layer is not present at birth but begins to form at 6 to 12 weeks of age. Deep to this layer is a fibrous tissue layer, through which run the conjunctival vessels and nerves. This layer varies in thickness and is very limited over the tarsus.

Over the globe, a layer of loose areolar tissue separates the conjunctiva from Tenon's layer,

also called the *episclera*. Tenon's layer contains branches of the anterior ciliary arteries, which have passed forward from the insertions of the extraocular muscles. Approximately 3 to 4 mm from the limbus, Tenon's layer and conjunctiva merge. The conjunctiva and its vessels can normally be moved freely over Tenon's layer and its vessels.

Two types of accessory lacrimal glands are present in the conjunctiva: Krause's glands and the glands of Wolfring. Their structures are similar to that of the lacrimal gland. Krause's glands are located in the upper fornix and in the caruncle in the submucosal connective tissue. The glands of Wolfring are located in the tarsi, at the upper border of the upper tarsus and the lower border of the lower tarsus (Fig. 1-4).

Vascular Supply and Lymphatic Drainage

The conjunctiva receives its blood supply from the muscular, medial palpebral, and lacrimal branches of the ophthalmic artery. The medial palpebral and lacrimal branches form the peripheral, or marginal, arcades of the lids, located between the tarsus and the orbicularis muscle (Fig. 1-5). Branches from these arcades pass through the tarsi to the conjunctiva at about the level of the subtarsal groove. They supply the entire conjunctiva except for the

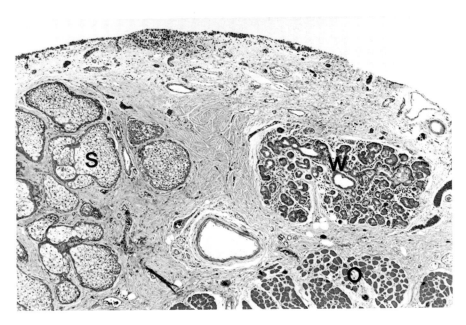

Figure 1-4
Accessory lacrimal gland of Wolfring (*W*). The tarsus and sebaceous glands (*S*) and orbicularis muscle (*O*) can also be seen. (Hematoxylin-eosin stain, ×80.) (Courtesy of Bruce L. Johnson, Pittsburgh.)

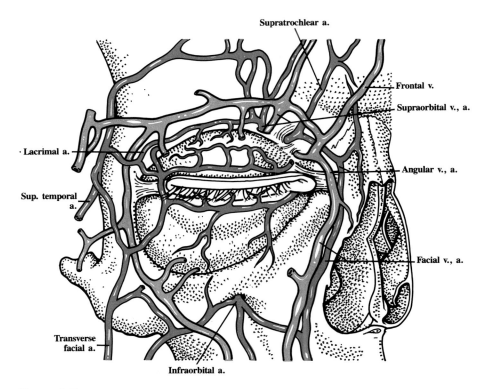

Figure 1-5
Vascular supply of the lids and conjunctiva, frontal view.

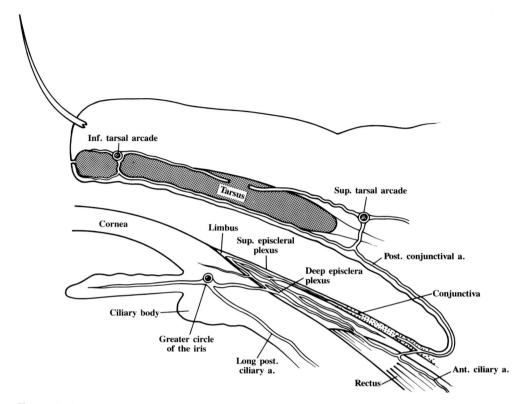

Figure 1-6
Vascular supply of the conjunctiva and cornea, sagittal view.

area lying within 3 to 4 mm of the limbus. In this area there is anastomosis of the conjunctival vessels with the branches of the anterior ciliary arteries in Tenon's layer (Fig. 1-6). The branches from the anterior ciliary artery appear darker than the superficial vessels and do not move with the conjunctiva.

The conjunctival capillaries are fenestrated, similar in structure to those found in the choroid. Under conditions of inflammation, the leakage through these fenestrations can exceed the rate at which the fluid can pass through the conjunctiva to the surface, resulting in chemosis.

Normally, no lymphatics are present in the cornea; however, the conjunctiva has a rich lymphatic network. The lymphatics arise approximately 1 mm from the limbus. Lymphatics in the lateral portions of the conjunctiva drain to the preauricular and intraparotid nodes, and in the medial portions they drain to the submandibular nodes.

Innervation
Sensory innervation of the conjunctiva is supplied by the ophthalmic division of the fifth cranial nerve. In general, the nerve supply of the conjunctiva is from the same source as that of the lid, except that the long ciliary nerves innervate the limbal conjunctiva. The only sensory modality perceived is pain, except for some pressure sensation in the marginal tarsal conjunctiva and the caruncle. Autonomic fibers are also present and are associated with blood vessels.

TEAR FILM

The integrity of the cornea depends on the presence of a precorneal tear film. This layer lubricates the surface of the cornea, is necessary for the health of the epithelial cells, and provides a smooth optic surface for good visual acuity.

The tear film, approximately 7 μm thick, is thickest immediately after a blink and thins progressively until the next blink, or until the tear film breaks up. It consists of three layers (Table 1-1). The outermost layer, the *lipid layer*, is approximately 0.5 μm thick and contains low-polarity lipids such as waxy and cholesterol

Table 1-1 Precorneal Tear Film		
Layer and Source	**Location**	**Function**
INNERMOST: MUCIN (0.2–0.5 μm)		
Conjunctival goblet cells	Most numerous over tarsi and on plica	Reduces surface tension between the epithelial surface and the tear film to enhance spreading of tear film. Lubricates the ocular surface; coats and traps debris
MIDDLE: AQUEOUS (6.5 μm)		
		Source of water, glucose, immunoglobulins, and antimicrobial enzymes
Lacrimal gland	Lacrimal fossa, superior temporal orbit; orbital and palpebral lobes; ducts enter cul-de-sac in superior temporal area	Lacrimal gland is source of reflex section
Accessory lacrimal glands of Krause	Upper conjunctival fornix and caruncle	Accessory glands are primary basal secretors
Accessory lacrimal glands of Wolfring	Adjacent to upper margin of upper tarsus and lower margin of lower tarsus	
SUPERFICIAL LAYER: LIPID (0.5 μm)		
Meibomian glands	About 25 in upper tarsus, 20 in lower tarsus; empty onto lid margin	Retards evaporation of aqueous layer
Gland of Zeis	Palpebral margin of each eyelid; empty directly onto lid margin	
Glands of Moll	Roots of eyelashes; empty into hair follicles	

Modified from Grayson M, Keates RH: *Manual of diseases of the cornea,* Boston, 1969, Little, Brown & Co.

esters.[3] Derived from the secretions of the meibomian glands, the lipid layer's primary function is to retard evaporation.

The *middle layer,* approximately 6.5 μm thick, consists of aqueous tear fluid and contains ions of inorganic salt, glucose, urea, and various proteins, including enzymes, immunoglobulins, complement, and albumin.[4] It is secreted by the main and accessory lacrimal glands. Numerous cells are present in the aqueous tears, derived from the corneal and conjunctival epithelium, the conjunctival lymphoid tissue, and the conjunctival vessels. Lymphocytes are most numerous, followed by desquamated epithelial cells and polymorphonuclear leukocytes.[5]

The third layer of the tear film is a *mucin layer,* which is 0.2 to 0.5 μm thick and coats the epithelial cell surfaces. It is derived from the conjunctival goblet cells. The mucin reduces the surface tension between the epithelial surface and the tear film, enhancing spread of the tear film. Mucus in the tear film also lubricates the ocular surface, reducing friction during lid or eye movement and coating and trapping debris.

CORNEA

Gross Anatomy

The *cornea* is the transparent, anterior portion of the outer shell of the eye, corresponding to a watch crystal. It is spheric but appears slightly elliptic anteriorly because the limbus is more prominent vertically. Anteriorly, the cornea measures about 12.5 × 11.5 mm (Fig. 1-7). It is thinnest centrally, averaging about 0.52 mm, whereas the periphery is approximately 0.65 mm thick. The central one third of the cornea, called the *optical zone,* is almost spheric, with an average radius of curvature of 7.8 mm. The peripheral cornea is less curved, but variably so. The posterior corneal surface is nearly spheric, and its radius of curvature has been estimated to be approximately 6.8 mm.[6] Using these

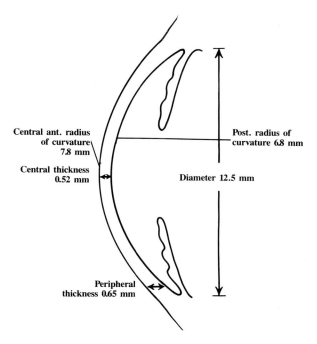

Figure 1-7
Corneal dimensions.

numbers, the refractive power of the anterior surface of the cornea is +48.8 D, and the posterior surface is −5.8 D. The net refractive power of the cornea, therefore, is 43 D, or 70% of the total refractive power of the eye.

In the newborn the cornea is relatively large, averaging 10 mm vertically. Its curvature is also steeper, approximately 51 D at term birth.[7] The average central thickness is approximately 0.585 mm, and the peripheral thickness averages 0.70 to 0.75 mm.[8] In premature infants the cornea is smaller in diameter and steeper in curvature. At 34 weeks, the corneal diameter averages 8.5 mm,[9-11] and corneal curvature averages 52 to 53 D. The cornea continues to grow in diameter and flatten with age, reaching close to adult measurements after the first year of life.[9,12]

Microscopic Anatomy

The cornea consists of five layers: epithelium, Bowman's layer, stroma, Descemet's membrane, and endothelium (Fig. 1-8). In the normal state it does not contain blood or lymphatic vessels.

Epithelium

The *corneal epithelium* is a stratified, squamous, nonkeratinizing epithelium. Approximately five cells deep, it is composed of three types of cells: columnar basal, polygonal wing, and flat

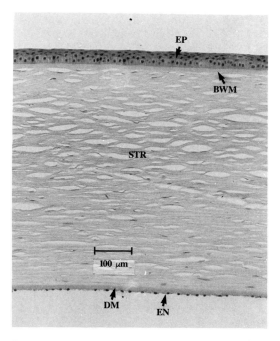

Figure 1-8
Photomicrograph of a cross-section of human cornea showing stratified squamous epithelium (*EP*), Bowman's layer (*BWM*), stroma (*STR*), Descemet's membrane (*DM*), and endothelium (*EN*). (Courtesy of Nirmala Sundar-Raj, Pittsburgh.)

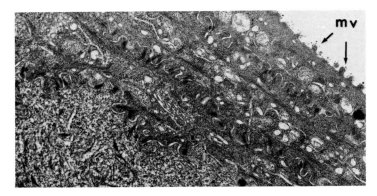

Figure 1-9
Superficial cells are flat, with microvilli (*mv*) on their surface. (From McTigue JW et al: *Clinical application of electron microscopy of the cornea: a course,* Chicago, 1968, American Academy of Ophthalmology and Otolaryngology.)

superficial. The superficial cells lie in two layers. On scanning electron microscopy, flat and mostly hexagonal epithelial cells are seen, attached to each other by straight cell boundaries.[13-15] They exhibit numerous microprojections (microvilli and microplicae) and have an extensive fibrillar glycocalyx, or buffy coat, on their surface membrane (Fig. 1-9). The microprojections enhance the adherence of the tear film to the glycocalyx. Tight junctions are present around the entire lateral borders of each cell, serving as an anatomic barrier to passage of substances into the intercellular space.

The wing cell layer is three cells deep; the more superficial the cell, the flatter its appearance. The nuclei of the wing cells lie parallel to the surface. There is extensive interdigitation of the wing cells, with numerous desmosomal attachments. Mats of tonofilaments, which maintain cell shape, are present.

The deeply situated basal cells compose the single layer of columnar cells that rest on the basement membrane. These cells are rounded on their anterior surface with oval nuclei arranged perpendicularly to the surface (Fig. 1-10). These cells are mitotically active, and the daughter cells that are produced move anteriorly to become wing cells. The basal cells also contain arrays of tonofilaments to maintain cell shape. Actin filaments are present and may play a role in cell migration, such as occurs during wound healing.[16] Unlike basal conjunctival cells, the basal surface of these cells is flat, which is thought to facilitate their adherence. Hemidesmosomes along the basal surface of these cells attach them to the basal lamina.

Other types of cells may be found among the basal epithelial cells. Slender cells with electron-dense cytoplasm and rich rough endoplasmic reticulum (RER) are occasionally seen and may be recently divided cells. Lymphocytes and small cells with dark nuclei and multiple dendritic processes are also found. Peripherally, Langerhans cells, which are antigen-presenting immune cells, are present.

The epithelial cells of the cornea are interdigitated and firmly attached to each other by many desmosomes. These junctions provide mechanical stability to the epithelial layer. Gap junctions are present between all adjacent cells in the epithelium. These serve as conduits through which small molecules may pass from one cell to another.

The cytoplasm of the epithelial cell exhibits a dense matrix containing many fine keratofibrils. The microorganelles generally are sparse but are more evident in basal cells than in wing or superficial cells. Mitochondria are small and not very abundant. The Golgi apparatus and RER are relatively small.

Glycogen particles are seen in the epithelial cells, particularly in basal cells. The amount present varies in different pathologic conditions; in disease, epithelial glycogen stores may be markedly depleted, and the glycogen particles may disappear from epithelial cells during acute wound healing.[17,18]

Epithelial cells appear to migrate centripetally across the corneal surface. Both basal and wing cells slide toward the inferocentral cornea as well as toward the surface, where desquamation occurs (the X-Y-Z hypothesis).[19-22] Thoft and Friend[19] proposed that the centripetal sliding of the basal epithelial cells is caused by a higher mitotic rate and lower superficial cell slough rate in the corneal periphery relative to

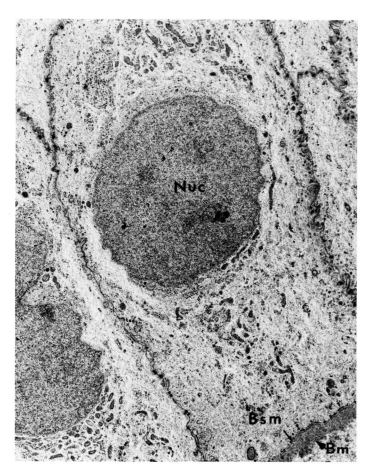

Figure 1-10
Basal cell of the epithelium. The nucleus (*Nuc*) is round, and the basement membrane of the cell (*Bsm*) borders on Bowman's layer (*Bm*). (From McTigue JW et al: *Clinical application of electron microscopy of the cornea: a course,* Chicago, 1968, American Academy of Ophthalmology and Otolaryngology.)

the inferocentral cornea. Stem cells appear to be located in the limbal cornea, especially superiorly (see Limbus). These cells probably give rise to transient amplifying cells, which move centrally and become fully differentiated cells. The basal epithelial nerves appear to move centrally with the epithelial cells.[23]

Beneath the basal layer of epithelial cells, and produced by these cells, is the basal lamina, or basement membrane. It is approximately 500 Å thick, and by electron microscopy is composed of an anterior clear zone, the lamina lucida, and a posterior dark zone, the lamina densa (Fig. 1-11). Biochemically, the epithelial basal lamina appears to be similar to skin basal lamina, containing type IV collagen,[24] laminin,[24,25] fibronectin, fibrin, and bullous pemphigoid antigen.[26,27] Basement membrane, together with its hemidesmosomes and anchor-

ing fibrils, participates in the adherence of the epithelial cells to the stroma (Fig. 1-12). Hemidesmosomes attach the basal epithelial cells to the basal lamina and to anchoring fibrils. Anchoring fibrils, composed of type VII collagen, extend from the basal lamina into the superficial stroma and end in localized plaques, composed of type IV and type VII collagen.[28]

Bowman's Layer
Bowman's layer is an acellular zone, 8 to 10 μm thick, beneath the epithelium. The anterior margin is limited anteriorly by the basement membrane of the epithelium, and the posterior border merges into the anterior stromal collagen fibers. Under the light microscope, Bowman's layer appears homogeneous, but by electron microscopy it is seen to consist of randomly arranged, short collagen fibrils (Fig.

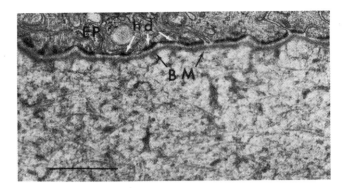

Figure 1-11
The basement membrane (*BM*) is made up of fine granular material and is composed of two layers: lamina lucida and lamina densa. Hemidesmosomes (*hd*) are noted. A basal epithelial cell can also be seen (*EP*). (From Kuwabara T: *Fine structure of the eye,* ed 2, Boston, 1970, Howe Laboratory of Ophthalmology, Harvard Medical School.)

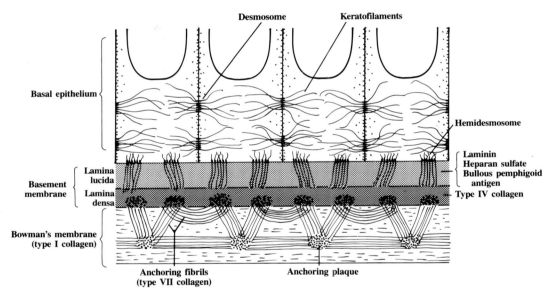

Figure 1-12
Schematic of the mechanism of adherence of the corneal epithelium.

1-13). The collagen fibrils are smaller in diameter, approximately two thirds that of stromal fibrils. In the deeper portions, these fibrils increase in diameter and length and gradually transform into the regular stroma.

Bowman's layer is often said to be resistant to trauma, offering a barrier to corneal invasion by microorganisms and tumor cells, but this has not been proven. Conversely, Bowman's layer is considered to have no regenerative capacity when damaged. A thin layer with a fine structure identical to that of Bowman's layer is formed during wound healing; however, this

secondary type of layer does not regain its original thickness.

Stroma

The *stroma,* which constitutes about 90% of the cornea, consists primarily of collagen fibers, stromal cells, and ground substance. It is approximately 78% water. The collagen fibrils account for about 80% of the dry weight of the cornea, the ground substance for about 15%, and cellular elements for only about 5%. It is well known that the collagen fibrils are arranged in 200 to 300 lamellae parallel to the

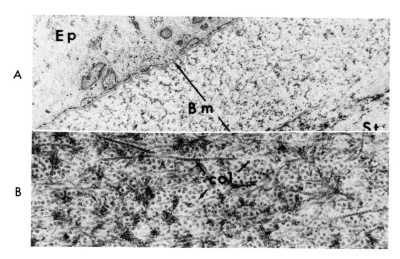

Figure 1-13
A, Bowman's layer (*Bm*) is a noncellular layer seen beneath the epithelium (*Ep*). **B,** Short and fine collagen fibril material (*col*) intermingling in Bowman's layer. (From McTigue JW et al: *Clinical application of electron microscopy of the cornea: a course,* Chicago, 1968, American Academy of Ophthalmology and Otolaryngology.)

tear surface (Fig. 1-14*A*). Interlacing lamellae cross each other in a highly regular fashion, at less than 90° in the anterior stroma and at nearly right angles in the posterior stroma. The lamellae run parallel to each other and to the surface of the cornea, each running the full length of the cornea. Therefore, a cross-section of the stroma will show some fibrils running nearly parallel to the section and some running nearly perpendicular (Fig. 1-14*A*). The layered arrangement of the fibrils facilitates lamellar dissection of the cornea.

The collagen fibrils of the corneal stroma are uniform and small, about 250 to 300 Å in diameter.[29] The fibrils in the stroma are the smallest of those in any tissue in the body, and they show bandings very similar to those of other collagen fibrils. Cross-section reveals that individual fibrils are composed of several subunits of extremely fine fibrils (Fig. 1-14*B*). Type I collagen is the predominant collagen found in the cornea. Types V and VI comprise 10% and 25%, respectively,[30] and type III may also be present.[31] The collagen is relatively stable, with little yearly turnover.[32]

The ground substance surrounding the collagen fibrils is composed primarily of proteoglycans. *Proteoglycans* are a type of glycoprotein composed of noncollagenous protein chains with covalently bound oligosaccharides and glycosaminoglycan (GAG) side chains. GAGs, previously known as mucopolysaccharides, are composed of repeating disaccharide units, typi-

cally a hexosamine plus a uronic acid. In the past, the GAG portions of the proteoglycans were much better characterized than the core proteins, so many proteoglycans were named according to the type(s) of GAG side chain (e.g., chondroitin sulfate proteoglycan). More information is now available about the structure of the core protein, and the nomenclature is changing. More often the proteoglycan is given a single simple name that reflects the properties of the core protein (e.g., aggrecan).

Keratan sulfate and chondroitin sulfate are the primary GAGs of the stroma, in a ratio of approximately 3:1.[33] The core protein that contains the chondroitin/dermatan sulfate chains is *decorin*,[34] which has also been found in other body tissues. The core protein of the proteoglycan containing keratan sulfate is similar to decorin and has been named *lumican*.[35] Lumican is also found in aorta and intestine.

The ground substance may play a role in maintaining the regular array of collagen fibrils. Both decorin and lumican inhibit fibril diameter growth.[36] The core proteins probably bind to the surface of the collagen fibrils and the GAG side chains extend out into the interfibrillar spaces, maintaining fibril spacing.[37] With stromal edema the individual collagen fibril size does not change, the volume of the ground substance increases, and the space between collagen fibrils increases.

The *keratocyte* is the predominant cell of the stroma. There are an average of 2430 kerato-

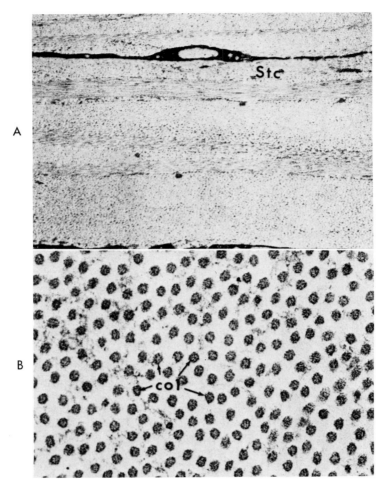

Figure 1-14
A, Corneal stroma consists of a regular arrangement of collagen fibrils parallel to the cell surface.
B, The regularity of a 300 Å diameter collagen fiber (*col*) is noted. *Stc,* Stromal cells. (From McTigue JW et al: *Clinical application of electron microscopy of the cornea: a course,* Chicago, 1968, American Academy of Ophthalmology and Otolaryngology.)

cytes in the cornea.[38] It is a large, flat cell with a number of large processes that extend out from the cell body in a stellate fashion. The cell bodies are seen between packed collagen lamellae, and their processes usually extend within or between the same lamellar planes. Occasionally, the tips of the processes touch neighboring cells. Their cytoplasm contains microorganelles, microtubules, some lysosomes, glycogen particles, lipid particles, and various inclusion bodies (Fig. 1-15). Keratocytes are probably derived from neural crest and maintain the collagen and extracellular matrix of the stroma. Small fibrillar bundles of recently synthesized collagen can be observed adjacent to keratocytes.[39]

In response to stromal injury, the keratocytes migrate into the wound area and undergo transformation into fibroblasts. These transformed cells have increased RER and Golgi complexes and reduced cytoplasmic processes. They contribute to scar formation by proliferation and collagen production.[18] The keratocyte can produce abundant basal lamina in endothelial dystrophy,[39] and in other pathologic conditions, inclusions (e.g., lipid droplets) can be present. The keratocytes accumulate metabolic products in many conditions, such as cystinosis, multiple myeloma, and lysosomal storage diseases, such as the mucopolysaccharidoses and sphingolipidoses. In addition to keratocytes, small numbers of polymorphonu-

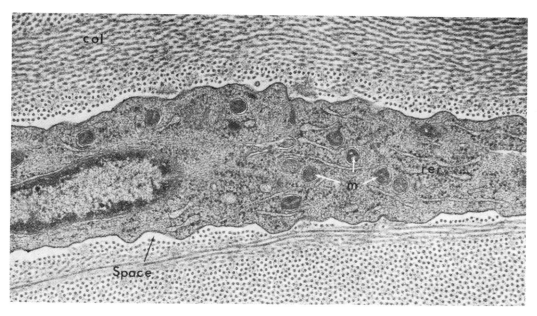

Figure 1-15
This keratocyte is rich in rough endoplasmic reticulum (*rer*) and mitochondria (*m*). A small space can be seen around the keratocyte as it borders stromal collagen (*col*). (From Kuwabara T: *Fine structure of the eye,* ed 2, Boston, 1970, Howe Laboratory of Ophthalmology, Harvard Medical School.)

clear leukocytes, plasma cells, and macrophages are seen in the normal stroma, located between the lamellae of the collagen fibers.

Descemet's Membrane

Descemet's membrane, which is approximately 10 μm thick in adults, is a thick basal lamina produced by the endothelium (Fig. 1-16). *Schwalbe's ring* marks the termination of Descemet's membrane peripherally. On electron microscopy, Descemet's membrane is composed of anterior banded and posterior homogeneous zones. The anterior zone is produced in utero, beginning at approximately 4 months of gestation. The posterior portion is produced after birth and thickens progressively with age. It contains type IV collagen,[40] type VIII collagen,[41] and fibronectin.[42] Peripherally, localized thickenings of Descemet's membrane, called *Hassall-Henle* bodies, are present in the normal eye.

In contrast to Bowman's layer, Descemet's membrane is easily detached from the stroma and regenerates readily after injury. In some pathologic conditions, metallic substances are deposited in Descemet's membrane (e.g., copper in Wilson's disease and silver in argyrosis; see Fig. 24-5). The endothelial cell, when stimulated by inflammation, trauma, or genetic disturbances, can produce excess abnormal basal lamina[43] (which also contains type I collagen[44,45]), causing a thickening of Descemet's membrane and Descemet's wart formation. Thus the multiple layers of Descemet's membrane can provide a morphologic record of previous episodes of disease.

Endothelium

A single layer of flat hexagonal cells lies posteriorly on Descemet's membrane. On scanning electron microscopy, the normal flat surface cells with sharply demarcated borders can be seen (Fig. 1-17). The endothelial cells, more cuboidal in shape and about 10 μm in height at birth, flatten with age to about 4 μm in adults. The endothelium is probably derived from neural crest cells. The cell density decreases from approximately 3500 to 4000 cells/mm² at birth to 2500 to 3000 cells/mm² in the adult cornea, for a total of about 400,000 cells.[46-48]

Generally, there is no mitotic activity in the endothelium after birth. Some endothelial cells die throughout life, resulting in a gradual decrease in the endothelial cell population with age. As cell loss occurs with aging or trauma, the neighboring cells spread out to cover the vacant areas. This results in an increase in cell area and a decrease in cell density. The endothelial cells are capable of preserving function despite tremendous enlargement and generally

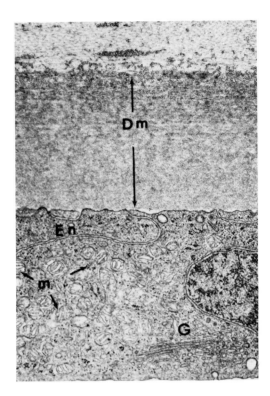

Figure 1-16
Descemet's membrane (*Dm*) is a basement membrane of endothelial cells (*En*). It is rich in Golgi apparatus (*G*) and mitochondria (*m*). (From McTigue JW et al: *Clinical application of electron microscopy of the cornea: a course,* Chicago, 1968, American Academy of Ophthalmology and Otolaryngology.)

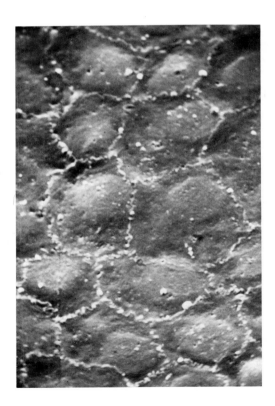

Figure 1-17
Normal orderly arrangement of endothelium with clear-cut cell borders. (From Grayson M: *Trans Am Ophthalmol Soc* 72:517, 1974.)

can maintain corneal function at cell densities as low as 300 to 600 cells/mm^2.

Histologically, these cells exhibit numerous large mitochondria, smooth endoplasmic reticula and RER, a well-developed Golgi apparatus, and free ribosomes. A microvillus may be seen occasionally, but usually the presence of microvilli denotes some pathologic state (Fig. 1-18). A central cilium is present in many endothelial cells; its function is unclear. There is elaborate interdigitation of the lateral walls of adjacent cells (Fig. 1-19), and multiple junctional complexes, including zonulae occludentes, maculae occludentes, and desmosomes are present. Apical focal junctions are not the classic tight junctions, not constituting complete zona occludens, and therefore permit the passage of fluid and molecules. However, there is some resistance to the intercellular passage of substances created by both the elaborate inter-digitation of the cell borders, which increases the distance substances must travel, and localized occlusive cell junctions.[49]

The endothelial cell can show great change in response to pathologic stimulation. Even minor corneal injury can elicit a response: The endothelial cells posterior to a corneal epithelial wound may become swollen and develop numerous protrusions immediately after injury. Following endothelial trauma, damaged endothelial cells slide over the injured area, acting as a reparative element, elaborating new Descemet's membrane where it is absent. In Fuchs' dystrophy the cell appears to have "collapsed," the border is irregular, and the nucleus stands out as a white, raised, fluffy structure. Where there is extreme stress, the endothelial cells may undergo transformation into fibroblast-like cells and elaborate an abnormal posterior collagenous layer (Fig. 1-20).[43]

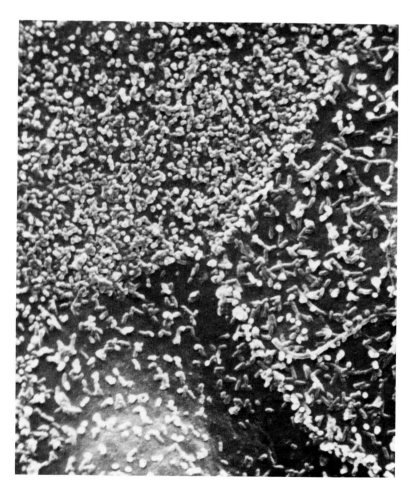

Figure 1-18
Microvilli noted on endothelial cells in pathologic states. (From Grayson M: *Trans Am Ophthalmol Soc* 72:517, 1974.)

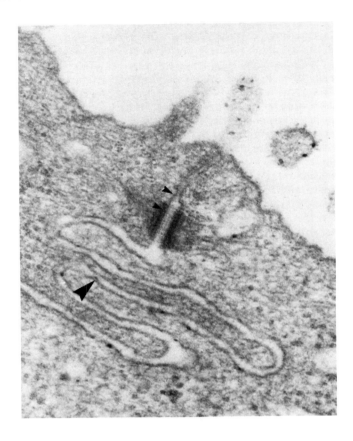

Figure 1-19
Interdigitation of cell borders is prominent (*large arrow*). Endothelial cells are joined by zonula occludens (*small arrows*).

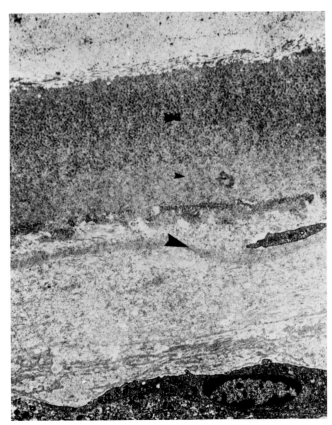

Figure 1-20
Descemet's membrane consists of an anterior banded layer (*medium arrow*) and a nonbanded area (*small arrow*). A multilaminar basement membrane is laid down by altered endothelial cells (*large arrow*).

Innervation

Sensory innervation of the cornea is supplied by the first division of the trigeminal nerve by way of the long ciliary and possibly the short ciliary branches of the nasociliary nerve (Fig. 1-21). The long ciliary nerves enter the eye near the optic nerve and pass anteriorly in the suprachoroidal space. They branch several times before reaching the limbus and may anastomose with branches from the short ciliary nerves, which enter the sclera a few millimeters posterior to the limbus. Recurrent branches pass out through the sclera to innervate the limbal conjunctiva and limbal corneal epithelium. About 70 nerve trunks pierce the cornea at the middle one third of its thickness. The nerves lose their myelin sheath after traversing 0.5 to 2.0 mm into the cornea and then continue as transparent axon cylinders.

The nerves find their way to beneath Bowman's layer where they form a dense subepithelial plexus. They then pierce Bowman's layer to terminate among the epithelial cells as simple axon terminals without specialized sensory organs. However, it appears that there is functional and structural differentiation of the free nerve endings. Nerves responding to mechanical, thermal, and chemical stimuli are found.[50,51] Many of the nerve fibers contain substance P or calcitonin gene-related peptide.[52-56] Adjacent nerves intermingle via numerous connecting elements. The basal epithelial cells are densely supplied with nerves; almost every cell is in contact with a nerve.[57] The basal epithelial nerves have varicosities, which are thought to be axonal efferent and sensory terminals.[45,58] Some nerve trunks proceed into the deep stroma, dividing in a manner similar to that of the superficial fibers, and end among the stromal cells.

Sympathetic fibers also innervate the cornea, although their role is unclear.[59,60] Their cell bodies lie in the superior cervical ganglion, and their axons are carried in the trigeminal nerve, passing with the sensory fibers to the corneal epithelium. β-adrenergic receptors are present on the cell membranes.[61,62] Activation of these receptors stimulates transport of chloride from the cells into the tears (see Chapter 2).

There is a relatively high concentration of extraaxonal acetylcholine in the epithelium, as well as acetylcholinesterase and choline acetyl transferase. Muscarinic cholinergic receptors have also been identified in the epithelial cells. The role of acetylcholine is not known.

After sectioning of the nerve trunks at the

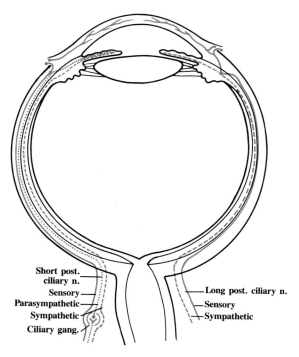

Figure 1-21
Corneal and conjunctival innervation.

limbus, there is a migration of neighboring intact nerves into the denervated area; regeneration of damaged fibers usually takes about 9 months. However, reinnervation after penetrating keratoplasty is limited, with central sensation severely reduced or absent even decades later.[63] Corneal sensitivity is much greater centrally than it is peripherally, and much greater peripherally than on the conjunctiva.

LIMBUS

The *limbus* is the semitransparent, vascularized transition zone between the conjunctiva and sclera on one side and the cornea on the other. Clinically, the peripheral corneal margin blends inconspicuously with the sclera, and the central extent of the limbus is reasonably defined by a line joining the ends of Bowman's layer and Descemet's membrane.

Several changes occur at the limbus. The stroma of the cornea loses its transparency, and the stromal lamellae lose their orderly arrangement. The individual collagen fibers become larger and varied in diameter and arrangement, acquiring the characteristics of the sclera. Bowman's layer terminates in a rounded end at the central margin of the limbus and gives rise to fibrous connective tissue, in which the subepithelial papillae develop in the zone of the palisade.

Clinically, the termination of Bowman's layer is approximately at the apices of the limbal blood vessels. The epithelium of the cornea becomes thicker at the limbus, containing about 12 cell layers (Fig. 1-22). The epithelium projects downward between the subepithelial papillae, which appear as white, radially oriented lines crossing the limbus every 1 to 2 mm. These clinically visible projections are known as the *palisades of Vogt*. Corneal and conjunctival epithelium contain different keratins, allowing for their immunohistochemical differentiation (Fig. 1-23).

The limbus appears to be very important in corneal epithelial regeneration. Limbal epithelium has greater proliferative potential than peripheral or central corneal epithelium[64] and appears to contain a population of stem cells whose daughter cells populate the cornea.[65,66] Stem cells are probably located at the base of the epithelial pegs and possibly in the peripheral superior cornea as well.[67,68] The superior limbus appears to have a larger pool of epithelial cells with stem cell–like characteristics.[69] If the limbus is totally destroyed, as in severe alkali burns or Stevens-Johnson syndrome, there is reduced capacity for epithelial regeneration.

SCLERA

The *sclera* is a roughly spherical shell that averages 22 mm in diameter.[70] The thickness of the sclera varies: It is 0.8 mm at the limbus, 0.4 to 0.5 mm at the equator, 1.0 mm near the optic nerve, 0.3 mm immediately behind the inser-

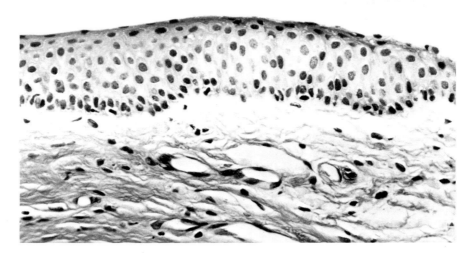

Figure 1-22
Limbal conjunctiva. The epithelium is approximately 12 layers in thickness. (Hematoxylin-eosin stain; ×500.) (Courtesy of Bruce L. Johnson, Pittsburgh.)

tions of the muscle tendons, and 0.6 mm where the tendons attach.[71]

Almost all of the sclera is derived from neural crest cells; a small temporal portion of the sclera is derived from mesoderm. The sclera contains collagen bundles, elastic fibers, fibroblasts, proteoglycans, and melanocytes. The sclera is approximately 68% water.[72] Collagen fibers constitute 75% of its dry weight. In contrast to those of the cornea, the scleral collagen fibrils and bundles vary in diameter and are interlaced in an irregular manner, rather than lying in orderly, regular lamellae.[73] The collagen bundles in the outer sclera are thinner than those in the inner sclera. The scleral collagen is predominantly type I, but types III, V, and VI are also found.[74-76] Less than 2% of the dry weight of the sclera is elastin.[77]

Dermatan sulfate, chondroitin sulfate, heparan sulfate, and hyaluronic acid are present in the ground substance of the sclera.[78] Dermatan sulfate is most common, followed by chondroitin sulfate.[76] Fibroblasts are relatively few in number.

The sclera can be divided into three layers: the episclera, the scleral stroma, and the lamina fusca. The *episclera* is the most superficial portion of the sclera. It is a thin fibrovascular layer, with loosely arranged bundles of collagen that are smaller in diameter and the ground substance more plentiful than in the scleral stroma. The vessels in the anterior episclera are derived mainly from the anterior ciliary arteries, whereas posterior to the insertions of the rectus muscles the episclera is supplied by the posterior ciliary arteries. The vessels are usually inconspicuous in the absence of inflammation. The innermost layer of the sclera is called the *lamina fusca* because of its faint brown color. There are a large number of melanocytes. The collagen bundles are smaller than in the scleral stroma, and some fibers cross the lamina fusca and suprachoroidal space, providing a weak attachment between sclera and choroid. These fibers are most numerous around the emissary canals for the major vessels and nerves.

Vascular Supply

The scleral stroma is relatively avascular. The anterior ciliary arteries run anteriorly from the insertions of the rectus muscles and pass through the sclera to the greater circle of the iris (Fig. 1-6). The anterior ciliary arteries anastomose through their lateral branches to form the anterior episcleral arterial circle. There are also anastomoses with the posterior conjunctival arteries, branches of the inferior and superior palpebral arcades that extend from the fornices in the bulbar conjunctiva. In this region the vessels form several closely connected plexuses: the limbal arcades, an anterior conjunctiva plexus, a superficial episcleral plexus, and a deep episcleral plexus (Fig. 1-6). These feed the limbal, anterior conjunctival, and anterior episcleral tissues.

Innervation

The sclera is densely innervated with branches of the posterior ciliary nerves. The short posterior ciliary nerves supply the posterior sclera, and the long posterior ciliary nerves supply the anterior portion.

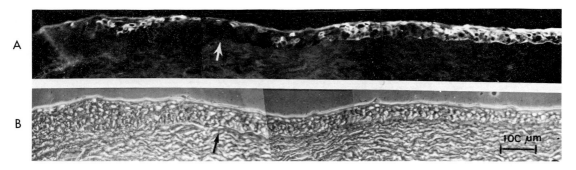

Figure 1-23
Differential distribution of an epithelial basic keratin (*K3*) in the human cornea and limbus, as determined by immunofluorescence staining with the monoclonal antibody AE5. **A,** Immunofluorescent staining. **B,** Corresponding phase contrast micrograph. *Arrows* point to the beginning of Bowman's layer. Note in the limbus (to the left of the arrow) K3 is not detectable in the basal and suprabasal cells. In the cornea (to the right of the arrow), K3 is detectable in all the layers in the central regions but is not detectable in the basal cells in the peripheral region. (Courtesy of Nirmala Sundar-Raj, Pittsburgh.)

REFERENCES

1. Ralph RA: Conjunctival goblet cell density in normal subjects and in dry eye syndromes, *Invest Ophthalmol* 14:299, 1975.
2. Nichols B, Dawson CR, Togni B: Surface features of the conjunctiva and cornea, *Invest Ophthalmol Vis Sci* 24:570, 1983.
3. Brown SI, Dervichian DG: The oils of the meibomian glands: physical and surface characteristics, *Arch Ophthalmol* 82:537, 1969.
4. Records R: *The tear film.* In Duane T, Jaeger E, editors: *Clinical ophthalmology,* vol 4, Philadelphia, 1988, Harper & Row.
5. Norn MS: The conjunctival fluid: its height, volume, density of cells, and flow, *Acta Ophthalmol* 44:212, 1966.
6. Katz M: *The human eye as an optical system.* In Tasman W, Jaeger EA, editors: *Duane's clinical ophthalmology,* vol 1, Philadelphia, 1989, JB Lippincott Co.
7. Donzis PB, Insler MS, Gordon RA: Corneal curvatures in premature infants, *Am J Ophthalmol* 99:213, 1988.
8. Remon L et al: Central and peripheral corneal thickness in full-term newborns by ultrasonic pachymetry, *Invest Ophthalmol Vis Sci* 33:3080, 1992.
9. Isenberg SJ: *The eye in infancy,* Chicago, 1989, Mosby–Year Book, Inc.
10. Tucker SM et al: Corneal diameter, axial length, and intraocular pressure in premature infants, *Ophthalmology* 99:1296, 1992.
11. Al-Umran KU, Pandolfi MF: Corneal diameter in premature infants, *Br J Ophthalmol* 76:292, 1992.
12. Gordon RA, Donzis PB: Refractive development of the human eye, *Arch Ophthalmol* 103:785, 1985.
13. Harding CV et al: A comparative study of corneal epithelial cell surfaces utilizing the scanning electron microscope, *Invest Ophthalmol* 13:906, 1974.
14. Hoffman F: The surface of epithelial cells of the cornea under the scanning electron microscope, *Ophthalmol Res* 3:207, 1972.
15. Pfister RR: The normal surface of corneal epithelium: scanning electron microscopic study, *Invest Ophthalmol* 12:654, 1973.
16. Gipson IL, Anderson RA: Actin filaments in normal and migrating corneal epithelial cells, *Invest Ophthalmol Vis Sci* 16:161, 1977.
17. Kuwabara T, Perkins DG, Cogan DG: Sliding of the epithelium in experimental corneal wounds, *Invest Ophthalmol* 15:4, 1976.
18. Robb RM, Kuwabara T: Corneal wound healing. I: The movement of polymorphonuclear leukocytes into corneal wounds, *Arch Ophthalmol* 68:632, 1962.
19. Thoft RA, Friend J: The X,Y,Z hypothesis of corneal epithelial maintenance, *Invest Ophthalmol Vis Sci* 24:1442, 1983.
20. Sharma A, Coles WH: Kinetics of corneal epithelial maintenance and graft loss: a population balance model, *Invest Ophthalmol Vis Sci* 30:1962, 1989.
21. Lemp MA, Mathers WD: Renewal of the corneal epithelium, *CLAO J* 17:258, 1991.
22. Lemp MA, Mathers WD: Corneal epithelial cell movement in humans, *Eye* 3:348, 1989.
23. Auran JD et al: Scanning slit confocal microscopic observation of cell morphology and movement within the normal human anterior cornea, *Ophthalmology* 102:33, 1995.
24. Madri JA et al: *The ultrastructural organization and architecture of basement membranes.* In Porter R, Whelan J, editors: *Basement membranes and cell movement,* CIBA Foundation Symposium, vol 108, London, 1984, Pitman Press.
25. Madri JA et al: Ultrastructural localization of fibronectin and laminin in the basement membrane of the murine kidney, *J Cell Biol* 86:682, 1980.
26. Masutani M et al: Detection of specific collagen types in normal and keratoconus corneas, *Invest Ophthalmol Vis Sci* 20:738, 1981.
27. Millin JA, Golub BM, Foster CS: Human basement membrane components of keratoconus and normal corneas, *Invest Ophthalmol Vis Sci* 27:604, 1986.
28. Gipson IK, Spurr-Michaud SJ, Tisdale A: Anchoring fibrils form a complex network in human and rabbit cornea, *Invest Ophthalmol Vis Sci* 28:212, 1987.
29. Komai Y, Ushiki T: The three-dimensional organization of collagen fibrils in the human cornea and sclera, *Invest Ophthalmol Vis Sci* 32:2244, 1991.
30. Doane KJ, Yang G, Birk DE: Corneal cell-matrix interactions: type IV collagen promotes adhesion and spreading of corneal fibroblasts, *Exp Cell Res* 200:490, 1992.
31. Freeman IL: Collagen polymorphism in mature rabbit cornea, *Invest Ophthalmol Vis Sci* 17:171, 1978.
32. Smelser GK, Pollack FM, Ozaniks V: Persistence of donor collagen in corneal transplants, *Exp Eye Res* 4:349, 1965.
33. Praus R, Brettschneider I: Glycosaminoglycans in embryonic and postnatal human cornea, *Ophthalmic Res* 7:542, 1975.
34. Li W et al: cDNA clone to chick corneal chondroitin/dermatan sulfate proteoglycan reveals identity to decorin, *Arch Biochem Biophys* 296:190, 1992.
35. Blochberger TC et al: cDNA to chick lumican (corneal keratan sulfate proteoglycan) reveals homology to the small interstitial proteoglycan gene family and expression in muscle and intestine, *J Biol Chem* 267:347, 1992.
36. Friend J, Hassal JR: *Biochemistry of the cornea.* In Thoft RA, Smolin G, editors: *The cornea: scientific foundations and clinical practice,* Boston, 1994, Little, Brown & Co.
37. Scott JE: Proteoglycan: collagen interactions and corneal ultrastructure, *Biochem Eye* 19:877, 1991.

38. Moller-Pederson T, Ledet T, Ehlers N: The keratocyte density of human donor corneas, *Curr Eye Res* 13:163, 1994.

39. Kuwabara T: Current concepts in anatomy and histology of the cornea, *Contact Intraocular Lens Med J* 4:101, 1978.

40. Kefalides N: Structure and biosynthesis of basement membranes, *Int Rev Connect Tissue Res* 6:63, 1973.

41. Kapoor R et al: Type VIII collagen has a restricted distribution in specialized extracellular matrices, *J Cell Biol* 107:721, 1988.

42. Newsome DA et al: Detection of specific collagen types in normal and keratoconus corneas, *Invest Ophthalmol Vis Sci* 20:738, 1981.

43. Waring GO, Laibson PR, Rodrigues M: Clinical and pathologic alterations of Descemet's membrane, with emphasis on endothelial metaplasia, *Surv Ophthalmol* 18:325, 1974.

44. Kenney C et al: Analyses of collagens from ultrastructurally pure Descemet's membrane and cultured endothelial cells, *Invest Ophthalmol Vis Sci* 17(suppl):253, 1978.

45. Perlman M, Baum JL, Kaye GI: Fine structure and collagen synthetic activity of monolayer cultures of rabbit corneal endothelium, *J Cell Biol* 63:306, 1974.

46. Nucci P et al: Normal endothelial cell density range in childhood, *Arch Ophthalmol* 108:247, 1990.

47. Laing RA et al: Changes in the corneal endothelium as a function of age, *Exp Eye Res* 22:587, 1976.

48. Laule A et al: Endothelial cell population changes of human cornea during life, *Arch Ophthalmol* 96:2031, 1978.

49. Kreutziger GO: Lateral membrane morphology and gap junction structure in rabbit corneal endothelium, *Exp Eye Res* 23:285, 1986.

50. Galar J et al: Response of sensory units with unmyelinated fibres to mechanical, thermal, and chemical stimulation of the cat's cornea, *J Physiol (Lond)* 468:609, 1993.

51. MacIver MB, Tanelian DK: Structural and functional specialization of A delta and C fiber free nerve endings innervating rabbit corneal epithelium, *J Neurosci* 13:4511, 1993.

52. Tervo K et al: Substance P-immunoreactive nerves in the human cornea and iris, *Invest Ophthalmol Vis Sci* 23:671, 1982.

53. LaVail JH, Johnson WE, Spencer LC: Immunohistochemical identification of trigeminal ganglion neurons that innervate the mouse cornea: relevance to intercellular spread of herpes simplex virus, *J Comp Neurol* 327:133, 1993.

54. Beckers HJ et al: Substance P in rat corneal and iridal nerves: an ultrastructural immunohistochemical study, *Ophthalmic Res* 25:192, 1993.

55. Stone RA, McGlinn AM: Calcitonin gene-related peptide immunoreactive nerves in human and rhesus monkey eyes, *Invest Ophthalmol Vis Sci* 29:305, 1988.

56. Ueda S et al: Peptidergic and catecholaminergic fibers in the human corneal epithelium: an immunohistochemical and electron microscopic study, *Acta Ophthalmol* 192(suppl):80, 1989.

57. Duke-Elder S, Wybar KC: *The anatomy of the visual system.* In Duke-Elder S, editor: *System of ophthalmology,* St. Louis, 1961, The CV Mosby Co.

58. Matsuda A: Electron microscopic study on the corneal nerve with special reference to its endings, *Jpn J Ophthalmol* 12:163, 1968.

59. Klyce SD et al: Distribution of sympathetic nerves in the rabbit cornea, *Invest Ophthalmol Vis Sci* 27(suppl):354, 1986.

60. Marfurt CF, Ellis LC: Immunohistochemical localization of tyrosine hydroxylase in corneal nerves, *J Comp Neurol* 336:517, 1993.

61. Canadia OA, Neufeld AJ: Topical epinephrine causes a decrease in density of beta adrenergic receptors and catecholamine stimulated chloride transport on the rabbit cornea, *Biochem Biophys Acta* 543:403, 1978.

62. Fogle JA, Neufeld AH: The adrenergic and cholinergic corneal epithelium, *Invest Ophthalmol Vis Sci* 18:1212, 1979.

63. Rao GN et al: Recovery of corneal sensitivity in grafts following penetrating keratoplasty, *Ophthalmology* 92:1408, 1985.

64. Ebato B, Friend J, Thoft R: Comparison of limbal and peripheral human corneal epithelium in tissue culture, *Invest Ophthalmol Vis Sci* 29:1533, 1988.

65. Schermer A, Galvlin S, Sun T: Differentiation-related expression of a major 64K corneal keratin in vivo and in culture suggests limbal location of corneal epithelial stem cells, *J Cell Biol* 103:49, 1986.

66. Thoft RA, Wiley LA, Sundar-Raj N: The multipotential cells of the limbus, *Eye* 3:109, 1989.

67. Lauweryns B, van den Oord JJ, Missotten L: A new epithelial cell type in the human cornea, *Invest Ophthalmol Vis Sci* 34:1983, 1993.

68. Lauweryns B, van den Oord JJ, Missotten L: The transitional zone between limbus and peripheral cornea: an immunohistochemical study, *Invest Ophthalmol Vis Sci* 34:1991, 1993.

69. Wiley L et al: Regional heterogeneity in human cornea and limbal epithelia: an immunohistochemical evaluation, *Invest Ophthalmol Vis Sci* 32:594, 1991.

70. Spencer WH: *Sclera.* In Spencer WH, editor: *Ophthalmic pathology,* ed 3, Philadelphia, 1985, WB Saunders Co.

71. Vannas S, Teir H: Observations on structure and age changes in the human sclera, *Acta Ophthalmol* 38:268, 1960.

72. Dische J: Biochemistry of connective tissues of the vertebrate eye, *Int Rev Connect Tissue Res* 5:209, 1970.

73. Komai Y, Ushiki T: The three-dimensional organization of collagen fibrils in the human cornea and sclera, *Invest Ophthalmol Vis Sci* 32:2244, 1991.

74. Keeley RW, Morin JD, Vesely S: Characterization of collagen from normal human sclera, *Exp Eye Res* 39:533, 1984.

75. Tengroth B, Rehnberg M, Amitzboll T: A comparative analysis of the collagen type and distribution in the trabecular meshwork, sclera, lamina cribrosa and the optic nerve in the human eye, *Acta Ophthalmol (Copenh)* 63(suppl 173):91, 1985.

76. Foster CS, Sainz de la Maza M: *The sclera,* New York, 1994, Springer-Verlag.

77. Moses RA et al: Elastic content of the scleral spur, trabecular meshwork, and sclera, *Invest Ophthalmol Vis Sci* 17:817, 1978.

78. Trier K, Olsen EB, Ammitzboll T: Regional glycosaminoglycan composition of the human sclera, *Acta Ophthalmol (Copenh)* 68:304, 1990.

Two

Physiology

METABOLISM

The cells of the cornea—epithelium, kerato-cytes, and endothelium—are metabolically active and require nutrients for their function. The metabolism of the corneal epithelium is most readily studied and therefore best understood.

Epithelium

The major nutrients required by the epithelium are glucose, oxygen, vitamins, and amino acids. The catabolism of glucose and glycogen is the main energy source for the epithelial cells. Most of the glucose is derived from the aqueous humor; 10% or less comes from the limbal vessels or tears. The epithelium is also able to store large amounts of glycogen, which can be mobilized when the supply of free glucose is insufficient (e.g., hypoxia and trauma), and can metabolize alanine (through gluconeogenesis) as well.[1]

Glucose is catabolized through both aerobic pathways, including the tricarboxylic acid (TCA) (Krebs') cycle and hexose monophosphate shunt, and anaerobic pathways (Fig. 2-1). The relative roles of these pathways have not been determined, but it is thought that the TCA cycle is not very active because it takes place in mitochondria, and mitochondria are not very abundant in the epithelium.[2,3] In vitro, 35% of the glucose used by the epithelium passes through the hexose monophosphate shunt. The catabolism of glucose through these pathways produces ATP and nicotinamide–adenine dinucleotide phosphate (NADPH), high-energy compounds that are then used in cellular processes.

Anaerobic glycolysis produces pyruvate and lactate, which, under aerobic conditions, can then be converted to carbon dioxide by the TCA cycle. The carbon dioxide is readily eliminated by diffusion across the endothelium and epithelium and by conversion to bicarbonate by the endothelium. Lactate cannot pass through the epithelium and must diffuse through the stroma and endothelium into the aqueous humor.[4] During hypoxia or other times of corneal stress, lactate accumulates and can cause localized acidosis and an increased

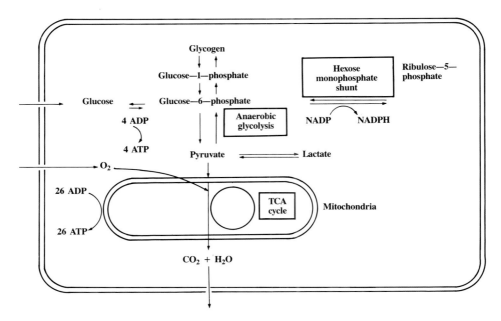

Figure 2-1
Epithelial glucose metabolism.

osmotic solute load. This effect can result in epithelial and stromal edema and possibly alter endothelial morphology and function.[4,5]

Most of the oxygen taken in by the cornea is consumed by the epithelium and the endothelium. Oxygen is supplied mainly by diffusion from the tear film. The oxygen tension in the aqueous humor is probably 30 to 40 mm Hg,[6] which is not sufficient to meet epithelial metabolic needs. When the eye is open, atmospheric oxygen enters the tears, and the partial pressure of oxygen is approximately 155 mm Hg. When the lids are closed, oxygen enters the tears only by diffusion from the conjunctival blood vessels, and the partial pressure falls to about 55 mm Hg.[7]

The use of contact lenses and intrastromal lenses for correction of refractive errors has increased our awareness of corneal oxygenation and nutrition. Successful contact lens wear requires an adequate supply of oxygen to the epithelium. With oxygen-impermeable (e.g., polymethylmethacrylate) lenses, tear flow beneath the lens must carry oxygenated tears to the central epithelium (Fig. 2-2B). Hydrophilic soft contact lenses and oxygen-permeable (e.g., silicone, fluoropolymer) rigid lenses supply oxygen both by diffusion through the lens and by tear flow (Fig. 2-2C,D). Oxygen supply is most limited beneath the upper lid and during sleep, when tear oxygen tension is reduced. When impermeable lenses such as polysulfone are placed in the corneal stroma, glucose and other nutrients must diffuse around the lens to reach the anterior epithelium and keratocytes. If the lenses are too large or too anterior, such that the supply of nutrients is inadequate, the anterior cornea melts. Amino acids, vitamins, and other nutrients are supplied to the epithelium principally by the aqueous humor.

Endothelium

The endothelium appears to contain the same aerobic and anaerobic glycolytic pathways as the epithelium, although their activities are lower. The major energy source is glucose, which is derived from the aqueous humor. The ability of the endothelium to store glycogen is not known. Unlike the epithelium, the endothelial oxygen need is met by the aqueous humor. Glutathione is also important for normal endothelial function.[8] Most likely it plays a role in the elimination of free radicals and toxic peroxides formed during light exposure.[9,10]

CONTROL OF STROMAL HYDRATION

The control of corneal stromal hydration is essential for transparency. Water accounts for 78% of the weight of the cornea, higher than most connective tissues elsewhere in the body. Hydration can also be described as the ratio of

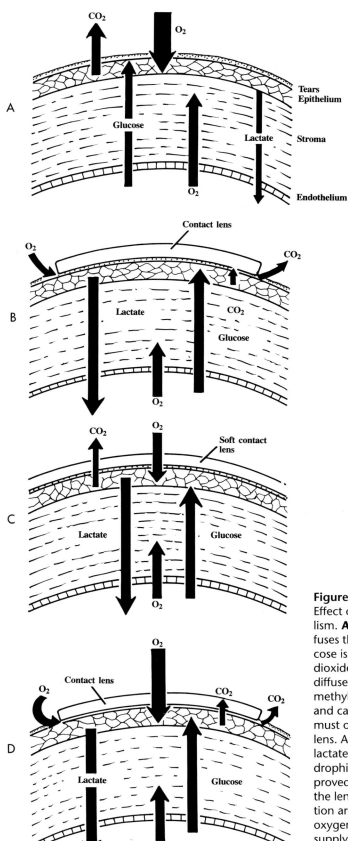

Figure 2-2
Effect of contact lens wear on epithelial metabolism. **A,** Normal state. Most of the oxygen diffuses through the tears from the atmosphere; glucose is supplied by the aqueous humor; carbon dioxide is released into the atmosphere; lactate diffuses into the aqueous humor. **B,** During polymethylmethacrylate lens wear, oxygen supply and carbon dioxide release are impaired and must occur through passage of tears beneath the lens. As a result of hypoxia, glucose demand and lactate production are increased. **C,** During hydrophilic contact lens wear, oxygen supply is improved because some oxygen can pass through the lens, but glucose demand and lactate production are increased moderately. **D,** With highly oxygen-permeable rigid contact lenses, oxygen supply, glucose demand, and lactate production are near normal.

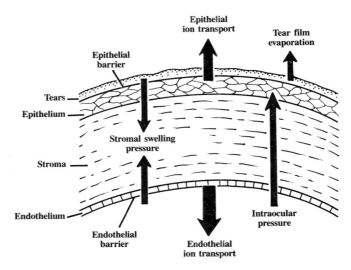

Figure 2-3
Control of stromal hydration.

water (by weight) to dry weight of tissue. The normal hydration of the cornea is 3.45. If the hydration is increased to 6.8, or 87% of the weight of the cornea, the thickness doubles.

Several mechanisms play a role in the regulation of corneal hydration (Fig. 2-3):

1. Barrier function of the epithelium and endothelium
2. Swelling pressure of the stroma
3. Ionic transport by the epithelium and endothelium
4. Intraocular pressure
5. Evaporation of water from the corneal surface

Barrier Function of the Epithelium and Endothelium

Both the epithelium and the endothelium act as barriers to the movement of water and ions into the stroma. The greatest resistance to electrolyte diffusion lies in the epithelium, primarily the surface layers.[11-13] The epithelial cell outer membranes are relatively impermeable to the passage of ions, and the epithelial cells are connected to surrounding cells by tight junctions, which, although not as effective as the cell membranes, also significantly impede ion flow.[14]

Comparatively, the endothelium is 200 times more permeable to electrolytes than is the epithelium, but it is still 10 times more resistant than the stroma.[11-13] The resistance to intercellular passage of ions is created by both the elaborate interdigitation of the cell borders, in-

creasing the distance substances must travel, and by localized occlusive cell junctions.[15]

Swelling Pressure of the Stroma

If the epithelium and endothelium are removed, the corneal stroma will swell to approximately twice its normal thickness as a result of imbibition of water by the stromal ground substance. The glycosaminoglycans of the ground substance are negatively charged and repel each other. They also have a tendency to take on cations to preserve ionic charge neutrality (Donnan's equilibrium). The stromal swelling pressure is approximately 50 to 60 mm Hg at normal thickness and decreases exponentially as the stroma swells.[16,17] Therefore, at normal thickness the stromal swelling pressure must be counterbalanced by a force that moves water out of the stroma.

Ionic Transport by the Epithelium and Endothelium

It was demonstrated in the 1950s that active metabolic processes are necessary for maintenance of normal stromal hydration.[18,19] Lowering corneal temperature, blocking anaerobic glycolysis, or depriving the cornea of oxygen or glucose will lead to stromal swelling. It was also suspected that the endothelium played the greater role, because its removal had the greater effect.

It is now well established that the endothelium is responsible for active dehydration of the cornea.[20] Although it was originally referred to as an endothelial "fluid pump," the mechanism appears to be one of active transport of ions from the stroma into the aqueous humor, with passive, secondary movement of water. The exact process remains unclear, but the endothelium actively transports bicarbonate[21,22] and sodium[23] from the stroma to the aqueous humor. The main pump enzymes, Na^+-K^+-ATPase and carbonic anhydrase, are located on the lateral plasma membranes of the endothelium. This ion transport creates an osmotic gradient (2 to 3 mOsm), which balances the swelling pressure of the corneal stroma.[24,25]

There is also evidence for ion transport in the corneal epithelium, which may also play a role, although certainly a much smaller one. The epithelium secretes chloride into the tears by active transport,[26,27] which is regulated by a β-adrenergic receptor and is mediated intracellularly by adenylate cyclase.[28] A Na^+-K^+-ATPase pump and Na^+-Cl^- cotransporter present in the basolateral epithelial cell membrane actively transport Na^+ and Cl^- into the cells. The sodium and chloride ions diffuse toward the apical surface and into the tears through gap junctions. Cyclic AMP increases the permeability of these junctions and the conductance of chloride molecules.[29]

The adrenergic receptors probably respond to catecholamines released by the sympathetic nerve fibers present in the epithelium and possibly also to other neurotransmitters.[30] In the frog[31] and in the rabbit[32] the corneal epithelium is capable both of secreting chloride and fluid and of thinning the stroma. However, this has not yet been demonstrated in primates.

The corneal epithelial cells also have a Na^+-H^+ exchanger and a lactate-H^+ cotransporter, which are active along the basal membrane.[33] They help regulate intracellular pH by transporting H^+ and lactate out of the cell.

Intraocular Pressure

In the normal eye, intraocular pressure (IOP) has little effect on stromal thickness. However, when the IOP exceeds the stromal swelling pressure, epithelial edema occurs. Thus epithelial edema occurs in the normal cornea when the IOP exceeds 55 mm Hg. However, if endothelial function decreases and the stroma thickens to 0.60 mm, epithelial edema will occur at an IOP of approximately 30 mm Hg. After penetrating keratoplasty, corneal thickness is much more responsive to IOP; increasing the IOP thins the donor cornea, whereas decreasing it thickens the donor. The mechanism for this process has not been established, but it is thought to be related to the anterior stromal lamellae bearing the stress of IOP.[34]

Evaporation of Water from the Corneal Surface

Evaporation of water from the tear film results in hypertonicity of the tears and draws water from the epithelial cells and subsequently from the stroma. Evidence for this effect is that the cornea is 5% thinner during waking hours than during sleep.[35] In addition, in patients with borderline endothelial function, vision is often worse in the morning and improves over the course of the day. However, the ability of tear evaporation to thin the stroma is normally quite limited because blinking and reflex tearing rapidly restore isotonicity. Only in eyes without normal tear flow or surfacing (e.g., dellen) can significant stromal thinning occur.

CORNEAL TRANSPARENCY

The cornea transmits approximately 90% of light in the visible spectrum. (However, all light with a wavelength of 300 nm or less, and the majority of light with a wavelength greater than 1400 nm, is absorbed.) The need for corneal transparency is obvious, but the mechanism by which this is achieved has long been obscure. The lack of blood and lymph vessels, the absence of myelin sheaths around the corneal nerves, and proper hydration of the stroma are certainly necessary. Why then is the corneal stroma transparent, whereas other tissues with similar mixtures of collagen fibrils and ground substance (e.g., sclera) are not? Dry collagen has a refractive index of 1.55, whereas the ground substance has a refractive index of 1.35; normally such disparity produces light scatter, and the tissue is opaque.

Maurice[36] suggested that the tight packing and regular lattice arrangement of the stromal collagen fibrils is responsible. Light scattered by individual fibers is cancelled by destructive interference with scattered light from neighboring fibers. As long as the fibers are arranged regularly and separated by less than a wavelength of light, the cornea will remain transparent. However, if the stroma is edematous, the space between the fibers increases, destructive interference no longer occurs, light is scattered, and corneal transparency is reduced.

More recently, it has been determined that a regular lattice arrangement of the collagen fibers is not necessary for transparency. In Bowman's layer the collagen fibrils are arranged irregularly, and the shark cornea also contains regions of disorganized collagen fibrils.[37] Goldman and Benedek[37,38] and others[39] concluded that appreciable light scattering does not occur unless regional fluctuations in refractive index exceed 2000 Å. (The wavelengths of visible light is 4000 to 7000 Å.) The corneal stroma does not scatter light because its collagen fibrils are small in diameter (approximately 300 Å) and closely spaced (approximately 550 Å). Corneal clouding occurs when variations in refractive index occur over areas greater than 2000 Å in diameter. Stromal swelling can increase interfibrillar distance to greater than this amount.[40]

DRUG PENETRATION

Mixing in the Tears

When drugs intended to act in the corneal stroma or anterior chamber are administered as drops, they must overcome several obstacles before they can exert their therapeutic effect. The penetration of any drug is affected by its concentration on the surface and the time of contact, that is, for topical ocular medications, the concentration achieved in tears and the persistence of the medication in the tears.

The volume of a drop from a standard medication bottle is approximately 40 μl, whereas the volume of tears on the surface of the eye is only about 10 μl.[41] Therefore, much of the medication is immediately lost onto the eyelashes. Some extra volume can be retained (up to 25 μl), but blinking or squeezing of the lids in response to the drop reduces the excess. In addition, the medication becomes diluted by the tears already in the eye to approximately 25% of that in the drop.[42] Therefore, both the volume and concentration of the drop are immediately reduced. Smaller, more concentrated drops of medication would be more effective, but they are not marketed because of increased manufacturing costs.

After initial mixing, the drug is diluted progressively by new tear secretion. In the normal eye, with a relatively nonirritating drug, the concentration is reduced about 90% by tearing alone in 20 minutes. Tear concentration is also reduced by absorption of the drug into the eye; and for some lipophilic drugs (e.g., pilocarpine), the combination of absorption and dilution reduced tear concentration to 10% of its starting value in only 4 minutes.[43] If the drop is irritating, reflex tearing occurs and the dilution is even more rapid. Irritation is caused primarily by a pH or osmolality far from that of the tears.

Ophthalmic ointments are composed of drug particles suspended in an oleaginous base. The purpose of ointment administration is to increase the time that drug is present in the tears. The ointment is retained in the cul-de-sac and gradually melts, releasing the drug into the tears. This theoretic advantage is not always realized, however; aqueous humor levels of tetracycline and chloramphenicol were found to be higher after administration of ointment preparations than solutions,[44,45] but levels of dexamethasone were much lower.[46]

Corneal Penetration

Topically applied drugs reach the corneal stroma and aqueous humor only through the cornea; nearly all of the drug penetrating the conjunctiva is carried away by blood vessels. To penetrate the cornea, a drug must pass through both the epithelium and the stroma, which are very different types of barriers. Because the epithelium is cellular and composed largely of lipid membranes, nonpolar substances penetrate readily, but polar, or hydrophilic, substances penetrate poorly. The stroma, on the other hand, is composed primarily of water, and polar groups pass through it more easily. Because drugs must pass through both barriers, those soluble in both lipid and water exhibit the best penetration. However, hydrophilic compounds of very low molecular weight penetrate rapidly, apparently in the intercellular spaces of the epithelium.[47,48]

Many ophthalmic medications are weak bases, which tend to penetrate well because they exist in an equilibrium between a neutral and an ionic form. The neutral form penetrates the epithelium well; once in the stroma the equilibrium shifts to favor the ionic form. The ions are able to pass through the stroma to the endothelium, where the reverse process occurs.

If the epithelium is not intact, such as after a corneal abrasion or during treatment of an infectious ulcer, hydrophilic drugs are much more effective. Inflammation also increases drug penetration, but to a lesser extent. Some preservatives and surfactants present in drug formulations, such as benzalkonium chloride, impair the integrity of the epithelial barrier and increase penetration.

REFERENCES

1. Gottsch JD et al: Corneal alanine metabolism demonstrated by NMR spectroscopy, *Curr Eye Res* 7:253, 1988.
2. Kinoshita JH: Some aspects of the carbohydrate metabolism of the cornea, *Invest Ophthalmol* 1:178, 1962.

3. Thoft RA, Friend J: Corneal epithelial glucose metabolism, *Arch Ophthalmol* 88:58, 1971.

4. Klyce SD: Stromal lactate accumulation can account for corneal edema osmotically following epithelial hypoxia in the rabbit, *J Physiol* 321:49, 1981.

5. Huff JW: Effects of sodium lactate on isolated rabbit corneas, *Invest Ophthalmol Vis Sci* 31:942, 1990.

6. Klyce SD, Beuerman RW: *Structure and function of the cornea.* In Kaufman HE et al, editors: *The cornea,* New York, 1988, Churchill Livingstone.

7. Efron N, Carney LG: Oxygen levels beneath the closed eyelid, *Invest Ophthalmol Vis Sci* 18:93, 1979.

8. Dikstein S, Maurice DM: The metabolic basis of the fluid pump of the cornea, *J Physiol (Lond)* 221:29, 1955.

9. Riley MV et al: Oxidized glutathione in the corneal endothelium, *Exp Eye Res* 30:607, 1981.

10. Ng MC, Riley MV: Relation of intracellular levels and redox state of reduced glutathione to endothelium function in the rabbit cornea, *Exp Eye Res* 30:511, 1980.

11. Maurice DM: The permeability to sodium ions of the living rabbit's cornea, *J Physiol (Lond)* 112:367, 1951.

12. Maurice DM: *Cornea and sclera.* In Davson H, editor: *The eye,* ed 3, New York, 1984, Academic Press.

13. Mishima S, Hedbys BO: The permeability of the corneal epithelium and endothelium, *Exp Eye Res* 6:10, 1967.

14. Marshall WS, Klyce SD: Cellular and paracellular pathway resistances in the "tight" Cl⁻-secreting epithelium of the rabbit cornea, *J Membr Biol* 73:275, 1983.

15. Kreutziger GO: Lateral membrane morphology and gap junction structure in rabbit corneal endothelium, *Exp Eye Res* 23:285, 1986.

16. Dohlman CH, Hedbys BO, Mishima S: The swelling pressure of the corneal stroma, *Invest Ophthalmol Vis Sci* 1:158, 1962.

17. Hedbys BO, Dohlman CH: A new method for the determination of the swelling pressure of the corneal stroma in vitro, *Exp Eye Res* 1:122, 1963.

18. Davson H: The hydration of the cornea, *Biochem J* 59:24, 1955.

19. Harris JE, Nordquist LT: The hydration of the cornea, *Am J Ophthalmol* 40:100, 1955.

20. Maurice DM: The location of the fluid pump in the cornea, *J Physiol (Lond)* 221:43, 1972.

21. Hodson S, Miller F: The bicarbonate ion pump in the endothelium which regulates the hydration of the rabbit cornea, *J Physiol* 263:563, 1976.

22. Hull DS et al: Corneal endothelium bicarbonate transport and the effect of carbonic anhydrase inhibitors on endothelial permeability and fluxes and corneal thickness, *Invest Ophthalmol Vis Sci* 16:883, 1977.

23. Lim JJ, Ussing HH: Analysis of presteady-state Na⁺ fluxes across the rabbit corneal endothelium, *J Membr Biol* 65:197, 1982.

24. Fischbarg J et al: The mechanism of fluid and electrolyte transport across corneal endothelium: critical revision and update of a model, *Curr Eye Res* 4:351, 1985.

25. Wiederholt M, Jentsch TJ, Keller SK: Electrical sodium-bicarbonate symport in cultured corneal endothelial cells, *Pflugers Arch* 405:S167, 1985.

26. Klyce SD, Neufeld AH, Zadunaisky JA: The activation of chloride transport by epinephrine and Db cyclic-AMP in the cornea of the rabbit, *Invest Ophthalmol* 12:127, 1973.

27. Wiederholt M: Physiology of epithelial transport in the human eye, *Klin Wochenschr* 58:975, 1980.

28. Klyce SD, Wong RKS: Site and mode of adrenaline action on chloride transport across the rabbit corneal epithelium, *J Physiol* 266:777, 1977.

29. Wolosin JM: Gap junctions in rabbit corneal epithelium: limited permeability and inhibition by cAMP, *Am J Physiol* 261:857, 1991.

30. Klyce SD, Beuerman RW, Crosson CE: Alteration of corneal epithelial transport by sympathectomy, *Invest Ophthalmol Vis Sci* 26:434, 1985.

31. Zadunaisky JA, Lande MA: Active chloride transport and control of corneal transparency, *Am J Physiol* 221:1837, 1981.

32. Klyce SD: Enhancing fluid secretion by the corneal epithelium, *Invest Ophthalmol Vis Sci* 16:968, 1977.

33. Bonano J: Regulation of corneal epithelial intracellular pH, *Optom Vis Sci* 68:856, 1991.

34. McPhee TJ, Bourne WM, Brubaker RF: Location of the stress-bearing layers of the cornea, *Invest Ophthalmol Vis Sci* 26:869, 1985.

35. Mishima S, Maurice DM: The effect of normal evaporation on the eye, *Exp Eye Res* 1:46, 1961.

36. Maurice DM: The structure and transparency of the cornea, *J Physiol* 136:263, 1957.

37. Goldman JN, Benedek GB: The relationship between morphology and transparency in the nonswelling corneal stroma of the shark, *Invest Ophthalmol* 6:574, 1967.

38. Benedek GB: Theory of transparency of the eye, *Appl Optics* 10:459, 1971.

39. Farrell RA, McCally RL, Tatham PER: Wavelength dependencies of light scattering in normal and cold swollen rabbit cornea and their structural implications, *J Physiol* 233:589, 1973.

40. Goldman JN et al: Structural alterations affecting transparency in swollen human corneas, *Invest Ophthalmol* 7:501, 1968.

41. Mishima S et al: Determination of tear volume and tear flow, *Invest Ophthalmol* 5:264, 1966.

42. Maurice DM: *Kinetics of topically applied ophthalmic drugs.* In Saettone MF, Bucci M, Speiser P, editors: *Ophthalmic drug delivery: biopharmaceutical, technological and clinical aspects,* New York, 1987, Springer-Verlag.

43. Sieg JW, Robinson JR: Mechanistic studies on transcorneal permeation of pilocarpine, *J Pharmacol Sci* 65:1816, 1976.

44. Hanna C et al: Ocular penetration of topical chloramphenicol in humans, *Arch Ophthalmol* 96:1258, 1978.

45. Massey JT et al: Effect of drug vehicle on human ocular retention of topically applied tetracycline, *Am J Ophthalmol* 81:151, 1976.

46. Cox WV, Kupferman A, Leibowitz HM: Topically applied steroids in corneal disease. II: The role of drug vehicle in stromal absorption of dexamethasone, *Arch Ophthalmol* 88:549, 1972.

47. Grass GM, Robinson JR: Mechanisms of corneal drug penetration. I: In vivo and in vitro kinetics, *J Pharmacol Sci* 77:3, 1988.

48. Grass GM, Robinson JR: Mechanisms of corneal drug penetration. II: Ultrastructural analysis of potential pathways for drug movement, *J Pharmacol Sci* 77:15, 1988.

Three

History and Examination

HISTORY

Because diagnosis can often be made by examination alone, ophthalmologists may neglect taking a thorough history. However, an organized and direct patient history can be very informative and can provide valuable clues to both the diagnosis and possible pitfalls in treatment. Specific forms may be used to facilitate the completion of a comprehensive external disease history and physical examination and can help ensure that necessary portions are not omitted. The forms I use are shown in Figs. 3-1 and 3-2. As in a general medical examination, the physician should first ask about the patient's chief complaint and record it in the patient's own words. The history of the present illness, past ocular history (including medications), general medical history (including systemic medications and allergies), and family history should then be obtained.

History of Present Illness

Triggering mechanisms, daily or seasonal variations, associated factors, and factors that improve or worsen the symptoms should be elicited. Following are some common symptoms and their associated diseases.

A sensation of dryness or burning in the eyes suggests keratoconjunctivitis sicca. This sensation may be associated with dryness of the mouth or other signs of Sjögren's syndrome. The ocular symptoms are usually worse in the afternoon. They may be aggravated in a dry atmosphere, such as inside a building with dry-air heat during the winter. Reading and watching television also tend to worsen the symptoms. The dry eye is prone to infection, delayed healing, and adverse effects from topical medications. Therefore, keratoconjunctivitis sicca must be considered and tested for in the presence of these problems.

A full description of the characteristics of ocular pain aids in determining the cause. The type of pain, chronicity, location, onset, frequency, duration, and aggravating and relieving conditions should be investigated. Sharp

Name _____ MR# _____
        Last,   First

Referring Doctor _____

Date First Seen _____ Allergies _____

Primary Ophthalmological Diagnoses

1. _____

2. _____

3. _____

4. _____

5. _____

6. _____

Eye Procedures (Dates)

Right Eye   Left Eye

1. _____   1. _____

2. _____   2. _____

3. _____   3. _____

4. _____   4. _____

5. _____   5. _____

Medical Diagnoses

1. _____

2. _____

3. _____

4. _____   _____

5. _____

Figure 3-1
Using a comprehensive form can aid in obtaining a complete patient background history.

Patient Name: _____ Date: _____

Referring Doctor: _____

HISTORY

Chief complaint:

Present Illness:

Past Ocular History:

Current Medications:

  Eye: General:

General Medical History:

Diabetes ☐	Hypertension ☐	Heart Failure ☐	Stroke ☐	Heart Attack ☐
Kidney Stones ☐	Asthma/COPD ☐	Gastric Ulcer ☐	Thyroid Disease ☐	Cancer ☐
Eczema ☐	Skin Condition ☐		Rheumatoid Arthritis ☐	

Family History:

Vision   cc

glasses   CL

Correction

Manifest

External: Pupils
                         EOM

Lids

Conjunctiva

Cornea

Sensation
R_____ L_____

Thickness
R_____ L_____

Tear Film   Schirmer R_____ L_____
                                              c   s

Tension _____   R_____ L_____

Anterior
Chamber

Figure 3-2
Using a comprehensive form can aid in the performance of a complete examination.

Iris

Lens

Fundus

Other

Assessment

Recommendations

Signature _____

pain followed by foreign body sensation, photophobia, and tearing may signal a corneal erosion. The symptoms can last minutes to days and can occur repeatedly. Spontaneous erosions occur most often during dreaming, probably from rapid eye movements, or upon awakening, but can occur at any time of the day.

Worsening of eye irritation in the morning is typical of blepharitis, nocturnal lagophthalmos, and floppy lid syndrome. The complaint of decreased vision in the morning that improves in the afternoon usually connotes early epithelial edema due to corneal decompensation.

Photophobia is a prominent complaint when there is infiltration of the cornea with inflammatory cells, an epithelial defect, or iritis. It is seen in phlyctenulosis, exposure to ultraviolet light (sunlamp), severe keratoconjunctivitis, corneal erosions or abrasions, and infectious keratitis. It may be observed in some systemic syndromes, such as Sjögren's or Richner-Hanhart syndrome, and with some intracranial lesions.

Itching, especially of the inner canthi, is an important complaint to note because of its association with allergic states. Seasonal variation is usually a hallmark of external inflammation due to airborne allergens such as pollen.

The presence and type of discharge are important clues to the nature of the underlying disease. If the eyelids are sealed in the morning, a polymorphonuclear response should be suspected. This response may occur not only in bacterial and chlamydial infections but also in viral conjunctivitis if the conjunctival inflammation is severe, such as when membranes are present. Purulent discharge suggests bacterial and chlamydial disease. A mucoid, ropy discharge is highly suggestive of an allergic condition or keratoconjunctivitis sicca.

Watery tearing and epiphora are common complaints. The patient may state that the "tears run down the face." Such tearing can be most annoying and may require constant wiping, which in itself is irritating to the skin of the lids. Usually, tearing is related to ocular irritation or inflammation, but blockage of the lacrimal drainage system must be considered. Examination of the lacrimal drainage system is also indicated in the presence of repeated episodes of bacterial conjunctivitis or when there are findings suggestive of canalicular or lacrimal sac inflammation.

A patient may report a newly noted pigmentation or mass of the lid, conjunctiva, cornea, or iris. Inquiry should be made as to the duration of its presence and whether it has increased in size, bled, become inflamed, or changed color. Obtaining old photographs of the patient may be helpful.

The patient's nutritional status can play a role in external disease. A nutritional history may be indicated, particularly in patients who are emaciated, severely debilitated, or impoverished. Faddish or other unusual dietary habits can lead to vitamin or protein insufficiency or hypervitaminosis.

Injury, present or past, and its nature must be thoroughly investigated. Inquiry as to where the injury occurred is important. If the injury occurred in a garden and the cornea was struck with vegetable matter and subsequently develops an infiltrate or ulcer, fungal keratitis must be suspected. If a liquid has been splashed in the eye, it is important to determine the exact chemical contents and concentrations in the liquid. The amount of the liquid, the duration of exposure, the amount of time that elapsed before irrigation, and the amount of irrigation should also be determined. Grant's[1] *Toxicology of the Eye* is very useful in determining the potential adverse effects of the chemicals involved.

If a foreign body is suspected, it is important to determine its composition, whether it is inert or toxic, and whether it carries infectious agents. Its size and the velocity on impact should also be estimated.

Contact lens wear is often associated with external disease. If a patient wears contacts, the types and age of the lenses, wearing pattern, cleaning and disinfection regimen, and solution types and ages should be investigated. Use of tap water, homemade saline solutions, and saliva are important to elicit because of their association with *Acanthamoeba* keratitis.

Medications

It is important to note what medications, both topical and systemic, have been used and for how long. It is also vital to determine all components of combined medications, including any preservatives. Topical therapy can mask underlying disease, interfere with laboratory testing, or be the cause of signs and symptoms. For example, topical antibiotic administration can prevent growth of causative organisms in culture. Steroid use can suppress a disease and make it more difficult to diagnose; they can also promote corneal ulceration, cataract development, and glaucoma. Common preservatives, such as thimerosal or benzalkonium chloride, can cause an allergic conjunctivitis, a toxic follicular reaction, or epithelial keratitis. Other drugs can cause follicular responses, calcific band keratopathy, conjunctival scarring, or pigmentation of the conjunctiva and cornea (see Chapter 25). Topical anesthetic agents are occasionally inappropriately prescribed or self-administered by patients and can result in severe corneal changes.

Systemically administered medications may cause conjunctival scarring (e.g., practolol), decrease tear production or blink rate, or cause deposits in the lens and cornea (see Chapter 26). Systemic immunosuppression predisposes to infection and probably to recurrence of herpes simplex or herpes zoster as well.

Past Ocular History

The past history of eye disease should be obtained, including previous episodes of inflammation and infection, surgery, and injury. As an example, the presence of inferior conjunctival scarring may suggest a diagnosis of cicatricial pemphigoid; however, the scarring may be the result of years of phospholine iodide use or an old alkali injury.

General Medical History

Investigation of a patient's past history of systemic disease should include skin, cardiovascular, neurologic, mucous membrane, collagen, metabolic, and immune diseases. Many external disease problems are associated with these entities, as will be seen in subsequent chapters. Determining whether the patient is an immunocompromised host is important, especially when treating an infection or contemplating surgery. For example, prior exposure of the lids or eyes to radiation treatment can contribute to keratinization, cicatrization, and telangiectasia of the conjunctiva, as well as to drying of the eye and epithelial disease.

Other History

Family history is important because a number of corneal conditions are hereditary. In some, such as the dystrophies, manifestations can be limited to the cornea. In addition, a large number of other hereditary conditions, primarily involving other organ systems, can cause external disease. Thus no external ocular problem should be handled without considering the patient's general health, capability of response to infection, family history, previous ocular history, and medication use.

CLINICAL EXAMINATION

The examination of the eyes is begun after establishing the history of the case. In making

this examination too much stress can not be laid upon the necessity of proceeding systematically, since otherwise important matters can very readily be overlooked. We first examine the patient with regard to his general physical condition as well as with regard to the expression of his countenance, and then, in observing the eyes themselves, proceed gradually from the superficial parts—lids, conjunctiva, and cornea—to the deeper portions (Fuchs E: *Textbook of Ophthalmology,* New York, 1892, D. Appleton & Co).

General Appearance

As stressed by Fuchs, it is important not to proceed directly to biomicroscopic examination of the eye, but instead first to observe the patient's general condition then the face and skin, and then to perform a flashlight examination of the lids and conjunctiva. Whether a patient is debilitated, has poor hygiene, or is obese should be noted. The patient's ability to provide an accurate history, to comprehend the nature of the disease, and to comply with therapy should be assessed.

Visual Acuity

Uncorrected and best-corrected vision should be determined. If normal vision cannot be obtained with the patient's correction, a pinhole test or refraction should be performed. Astigmatism, regular or irregular, is often overlooked as a cause of unexplained decreased vision and can be diagnosed with a keratometer or corneal topography device, as described below, or by a temporary hard contact lens fitting. A hard contact lens will correct astigmatism and indicate how much of the decreased vision can be attributed to this mechanism. A number of devices, such as the blue-field entoscope, Potential Acuity Meter (Mentor, Norwell, MA) and laser interferometer, can help determine visual impairment due to corneal and lenticular opacities.

Skin

Skin diseases, particularly those involving the face, commonly cause external disease of the eye. Acne rosacea and eczema are common diseases that can easily be overlooked, particularly when examining a patient in a darkened room. Discoid lupus, bullous pemphigoid, epidermolysis bullosa, and seborrheic dermatitis are other examples of skin diseases associated with external eye disease.

Lymph Nodes

Both palpable and grossly visible preauricular and submandibular nodes should be sought.

Small palpable preauricular nodes are seen in the following conditions:

1. Trachoma
2. Vaccinia
3. Inclusion conjunctivitis
4. Primary herpes simplex
5. Adenoviral conjunctivitis
6. Hyperacute conjunctivitis (*Neisseria*)
7. Lid conditions such as hordeolum, impetigo, and cellulitis
8. Dacryoadenitis
9. Toxic reaction to drugs such as idoxuridine
10. Newcastle disease

It is rare for a routine bacterial conjunctivitis to produce a preauricular node. The only exception is hyperacute conjunctivitis. Grossly visible preauricular nodes are usually associated with localized conjunctival nodules or ulcerations (Parinaud's oculoglandular syndrome) or a follicular conjunctival response (see Chapter 6). Rarely, enlarged nodes are produced by lymphatic spread of ocular surface tumors.

Lids

The lid margins, bases of the lashes, and meibomian gland orifices should be examined routinely for signs of inflammation. Yellowish collars surrounding a lash (see Fig. 13-1) suggest staphylococcal blepharitis. Staphylococcal infection of the lids is one of the most common causes of a chronic red eye. A small ulcerated area around the base of the lash may be seen. In chronic staphylococcal blepharitis, other lid margin problems, such as broken lashes, loss of lashes, and thickening of the lid margins, may be present. The cornea is often affected, most commonly with an inferior epithelial keratitis. Less often an acutely inflamed eye, marginal corneal infiltrates, superficial corneal vascularization, or phlyctenules may develop. These problems are discussed at greater length in other chapters.

Large greasy scales (scurf) attached to the lashes (see Fig. 13-5) indicate seborrheic blepharitis, which is noninfectious and commonly associated with seborrheic dermatitis. It can also be associated with conjunctival and corneal inflammation. Blepharitis can be associated with ulceration of the skin of the lid margin. Ulcerative blepharitis most commonly occurs at the lateral canthus, when it is called *angular blepharitis* (see Fig. 6-8). A number of infectious agents can produce this situation, including *Moraxella*. In meibomitis, inflammation is noted around the orifices of the meibomian glands, and the secretions are thickened (see Fig. 13-6). Corneal and conjunctival in-flammation can occur. A more thorough discussion of blepharitis and meibomitis can be found in Chapter 13.

Many tumors may arise from the lids, and some of these may be associated with corneal disease. *Molluscum contagiosum* lesions (see Fig. 13-9) are easy to overlook and can be associated with a chronic follicular conjunctivitis. Commonly, acute and chronic inflammatory masses arise from inflammation of skin structures at the lid margin. A *hordeolum* is an acute nodular inflammation of the eyelid. It may be infectious, usually caused by *Staphylococcus aureus*, or sterile. External hordeola involve the anterior lamellae of the lid and may arise from the Zeis glands, sweat glands, or hair follicles. Internal hordeola affect the posterior lamellae and arise from the meibomian glands. In contrast to these, a *chalazion* is a relatively quiet, chronic granulomatous reaction to sebaceous material extruded from a Zeis or meibomian gland.

It is important to assess lid function. Incomplete blinking (*lagophthalmos*) or a decreased blink rate may not be noted unless specifically tested for. Lagophthalmos may result in corneal drying and subsequent irritation, infection, vascularization, or ulceration. Lagophthalmos can occur only during sleep and often must be inferred from observation of corneal changes. Ectropion (Fig. 3-3) and entropion often cause corneal or conjunctival disease and should be noted.

Conjunctiva

The most common signs of conjunctival disease are chemosis, papillae, follicles, membranes, and scarring. These are briefly discussed here, and together with other conjunctival findings are discussed in more detail in Chapter 6.

Chemosis

Chemosis is accumulation of fluid within or beneath the conjunctiva (Fig. 3-4). It is caused most commonly by allergic conjunctivitis but can result from orbital inflammation or severe intraocular inflammation (e.g., endophthalmitis), or may be seen in conjunction with severe infectious conjunctivitis, such as the hyperacute conjunctivitis of gonorrhea or epidemic keratoconjunctivitis.

Papillae

Papillae and follicles in the conjunctiva must be identified and differentiated to diagnose inflammatory external disease. The characteristics of papillae and follicles are given in Table 3-1.

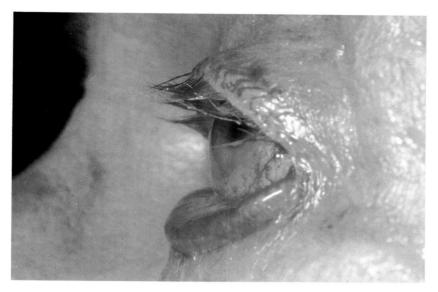

Figure 3-3
Ectropion. (Courtesy of Diane Curtin, Pittsburgh, PA.)

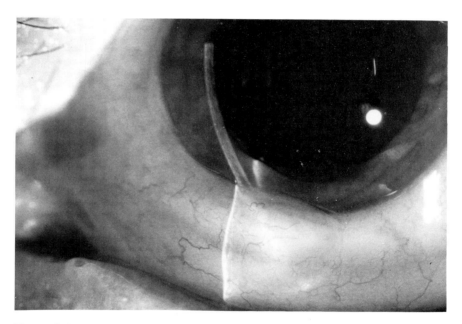

Figure 3-4
Chemosis.

Papillae can occur only where the conjunctiva is fastened down to the underlying tissue by anchoring septae, such as over the tarsi and at the bulbar limbus. The anchoring septae normally divide the conjunctiva into a mosaic pattern of polygonal papillae, each less than 1 mm in diameter. A central fibrovascular core is present within each papilla.

A *papillary response* is a nonspecific sign of conjunctival inflammation and results from edema and polymorphonuclear cell infiltration of the conjunctiva (Fig. 3-5). Giant papillae result from breakdown of the fine fibrous strands that compose the anchoring septae. With the breakdown of the attachments, larger papillae (> 1 mm) may develop, most commonly in the

Table 3-1	Characteristics of Papillae and Follicles	
Follicle	**Papilla**
Discrete, round, elevated lesion of conjunctiva	Elevated polygonal hyperemic areas separated by paler areas
Diameter of 0.5 to 5.0 mm	Diameter of 0.3 to 2.0 mm; "giant" if > 1.0 mm
Usually located in the inferior palpebral conjunctiva, although they can be seen superiorly	May be seen anywhere on the conjunctiva, or limbus; giant papillae are usually seen over the superior tarsus
Vascular network grows around follicle; vessels disappear toward center of follicle	Central fibrovascular core noted in each papilla with central blood vessel, which, when reaching surface, forms arborized vascular figure
Represents new formation of lymphoid tissue	Histopathologically composed of lymphocytes, macrophages, and plasma cells; may form lymphoid follicles
No histologic difference between follicles caused by irritants, infections, or in folliculosis	Composed of polymorphonuclear leukocytes and other acute inflammatory cells; epithelial hypertrophy
	Connective tissue septae are anchored into deeper tissues, resulting in polygonal outline; giant papillae occur when these septae rupture

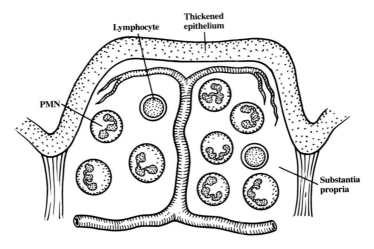

Figure 3-5
Schematic diagram of a papilla.

upper tarsal conjunctiva. Papillae in the tarsal conjunctiva tend to be flat-topped, whereas those found at the limbus are more dome-shaped (Fig. 3-6). Small white dots (*Trantas' dots*), composed of eosinophils, may be seen on the surface of limbal papillae in vernal conjunctivitis (see Fig. 8-6). When the everted upper tarsal conjunctiva is examined, the superior edge often appears to contain large papillae. This finding is normal, resulting from the decrease in the density of the anchoring septae. Giant papillae in the remaining tarsal conjunctiva can be seen in vernal conjunctivitis, atopic

keratoconjunctivitis, and as a reaction to foreign material, such as contact lenses, prostheses, and suture material (Fig. 3-7).

Follicles

Follicles may be seen in the normal conjunctiva, particularly in younger patients. Follicles are produced by a lymphocytic response, sometimes with a germinal center (Fig. 3-8). Newborns are incapable of developing a follicular response for the first 6 to 12 weeks of life. Follicles appear as smooth, translucent elevations of the conjunctiva, sometimes with vessels over

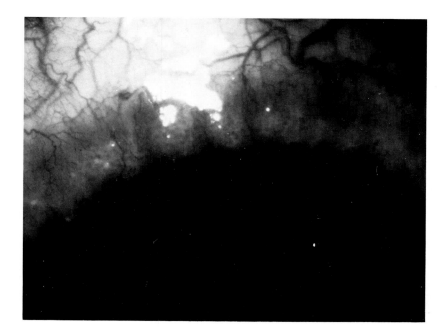

Figure 3-6
Limbal papillae in vernal catarrh.

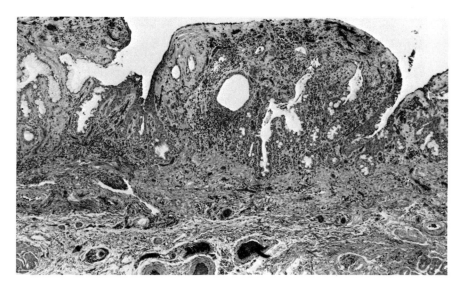

Figure 3-7
Papilla of the superior tarsal conjunctiva in vernal conjunctivitis showing proliferation of fibrovascular connective tissue and chronic inflammatory infiltrate. (Hematoxylin-eosin stain, ×80.) (Courtesy of Bruce L. Johnson, Pittsburgh.)

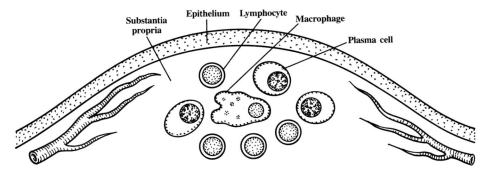

Figure 3-8
Schematic diagram of a follicle.

the peripheral surface (see Fig. 7-12). They are most easily appreciated in the upper tarsal conjunctiva and the lower cul-de-sac, the latter usually exhibiting the greater response. However, they can also be seen at the limbus. It is extremely important for the ophthalmologist to determine if a significant follicular response is present, because it is a relatively specific inflammatory response and helps define the differential diagnosis.

Membranes

Membranes of the conjunctiva are striking clinical signs (Fig. 3-9). Membranes are composed primarily of fibrin that has coagulated on the epithelial surface. Little distinction exists between pseudomembranes and true membranes, except when true membranes are peeled off a raw surface and bleeding might result, thus signifying more intense conjunctival inflammation. A variety of infectious agents can produce

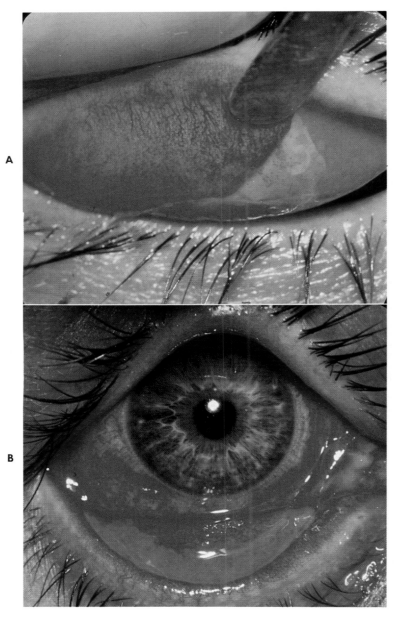

Figure 3-9
Membrane formation on the tarsal conjunctiva in a case of epidemic keratoconjunctivitis. **A,** Upper lid. **B,** Lower lid.

pseudomembranous or membranous conjunctivitis. Formerly it was caused principally by *Corynebacterium diphtheriae* and β-hemolytic streptococci; but now, in this country, adenoviral conjunctivitis is the most common cause, followed by primary herpetic conjunctivitis.

Scarring

Ordinary acute or chronic conjunctivitis heals without cicatrization. In fact, the epithelium can be severely damaged without provoking the formation of scar tissue. Scars form only when there is destruction of stromal tissue. There may be severe infiltration and edema of the stroma, as in gonococcal ophthalmia in adults, without scar formation.

Nontraumatic conjunctival scarring can result from a variety of conjunctival and systemic inflammatory diseases, including any disease that causes membranous conjunctivitis. Scarring after membranous conjunctivitis tends to be diffuse and nonspecific in appearance, with no predilection for the conjunctiva of either the upper or lower lid.

Special types of scarring, with characteristic morphologic features and locations, are seen in trachoma, ocular cicatricial pemphigoid, and atopic keratoconjunctivitis. Severe shrinkage, such as in cicatricial pemphigoid, also occurs occasionally in a few other diseases.

Tear Film and Lacrimal System

Examination of the tear film is extremely important. Keratoconjunctivitis sicca is very common and often overlooked. It should be considered in cases of unexplained conjunctival injection, corneal thinning, persistent epithelial defect, or poor wound healing. The tear meniscus, tear breakup time, and Schirmer's tests may be used to facilitate diagnosis, as discussed in Chapter 14.

Attention should be focused next on the lacrimal drainage system. Canaliculitis or dacryocystitis should be suspected if there is a complaint of discharge from the eye and if pouting of the punctum is present on examination, or if tenderness and swelling are noted in the area of the canaliculi or lacrimal sac (Fig. 3-10). An attempt should be made to express purulent material from the canaliculus and sac. *Canaliculitis* is usually caused by *Actinomyces israelii*, a gram-positive, branching filamentous bacterium, whose unusual structure facilitates its lodging in the canaliculus. Curettage, with or without canaliculotomy, is necessary to remove concretions formed during infection.[2]

The following organisms are most likely to cause canaliculitis:

1. *Actinomyces israelii*
2. *Candida albicans*
3. *Aspergillus niger*
4. Primary herpes simplex
5. Herpes zoster
6. Vaccinia
7. Syphilis
8. Tuberculosis

Swelling, inflammation, and tenderness over

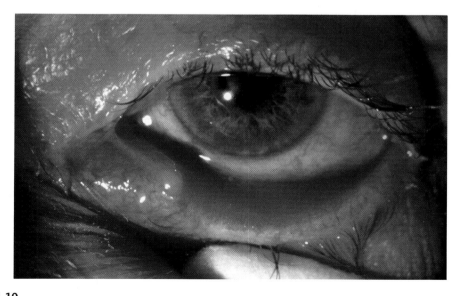

Figure 3-10
Canaliculitis. The nasal lid margin is thickened and injected. Purulent material can be expressed from the punctum.

the lacrimal sac area (below the medial canthus) are seen in *dacryocystitis.* This condition is usually accompanied by pain, tearing, and purulent discharge, but the only symptom may be occasional epiphora. In any patient with such a complaint or with recurrent conjunctivitis, pressure should be applied over the lacrimal sac to look for reflux of mucopurulent material. The following organisms are most likely to cause dacryocystitis:

Acute dacryocystitis

1. *S. aureus*
2. β-hemolytic streptococcus

Chronic dacryocystitis

1. *Streptococcus pneumoniae*
2. *Haemophilus influenzae*

Cornea
Superficial Vascularization
Superficial limbal vessels do not normally extend onto the cornea for more than 1 mm. Any growth beyond the normal limbal arcade is called *pannus.* Pannus may be accompanied by subepithelial fibrous tissue or stromal scarring, in which case the clarity of the stroma is reduced. Vascular pannus can be divided into *micropannus,* where vessels extend only 1 to 2 mm beyond the normal arcade, and *gross pannus,* where they extend more than 2 mm. The most common causes are listed in Table 3-2.

Stains
Fluorescein and rose bengal dyes should be applied routinely when diagnosing corneal and conjunctival diseases. Fluorescein will travel wherever water can enter the cornea (i.e., wherever there is bare stroma or where the barrier function of the surface epithelium is lost). Rose bengal stain is a red aniline dye chemically related to fluorescein. It stains cells lacking protection by the precorneal tear film.[3,4] Albumin, mucin, and carboxycellulose prevent rose bengal staining of cells. Rose bengal is particularly useful in keratoconjunctivitis sicca and superior limbal keratoconjunctivitis and in any eye with milder epithelial injury. It produces irritation, so it is best applied after topical anesthesia. It stains the skin and clothing, so care must be taken in application. To reduce the volume instilled, a wooden applicator stick can be broken and a drop placed on the obliquely broken surface or some of the dye can be taken up into the hollow end of a plastic applicator stick. Rose bengal strips are best placed in a container with a few drops of sterile saline before application. Testing of sensation, Schirmer's test, or applanation tonometry should be avoided before evaluating the ocular surface with these dyes.

Epithelial Staining
Punctate epithelial keratitis can result from any disease of the corneal epithelium. Some of the more common causes are given in Tables 3-3, 3-4, and 3-5.

Punctate epithelial keratitis may be visible with illumination or only after instillation of fluorescein or rose bengal. The pattern of the staining, both on the conjunctiva and on the cornea, may be suggestive of an etiology, but often a systematic history and examination are required to determine the cause. Some common staining patterns are illustrated in Fig. 3-11.

Focal epithelial keratitis is a term that can be used to describe the coarser or grouped epithelial lesions, which may be seen in a number of diseases (Fig. 3-12). These lesions appear like the cytopathologic effect caused by some viruses in culture, and in many cases represent a similar process occurring in the corneal epithelium. Viral infections are usually responsible (see Chapter 9).

Other characteristic epithelial lesions include the following:

1. Syncytial: Vernal keratoconjunctivitis
2. Dendritic: Herpes simplex, herpes zoster, mucoid plaque, healing epithelial defect, acanthamoeba, tyrosinosis
3. Stellate: Herpes zoster and herpes simplex
4. Linear: Foreign body, trichiasis

Table 3-2 Causes of Pannus

Gross Pannus
- Trachoma
- Phlyctenulosis
- Acne rosacea
- Atopic keratoconjunctivitis
- Contact lens wear
- Staphylococcal blepharitis
- Herpes simplex keratitis
- Trauma
- Previous bacterial ulceration

Micropannus
- Inclusion conjunctivitis
- Childhood trachoma
- Staphylococcal blepharitis
- Contact lens wear
- Superior limbal keratoconjunctivitis
- Vernal conjunctivitis

Table 3-3 Common Causes of Punctate Epithelial Keratitis	
General Grouping	**Specific Disease**
Viral	Herpes simplex
	Herpes zoster
	Molluscum contagiosum
	Measles
	Mumps
	Infectious mononucleosis
	Adenoviral disease
	Vaccinia
	Newcastle disease
Chlamydial	Trachoma
	Adult inclusion conjunctivitis
Bacterial	Staphylococcal blepharitis
	Bacterial conjunctivitis
Systemic inflammatory disease	Sjögren's syndrome
	Systemic lupus erythematosus
Traumatic	Post corneal erosion
	Chemical burn
	Radiation
Lid disease	Blepharitis
	Meibomitis
	Exposure
	Trichiasis
Allergy	Vernal keratoconjunctivitis
Nutritional	Vitamin A deficiency
Toxic	Medicamentosa
Neurologic	Neurotrophic keratitis
Unknown	Superior limbal keratoconjunctivitis
	Thygeson's superficial punctate keratitis

Subepithelial Nummular Opacities

Subepithelial nummular opacities that do not stain can follow active epithelial lesions, or they may occur without clinical epithelial involvement. They are discussed in detail in Chapter 9. Table 3-6 lists some of the common causes.

Filaments

Filaments are small mucoid deposits adherent to the corneal surface (Fig. 3-13). They stain with fluorescein and rose bengal. The mechanism of their formation is controversial. Filaments consist of a coil of epithelial cells attached to the cornea at one end, with adherent mucus and other debris. Filamentary keratitis is discussed in Chapter 9.

Sensation

It is important to recognize decreased corneal sensation because it frequently results in corneal disease and because its presence has etiologic significance. Corneal sensation can be de-

termined qualitatively with a cotton applicator, or quantitatively with an esthesiometer, such as that devised by Cochet and Bonnet[5] (Fig. 3-14). The cornea should be examined with fluorescein before corneal sensation is tested because this testing may leave punctate or even linear staining. What appears to be an infected area of the cornea should never be touched before touching an uninvolved area of the cornea with the same testing device; a separate cotton applicator should be used for each eye when there is infection.

Measurement of corneal sensitivity with the Cochet-Bonnet esthesiometer is performed as follows: With the patient fixating straight ahead, the nylon filament is moved perpendicularly toward the cornea until it hits the cornea and begins to bend. This is repeated with progressively shorter lengths of filament until a response is obtained in 50% of stimulations.

Injury to the fifth cranial nerve from any cause may decrease corneal sensation, but herpes simplex and herpes zoster infections are

Table 3-4	Findings Associated with Superficial Epithelial Keratopathy
Lid Disease	**Conjunctival Lesions**
Blepharitis	Follicles
Meibomitis	Adenovirus
Lid position abnormalities	Trachoma
Entropion	Molluscum contagiosum
Ectropion	Primary herpes simplex
Lagophthalmos	Herpes zoster
Ichthyosis	Adult chlamydial keratoconjunctivitis
Urbach-Wiethe disease	Drug toxicity
Lid warts	
Molluscum contagiosum	Giant papillae
Ulcers or vesicles of lid, as seen in herpes simplex,	Vernal catarrh
herpes zoster, and vaccinia	Contact lens wear
Psoriasis	
	Membrane
	Epidemic keratoconjunctivitis
	Hyperacute conjunctivitis
	Ligneous conjunctivitis
	Stevens-Johnson syndrome
	Scarring
	Pemphigoid
	Trachoma
	Epidemic keratoconjunctivitis
	Atopic disease
	Lye burns
	Stevens-Johnson syndrome
	Lyell's disease (Ritter) (toxic
	epidermal necrolysis)

Figure 3-11

Staining patterns (usually more prominent with rose bengal than with fluorescein) of various conditions. **A,** Drug-induced toxicity or allergy. **B,** Keratoconjunctivitis sicca. **C,** Keratoconjunctivitis sicca with superimposed drug toxicity or allergy. **D,** Contact lens–induced keratoconjunctivitis. **E,** Perilimbal staining in a soft contact lens wearer without papillary keratoconjunctival reaction. **F,** Typical hard contact lens–induced staining. **G,** Staining caused by inferonasal gravitation of increased amounts of conjunctival mucus, especially in patients who rub their eyes. **H,** Staining from a recent Schirmer's test strip. **I,** Factitious (self-induced) conjunctivitis from rubbing or scraping of inferior conjunctiva or from instillation of an irritating substance into the lower cul-de-sac. **J,** Superior limbic keratoconjunctivitis. **K,** Fine punctate epithelial keratopathy, worse above, of vernal catarrh, "floppy eyelid" syndrome, or early contact lens–induced keratoconjunctivitis. **L,** Staphylococcal blepharokeratoconjunctivitis. **M,** Lagophthalmos. **N,** Focal epithelial keratitis, as caused by adenovirus, molluscum contagiosum, rubeola, inclusion conjunctivitis, or Thygeson's superficial punctate keratitis. (Modified from Wilson FM: *Trans Am Ophthalmol Soc* 81:854, 1983.)

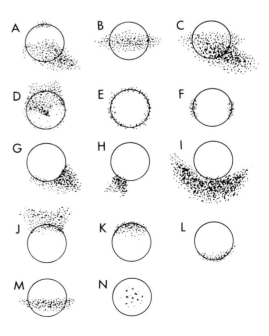

Table 3-5	Characteristic Distributions of Superficial Keratopathy
Location	**Causes**
Lower third	Staphylococcal and seborrheic blepharitis
	Exposure
	Entropion
	Drug toxicity
	Acne rosacea
Interpalpebral	Bacterial conjunctivitis
	Keratitis sicca
	Neurotrophic keratitis
	Exposure keratitis
	Ultraviolet exposure
Upper third	X-ray exposure
	Trachoma
	Inclusion conjunctivitis
	Superior limbal keratoconjunctivitis
	Vernal catarrh
	Molluscum contagiosum
	Verruca of lid
Central	Epidemic keratoconjunctivitis
	Inclusion conjunctivitis
	Contact lens keratopathy
	Meesmann's dystrophy
	Verruca vulgaris
Diffuse	Molluscum contagiosum
	Mumps
	Infectious mononucleosis
	Acute conjunctivitis—bacterial and viral
	Drug toxicity
	Severe vernal keratoconjunctivitis
	Staphylococcal blepharitis
	Keratoconjunctivitis sicca (severe)
	Vitamin A deficiency
Random	Edema of epithelium
	Erosion
	Trichiasis
	Foreign body
	Chemical injury
	Herpes simplex keratitis

Inferior staining is characteristic of staphylococcal blepharitis, exposure, and rosacea. Interpalpebral staining is characteristic of keratoconjunctivitis sicca, medicamentosa, lagophthalmos, neurotrophic keratitis, and ultraviolet exposure. Staining in the superior portion of the cornea usually occurs in vernal catarrh, in superior limbal keratoconjunctivitis, and in the presence of a foreign body in the upper lid. Causes of sectoral staining include trichiasis and trauma.

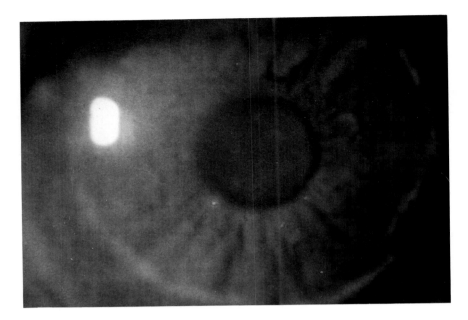

Figure 3-12
Focal epithelial keratitis.

Table 3-6	Common Causes of Subepithelial Nummular Opacities
Etiologic Agent	**Specific Entity**
Viral	Herpes simplex
	Herpes zoster (round irregular)
	Epidemic keratoconjunctivitis
	Acute hemorrhagic conjunctivitis
	Newcastle disease
Unknown	Nummular (Dimmer)
	Padi keratitis
Rare forms	Leprosy (rare)
	Onchocerciasis (more common)
Chlamydia	Trachoma
	Inclusion conjunctivitis (round, as seen in epidemic keratoconjunctivitis)

probably the most common causes. A more complete discussion is provided in Chapter 15.

Increased Visibility of Corneal Nerves

The corneal nerves may be seen in normal eyes as fine branching white lines that originate at the limbus in the midstroma and become more anterior centrally (Fig. 3-15). Some of the conditions associated with increased visibility of the corneal nerves are listed in Table 3-7.[6]

Corneal nerves may become thickened secondarily as a consequence of injury (hyper-regeneration). This condition was described by Wolter[10-12] and is seen with trauma, keratoplasty, granulomatous uveitis, congenital glaucoma, retinopathy of prematurity, congenital cataract, intraocular foreign bodies, phthisis bulbi, band keratopathy, and increased age. In these conditions the nerve fibers are irregularly thickened and course irregularly through the stroma into the epithelium. Inflammation of one or several corneal nerves, with stromal infiltration surrounding them, has been called *radial keratoneuritis* and can be seen in *Acanthamoeba* keratitis (see Fig. 11-15).

Verticillata

Verticillata, whorllike opacities that are occasionally seen in the corneal epithelium, result from accumulation of substances within the corneal epithelium. The vortex pattern (see Fig. 24-11) reflects the growth pattern of the epithelial cells. Cells move centrally from the limbus and desquamate slightly below the center of the cornea. Materials that progressively accumulate in epithelial cells are seen in highest concentration centrally, and least near the limbus. Corneal verticillata are discussed in more detail in Chapter 9.

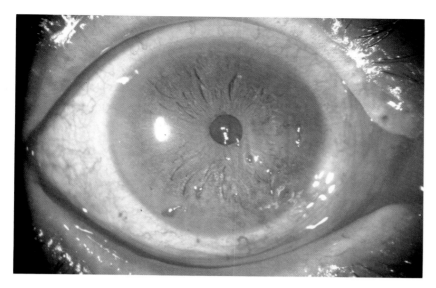

Figure 3-13
Corneal filaments stained with rose bengal.

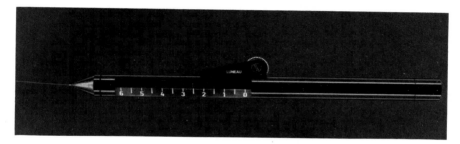

Figure 3-14
Cochet-Bonnet esthesiometer.

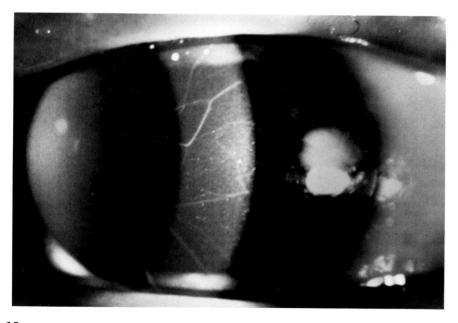

Figure 3-15
Increased visibility of corneal nerves in multiple endocrine neoplasia type IIb. (Courtesy of Richard W. Yee, San Antonio.)

Table 3-7	Conditions Associated with Increased Visibility of the Corneal Nerves
Fuchs' dystrophy	
Keratoconus	
Neurofibromatosis	
Refsum's syndrome[7]	
Ichthyosis	
Leprosy	
Congenital glaucoma	
Failed corneal graft	
Multiple endocrine neoplasia[8]	
Use of *Cannabis sativa* (marijuana)[9]	
Deep filiform dystrophy	
Aging	
Ectodermal dysplasia	
Posterior polymorphous dystrophy	
Primary amyloidosis	
Siemen's disease (keratosis follicularis spinulosa decalvans)	

Table 3-8	Conditions Associated with Corneal Crystals
Schnyder's crystalline dystrophy	
Lecithin cholesterol-acyltransferase deficiency	
Tangier disease	
Secondary lipid keratopathy	
Band keratopathy	
Cystinosis	
Tyrosinosis	
Hyperuricemia (gout)	
Multiple myeloma and other dysproteinemias (see Fig. 19-21)	
Porphyria	
Marginal crystalline dystrophy of Bietti	
Diffenbachia plant (calcium oxalate)[13]	

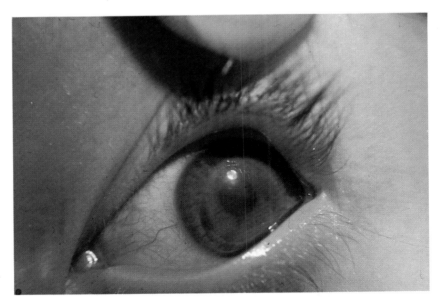

Figure 3-16
Ring infiltrate. The reaction is similar to that with the Wessely ring.

Crystals

Although uncommon, crystals in the cornea are a striking finding and have great diagnostic significance. Conditions in which crystals are found in the cornea are listed in Table 3-8.

Ring Infiltrates

Partial or complete ring-shaped stromal infiltrates (Fig. 3-16) can be seen in a number of conditions. The classic form of ring infiltration is the Wessely ring reaction, which is seen 10 to 12 days after experimental introduction of antigen into the cornea. The ring, which consists primarily of antigen-antibody complexes, complement, and polymorphonuclear leukocytes, slowly migrates centripetally and diminishes in intensity until the cornea is clear. Occasionally, pannus can result. This type of ring infiltrate, presumably also the result of an immunologic response, can be seen in patients with

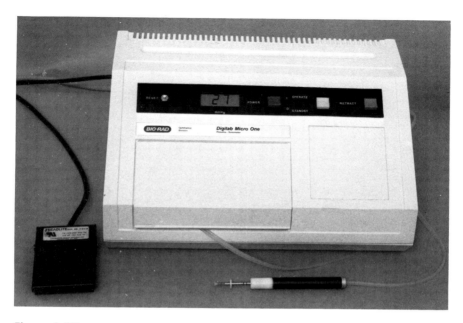

Figure 3-17
Pneumotonometer.

severe corneal burns; corneal foreign bodies; bacterial (especially *Pseudomonas*), herpetic, *Acanthamoeba,* or fungal keratitis; and abuse of topical anesthetic agents.

Intraocular Pressure Measurement

Applanation tonometry may be inaccurate when there is corneal surface irregularity or astigmatism. Errors in astigmatic corneas are reduced by measuring the pressure with the tonometer mires divided in the axis halfway between the steeper and flatter axes. With marked corneal irregularity, a MacKay-Marg tonometer or pneumotonometry (Fig. 3-17) is necessary. I have found the MacKay-Marg tonometer to be more accurate, but these units are no longer available. Both devices tend to give a higher reading than with applanation and can give a minimum reading of 4 to 10 mm even in the presence of an open eye. A hand-held device, the Tono-Pen (Bio-Rad, Santa Anna, CA) appears to be as accurate as a MacKay-Marg tonometer.[14] These devices can measure intraocular pressure fairly accurately with a soft contact lens in place, as long as it is not an aphakic lens.[15,16]

Measurement of Corneal Thickness

The normal central corneal thickness is 0.52 mm; any greater thickness indicates endothelial dysfunction. Measurement of corneal thickness is therefore valuable in determining the functional status of the endothelium, such as in assessing risk of corneal decompensation before cataract surgery, determining the health of a corneal graft, or guiding treatment of a case of herpetic disciform edema. With practice, fairly accurate corneal thickness measurements can be obtained with an optical pachymeter attached to the slit-lamp microscope (Fig. 3-18). Ultrasonic pachymeters (Fig. 3-19) can give rapid measurements and can yield peripheral thicknesses more easily. When a given cornea is tested with multiple ultrasonic devices, the measurements vary considerably, but most units are internally consistent.[17] Pachymetry can also be obtained with some specular microscopes.

Specular Microscopy

A specular microscope (Fig. 3-20) permits visualization and photography of the endothelial cell layer. Endothelial cell density can be estimated from these photographs. Corneal thickness generally does not begin to increase until there has been considerable loss of endothelial cells; lesser degrees of endothelial cell loss and qualitative changes can be determined by specular microscopy (Fig. 3-21). Repeated endothelial cell counts are useful to assess the effect of different types of injury, such as cataract extraction, vitreous touch, intraocular lens implants, or corneal transplantation. Specular microscopy is used routinely to evaluate donor tissue

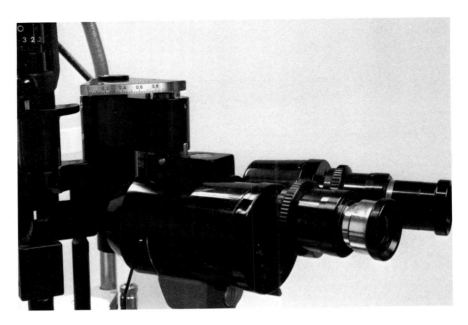

Figure 3-18
Haag-Streit optical pachymeter attached to slit-lamp microscope.

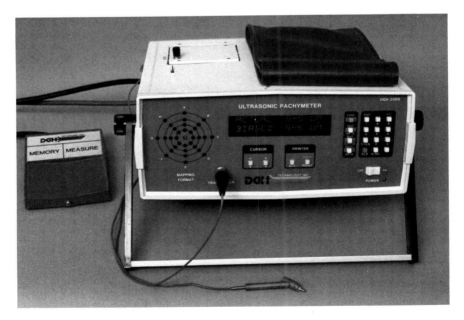

Figure 3-19
Ultrasonic pachymeter.

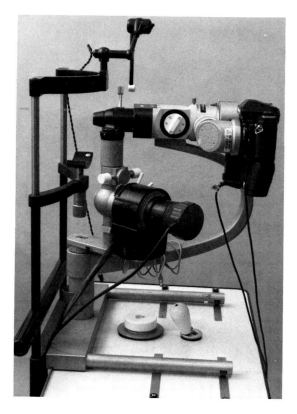

Figure 3-20
Specular microscope.

for suitability for transplantation. It may be useful in assessing the ability of the cornea to withstand intraocular procedures such as cataract surgery or secondary lens implantation.

Confocal Microscopy

The confocal microscope (Fig. 3-22) allows noninvasive optical imaging of living tissues. Both the light source and the microscope objective lens are focused on a small area within the tissue (hence the term *confocal*). This is accomplished via a rotating disk (Nipkow disk) that focuses light at a thin object plane and accepts light back only from this plane. The point of focus can be moved in three dimensions, permitting examination of all layers of the tissue. The microscope has been adapted and approved by the Food and Drug Administration for clinical corneal use.[18] Corneal epithelial cells, stromal keratocytes, nerves, and endothelium can be examined (Fig. 3-23), and abnormal images have been observed in disease processes such as corneal dystrophies and infections. The confocal microscope is superior to the specular microscope in visualizing the endothelium through a hazy or edematous cornea. Infectious organisms, such as amoebae, bacteria, and fungi, can also be detected.[18-20]

Corneal Topography

The corneal surface, or more accurately, the air-tear interface, is the most powerful refractive surface of the eye, accounting for approxi-

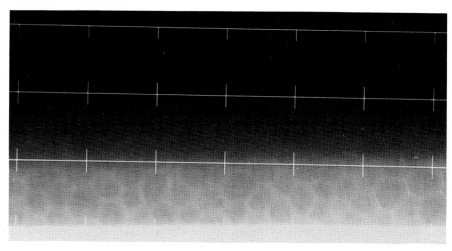

Figure 3-21
Specular photograph of endothelium showing polymegathism.

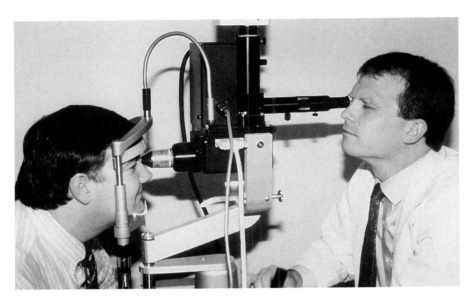

Figure 3-22
A tandem scanning confocal microscope adapted for use in ophthalmology (Tandem Scanning Corp, Reston, Virginia). (From Petroll WM, Jester JV, Cavanagh JV: Confocal microscopy, *Cornea*, 1995, in press.)

mately two thirds of the eye's total refractive power. The power of the surface is inversely proportional to its radius of curvature, which is determined optically by the keratometer to estimate the refractive power of the cornea. An illuminated ring is placed at a fixed distance from the corneal surface, and the size of the reflected image of the ring is determined by the curvature of the corneal surface. Measurement in different meridians can indicate the axis and amount of corneal astigmatism. Knowledge of the corneal curvature is important in fitting contact lenses, measuring and correcting astigmatism, calculating intraocular lens implant power, and planning and analyzing refractive surgical procedures. The keratometer may also be used to observe corneal surface irregularity.

The keratometer measures the corneal curvature at approximately 1.5 mm from the visual axis. In most cases the curvature over the visual axis is fairly uniform, and this single measurement is sufficiently descriptive. However, if the cornea does not have regular astigmatism, with the major axes 90° apart, its accuracy is reduced. In addition, keratometry does not provide information about the shape of the peripheral cornea.

Keratoscopy is a means of getting information about the shape of the entire cornea. This method was originally devised by Placido,[21] and the simplest device for obtaining these images

is called Placido's disk. A series of concentric illuminated white rings are placed on a disk that is held in front of the cornea (Fig. 3-24). When the examiner looks through the window in the center of the disk, he or she sees the reflections of the rings, and the position, size, and spacing of these rings are determined by the corneal shape. A photokeratoscope permits photography of the reflected images, and several commercial systems are available (Figs. 3-25 and 3-26). Photokeratoscopy is useful in diagnosing and staging keratoconus[22-24] and other corneal thinning disorders, guiding suture removal after cataract and corneal transplant surgery,[25] observing and treating corneal astigmatism, and planning and evaluating other refractive procedures.[26-28]

Quantitative data about the corneal curvature can be obtained by computer analysis of the Placido's disk images.[29] One such device is shown in Fig. 3-27. Current computer-assisted topography devices also provide information from a larger portion of the corneal surface than photokeratoscopy devices.

Various displays can be created and descriptive indices derived from the quantitative data. The accuracy of the derived corneal refractive powers is unclear. Measurements of test spheres are fairly accurate, but measurements of aspheric surfaces are less so, particularly peripherally.[30-33] In addition, the relationship between

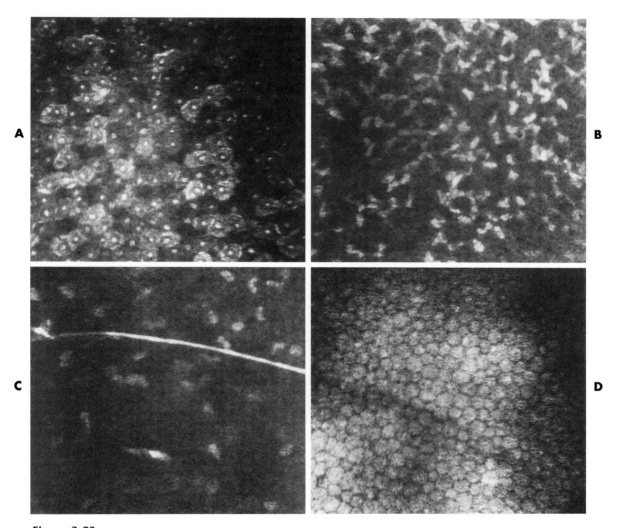

Figure 3-23
A, With the tandem scanning confocal microscope (TSCM) focal plane set to the level of the superficial epithelium, an en face image similar to that of a scanning electron micrograph is obtained. The borders of the epithelial cells are readily seen, as are the cell nuclei (*arrows*). **B,** Anterior stroma just below Bowman's layer. Note the large number of keratocyte nuclei (*arrows*) detected using the TSCM. **C,** Midstroma with a nerve fiber (*curved arrow*) between keratocyte nuclei (*arrows*). Note the decreased density of the keratocyte nuclei as compared with **B. D,** Normal endothelium. Horizontal field width = 400 μ. (From Cavanagh HD et al: *Ophthalmology* 100:1444, 1993.)

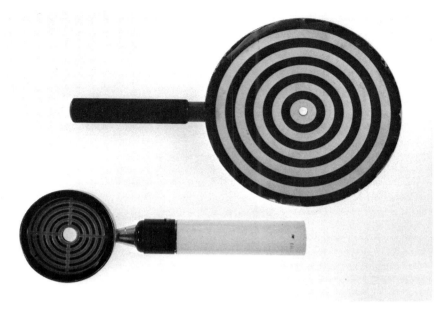

Figure 3-24
Placido's disk devices.

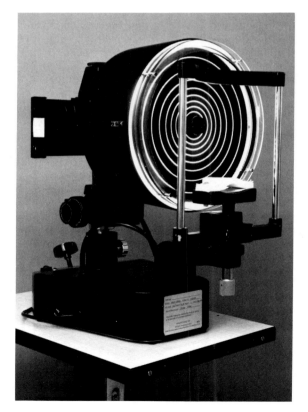

Figure 3-25
Photokeratoscope.

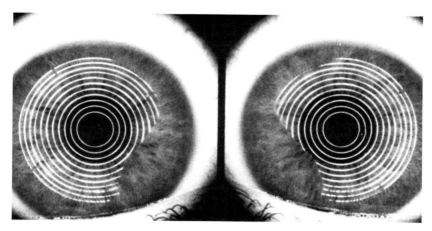

Figure 3-26
Photokeratoscopic picture of normal corneas.

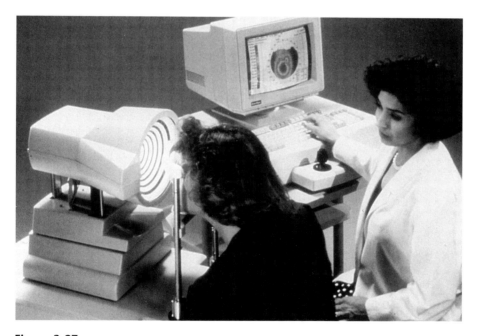

Figure 3-27
Eyesys videokeratography device (Eyesys, Houston, TX).

corneal curvature and refractive power differs peripherally due to the effect of spherical aberration, but most devices do not take this into account.[34] Nevertheless, computer-assisted topography devices allow a much more sensitive analysis, which has expanded our knowledge of topography in normal eyes and the effects of corneal disease and surgery. The topographic patterns seen in corneal disease will be described in more detail in the chapters dedicated to those diseases. A general description of computer-assisted corneal topography is provided here.

The most commonly used display is a color-coded map of corneal curvature (Fig. 3-28). Colors in the red spectrum are typically used to indicate steeper portions of the cornea and colors in the blue spectrum to indicate flatter areas. The scales are not standardized and must therefore be examined in each map in order to determine the powers represented by each color and the difference between color steps. In general it is best to use steps of 1.0 to 1.5 D.

The normal cornea (Fig. 3-28) is aspheric, flattening from center to periphery. The degree of flattening is variable and tends to be

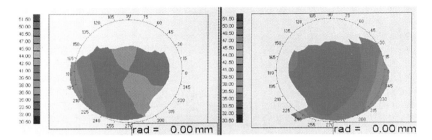

Figure 3-28
Normal corneal curvature map. Note that corneas are aspheric, flattening from center to periphery, more nasally than temporally. The right and left eyes have similar central patterns, with mirror-image symmetry.

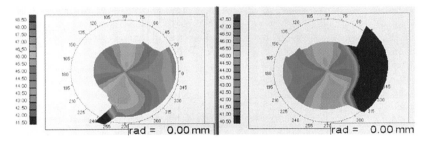

Figure 3-29
Appearance of naturally occurring astigmatism with videokeratoscopy. Note the symmetric bow-tie patterns, with mirror-image symmetry between the right and left eyes.

closer to the central cornea nasally than temporally.[35-39] The right and left eyes tend to have similar central patterns, with mirror-image symmetry. Naturally occurring astigmatism is nearly always with-the-rule. A bow-tie–shaped pattern is seen on the color map (Fig. 3-29).[40,41] The areas of steepening are usually orthogonal and symmetrically distributed above and below fixation. Deviation from this pattern in a cornea that appears normal on biomicroscopy may be caused by keratoconus or contact lens–induced corneal warpage (see Chapter 17).

With all the data provided by these systems, a good deal of knowledge and experience is required to interpret them. To make this easier and more objective, quantitative indices have been developed. The surface asymmetry index (SAI) and surface regularity index (SRI) were developed by Klyce and associates.[42] The SAI is a measure of the central corneal symmetry. It is a centrally weighted summation of differences in corneal power between corresponding points 180° apart on the four central photokeratoscope mires. The SAI approaches zero for a radi-

ally symmetric surface and increases with more asymmetric contour. The SRI is a measure of the point-to-point fluctuation in power over the surface. The SRI increases with increasing irregular astigmatism, and there is a high correlation between the SRI and spectacle-corrected visual acuity.[43]

An automated system for detection of keratoconus has been developed.[44] This system can differentiate between normal, keratoconus, and other abnormal topography patterns with high sensitivity and specificity.

The topography devices discussed above are all based on Placido's disk images. These require a smooth reflective corneal surface, and therefore will not obtain images from corneas with epithelial defects, scarring, or marked irregularity. In addition, information about the most central cornea is limited, and these devices measure corneal curvature, not elevation. Another method of corneal topography analysis, which measures corneal elevation and is not dependent on the reflectivity of the corneal surface, has been developed. In *rasterstereography,*

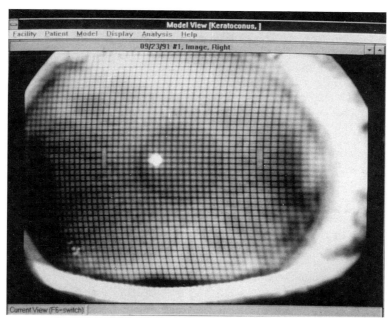

Figure 3-30
Rasterstereography, with the projection of grid pattern on the cornea.

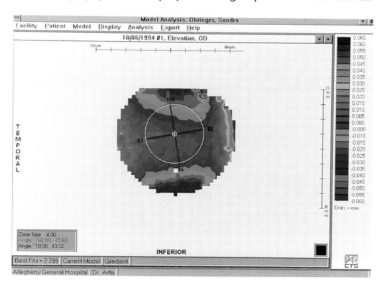

Figure 3-31
With-the-rule astigmatism with rasterstereography. Pattern shows deviation from a perfect sphere. Blue areas are depressed below a spherical surface as a result of steeper curvature in that axis.

a grid of parallel lines is projected onto the corneal surface, and the distortion of the grid by the cornea is viewed from a fixed angle (Fig. 3-30).[45,46] Astigmatism is seen as a relative depression of the steep axis (Fig. 3-31). Surface irregularities do not degrade the image. This device appears to be less sensitive to improper alignment or focusing.[47] It has also been adapted for use on an operating microscope.[48] Whether this system will prove clinically more useful than Placido's disk–based systems is still unclear.

Other Ocular Structures

It is essential to perform a complete ocular examination even if pathology initially appears to be isolated to the cornea because other, unrelated diseases can be present. More relevant, however, is the frequent presence of other signs that provide clues to the diagnosis of corneal disorders. For instance, the association of iritis with noninfiltrative stromal and epithelial disease is suggestive of herpes viruses; sectoral iris atrophy suggests herpes zoster; in the presence of corneal decompensation, corectopia, polycoria, and peripheral anterior synechiae suggest the iridocorneal endothelial syndrome; and an anterior subcapsular cataract suggests atopic keratoconjunctivitis.

REFERENCES

1. Grant WM: *Toxicology of the eye,* ed 3, Springfield, IL, 1986, Charles C Thomas.
2. Pavilack MA, Frueh BR: Thorough curettage in the treatment of chronic canaliculitis, *Arch Ophthalmol* 110:200, 1992.
3. Feenstra RPG, Tseng SCG: Comparison of fluorescein and rose bengal staining, *Ophthalmology* 99:605, 1992.
4. Feenstra RPG, Tseng SCG: What is actually stained by rose bengal? *Arch Ophthalmol* 110:984, 1992.
5. Cochet P, Bonnet R: L'esthesie corneenne, *Clin Ophthalmol* 4:12, 1960.
6. Mensher JH: Corneal nerves, *Surv Ophthalmol* 19:1, 1974.
7. Baum JL, Tannenbaum M, Kolodny EH: Refsum's syndrome with corneal involvement, *Am J Ophthalmol* 60:699, 1965.
8. Colombo CG, Watson AG: Ophthalmic manifestations of multiple endocrine neoplasia, type three, *Can J Ophthalmol* 11:290, 1976.
9. Dawson WW: Cannabis and eye function, *Invest Ophthalmol* 15:243, 1976.
10. Wolter JR: Regeneration and hyper-regeneration of corneal nerves, *Ophthalmologica* 151:588, 1960.
11. Wolter JR: Hyper-regeneration of corneal nerves in bullous keratopathy, *Am J Ophthalmol* 58:31, 1964.
12. Wolter JR: Hyper-regeneration of corneal nerves in a scarred transplant, *Am J Ophthalmol* 61:880, 1966.
13. Ellis W, Barfort P, Mastman GJ: Keratoconjunctivitis with corneal crystals caused by the diffenbachia plant, *Am J Ophthalmol* 76:143, 1973.
14. Rootman DS et al: Accuracy and precision of the Tono-Pen in measuring intraocular pressure after keratoplasty and epikeratophakia and in scarred corneas, *Arch Ophthalmol* 106:1697, 1988.
15. Rubenstein JB, Deutsch TA: Pneumotonometry through bandage contact lenses, *Arch Ophthalmol* 103:1660, 1985.
16. Meyer RF, Stanifer RM, Bobb KC: MacKay-Marg tonometry over therapeutic soft contact lenses, *Am J Ophthalmol* 86:19, 1978.
17. Reader A, Salz JJ: Differences among ultrasonic pachymeters in measuring corneal thickness, *J Refract Surg* 3:7, 1987.
18. Cavanagh HD et al: Clinical and diagnostic use of in vivo confocal microscopy in patients with corneal disease, *Ophthalmology* 100:1444, 1993.
19. Chew SJ et al: Early diagnosis of infectious keratitis with in vivo real time confocal microscopy, *CLAO J* 18:197, 1992.
20. Auran JD et al: In vivo scanning slit confocal microscopy of *Acanthamoeba* keratitis: a case report, *Cornea* 13:183, 1994.
21. Duke-Elder S, Abrahms D: *The dioptric imagery of the eye.* In Duke-Elder S, Leigh AG, editors: *System of ophthalmology,* vol 5, *Ophthalmic optics and refraction,* St Louis, 1970, Mosby–Year Book, Inc.
22. Rowsey JJ, Reynold AE, Brown R: Corneal topography, *Arch Ophthalmol* 99:1093, 1981.
23. Maguire LJ, Bourne WD: Corneal topography of early keratoconus, *Am J Ophthalmol* 108:107, 1989.
24. Rabinowitz YS, McDonnell PJ: Computer-assisted corneal topography in keratoconus, *J Refract Corneal Surg* 5:400, 1989.
25. Binder PS: Selective suture removal can reduce postkeratoplasty astigmatism, *Ophthalmology* 92:1412, 1985.
26. Rowsey JJ et al: PERK corneal topography predicts refractive results in radial keratotomy, *Ophthalmology* 93(suppl):94, 1986.
27. Maguire LJ et al: Corneal topography in myopic patients undergoing epikeratophakia, *Am J Ophthalmol* 103:404, 1987.
28. Maguire LJ: Corneal topography of patients with excellent Snellen visual acuity after epikeratophakia for aphakia, *Am J Ophthalmol* 109:162, 1990.
29. Klyce SD: Computer-assisted corneal topography: high resolution graphic presentation and analysis of keratoscopy, *Invest Ophthalmol Vis Sci* 25:1426, 1984.
30. Hannush SB et al: Accuracy and precision of keratometry, photokeratoscopy, and corneal modeling on calibrated steel balls, *Arch Ophthalmol* 107:1235, 1989.
31. Hannush SB et al: Reproducibility of normal corneal power measurements with a keratometer, photokeratoscope, and video imaging system, *Arch Ophthalmol* 108:539, 1990.
32. Legeais JM, Ren Q, Simon G et al: Computer-assisted corneal topography: accuracy and reproducibility of the topographic modeling system, *Refract Corneal Surg* 9:347, 1993.
33. Maguire LJ et al: Evaluating the reproducibility of topography systems on spherical surfaces, *Arch Ophthalmol* 111:259, 1993.
34. Roberts C: The accuracy of 'power' maps to display curvature data in corneal topography, *Invest Ophthalmol Vis Sci* 35:3525, 1994.

35. Knoll HA: Corneal contours in the general population as revealed by the photokeratoscope, *Am J Optom* 38:389, 1961.

36. Clark BAJ: Mean topography of normal corneas, *Aust J Optom* 57:107, 1974.

37. Dingeldein SA, Klyce SD: The topography of normal corneas, *Arch Ophthalmol* 107:512, 1989.

38. Rowsey JJ, Balyeat HD, Monlux R et al: Prospective evaluation of radial keratotomy: photokeratoscope corneal topography, *Ophthalmology* 95:322, 1988.

39. Bogan DJ, Waring GO, Ibrahim O et al: Classification of normal corneal topography based on computer-assisted videokeratography, *Arch Ophthalmol* 108:945, 1990.

40. Rabinowitz YS, Garbus J, McDonnell PJ: Computer-assisted corneal topography in family members of patients with keratoconus, *Arch Ophthalmol* 108:365, 1990.

41. McClusky DJ, Villaseňor R, McDonnell PJ: Prospective topographic analysis in peripheral arcuate keratotomy for astigmatism, *Ophthalmic Surg* 21:464, 1990.

42. Dingeldein SA, Klyce SD, Wilson SE: Quantitative descriptors of corneal shape from computer-assisted analysis of photokeratographs, *Refract Corneal Surg* 5:372, 1989.

43. Wilson SE, Klyce SD: Quantitative descriptors of corneal topography: a clinical study, *Arch Ophthalmol* 109:349, 1991.

44. Maeda N et al: Automated keratoconus screening with corneal topography analysis, *Invest Ophthalmol Vis Sci* 35:2749, 1994.

45. Warnicki JW et al: Corneal topography using computer analyzed rasterstereographic images, *Appl Optics* 27:1135, 1988.

46. Warnicki JW et al: *Corneal topography using a projected grid*. In Schanzlin DJ, Robin JB, editors: *Corneal topography: measuring and modifying the cornea,* New York, 1992, Springer-Verlag.

47. Belin MW, Zloty P: Accuracy of the PAR corneal topography system with spatial misalignment, *CLAO J* 19:64, 1993.

48. Belin MW: Intraoperative raster photogrammetry: the PAR corneal topography system, *J Cataract Refract Surg* 19(suppl):188, 1993.

Four

Laboratory Evaluation

CYTOLOGY

Cytology is a relatively underused aid in the diagnosis of external ocular disease. In infectious diseases, the responsible organisms can frequently be seen, and in many diseases clues may be obtained from the types of inflammatory cells present and from changes in the conjunctival epithelial cells. For example, the presence of eosinophils in a specimen is a fairly specific finding that limits the differential to a few diseases, including allergic diseases such as hay fever conjunctivitis, atopic keratoconjunctivitis, and vernal conjunctivitis. In conjunctival or corneal infections, isolation and identification of the organism by culture is the primary goal; however, this is not always possible. In some cases, culture of the organism is difficult, such as with chlamydia, syphilis, or mycobacteria, or requires a prolonged period of incubation, as with some fungi. Pretreatment with antibiotics may prevent growth in culture, and cytologic examination of specimens may be the only way to identify the responsible organism. In addition, in some cases, such as with *Pseudomonas* keratitis, *Neisseria gonorrhoeae* conjunctivitis, or endophthalmitis, extensive ocular damage may occur before the organism can be identified in culture. Rarely, malignancy may be an unidentified cause of chronic conjunctivitis, and it can be detected with cytology.

Technique

Specimens should be taken from the site of most active inflammation. Any portion of the ocular surface can be scraped to yield an adequate specimen. In most cases either the conjunctiva will be uniformly affected or the inferior fornix will be most involved, so specimens are obtained from the inferior fornix. Other sites, however, such as the upper tarsal conjunctiva in trachoma and the limbal conjunctiva in limbal vernal conjunctivitis, often yield more information.

Topical anesthesia with proparacaine is usually sufficient, but additional anesthesia is sometimes required for conjunctival speci-

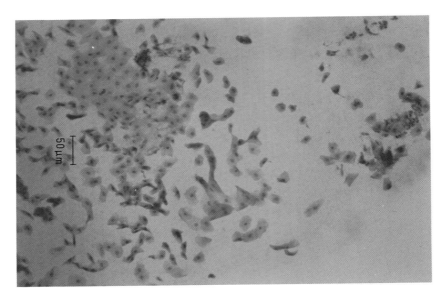

Figure 4-1
Impression cytology. Normal cells are on the left with blue cytoplasm and diffusely staining nuclei. Squamous metaplasia can be seen on the right with larger cells, smaller, more densely staining (pyknotic) nuclei, and red-staining cytoplasm. (Courtesy of Melvin I. Roat, Pittsburgh.)

mens. In those cases a pledget soaked in proparacaine can be applied to the site before scraping. Local application of tetracaine or cocaine can also be used. A platinum spatula, such as a Kimura spatula, is held at 45° to the surface and is passed several times in the same direction until sufficient material is obtained. Enough pressure is applied to blanch the conjunctival vessels. If membranes are present, they should be stripped from the area first and placed on a slide, and then the bed should be scraped. For corneal ulcers, all loose material should be removed first, and then the bed should be scraped. Jeweler's forceps may be helpful in obtaining infected stroma. The sample is smeared on a glass slide that has been cleaned with alcohol. If possible, a specimen 10 mm in diameter is obtained. At least two specimens should be obtained—more if specific stains or tests will be required.

Impression Cytology

Surface epithelial cells will adhere to a piece of cellulose acetate filter paper pressed against the conjunctiva when the paper is removed. The filter paper can be stained and the morphology of the surface epithelium examined. This simple, noninvasive method can be used to assess goblet cell density and epithelial cell differentiation (Fig. 4-1).[1-3] With this technique, squamous metaplasia and goblet cell loss have been demonstrated in cicatricial pemphigoid and keratitis sicca.[4,5] It also can be used in place of conjunctival scraping to diagnose infectious conjunctivitis, allergic conjunctivitis, and mucopolysaccharidosis.[6]

Follicular Expression

One may express follicles with the use of ring forceps. This method is valuable in differentiating trachomatous from nontrachomatous follicles. Trachomatous follicles are soft and express easily. They contain lymphocytes, plasma cells, monocytes, macrophages, and Leber cells.

Exudate Smear

An exudate smear is easier than a scraping to obtain but does not provide as much information. Obtaining an exudate smear requires removing the exudate present on the lid margin or within the conjunctival sac with a glass rod or the wooden end of an applicator stick and smearing it onto a microscope slide. The exudate smear contains only cells that have been sloughed from the conjunctiva, such as aged or keratinized epithelial cells, inflammatory cells, and occasionally organisms. This technique is especially good for demonstrating eosinophils; occasionally, eosinophils may be found in an exudate smear when they are not seen in a scraping.

Stain	Time	Uses	Comments
Gram's	10 min	Bacteria, yeasts	Differentiates gram-positive and gram-negative bacteria
Giemsa (see Fig. 11-2)	45–60 min	Cytology, fungi, chlamydial inclusions, bacteria (all stain blue)	Does not reveal intranuclear inclusions
Wright	15 min	Cytology, especially hematologic	Not as good as Giemsa for cytology
Papanicolaou	30 min	Tumor cells, inclusions	Relatively complicated
Periodic acid-Schiff (see Fig. 11-8)	25 min	Fungi	
Calcofluor white (Fig. 4-2)	1 min	Fungi,[7,8] *Acanthamoeba*[9]	Requires fluorescence microscope; may be difficult to interpret
Acridine orange (Fig. 4-3)	1 min	Fungi, bacteria, *Acanthamoeba*	Requires fluorescence microscope
Methenamine silver[14] (Fig. 4-4)	1–2 hr	Fungi	Relatively complicated; gelatin-coated slides for modified technique
Potassium hydroxide/ink–potassium hydroxide[8,15] (Fig. 4-5)	5 min–12 hr	Fungi	Difficult to read early
Acid fast (Ziehl-Nielsen)	10 min	Mycobacteria, *Nocardia*, *Actinomyces*	

Table 4-1   Stains for Corneal and Conjunctival Cytology

Staining

A great number of stains are available for examination of specimens, but in most cases Gram's or Giemsa stains are used. Gram's stain is generally used to identify bacteria, and Giemsa is used for cellular identification and morphology, fungi, and chlamydial inclusions. These and other commonly used stains are described in Table 4-1.

Calcofluor white[7-10] and acridine orange[11-13] stains have been used with increasing frequency, particularly for detection of *Acanthamoeba* and fungi (Figs. 4-2 and 4-3). These organisms can be missed easily with other stains, both in cytologic and histologic sections. Both stains require fluorescence microscopy but are very rapid and easy to perform. In one series calcofluor white was significantly more sensitive than potassium hydroxide wet mount in demonstrating fungal pathogens.[16]

Immunologically based methods have recently been developed for identification of organisms in scrapings. These are described later in this chapter.

Cells

The important types of cells seen and their significance are described in this section.[17] Unless otherwise indicated, the cells are described as they appear with Giemsa staining. The conditions associated with various cell types are summarized in the box on page 67.

Normal Conjunctival Epithelium

With scraping of a normal conjunctiva, epithelial cells come off in sheets. The cells have large central nuclei, which are oval and uniform in size and may have prominent nucleoli (Fig. 4-6). With the Giemsa stain, the nuclei are dark blue to purple, and the cytoplasm is pale blue and slightly granular. The nucleus to cytoplasm ratio is approximately 1:2. Keratin is not normally visible in the cytoplasm.

Keratinization and Pyknosis of Epithelial Cells

Epithelial cells become keratinized with exposure, drying, or mechanical trauma. Keratinization also occurs with conjunctival scarring, as in cicatricial pemphigoid, erythema multiforme, trachoma, vitamin A deficiency, superior limbal keratitis, and after irradiation. Keratinization is identified by the presence of faint red granules in the cytoplasm and increasing eosinophilia of the cytoplasm. With increasing cellular injury and degeneration, the cell becomes pyknotic. The cytoplasm and nucleus shrink and become increasingly basophilic, and eventually the nucleus is lost (Fig. 4-7).

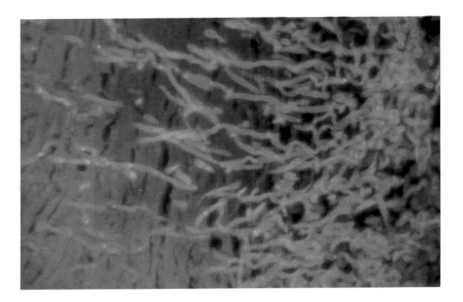

Figure 4-2
Fungal keratitis stained with calcofluor white.

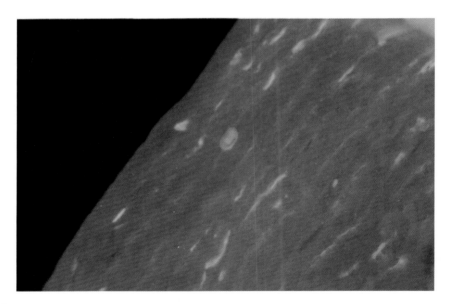

Figure 4-3
Acanthamoeba cyst (orange) stained with acridine orange. (Courtesy of Regis P. Kowalski, Pittsburgh.)

Leukocytes

The polymorphonuclear leukocyte (PMN) is the most common inflammatory cell in ocular specimens. The nucleus, which is basophilic, is segmented into two to five portions. The cytoplasm may stain pink or blue and may contain bluish granules.

All bacterial infections except those caused by *Moraxella (Branhamella) catarrhalis* evoke a polymorphonuclear response. PMNs also are seen in the presence of membranes or necrosis of the conjunctiva, whatever the cause. They are also prominent in trachoma, inclusion conjunctivitis, lymphogranuloma venereum, psit-

Cytology of Conjunctival Scrapings

Polymorphonuclear Cells
Bacterial infection, except *Moraxella (Branhamella)*
  catarrhalis
Fungal infection
Chlamydial infection
Membranous conjunctivitis (any cause)
Necrosis of conjunctiva (any cause)
Staphylococcal conjunctival phlyctenulosis

Mononuclear Cells (Lymphocytes)
Viral infection
Thyroid conjunctival hyperemia

Mixed, Polymorphonuclear Cells Predominate
Chlamydial infection, chronic
Most cases of chronic conjunctivitis
Catarrhal ulcers
Superior limbal keratoconjunctivitis
Pemphigoid
Erythema multiforme
Reiter's syndrome
Acne rosacea
Chemical burns
Some drug reactions

Mixed, Lymphocytes Predominate
Early viral infections
Viral infections with membranes
Most drug reactions
Keratoconjunctivitis sicca
Tuberculous conjunctivitis
Syphilitic conjunctivitis

Basophils
Trachoma
Vernal catarrh
Chronic conjunctivitis

Eosinophils
Vernal catarrh
Atopic keratoconjunctivitis
Hay fever conjunctivitis
Occasionally in drug allergies
Erythema multiforme
Pemphigoid

Plasma Cells
Trachoma

Keratinized Epithelial Cells
Keratoconjunctivitis sicca
Pemphigoid
Chemical burns
Erythema multiforme
Superior limbal keratoconjunctivitis
Squamous metaplasia
Vitamin A deficiency
Trachoma
Radiation
Severe membranous conjunctivitis
Some drug reactions

Goblet Cells
Keratoconjunctivitis sicca
Chronic conjunctivitis

Multinucleated Epithelial Cells
Herpes simplex infection
Varicella zoster infection
Chlamydial infection
Measles
Cytomegalovirus infection
Newcastle virus conjunctivitis
Squamous neoplasia
Radiation

tacosis, Reiter's syndrome, psoriasis, erythema multiforme, and drug toxicity. Phlyctenulosis of the conjunctiva characteristically shows little exudate unless it is caused by staphylococci, in which case PMNs will be the predominant cell type.

The intensity of the polymorphonuclear response may vary according to the stage of disease. For example, in acute gonococcal conjunctivitis an intense PMN response occurs, with marked fibrin formation; but in later stages, while the PMNs continue to predominate, there is an increased number of mononuclear cells. In very early viral conjunctivitis, PMNs may predominate. Generally, however, in chronic infections PMNs will predominate, with mononuclear cells present in a moderate amount. The exception is staphylococcal conjunctivitis, in which the PMNs are present in marked numbers, even in chronic conjunctivitis.

Lymphocytes are smaller cells, with a nonsegmented, dark-staining nucleus and scant bluish cytoplasm (Fig. 4-8). They are the predominant cells in viral conjunctivitis. They also are common in chronic conjunctivitis, chlamydial infections, and hypersensitivity diseases; but PMNs are usually more plentiful. Rarely, they may be the predominant cells in tuberculosis, syphilis, and trachoma.

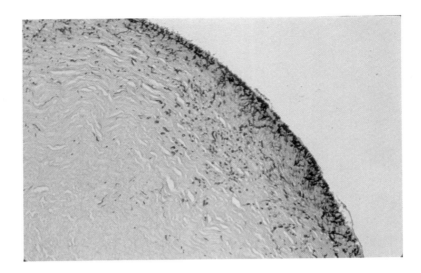

Figure 4-4
Actinomyces keratitis stained with methenamine silver. (Courtesy of Michael W. Belin, Albany, NY.)

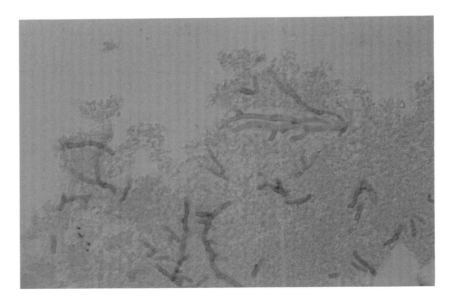

Figure 4-5
Fungi in scraping stained with ink–potassium hydroxide.

Monocytes are larger mononuclear cells, with a folded, kidney-bean–shaped nucleus and abundant cytoplasm. Like lymphocytes, they are usually found in viral infections.

Plasma cells are lymphocytes that actively produce antibody. They have an eccentric dark nucleus, with a cartwheel chromatin pattern (Fig. 4-8). There is a clear halo adjacent to the nucleus and they contain an eccentric, basophilic cytoplasm. Although these are promi-

nent subepithelially in many types of conjunctivitis and are associated with immune-mediated disorders, they are rarely present in scrapings. They are found in trachoma because in this condition the follicles readily rupture with scraping and plasma cells are released.

Eosinophils are never seen in scrapings from a normal eye. They are leukocytes with bilobed nuclei and pink granules in the cytoplasm (Fig. 4-9). The cells are quite fragile, and frequently

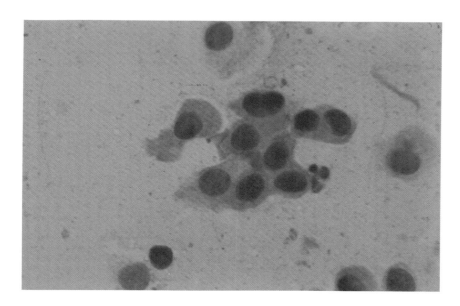

Figure 4-6
Scraping containing normal conjunctival epithelium (Giemsa stain). (Courtesy of Regis P. Kowalski, Pittsburgh.)

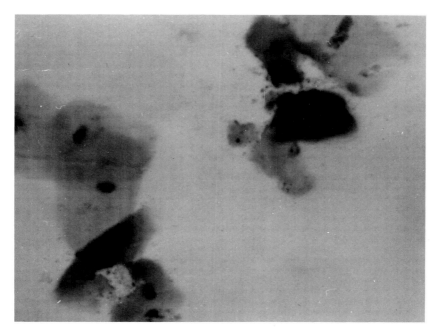

Figure 4-7
Keratinized epithelial cells (Giemsa stain).

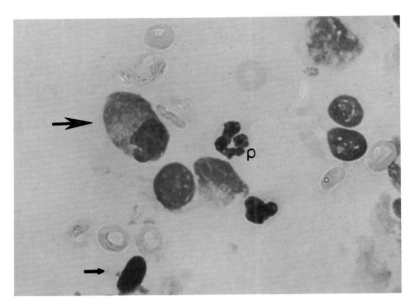

Figure 4-8
Conjunctival scraping containing mononuclear cells (*small arrow*), polymorphonuclear cells (*P*), and plasma cells (*large arrow*) (Giemsa stain). (Courtesy of Regis P. Kowalski, Pittsburgh.)

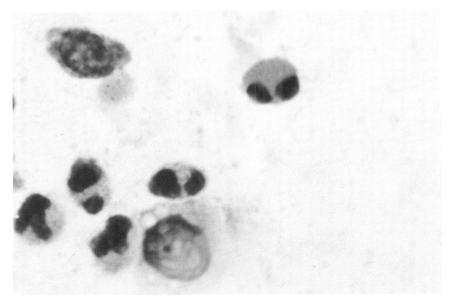

Figure 4-9
Conjunctival scraping showing eosinophils in a case of cicatricial pemphigoid (Giemsa stain).

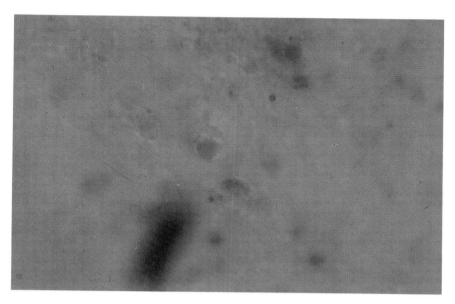

Figure 4-10
Mast cells (Unna's stain, ×1000).

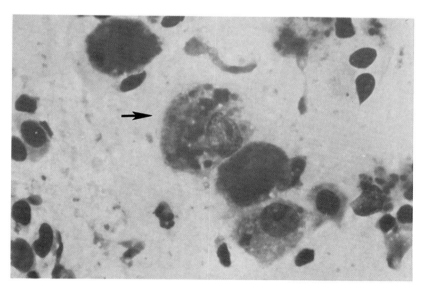

Figure 4-11
Leber cell (*arrow*) (Giemsa stain). (Courtesy of Regis P. Kowalski, Pittsburgh.)

only broken cell remnants and free granules are observed. Eosinophils usually indicate allergic inflammation—hay fever, atopic dermatitis, or vernal conjunctivitis. A few eosinophils are seen in drug and cosmetic allergies, except for phospholine iodide or pilocarpine sensitivity. Eosinophils also may be observed in ocular cicatricial pemphigoid.

Basophils (mast cells) are small bluish cells that contain large, dark blue cytoplasmic gran-

ules (Fig. 4-10). They are also seen in allergic disorders, particularly vernal conjunctivitis. Small numbers of basophils may be present in trachoma.

Leber cells are very large macrophages. They are often several times the size of epithelial cells and contain phagocytized cellular debris (Fig. 4-11). They are more numerous in trachoma but may be seen in other types of conjunctivitis.

Goblet Cells

Goblet cells contain a large, pink-staining mass of mucoid material. The nucleus is pushed aside to the cell wall and is purple. Goblet cells may be observed in scrapings from normal eyes and are increased in scrapings in keratoconjunctivitis sicca.

Multinucleated Epithelial Cells

Multinucleated epithelial cells may result from either failure of the nucleus to completely divide during mitosis or fusion of several cells. In the former, they tend to be close to normal in size and are seen in many forms of conjunctival inflammation, including viral and chlamydial infections, allergy, and after irradiation. Fusion of multiple cells produces giant cells, which contain 5 to 20 nuclei. These are seen only in simplex or zoster herpetic infections (see Fig. 12-20). Tumor cells also may be multinucleated, but these usually exhibit other abnormal characteristics, as described later.

Epithelial Cell Inclusions

Epithelial cell inclusions occur in viral and chlamydial infections and can be diagnostic. The types of inclusions seen in external ocular infections are listed in Table 4-2. Viral inclusions are best demonstrated with Papanicolaou (PAP) staining, and even then can be difficult to appreciate. Inclusions in molluscum contagiosum are readily appreciated with hematoxylin and eosin staining of specimens from skin lesions. They appear as eosinophilic cytoplasmic masses (Fig. 4-12).

The inclusions of trachoma and inclusion conjunctivitis are readily identifiable with Giemsa staining. The classic chlamydial inclusion, Halberstaedter-Prowazek, is seen as a mass of basophilic granules capping the nucleus (see Fig. 8-3). It is composed of elementary bodies (the infectious form of the organism) containing DNA. Individual elementary bodies may also be seen as uniform, round, reddish-blue or purple granules, 0.3 μm in size, in epithelial cells, PMNs, or extracellularly. These swell to 1 μm, or about the size of a staphylococcus, when they enter an epithelial cell and produce RNA, after which they are called *reticulate* or *initial bodies*.

Melanin granules, 0.3 to 1.0 μm in diameter, may be seen within epithelial cells. They are deep brown in an unstained slide and greenish-black after Giemsa staining. Mascara may also be seen as pigmented granules within epithelial cells. Nuclear debris may be phagocytosed by epithelial cells, and this stains a uniform dark blue with a clear, circumscribed border.

Tumor Cells

Several morphologic abnormalities are suggestive of neoplasia (Fig. 4-13):

1. Increased nucleus-to-cytoplasm ratio
2. Increase in chromatin content, producing hyperchromatism (may also be seen in pyknosis or if the slide is overstained)
3. Aberrant chromatin pattern, with elongation and irregularity in outline

Table 4-2 Viral and Chlamydial Inclusions					
	Location		Staining (Giemsa)		
Disease	Cytoplasmic	Nuclear	Eosinophilic	Basophilic	Iodine Stain
Herpes simplex (Cowdry's type A)	−	+	+	−	
Varicella zoster (Lipschütz)	−	+	+	−	
Variola (Guarnieri)	+	+	+	−	
Vaccinia (Guarnieri)	+	−	+	−	
Newcastle	+	−	+	−	
Molluscum (Henderson-Paterson)	+	−	+	−	
Adenovirus	−	+	+(early)	+(late)	
Trachoma	+	−	−	+	+
Inclusion conjunctivitis (Halberstaedter-Prowazek)	+	−	−	+	+
Lymphogranuloma venereum	+	−	−	+	−
Psittacosis	+	−	−	+	

4. Enlarged or increased nucleoli (usually four or more)
5. Increased and abnormal mitotic figures
6. Multinucleated cells with associated nuclear changes
7. Bizarre cell shapes
8. Irregularity of cells, variable cell size, and lack of distinct cell boundaries

A PAP stain is preferable for evaluation of these characteristics in cytology specimens. However, if a tumor is suspected, a biopsy should be performed; cytology alone is not sufficient for diagnosis.

Organisms

The Gram's stain characteristics of the most common ocular pathogens are as follows:

Bacteria	Distinguishing Characteristics
Gram-positive cocci	
Staphylococci	Irregular groups or clusters of spheres that may vary in size and staining qualities
Streptococcus pneumoniae	Lancet-shaped diplococci; may see capsule
Other streptococci	Usually oval or elliptic cocci; often in chains
Micrococci	Usually in tetrads
Peptostreptococcus, Peptococcus	May occur in pairs or chains
Gram-positive rods*	
Corynebacteria	Club-shaped bacillus, often with barred metachromatic granules or terminal masses at the poles
Propionibacterium	Pleomorphic
Clostridia	Slender, motile rods
Gram-positive filaments	
Actinomyces	Intertwining, branching filaments with or without clubs and diphtheroid forms
Nocardia	Intertwining, branching filaments without terminal clubs
Gram-negative rods	
Pseudomonas aeruginosa	Slender, motile rod with straight parallel sides and curved ends
Klebsiella pneumoniae	Short, fat rod with capsule, often diplobacilli
Bacteroides	Thin, filamentous rods
Haemophilus influenzae	Small coccobacillary rods, may have capsules
Moraxella	Diplobacilli, plump rods arranged end-to-end; polar staining, round or rectangular ends; largest of the gram-negative rods
Escherichia coli	Rods without distinguishing characteristics
Proteus	
Serratia	
Citrobacter	
Enterobacter	
Azotobacter	
Acinetobacter	
Gram-negative cocci*	
Neisseria	Kidney-shaped diplococci; often intracellular; may not decolorize well after antibiotic exposure

*Gram-positive rods and gram-negative cocci are relatively uncommon, and incorrect staining should be suspected.

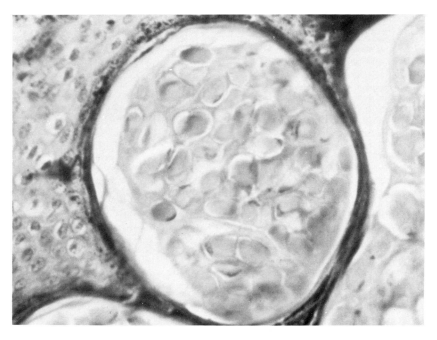

Figure 4-12
Molluscum bodies (Hematoxylin-eosin stain).

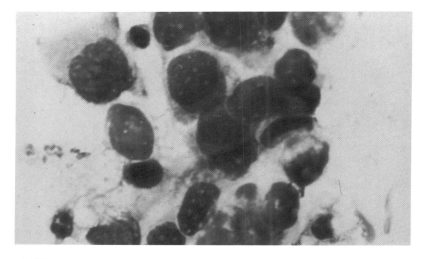

Figure 4-13
Malignant cells in a scraping (Giemsa stain). (Courtesy of Regis P. Kowalski, Pittsburgh.)

CULTURE

Diagnosis and appropriate treatment of conjunctival and corneal infections require isolation and identification of the causative organism(s).

Media

Different media must be used because of the varying requirements of ocular pathogens.

Commonly used media are described in Table 4-3. Eye cultures should be inoculated directly onto the culture media, rather than into a carrier, because the sample size is small, and many eye pathogens are fastidious organisms.

Mannitol-salt agar plates are helpful to the microbiologist in the preliminary identification of staphylococci. Nearly all *Staphylococcus aureus* isolates will ferment mannitol, whereas many nonaureus species will not. Therefore

Table 4-3 Common Media

Media	Organisms	Comments
Blood agar (5% sheep's blood)	Majority of aerobic bacteria; saprophytic fungi	Room temperature for fungi
Chocolate agar	*Haemophilus, Neisseria, Moraxella*	5%–10% carbon dioxide
Sabouraud dextrose agar	Fungi	Room temperature
Mannitol-salt agar	Staphylococci, diphtheroids, *Proteus*	37°C air
Thayer-Martin agar	*Neisseria*	10% carbon dioxide
Löwenstein-Jensen culture	Mycobacteria, *Nocardia*	
Middlebrook-Cohn agar	Mycobacteria, *Nocardia*	
Escherichia coli seeded agar (nonnutrient agar with *E. coli* overlay)	*Acanthamoeba*	
Centers for Disease Control anaerobic blood agar	Bacterial anaerobes	Incubate in anaerobic chamber
Enriched thioglycollate broth	Aerobic and anaerobic bacteria	Better than blood agar for anaerobes and small inoculums
Brain-heart infusion	Bacteria, fungi	Fastidious organisms
Chopped meat-glucose	Anaerobes, particularly clostridia	
Loeffler's media	*Corynebacterium diphtheria*	

only mannitol-positive isolates are tested for coagulase or protein A, for identification of *S. aureus*, which saves time and expense.

Blood agar, mannitol-salt agar, and chocolate agar are normally used for lid and conjunctival cultures. If a specific organism is suspected, other media may be necessary.

In general, two blood agar plates and one each of chocolate agar, mannitol-salt agar, Sabouraud dextrose agar, and enriched thioglycollate broth are inoculated for corneal ulcers. One blood agar plate and the chocolate agar are incubated in 5% carbon dioxide at 37°C, and the mannitol-salt plate and enriched thioglycollate broth are incubated in air at 37°C. Another blood agar and the Sabouraud plate are left at room temperature. If another organism is suspected, or if an infection is not responding to therapy, other media are used.

Chlamydial and viral isolation is more difficult, more expensive, and not as widely available as bacterial cultures. However, if available, they can be useful in some patients. For viral and chlamydial cultures, transport media are required. The viral transport media may not be usable for chlamydia because they often contain antibiotics that inhibit their growth. Chlamydial media, however, can usually be used for both viral and chlamydial transport.

Chlamydiae are normally grown in cultures of cycloheximide-treated McCoy cells. After inoculation with a specimen, the culture is incubated for 48 to 72 hours and then examined for cytoplasmic inclusions using Giemsa staining. This can be facilitated by using fluorescein-tagged monoclonal antibodies to the chlamydia.[18]

Viruses must also be grown in cell cultures. A large number of cell lines are available for different viruses. Currently, in Pittsburgh's Campbell laboratory cell lines A549 and MRC5 are used because they support growth of herpes simplex, herpes zoster, adenoviruses, and cytomegalovirus as well as other, less common ocular pathogens. The tissue cultures must be examined several times per week for up to 4 weeks for evidence of cellular damage resulting from viral reproduction (cytopathic effect). Once growth is observed, the causative virus must be identified by other means.

Technique
Conjunctiva and Lids
Anesthesia with topical proparacaine is sufficient. A cotton-tipped or calcium alginate swab is used. These swabs should be moistened with a broth, such as Mueller-Hinton or trypticase soy, or with sterile saline because doing so increases the recovery of organisms. For lid cultures the anterior margins of the upper and lower lids are swabbed several times. The swab is then rolled onto the media. There is no need

to culture the upper and lower lids on separate media.

Conjunctival cultures are usually obtained from the tarsal surface of the lower lid. The patient is told to look up, the lower lid is pulled down, and a moistened applicator is used to swab back and forth over the tarsal conjunctiva.

Both eyes are routinely cultured, even if only one is affected. It is convenient and economical to use only one plate for lid and conjunctival cultures from both eyes. A patterned inoculation facilitates this procedure. For viral cultures a sterile plastic-handled cotton or Dacron swab (calcium alginate should not be used because it binds and inactivates some viruses[19]) should be moistened with the viral transport medium and rubbed against the superior and inferior tarsal conjunctiva. The tip of the swab is then broken off and placed in the transport medium. Rose bengal should not be applied before obtaining viral cultures because it markedly reduces viral titers.[20]

Cornea

Corneal cultures are best obtained with the aid of a slit-lamp or operating microscope. Proparacaine should be used for anesthesia because cocaine and tetracaine are more bactericidal. Specimens can be obtained with either a platinum spatula or a broth-moistened swab. In one report, the spatula and a calcium alginate swab moistened with trypticase soy broth were similar in yield.[21] The recommended spatula technique is as follows: A flamed and cooled platinum spatula is used to scrape the leading edge and bed of the ulcer. If loose material is present on the surface, it should be removed first and placed on a slide. A jeweler's forceps or hypodermic needle can sometimes yield a better specimen, particularly for smaller lesions. The specimens are first applied to microscope slides for examination. As discussed earlier, at least two slides should be prepared, and they should be cleaned and dried before use. Multiple areas of a large ulcer should be scraped. The spatula is flamed and cooled again, and the media are inoculated. Each scraping should be used to inoculate one medium; multiple C streaks are used on the agar plates. For viral cultures of corneal lesions it is best to scrape the lesion and transfer the material to a cotton swab, which is then placed in the transport medium.

Interpretation

The growth of aerobic bacteria from conjunctiva or cornea usually becomes apparent on standard media within 48 hours and often is evident after only 12 hours. A sample can be taken and examined with Gram's stain to give a preliminary identification.

It is often difficult to tell whether an organism in culture is responsible for ocular infection. One clue is that any organism growing outside the C streaks on solid media should be considered a contaminant. Some criteria have been recommended for distinguishing pathogens from nonpathogens. First, clinical signs of infection should be present. Then, according to Liesegang and Forster,[15] one of the following must be present: (1) growth of an organism in two or more media, (2) confluent growth of a known ocular pathogen in one solid medium, or (3) growth in one medium of an organism identified in cytology. Jones[22] recommends that 10 or more colonies of bacterial growth be present on one solid medium, and that for fungi any detectable growth on any two media or growth on one medium with positive cytology is sufficient.

These recommendations have limitations, however, because often only one medium is suitable for a pathogen and only a few viable organisms of a pathogen may be obtained. Therefore, clinical judgment must often be used. The likelihood of an organism to be a pathogen, the likelihood of it producing the observed clinical picture, and the relative risk of treatment versus not treating a pathogen should be considered. Bacterial and fungal organisms present in normal conjunctiva and their approximate incidences are as follows:[23-29]

Bacterial and Fungal Organisms in Normal Conjunctiva	
Organism	**Incidence (%)**
Staphylococcus epidermidis	75-90
Propionibacteria	80
Diphtheroids	35-55
Staphylococcus aureus	5-20
α-Hemolytic streptococci	2-7
Pseudomonas	0-6
Haemophilus influenzae	1.5-3
Streptococcus pneumoniae	1-4
Other gram-negative rods	4-7
Total fungi*	10-20
Aspergillus	1-7
Candida	0.5-3

*There is a higher rate of positive fungal cultures in warmer climates (e.g., the Philippines and India).

Many organisms that are commensals under some circumstances or in some individuals can produce serious disease in other individuals or under different conditions.

BIOPSY

Indications
Conjunctiva

Tissue specimens are often valuable in the diagnosis of ocular and systemic disease. The most obvious indication for biopsy is when there is a question of malignancy. Because conjunctival malignancies may be subtle, a biopsy should be considered in any case of chronic conjunctivitis of undetermined etiology. Sarcoid commonly produces conjunctival granulomas, and a biopsy of suspicious lesions may prove diagnostic and prevent more invasive procedures. Several infectious diseases, including tuberculosis, leprosy, and syphilis, can produce conjunctival granulomas, sometimes in association with visible enlargement of preauricular nodes (i.e., Parinaud's oculoglandular syndrome; see Chapter 7). The causative organisms can often be identified in conjunctival biopsy specimens.

Dermatologic diseases affect the conjunctiva and may be diagnosed from conjunctival biopsies are listed below.

In most cases, diagnosis requires immunopathologic examination for antibodies or complement components.

Some of the many metabolic diseases that exhibit characteristic changes in the conjunctiva[44,45] are listed below.

Conjunctival goblet cell content and mitotic rate may be important in ocular surface diseases such as cicatricial pemphigoid, vitamin A deficiency, erythema multiforme, and keratoconjunctivitis sicca. In each of these diseases there is loss of goblet cells. In cicatricial pemphigoid, vitamin A deficiency, and atopic dermatitis, an increase in the normal mitotic rate of the conjunctival epithelium has been observed.[36,64] In contrast to the other diseases, increased goblet cell density is found in atopic dermatitis.[65]

Dermatologic Diseases and Immunopathologic Findings

Disease	Immunopathologic Findings
Cicatricial pemphigoid	Antibody deposited on epithelial basement membrane: IgG, IgA, IgM, complement[30-35]
	Increased epithelial mitotic rate[36]
Erythema multiforme	C3, IgM, fibrin in vessel walls[37]
Epidermolysis bullosa acquisita*	IgG, IgA, IgM, complement deposits in epithelial BM[38-41]
Pemphigus vulgaris	Epithelial intercellular IgG, IgA, IgM, complement[42]
Adult linear IgA disease	Linear deposits of IgA, IgG along epithelial BM[43]
Toxic epidermal necrolysis	Intercellular IgG, IgM, C3[35]
Molluscum contagiosum	Eosinophilic cytoplasmic inclusions

*Immunopathologic changes demonstrated in skin and conjunctival involvement are common, but immunopathologic examination of conjunctiva has not been reported.

Metabolic Diseases

Disease	Findings
Cystinosis	Intracellular crystals[46,47]
Oxalosis	Crystals
Primary familial amyloidosis (rarely secondary systemic)	Amyloid[48]
Fabry's disease	Intracytoplasmic lamellar inclusions[49-51]
Mucolipidoses	Vacuolization of epithelium; intracytoplasmic lamellar or fibrillogranular inclusions[52-57]
Mucopolysaccharidoses	Intracytoplasmic accumulation of acid mucopolysaccharide[58-60]
Tyrosinemia, type II	Intracytoplasmic whorled membranous inclusions[61]
Fucosidosis	Intracytoplasmic multilaminate inclusions in epithelium[62,63]

Cornea

Corneal stromal biopsies are not often performed because of their destructive effect. However, if an unidentified destructive corneal process is progressing despite current treatment, biopsy is indicated to attempt to make the diagnosis. Obviously, reluctance to remove tissue is much greater when the process involves the visual axis, but biopsy is still indicated in some cases. For example, infections due to fungi,[66] Acanthamoeba,[67,68] and atypical mycobacteria[69] can be diagnosed by biopsy when cultures and scrapings do not reveal the organism.

Technique

It is often best to check with the pathologist to determine the optimum handling and fixation method before obtaining a specimen. These procedures vary greatly depending on the studies required.

Conjunctiva

Sufficient anesthesia usually can be obtained with a proparacaine-soaked pledget held against the biopsy site. The specimen should be handled as little as possible because crushing the tissue prevents histologic analysis. One edge of the area is picked up with toothed forceps, tenting the tissue, and Wescott scissors are used to snip off a specimen. Multiple pieces may be obtained; if they are from different areas, they should be fixed and labeled individually. If malignancy is suspected, a map of the lesion and location of biopsies should be made.

Cornea

Limited biopsies may be performed at the slit-lamp microscope with a sharp blade and fine forceps. Topical anesthesia is administered, and the lids are held open manually or with a speculum. At the base of the ulcer a piece of infiltrated tissue is grasped and cut free with the blade. Several small pieces can be removed for culture and staining.

If these procedures are insufficient, or if no ulceration is present, lamellar keratectomy is required. Keratectomy must be performed in the operating room and involves removal of a section 2 to 5 mm in diameter, one third to one half of the stromal depth.[70]

Fixation

Most specimens will be examined only histologically with light microscopy and can be fixed in 10% formalin. These small specimens tend to curl up in solution, so it is best to lay them flat on a carrier before placing them in the formalin. A wet cellulose sponge or a tongue blade may be used for this purpose. Some have recommended dried cucumber slices, to which the biopsy specimen is attached by albumin fixative.[71,72]

Several diseases are characterized by the presence of crystal in the conjunctiva, and in two of the diseases, cystinosis and oxalosis, the crystals are soluble in formalin. (Also, in advanced gout, crystals may be found in the subcutaneous tissue of the lids, and these crystals are also soluble in formalin). Therefore, if a biopsy is performed for diagnosis of one of these diseases the tissue should be fixed in absolute alcohol.

Tissues on which immunopathologic examination is planned should be placed in a Petri dish, with a small amount of saline solution. They must be fresh-frozen in a special mounting medium, such as "optimal cutting temperature," a procedure that should be performed by the laboratory. For electron microscopy, glutaraldehyde solutions are recommended.

IMMUNOPATHOLOGIC TESTS

Many tests have been developed to detect specific antigens in specimens using monoclonal antibodies. These tests are becoming more widely available, more specific, and easier to perform. Commercial tests are now available for detection of a number of ocular pathogens, particularly viruses and chlamydia (described in sections on specific pathogens). A specific antibody is allowed to react with the specimen, and detection of antibody attachment is accomplished by one of several methods. Immunoperoxidase techniques are probably most common today. The monoclonal antibody is labeled with peroxidase, and the presence of the enzyme is detected by its reaction with chromogens, which can be observed with light microscopy. Another common method is by fluorescence; the monoclonal antibody is labeled with fluorescein, and the amount and location of antibody binding is determined with a fluorescence microscope.

Serologic tests are also available for most viruses and for chlamydia. Patient antibodies against an agent can be detected and quantified. Single measurements of titers may be useful, but usually both acute and convalescent titers are required to make the diagnosis of an acute infection. Obviously, this method is not useful in recurrent or longstanding disease.

Dermatologic Disorders

As mentioned previously, immunopathologic techniques can help diagnose a number of dermatologic disorders associated with conjunctival scarring (see the box on page 77).

Lymphoid Lesions

Immunopathologic techniques have been used to distinguish reactive lymphoid hyperplasia from lymphoma and to classify lymphomas. Light chain monoclonality suggests lymphoma, whereas polyclonality suggests lymphoid hyperplasia.[73] Knowles et al.[74] present a good review of the characterization of lymphoid tumors.

Infectious Diseases
Chlamydia

It is often difficult to establish the diagnosis of chlamydial infection, particularly in adults. Chlamydial cultures are not widely available and are frequently negative despite the presence of infection.[75,76] Typical inclusions in Giemsa-stained specimens, while diagnostic, are rarely seen in adults. Equal difficulty has been encountered in the diagnosis of genital infections, and much of the development in techniques has been performed by researchers in this field.[77]

Two direct tests are commercially available for examining conjunctival specimens: (1) Microtrak (Syva, Palo Alto, CA), a fluorescein-tagged monoclonal antibody, and (2) Chlamydiazyme (Abbott Laboratories, North Chicago, IL), an enzyme immunosorbent assay (EIA). In Microtrak, the fluorescein-tagged antibodies are reacted with a smear, and the slide is then examined with a fluorescence microscope for fluorescent chlamydial elementary bodies. The test is relatively easy to perform but requires experience to interpret accurately. In reported series the sensitivity has varied from 60% to 100%, and specificity from 50% to 100%.[75,76,78-81] In our experience this test is difficult to interpret and should be read only by those with a great deal of experience.

In the EIA, the swab is placed in a solution and reacted with peroxidase-labeled antibodies. The presence of chlamydial antigen is indicated by a change in the color of the solution after the addition of a chromogen substrate of the peroxidase. In a report of adult chlamydial conjunctivitis, this test had a sensitivity of 71% and a specificity of 97%, which was better than the direct fluorescent test.[81] This test is easy to interpret but relatively difficult to perform. An-

other EIA, the Kodak Surecell *Chlamydia* test (Kodak Clinical Products, Rochester, NY), was found to be easy to perform and 100% specific, but only 40% sensitive.[82] In patients with active trachoma, both of these tests have been less sensitive, particularly in those with mild disease.[83,84]

Serum assays for chlamydial antibodies are also available and may be useful in the diagnosis of ocular disease.[85,86] As mentioned earlier, an acute rise in titer is the most accurate means of serum diagnosis, but single high titers are suggestive. In a recent study[87] a single serum titer 1:28 (Pharmacia Diagnostics [Electronucleosis], Columbia, MD) had a sensitivity of 90% and a specificity of 76% compared with culture.

Viruses

Several immunologic tests are available for detection of herpes simplex types I and II in ocular specimens. Probably the most accurate of these is the enzyme immunosorbent assay, Herpcheck (Dupont–New England Nuclear Division, Billerica, MA), which has been approved by the Food and Drug Administration.[88,89] Unfortunately, this test is both expensive and time consuming (5 hours). Immunocytologic staining can also be performed on impression cytology specimens obtained from epithelial dendrites. In one study it was as sensitive as tissue culture.[90]

An EIA for adenovirus (Adenoclone Test; Cambridge Bioscience, Worcester, MA) was found to have a sensitivity of 81% and a specificity of 100% for specimens taken within 1 week of the onset of symptoms.[91] An immunofiltration system, designed by Cleveland and Richman[92] (V & P Scientific, San Diego, CA), appears to be nearly as accurate and much more practical, and it can also be used for detection of chlamydia and adenovirus.

Polymerase Chain Reaction. The polymerase chain reaction (PCR) is a method of detecting very small quantities of specific DNA or RNA segments in samples. Any DNA or RNA that matches the probe DNA or RNA sequence is amplified in vitro up to 1 million times. Theoretically, this technique could be applied to the detection of all microorganisms as well as to the detection of genetic disease. Appropriate probes must be determined for each organism tested. The DNA or RNA sequences of the probes must be unique to the organism. Currently, the technique is relatively complicated and time consuming, and is therefore performed in few clinical laboratories, but it is becoming increasingly common.

Polymerase chain reaction appears to be as or more sensitive than culture and immunofluorescence techniques for the diagnosis of chlamydial conjunctivitis.[93-97] A new commercially available PCR test for chlamydia (Amplicor; Diagnostics, Branchburg, NJ) was found to be 88% sensitive and 100% specific.[98] PCR appears to be as or more sensitive than culture and enzyme immunoassay for herpes simplex keratitis.[99-102] The PCR technique also appears to be applicable to the detection of adenovirus in ocular swabs.[103]

OTHER TESTS

Limulus Lysate Test

The *limulus lysate test* is a simple, quick, and fairly accurate method for detecting endotoxin in corneal specimens.[15,104,105] Endotoxin is lipopolysaccharide in the cell wall of gram-negative enteric organisms, and its detection would therefore indicate that one of these organisms was present in the specimen. The horseshoe crab *Limulus polyphemus* produces cells, coelomic amebocytes, which cause clotting when exposed to endotoxin. The natural response of this organism to gram-negative bacterial infection is disseminated intravascular coagulation. This endotoxin activation of the coagulation pathway has been adapted as a sensitive in vitro assay for the presence of bacterial lipopolysaccharide. It becomes positive earlier than bacterial cultures and is unaffected by the presence of antibiotics; therefore, it theoretically allows accurate diagnosis of partially treated patients with gram-negative corneal infections. The test cannot be used to assess the effectiveness of antibacterial therapy because endotoxin persists in the corneal debris for several days despite negative cultures taken from ulcerated areas.[105] To perform the test, material from corneal scrapings is emulsified in a test tube with the amebocyte lysate reagent. If endotoxin is present, a visible clot is formed. In our experience at the University of Pittsburgh, this test has produced many false-positive results.

REFERENCES

1. Egbert PR, Lauber S, Maurice DM: A simple conjunctival biopsy, *Am J Ophthalmol* 84:793, 1977.
2. Tseng SCG: Staging of conjunctival squamous metaplasia by impression cytology, *Ophthalmology* 92:728, 1985.
3. Vadreyu VL, Fullard RJ: Enhancements to the conjunctival impression cytology technique and examples of applications in a clinico-biochemical study of dry eye, *CLAO J* 20:59, 1994.
4. Nelson JD, Havener VR, Cameron JD: Cellulose acetate impressions of the ocular surface: dry eye states, *Arch Ophthalmol* 101:1869, 1983.
5. Nelson JD, Wright JC: Conjunctival goblet cell densities in ocular surface disease, *Arch Ophthalmol* 102:1049, 1984.
6. Maskin SL et al: Diagnostic impression cytology for external eye disease, *Cornea* 8:270, 1989.
7. Sutphin JE et al: Improved detection of oculomycoses using induced fluorescence with Cellufluor, *Ophthalmology* 93:416, 1986.
8. Arffa RC et al: Calcofluor white and ink-potassium hydroxide preparations for identifying fungi, *Am J Ophthalmol* 100:719, 1985.
9. Wilhelmus KR et al: Rapid diagnosis of *Acanthamoeba* keratitis using calcofluor white, *Arch Ophthalmol* 104:1309, 1986.
10. Marines HM, Osato MS, Font RL: The value of calcofluor white in the diagnosis of mycotic and *Acanthamoeba* infections of the eye and adnexa, *Ophthalmology* 94:23, 1987.
11. Groden LR et al: Acridine orange and Gram stains in infectious keratitis, *Cornea* 9:122, 1990.
12. Mattman LH: *Cell wall deficient forms*, Cleveland, 1974, CRC Press.
13. Gomez JT et al: Comparison of acridine orange and Gram stains in bacterial keratitis, *Am J Ophthalmol* 106:735, 1988.
14. Forster RK et al: Methenamine silver–stained corneal scraping in keratomycosis, *Am J Ophthalmol* 82:261, 1976.
15. Liesegang TJ, Forster RF: Spectrum of microbial keratitis in South Florida, *Am J Ophthalmol* 90:38, 1980.
16. Chander J et al: Evaluation of calcofluor staining in the diagnosis of fungal corneal ulcer, *Mycoses* 36:243, 1993.
17. Stenson S: *Cytologic diagnosis*. In Karcioglu ZA, editor: *Laboratory diagnosis in ophthalmology*, New York, 1987, Macmillan.
18. Munday PE et al: A comparison of the sensitivity of immunofluorescence and Giemsa for staining *Chlamydia trachomatis* inclusions in cycloheximide-treated McCoy cells, *J Clin Pathol* 33:177, 1980.
19. Bettoli EJ et al: The role of temperature and swab materials in the recovery of herpes simplex virus from lesions, *J Infect Dis* 145:399, 1982.
20. Roat MI et al: The antiviral effects of rose bengal and fluorescein, *Arch Ophthalmol* 105:1415, 1987.
21. Benson WH, Lanier JD: Comparison of techniques for culturing corneal ulcers, *Ophthalmology* 99:800, 1992.

22. Jones DB: Polymicrobial keratitis, *Trans Am Ophthalmol Soc* 79:95, 1975.
23. Reyes AC, Punsaland AP, Sulit HL: Mycotic flora of the conjunctiva, *Philippine J Ophthalmol* 2:119, 1970.
24. Pardos GJ, Gallagher MA: Microbial contamination of donor eyes: a retrospective study, *Arch Ophthalmol* 100:1611, 1982.
25. McCulley JP, Dougherty JM, Deneau DG: Classification of chronic blepharitis, *Ophthalmology* 89:1173, 1982.
26. Allansmith MR, Ostler HB, Butterworth M: Concomitance of bacteria in various areas of the eye, *Arch Ophthalmol* 82:37, 1969.
27. Locatcher-Khorazo D, Shegal BC: *Microbiology of the eye*, St Louis, 1972, Mosby–Year Book, Inc.
28. Ainley R, Smith B: Fungal flora of the conjunctival sac in healthy and diseased eyes, *Br J Ophthalmol* 49:505, 1965.
29. Hammeke JC, Ellis PP: Mycotic flora of the conjunctiva, *Am J Ophthalmol* 49:1174, 1960.
30. Griffith MR et al: Immunofluorescent studies in mucous membrane pemphigoid, *Arch Dermatol* 109:195, 1974.
31. Furey N et al: Immunofluorescent studies of ocular cicatricial pemphigoid, *Am J Ophthalmol* 80:825, 1975.
32. Mondino BJ, Brown SI, Rabin BS: Autoimmune phenomena of the external eye, *Ophthalmology* 85:801, 1978.
33. Mondino BJ et al: Autoimmune phenomena in ocular cicatricial pemphigoid, *Am J Ophthalmol* 83:443, 1977.
34. Rogers RS et al: Immunopathology of cicatricial pemphigoid: studies of complement deposition, *J Invest Dermatol* 68:39, 1977.
35. Proia A, Foulks GN, Sanfilippo FP: Ocular cicatricial pemphigoid with granular IgA and complement deposition, *Arch Ophthalmol* 103:1669, 1985.
36. Thoft RA et al: Ocular cicatricial pemphigoid associated with hyperproliferation of the conjunctival epithelium, *Am J Ophthalmol* 98:37, 1984.
37. Kasmierowski JA, Wuepper KD: Erythema multiforme: immune complex vasculitis of the superficial cutaneous microvasculature, *J Invest Dermatol* 71:366, 1978.
38. Richter BJ, McNutt NS: The spectrum of epidermolysis bullosa acquisita, *Arch Dermatol* 115:1325, 1979.
39. Yaoita H et al: Epidermolysis bullosa acquisita: ultrastructural and immunologic studies, *J Invest Dermatol* 76:288, 1981.
40. Woodley D et al: Identification of the skin basement autoantigen in epidermolysis acquisita, *N Engl J Med* 310:1007, 1984.
41. Woodley D: Epidermolysis bullosa acquisita, *Prog Dermatol* 22:1, 1988.
42. Bean SF, Halubar KK, Gillett RB: Pemphigus involving the eyes, *Arch Dermatol* 111:1484, 1975.
43. Leonard JN et al: The relationship between linear IgA disease and benign mucous membrane pemphigoid, *Br J Dermatol* 110:307, 1984.
44. Libert J: Diagnosis of lysosomal storage diseases by the ultrastructural study of conjunctival biopsies, *Pathol Annu* 15(part 1):37, 1980.
45. Van Hoof F et al: The assay of lacrimal tear enzymes and the ultrastructural analysis of conjunctival biopsies: new techniques for the study of in-born lysosomal diseases, *Metab Ophthalmol* 1:165, 1977.
46. Kenyon KR, Sensenbrenner JA: Electron microscopy of cornea and conjunctiva in childhood cystinosis, *Am J Ophthalmol* 78:68, 1974.
47. Sanderson PO et al: Cystinosis: a chemical, histopathologic, and ultrastructural study, *Arch Ophthalmol* 91:270, 1974.
48. Blodi FC, Apple DJ: Localized conjunctival amyloidosis, *Am J Ophthalmol* 88:346, 1979.
49. Riegel EM et al: Ocular pathology of Fabry's disease in a hemizygous male following renal transplantation, *Surv Ophthalmol* 26:247, 1982.
50. Weingeist TA, Blodi FC: Fabry's disease: ocular findings in a female carrier. A light and electron microscopic study, *Arch Ophthalmol* 85:169, 1971.
51. Frost P, Tanaka Y, Spaeth GL: Fabry's disease-glycolipid lipidosis: histochemical and electron-microscopic studies of two cases, *Am J Med* 40:618, 1966.
52. Kenyon KR, Sensenbrenner JA: Mucolipidosis II (I-cell disease): ultrastructural observations of conjunctiva and sclera, *Invest Ophthalmol* 10:555, 1971.
53. Libert J et al: Ocular findings in I-cell disease (mucolipidosis type II), *Am J Ophthalmol* 83:17, 1977.
54. Quigley HA, Goldberg MF: Conjunctival ultrastructure in mucolipidosis 3 (pseudo Hurler polydystrophy), *Invest Ophthalmol* 10:568, 1971.
55. Kenyon KR et al: Mucolipidosis IV: histopathology of conjunctiva, cornea and skin, *Arch Ophthalmol* 97:1106, 1979.
56. Zwann J, Kenyon KR: Two brothers with presumed mucolipidosis IV, *Birth Defects* 18:381, 1982.
57. Riedel KG et al: Ocular abnormalities in mucolipidosis IV, *Am J Ophthalmol* 99:125, 1985.
58. Kenyon KR et al: Ocular pathology of the Maroteaux-Lamy syndrome (systemic mucopolysaccharidosis type VI): histologic and ultrastructural report of two cases, *Am J Ophthalmol* 73:718, 1972.
59. Quigley HA, Goldberg MF: Scheie syndrome and macular corneal dystrophy: an ultrastructural comparison of conjunctiva and skin, *Arch Ophthalmol* 85:553, 1971.
60. Kenyon KR et al: The systemic mucopolysaccharidoses: ultrastructural and histological studies of conjunctiva and skin, *Am J Ophthalmol* 73:811, 1972.

61. Charlton KH et al: Pseudodendritic keratitis and systemic tyrosinemia, *Ophthalmology* 88:355, 1981.

62. Libert J, Van Hoof F, Tonduer M: Fucosidosis: ultrastructural study of conjunctiva and skin and enzyme analysis of tears, *Invest Ophthalmol* 15:626, 1976.

63. Hoshino M et al: Fucosidosis: ultrastructural study of the eye in an adult, *Graefes Arch Clin Exp Ophthalmol* 227:162, 1989.

64. Rao V et al: Conjunctival goblet cells and mitotic rate in children with measles and vitamin A deficiency, *Arch Ophthalmol* 105:378, 1987.

65. Roat MI, Sossi G, Thoft RA: Increased conjunctival epithelial mitosis and goblet cell frequency in atopic keratoconjunctivitis, *Invest Ophthalmol Vis Sci* 30(suppl):83, 1989.

66. Ishibashi Y, Hommura S, Matsumoto Y: Direct examination vs culture of biopsy specimens for the diagnosis of keratomycosis, *Am J Ophthalmol* 103:636, 1987.

67. Moore BM et al: *Acanthamoeba* keratitis associated with soft contact lenses, *Am J Ophthalmol* 100:396, 1985.

68. Moore MB et al: Radial keratoneuritis as a presenting sign in *Acanthamoeba* keratitis, *Ophthalmology* 93:1310, 1986.

69. Moore MB, Newton C, Kaufman HE: Chronic keratitis caused by *Mycobacterium gordonae*, *Am J Ophthalmol* 102:516, 1986.

70. Newton C, Moore MB, Kaufman HE: Corneal biopsy in chronic keratitis, *Arch Ophthalmol* 105:577, 1987.

71. Erie JC, Collyer SK, Campbell RJ: Dehydrated cucumber slices as a mount for conjunctival biopsy specimens, *Am J Ophthalmol* 99:539, 1985.

72. Campbell RJ: *Tissue diagnosis: eyelid and conjunctiva.* In Karcioglu ZA, editor: *Laboratory diagnosis in ophthalmology,* New York, 1987, Macmillan.

73. Levy N et al: Reactive lymphoid hyperplasia with single class (monoclonal) surface immunoglobulin, *Am J Clin Pathol* 80:300, 1983.

74. Knowles DM et al: The application of monoclonal antibodies to the characterization and diagnosis of lymphoid neoplasms: a review of recent studies, *Diagn Immunol* 1:142, 1983.

75. Schachter J et al: Evaluation of laboratory methods for detecting acute TRIC agent infection, *Am J Ophthalmol* 70:377, 1970.

76. Taylor HR, Agarwala N, Johnson SL: Detection of experimental *Chlamydia trachomatis* eye infection on conjunctival smears and in tissue culture by use of fluorescein-conjugated monoclonal antibody, *J Clin Microbiol* 20:391, 1984.

77. Stamm WE, Holmes KK: Chlamydial infections: what should we do while waiting for a diagnostic test?, *West J Med* 135:226, 1981.

78. Potts MJ et al: Rapid diagnosis of *Chlamydia trachomatis* infection in patients attending an ophthalmic casualty department, *Br J Ophthalmol* 70:677, 1986.

79. Hawkins DA et al: Rapid, reliable diagnosis of chlamydial ophthalmia by means of monoclonal antibodies, *Br J Ophthalmol* 69:640, 1985.

80. Bialasiewicz AA, Jahn GJ: Evaluation of diagnostic tools for adult chlamydial keratoconjunctivitis, *Ophthalmology* 94:532, 1987.

81. Sheppard JD et al: Immunodiagnosis of adult chlamydial conjunctivitis, *Ophthalmology* 95:434, 1988.

82. Tantisira JG, Kowalski RP, Gordon YJ: Evaluation of the Kodak Surecell *Chlamydia* test for the laboratory diagnosis of adult inclusion conjunctivitis, *Ophthalmology* 102:1035, 1995.

83. Tabbara KF, Rahi A: Enzyme immunoassay in the detection of chlamydial antigens in patients with trachoma, *Ophthalmology* 94(suppl):123, 1987.

84. Taylor PB, Burd EM, Tabbara KF: Comparison of diagnostic laboratory techniques in the various stages of trachoma, *Ophthalmology* 94(suppl):123, 1987.

85. Darougar S et al: Rapid serological test for diagnosis of chlamydial ocular infections, *Br J Ophthalmol* 62:503, 1978.

86. Wang S, Grayston J: Immunologic relationship between genital TRIC, lymphogranuloma venereum, and related organisms in a new microtiter indirect immunofluorescence test, *Am J Ophthalmol* 70:367, 1970.

87. Arffa RC, Kowalski RP, Springer DS: The value of serology in the diagnosis of adult chlamydial keratoconjunctivitis, *Ophthalmology* 95(suppl):145, 1988.

88. Kowalski RP, Gordon YJ: Evaluation of immunologic tests for the detection of ocular herpes simplex virus, *Ophthalmology* 96:1583, 1989.

89. Lee AF et al: Comparative laboratory diagnosis of experimental herpes simplex keratitis, *Am J Ophthalmol* 109:8, 1990.

90. Simon MW et al: Comparison of immunocytology to tissue culture for diagnosis of presumed herpesvirus dendritic epithelial keratitis, *Ophthalmology* 99:1408, 1992.

91. Kowalski RP, Gordon YJ: Comparison of direct rapid tests for the detection of adenovirus antigen in routine conjunctival specimens, *Ophthalmology* 96:1106, 1989.

92. Cleveland PH, Richman DD: Enzyme immunofiltration staining assay for the immediate diagnosis of herpes simplex virus and varicella-zoster virus directly from clinical specimens, *J Clin Microbiol* 25:416, 1987.

93. Bobo L et al: Diagnosis of Chlamydia trachomatis eye infection in Tanzania by polymerase chain reaction/enzyme immunoassay, *Lancet* 338:847, 1991.

94. Tabrizi SN, Lees MI, Garland SM: Comparison of polymerase chain reaction and culture techniques for detection of Chlamydia trachomatis, *Mol Cell Probes* 7:357, 1993.

95. Talley AR et al: The use of polymerase chain re-

action for the detection of chlamydial kerato-conjunctivitis, *Am J Ophthalmol* 114:685, 1992.

96. Talley AR et al: Comparative diagnosis of neonatal chlamydial conjunctivitis by polymerase chain reaction and McCoy cell culture, *Am J Ophthalmol* 117:50, 1994.

97. Bailey RL et al: Polymerase chain reaction for the detection of ocular chlamydial infection in trachoma-endemic communities, *J Infect Dis* 170:709, 1994.

98. Kowalski RP et al: Evaluation of the polymerase chain reaction test for detecting chlamydial DNA in adult chlamydial conjunctivitis, *Ophthalmology* 102:1016, 1995.

99. Kowalski RP et al: A comparison of enzyme immunoassay and polymerase chain reaction with the clinical examination for diagnosing ocular herpetic disease, *Ophthalmology* 100:530, 1993.

100. Dumas AL, de Ancos E, Herbort CP: Evaluation of the method of DNA amplification (PCR,

polymerase chain reaction) for diagnosis of superficial ocular herpes, *Klin Monatsbl Augenheilkd* 200:472, 1992.

101. Xu W et al: Detection of the direct genotyping of HSV by PCR and its primal usage in ophthalmology, *Yen Ko Hsueh Pao* 9:163, 1993.

102. Yamamoto S et al: Detection of herpes simplex virus DNA in human tear film by the polymerase chain reaction, *Am J Ophthalmol* 117:160, 1994.

103. Kinchington PR et al: Use of polymerase chain amplification reaction for the detection of adenoviruses in ocular swab specimens, *Invest Ophthalmol Vis Sci* 35:4126, 1994.

104. McBeath J, Forster RK, Rebell G: Diagnostic limulus lysate assay for endophthalmitis and keratitis, *Arch Ophthalmol* 96:1265, 1978.

105. Walters RW et al: Limulus lysate assay for early detection of certain gram-negative corneal infections, *Arch Ophthalmol* 97:875, 1979.

Five

Congenital Anomalies

This chapter describes the more common congenital anomalies of the anterior segment of the eye. These are characterized by alterations in structure caused by abnormalities in development. The abnormalities are present at birth, differentiating them from most corneal dystrophies and systemic disorders of metabolism. The etiology can be genetic, infectious, traumatic, toxic, or a combination of these influences. Most often these etiologic factors affect development between the 6th and 16th weeks of gestation, when differentiation of the anterior segment occurs. Developmental anomalies generally fall into three categories: developmental arrest, abnormal differentiation, or a combination of the two.

DYSGENESIS OF THE LIDS

Cryptophthalmos
Cryptophthalmos is a rare condition in which the lids fail to form and the exposed corneal and conjunctival epithelium undergo metaplasia into skin (dermoid transformation). There are no lashes or brows, and in many cases the lacrimal gland and canaliculi also are absent.[1,2] Other anterior segment abnormalities are usually present as well. Incomplete forms occur, with nasal or superior involvement only. An *abortive form* also has been seen, with replacement of the upper eyelid with a fold of skin that is adherent to the upper third of the cornea, but a normal lower lid.[2] Movement of a microph-

thalmic globe can be seen beneath the skin. The structure of the globe can be observed with B-scan ultrasonography. There is no treatment; an incision into the skin would enter the globe.

This condition is usually inherited as an autosomal recessive trait and may be unilateral or bilateral. It can be associated with systemic abnormalities, including craniofacial anomalies, syndactyly, cardiac anomalies, genitourinary anomalies, and mental retardation.[1-7] Renal agenesis has been reported in siblings of patients with this condition.[2]

Ankyloblepharon

In some cases the upper and lower lids are formed but fused in front of a normal cornea. Brows and lashes are present in ankyloblepharon, in contrast to cryptophthalmos. The lids can be incised, although they may fuse again.[8,9]

ABNORMALITIES OF CORNEAL SIZE

Megalocornea

Megalocornea is defined as an adult cornea that measures 13 mm or more in horizontal diameter (Fig. 5-1) or a newborn cornea 12 mm or more in diameter. It is not associated with congenital glaucoma and is nonprogressive. The condition is usually bilateral and transmitted as a sex-linked recessive trait; 90% of affected patients are male. The gene locus for the X-linked form is the X12-q26 region, near the locus described for Aarskog syndrome (Xq12-13).[10,11] Occasionally it is transmitted as an autosomal dominant trait,[12] and rarely as an autosomal recessive trait.

The cornea is clear and histologically normal. Often the anterior chamber is deep, and the ciliary body and lens are enlarged.[13] High myopia, resulting from increased corneal curvature, and with-the-rule astigmatism can be present. Megalocornea can be associated with other ocular abnormalities, including anterior embryotoxon, pigment dispersion with Kru-

kenberg's spindle,[14,15] hypoplasia of the iris stroma, polycoria, mosaic corneal dystrophy,[16,17] miosis, and heavy pigmentation of the trabecular meshwork. Eyes with megalocornea are prone to ectopia lentis and glaucoma. Cataracts frequently appear prior to 40 years of age. Megalocornea can also be associated with systemic syndromes, including Marfan syndrome, Apert syndrome,[18] and mucolipidosis type II.[19] Megalocornea mental retardation syndrome, also known as Neuhaser's syndrome, appears to encompass a variety of familial and sporadic cases.[20] Iris hypoplasia, growth retardation, macrocephaly, hypotonia, camptodactylia, scoliosis, and other abnormalities may be seen.[21-24]

Megalocornea may result from failure of the anterior tips of the optic cup to grow far enough toward each other, allowing the large remaining space to be occupied by the cornea. It may also reflect an exaggeration of the normal tendency for the cornea to be relatively large, compared with the rest of the eye, from embryonic life to 7 years of age. Finally, megalocornea may result from a spontaneously arrested congenital glaucoma. It is interesting to note that megalocornea and congenital glaucoma can occur in different members of the same family, and, rarely, megalocornea can occur in one eye of a patient and congenital glaucoma in the other.[25]

Microcornea

The term *microcornea* is used when the corneal diameter in an otherwise normal-sized eye is 10 mm or less.[26] If the entire eye is small but otherwise normal, the condition is called *nanophthalmos;*[27] if the entire eye is small and malformed, *microphthalmos* is said to exist.

Microcornea occurs unilaterally and bilaterally at the same rate (Fig. 5-2). It can be transmitted as an autosomal dominant or recessive trait. The cornea is usually clear, and if the globe is otherwise normal, visual acuity can be good. The corneal curvature can be flat or steep, and because the axial length also varies greatly,

Figure 5-1
Infant with bilateral megalocornea. (Courtesy of Diane Curtin, Pittsburgh, PA.)

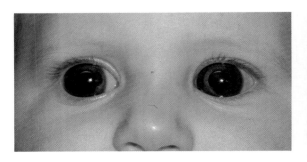

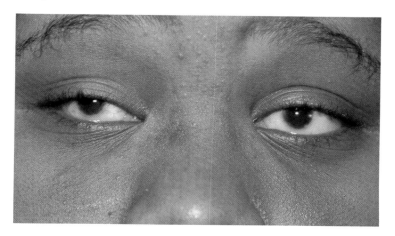

Figure 5-2
Bilateral microcornea.

Table 5-1	Conditions Associated with Microcornea	
Ocular	**Systemic Syndromes[29]**	
Microblepharon	Ehlers-Danlos[30]	
Corneal leukoma	Weill-Marchesani[31]	
Cornea plana	Rieger's[32]	
Iris coloboma	Waardenburg's[33]	
Aniridia	Norrie's	
Corectopia	Turner's[34]	
Persistent pupillary	Trisomy 13-15[35]	
membrane	Alagille syndrome[36]	
Microphakia	Meyer-Schwickerath	
Congenital cataract	and Weyers	
Congenital glaucoma	Nance-Horan	
Angle-closure glaucoma	(cataract-dental)[37]	
Open-angle glaucoma	Progeria	
	Rubella[38]	

any refractive error can exist. To differentiate microcornea from sclerocornea or cornea plana, where the limbus is indistinct, the true limbus can be identified by transillumination, which will highlight the ciliary ring.

Glaucoma can occur congenitally or in adulthood, secondary to angle closure, with the crowded anterior segment, or with goniodysgenesis. Patients with microphthalmos associated with cataract, chorioretinal coloboma, or markedly reduced corneal diameter (6 mm or less) are most likely to have severe visual impairment.[28] Microcornea has been associated with a wide variety of ocular and systemic conditions (Table 5-1). The etiology is unknown but may be an overgrowth of the anterior tips of the optic cup, leaving less than the normal space for the cornea.

ABNORMALITIES OF CORNEAL SHAPE AND CURVATURE

Cornea Plana

In cornea plana corneal curvature is 38 D or less, most commonly 30 to 35 D. The curvature is the same or less than that of the sclera. In fact, cornea plana may be a form of sclerocornea: Some peripheral scleralization of the cornea occurs in all cases, making the limbus indistinct.[39-43] The central cornea is usually clear, but diffuse opacification of the cornea may be seen. The condition is commonly associated with microcornea and other ocular and systemic conditions (Table 5-2).

The anterior chamber is usually shallower than normal, but glaucoma does not appear to be frequent. Despite the flattened cornea the refractive error is not consistently hyperopic because the axial length varies. The refractive error can be corrected with spectacles or contact lenses.[44]

Cornea plana can be inherited as an autosomal dominant or recessive trait; the recessive form is more severe. It is thought to result from a developmental arrest in the 4th month of gestation, at which time the cornea begins to increase its curvature relative to the sclera.

Oval Cornea

A vertically oval cornea may be seen in Turner's syndrome,[34] in Rieger's anomaly, and in microphthalmos with coloboma.[29] It can also develop after intrauterine interstitial keratitis (usually luetic). The cornea normally appears to be slightly oval horizontally as a result of the extension of the limbus onto the cornea vertically. This condition is exaggerated in sclerocornea.

Table 5-2	Conditions Associated with Cornea Plana
Ocular	**Systemic**
High refractive errors (particularly hyperopia)	Osteogenesis imperfecta
Pseudoptosis	Hurler's syndrome
Microcornea	Trisomy 13
Microphthalmos	Epidermolysis bullosa dystrophica[45]
Blue sclera	
Iris coloboma	
Anterior segment dysgenesis	
Aniridia	
Congenital cataract	
Ectopia lentis	
Retinal aplasia	
Choroidal coloboma	

Keratectasia

Keratectasia is a bulging, opaque cornea that protrudes through the palpebral aperture. The stroma is variably thinned and scarred. Usually unilateral, most cases probably result from an intrauterine keratitis with perforation. The corneal tissue subsequently undergoes metaplasia to skinlike tissue (dermoid transformation). Keratectasia may also be caused by a failure of mesenchyme to migrate into the developing cornea, with subsequent thinning, bulging, and metaplasia. *Congenital anterior staphyloma* is similar to keratectasia, but uveal tissue lines the ectatic cornea, giving it a bluish color.[46]

GENERALIZED POSTERIOR KERATOCONUS

Generalized posterior keratoconus is a rare congenital condition in which the entire posterior surface of the cornea is more curved than normal.[8,47-49] Central corneal thinning can result, but the anterior surface is normal. The cornea is usually clear and vision is normal, but stromal haze can be present. The condition is usually unilateral and nonprogressive, and there is no evidence of hereditary transmission. All reported cases have occurred in women.

The condition is probably a developmental arrest, because the posterior corneal curvature is usually more marked in the embryonic cornea. This should not be confused with circumscribed posterior keratoconus, in which there is a localized craterlike defect in the posterior corneal surface and frequent stromal opacity.

CORNEAL ASTIGMATISM

Most cases of primary corneal astigmatism are minor and accompany myopia. However, high degrees of idiopathic astigmatism can occur in a hereditary pattern, usually autosomal dominant.[50] The correlation in the amount of astigmatism between monozygotic twins is not higher than that between dizygotic twins, suggesting that genetic factors are not the major determinant.[51]

ANTERIOR SEGMENT DYSGENESIS

Anterior segment dysgenesis (ASD) is a spectrum of corneal, iris, angle, and lens abnormalities that appear to be related to abnormal development of the mesenchyme forming the anterior segment of the eye.[52,53] These abnormalities were previously referred to as *mesodermal dysgenesis* or *anterior chamber cleavage syndrome*, but Wilson[54] has suggested the term ASD because the embryonic mesenchyme is probably derived from neural crest cells, not mesoderm, and anterior chamber cleavage probably does not occur during development. Most likely, ASD represents abnormal migration or differentiation of the secondary mesenchyme.[55]

During early development of the embryo, primary mesenchyme separates the surface ectoderm and the lens vesicle. The paraxial (secondary) mesenchyme then migrates centrally across the opening of the optic cup in three successive waves. The first wave gives rise to the corneal endothelium, the second to the corneal stroma, and the third to the iris stroma. The anterior chamber is absent, with the space being filled with primary or secondary mesenchyme. This tissue gradually recedes, forming the anterior chamber, pupillary aperture, and last, the angle recess. Throughout most of corneal development the vascular pupillary membrane is closely associated with the developing endothelium.[56]

Incomplete migration of the secondary mesenchyme across the front of the eye or incomplete recession of the mesenchyme could be responsible for the following disorders: posterior embryotoxon, Axenfeld's anomaly, Rieger's anomaly, Peters' anomaly, congenital peripheral anterior synechiae, and posterior keratoconus. Abnormal differentiation of the mesenchyme could lead to congenital hereditary endothelial dystrophy, congenital hereditary stromal dystrophy, posterior polymorphous

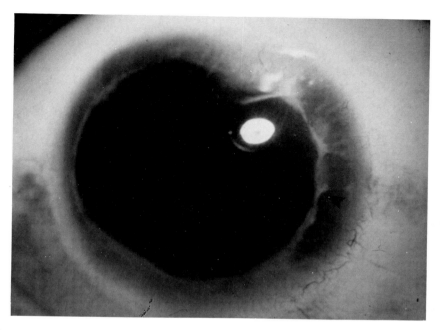

Figure 5-3
Posterior embryotoxon is thick, centrally displaced anterior border ring of Schwalbe (*arrow*).

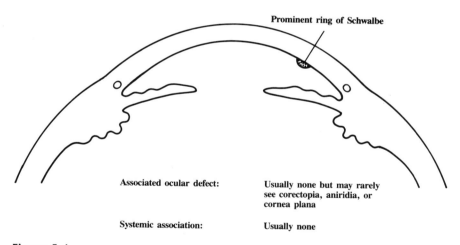

Figure 5-4
Posterior embryotoxon in an otherwise normal eye.

dystrophy, sclerocornea, and congenital cornea guttata.

The conditions described in the next sections are separated relatively arbitrarily based on common combinations of findings and historical appellations. Because these diseases occur as a spectrum of anterior segment changes, many cases will not fit into a specific category. Nevertheless, it is useful for instruction and recognition to review the traditional descriptions.

Posterior Embryotoxon

Posterior embryotoxon is a thickened and centrally displaced anterior border Schwalbe's ring (Figs. 5-3 and 5-4). *Schwalbe's ring* is a circumferential collagenous band, located peripherally on the posterior surface of the cornea, at the juncture of Descemet's membrane and the trabecular meshwork. In most people it is visible only on gonioscopy, but in approximately 15% of otherwise normal eyes it is sufficiently anteriorly displaced to become visible.[57] It is seen as a reluccent irregular line or ridge up to 2 mm central to the limbus, and the posterior corneal surface between the line and the limbus is translucent. It is most often seen temporally and nasally. Occasionally it is dislocated from

the cornea and hangs in the angle area.

Posterior embryotoxon is often inherited as an autosomal dominant trait. The eye is usually otherwise normal, but other signs of ASD, including Axenfeld's anomaly, cornea plana, corectopia, and aniridia may be present.

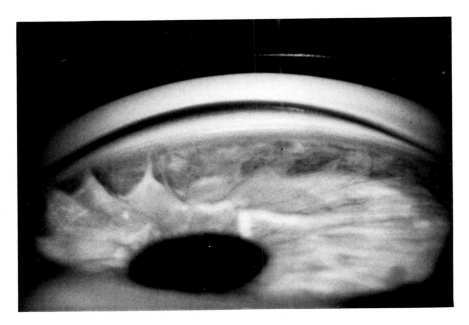

Figure 5-5
Gonioscopic photograph of Axenfeld's anomaly with iris adhesions to the prominent Schwalbe's ring.

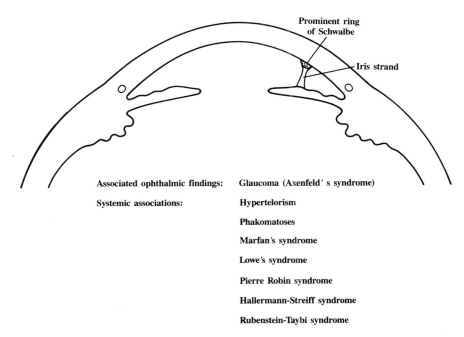

Figure 5-6
Axenfeld's anomaly.

Axenfeld's Anomaly and Syndrome

In Axenfeld's anomaly, iris strands extend across the angle to insert into a prominent Schwalbe's ring (Figs. 5-5 and 5-6). About 50% of these patients develop glaucoma, in which case it is called *Axenfeld's syndrome*.[58] The glaucoma most often appears during childhood or young adulthood but may develop during infancy. Both Axenfeld's anomaly and Axenfeld's syndrome are dominantly inherited. Skeletal anomalies, such as hypertelorism, facial asym-

metry, and hypoplastic shoulder, are occasionally present.[40] Axenfeld's anomaly can rarely be associated with systemic disease.[59]

Rieger's Anomaly and Syndrome

In Rieger's anomaly, a prominent Schwalbe's ring, iris strands extending to Schwalbe's ring, and hypoplasia of the iris stroma can be seen (Figs. 5-7 and 5-8).[52,60,61] The iris abnormalities range from mild stromal thinning to marked hypoplasia and hole formation. In some cases

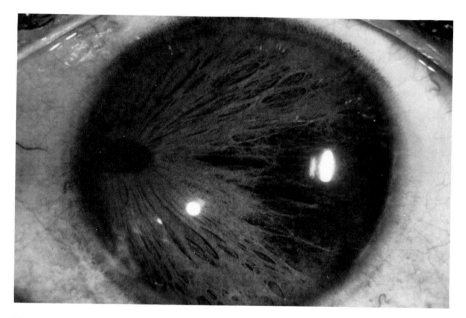

Figure 5-7
Rieger's anomaly.

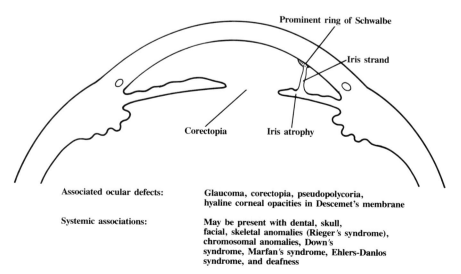

Prominent ring of Schwalbe
Iris strand
Corectopia
Iris atrophy

Associated ocular defects: Glaucoma, corectopia, pseudopolycoria, hyaline corneal opacities in Descemet's membrane

Systemic associations: May be present with dental, skull, facial, skeletal anomalies (Rieger's syndrome), chromosomal anomalies, Down's syndrome, Marfan's syndrome, Ehlers-Danlos syndrome, and deafness

Figure 5-8
Rieger's anomaly.

the sphincter is easily seen, and there are no crypts, furrows, or collarette. The deep iris stroma may appear to be made up of delicate radial fibrils, which give the iris a gray-brown, stringy appearance. An abnormality of the shape of the pupil is present in approximately 70% of cases.[62] The iris abnormalities are usually stable, but in a small percentage of patients they will progress.[63-66] Glaucoma occurs in 50% to 60% of these patients and usually develops between 5 and 30 years of age.

Iridodysgenesis with cataract is a variation of Rieger's anomaly in which posterior embryotoxon is absent, juvenile cataract is present, and the inheritance is autosomal recessive.[52,60] *Goniodysgenesis with glaucoma* is Rieger's anomaly without posterior embryotoxon.[52,60]

Rieger's syndrome is the combination of Rieger's anomaly and nonocular developmental anomalies, particularly skeletal anomalies. Maxillary hypoplasia, a broad, flat nasal root, and microdontia or anodontia can be associated with Rieger's syndrome. Other associated systemic abnormalities include malformations of the limbs and spine, deafness, mental retardation, osteogenesis imperfecta, and Marfan, Down's, and Ehlers-Danlos syndromes.[59,62,67]

Rieger's anomaly and syndrome are inherited as an autosomal dominant trait in about 75% of cases with 95% penetrance and extreme variation in expressivity.[60,61] In one case there was presumptive isochromosome of the long arm of chromosome 6,[68] and another had a pericentric inversion of chromosome 6.[69] Both Axenfeld's and Rieger's anomalies have been described in the same pedigree.[70,71]

In view of the similarity of these two conditions, a single term—*Axenfeld-Rieger syndrome*—has been proposed to encompass the spectrum of changes seen in both.[63,72] However, other disorders such as Peters' anomaly, posterior embryotoxon, and posterior keratoconus are probably part of the same spectrum, which is better described by the term ASD.

Circumscribed Posterior Keratoconus

Circumscribed posterior keratoconus is a rare disorder characterized by one or more localized crater defects on the posterior corneal surface with a concavity facing toward the anterior chamber[49,52,73-75] (Fig. 5-9). The lesion is usually unilateral, single, and central, but bilateral, eccentric, and multiple lesions can be present.[49] A nebular stromal haze can overlie the involved area. The anterior surface is normal, visual acuity is usually not affected, and progression does not occur.

Descemet's membrane and endothelium are present in the involved area; however, Descemet's membrane may show abnormal anterior banding, a multilayered configuration, and posterior excrescences.[74] These findings suggest an early onset, probably before the 6th month of gestation.[76] Most likely it is the result of abnormal migration or differentiation of the secondary mesenchyme that forms the corneal stroma.[54]

Circumscribed posterior keratoconus may accompany other anterior segment anom-

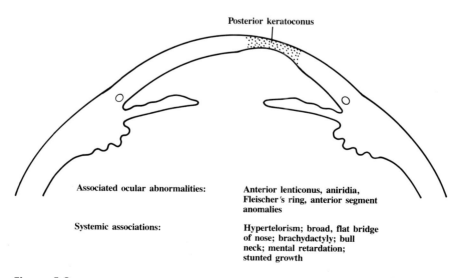

Figure 5-9
Posterior keratoconus.

alies, including aniridia, anterior lenticonus, Fleischer ring, and other signs of ASD. Associated systemic findings can include hypertelorism, poorly developed nasal bridge, brachydactyly, bull neck, mental retardation, and growth retardation.

Most cases are sporadic, but familial cases have been reported.[77] Similar findings can be seen after trauma. In the past, some have used the term *von Hippel's internal ulcer* synonymously with posterior keratoconus. However, in the former, Descemet's membrane and endothelium are absent in the crater, and vascularization and anterior synechiae may be present. These cases may be a form of Peters' anomaly, caused by intrauterine infection or more extensive anterior segment dysgenesis.

Peters' Anomaly

Peters' anomaly refers to a central corneal opacity (corneal leukoma) associated with a posterior corneal defect.[78-80] It encompasses a variety of abnormalities and probably can result from multiple etiologies. In some cases the central leukoma and adherent iris strands are the only signs, and the lens is clear (Figs. 5-10*A* and 5-11); this has been called the mesodermal form of Peters' anomaly. The iris adhesions usually arise from the iris collarette and extend to the margin of the leukoma. This form is rarely associated with the types of peripheral anomalies seen in Axenfeld's and Rieger's syndromes (Fig. 5-10*C*). Microcornea, sclerocornea, and infantile glaucoma can be present. Peters' anomaly can be bilateral or unilateral and is sporadic, al-

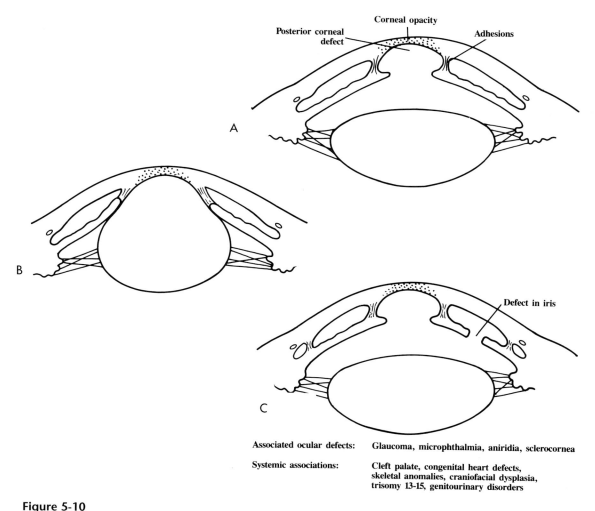

Associated ocular defects: Glaucoma, microphthalmia, aniridia, sclerocornea

Systemic associations: Cleft palate, congenital heart defects, skeletal anomalies, craniofacial dysplasia, trisomy 13-15, genitourinary disorders

Figure 5-10
Peters' anomaly. All forms have central corneal opacity and a posterior defect as well as central iris adhesions. **A,** With a normal lens. **B,** With keratolenticular contact and/or cataract. **C,** With peripheral anomalies seen in Axenfeld's and Rieger's syndromes.

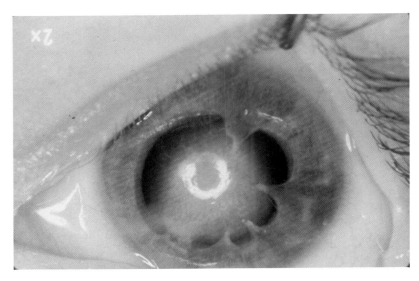

Figure 5-11
Peters' anomaly. Note the central corneal opacity with adherent iris strands.

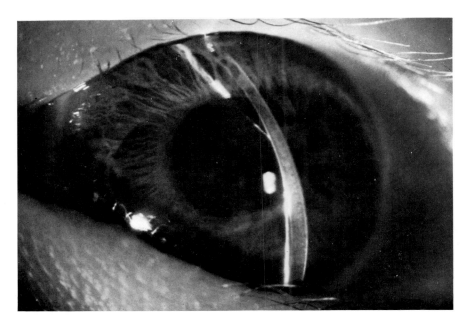

Figure 5-12
Peters' anomaly with lens-cornea touch. (Courtesy of Diane Curtin, Pittsburgh, PA.)

though recessive and dominant pedigrees have been reported.[81,82]

In other cases the lens is cataractous or is apposed to the leukoma (Figs. 5-10B and 5-12). The corneal opacity tends to be denser than in the previously mentioned cases, and associated ocular and systemic abnormalities are more frequent. These abnormalities include aniridia, sclerocornea, microphthalmos with choroidal coloboma, trisomy 13-15, congenital heart defects, genitourinary disorders, mental retardation, cleft lip and palate,[83] and skeletal anomalies.[62,84,85]

In all cases Descemet's membrane and endothelium are absent in the area of the opacity.[79-81,86] Bowman's layer may also be absent centrally. In cases in which the lens is adherent to the corneal stroma, the lens capsule

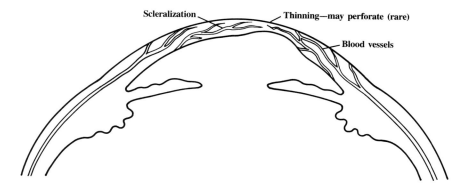

Figure 5-13
Sclerocornea.

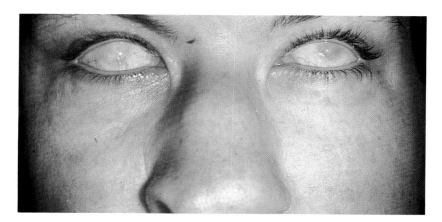

Figure 5-14
Sclerocornea involving the entire corneal area.

can be present or absent. Histochemically, corneas with Peters' anomaly contain much more fibronectin than normal.[87]

A number of pathogenetic mechanisms have been proposed. Dysgenesis of the mesenchymal tissue forming the central iris, endothelium, and corneal stroma may cause the form of Peters' anomaly that is limited to the cornea and iris. Intrauterine inflammation could interfere with development of the regional surface ectoderm and neuroectoderm or even cause perforation. Evidence of inflammation is present in some cases, as was described for posterior keratoconus, and the term *von Hippel's internal corneal ulcer* also can be applied to these cases. Faulty separation of the lens vesicle from the surface ectoderm can be responsible for some cases of lens-cornea adhesion (surface ectodermal Peters' anomaly). However, histologic studies suggest that in most cases the lens develops normally and later advances forward.[80,86,88] This movement may result from dislocation of an abnormal lens, as in aniridia and microphthalmos with coloboma, or from displacement by a retrolenticular mass, as in microphthalmos with persistent hyperplastic primary vitreous.

Sclerocornea

Sclerocornea is a congenital anomaly characterized by nonprogressive, noninflammatory opacification of the peripheral or entire cornea with vascularization[89,90] (Fig. 5-13). The sclera appears to extend onto the cornea, with opacification and deep or superficial vascularization. It can involve only the peripheral cornea or the entire cornea (total sclerocornea) (Fig. 5-14). When the condition is total the central cornea is slightly less opaque than the periphery. Involved areas have fine, superficial, uninflamed vessels that are extensions of the normal episcleral and conjunctival vessels. In most cases the corneal curvature is flattened (cornea plana). Visual acuity can be severely reduced when the central cornea is involved.

Table 5-3	Conditions Associated with Sclerocornea	
Ocular	**Systemic[93–95]**
Microphthalmos	Cerebellar anomalies
Blue sclera	Mental retardation
Cornea plana	Cranial anomalies
Angle anomalies	Cardiac malformations
(anterior segment	Decreased hearing
dysgenesis)	(Lobstein's syndrome)[40]
Aniridia	Deformities of the hands
Iris coloboma	and feet
Cataract	Cryptorchidism
Glaucoma (open-	Occult spina bifida
and closed-angle)	Hereditary
Choroidal coloboma	osteoonychodysplasia[96]
	Hallermann-Streiff
	syndrome
	Mieten's syndrome[97]
	Monosomy[98]
	Osteogenesis imperfecta
	Others

Sclerocornea is usually bilateral and affects males and females equally. Most cases are sporadic, but it can be inherited as an autosomal dominant or recessive trait; the dominant forms are less severe.[91,92] It can be associated with the ocular and systemic abnormalities listed in Table 5-3.

Histologic examination demonstrates collagen fibers of increased diameter in the superficial stroma, greater than in the posterior stroma, which is typical of sclera but not of the normal cornea.[100] Bowman's layer is usually absent, and Descemet's membrane and the endothelium can be normal, abnormal, or absent.[92,93,97,100] Anterior chamber angle abnormalities, such as anterior synechiae, are frequently present.[93,101]

Most likely, the wave of mesenchymal tissue that normally forms the corneal stroma forms tissue resembling sclera instead. The tissue destined to become sclera and cornea is a homogeneous sheet until the limbal anlage develops during the 7th to 10th weeks of gestation. The limbal anlage appears to be necessary for development of the increased curvature of the corneal surface. Lack of formation of the limbal anlage or its central displacement may be responsible for sclerocornea.[99]

Penetrating keratoplasty can be performed, particularly if the condition is total bilaterally. Glaucoma is a relatively frequent postoperative complication and bodes a poor prognosis.

Congenital Cornea Guttata

Corneal guttae are rarely seen as a congenital anomaly. The condition is stationary but can be associated with deep stromal opacification. It sometimes occurs as a familial condition. Two different dominant pedigrees have been described in which congenital cornea guttata was associated with other congenital malformations: in one with anterior polar cataract[102] and in another with mandibulofacial dysostosis, a condition thought to result from a defect in neural crest cell migration during the 4th week of gestation.[103] Both associations suggest that congenital cornea guttata is related to abnormal cellular migration in the anterior chamber during early development.

Congenital Hereditary Endothelial Dystrophy

Congenital hereditary endothelial dystrophy (CHED) is characterized by bilateral diffuse corneal edema that is present at birth or develops within a few years of life. It can be inherited either as an autosomal dominant or autosomal recessive trait. It may be classified as a form of anterior segment dysgenesis. CHED is discussed further in Chapter 18. Differentiating characteristics of CHED and other causes of corneal clouding at birth are presented in Table 5-4.

CONGENITAL HEREDITARY STROMAL DYSTROPHY

Congenital hereditary stromal dystrophy is a rare condition that is inherited as an autosomal dominant trait.[104] It is present at birth and is nonprogressive. The corneal stroma exhibits a flaky, feathery cloudiness, which is more prominent centrally and fades peripherally. The stromal collagen fibrils are abnormal in form, size, and arrangement.[105]

POSTERIOR POLYMORPHOUS DYSTROPHY

Posterior polymorphous dystrophy (PPD) is often seen as a congenital anomaly. Most often present are localized endothelial abnormalities, which are stable or slowly progressive. Occasionally, patients have cloudy corneas at birth. PPD can be associated with the types of iris and angle anomalies seen in ASD.[105] PPD is discussed further in Chapter 18.

Table 5-4　Causes of Corneal Clouding at Birth

	Congenital Hereditary Endothelial Dystrophy	Congenital Hereditary Stromal Dystrophy	Posterior Polymorphous Dystrophy	Peters' Anomaly	Sclerocornea	Congenital Glaucoma	Birth Trauma	Congenital Rubella	Congenital Syphilis
Inheritance	Autosomal recessive (most common)	Autosomal dominant	Autosomal dominant	Usually none	Usually none	Usually none	None	None	None
Laterality	Bilateral	Bilateral	Bilateral	Unilateral or bilateral	Usually bilateral	Unilateral 25%, bilateral 75%	Unilateral	Bilateral	Bilateral
Progression	May regress	No	Yes	May regress	No	May worsen or improve	Improves	No	No
Thickness	Increased	Normal	Increased	Normal or increased	Normal	Increased	Increased	Variable	Variable
Vascularization	No	No	No	No	Yes	No	No	Yes	Yes
Inflammation	No	No	No	No	No	No	Yes	Yes	Yes
Location of greatest opacity	Central	Central	Central	Central	Peripheral	Central	Localized	Variable	Variable
Other signs that may be present	—	—	Endothelial vesicles or bands	Cataract; iris adhesions	Flat curvature	Elevated pressure; enlarged globe	History of forceps use; may see ruptures	Cataract, microphthalmia, miosis, iritis, glaucoma, retinopathy	Retinopathy

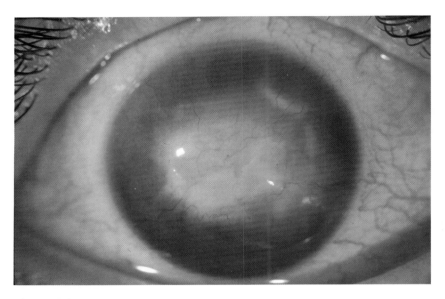

Figure 5-15
Corneal scarring and cataract formation in aniridia.

ANIRIDIA

Aniridia is a congential hypoplasia of the iris that can be hereditary (autosomal dominant) or sporadic. It is associated with glaucoma, cataracts, foveal hypoplasia, ectopia lentis, and Wilms' tumor (in the sporadic cases).[106] It is also often associated with corneal opacification.[107,108] Beginning after 2 years of age, bilateral superficial vascularization and opacification can be seen at the limbus in one or more locations, usually in the vertical meridians. This phenomenon progresses slowly, extending centrally and circumferentially, and can involve the visual axis, reducing vision (Fig. 5-15). Clinically, the palisades of Vogt appear to be absent, and impression cytology demonstrates many goblet cells in the peripheral corneal epithelium.[109] The cause of the corneal changes is not known. Schirmer's tests are abnormal in many of the patients,[107] but this is not sufficient to explain the corneal disease. It is more likely that the cause is a congenital deficiency of corneal epithelial stem cells.[110]

There is no known treatment for the corneal opacification. Lamellar or penetrating keratoplasty can be performed, but they can be complicated by management of glaucoma, difficulties with epithelial healing, and recurrent scarring.[111] Penetrating keratoplasty appears to have a higher rate of success than lamellar keratoplasty. Corneal epithelial transplantation is another option.

CONGENITAL MASS LESIONS OF THE CORNEA

Dermoids

Dermoids are choristomas—congenital masses of tissue not normally present in the location in which they are found.[112,113] (This is in contrast to hamartomas, which are abnormal growths of tissue normally present at the site.) Most likely, tissue destined to become skin is displaced to the surface of the eye during fetal development. Dermoids can occur over the cornea, limbus, or conjunctiva.[112,114] They are seen most commonly at the limbus, particularly inferotemporally. They are round or ovoid, yellowish-white, solid, vascularized, and domelike (Fig. 5-16). They can involve the central or entire cornea or form a ring around the circumference of the limbus.[115,116] Hairs can protrude from the mass.

These lesions are present at birth, and they occasionally enlarge, especially at puberty. They can decrease vision by covering the visual axis or by inducing astigmatism. Often a line of lipid material develops along the central edge of the tumor, and this can also impair vision.

The tumors are of dermal origin, composed of dermislike collagen, and can contain cutaneous adnexal structures, such as sebaceous glands, sweat glands, hairs, and fat. A *dermolipoma* is a dermoid in which fat is prominent, and the cutaneous adnexal structures are usually absent. Limbal and corneal dermoids al-

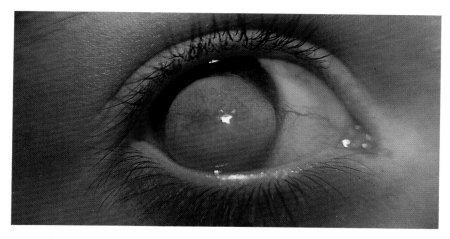

Figure 5-16
Dermoid of cornea.

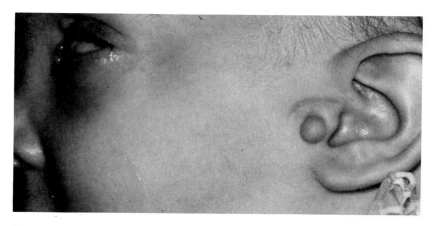

Figure 5-17
Pretragal appendage in Goldenhar's syndrome.

ways extend into the corneal stroma and can extend into the anterior chamber.

Approximately 30% of individuals with Goldenhar's syndrome (oculoauricolovertebral dysplasia) have epibulbar dermoids.[117] They most commonly occur unilaterally and at the inferotemporal limbus. Other ocular findings of Goldenhar's syndrome include lid colobomas, microphthalmos, iris coloboma, aniridia, Duane's syndrome, and miliary aneurysms of the retina.[112, 117, 118] Abnormalities of the structures derived from the first and second branchial arches are common: preauricular appendages (Fig. 5-17), pretragal fistulas, vertebral anomalies, mandibular and malar hypoplasia, and hemifacial microsomia can be seen. Other systemic abnormalities may also be present.[112,117] Other systemic syndromes associated with epibulbar dermoids include Franceschetti

(or Treacher Collins) syndrome, incontinentia pigmenti (Bloch-Sulzberger syndrome), encephalocraniocutaneous lipomatosis, linear sebaceous nevus syndrome, and cri du chat syndrome.[112]

Due to the posterior extension of corneal dermoids, they cannot be totally excised without deep lamellar or penetrating keratoplasty. Shaving of the elevated portion can reduce astigmatism and improve cosmesis but will not remove the opacity.[119]

Other Choristomas

Lacrimal tissue also can be displaced to the ocular surface during fetal development (ectopic lacrimal gland).[120] Sweat glands, hairs, smooth muscle, and sebaceous gland tissue can be present in the mass. Ectopic lacrimal glands tend to be fleshy, with raised translucent nodules and abundant vascularization. Like dermoids, they can extend into the corneal stroma and can exhibit slow growth, particularly during puberty. Surgical removal can be complicated by the presence of soft lacrimal tissue in the corneal stroma.

Osseous and neuroglial choristomas also can be found on the bulbar surface.[121] Osseous choristomas are usually located in the upper temporal quadrant, tend to have sharp edges, and often spare the cornea.

Keloids

A *keloid* is an exuberant growth of fibrous tissue that occurs in response to injury or as a congenital corneal mass.[122,123] They are chalky white, glistening solid tumors that show variable posterior extension.[124]

OTHER CAUSES OF CORNEAL OPACIFICATION AT BIRTH

Many of the conditions discussed previously cause corneal opacification at birth. Other conditions can also cause diffuse corneal opacification at birth or during infancy and must be included in the differential diagnosis. Other

Table 5-5	Causes of Early Corneal Opacification
Condition	**Characteristics**
Progressive Opacification, Can Be Evident Before 6 Months	
Cystinosis	Bilateral, stromal crystals, renal disease, autosomal recessive
Mucopolysaccharidosis: Hurler's (MPS1-H) and Scheie's (MPS1-S) syndrome	Bilateral, diffuse corneal clouding, abnormal facies, skeletal dysplasia, ± optic atrophy, ± retinopathy, autosomal recessive
Fabry's disease	Bilateral, superficial whorllike opacities, renal failure, skin lesions, X-linked recessive
Mucolipidosis, especially types II and IV	Bilateral, may have abnormal facies, macular cherry-red spot, autosomal recessive

conditions that can cause corneal opacification at birth are listed in Table 5-4. Conditions that can cause progressive opacification beginning in infancy are listed in Table 5-5.

In addition to rubella and syphilis, many other infectious agents can cause intrauterine keratitis, including *Neisseria gonorrhoeae*, staphylococci, herpes simplex, and influenza virus. The process can still be active at birth, or it may be resolved, leaving a leukoma, keratectasia, or congenital anterior staphyloma. Zellweger syndrome (see Chapter 21) and G_{M1} gangliosidosis also can present with early corneal clouding.

PENETRATING KERATOPLASTY FOR CONGENITAL CORNEAL OPACITIES

Penetrating keratoplasty can be successful in infants (Fig. 5-18), but the surgery and the postoperative care can be more demanding.[125-132] Other ocular abnormalities, such as glaucoma, strabismus, and aphakia, often complicate management and interfere with vision. Frequent examinations with the infant under anesthesia are required, and the sutures must be removed 4 to 6 weeks after surgery. If a clear graft is obtained, refractive correction and amblyopia therapy are essential for visual rehabilitation. In one recent report only 4 of 16 eyes obtained clear grafts (with a total of 26 grafts).[132] Glaucoma was highly correlated with graft failure. The Emory group[129] reported that 60% of grafts were clear at 1 year. However, the visual results were more disappointing. For patients with Peters' anomaly the probability of survival of a first graft was 40% at 10 years, and regrafts had a very low likelihood of success.[110] Visual acuity was 20/100 or better in 19% of eyes. Preoperative vascularization and the necessity for lensectomy and vitrectomy correlate with poor graft survival.

The decision to perform surgery should take into consideration whether retinal, lens, or angle abnormalities are present, whether the disease is unilateral or bilateral, and whether the family can cooperate with the taxing regimens required. In bilateral cases surgery is indicated in an attempt to obtain some useful vision. Surgery can be performed for unilateral disease, particularly if conditions are favorable, but in most cases it is not worthwhile.

CHROMOSOMAL ABERRATIONS

Corneal diseases are rarely associated with a chromosomal aberration, and most chromo-

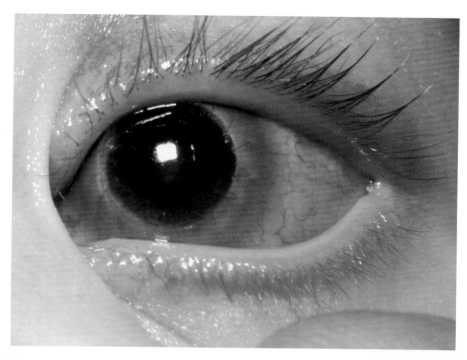

Figure 5-18
Penetrating keratoplasty in an infant with Peters' anomaly. (Courtesy of Diane Curtin, Pittsburgh, PA.)

somal aberrations are not associated with corneal disease.[133] Most associations have been noted in only a few cases; however, a few associations occur often enough to be worth mentioning. Trisomy 21 (Down's syndrome) is the most common of all chromosomal disorders, and is frequently associated with keratoconus.

Trisomy 17-18 (Edwards' syndrome) is associated with anterior corneal opacities, cataracts, and pupillary abnormalities.[134,135] Three different types of chromosome 18 deletion defects can be associated with corneal abnormalities: short arm deletion with posterior keratoconus; long arm deletion with microcornea, corneal opacities, Peters' anomaly, oval cornea, and ASD;[136] and ring chromosome with corneal leukomas.[137]

In trisomy 13 (Bartholin-Patau syndrome), dysgenesis of the cornea, iris, and anterior chamber angle and retinal dysplasia are seen. The cornea can be poorly defined, with opacification or scleralization. Nonspecific, spotty corneal opacities may be present.[138,139] Turner's syndrome (XO) can be associated with blue sclera, oval cornea, corneal opacities, or cataracts.[34]

REFERENCES

1. Goldhammer Y, Smith JL: Cryptophthalmos syndrome with basal encephaloceles, *Am J Ophthalmol* 80:146, 1975.
2. Codère F, Brownstein S, Chen MF: Cryptophthalmos syndrome with bilateral renal agenesis, *Am J Ophthalmol* 91:737, 1981.
3. Ide CH, Wollschlaeger PB: Multiple congenital abnormalities associated with cryptophthalmos, *Arch Ophthalmol* 81:638, 1969.
4. Bergsma D, editor: *Birth defects: atlas and compendium*, Baltimore, 1973, Williams & Wilkins Co.
5. Sugar HS: The cryptophthalmos-syndactyly syndrome, *Am J Ophthalmol* 66:897, 1968.
6. Waring GO, Shields JA: Partial unilateral cryptophthalmos with syndactyly, brachycephaly, and renal anomalies, *Am J Ophthalmol* 79:437, 1975.
7. Francois J: Syndrome malformatif avec cryptophthalmie, *Acta Genet Med Gemellol* 18:18, 1969.
8. Duke-Elder S: *System of ophthalmology*, vol 3, part 2, *Normal and abnormal development: congenital deformities*, St Louis, 1964, Mosby–Year Book, Inc.
9. Reinecke RD: Cryptophthalmos, *Arch Ophthalmol* 85:376, 1971.
10. Mackey DA et al: Description of X-linked megalocornea with identification of the gene locus, *Arch Ophthalmol* 109:829, 1991.

11. Meire FM et al: X-linked megalocornea: ocular findings and linkage analysis, *Ophthalmic Paediatr Genet* 12:153, 1991.

12. Rogers GL, Polomeno RC: Autosomal dominant inheritance of megalocornea associated with Down's syndrome, *Am J Ophthalmol* 78:526, 1974.

13. Vail DT: Adult hereditary anterior megalophthalmos sine glaucoma: a definite disease entity, *Arch Ophthalmol* 6:39, 1931.

14. Friede R: Megalocornea congenita, a phylogenetic anomaly, *Graefes Arch Clin Ophthalmol* 148:716, 1948.

15. Vail DT: Adult hereditary anterior megalophthalmos glaucoma: a definite disease entity, *Arch Ophthalmol* 6:38, 1931.

16. Malbran E: Megalocornea with mosaic-like dystrophy, *Arch Ophthalmol* 74:130, 1965.

17. Young AI: Megalocornea and mosaic dystrophy in identical twins, *Am J Ophthalmol* 66:734, 1968.

18. Calamandrei D: Megalocornea in due pazienti con syndrome craniosinotoscia, *Q Ital Ophthalmol* 3:278, 1950.

19. Libert J et al: Ocular findings in I cell disease (mucolipidosis type II), *Am J Ophthalmol* 83:617, 1977.

20. Verloes A et al: Heterogeneity versus variability in megalocornea-mental retardation (MMR) syndromes: report of new cases and delineation of 4 probable types, *Am J Med Genet* 46:132, 1993.

21. Grnbech-Jensen M: Megalocornea and mental retardation syndrome: a new case, *Am J Med Genet* 32:468, 1989.

22. Frydman M et al: Megalocornea, macrocephaly, mental and motor retardation (MMMM), *Clin Genet* 38:149, 1990.

23. Santolaya JM et al: Additional case of Neuhauser megalocornea and mental retardation syndrome with congenital hypotonia, *Am J Med Genet* 43:609, 1992.

24. Gibbs ML et al: Megalocornea, developmental retardation and dysmorphic features: two further patients, *Clin Dysmorphol* 3:132, 1994.

25. Malbran E, Dodds R: Megalocornea and its relation to congenital glaucoma, *Am J Ophthalmol* 49:908, 1960.

26. Dinno ND et al: Bilateral microcornea, coloboma, short stature and other skeletal anomalies: a new hereditary syndrome, *Birth Defects* 8:109, 1976.

27. Cross HE, Yoder F: Familial nanophthalmos, *Am J Ophthalmol* 81:300, 1976.

28. Elder MJ: Aetiology of severe visual impairment and blindness in microphthalmos, *Br J Ophthalmol* 78:332, 1994.

29. Warburg M: *The heterogeneity of microphthalmia in the mentally retarded*. In Bergsma D, editor: *The eye*, vol 7, Baltimore, 1971, Williams & Wilkins Co.

30. Durham DG: Cutis hyperelastica (Ehlers-Danlos syndrome) with blue scleras, microcornea, and glaucoma, *Arch Ophthalmol* 49:220, 1953.

31. Feiler-Ofry V, Stein R, Godel V: Marchesani's syndrome and chamber angle anomalies, *Am J Ophthalmol* 65:862, 1968.

32. Henkind P, Siegel IM, Carr RE: Mesodermal dysgenesis of the anterior segment: Rieger's anomaly, *Arch Ophthalmol* 73:810, 1965.

33. Goldberg G: Waardenburg's syndrome with fundus and other anomalies, *Arch Ophthalmol* 76:797, 1966.

34. Lessel S, Forbes AP: Eye signs in Turner's syndrome, *Arch Ophthalmol* 76:211, 1966.

35. Ginsberg J, Boue KE: Ocular pathology of trisomy 13, *Ann Ophthalmol* 6:113, 1974.

36. Brodsky MC, Cunniff C: Ocular anomalies in the Alagille syndrome (arteriohepatic dysplasia), *Ophthalmology* 100:1767, 1993.

37. Lewis RA, Nussbaum RL, Stambolian D: Mapping X-linked ophthalmic diseases IV: provisional assignment of the locus for X-linked congenital cataracts and microcornea (the Nance-Horan syndrome) to Xp22.2-p22.3, *Ophthalmology* 97:110, 1990.

38. Boniuk V, Boniuk M: Congenital rubella syndrome, *Int Ophthalmol Clin* 8:487, 1968.

39. Larsen V, Eriksen A: Cornea plana, *Acta Ophthalmol* 27:275, 1949.

40. Desvignes P et al: Aspect iconographique d'une cornea plana dans une maladie de Lobstein, *Arch Ophthalmol (Paris)* 27:585, 1967.

41. Erikkson AW, Lehmann E, Forsius H: Congenital cornea plana in Finland, *Clin Genet* 4:301, 1973.

42. Forsius H: Studien über cornea plana congenita. Bei 19 kranken in 9 familien, *Acta Ophthalmol (Copenh)* 39:203, 1961.

43. Felix CH: Kongenitale familiäre cornea plana, *Klin Monatsbl Augenheilkd* 74:710, 1925.

44. Dada VK, Verma LK, Sachdev MS: Comprehensive visual and cosmetic rehabilitation of cornea plana, *Cornea* 7:102, 1988.

45. Sharkey JA et al: Cornea plana and sclerocornea in association with recessive epidermolysis bullosa dystrophica: case report, *Cornea* 11:83, 1992.

46. Olson JA: Congenital anterior staphyloma: report of two cases, *J Pediatr Ophthalmol* 8:177, 1971.

47. Ross JVM: Keratoconus posticus generalis, *Am J Ophthalmol* 33:801, 1950.

48. Jacobs HB: Posterior conical cornea, *Br J Ophthalmol* 41:31, 1957.

49. Collier J: Le keratocone posterieur, *Arch Ophthalmol (Paris)* 22:376, 1962.

50. Francois J: *Heredity in ophthalmology*, St Louis, 1971, Mosby–Year Book, Inc.

51. Teikari JM, O'Donnell JJ: Astigmatism in 72 twin pairs, *Cornea* 8:263, 1989.

52. Waring GO, Rodrigues MM, Laibson PR: Anterior chamber cleavage syndrome: a stepladder classification, *Surv Ophthalmol* 20:3, 1975.

53. Reese AB, Ellsworth RM: The anterior chamber

cleavage syndrome, *Arch Ophthalmol* 75:307, 1966.

54. Wilson FM: *Congenital anomalies.* In Smolin G, Thoft RA, editors: *The cornea: scientific foundations and clinical practice,* Boston, 1983, Little, Brown & Co.

55. Bahn CF et al: Classification of corneal endothelial disorders based on neural crest origin, *Ophthalmology* 91:558, 1984.

56. Cintron C, Covington HI, Kublin CL: Morphogenesis of rabbit corneal endothelium, *Curr Eye Res* 7:913, 1988.

57. Forsius H, Erikksson A, Fellman J: Embryotoxon corneae posterius in an isolated population, *Acta Ophthalmol* 42:42, 1964.

58. Sugar HS: Juvenile glaucoma with Axenfeld syndrome, *Am J Ophthalmol* 9:1012, 1969.

59. Brear DR, Insler MS: Axenfeld's syndrome associated with systemic abnormalities, *Ann Ophthalmol* 17:291, 1985.

60. Henkind P, Friedman AH: Iridogoniodysgenesis with cataract, *Am J Ophthalmol* 72:949, 1971.

61. Henkind P, Siegel IM, Carr RE: Mesodermal dysgenesis of the anterior segment: Rieger's anomaly, *Arch Ophthalmol* 73:810, 1965.

62. Alkemade PPH: *Dysgenesis mesodermalis of the iris and the cornea,* Springfield, Ill, 1969, Charles C Thomas, Publishers.

63. Shields MB: Axenfeld-Rieger syndrome: a theory of mechanism and distinctions from the iridocorneal endothelial syndrome, *Trans Am Ophthalmol Soc* 81:736, 1983.

64. Cross HE, Maumenee AE: Progressive spontaneous dissolution of the iris, *Surv Ophthalmol* 18:186, 1973.

65. Judisch GF, Phelps CD, Hanson J: Rieger's syndrome: a case report with a 15-year follow-up, *Arch Ophthalmol* 97:2120, 1979.

66. Gregor S, Hitchings RA: Rieger's anomaly: a 42-year follow-up, *Br J Ophthalmol* 64:56, 1980.

67. Dark AJ, Kirkham TH: Congenital opacities: patient with Rieger's anomaly and Down's syndrome, *Br J Ophthalmol* 52:631, 1968.

68. Tabbara KF, Khouri FP, der Kaloustian VM: Rieger's syndrome with chromosomal anomaly: report of a case, *Can J Ophthalmol* 8:488, 1973.

69. Heinemann M, Breg R, Cotlier E: Rieger's syndrome with pericentric inversion of chromosome 6, *Br J Ophthalmol* 63:40, 1979.

70. Falls JF: A gene producing various defects of the anterior segment of the eye, *Am J Ophthalmol* 32:41, 1949.

71. Pearce EH, Kerr CB: Inherited variations in Rieger's malformation, *Br J Ophthalmol* 49:530, 1969.

72. Shields MB et al: Axenfeld-Rieger syndrome: a spectrum of developmental disorders, *Surv Ophthalmol* 29:387, 1985.

73. Townsend WM, Font RL, Zimmerman LE: Congenital corneal leukomas. III: Histopathologic findings in 13 eyes with paracentral defect in Descemet's membrane, *Am J Ophthalmol* 77:400, 1974.

74. Wolter FR, Haney WP: Histopathology of keratoconus posticus circumscriptus, *Arch Ophthalmol* 69:357, 1963.

75. Butler TM: Keratoconus posticus, *Trans Ophthalmol Soc UK* 50:551, 1930.

76. Krachmer F, Rodrigues MM: Posterior keratoconus, *Arch Ophthalmol* 96:1867, 1978.

77. Haney WP, Falls HF: The occurrence of congenital keratoconus posticus circumscriptus in two siblings presenting a previously unrecognized syndrome, *Am J Ophthalmol* 52:53, 1961.

78. Peters A: Über Angeborene Defektbildung der Descemetschen Membran, *Klin Monatsbl Augenheilkd* 44:27, 1906.

79. Townsend WM: Congenital corneal leukomas. I: Central defect in Descemet's membrane, *Am J Ophthalmol* 77:80, 1974.

80. Townsend WM, Font RL, Zimmerman LE: Congenital corneal leukomas. II: Histopathologic findings in 19 eyes with central defect in Descemet's membrane, *Am J Ophthalmol* 77:192, 1974.

81. Stone DL et al: Congenital central and corneal leukoma (Peters' anomaly), *Am J Ophthalmol* 81:173, 1976.

82. Holmstrom GE et al: Heterogeneity in dominant anterior segment malformations, *Br J Ophthalmol* 75:591, 1991.

83. Ide CH et al: Dysgenesis mesodermalis of the cornea (Peters anomaly): associated cleft lip and palate, *Ann Ophthalmol* 98:1059, 1980.

84. Kivlin JD et al: Peters anomaly as a consequence of genetic and nongenetic syndromes, *Arch Ophthalmol* 104:61, 1986.

85. Hennekam RC et al: The Peters'-Plus syndrome: description of 16 patients and review of the literature, *Clin Dysmorphol* 2:283, 1993.

86. Nakaniski I, Brown SI: The histopathology and ultrastructure of congenital central corneal opacity (Peters' anomaly), *Am J Ophthalmol* 72:801, 1971.

87. Lee CF et al: Immunohistochemical studies of Peters' anomaly, *Ophthalmology* 96:958, 1989.

88. Heckenlively J, Kielar RP: Congenital perforated cornea in Peters' anomaly, *Am J Ophthalmol* 88:63, 1979.

89. Goldstein JE, Cogan DH: Sclerocornea and associated congenital anomalies, *Arch Ophthalmol* 67:761, 1962.

90. Howard RO, Abrahams IW: Sclerocornea, *Am J Ophthalmol* 71:1254, 1971.

91. Block N: Les differents types de sclerocornée, leurs modes d'heredité et les malformations congénitales concomitantes, *J Genet Hum* 15:133, 1965.

92. Rodrigues MM, Calhoun J, Weinreb S: Sclerocornea with an unbalanced translocation (17p, 10q), *Am J Ophthalmol* 78:49, 1974.

93. Friedman AH et al: Sclerocornea and defective mesodermal migration, *Br J Ophthalmol* 59:683, 1975.

94. Traboulsi EI, Maumenee IH: Peters' anomaly and associated congenital malformations, *Arch Ophthalmol* 110:1739, 1992.

95. Heon E et al: Peters' anomaly: the spectrum of associated ocular and systemic malformations, *Ophthalmic Paediatr Genet* 13:137, 1992.

96. Fenske HD, Spitalny LA: Hereditary osteo-onychodysplasia, *Am J Ophthalmol* 70:604, 1970.

97. Waring GO, Rodrigues MM: Ultrastructure and successful keratoplasty of sclerocornea in Mieten's syndrome, *Am J Ophthalmol* 90:469, 1980.

98. Doane JF, Sajjadi H, Richardson WP: Bilateral penetrating keratoplasty for sclerocornea in an infant with monosomy 21, *Cornea* 13:454, 1994.

99. Kanai A et al: The fine structure of sclerocornea, *Invest Ophthalmol* 9:687, 1971.

100. Wood TO, Kaufman HE: Penetrating keratoplasty in an infant with sclerocornea, *Am J Ophthalmol* 70:609, 1970.

101. Goldstein JE, Cogan DG: Sclerocornea and associated congenital anomalies, *Arch Ophthalmol* 67:761, 1962.

102. Dohlman CH: Familial congenital cornea guttata in association with anterior polar cataract, *Acta Ophthalmol (Copenh)* 29:445, 1951.

103. Nucci P et al: Mandibulofacial dysostosis and cornea guttata, *Am J Ophthalmol* 108:204, 1989.

104. Witschel H et al: Congenital hereditary stromal dystrophy, *Arch Ophthalmol* 96:1043, 1978.

105. Grayson M: The nature of hereditary deep polymorphous dystrophy of the cornea: its association with iris and anterior chamber dysgenesis, *Trans Am Ophthalmol Soc* 72:516, 1974.

106. Nelson LB et al: Aniridia: a review, *Surv Ophthalmol* 28:621, 1984.

107. Mackman G, Brightbill FS, Optiz JM: Corneal changes in aniridia, *Am J Ophthalmol* 87:497, 1979.

108. Grove JH, Shaw MW, Bourque G: A family study of aniridia, *Arch Ophthalmol* 65:81, 1961.

109. Nishida K et al: Ocular surface abnormalities in aniridia, *Am J Ophthalmol* 120:368, 1995.

110. Yang LL-H et al: Penetrating keratoplasty in infants and children with Peters' anomaly, *Ophthalmology* 102(suppl):122, 1995.

111. Kremer I et al: Results of penetrating keratoplasty in aniridia, *Am J Ophthalmol* 115:317, 1993.

112. Benjamin SN, Allen F: Classification of limbal dermoid choristomas and branch arch anomalies, *Arch Ophthalmol* 87:305, 1927.

113. Mansour AM et al: Ocular choristomas, *Surv Ophthalmol* 33:339, 1989.

114. Daily EG, Lubowitz RM: Dermoids of the limbus and cornea, *Am J Ophthalmol* 53:661, 1962.

115. Mattos J, Contreras F, O'Donnell FE: Ring dermoid syndrome: a new syndrome of autosomal dominantly inherited bilateral, annular limbal dermoids with corneal and conjunctival extension, *Arch Ophthalmol* 98:1059, 1980.

116. Henkind P et al: Bilateral corneal dermoids, *Am J Ophthalmol* 76:972, 1973.

117. Baum JL, Feingold M: Ocular aspects of Goldenhar's syndrome, *Am J Ophthalmol* 75:250, 1973.

118. Mansour AM et al: Ocular findings in the facio-auriculovertebral sequence (Goldenhar-Gorlin syndrome), *Am J Ophthalmol* 100:555, 1985.

119. Panton RW, Sugar J: Excision of limbal dermoids, *Ophthalmic Surg* 21:85, 1990.

120. Pokorny KS et al: Epibulbar choristomas containing lacrimal tissue: clinical distinction from dermoids and histologic evidence of an origin from the palpebral lobe, *Ophthalmology* 94:1249, 1987.

121. Boniuk M, Zimmerman LE: Epibulbar osteoma (episcleral osseous choristoma), *Am J Ophthalmol* 53:290, 1962.

122. Smith HC: Keloid tumors of the cornea, *Trans Am Ophthalmol Soc* 38:519, 1940.

123. O'Grady RB, Kirk HQ: Corneal keloids, *Am J Ophthalmol* 73:206, 1972.

124. Weizenblatt S: Congenital malformations of cornea associated with embryonic arrest of ectodermal and mesodermal structures, *Arch Ophthalmol* 52:415, 1954.

125. Picetti B, Fine M: Keratoplasty in children, *Am J Ophthalmol* 61:782, 1966.

126. Brown SI: Corneal transplantation of the infant cornea, *Trans Am Acad Ophthalmol Otolaryngol* 78:OP461, 1974.

127. Waring GO, Laibson PR: Keratoplasty in infants and children, *Trans Am Acad Ophthalmol Otolaryngol* 83:OP283, 1977.

128. Schanzlin DJ, Goldberg DB, Brown SI: Transplantation of congenitally opaque corneas, *Ophthalmology* 87:1253, 1980.

129. Stulting RD et al: Penetrating keratoplasty in children, *Ophthalmology* 91:1222, 1984.

130. Cowden JW: Penetrating keratoplasty in infants and children, *Ophthalmology* 97:324, 1990.

131. Dana M-R et al: The indications for and outcome in pediatric keratoplasty: a multicenter study, *Ophthalmology* 102:1129, 1995.

132. Parmley VC, Stonecipher KG, Rowsey JJ: Peters' anomaly: a review of 26 penetrating keratoplasties in infants, *Ophthalmic Surg* 24:31, 1993.

133. Jay M: *The eye in chromosome duplications and deficiencies,* New York, 1977, Marcel Dekker.

134. Ginsberg J, Perin EV, Sueoka ET: Ocular manifestations of trisomy 18, *Am J Ophthalmol* 66:59, 1968.

135. Mullaney J: Ocular pathology in trisomy 18 (Edward's syndrome), *Am J Ophthalmol* 76:246, 1973.

136. Izquierdo NJ, Maumenee IH, Traboulsi EI: Anterior segment malformations in 18q- (de Grouchy) syndrome, *Ophthalmic Paediatr Genet* 14:91, 1993.

137. Yanoff M, Rorke LB, Niederer BS: Ocular and cerebral abnormalities in chromosome 18 deletion defect, *Am J Ophthalmol* 70:391, 1970.

138. Apple DJ, Holden JD, Stallworth B: Ocular pathology of Patau's syndrome with unbalanced O-D translocation, *Am J Ophthalmol* 70:383, 1970.

139. Roch LM, Petrucci JV, Varaber AB: Studies on the development of the eye in 13-15 trisomy syndrome, *Am J Ophthalmol* 60:1067, 1965.

Six

Approach to Patients with Conjunctival Disease

ACUTE CONJUNCTIVITIS
Acute Follicular Conjunctivitis
Acute Membranous or Ulcerative Conjunctivitis
Acute Granulomatous Conjunctivitis
Other Causes of Acute Conjunctivitis

CHRONIC CONJUNCTIVITIS
Chronic Follicular Conjunctivitis
Giant Papillary Conjunctivitis
Chronic Membranous Conjunctivitis
Chronic Granulomatous Conjunctivitis
Cicatricial Conjunctivitis
Other Causes of Chronic Conjunctivitis

RECURRENT ACUTE CONJUNCTIVITIS

OTHER CONJUNCTIVAL CONDITIONS
Chemosis
Keratinization
Telangiectasia and Sludging
Others

Patients with conjunctivitis can pose one of the most difficult diagnostic dilemmas in ophthalmology. There are numerous possible etiologies, and the clues are often subtle. However, with a systematic approach the cause or causes can be found in most cases. The first step is to limit the differential based on certain key findings, including the duration of symptoms, the type of discharge, and the presence or absence of giant papillae, follicles, membranes, ulcerations, granulomas, and scarring (Table 6-1). A list of the conjunctival diseases associated with each type of discharge is given in Table 6-2. It is also helpful to differentiate unilateral from bilateral disease (Table 6-3). Neonatal conjunctivitis (ophthalmia neonatorum) is considered in a separate section, because the causes, manifestations, and treatment are different than in older children and adults.

Conjunctivitis is considered acute if the duration is less than 3 weeks and chronic if it has been present longer. All chronic cases must have been acute at one time, but often the onset is insidious and the patient does not present to the eye doctor until several weeks have passed. Most cases of acute conjunctivitis will resolve, even without treatment, in less than 3 weeks. Nearly all cases of conjunctivitis will exhibit a papillary response, although in some cases it is obscured by the presence of inflammatory membranes. However, giant papillae (> 1 mm in diameter) occur in only a limited number of conditions. The differentiation of follicles and papillae was discussed in Chapter 3. Granulomatous lesions must also be differentiated. Figure 6-1 shows the solitary, solid, raised, rounded, opaque appearance of a sarcoid granuloma.

ACUTE CONJUNCTIVITIS

Acute Follicular Conjunctivitis

Acute follicular conjunctivitis is caused by viral or chlamydial infection (Table 6-4). The con-

junctivitis usually has a rapid onset and is often unilateral early in the infection. The second eye usually becomes involved within a week. Preauricular lymphadenopathy is often present. Most of the infections causing acute follicular conjunctivitis have extraocular manifestations. Many of the infections can be differentiated based on these extraocular manifestations. It is probably most important to diagnose chlamydial infection, because without systemic treatment it can become chronic with vascularization and scarring, and herpes simplex, in order to avoid exacerbating the infection with topical corticosteroid treatment.

Differentiation between epidemic keratoconjunctivitis (EKC), adult chlamydial keratoconjunctivitis, and primary herpetic conjunctivitis can be difficult. Chlamydial conjunctivitis is more likely to be unilateral and have a mucopurulent discharge than EKC and occurs only in individuals who are sexually active. Primary herpes simplex conjunctivitis usually occurs before 25 years of age, is usually unilateral, is often accompanied by systemic symptoms, such as fever and upper respiratory tract inflammation, and is often associated with vesicular skin lesions and corneal dendrites. However, the

Table 6-1   Conjunctivitis Classification

Acute
  Ophthalmia neonatorum
  Follicular
  Membranous/ulcerative
  Granulomatous
  Others
    Purulent discharge
    Mucopurulent discharge
    Mucoid/watery discharge
Chronic
  Follicular
  Giant papillary
  Membranous
  Granulomatous
  Cicatricial
  Others
    Mucopurulent discharge
    Mucoid/watery discharge

Table 6-2   Classification of Conjunctivitis by Discharge

Purulent	Mucopurulent	Mucoid/Watery
Bacteria	Most bacterial cases, acute and	Viral
Neisseria gonorrhoeae (hyperacute)	chronic, including all those listed	Adenovirus
Neisseria meningitidis (hyperacute)	to the left plus	Varicella
Staphylococci	*Moraxella (Branhamella) catarrhalis*	Herpes zoster
Streptococcus pneumoniae	Viral	Herpes simplex
Streptococcus pyogenes	Adenoviral infections	Cytomegalovirus
Haemophilus influenzae	Herpes simplex	Infectious mononucleosis
Haemophilus aegyptius	Varicella	Measles
Pseudomonas aeruginosa	Herpes zoster	Mumps
Escherichia coli	Infectious mononucleosis	Newcastle conjunctivitis
Corynebacterium diphtheriae	Cytomegalovirus	Influenza
Bacillus spp.	Influenza	Molluscum contagiosum
Viral conjunctivitis with	Canaliculitis	Fungi
membranes	Chlamydial conjunctivitis	Parasites
Fungi	Parinaud's oculoglandular	Medication toxicity or allergy
Blastomycosis (rare)	syndrome	Conjunctival neoplasia
Sporotrichosis	Vincent's infection	Allergy, including vernal, atopic
		Superior limbal keratoconjunctivitis
		Cicatricial pemphigoid
		Blepharitis
		Acne rosacea
		Floppy eyelid syndrome
		Conjunctival papilloma

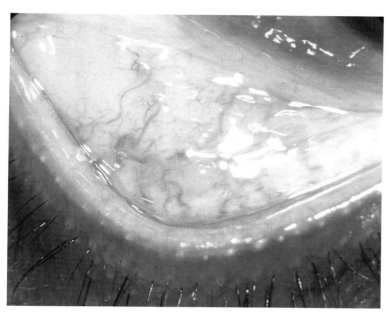

Figure 6-1
Sarcoid granuloma of the conjunctiva.

Table 6-3   Causes of Unilateral Conjunctivitis
Viral
Cytomegalovirus
Infectious mononucleosis
Adenovirus*
Herpes simplex*
Molluscum*
Herpes zoster
Papilloma*
Bacterial*
Parinaud's oculoglandular syndrome
Foreign body
Medication*
Masquerade syndrome
Canaliculitis
Lacrimal drainage obstruction*
Chlamydial*
Floppy eyelid syndrome
Vincent's infection

*Can be bilateral.

Table 6-4   Causes of Acute Follicular Conjunctivitis
Viral
Adenovirus
Epidemic keratoconjunctivitis
Pharyngoconjunctival fever
Primary herpes simplex
Acute hemorrhagic keratoconjunctivitis
(picornavirus)
Newcastle disease conjunctivitis
Influenza virus
Varicella
Herpes zoster
Cytomegalovirus
Epstein-Barr virus
Rubella
Chlamydial
Adult chlamydial keratoconjunctivitis
(inclusion conjunctivitis)
Acute trachoma

three diseases can be clinically indistinguishable. Laboratory testing, particularly Giemsa staining of scrapings and cultures, may be necessary.

The viral diseases are considered in further detail in Chapter 12 and the chlamydial diseases in Chapter 7. The chief characteristics of most of the diseases are given in Table 6-5.

Acute Membranous or Ulcerative Conjunctivitis

Membranes are collections of fibrin and exudate on the conjunctival surface. They occur when conjunctival inflammation is severe and in areas of ulceration. Pain, marked eyelid swelling, and mucopurulent or purulent discharge are often present. Stripping of the membranes

Table 6-5 Diagnostic Features of Acute Follicular Conjunctivitis*

Disease	Discharge and Conjunctival Appearance	Cornea	Laboratory Findings	Etiologic Factors	Epidemiologic and Other Characteristics
EKC†	Watery discharge Hyperemia and chemosis Membranes in one third of cases, which may result in scars Course of 7 to 14 days Often subconjunctival hemorrhages Follicular response, mostly lower fornix Rare chronic papillary conjunctivitis	Fine, diffuse, punctate keratitis early; may persist 3 weeks Focal epithelial keratitis on 7th to 13th day Subepithelial opacities (14th to 20th day) at sites of epithelial lesions in 50% of cases; may last months (usually) or years May have stromal infiltration and edema, severe keratitis No pannus (no vascularization)	Mononuclear response except for polymorphonuclear leukocytes with membranes EIA‡ test specific and sensitive first week Fourfold increase of antibody titer between acute and convalescent sera Adenovirus can be recovered in cell culture up to 2 weeks after onset, rarely longer	Adenovirus, most commonly types 8 and 19 Transmission from respiratory tract to eye, eye to eye, hand or instrument to eye; frequently acquired from eye care personnel Incubation period is 2 to 14 days Other eye usually involved in 2 to 7 days	Age group: 20 to 40 years Eye is infectious up to 14 days Acute systemic symptoms only in children; hyperacute eye involvement Lymph nodes; prominent palpable, tender, and occasionally visible (90% of cases) Vision may be decreased
Pharyngoconjuncti-val fever	Scant watery discharge Hyperemia, chemosis Follicular; may have papillary reaction in upper and lower fornices No scars	Fine epithelial keratitis affecting entire cornea Occasionally subepithelial infiltrates (especially types 3, 4, and 7) but milder and smaller than in EKC No pannus	Same as above	Adenovirus, most commonly types 3 and 7 Transmission mainly via respiratory secretions, but also by contaminated swimming pools Incubation period is 3 to 14 days	Pharyngitis and fever Lymph nodes small and palpable but not visible or tender (90% of cases) Occurs in schools and swimming pools Lasts 7 to 14 days No sequelae

Acute trachoma* (usually occurs in children)	Diffuse follicular response typically most prominent on upper tarsal plate, often seen at limbus; trachoma follicles soft, can be necrotic. Papillary hypertrophy. Conjunctival scarring, especially of upper lid. Pain, mucopurulent discharge, photophobia	Fine epithelial keratitis; fine punctate, subepithelial infiltrates; fine keratitis may last until disease subsides. Superior pannus (2 to 3 mm early). Marginal corneal infiltrates. Occasionally dense focus of cellular infiltrates (trachoma pustule). Cicatrized limbal follicles (Herbert's pits)	Basophilic, cytoplasmic epithelial inclusions (infrequent). Mainly polymorphonuclear response; may have equal numbers of polymorphonuclear and mononuclear cells in chronic phase. Cytologic findings of expressed follicle; Leber cell (macrophages), Plasma cells, Lymphoblasts. Fluorescent antibody-stained conjunctival scrapings, culture, polymerase chain reaction, and serum titers may be helpful	Chlamydia types A–C. Incubation period 1 to 3 weeks. Secondary bacterial infection common in endemic areas	Well described since 1500 B.C. Other complications are trichiasis, distichiasis, keratitis sicca. Preauricular nodes: palpable, rarely tender or visible. Most commonly eye-to-eye transmission. Multiple reinfections and bacterial superinfections important in pathogenesis of severe disease
Adult chlamydial keratoconjunctivitis (inclusion conjunctivitis)*	Mild to moderate mucopurulent discharge. Never membranous in adults. Worse below. No conjunctival cicatrization. Redness, chemosis. Follicular reaction	Superficial punctate to slightly coarse epithelial keratitis. Sometimes subepithelial infiltrates (smaller than in EKC), which may leave scars. Superior micropannus	Polymorphonuclear response. May have 50% polymorphonuclear and 50% mononuclear cells in chronic phase. Basophilic, intracytoplasmic, epithelial inclusions. Fluorescent antibody-stained conjunctival scrapings, culture, polymerase chain reaction, and serum titers may be helpful	C. trachomatis (types D–K). Incubation period 2 to 19 days	Venereal, hand-to-eye transmission. Persists for 3 to 12 months in untreated cases. Lymph nodes: palpable, sometimes tender or visible. Otitis media in 15% of cases. Rarely swimming pool transmission (chlorine inhibits agent)

Continued

Table 6-5 Diagnostic Features of Acute Follicular Conjunctivitis—cont'd

Disease	Discharge and Conjunctival Appearance	Cornea	Laboratory Findings	Etiologic Factors	Epidemiologic and Other Characteristics
Herpes simplex virus primary (nonneonatal)	Usually unilateral Scant watery discharge unless membranous (50% of cases) Follicles often masked by membrane May have conjunctival scars after membrane formation Pain, photophobia	Fine epithelial keratitis (punctate, stellate) Dendrites after 7 days Decreased corneal sensitivity Stromal disease can develop Pannus extremely uncommon	Mononuclear cells; polymorphonuclear leukocytes when membranes are present Multinucleated giant cells Virus can be isolated in cell culture Direct immunologic or serologic tests may be helpful	Herpes simplex virus, usually type I	Usually occurs in children but can occur in adults Type I: direct transfer from relatives and friends, blister to eye Vesicles on lid Ulcerative blepharitis Lymph nodes; small, palpable, occasionally tender or visible Duration: 2 weeks
Newcastle disease	Scant watery discharge Primarily affects inferior conjunctiva May have papillary or follicular conjunctivitis If present, follicles are prominent on lower lid Usually unilateral Pain, redness, tearing	Cornea rarely affected, but fine punctate epithelial keratitis and occasionally small subepithelial infiltrates can be seen No pannus	Mononuclear response	Newcastle disease virus (a paramyxovirus)	Droplet (finger to eye) transmission from poultry to human: occurs with occupational exposure (poultry workers, veterinarians, laboratory workers) Lymph nodes: palpable, small, sometimes tender No sequelae Duration: 7 to 10 days

Acute hemorrhagic conjunctivitis	Serous to mucoid discharge Chemosis early, in first 24 hours Bilateral subconjunctival pinpoint hemorrhages in upper palpebral or bulbar conjunctiva; becomes more profuse temporally on bulbar conjunctiva; takes 1 to 2 weeks to absorb Follicles, but not prominent No pseudomembranes Pain, photophobia, redness	May have fine keratitis	Mononuclear response in early stages, polymorphonuclear in later stage Virus can be isolated during first 2 days	Enterovirus: most commonly enterovirus type 70, coxsackie type A24	Massive epidemics in Asia, Africa, and Americas Hand-to-eye transmission Incubation period less than 24 hours Small preauricular node (sometimes absent) No ocular sequelae, rarely neurologic complications (radiculomyelitis) Anterior uveitis Lasts 10 days or less
Infectious mononucleosis (Epstein-Barr virus)	Acute conjunctivitis Membranous or follicular Subconjunctival hemorrhage Rarely nodules	Fine epithelial keratitis; microdendrites Nummular keratitis: lesions are in the peripheral cornea, at all levels; may become confluent or vascularized	Serum antibody titers	Epstein-Barr virus	Uveitis, episcleritis, retinal hemorrhages, papillitis, and retinal edema

*These entities also can be classified with chronic follicular conjunctivitis.

†Epidemic keratoconjunctivitis.

‡EIA = Enzyme immunoassay (Adenoclone, Cambridge Bioscience, Worcester, MA).

can result in bleeding. With time the membrane can resorb or slough, leaving a bed of granulation tissue. Healing can occur with scar formation, which can lead to symblepharon, entropion, trichiasis, mucus deficiency, and keratoconjunctivitis sicca. Orbital abscess formation and gangrene of the eyelids have occurred.[1] Membranous conjunctivitis can also be associated with corneal ulceration and perforation. In all cases efforts should be made to minimize conjunctival scarring and corneal injury.

All diseases that cause membranous conjunctivitis can also cause conjunctival ulceration. Conjunctival ulceration also occurs in viral and skin diseases that cause formation of conjunctival vesicles or blisters, such as pemphigus vulgaris, cicatricial pemphigoid, varicella (discussed below), Behçet's disease, trauma, and granulomatous conjunctivitis (discussed below).

The first step is to determine the etiology of the conjunctival inflammation (Table 6-6). Specimens should be obtained for Gram's stain and bacterial culture. The most common cause is adenoviral infection. The infection is usually bilateral and is associated with adenopathy but no systemic disease. Primary herpes simplex

usually occurs before 25 years of age and is usually unilateral. Adenopathy is usually present, and lid vesicles and corneal dendrites may be seen. Systemic symptoms, such as fever and upper respiratory tract inflammation, are common.

There are no distinguishing features of most of the bacterial causes of acute membranous conjunctivitis. *Streptococcus pyogenes* and *Staphylococcus aureus* are the most common agents.[2] *Corynebacterium diphtheriae* was the most frequent cause before immunization was common. Neisserial infections can usually be distinguished by the hyperpurulent nature of the conjunctivitis. Vincent's infection of the conjunctiva is a rare condition that occurs in patients with trench mouth. The conjunctivitis is usually unilateral, arising either by extension of the infection from the lacrimal sac or canaliculus or from direct inoculation.[3] In primary syphilis conjunctival chancres can form. These are localized areas of inflammation that begin as a hard nodule that expands and ulcerates, forming a membrane in an area of ulceration. Dull erythematous patches, erosions with overlying exudate, or a fleshy mass can also be seen in syphilis.

Cases of herpes zoster, toxic epidermal necrolysis, and erythema multiforme major (Stevens-Johnson syndrome) are easy to identify because of the skin lesions. Cytomegalovirus infection may occur with or without systemic symptoms or signs. In the absence of systemic involvement the conjunctivitis has no distinguishing characteristics.

Specific antibiotic or antiviral treatment should be given if possible. In addition, topical corticosteroid treatment, such as prednisolone acetate 1% four times daily, can reduce inflammation and scarring. Peeling of membranes can relieve discomfort. It is also best to separate symblepharon as it forms, with a glass rod or cotton-tipped applicator.

Acute Granulomatous Conjunctivitis

Conjunctival granulomas are highly vascularized sessile or polypoid masses that can be found on any part of the conjunctival surface. They are usually elevated, may be multiple (usually clustered), and may be associated with ulceration and necrosis of the conjunctiva. Parinaud's oculoglandular syndrome is the association of conjunctival granulomas or ulceration with a grossly visible preauricular node. It usually begins acutely but can last for months. Most forms of granulomatous conjunctivitis typically present as Parinaud's oculoglandular syndrome, and are discussed in Chapter 7. How-

Table 6-6	Causes of Acute Membranous Conjunctivitis

Viral
  Adenoviral keratoconjunctivitis, commonly type 8
  Primary herpes simplex
  Herpes zoster
  Cytomegalovirus
Bacterial
  Corynebacterium diphtheriae
  Streptococcus pyogenes
  Staphylococcus aureus
  Neisseria meningitidis
  Neisseria gonorrhoeae
  Moraxella (Branhamella) catarrhalis
  Pseudomonas aeruginosa
  Escherichia coli
  Shigella spp.
  Salmonella spp.
  Primary syphilis
  Vincent's infection
Others
  Candida
  Chemical burns
  ? Cicatricial pemphigoid
  Stevens-Johnson syndrome
  Lyell's disease (toxic epidermal necrolysis)

ever, the regional nodes are not always grossly enlarged.

Conjunctival granulomata, which usually occur in the absence of grossly enlarged nodes, include ophthalmia nodosum and other foreign body granulomas, rhinosporidiosis, Churg-Strauss syndrome, and sarcoid granulomas. Pyogenic granulomas can resemble a true granuloma but occur after trauma or surgery and are not associated with adenopathy.

Other Causes of Acute Conjunctivitis

Other types of acute conjunctivitis can be divided according to the type of discharge they produce—purulent, mucopurulent, or mucoid/watery (Table 6-7). Purulent discharge, in the absence of membranes, indicates bacterial infection. Hyperacute purulent conjunctivitis is characterized by profuse grossly purulent exudate and is nearly always caused by either *Neisseria gonorrhoeae* or *Neisseria meningitidis*. Bacterial conjunctivitis is discussed below.

A variety of diseases can cause acute conjunctivitis with mucopurulent discharge. Most cases of bacterial conjunctivitis will have mucopurulent discharge. Some viral infections can present without follicles and with a mucopurulent discharge. These include varicella, herpes zoster, influenza, cytomegalovirus, and Epstein-Barr virus (infectious mononucleosis). Reiter's syndrome and canaliculitis can present with acute mucopurulent conjunctivitis.

In addition to the virus infections listed above, measles, mumps, papillomavirus, and rubella can present without follicles and with mucoid/watery discharge. Parasitic infections, such as *Enterobius vermicularis* and fly larvae (myiasis), can present with an acute watery/mucoid conjunctivitis. In most cases the parasite is visible in the conjunctiva. Contact dermatitis can involve the conjunctiva. Eczematoid dermatitis is usually found on the lids, and itching and chemosis are usually prominent. An acute allergic reaction (anaphylactoid blepharoconjunctivitis) can develop after conjunctival exposure to a medication or other antigen to which the patient has already been sensitized. It is characterized by intense itching, urticaria or angioedema of the eyelids, and chemosis of the conjunctiva. Toxic papillary reactions to medications can also develop after less than 3 weeks of treatment. These are diagnosed by the history of medication use and characteristic inferonasal conjunctival staining with rose bengal.

Table 6-7	Other Causes of Acute Conjunctivitis

Purulent Discharge
Hyperpurulent
  Neisseria gonorrhoeae
  Neisseria meningitidis
Bacterial conjunctivitis

Mucopurulent Discharge
Most bacterial infections
  Lyme disease
Viral
  Herpes zoster
  Cytomegalovirus
  Infectious mononucleosis
  Influenza
  Reiter's syndrome

Watery/Mucoid Discharge
Viral infections
  Varicella
  Herpes zoster
  Cytomegalovirus
  Infectious mononucleosis
  Papilloma
  Rubeola
  Mumps
  Influenza
  Rubella
Parasites
  Enterobius vermicularis
  Myiasis
Anaphylactoid blepharoconjunctivitis
Contact dermatitis
Toxic papillary conjunctivitis

CHRONIC CONJUNCTIVITIS

Chronic Follicular Conjunctivitis

Chronic follicular conjunctivitis can be diagnosed in cases in which symptoms persist for longer than 3 weeks. These patients may report an acute onset, with persistent or insidious disease development. The conjunctivitis can continue for months or years. Diseases and related conditions that should be considered are as follows:

Chlamydial
  Trachoma
  Adult chlamydial keratoconjunctivitis
  Feline pneumonitis
  Psittacosis
  Lymphogranuloma venereum
Viral
  Molluscum contagiosum
Bacterial
  Moraxella
  Streptococcus
  Haemophilus

Drug-induced conjunctivitis (eserine, idoxuridine, and eye cosmetics)

Unknown etiology

    Axenfeld's chronic follicular conjunctivitis (orphan conjunctivitis)

    Chronic follicular conjunctivitis of Merrill-Thygeson type

Folliculosis of childhood

Table 6-8 offers pertinent details of most of the diseases listed above. Patients should be questioned about recent sexual activity, genital symptoms, and contact with birds or cats (chlamydia). The lids should be examined carefully for molluscum lesions. Topical agents that can cause follicular conjunctivitis should be discontinued. Laboratory testing is useful in diagnosis. Conjunctival scrapings, Gram's- and Giemsa-stained, and bacterial cultures should be performed. Immunologic testing for chlamydia and for viral and chlamydial cultures can also be helpful.

Giant Papillary Conjunctivitis

Giant papillae are greater than 1 mm in diameter and are usually found on the superior tarsal conjunctiva. They are seen in reactions to contact lens wear, vernal keratoconjunctivitis, atopic conjunctivitis, and reactions to foreign material (ocular prosthesis, corneal shells, exposed nylon sutures, cyanoacrylate glue, and extruded scleral buckles). Giant papillae are uncommon in atopic conjunctivitis. They are usually found in the inferior tarsal conjunctiva. Giant papillae are common in vernal keratoconjunctivitis, where they are usually present on the superior tarsal conjunctiva.

Chronic Membranous Conjunctivitis

The only chronic form of membranous conjunctivitis is *ligneous conjunctivitis,* in which prominent, hard membranes form on the tarsal conjunctival surfaces. It usually affects children between 2 and 6 years of age and is usually bilateral. The membranes can persist for months or years, and treatment is often ineffective. Ligneous conjunctivitis is discussed in more detail in Chapter 7.

Chronic Granulomatous Conjunctivitis

The differential diagnosis of chronic granulomatous conjunctivitis is the same as that of acute granulomatous conjunctivitis, which was discussed earlier (see Parinaud's syndrome, Chapter 7).

Cicatricial Conjunctivitis

A variety of diseases can cause conjunctival scarring (Table 6-9).

The scar pathognomonic of trachoma is at the limbus. It is called *Herbert's peripheral pit* and is the cicatricial remains of a limbal follicle (see Fig. 7-17). Less characteristic but still diagnostically important are the stellate scars resulting from cicatrization of necrotic conjunctival follicles. Diffuse scarring may also occur, leading to bowing of the upper tarsus or ectropion if severe enough. *Arlt's line,* a cicatricial line near the lid border of the upper tarsus, can occur in other diseases, but also suggests trachoma, as does an S curve of the upper lid border caused by cicatrization. In trachoma, scarring is always more prominent on the upper lid than on the lower lid.

In atopic keratoconjunctivitis the scars are focal and tend to occur in the centers of the giant papillae. There also can be diffuse shrinkage of the lower fornix, but even in this instance symblepharon, entropion, and trichiasis tend not to occur. Vernal conjunctivitis does not normally scar the conjunctiva, but radical treatment of the disease frequently does.

In cicatricial pemphigoid the scarring is progressive and affects primarily the inferior fornix. Progressive scarring also occurs in all of the chronic skin diseases, rarely after erythema multiforme major, in trachoma, with continued administration of causative topical or systemic medications, and after irradiation.

Every possible effort should be made to prevent conjunctival cicatrization because of its long-term complications. Entropion, trichiasis, mucus deficiency from loss of conjunctival goblet cells, and closure of lacrimal ducts can occur. Recurrent inflammation can occur from these complications, as can recurrent bacterial infection.

Other Causes of Chronic Conjunctivitis

A wide variety of conditions can cause chronic papillary conjunctivitis, and it is difficult to classify them clinically. Probably the best way is to divide them according to whether or not they have distinct findings on examination that permit clinical diagnosis (Table 6-10). It is also useful to divide the diseases according to type of exudate (Table 6-2) and whether they are unilateral or bilateral (Table 6-3).

In superior limbal keratoconjunctivitis, contact lens–induced keratoconjunctivitis, vernal keratoconjunctivitis, floppy lid syndrome, and lid imbrication, the inflammation primarily affects the superior conjunctiva. Giant papillae

Table 6-8 Diagnostic Features of Chronic Follicular Conjunctivitis and Related Conditions					
Disease	**Conjunctiva**	**Cornea**	**Cytologic Findings**	**Etiologic Factors**	**Remarks**
Molluscum contagiosum	Conjunctival scarring Follicular conjunctivitis Occlusion of punctum May have molluscum on conjunctiva	Fine epithelial keratitis superiorly Superior pannus	Molluscum bodies (eosinophilic, cytoplasmic inclusions) in biopsy of lid margin nodule Mononuclear response	Molluscum contagiosum virus (a poxvirus) White painless lid lesions with umbilicated center Incubation period 14 to 50 days	Molluscum of lid should be eradicated by curetting of lesion Often in adolescents and young adults with molluscum on other parts of body as well as lids; may spread venereally Self-limited unless cellular immunity is depressed, but ocular disease may persist for months and can result in visual loss No lymph node enlargement

Continued

Table 6-8 Diagnostic Features of Chronic Follicular Conjunctivitis and Related Conditions—cont'd

Disease	Conjunctiva	Cornea	Cytologic Findings	Etiologic Factors	Remarks
Adult chlamydial keratoconjunctivitis	Mild to moderate mucopurulent discharge Never membranous in adults Worse below No conjunctival cicatrization Redness, chemosis Follicular reaction	Superficial punctate to slightly coarse epithelial keratitis Sometimes subepithelial infiltrates (smaller than in EKC), which may leave scars Superior micropannus	Polymorphonuclear response May have 50% polymorphonuclear and 50% mononuclear cells in chronic phase Basophilic, intracytoplasmic, epithelial inclusions Fluorescent antibody-stained conjunctival scrapings, culture, polymerase chain reaction, and serum titers may be helpful	C. trachomatis (types D–K) Incubation period 2 to 19 days	Venereal, hand-to-eye transmission Persists for 3 to 12 months in untreated cases Lymph nodes: palpable, sometimes tender or visible Otitis media in 15% of cases Rarely swimming pool transmission (chlorine inhibits agent)
Drug-induced follicular conjunctivitis	Keratinization Drying Follicles mainly inferior fornix	Fine or blotchy epithelial keratitis Pseudodendrite Keratinization Pannus Limbal follicles can occur with idoxuridine No Herbert's pits, as in trachoma	Polymorphonuclear leukocytes and lymphocytes	"Toxic" reaction Agents include idoxuridine, miotics, dipivafrin epinephrine, atropine, adenine arabinoside, neomycin, gentamicin, tobramycin, and preservatives	Seen after prolonged use of medicines May see follicles without germinal centers with atropine Palpable preauricular adenopathy occurs rarely (idoxuridine) Epithelial keratitis may last several weeks after stopping medication

Axenfeld's chronic follicular conjunctivitis	No bulbar conjunctival follicles Follicles mainly on lower fornix and tarsus, but also on upper tarsus Heals in 1 to 2 years without scars	No keratitis No pannus	Mononuclear	May be a slow virus	Seen in orphanages No symptoms No lymph node enlargement
Merrill-Thygeson chronic follicular conjunctivitis	Follicles mainly on lower fornix and tarsus, but also on upper tarsus Heals in 4 to 5 months without scars	Epithelial keratitis, mainly above Micropannus in some cases	Mononuclear	Unknown	Cannot transfer to monkeys or rabbits May be transmitted by sharing of eye makeup No lymph node enlargement
Oculoglandular (Parinaud's) syndrome	Focal granulomatous conjunctivitis Granulomas may be surrounded by follicles May have conjunctival ulcers	Usually no involvement; however, it depends on etiology	Mixed mononuclear and polymorphonuclear leukocytes	Cat-scratch disease (*Bartonella henselae*) most common Others: tularemia, sporotrichosis, tuberculosis, sarcoid (node rarely enlarged), coccidioidomycosis, lues	May have contact with kitten Lymph node visibly enlarged May have fever, malaise Serum and skin tests, plus anaerobic and aerobic cultures (Gram's, Giemsa, and acid-fast stains), chest radiography

Continued

Table 6-8   Diagnostic Features of Chronic Follicular Conjunctivitis and Related Conditions—cont'd

Disease	Conjunctiva	Cornea	Cytologic Findings	Etiologic Factors	Remarks
Moraxella	Tarsal follicles Subacute conjunctivitis with moderate discharge Angular blepharoconjunctivitis	Occasionally marginal (catarrhal) infiltrate	Gram-negative diplobacilli on smear Much fibrin and only scant polymorphonuclear leukocytes	*Moraxella lacunata*	Adolescent patient Most common in southwestern United States Other bacteria, especially those in lacrimal system (that is, *Streptococcus* and *Haemophilus*), occasionally cause follicular conjunctivitis No lymph node enlargement
Eye makeup–induced follicular conjunctivitis	Insidious or asymptomatic Pigment (mascara) in "follicles" on tarsal and forniceal conjunctiva	No keratitis	Pigment granules only	Incorporation of makeup granules in conjunctival cysts: uncertain whether true follicles develop	In user of cosmetics No lymph node enlargement
Folliculosis of childhood	No inflammation Upper lid can be mildly involved Semilunar fold is spared Follicles tend to be prominent in fornix and fade out toward lid margins	No corneal disease	Mononuclear cells occasionally	Physiologic change of childhood and adolescence	Seen in children and can be associated with generalized lymphoid hyperplasia Newborn cannot have follicles until 6 weeks of age

Table 6-9 Causes of Conjunctival Scarring
Any cause of membranous conjunctivitis (see Table 6-6)
Chlamydial infections
Inclusion conjunctivitis of the newborn
Trachoma
Lymphogranuloma venereum
Skin diseases
Erythema multiforme major
Toxic epidermal necrolysis
Atopic dermatitis (atopic keratoconjunctivitis)
Cicatricial pemphigoid
Pemphigus vulgaris
Epidermolysis bullosa
Dermatitis herpetiformis
Poikiloderma atrophicans vasculare
Discoid lupus erythematosus
Exfoliative dermatitis
Lichen planus
Ectrodactyly-ectodermal dysplasia-cleft lip/palate syndrome
Trauma
Surgical
Injuries
Chemical
Irradiation
Drugs
Topical
Phosphodiesterase inhibitors
Pilocarpine
Idoxuridine
Atropine
Epinephrine
Dipivefrin
Systemic
Practolol
Penicillamine
5-Fluorouridine

Table 6-10 Causes of Chronic Papillary Conjunctivitis	
Distinct Clinical Findings	**Subtle or No Distinct Findings**
Superior limbal keratoconjunctivitis	Keratoconjunctivitis sicca
	Blepharitis/meibomitis
Contact lens–induced keratoconjunctivitis	Nocturnal lagophthalmos
	Acne rosacea
Vernal keratoconjunctivitis	Medication toxicity
	Airborne allergy
Atopic keratoconjunctivitis	Chronic bacterial infection
Lid position abnormalities	*Staphylococcus aureus*
	Moraxella (Branhamella) catarrhalis
Floppy eyelid syndrome	*Moraxella* spp.
Entropion	*Streptococcus pyogenes*
Ectropion	*Streptococcus pneumoniae*
Lagophthalmos	
Lid imbrication	*Neisseria gonorrhoeae*
Masquerade syndrome	Dacryocystitis
	Reaction to systemic drugs
Lid veruccae	Adriamycin
Canaliculitis	Alkylating agents
Ophthalmia nodosum	Cytarabine
	Diethylcarbamazine
Parasitic infection	Fluorouracil
	Indomethacin
	Methotrexate
	Practolol
	Retinoids

may be present on the superior tarsal surface in contact lens–induced and vernal keratoconjunctivitis. In atopic keratoconjunctivitis typical eczematoid dermatitis is present, often affecting the lids. Diagnosis of lid position abnormalities may require specific testing, such as asking the patient to squeeze the lids or to lie back and gently close his or her eyes, while checking for any separation with a flashlight.

Masquerade syndrome typically affects either the upper or lower lid, is unilateral, and exhibits abnormalities of the lid margin and conjunctival surface. In canaliculitis, unilateral swelling and tenderness of the medial lid margin are present. Mucopurulent material and concretions usually can be expressed from the punctum. Dacryocystitis is characterized by re-

current mucopurulent conjunctivitis. Tenderness, redness, and swelling may be present in the medial canthal region. Purulent material is expressed from the punctum when the lacrimal sac is compressed.

Examination of the lid margins for blepharitis and meibomitis and Schirmer's testing should be performed in all cases of chronic conjunctivitis. Bacterial cultures and scrapings are helpful in the absence of a clear diagnosis. Multiple conjunctival biopsies should be performed if malignancy is suspected.

These diseases are discussed in more detail in the remainder of this chapter and in Chapter 7. Conjunctival inflammation due to topical medications is discussed in Chapter 25.

RECURRENT ACUTE CONJUNCTIVITIS

There are a few conditions that create a predisposition to recurrent bacterial conjunctivitis. These include nasolacrimal duct obstruction, congenital absence of the nasolacrimal duct, dacryocystitis, dry eye, ectropion, entropion, and exposure. Extensive conjunctival scarring from cicatricial pemphigoid, erythema multiforme, trachoma, chemical burns, and other diseases can be associated with dry eye and lid position abnormalities and are commonly associated with recurrent bacterial conjunctivitis.

Herpes simplex conjunctivitis and keratitis are often recurrent, and lid or conjunctival vesicles and epithelial dendrites should be sought in anyone with recurrent conjunctivitis. Many skin diseases can be associated with recurrent episodes of conjunctivitis. These include cicatricial pemphigoid, atopic dermatitis, acne rosacea, psoriasis, epidermolysis bullosa, discoid lupus erythematosus, and porphyria.

OTHER CONJUNCTIVAL CONDITIONS

Chemosis

Chemosis is caused most commonly by allergic conjunctivitis but can result from orbital inflammation or tumor, severe intraocular in-

Table 6-11	Causes of Telangiectasia of Conjunctival Vessels

Ataxia-telangiectasia
Diabetes mellitus
Fabry's disease (see Fig. 21-14)
Sickle cell anemia
Degos' syndrome
Osler-Weber-Rendu disease
Polycythemia vera
Radiation (late)
Arteriosclerosis
Fucosidosis
G_{M1} gangliosidosis
Antiphospholipid syndrome
Xeroderma pigmentosum

Table 6-12	Conditions Associated with Conjunctival Vesicles and Blisters

Viral
Varicella
Herpes zoster
Herpes simplex
Variola (smallpox)

Bullous Skin Diseases
Cicatricial pemphigoid
Erythema multiforme
Pemphigus vulgaris
Linear IgA
Epidermolysis bullosa
Chronic bullous disease of childhood

Other Skin Diseases
Hydroa vacciniforme
Dyskeratosis congenita

Table 6-13	Conditions Associated with Conjunctival Deposits
Condition	**Appearance**
Topical exposure	
Epinephrine	Discrete subepithelial dark brown-black deposits, 1-3 mm
Silver	Silver coloration (argyrosis)
Mercury	Perivascular bluish-gray deposits
Local disease	
Spheroidal degeneration	Interpalpebral subepithelial spherical golden brown translucent drops
Localized amyloidosis	Pink to yellow-white fleshy, waxy subconjunctival nodules
Systemic drugs	
Clofazimine	Reddish pigmentation
Antacids	Bluish pigmentation
Quinacrine	Yellow, white, brown, blue, or gray deposits
Phenothiazine	Yellow-brown interpalpebral granules
Gold therapy	Gold granules
Systemic diseases	
Ochronosis	Bluish-gray or black pigmentation, interpalpebral
Tangier disease	Yellow-orange tinge
Gaucher's disease	Brown pingueculum
Hypercalcemia	Calcium deposition (granular appearance)
Hypophosphatasia	Calcium deposition (granular appearance)
Cystinosis	Crystals (ground glass appearance)
Multiple myeloma	Crystals (ground glass appearance)

flammation (e.g., endophthalmitis), or with severe infectious conjunctivitis. Graves' disease, trichinosis, exposure, radiation, and arteriovenous fistula are causes of chemosis. In addition, any condition that leads to impairment of lymphatic drainage can lead to chemosis, including trauma, surgery, radiation, neoplasm, or primary lymphedema.[4] In some cases the chemosis is not associated with conjunctival inflammation or injection.

Keratinization

Keratin may be seen in conditions of drying (exposure), mechanical irritation, superior limbal keratoconjunctivitis, vitamin A deficiency, and squamous neoplasia. Keratinized conjunctival lesions also occur in hereditary benign intraepithelial dyskeratosis, hereditary mucoepithelial dysplasia, acanthosis nigricans, and pityriasis rubra pilaris.

Telangiectasia and Sludging

Telangiectasia and sludging of the circulation of the conjunctival vessels can occur in a number of systemic diseases (Table 6-11). Sludging within conjunctival vessels occurs in multiple myeloma and sickle cell disease. Engorgement of conjunctival veins may be seen in cavernous sinus thrombosis, or with arteriovenous fistulas affecting the orbital circulation.

Others

Conjunctival *vesicles* and *blisters* are unusual signs that occur in skin diseases and viral infections (Table 6-12). In nearly all of these conditions vesicular or bullous disease also affects the skin, and the nature of the disease can be discerned from the systemic involvement.

Localized *infiltrates,* usually on an erythematous base, are seen in measles (Koplik spots), varicella, molluscum contagiosum, and conjunctival phlyctenulosis. A wide variety of *depositions* can affect the conjunctiva (Table 6-13). These can be related to topical or systemic medication or systemic disease. Avascular conjunctival patches can be seen in malignant atrophic papulosis. Epithelial hypertrophy and hyperkeratosis can be seen in acanthosis nigricans. Yellow plaquelike lesions occur in psoriasis, and pale yellow, waxy, raised, and very friable lesions have been reported in polyarteritis nodosa. Conjunctival tumors are discussed in Chapter 27.

REFERENCES

1. Duke-Elder S: *System of ophthalmology,* vol VIII, *Diseases of the outer eye,* part I, St Louis, 1965, CV Mosby.
2. Locatcher-Khorazo D, Seegal BC: *Microbiology of the eye,* St Louis, 1972, CV Mosby.
3. Givner I: *Purulent, membranous and pseudomembranous conjunctivitis.* In Allen HF et al, editors: *Infectious diseases of the conjunctiva and cornea,* St Louis, 1963, CV Mosby.
4. Tabbara KF, Baghdassarian SA: Chronic hereditary lymphedema of the legs with congenital conjunctival lymphedema, *Am J Ophthalmol* 73:531, 1972.

Seven

Infectious Conjunctivitis

OPHTHALMIA NEONATORUM

Conjunctivitis in neonates should be considered separately from that in older patients because the causes and presentations differ in these groups. The infections are usually acquired from the birth canal, and this is reflected in the types of agents seen. The relative frequency of different causes varies, depending on the prevalence of the organisms in the birth canal (of different venereal diseases) and the type of prophylaxis used.

The prevalence of neonatal conjunctivitis is approximately 0.9% in the United States.[1] The Centers for Disease Control and Prevention reported 900,000 cases in 1986. The two most important infectious causes are chlamydia and gonococcus; most commonly, however, no infectious cause is identified. Some of these cases are chemical, whereas others may be undiagnosed chlamydial infection. The neonatal conjunctiva rapidly acquires an indigenous flora, and most bacterial species are equally likely to be present in inflamed and quiet eyes.[2-4] In one study, 75% of newborns had positive cultures, and 78% of the organisms were nonaerobic—mainly lactobacilli and diphtheroids.[5] Therefore, it is difficult to determine even whether a cultured organism is the cause of clinical disease. Most cases of ophthalmia neonatorum are self-limited and leave no permanent sequelae even if untreated. However, it is probably wise to treat any potential pathogen with appropriate antibiotics.

The most important bacterial agents to recognize are *Neisseria gonorrhoeae* and *Pseudomonas* spp., because they can rapidly cause extensive ocular injury and, in the case of *Pseudomonas* infections, even death. It is also important to recognize herpes simplex conjunctivitis because it often is associated with disseminated disease, which has a high rate of morbidity and mortality. Early treatment with systemic antiviral therapy can greatly improve the outcome.

The most common agents, typical presentations, and current recommendations for treatment are provided in Table 7-1. Although clinical criteria are helpful in differentiating be-

Table 7-1 Differential Diagnosis and Treatment of Ophthalmia Neonatorum

Agents	Day of Onset After Exposure	Type of Discharge	Presence of Membrane	Presence of Follicles	Corneal Involvement	Laboratory Findings	Recommended Treatment
Neonatal inclusion disease (*Chlamydia trachomatis* types D–K)	4–12 days	Purulent or mucopurulent	+/– May result in conjunctival scars	None in newborn; may develop in 6–12 weeks	Superior micropannus in treated cases; Fine epithelial keratopathy	Polymorphonuclear cells; Basophilic cytoplasmic inclusions; Positive FA test	Erythromycin 12.5 mg/kg every 6 hours for 14 days; Topical tetracycline four times a day for 2 weeks
Silver nitrate irritation (Credé method)	< 24 hours	Purulent in severe cases	+ In severe cases	—	If severe, may have keratopathy or corneal scarring	Polymorphonuclear cells	Proper administration of drug (1%); Clear discharge away; Do not use stock bottles of silver nitrate; concentration of drug may be 90%
Neisseria gonorrhoeae	3–5 days; shorter if very severe; After 5 days indicates exposure after birth	Mucopurulent to purulent	+/–	—	Marginal or central ulcer or ring abscess; Perforation	Intraepithelial gram-negative diplococci	For conjunctivitis: Intramuscular ceftriaxone, 50 mg/kg (one dose); Also, topical saline lavage and erythromycin ointment (0.5%) four times daily
Staphylococcus aureus	5+ days, average 16 days	Catarrhal to mucopurulent	—	—	Punctate keratopathy	Gram-positive cocci and polymorpho-nuclear cells	Erythromycin ointment (0.5%) six times daily for 2 or 3 weeks

Streptococcus pneumoniae	5+ days	Purulent	–	–	–	Ulcer or punctate keratopathy may develop, resembling staphylococcal keratitis	Gram-positive cocci in chains and polymorphonuclear cells	Erythromycin ointment (0.5%) or sulfacetamide sodium (10%) six times daily
Haemophilus	5+ days	Catarrhal, in severe cases purulent	–	–	–	Rare, but may develop punctate keratopathy, especially with *H. aegyptius* (Koch-Weeks conjunctivitis)	*H. aegyptius:* long, fine, gram-negative bacilli / *H. influenzae:* gram-negative coccobacillus	*H. aegyptius* and *H. influenzae:* chloramphenicol (0.5%) or 10% sulfacetamide every hour first day, then four times daily
Coliform species	5+ days	Copius Purulent	–	–	–	Rare	Gram-negative nonencapsulated rods in and among polymorphonuclear cells	Irrigation of conjunctival sac Gentamicin (0.3%) or polymyxin B six times daily
Primary herpes (type II)	3–15 days	Nonpurulent Watery	±	–	May develop in 6–12 weeks	Epithelial or stromal disease	Multinucleated giant cells Positive Fluorescent Antibody test	Debridement and patching Topical trifluoro-thymidine nine times daily Intravenous acyclovir (250 mg/m^2) every 8 hours
Candida	5+ days	– Sometimes conjunctival necrosis	–	–	–	Occasional marginal corneal ulcer	Pseudohyphal budding yeast forms Polymorphonuclear cells	5% natamycin, 1% miconazole drops, or nystatin ointment (100,000 units/gram)

tween the various agents and in determining initial therapy, laboratory diagnosis is essential. Clinical signs are often nonspecific, and follicles and adenopathy cannot develop in the newborn for 6 to 12 weeks. The time of onset of clinical disease is approximate and is determined by the time and duration of exposure, the size of the inoculum, the incubation period of the organism, and the effectiveness of the prophylaxis. Ocular exposure can occur prior to birth if membranes are broken before delivery, if there is an ascending infection, or if endometritis is present. In these cases the time before onset of clinical signs is shorter. Conjunctival infections can also occur in babies delivered by cesarean section, either by previous exposure or by postnatal inoculation.

The most common prophylaxis today is probably still Credé's method, using silver nitrate 1%.[6] This treatment was initiated in the 1880s, primarily to prevent infection with *N. gonorrhoeae*. However, its effectiveness in preventing *Chlamydia trachomatis*, which is currently the most common cause of infectious neonatal conjunctivitis, is unclear. The silver nitrate treatment also frequently causes a chemical conjunctivitis (discussed later in this chapter) and it can cause corneal injury if accidentally administered in a stronger solution. Consequently, many have suggested the use of other agents, particularly tetracycline and erythromycin ointments.[7-10] Even if tetracycline and erythromycin are no more effective than silver nitrate in preventing transmission of disease, they are probably preferable because they are nontoxic.

The American Academy of Pediatrics recommends prophylaxis with 1% silver nitrate solution, 1% tetracycline ointment, or 0.5% erythromycin instilled without subsequent irrigation in all infants.[1] The face and eyelids should be cleaned at birth. Prophylaxis should be delayed by no more than 1 hour. Infants delivered by cesarean section should also receive prophylaxis because of the possibility of ascending infection, even without rupture of membranes.

Scrapings and cultures are necessary (see Chapter 4). Giemsa-stained scrapings are most useful for diagnosing chlamydia infection, but culture, direct fluorescent monoclonal antibody testing, enzyme immunosorbent assay, and polymerase chain reaction may also be used. Gram-stained scrapings and culture, including blood agar and chocolate or Thayer-Martin media, are necessary for bacterial identification. It is absolutely imperative to rule out *N. gonorrhoeae* and *Neisseria meningitidis,* and these laboratory tests aid in their diagnosis.

Chemical Conjunctivitis
Chemical conjunctivitis occurs in most infants who receive silver nitrate prophylaxis. It is mild, lasts only a few days, and appears within hours after instillation of silver nitrate. Mucopurulent discharge, mild to moderate hyperemia, and mild to moderate lid edema may be present. Accidental instillation of higher concentrations of silver nitrate (10% to 20%) can cause conjunctival ulceration, corneal scarring, and cataracts.

Inclusion Conjunctivitis of the Newborn
Inclusion conjunctivitis of the newborn (inclusion blennorrhea) is caused by infection with *C. trachomatis,* serotypes D through K. The reservoir of infection with *C. trachomatis* types D through K is the urethra or cervix; the disease is transmitted venereally. The infant is infected during passage through the birth canal.[11,12] Inclusion conjunctivitis is the result of contamination of the eye by genital secretions. The disease may be transmitted to the eye by fingers or fomites and often occurs in those who harbor the genital infection. Eye-to-eye transmission is extremely rare.

Inclusion conjunctivitis in the newborn is the most common infectious type of ophthalmia neonatorum, affecting as many as 3% of all newborns according to some publications.[13,14] More likely the incidence of chlamydial infection is between 1.4 and 4.4 per 1000 births.[4,15,16] This is because approximately 5% to 13% of pregnant women have chlamydial infection of the cervix, and 30% to 40% of their babies will develop conjunctivitis.[12,17,18] An even higher percentage of these babies develop serologic or other systemic evidence of chlamydial infection, indicating that subclinical systemic spread via conjunctiva or other mucous membranes occurs.

Inclusion conjunctivitis appears as a purulent or mucopurulent papillary conjunctivitis.[19,20] The incubation period usually is 5 days but can vary from 4 to 12 days. No follicles appear in the newborn state, but they can develop if the disease persists, usually between 6 weeks and 3 months of age. Preauricular adenopathy does not appear unless the infection persists. Swelling of the lids and conjunctiva is common. A conjunctival pseudomembrane may be present. Superficial vascularization of the cornea as a micropannus can be seen, as well as a fine epithelial keratitis and, on occasion, underlying areas of stromal haze and infiltrate. Although these areas can occur anywhere in the cornea, they usually are more numerous in the periphery. Mild scarring of the conjunctiva is

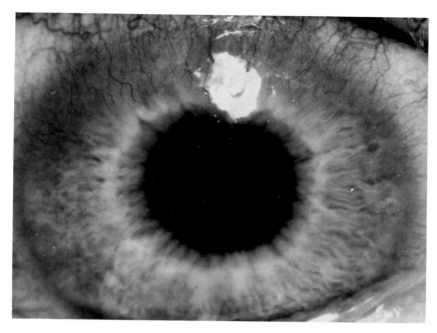

Figure 7-1
Micropannus in an untreated case of inclusion conjunctivitis in a newborn.

seen if conjunctival disease has been membranous.[14,21] If left untreated the disease may resolve in 3 to 4 weeks or may last for months or years. In one study the average duration was 4.5 months.[12] Persistent neonatal infection with *C. trachomatis* has been documented in children up to 6 years of age.[22,23] The longer the disease remains untreated, the greater the possibility that the patient will be left with a micropannus (Fig. 7-1) or subepithelial corneal scar.[21,24,25]

Systemic disease can also develop, particularly pneumonitis, which occurs in 10% to 20% of infants with inclusion conjunctivitis.[26-28] Chlamydial pneumonia usually develops at 2 to 3 months of age, and preceding or concurrent conjunctivitis is present in half of these infants.[27] Rhinitis,[24] otitis, vaginitis,[24] and hearing loss[29] have also been reported.

Laboratory diagnosis of chlamydial conjunctivitis is reviewed in Chapter 8. In children, Giemsa-stained scrapings and direct fluorescent antibody testing are more helpful because epithelial cell inclusions are present in greater numbers. The recommended treatment is oral erythromycin, 50 mg/kg/day, in four divided doses for 10 to 14 days.[30] This is effective in approximately 80% to 90% of cases.[31,32] Therefore, smears or cultures should be repeated after treatment. Patients who are intolerant or resistant to erythromycin treatment can be treated with trimethoprim/sulfamethoxazole, 0.5 mg/kg/day, in two divided doses for 14 days.

Gonococcal Conjunctivitis

In every case of ophthalmia neonatorum, gonococcal infection must be ruled out because of the possibility of blinding complications. In the last century, neonatal gonococcal conjunctivitis accounted for up to 25% of the inmates in institutions for the blind.[33] The advantage of prophylactic treatment with silver nitrate was first demonstrated by Credé in 1881.[6] This treatment, combined with better recognition and treatment of gonococcal venereal infection, has reduced the incidence in the United States to approximately 0.06%.[8] Untreated, approximately 40% of newborns exposed to *N. gonorrhoeae* will develop conjunctivitis.[9] Infection can occur in a number of ways: despite prophylaxis or if prophylaxis is incorrectly performed or delayed; as a result of prolonged exposure stemming from premature rupture of membranes; or through postnatal inoculation.

The incubation period for this infection usually is 3 to 5 days. However, with premature rupture of the membranes the infant can be infected in utero, and conjunctivitis will become evident earlier. Later infections are usually acquired after birth. Approximately 75% of cases are bilateral. The disease is usually less severe in children than in adults. Edema of the lids with severe chemosis and watery or serosanguineous exudate may occur. Subconjunctival hemorrhages, membranes, or pseudomembranes can develop. If untreated, copious purulent discharge often develops after 4 to 5 days. After 7 to 10 days, the conjunctivitis gradually diminishes. Healing continues over several weeks, commonly accompanied by formation of diffuse, flat, conjunctival scars.

The organism can penetrate intact corneal epithelium. The more severe the conjunctivitis and the longer it is left untreated, the more likely the cornea will be affected. The cornea may break down, with ulceration either centrally or marginally. Several peripheral ulcers can become confluent and form a ring abscess.

Gram's stain is about as sensitive as culture, and cases are often diagnosed by Gram's stain but are culture negative.[21] Therefore, both tests are required. Systemic treatment is required and is probably sufficient. The current recommended treatment for conjunctivitis is intramuscular ceftriaxone, 25 to 50 mg/kg, not to exceed 125 mg, daily, for 7 to 10 days.[34-36] Topical treatment can be used in addition (Table 7-1). Intramuscular cefotaxime, 50 mg/kg, is also effective. Infants with disseminated infection should receive intravenous or intramuscular ceftriaxone, 25 to 50 mg/kg/day, in single daily doses, or intravenous or intramuscular cefotaxime, 25 mg/kg, every 12 hours. The case should be reported to the Centers for Disease Control and Prevention, and both parents should be evaluated for sexually transmitted disease.

Meningococcal Conjunctivitis

N. meningitidis can cause a hyperpurulent conjunctivitis, which is clinically indistinguishable from gonorrheal ophthalmia. Keratitis or corneal ulceration has been reported in 15.5% of cases of *N. meningitidis* conjunctivitis.[37] The Gram's stain appearance is also identical, with intracellular diplococci and many polymorphonuclear leukocytes. Differentiation must be made by laboratory testing. Meningococcal conjunctivitis usually occurs by endogenous spread in patients with meningococcal septicemia. However, patients who present with primary conjunctival infection often develop meningococcemia or meningitis (10% to 28% of patients[37,38]). Therefore, rapid diagnosis and institution of systemic treatment is mandatory. Penicillin G is the drug of choice for topical treatment (100,000 U/ml every few minutes for several hours, then hourly) and systemic treatment (400,000 U/kg/day or 16 million U/m²/ day).

Other Bacteria

Certain bacteria are isolated more frequently from eyes with conjunctivitis than from noninflamed eyes, including *Staphylococcus aureus, Streptococcus pneumoniae, Haemophilus, Streptococcus viridans, Escherichia coli,* and *Pseudomonas aeruginosa.*[2,25] Any of these, and most likely other bacteria, can cause neonatal conjunctivitis. The clinical characteristics are usually nonspecific (Fig. 7-2), and each can be difficult to differentiate from gonococcal infection. However, some points can be made.

S. aureus conjunctivitis is common and may become serious because of the immature immunity of infants. The disease usually occurs initially as a mild conjunctivitis with hyperemia and mucoid or mucopurulent secretion.[19] It develops an average of 16 days after birth.[39] There may be some edema of the lids. A fine epithelial keratopathy can be present. Scrapings will show gram-positive cocci with polymorphonuclear cells. Unlike in the adult disease, staphylococcal conjunctivitis does not become chronic in newborns.

The conjunctivitis caused by *H. influenzae* is usually a severe purulent conjunctivitis with edema of the lids, in contrast to the conjunctivitis caused by *H. aegyptius,* which is usually a mild disease with only a small amount of mucoid exudate. *H. influenzae* conjunctivitis presents an average of 16 days following birth. It is often associated with otitis media and dacryocystitis.[40] On Gram's stain, *H. influenzae* are tiny gram-negative coccobacilli and *H. aegyptius* are long, fine, gram-negative bacilli. The preferred treatment is with topical chloramphenicol (0.5%) hourly the first day and then four times daily. Gentamicin is another alternative. Systemic treatment is indicated when there are signs of extraocular infection.

E. coli is the most common of the coliform bacteria to cause neonatal conjunctivitis. The disease is usually an acute, purulent conjunctivitis with severe chemosis of the conjunctiva, swelling of the lids, and copious purulent secretion. Topical gentamicin, tobramycin, or polymyxin B is effective. *S. pneumoniae* and *Streptococcus agalactiae* (group B streptococcus) produce a similar picture. *S. pneumoniae* has been reported to account for over 10% of cases of purulent conjunctivitis.[41] Because *S. agalactiae* can cause meningitis and sepsis in the newborn, some recommend parenteral penicillin G in all cases from which gram-positive cocci are seen on smear.[42]

Pseudomonas aeruginosa is an uncommon but important cause of neonatal conjunctivitis. In premature infants in a neonatal care unit, it

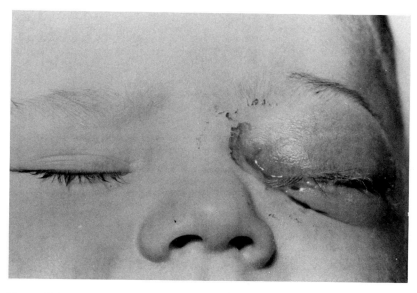

Figure 7-2
Neonatal bacterial conjunctivitis. (Courtesy of Kenneth Cheng, Pittsburgh, PA.)

may cause keratitis, endophthalmitis, septicemia, and even death.[43] The conjunctivitis can be purulent and membranous. However, it also can cause a mild conjunctivitis or even be isolated from noninflamed eyes.

Herpes Simplex

Herpes simplex virus (HSV) is an uncommon cause of conjunctivitis in newborns. Usually HSV type II is responsible, but in rare cases type I can be the cause. The conjunctivitis can be seen in isolation, combined with other ocular lesions, or with disseminated disease. It can be associated with vesicular blepharitis, corneal epithelial lesions, stromal keratitis, cataracts, or necrotizing chorioretinitis.[44,45] Conjunctivitis is occasionally the first sign of disease in a neonate who subsequently develops disseminated HSV, but it occurs more commonly in isolation or several days after manifestations of infection develop at other sites. Overall, conjunctivitis is seen in about 5% to 20% of cases of neonatal herpes.[44-47] In King County, Washington, the incidence of neonatal HSV infection was 28.2 per 100,000 births in 1982.[48]

The conjunctivitis can begin anywhere from 3 days to 2 weeks after birth, with 7 days being the average. The clinical appearance is not distinctive. There is moderate injection, lid edema, and in most cases a nonpurulent exudate with a mononuclear response (see Fig. 12-1). However, if a membrane is present, numerous polymorphonuclear leukocytes are

seen. In some cases a serosanguineous discharge is seen. Follicles are not present. Typical skin lesions are present somewhere on the body in one third to one half of patients with eye disease,[45] sometimes as a vesicular blepharitis.

Corneal involvement is also seen in about 10% of cases. Geographic epithelial lesions are most common, but dendrites and diffuse stromal keratitis have also been seen.[46] Necrotizing chorioretinitis and cataracts also can occur. In one case the virus was cultured from the lens 18 months after neonatal infection.[49]

If a herpetic infection is suspected, scrapings may be examined for multinucleated epithelial cells and intranuclear inclusions, and culture and immunopathologic studies may be performed. The finding of typical herpetic skin or corneal involvement can also aid in the diagnosis. The conjunctival inflammation of neonatal HSV resolves spontaneously in 2 to 3 weeks. Systemic and topical antiviral treatment is indicated. Intravenous acyclovir, 250 mg/m^2 is given every 8 hours, and topical trifluorothymidine is given nine times daily (Table 7-1).

PARINAUD'S OCULOGLANDULAR SYNDROME

In 1889, Parinaud, a Parisian ophthalmologist, described three butchers who developed a self-limited disease characterized by conjunctival "granulations" and suppurative preauricular

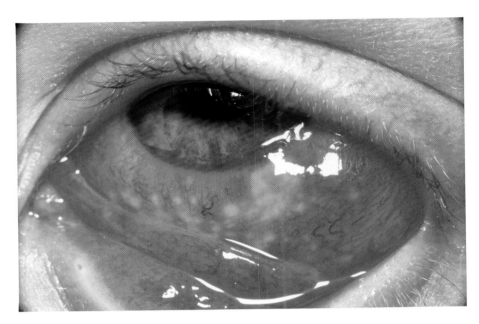

Figure 7-3
Conjunctival ulcerations in Parinaud's oculoglandular syndrome.

adenopathy that he believed was caused by an infectious agent transmitted by animals.[50] In 1913, Verhoeff, an American ophthalmologist, reported that a filamentous organism, *Leptothrix*, was present in the conjunctiva of patients with Parinaud's syndrome,[51] and he later isolated the organism.[52] Since that time it has become evident that the cases described by Parinaud and Verhoeff were most likely manifestations of cat-scratch disease (CSD), an infectious disease acquired from cats and caused by *Bartonella henselae*, a newly described rickettsia. However, the term *oculoglandular syndrome* has become more broadly applied, and its definition varies depending on the source. It is most commonly used to describe any condition in which conjunctival granulomas or ulcerations are associated with preauricular or submandibular adenopathy (Fig. 7-3).

Such a broad definition encompasses a spectrum of diseases, as shown in Table 7-2, but the most common remains CSD. The manifestations vary, depending on the etiologic agent, but usually are not specific enough to permit diagnosis without laboratory identification.

Diagnostic Evaluation

Which procedures are performed depends on which of the possible causative agents are suspected, based on history and examination. As a minimum, conjunctival scrapings and culture should be performed. Special media are required for many of the agents, such as blood-dextrose-cysteine agar for *Francisella tularensis*, Löwenstein-Jensen for mycobacteria, and Sabouraud agar for *Sporotrichum schenckii*. Biopsy of the conjunctival lesion for culture and examination is frequently helpful. Skin tests are available for CSD, lymphogranuloma venereum, coccidioidomycosis, glanders, and tuberculosis. Serologic tests are useful in tularemia, syphilis, infectious mononucleosis, rickettsial infection, and coccidioidomycosis.

Cat-Scratch Disease

Cat-scratch disease appears to be a relatively common disorder that often goes unrecognized. Eye involvement, manifested as Parinaud's oculoglandular syndrome, occurs in approximately 4% of patients.[53] It is caused by an infectious agent similar to that described by Verhoeff,[52] a newly described rickettsia named *B. henselae*.[54-56] The disease is transmitted by cats, usually immature ones, through a scratch or bite, contact with an open wound, or direct inoculation of mucous membranes. Person-to-person transmission does not appear to occur. Patients with Parinaud's syndrome probably inoculate the eye with their hand after touching a cat, but a cat may also contact the eye directly. It usually occurs in children and adolescents.

Table 7-2	Causes of Parinaud's Oculoglandular Syndrome

Common
Cat-scratch disease
Tularemia
Sporotrichosis

Occasional
Tuberculosis
Syphilis
Coccidioidomycosis

Rare
Chancroid
Pasteurella multocida
Yersinia pseudotuberculosis
Yersinia enterocolitica
Leprosy
Glanders
Lymphogranuloma venereum
Listeria monocytogenes
Actinomycosis
Blastomycosis
Mediterranean fever
Mumps
Infectious mononucleosis
Caterpillar hair
Rickettsia conorii (boutonneuse fever)
Sarcoid

From Chin GN, Hyndiuk RA: *Parinaud's oculoglandular conjunctivitis.* In Duane TA, Jaeger EA, editors: *Clinical ophthalmology,* vol 4, Philadelphia, 1988, Harper & Row, Publishers Inc. Used with permission of Lippincott-Raven Publishers; and Chin GN, Noble RC: Ocular involvement in *Yersinia enterocolitica* infection presenting as Parinaud's oculoglandular syndrome, *Am J Ophthalmol* 83:19, 1977.

Three to 5 days after inoculation of the skin, a papule develops. This becomes vesicular, crusts, and resolves, leaving a macule similar to that seen after chickenpox. Seven to 14 days after conjunctival inoculation, a soft, granulomatous nodule develops in the palpebral conjunctiva (Fig. 7-4). It usually is surrounded by follicles and associated with injection, chemosis, and watery discharge. Involvement is unilateral. The patient reports photophobia, irritation, and foreign body sensation.

Regional lymphadenopathy develops within 1 to 2 weeks, usually involving two to three nodes that are firm and usually nontender. The nodes typically regress over weeks to months, but 10% to 30% progress to suppuration. In most cases a mild systemic illness occurs, with aching, malaise, anorexia, and mild temperature elevation. In rare cases more severe complications occur, such as encephalopathy, pneumonia, or thyroiditis. The conjunctival granuloma may ulcerate, but it usually disappears over a few weeks, leaving no scar.[57] In one case *B. henselae* was detected by polymerase chain reaction analysis.[58] No treatment is necessary, but certain antibiotics appear to shorten the course and may be warranted in severe disease. Rifampin, ciprofloxacin, and gentamicin appear to be most effective.[59-61] Excision of large granulomas may also shorten the course of the disease.

The CSD skin test is very helpful in diagnosis: It is positive in 99% of patients with the disease versus positivity in approximately 4% of the general population.[53] Conjunctival or lymph node biopsy specimens should be examined with Warthin-Starry stain to observe the organism.[62]

Tularemia

Tularemia is acquired through bites from infected ticks or deer flies, by handling or ingesting infected animal tissue, or by inhaling infected aerosols. All rodents can be sources of infection, but rabbits are the most common source. In most cases a focal ulcer forms at the site of inoculation, with enlargement of local lymph nodes and a systemic reaction that includes fever, myalgia, headache, and malaise. Systemic spread of infection occurs, resulting in granulomatous lesions throughout the reticuloendothelial system and causing pneumonia in a significant percentage of patients. In rare cases, pericarditis, meningitis, and death can occur.

Eye involvement is characterized by necrotizing conjunctivitis with tender lymphadenopathy.[63,64] It is unilateral in about 90% of cases. The incubation period averages 3 days, but ranges from 1 to 14 days. The patient reports pain, photophobia, itching, tearing, chemosis, and mucopurulent discharge. Several small yellowish conjunctival nodules appear and develop shallow ulcerations. They usually are located on the tarsal conjunctiva. The nodules are covered by a gray, necrotic membrane and occasionally grow large. The enlarged regional nodes may suppurate and require incision and drainage. Systemic symptoms are more prominent than in CSD. In addition, more severe ocular complications can occur, including corneal ulceration, optic neuritis, panophthalmitis, and dacryocystitis.[63]

Diagnosis is made by culture of *F. tularensis,* a gram-negative coccobacillus, from the skin or

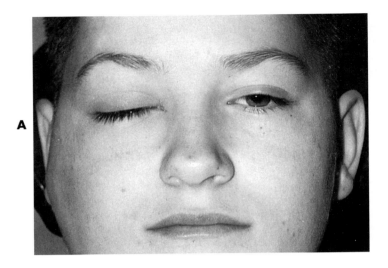

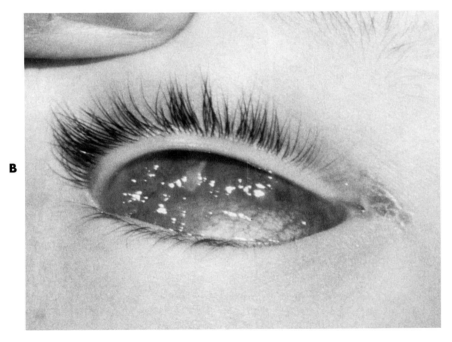

Figure 7-4
Child with Parinaud's oculoglandular syndrome due to cat-scratch disease. **A,** Visible preauricular adenopathy. **B,** Nodular inflammation in the superior fornix.

conjunctival lesion, affected lymph node, or serum. Blood-glucose-cysteine agar or another specific media must be used. The Foshay skin test is highly specific. Serologic diagnosis can be made by demonstrating rising titers.

The recommended treatment is intramuscular streptomycin, 1 g/day, for 7 days. Tetracycline, 25 mg/kg/day in three to four divided doses, or chloramphenicol, 50 mg/kg/day in three to four divided doses, may be used but are less effective.[64a] Topical gentamicin, tetracycline, or chloramphenicol every 2 to 3 hours may also be beneficial.

Sporotrichosis

Sporotrichosis results from inoculation of the skin or mucous membrane with *S. schenckii*. This organism is found in soil and decaying vegetation and on thorns. The most common means of acquiring the infection is through injury by a thorn, cactus, or brier. Nodular reactions are seen at the site of inoculation and along the draining lymphatics. The organism is a rare cause of Parinaud's syndrome.[65-67] The incubation period for conjunctival disease is 11 to 17 days. Small yellow nodules are seen that progress to ulceration and then granuloma formation. Conjunctival scarring can occur. Large subcutaneous nodules may occur in the eyelid skin; these break down and form deep ulcers. Painful adenopathy also is present.[33] Generalized symptoms are rare. Diagnosis is based on culture of the fungus from the conjunctiva or lymphatic lesions. The organism grows on all media commonly used for fungal culture. Treatment is with oral iodide. Potassium iodide (up to 4.5 to 9 ml of a saturated solution per day in divided doses) is given until 1 to 2 months after resolution of signs and symptoms.[68]

Tuberculosis

The conjunctiva may be the primary site of tuberculosis infection or may become involved secondarily from the spread of extraocular disease. Most cases occur in individuals younger than 20 years of age. A wide range of manifestations can be seen, and these have been well described.[33,69-71] An acute conjunctivitis may occur with purulent discharge, and membranes can develop. The conjunctiva can instead be relatively quiet and contain yellow or gray nodules surrounded by follicles, pedunculated growths, or small miliary ulcers. Regional adenopathy may be present, particularly in primary cases, and the nodes can suppurate. The diagnosis is made by biopsy of the conjunctiva or node, with demonstration of acid-fast organisms or growth of the organism in culture. Once the diagnosis is made, systemic treatment is administered. Excision of larger conjunctival masses can also be helpful.

Syphilis

Direct inoculation of the organism into the conjunctiva can result in primary conjunctival syphilis. The lesion appears similar to chancres occuring elsewhere: After an incubation period of 2 to 4 weeks, an indurated papule develops, ulcerates, and gradually enlarges with surrounding induration. There is little pain or discharge, but the lids become swollen, and the preauricular nodes enlarge and harden.[33,72]

Conjunctivitis or scleritis can be seen in secondary syphilis.[73] Simple papillary conjunctivitis, granular conjunctivitis, and mucus patches can be seen. The granular conjunctivitis is characterized by a uniform gelatinous, rose-colored thickening of the bulbar conjunctiva and upper fornix.[74] Relatively clear follicle-like lesions are seen on the superior tarsal surface. Superior pannus and regional lymphadenopathy are common. Mucus patches are a form of papular lesions (papulary syphilid) that affect the skin in secondary syphilis. They appear as dull erythematous patches, as a gray exudate overlying an erosion, or as an exuberant fleshy mass. In tertiary syphilis a gumma can involve the conjunctiva, most commonly the bulbar conjunctiva near the limbus. Keratitis, scleritis, and perforation of the globe can occur.[73,74]

Coccidioidomycosis

Conjunctival granulomas may develop in patients with secondary coccidioidomycosis (disseminated infection with *Coccidioides immitis*). They are usually found on the palpebral conjunctiva and may resemble a chalazion. They may be multiple, may be associated with follicular conjunctivitis, and are usually accompanied by a grossly enlarged preauricular node.[75,76] A conjunctival or corneal phlyctenule can develop in primary coccidioidomycosis.

Other Causes

Chancroid is a sexually transmitted disease caused by *Haemophilus ducreyi,* a gram-negative bacteria. Rarely it will infect the conjunctiva, beginning as an erythematous lesion that pustulates and then ulcerates. The ulcer bed is covered by a dirty-gray membrane. Preauricular and cervical adenopathy are usually present.

Limbal and tarsal subconjunctival granulomas can develop in lepromatous leprosy (Fig. 7-5).[77] The limbal granulomas are most common in the upper temporal quadrant but can spread posteriorly, anteriorly over the cornea, or circumferentially. They can ulcerate with a raised indurated border and a necrotic base.

Rarely, *Actinomyces* spp. can primarily infect the conjunctiva. The salient feature is scattered tiny yellow granulomatous nodules that may be pedunculated. Preauricular adenopathy is usually present. The nodes may be grossly visible and may suppurate and drain.

Conjunctival involvement can occasionally be seen in lymphogranuloma venereum. A small conjunctival nodule or ulcer may be present, or papillary, follicular, or granulomatous conjunctivitis can occur. Regional adenopathy is often present.

Pseudomonas pseudomallei (glanders) is acquired from diseased horses. Severe ulcerative or granulomatous conjunctivitis is associated with adenopathy, nose and mouth inflammation, preauricular adenopathy, and manifestations of septicemia. *Pasteurella multocida* and

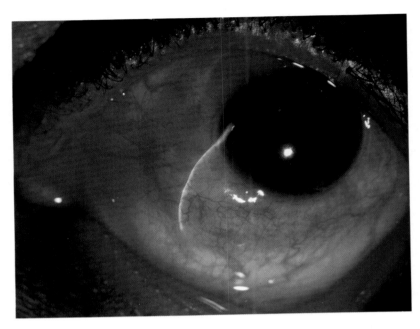

Figure 7-5
Nodular conjunctival leproma in leprosy.

Y. pseudotuberculosis conjunctival infections are associated with yellowish granulomas and preauricular adenopathy.

BACTERIAL CONJUNCTIVITIS

Pathogenesis

The ocular surface resists infections through several mechanisms. The mechanical action of the lids and the washing effect of tear flow help by physically removing pathogens. Antimicrobial enzymes, including lysozyme, lactoferrin, and beta-lysin, are present in the tears, as well as secretory IgA antibody. Ceruloplasmin, IgG, and IGM may also play a role.[78,79] The intact epithelial surfaces serve as mechanical barriers that inhibit penetration by organisms. The normal, nonpathogenic flora of the ocular surface inhibits growth of foreign bacteria and limits their own population size. This may be accomplished through release of antibiotic-like substances or by means of acidic metabolic endproducts.[80] The rich blood supply and the lymphoid layer of the conjunctiva provide a rapid and abundant supply of inflammatory cells and mediators.

Conjunctival infection occurs when an organism is able to overcome the host resistance; this depends on the virulence of the organism and the status of host resistance. A less virulent organism may exist as a commensal in one person's eye and cause a conjunctivitis in another person's eye; this has been demonstrated for *S. aureus*.[81]

Each of the mechanisms of resistance can be impaired in disease states. Decreased tear production occurs in keratoconjunctivitis sicca, and tear stagnation occurs with lacrimal duct obstruction. Exposure or poor lid function can lead to localized drying and impairment of the mechanical barrier of the surface. Trauma, including contact lens wear, scarring, or severe nutritional deficiency (particularly vitamin A), also makes the surface less resistant to infection. Antibiotic use can alter the normal flora and allow growth of pathogens that are resistant to the antibiotic. Local and systemic immunosuppression impairs the host's ability to respond to infection. Poor hygiene may lead to frequent inoculation with pathogenic organisms.

The virulence of an organism also determines how often it produces disease and the severity of the disease. Virulence is related to the organism's ability to adhere to the surface, to resist the tear enzymes, to penetrate the epithelium, and to destroy tissue and spread within it. Many bacteria elaborate toxins that impair host response and contribute to the signs and

Table 7-3   Bacterial Conjunctivitis

Acute conjunctivitis
  Staphylococcus aureus
  Haemophilus aegyptius
  Haemophilus influenzae
  Streptococcus pneumoniae
  Streptococcus pyogenes
  Pseudomonas aeruginosa
  Escherichia coli
  Corynebacterium diphtheriae
  Branhamella catarrhalis
  Neisseria gonorrhoeae
  Neisseria meningitidis

Hyperacute conjunctivitis
  N. gonorrhoeae
  N. meningitidis

Chronic conjunctivitis
  S. aureus
  Branhamella
  B. catarrhalis
  E. coli
  S. pyogenes
  S. pneumoniae
  N. gonorrhoeae
  Acinetobacter (Mimeae)
  E. coli, Klebsiella, and other coliforms
  Proteus
  Pseudomonas

symptoms of disease (see Chapter 9). For example, gonococci are able to invade normal epithelium because of pili that attach to sugar chains on the epithelial cell surface.[82] The epithelial cell phagocytoses the bacteria, and the bacteria multiply intracellularly, resulting in destruction of the cell and eventual subepithelial invasion. *L. monocytogenes, Corynebacterium diphtheriae,* and *Haemophilus* spp. are also able to penetrate conjunctival epithelium.

Clinical Manifestations

The manifestations of bacterial conjunctivitis depend on the virulence of the organism, as previously described, and the host's response. Fortunately, bacterial conjunctivitis is self-limiting in most cases: The host can overcome the infecting agent, and there are no sequelae. However, some agents can cause more severe disease and result in conjunctival or corneal scarring.

Bacterial conjunctivitis is commonly divided into acute, hyperacute, and chronic forms. Hyperacute infections are distinguished from acute infections by the presence of copious purulent discharge and lid swelling. The bacteria

commonly associated with these forms of conjunctivitis are shown in Table 7-3.

Acute Bacterial Conjunctivitis

Patients with acute bacterial conjunctivitis usually develop watering and irritation of the eyes, followed shortly by mucopurulent discharge and sticking together of the lids in the morning (Fig. 7-2). Most often both eyes are involved, although symptoms in one may precede those in the other by 1 to 2 days. On examination, the conjunctiva is diffusely injected, and the mucopurulent exudate may be seen in the fornix or inspissated on the lid margin. Petechial hemorrhages may be present, particularly in *S. pneumoniae* or *Haemophilus* infections. A diffuse, punctate keratopathy can be seen during the first 2 to 3 days of infection. Marginal corneal infiltrates may be present, more commonly in infections caused by *Haemophilus.*[83] Preauricular adenopathy is not present. Giemsa-stained scrapings typically reveal a predominantly polymorphonuclear response (except in infections caused by *Branhamella catarrhalis*). Gram's stain may reveal the causative organism. Cultures will isolate the pathogen and guide specific therapy. However, in most cases the cost and inconvenience of obtaining cultures exceed the benefit. If the conjunctivitis is more severe or prolonged or if the eye has been compromised, cultures should be obtained.

Pneumococcal conjunctivitis is more common in children and in colder climates. Subconjunctival hemorrhages are often present, especially in the upper tarsal and bulbar conjunctiva.[84] Without treatment it resolves after 7 to 11 days, leaving no sequelae.[33] *H. influenzae* conjunctivitis is relatively more common in young children (under 5 years of age), but it may be seen at any age (Table 7-4). It also is more common in the warmer regions of the United States, and can occur in epidemics. *H. influenzae* conjunctivitis lasts 9 to 15 days and tends to be more severe than that caused by *Pneumococcus.* In young children (under 36 months of age), otitis media is common. A severe preseptal cellulitis, with swelling and a bluish discoloration of the lids, can also develop.[85] It is important to recognize this condition, because septicemia, meningitis, septic arthritis, and endogenous endophthalmitis can occur. Systemic treatment is indicated to prevent these complications.

H. aegyptius conjunctivitis is similar to that caused by *H. influenzae,* but more commonly occurs in epidemic form. It can cause marginal

Table 7-4   Isolates in Bacterial Conjunctivitis at The Campbell Laboratory, Eye and Ear Hospital of Pittsburgh, 1983–1986*

Organism	Patient Age (Years)			
	0–10	11–60	>60	Total (%)
Staphylococcus aureus	23	86	45	154 (34.1%)
Haemophilus spp.	55	53	12	120 (26.6%)
Streptococcus pneumoniae	21	54	3	78 (17.3%)
Moraxella spp.	3	29	1	33 (7.3%)
Alpha-hemolytic streptococci	8	17	0	25 (5.5%)
Pseudomonas spp.	2	3	5	10 (2.2%)
Proteus spp.	0	3	4	7 (1.6%)
Acinetobacter spp.	3	2	1	6 (1.3%)
Beta-hemolytic streptococci	1	2	2	5 (1.1%)
Neisseria spp.	0	1	0	1 (0.2%)
Others†	2	3	7	12 (2.7%)
Total	118	253	80	451 (100%)

*Includes only cases in which the patient's age was known.

†*Bacillus* spp., *Enterobacter* spp., *Escherichia coli, Klebsiella* spp., *Serratia* spp., fewer than five isolates each.

corneal infiltration or ulceration and limbal phlyctenules. *P. aeruginosa* is a common cause of conjunctivitis in hospitalized patients, particularly those with tracheostomies, endotracheal tubes, or suctioning.[86]

Streptococcus pyogenes and *C. diphtheriae* can produce a severe conjunctivitis with membrane formation. Conjunctivitis is the most common ocular complication of Lyme disease and may be an early sign of that disorder.[87-89] In one study conjunctivitis was observed in 11% of patients with erythema chronicum migrans.[87] There can be a follicular response.

Treponema pallidum (syphilis), *H. ducreyi* (chancroid), *L. monocytogenes* (listeriosis), *Mycobacterium leprae* (leprosy), *P. multocida* (pasteurellosis), *Y. pseudotuberculosis* (pasteurellosis), *Pseudomonas mallei* (glanders), and *Actinomyces israelii* can cause conjunctivitis with granulomas or ulceration and preauricular adenopathy. They are discussed in the section on Parinaud's oculoglandular syndrome.

M. tuberculosis (tuberculosis) can infect the conjunctiva primarily or secondarily, by extension from adjacent lesions or by hematogenous spread. Primary conjunctival tuberculomas cause Parinaud's syndrome, and are discussed in that section. Lupus vulgaris, a slowly progressive chronic tuberculous skin infection, can affect the conjunctiva by extension from lesions on the lids.[90] Conjunctival tuberculids occur following the establishment of infection in some other part of the body. They are small evanescent nodules that spontaneously resolve. They are thought to result from hematogenous spread of organisms, which elicit a local hypersensitivity reaction. Papulonecrotic tuberculids of the bulbar conjunctiva also occur and are often associated with interstitial keratitis. Conjunctival and corneal phlyctenules commonly occur in tuberculosis.

Hyperacute Bacterial Conjunctivitis

Hyperacute conjunctivitis is typically caused by either *N. gonorrhoeae* or *N. meningitidis*, of which the former is by far the most common. It usually is acquired by autoinoculation from infected genitalia and therefore is seen most often in adolescents and young adults although it can occur at any age. It appears to be more common in warmer months.[91]

As with acute conjunctivitis, hyperacute conjunctivitis typically begins as redness and irritation but rapidly progresses to copious purulent discharge, swelling of the lids, pain, and tenderness (Figs. 7-6 and 7-7). There is marked hyperemia and chemosis of the conjunctiva, and membranes may form. Tender preauricular adenopathy can be present. Unilateral and bilateral involvement are equally common. Corneal involvement is common, with punctate keratopathy the most frequent finding. Stromal infiltration or ulceration most often develops in the periphery, beneath an overlying fold of edematous conjunctiva. Corneal involvement can occur at any time, even within 24 hours, but is more common the longer the infection is left untreated. Ulceration can progress and perforation can occur despite topical antibiotic treatment, and early peripheral corneal infil-

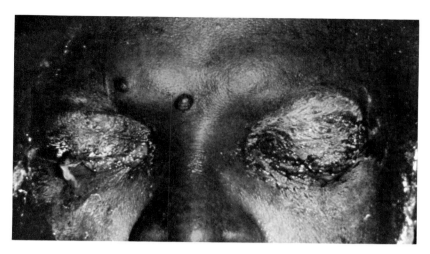

Figure 7-6
Discharge-coated lids in gonococcal conjunctivitis. (Courtesy of Thomas Roussel, Miami, FL.)

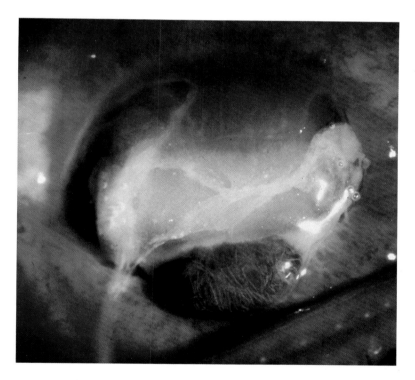

Figure 7-7
Corneal ulceration in gonococcal keratoconjunctivitis. (Courtesy of Thomas Roussel, Miami, FL.)

tration can develop during the first 1 to 3 days of parenteral therapy.[91,92] It is not clear whether the corneal ulceration is caused by invasion by the organism or is noninfectious, resulting from bacterial toxins or products of inflammation.[92]

In conjunctival scrapings the exuberant polymorphonuclear response is evident. Gram-negative diplococci are seen within the inflammatory cells. Culture on chocolate agar or Thayer-Martin media is indicated to isolate the organism and determine antibiotic sensitivity.

With appropriate therapy the discharge abates within 48 hours, and the other signs gradually resolve over 1 to 2 weeks. Corneal and conjunctival scarring can result.

CHRONIC BACTERIAL CONJUNCTIVITIS

Staphylococcal blepharoconjunctivitis is a common disease with many manifestations. Chronic conjunctival seeding occurs, and conjunctival cultures often yield the organism, but most of the bacteria reside on the lid. Conjunctival and corneal inflammation are probably related to the toxins produced by the staphylococci and the body's immunologic response to the organism and these toxins. These topics are considered in Chapters 13 (blepharitis) and 19 (immunologic diseases).

A number of other bacteria can cause a chronic conjunctivitis.[83,93] *Moraxella* organisms are probably the most common cause and are seen mainly in young adults. The infection can manifest itself either as a chronic follicular conjunctivitis or as an angular blepharoconjunctivitis (Fig. 7-8). The latter is characterized by ulceration of the lateral lid margins and conjunctival injection, which is most evident laterally. The ulceration is thought to be caused by a proteolytic enzyme produced by the *Moraxella* bacteria. *Proteus* is the only member of the enteric species that produces a marked conjunctival response.[93]

The symptoms of chronic bacterial conjunctivitis are relatively nonspecific. Irritation, redness, and mild mattering of the lids are the most common complaints. The findings include injection, mild papillary response, and mucoid or mucopurulent exudate. If staphylococcal blepharitis is present, additional findings may include redness and maceration of the lid margins, crusting, collarettes, inferior punctate keratitis, catarrhal infiltrates, and phlyctenulosis.

Treatment

For most cases of bacterial conjunctivitis, topical antibiotic therapy is sufficient. As mentioned previously, antibiotic selection is based ideally on isolation of the causative organism and determination of sensitivity. However, in most cases this is not necessary, and broad-spectrum antibiotic administration is sufficient. Using drops or ointment four times per day is usually sufficient. Sulfacetamide 10% to 15% and neomycin-polymyxin B combination are good broad-spectrum agents, although the latter has a relatively high rate of allergic reactions. Polysporin, a combination of bacitracin and polymyxin B; polytrim, a combination of trimethoprim and polymyxin B; and the fluoroquinolones norfloxacin, ciprofloxacin, and ofloxacin are also effective agents.[94-98] The amino-glycosides gentamicin and tobramycin are less appropriate: They are ineffective against *S. pneumoniae* and 7% to 8% of *S. aureus* and are associated with a significant risk of hypersensi-

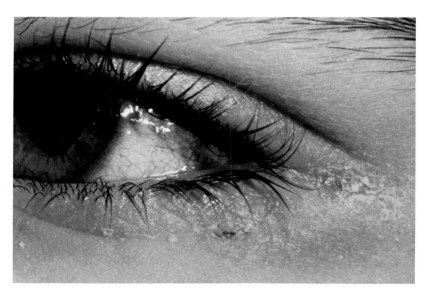

Figure 7-8
Angular blepharitis caused by *Branhamella* infection.

tivity and toxicity. Chloramphenicol has broad-spectrum activity, but its use is discouraged because of the very rare risk of aplastic anemia.[99] Treatment should be continued for at least 2 days after symptoms and signs resolve, usually 5 to 7 days.

Hyperacute conjunctivitis caused by *Neisseria* requires systemic therapy. Whenever it is suspected, systemic therapy should be initiated immediately and not delayed until culture confirmation is obtained.

The Centers for Disease Control and Prevention recommends the following treatments for gonococcal conjunctivitis in adults and children over 20 kg: intramuscular ceftriaxone, 125 mg; oral cefixime, 400 mg; oral ciprofloxacin, 500 mg; oral ofloxacin, 400 mg plus oral azithromycin 1 g; or oral doxycycline, 100 mg twice daily for 7 days. If keratitis or disseminated disease is present, a multidose regimen is probably safer:[36] intravenous ceftriaxone, 1 g (25 to 40 mg/kg) every 12 hours for 3 days (in patients allergic to penicillin, intramuscular spectinomycin, 2 g every 12 hours for 2 days, is substituted).

In all cases topical saline lavage, initially every hour, is helpful to remove the purulent discharge and toxic by-products. The value of topical antibiotic administration is unclear, but it is certainly not necessary. Ciprofloxacin is probably most effective. Bacitracin, erythromycin, and penicillin are also effective topical agents. Routine treatment for chlamydial infection is recommended by some because of the high incidence of coinfection.

When staphylococcal blepharoconjunctivitis is present, lid scrubs followed by application of bacitracin, erythromycin, or sulfacetamide ointment are performed once or twice daily for at least 1 month (see Chapter 13).

FUNGAL CONJUNCTIVITIS

Fungal conjunctivitis is uncommon. In most cases the findings are fairly specific and suggestive of the diagnosis. The exception is the conjunctivitis seen in primary coccidioidomycosis, which can be acute or chronic follicular.

Candidiasis
Candida spp. can be recovered from the conjunctiva in a small percentage of normal eyes (see Chapter 4). A thrushlike conjunctivitis can occur, particularly in immunosuppressed or debilitated patients. Raised white patches develop on the palpebral conjunctiva. When the patches are removed a red base is seen. Follicular and ulcerative conjunctivitis can also occur.[100]

The diagnosis can be made by examination of scrapings or culture. *Candida* organisms grow readily on blood agar and Sabouraud's medium at room temperature. Treatment is with topical amphotericin B 0.15%, miconazole 1%, or nystatin ointment, 100,000 U/g, four times daily.

Rhinosporidiosis
Rhinosporidium seeberi causes a chronic granulomatous mucocutaneous disease called *rhinosporidiosis*. The infection is seen most commonly in India and southeast Asia but occurs in most parts of the world. The conjunctiva is the second most common site of infection, after the nasal mucosa. A red, friable, papillomatous, pedunculated polyp is seen.[101] It is most commonly attached to the palpebral surface but can occur anywhere on the conjunctiva. Numerous whitish specks are present on the surface of the lesion. Usually only one lesion is present, but bilateral cases can occur.[102] Most patients are between 20 and 40 years of age. They usually have no complaint other than the presence of the mass. Diagnosis is by demonstration of 300-μm spherules with numerous large endospores in the tissue.[103] Treatment is by excision of the lesion.

Coccidioidomycosis
Coccidioidomycosis is a systemic infection caused by *C. immitis*. It is endemic in the geologic Lower Sonoran Desert Life Zone, which includes parts of the southwestern United States. The disease begins as a pulmonary infection following the inhalation of spores. In about 60% of cases the infection is asymptomatic; in the remainder mild to severe respiratory symptoms develop. In approximately 0.5% of symptomatic patients, disseminated disease, called *secondary coccidioidomycosis*, occurs. This can be acute or chronic. It is 5 to 10 times more common in blacks and Filipinos than in whites. An immune hypersensitivity reaction occurs in 10% of patients with acute primary infection. This is manifest most commonly as erythema nodosum, but erythema multiforme, arthralgias, and arthritis can occur. Episcleritis, scleritis, and phlyctenular keratoconjunctivitis can also occur as part of this condition.[104]

A mild to moderate acute or chronic follicular conjunctivitis can develop during primary coccidioidomycosis. The conjunctivitis is self-limited. Conjunctival granulomas can develop in secondary coccidioidomycosis. They are usually found on the palpebral conjunctiva, where they can resemble a chronic chalazion. The granulomas can be single or multiple and can be associated with a follicular conjunctivitis. They are commonly associated with a grossly enlarged preauricular node, and therefore are part of the differential diagnosis of Parinaud's syndrome.

Others

Conjunctival granulomas can occur in sporotrichosis, and these are discussed in the section on Parinaud's syndrome. Blastomycosis usually involves the conjunctiva in extension from lid lesions. However, noncontiguous conjunctival lesions may be seen.[105,106] They may be ulcerative, pseudomembranous, or granulomatous.

PARASITIC CONJUNCTIVITIS

Parasitic infection of the conjunctiva is uncommon, particularly in the United States. In most cases a worm or larva is present on the conjunctival surface or in the subconjunctival space. Localized inflammation is seen around the organism, with redness, irritation, and tearing. *Thelazia callipaeda, Loa loa,* the larvae of *Taenia solium* (cysticercosis), the larvae of *Spirometra* (sparganosis), and *Philophthalmas lachramosus broun* can invade the conjunctiva. *Thelazia californiensis* does not invade and is found on the conjunctival surface.

In trichinosis, localized yellowish conjunctival chemosis occurs, usually over the insertions of the lateral and medial recti. Chronic conjunctivitis can occur in onchocerciasis as a result of invasion of the conjunctiva with microfilariae. Lid edema, chemosis, limbal swelling, and mild injection are typical. Limbal pigmentation and lesions resembling conjunctival phlyctenules can also occur.

Fly larvae are occasionally deposited in the conjunctival sac. The fly can deposit the larvae while in flight.[107] The larvae can cause an acute conjunctivitis with foreign body sensation, burning, itching, pain, and watering. Elongated small active motile larvae 1 to 2 mm in length are seen on the conjunctival surface. They can avoid light and forceps removal. Instillation of cocaine paralyzes them or loosens their hold so that they can be removed. Lid or subconjunctival infestations can also occur (Fig. 7-9).

Follicular conjunctivitis can occur in children and young adults with pediculosis of the lashes. The larval form of *Amblyomma americanum,* a hard tick found in the southern United States and northern Mexico, can become attached to the conjunctiva. Conjunctival and corneal infection with microsporidia,

unicellular obligate intracellular protozoa, occurs primarily in AIDS patients, and is discussed in Chapter 11.

CHLAMYDIAL INFECTIONS

Chlamydial infections (Table 7-5) are some of the most common diseases affecting humans. Trachoma, a chlamydial ocular disease, affects approximately one seventh of the world's population and is the greatest cause of preventable vision loss. Trachoma is rare in the United States, but adult and neonatal inclusion conjunctivitis is commonly seen. Chlamydial conjunctivitis is commonly misdiagnosed in adults; suspicion of the disease and awareness of its clinical features are necessary for recognition.

The Organism

The chlamydiae have been classified in a separate section, as members of the order Chlamydiales. Like bacteria, they contain both DNA and RNA, divide by binary fission, are inhibited by sulfonamides and other antibiotics, and contain muramic acid in their cell walls; like true viruses, they are obligate, intracellular parasites. The family is called Chlamydiaceae, the genus, *Chlamydia.* The genus comprises two species, *C. trachomatis,* which causes eye disease, and *C. psittaci,* which primarily infects nonhuman species, particularly birds. *C. trachomatis* strains contain glycogen, produce iodine-staining intracytoplasmic inclusions, and are sensitive to sulfonamides, whereas *C. psittaci* strains do not contain glycogen, do not produce iodine-staining inclusions, and are not sensitive to sulfonamides. Eighteen serotypes of *C. trachomatis* have been identified. Strains A, B, Ba, and C are usually associated with trachoma, strains D through F with venereal disease and inclusion conjunctivitis, and strains L1, L2, L2a, and L3 with lymphogranuloma venereum.

Chlamydiae have a unique developmental cycle. The infectious organism exists in a form called an *elementary body* (EB), which is approximately 300 nm in diameter and has a rigid cell wall. The EB attaches to and is phagocytosed by an epithelial cell. Once in the cell it transforms into a larger particle, approximately 1000 nm in diameter, which is called a reticulate or initial body (RB). Over the next 48 hours the RB multiplies by binary fission to produce an aggregate of EBs. Hundreds to thousands of elementary bodies can be produced in an infected cell. These are located in the cytoplasm, usually near the nucleus, and can be seen in cytology

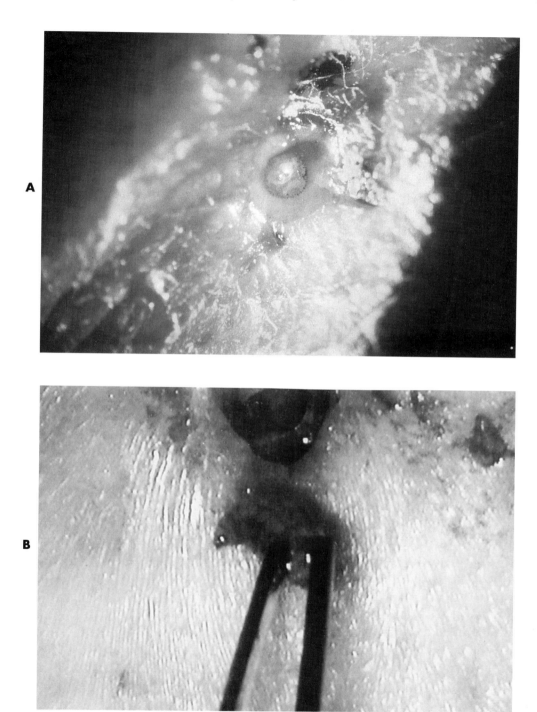

Figure 7-9
Fly larva in the lower lid. **A,** Larva can be seen protruding through tract in lid skin. **B,** Larva after removal from the lid.

Table 7-5   Features of Chlamydial Conjunctivitis

Feature	Acute Trachoma	Adult Chlamydial Keratoconjunctivitis	Lymphogranuloma Venereum	Chlamydia Psittaci
Incidence	Regional, endemic	Common	Uncommon	Rare
Onset	Insidious in children, acute in adults	Acute or subacute	Subacute	Acute or subacute
Duration (untreated)	Months to years	3 to 12 months	Usually 3 to 4 weeks, rarely years	?3 months
Laterality	Bilateral	Unilateral more common	Unilateral	?Unilateral
Adenopathy	Small, usually nontender	Small, usually nontender	Large	Small
Conjunctival response	Follicular, mainly superior Limbal follicles common Follicles can be expressed	Follicular, mainly inferior	Follicular Granulomatous	Follicular
Pannus	Superior 1–3 mm Common early	Superior 1 to 2 mm Occasionally	Uncommon but can be severe	No
Epithelial lesions	Superior punctate keratitis	Punctate keratitis Focal epithelial keratitis More common peripherally, especially superiorly	Minimal	Diffuse, fine keratitis
Subepithelial infiltrates	Occasional Superior	Occasional	Superior infiltration, can lead to diffuse vascularization	Can occur Superior
Sequelae	With chronic disease, reinfection, corneal and conjunctival scarring develop	None	Can lead to severe corneal and conjunctival scarring	None
Transmission	Eye to eye	Genital to eye	Genital to eye	Cat to human

as an inclusion body. The new EBs are released to infect other epithelial cells. Chlamydial infection in the newborn is covered above.

Adult Chlamydial Keratoconjunctivitis
Epidemiology
Ocular infection after the newborn period results from venereal disease. Chlamydia is a common venereal disease, with 3 to 5 million new cases diagnosed each year in the United States.[108,109] It accounts for 35% to 50% of cases of nongonococcal urethritis in men and is recovered from the cervix in 20% to 33% of women seen in clinics for sexually transmitted diseases.[108,110-112] Ocular inoculation may occur by spread from the genitalia to the fingers to the eye, from the genitalia directly to the eye, or from the genitalia to fomites to the eye. Autoinoculation is most common; eye-to-eye transmission is unusual. Inclusion conjunctivi-

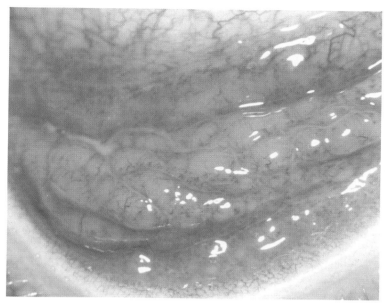

Figure 7-10
Marked follicular response in the inferior conjunctival fornix in an adult with chlamydial keratoconjunctivitis. (Courtesy of F. Wilson II, Indianapolis, IN.)

tis can also be transmitted in swimming pools with inadequately prepared chlorination.[113] (Most conjunctivitis from swimming pools is caused by the chlorine-resistant adenoviruses.)

Clinical Manifestations

The incubation period averages 5 days, but ranges from 2 to 19 days. Unilateral disease is more common than bilateral disease. The onset is typically subacute but may be acute. The patient complains of foreign body sensation, tearing, photophobia, redness, and lid swelling. The eye is mildly irritated and injected, and a scant mucopurulent discharge is present. Follicular hypertrophy is more marked in the lower tarsal conjunctiva (Fig. 7-10) and may take 2 to 3 weeks to appear. In contrast, follicular hypertrophy in trachoma is more marked in the supitarsal conjunctiva. No pseudomembranes are present, but a small, preauricular, tender node may develop. A pseudoptosis is often seen. Epithelial keratitis can be present, consisting of small, focal epithelial lesions that stain with fluorescein and tend to be more common in the periphery. Subepithelial infiltrates can occur, usually 2 to 3 weeks after the onset of the conjunctivitis; they tend to be smaller than those seen in adenovirus (Fig. 7-11). A superior corneal micropannus can be seen (Fig. 7-1). Small marginal corneal abscesses also can occur.[114]

Otitis media has been reported to occur on the same side as the involved eye in as many as 14% of cases.[115] A mild iritis also can be seen.

If left untreated, inclusion conjunctivitis can persist for 6 to 18 months. When a conjunctivitis persists for longer than 6 weeks in a sexually active person, one should be suspicious of the possibility of inclusion conjunctivitis.

A comparison of the features of adult chlamydial conjunctivitis (ACK) and adenoviral epidemic keratoconjunctivitis is given in Table 7-6.

Diagnosis

Scrapings of the conjunctival epithelium with Giemsa or Wright stain can be of immense value.[116] The predominant inflammatory cells are polymorphonuclear leukocytes. Cytoplasmic inclusions, plasma cells, Leber cells, and free EBs can also be present. Inclusions can be seen with Giemsa stain or with fluorescent antibody staining of conjunctival scrapings. The inclusions, which are basophilic and located in the cytoplasm of the epithelial cells (Fig. 7-12), are identical to the inclusions (Halberstaedter-Prowazek bodies) found in trachoma. The inclusion bodies are located immediately above the nucleus and form a small cap that sits on the nucleus. The inclusion consists of infectious EBs that are round, appear to be equal in size, have sharp-edged cell walls, and are light purple when stained with Giemsa

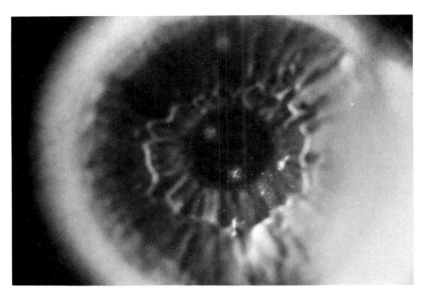

Figure 7-11
Subepithelial infiltrates in an adult with chlamydial keratoconjunctivitis. (Courtesy of Diane Curtin, Pittsburgh, PA.)

Table 7-6	Comparison of Adult Chlamydial Keratoconjunctivitis (ACK) and Adenoviral Epidemic Keratoconjunctivitis (EKC)	
Feature	**ACK**	**EKC**
Laterality	Unilateral more common	Bilateral more common
Discharge	Mucopurulent	Watery
Follicles	Present	Present
Adenopathy	Small, sometimes tender node	Prominent, tender node
Membranes	No	Occasionally
Focal epithelial keratitis	Occasionally, more common peripherally and superiorly	Usually, more common centrally
Subepithelial infiltrates	Occasionally, smaller than in EKC	Common
Associated findings	Otitis media, urethritis	None
Duration	Can last longer than a year	Conjunctivitis lasts 2 to 3 weeks
Cytology	Mixed mononuclear and polymorphonuclear cells; occasionally inclusions	Mononuclear cells (polymorphonuclear cells if membranes present)

stain. One must make sure when viewing the slide that true inclusion bodies are not mistaken for pseudoinclusions such as bacteria, extrusions of nuclear chromatin granules, or pigment granules. In addition to the EBs, RBs may be found. The RB is larger than the EB and stains dark blue, often in a bipolar fashion. Inclusion bodies are seen much more frequently in chlamydial conjunctivitis in infants; they may be difficult to find in adults.

McCoy cell tissue culture is the definitive means of diagnosis but is not widely available.

It also can be negative in up to half of cases and is impaired by antibiotic treatment.[117,118]

Because of the difficulties with these traditional tests, immunologic tests have been developed for diagnosing chlamydial infection. Both direct tests (examination of ocular specimens for chlamydial antigen) and indirect tests (testing of serum for antichlamydial antibodies) have been devised. A fluorescein-conjugated monoclonal antibody direct test is commercially available and has been reported to be highly sensitive and specific.[118-121] In my

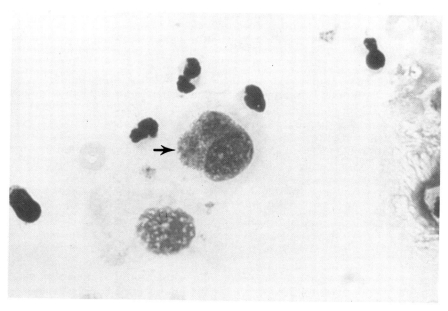

Figure 7-12
Intracytoplasmic inclusion (*arrow*) in chlamydial conjunctivitis. (Courtesy of Regis P. Kowalski, Pittsburgh, PA.)

experience this test is difficult to interpret and should be read only by those with a great deal of experience. An enzyme immunosorbent assay (Chlamydiazyme; Abbott Laboratories, North Chicago, IL) was found to be fairly sensitive and specific (71% and 97%, respectively).[121] Assay of antichlamydial tear s-IgA was found to be highly sensitive and specific in one study.[122]

Serum titers also can be useful. Commercial tests for antichlamydial IgG and IgA antibody titers are available and are relatively easy to perform.[120,122-124] Repeated tests showing a rising titer are diagnostic for recent infection, but single highly elevated titers suggest acute infection. Of course, antibodies can be present as a result of previous or nonocular infection.[125] Polymerase chain reaction appears to be as or more sensitive than culture and immunofluorescent techniques for the diagnosis of chlamydial conjunctivitis.[126-128]

Treatment

Topical treatment is not sufficient because it is not curative and frequently extraocular infection is also present. The treatment choices are oral tetracycline, 500 mg every 6 hours for 7 days; oral doxycycline, 100 mg twice daily for 7 days; oral azithromycin, 1 g;[129] oral erythromycin base, 500 mg four times daily for 7 days; oral erythromycin ethylsuccinate, 800 mg four times daily for 7 days; or oral ofloxacin, 300 mg twice daily for 7 days. Tetracycline and doxycy-cline should be taken on an empty stomach, and the patient should avoid milk products and antacids, which can prevent absorption of the drug. Pregnant women or children under 7 years of age should not be given tetracyclines. It is crucial to treat the patient's sexual partner to prevent reinfection.

Trachoma
Epidemiology

Trachoma has existed for 3000 years, if not longer, and has ravaged a good part of the world. Even today it is a major cause of preventable blindness. Around the world, 700 million cases are estimated, about 200 million of which involve blindness or significantly decreased visual acuity. Trachoma is endemic in parts of Africa, particularly North Africa, the Middle East, South America, and South Asia. In the United States trachoma is prevalent among the American Indians of the Southwest, and many cases are found in the "trachoma belt" of Arkansas, Missouri, Oklahoma, West Virginia, and Kentucky.

The disease is spread from eye to eye by way of fingers, fomites, water, and occasionally by flies. Mother-to-child transfer of infection is common. The highest incidence of trachoma is in unhealthy, dirty, crowded conditions, primarily in the low socioeconomic stratum of society. Even in endemic areas, the disease is associated with poorer personal hygiene, particularly decreased face washing, and improved hygiene has dramatically lowered the prevalence of disease.[130-132] One study in Tanzania found that the risk of trachoma was correlated with the presence of one or more flies on a child's face during a house visit.[133]

It is the childhood form that is important in the spread of disease in both the family and the community. In endemic areas preschool children serve as a reservoir of acute infection. Virtually all children are infected by 2 years of age, and acute infection is uncommon in adults.

Cultural customs can play an important role. In many endemic areas a mixture of lampblack and castor oil called kohl is applied around the eyes of all young children to ward off eye infections.[134] The same applicator is used on all female family members. Thus the infection is repeatedly transferred between mother and daughters, resulting in a higher incidence of acute disease and blindness in women. Jones described the situation in which trachoma arises as a disease of "ocular promiscuity," which entails "conditions that favor the frequent, unrestricted, and indiscriminate mixing of ocular contacts or of ocular discharges."[135]

A failure to induce immunity in trachoma may occur and may account for the long duration of disease and for the reinfections that are so common among school children who have been treated successfully during the school year. Repeated inoculation with chlamydia is probably necessary for development of trachoma.[136] Host inflammatory responses to the organism are more important than the cytopathic effect of the chlamydia on the conjunctival epithelium.[137]

Bacterial conjunctivitis is also very common in these populations and can play an important role in the pathogenesis of the scarring and blinding complications. Seasonal epidemics of bacterial conjunctivitis occur in many endemic areas, usually in spring and fall. Flies are a major vector in the spread of bacteria in these epidemics. Eyes already affected by trachoma are more likely to sustain serious complications from bacterial conjunctivitis. Although serotypes A through C are usually associated with trachoma, clinically typical cases of trachoma can develop from venereal infection with serotypes D through K.

Clinical Manifestations

Acute infection with trachoma can be seen in children or can be mild and go unrecognized. Approximately 5 days after inoculation, the child develops bilateral conjunctival injection, tearing, photophobia, and mucopurulent discharge. A tender preauricular node may be present. About 3 weeks later follicles may develop in the upper tarsal conjunctiva and sometimes at the limbus.

MacCallan[138] has divided the clinical features of trachoma into four stages. This system describes the course of trachoma but is not useful in estimating the intensity of disease, which is important in determining the outcome.[139] Therefore, another classification has been developed to score the intensity of inflammation.[139,140]

In the MacCallan classification, *stage I* is called incipient trachoma, with signs and symptoms similar to those of acute infection. This stage is characterized by the presence of immature follicles in the upper tarsal conjunctiva. These follicles are soft and easily expressible, unlike those of nontrachomatous follicular conjunctivitis. Follicles may also be seen at the limbus and on the caruncle. A minimal exudate usually occurs; however, if a secondary infection is present, greater exudation is seen. Intense cellular infiltration of the conjunctiva can occur; the subepithelial tissue of the conjunctiva is edematous and infiltrated with round inflammatory cells, mainly lymphocytes and plasma cells. Papillary hypertrophy also occurs, and the follicles may be buried as a result. In this stage of early formation of conjunctival follicles, one may see a diffuse punctate keratitis and early formation of a superior corneal pannus. Fibrovascular tissue may grow into the cornea underneath the epithelium and destroy Bowman's layer.

MacCallan's *stage II* is considered established trachoma and is characterized by mature follicles and more advanced keratitis. This stage is divided into *IIa*, in which the follicular response is predominant (Fig. 7-13), and *IIb*, in which follicles are seen but are largely obscured by a rather intense papillary response. Stage IIb is primarily a florid inflammation of the upper tarsal conjunctiva, with more acute inflammation and cellular infiltration. Larger, "mature" follicles have the appearance of "sago" grains (tapioca) and can undergo central necrosis. These follicles rupture easily with pressure, and the contents can occasionally extrude spontaneously. Limbal follicles can also occur, most commonly superiorly and at the corneoscleral junction. However, they can also occur on the cornea proper. Limbal follicles are only slightly elevated and are translucent. The corneal pannus as well as the subepithelial edema and round cell infiltration may increase. Large macrophages with phagocytosed debris (Leber cells)

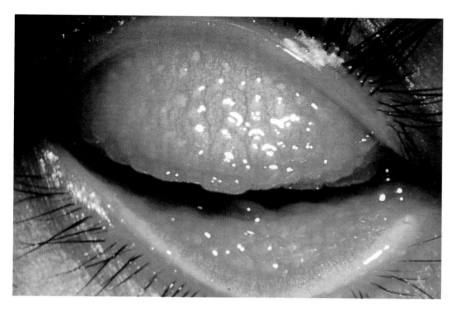

Figure 7-13
Stage IIa trachoma.

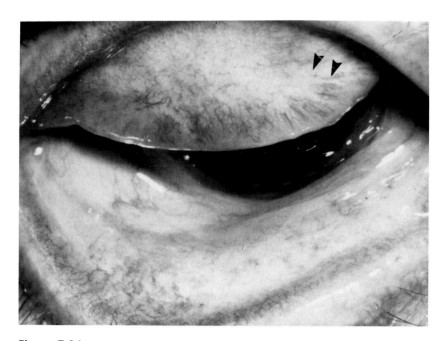

Figure 7-14
Scarring of the conjunctiva of the upper tarsus (*double arrow*) in stage III trachoma.

appear in the conjunctival substantia propria (see Fig. 4-11). At this stage the follicles cannot be differentiated histologically from lymphoid follicles secondary to other causes.

Stage III brings about variable amounts of scarring and cicatrization (Fig. 7-14). The lim-

bal corneal follicles, if present, cicatrize, and the area is covered with thickened transparent epithelium (*Herbert's pits*) (Fig. 7-15). They are seen as clear, round, or scalloped areas within a more opaque limbus. They appear depressed, but in most cases are filled with thickened epi-

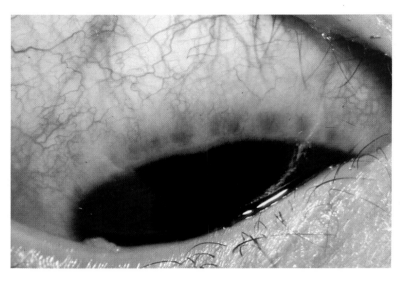

Figure 7-15
Herbert's pits in stage III trachoma.

thelium. These pits are pathognomonic of trachoma. Scarring also occurs in the palpebral
conjunctiva and is manifested clinically by the
appearance of fine linear scars on the tarsal
conjunctiva and sometimes in the bulbar conjunctiva. Individual follicles leave stellate scars.
Horizontal, sometimes criss-crossing, linear
scars also develop in the tarsal conjunctiva.
Arlt's line is a dense linear scar in the upper tarsal conjunctiva, located 2 to 3 mm above lid
margin. Cicatrization of the lids, symblepharon, trichiasis, and other lid distortions begin
to develop. Immunohistochemical staining
demonstrates that the inflammatory infiltrate
of the tarsal conjunctiva in cicatricial trachoma
is comprised predominantly of T cells.[141]

Each of the first three stages may last for
months or years. In *stage IV*, or healed trachoma, the conjunctival and corneal inflammation has subsided. Follicles and papillae are
no longer present, and there is no inflammatory infiltration of the cornea. The amount of
residual scarring is determined by the severity
of the inflammation in the previous stages.[139]
The scarring produces dry eyes, entropion, and
trichiasis. It is the complications of these disorders, and of superimposed bacterial conjunctivitis and keratitis, that lead to blindness.

The World Health Organization Committee
for Trachoma developed a severity classification
of trachoma.[142] Follicles, papillae, and scarring
are each graded on a scale of 0 to 3 (Table 7-7).

Corneal findings can include epithelial and
subepithelial keratitis, gross pannus of the up-

per portion of the cornea, and corneal ulceration. Early in the disease the superior epithelium is hazy and exhibits punctate staining
with fluorescein. Subepithelial infiltrates can
develop. With continued disease a fibrovascular
pannus extends centrally from the superior
limbus. It can invade Bowman's layer. Central
to the pannus the epithelium is hazy and exhibits punctate staining. Pinpoint, focal, or annular areas of superficial stromal infiltration
can develop central to the pannus. Corneal
scarring, opacification, and vascularization can
be so severe that vision is markedly impaired
(Fig. 7-16). The corneal findings are more prominent in the superior cornea.

Softening of the tarsus occurs as a result of
chronic inflammation. Infiltration by lymphocytes and mast cells is seen histologically. The
softened tarsus is especially susceptible to distortion by scarring of the lid margin and conjunctiva. Atrophy and distortion of the meibomian glands, meibomian gland retention cysts,
distichiasis, poliosis, blepharophimosis, and
elephantiasis can develop. Lacrimal complications such as punctal phimosis, punctal
occlusion, canaliculitis, canalicular occlusion,
nasolacrimal obstruction, dacryocystitis, dacryoadenitis, and fistulae in the skin have been
reported in trachoma.[143]

Diagnosis
The diagnosis of trachoma is usually made clin-
ically in endemic areas. Limbal follicles and
Herbert's pits are pathognomonic.

Table 7-7	World Health Organization Classification of Trachoma Severity

Follicles
Zone 1: Upper third of the upper lid
Zone 2: Middle third of the lid
Zone 3: Lower third of the lid (near lid border)
F0. No follicles on the upper tarsus
F1. Fewer than five follicles in zones 2 and 3
F2. More than five follicles in zones 2 and 3 but fewer than five follicles in zone 3
F3. Five or more follicles in each zone

Papillae
P0. Refers to a normal conjunctiva; the underlying vessels are clearly seen
P1. Minimal obscuration of the underlying conjunctival vessels by papillae
P2. More than half of the underlying conjunctival vessels partially obscured by papillae
P3. Diffuse conjunctival infiltration and papillary hypertrophy completely obscures over half of the underlying conjunctival vessels.

Scarring
S0. No scarring
S1. Stellate scars or small linear scars
S2. Large flat scars without lid distortion
S3. Conjunctival scarring with distortion of the lid, resulting in trichiasis or entropion

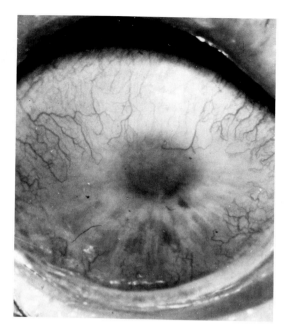

Figure 7-16
Scarring, vascularization, and corneal opacification in stage IV trachoma.

The primary inflammatory reaction may be a polymorphonuclear response; however, lymphocytes, plasma cells, lymphoblasts, Leber cells (large debris-filled macrophages), necrotic epithelial cells, and multinucleated giant epithelial cells may be seen in smears. Basophilic, intracytoplasmic, epithelial inclusion bodies (Halberstaedter-Prowazek bodies) identical to those described in inclusion conjunctivitis are diagnostic. The frequency of their presence depends on the stage of the trachoma, with up to 40% of smears positive in moderate cases.[144,145]

The diagnostic tests for chlamydial infection in trachoma are the same as those for adult inclusion conjunctivitis, as discussed previously. Their usefulness appears similar in the two conditions. Fluorescent monoclonal antibody staining of conjunctival smears is slightly less specific but more sensitive than Giemsa staining of smears.[144,146] In one study an enzyme immunoassay was found to be more specific than fluorescent monoclonal antibody or Giemsa staining.[147] Polymerase chain reaction appears to be the most sensitive means of detection.[148,149]

Treatment

The ideal treatment is with a full, oral dose of tetracycline, sulfonamide, or erythromycin for at least 3 weeks. If tetracycline is the drug given, the dosage should be 500 mg orally three times a day for at least 3 weeks. This medication should be taken 1 hour before or 2 hours after meals with water or juice but no milk. Tetracycline is not to be used in pregnant women or in children younger than 7 years of age.

Trisulfapyrimidines (triple sulfa) may be used. In adults the dose is 2 to 4 g immediately followed by a maintenance dosage of 2 to 4 g daily in three or four divided doses for at least 3 weeks. In children, a loading dose of half of the 24-hour dose is followed by a maintenance dosage of 150 mg/kg/24 hours in three or four doses for at least 3 weeks. Trisulfapyrimidines are not to be used in pregnant women, nursing mothers, or infants younger than 2 months of age.

This systemic treatment is most effective in sporadic cases in nonendemic areas. In hyperendemic areas in which half or more of the children have active disease, and seasonal epidemics of bacterial conjunctivitis are present, reinfection and recurrent bacterial infection prevent elimination of the disease. Elimination of the reservoir of the organism by mass treatment with systemic antibiotics is not practical. Therefore, the aim of the therapy instead is to avoid blinding complications. Topical tetracycline twice a day, given as a continuous 6-week course, appears to reduce or eliminate blinding complications. Similar results were achieved with a 5-day course of topical tetracycline repeated once monthly for 6 months.[150,151] A single dose of oral azithromycin, 20 mg/kg, appears to be as effective as the 6-week course of topical tetracycline.[152]

Topical medication may act by reducing the intensity of the disease, the rate of transmission, and the bacterial flora and seasonal conjunctivitis that contribute to the gravity of trachoma in these areas. Oral antibiotic therapy is recommended as an adjunct in children with moderate to severe trachoma to improve the outcome.[153] Surgical treatment is also important to correct entropion, trichiasis, and lacrimal disorders.

Other Chlamydial Infections
C. Psittaci

C. psittaci produces an infection of birds, with occasional transmission to humans. Its name comes from the Greek word for parrot (*psittakos*), which was the vector for the first recognized cases in humans. It can cause an asymptomatic infection, mild influenza-like illness, or serious pneumonia. Rare cases of conjunctivitis have been reported.[154,155] An acute or chronic follicular conjunctivitis can occur that may be similar to adult inclusion conjunctivitis. A diffuse follicular response, mild preauricular adenopathy, and mucopurulent discharge can be seen. There is no scarring of the conjunctiva. A diffuse epithelial keratitis and subepithelial infiltration can occur; however, no pannus is noted. No inclusions can be found on scrapings. There are no sequelae of any importance, and the disease apparently responds to tetracycline.

Feline pneumonitis is also caused by *C. psittaci*. Rarely, people in contact with an infected cat develop conjunctivitis. The findings are similar to those described above. Treatment for both conditions is a 6-week regimen of tetracycline, 500 mg four times daily, doxycycline, 100 mg twice daily, or erythromycin, 250 mg four times daily.

Lymphogranuloma venereum is transmitted venereally and usually is manifested by genital lesions followed by lymphadenitis and febrile systemic illness. Infection of the eye can occur by spread from the genital tract on fingers. A follicular conjunctivitis or granulomatous reaction associated with preauricular adenopathy (Parinaud's oculoglandular syndrome) can occur.[156] The conjunctivitis usually resolves after 3 to 4 weeks but can persist for years. Elephantiasis of the lids can occur in chronic cases as a result of blockage of lymphatic drainage. Corneal involvement is uncommon but can be severe. Spotty marginal corneal infiltration, usually superior, becomes deep and confluent and spreads centrally.[157,158] Superficial vascularization can ensue and may become so profuse that it resembles an epaulet.[159] Episcleritis, sclerokeratitis, and interstitial keratitis have also been seen. Chlamydial inclusions often are found on conjunctival scrapings. The Frei test is positive in half of these patients. Optic neuritis and anterior uveitis are seen occasionally,[159] and the orbit also may be involved.[160]

REFERENCES

1. American Academy of Pediatrics: *Sexually transmitted diseases.* In Peter G et al, editors: *1994 Red book: report of the infectious diseases,* ed 23, Elk Grove Village, IL, 1994.
2. Prentice MJ, Hutchinson GR, Taylor-Robinson D: A microbiological study of neonatal conjunctivae and conjunctivitis, *Br J Ophthalmol* 61:601, 1977.
3. Molgaard IL, Nielsen PB, Kaern J: A study of the incidence of neonatal conjunctivitis and of its bacterial causes including *Chlamydia trachomatis:* clinical examination, culture and cytology of tear fluid, *Acta Ophthalmol (Copenh)* 62:461, 1984.
4. Pierce JM, Ward ME, Seal V: Ophthalmia neonatorum in the 1980's: incidence, aetiology and treatment, *Br J Ophthalmol* 66:728, 1982.
5. Isenberg SJ et al: Bacterial flora of the conjunctiva at birth, *J Pediatr Ophthalmol Strabismus* 23:284, 1986.
6. Crede CSF: Die verhutung der augenentzundung der neugeborenen, *Arch Gynak* 21:179, 1881.
7. American Academy of Pediatrics: Prophylaxis and treatment of neonatal gonococcal infections, *Pediatrics* 65:1047, 1980.
8. Rothenberg R: Ophthalmia neonatorum due to *Neisseria gonorrhoeae:* prevention and treatment, *Sex Transm Dis* 6(suppl):187, 1979.
9. Laga M et al: Prophylaxis of gonococcal and chlamydial ophthalmia neonatorum: a comparison of silver nitrate and tetracycline, *N Engl J Med* 318:653, 1988.
10. Hammerschlag MR et al: Erythromycin ointment for ocular prophylaxis of neonatal chlamydial infection, *JAMA* 177:2142, 1980.
11. Schachter J: Reply to letter to editor, *JAMA* 234:592, 1975.
12. Thygeson P, Stone W Jr: Epidemiology of inclu-

sion conjunctivitis, *Arch Ophthalmol* 27:91, 1942.

13. Burns RP, Florey MJ: Conjunctivitis caused by Mimeae, *Am J Ophthalmol* 56:386, 1963.
14. Hansman D: Inclusion conjunctivitis, *Med J Aust* 1:151, 1969.
15. Stenson S, Newman R, Fedukowicz H: Conjunctivitis in the newborn: observations on incidence, cause and prophylaxis, *Ann Ophthalmol* 13:329, 1981.
16. Sandstrom KI et al: Microbial causes of neonatal conjunctivitis, *J Pediatr* 105:706, 1984.
17. Schachter J et al: Prospective study of perinatal transmission of *Chlamydia trachomatis, JAMA* 255:3374, 1986.
18. Hammerschlag MR et al: Prospective study of maternal and infantile infection with *Chlamydia trachomatis, Pediatrics* 64:142, 1979.
19. Ostler HB: Oculogenital disease, *Surv Ophthalmol* 20:233, 1976.
20. Hobson D, Rees E, Viswalingam ND: Chlamydial infections in neonates and older children, *Br Med Bull* 39:128, 1983.
21. Forster RK, Dawson CR, Schachter J: Late follow-up of patients with neonatal inclusion conjunctivitis, *Am J Ophthalmol* 69:467, 1970.
22. Stenberg KL, Mardh P-A: Persistent neonatal chlamydial infection in a 6-year-old girl, *Lancet* 2:1278, 1986.
23. Bell TA et al: Chronic *Chlamydia trachomatis* infections in infants, *JAMA* 267:400, 1992.
24. Mordhorst CH, Dawson C: Sequelae of inclusion conjunctivitis and associated disease in parents, *Am J Ophthalmol* 71:861, 1971.
25. Persson K et al: Neonatal chlamydial eye infection: an epidemiological and clinical study, *Br J Ophthalmol* 67:700, 1983.
26. Schacter J, Dawson C: Is trachoma an ocular component of a more generalized chlamydial infection?, *Lancet* 1:702, 1979.
27. Beem MO, Saxon EM: Respiratory tract colonization and a distinctive pneumonia syndrome in infants infected with *Chlamydia trachomatis, N Engl J Med* 296:306, 1977.
28. Harrison JR et al: *Chlamydia trachomatis* infant pneumonitis, *N Engl J Med* 298:702, 1978.
29. Gow JA, Ostler HB, Schachter J: Inclusion conjunctivitis with hearing loss, *JAMA* 229:519, 1974.
30. Sandstrom I: Treatment of neonatal conjunctivitis, *Arch Ophthalmol* 105:925, 1987.
31. Oriel JD: Ophthalmia neonatorum: relative efficacy of current prophylactic practices and treatment, *J Antimicrob Chemother* 14:209, 1984.
32. Rees E et al: Persistence of chlamydial infection after treatment for neonatal conjunctivitis, *Arch Dis Child* 56:193, 1981.
33. Duke-Elder S, Leigh AG: *System of ophthalmology,* vol 8, *Diseases of the outer eye,* St Louis, 1965, Mosby–Year Book.
34. Lepage P et al: Single-dose cefotaxime intramuscularly cures gonococcal ophthalmia neonatorum, *Br J Ophthalmol* 72:518, 1988.

35. Haimovici R, Roussel TJ: Treatment of gonococcal conjunctivitis with single-dose intramuscular ceftriaxone, *Am J Ophthalmol* 107:511, 1989.
36. Ullman S, Roussell TJ, Forster RK: Gonococcal keratoconjunctivitis, *Surv Ophthalmol* 32:199, 1987.
37. Santer DM, Myhre JA, Yogev R: Primary group Y meningococcal conjunctivitis and occult meningococcemia, *Pediatr Infect Dis J* 11:54, 1992.
38. Moraga FA et al: Invasive meningococcal conjunctivitis, *JAMA* 264:333, 1990.
39. Fox KR, Golomb HS: Staphylococcal ophthalmia neonatorum and staphylococcal scalded skin syndrome, *Am J Ophthalmol* 88:1052, 1979.
40. Cohen KL, McCarthy LR: *Haemophilus influenzae* ophthalmia neonatorum, *Arch Ophthalmol* 98:1214, 1980.
41. Sandstrom KI et al: Microbiological causes of neonatal conjunctivitis, *J Pediatr* 105:706, 1984.
42. Ostler HB: *Diseases of the external eye and adnexa,* Baltimore, 1993, Williams & Wilkins.
43. Burns RP, Rhodes DH: *Pseudomonas* eye infection as a cause of death in premature infants, *Arch Ophthalmol* 65:517, 1961.
44. Hagler WS, Walters PV, Nahmias AJ: Ocular involvement in neonatal herpes simplex virus infection, *Arch Ophthalmol* 82:169, 1969.
45. Nahmias AJ, Hagler WS: Ocular manifestations of herpes simplex in the newborn (neonatal ocular herpes), *Int Ophthalmol Clin* 12:191, 1972.
46. Hutchinson DS, Smith RE, Haughton PB: Congenital herpetic keratitis, *Arch Ophthalmol* 93:70, 1975.
47. Whitley RJ et al: The natural history of herpes simplex virus infection of mother and newborn, *Pediatrics* 66:489, 1980.
48. Sullivan-Bolyai J et al: Neonatal herpes simplex virus infection in King County, Washington: increasing incidence and epidemiologic correlates, *JAMA* 250:3059, 1983.
49. Cibis A, Burde RM: Herpes simplex virus–induced congenital cataracts, *Arch Ophthalmol* 85:220, 1971.
50. Parinaud H: Conjonctivite infectieuse paraissant transmise a l'homme par les animaux, *Recueil Ophthalmol* 11:176, 1889.
51. Verhoeff FH, King MJ: Parinaud's conjunctivitis: a mycotic disease due to a hitherto undescribed filamentous organism, *Arch Ophthalmol* 42:345, 1913.
52. Verhoeff FH, King MJ: Leptotrichosis conjunctivae (Parinaud's conjunctivitis): artificial cultivation of the leptotriches in three of four cases, *Arch Ophthalmol* 9:701, 1933.
53. Carithers HA: Cat-scratch disease: an overview based on a study of 1200 patients, *Am J Dis Child* 139:1124, 1985.
54. English CK et al: Cat-scratch disease: isolation

and culture of the bacterial agent, *JAMA* 259:1347, 1988.

55. Wear DJ et al: Cat-scratch disease bacilli in the conjunctiva of patients with Parinaud's syndrome, *Ophthalmology* 92:1282, 1985.

56. Anderson B et al: Detection of *Rochalimaea henselae* in cat-scratch disease skin test antigens, *J Infect Dis* 168:1034, 1993.

57. Cassady JV, Culbertson CS: Cat scratch disease and Parinaud's oculoglandular syndrome, *Arch Ophthalmol* 50:68, 1953.

58. Le HH et al: Conjunctival swab to diagnose ocular cat scratch disease, *Am J Ophthalmol* 118:249, 1994.

59. Margileth AM: Antibiotic therapy for cat-scratch disease: clinical study of therapeutic outcome in 268 patients and a review of the literature, *Pediatr Infect Dis J* 11:474, 1992.

60. Holley HP: Successful treatment of cat-scratch disease with ciprofloxacin, *JAMA* 265:1563, 1991.

61. Bogue C et al: Antibiotic therapy for cat-scratch disease?, *JAMA* 262:813, 1989.

62. Luna LB: *Manual of histologic staining methods of the Armed Forces Institute of Pathology*, ed 3, New York, 1968, McGraw-Hill.

63. Francis E: Oculoglandular tularemia, *Arch Ophthalmol* 28:711, 1942.

64. Anderson R: Oculoglandular tularemia, *J Iowa Med Soc* 60:21, 1970.

64a. Kaye D: *Tularemia*. In Braunwald E et al, editors: *Harrison's principles of internal medicine*, ed 11, New York, 1987, McGraw-Hill.

65. Gordon DM: Ocular sporotrichosis, *Arch Ophthalmol* 37:56, 1947.

66. McGrath H, Singer JI: Ocular sporotrichosis, *Am J Ophthalmol* 35:102, 1952.

67. Raul AG, Lopez-Villegas A: Primary ocular sporotrichosis, *Am J Ophthalmol* 62:150, 1966.

68. Bennett JE: *Fungal infections*. In Braunwald E et al, editors: *Harrison's principles of internal medicine*, ed 11, New York, 1987, McGraw-Hill.

69. Archer D, Bird A: Primary tuberculosis of the conjunctiva, *Br J Ophthalmol* 51:679, 1967.

70. Anhalt EF, Chang G, Byron HM: Conjunctival tuberculosis, *Am J Ophthalmol* 50:265, 1965.

71. Juler F: Primary tuberculosis of conjunctiva treated with streptomycin, *Trans Ophthalmol Soc UK* 69:297, 1949.

72. Maxey EE: Primary syphilis of the palpebral conjunctiva, *Am J Ophthalmol* 65:13, 1965.

73. Wilhelmus KR, Yokoyama CM: Syphilitic episcleritis and scleritis, *Am J Ophthalmol* 104:595, 1987.

74. von Popolczy F: Syphilis of the conjunctiva, *Arch f Augenh* 108:334, 1933.

75. Trowbridge DH: Ocular manifestations of coccidioidomycosis, *Trans Pacific Coast Otoophthalmol* 33:229, 1952.

76. Wood TR: Ocular coccidioidomycosis: report of a case presenting as Parinaud's oculoglandular syndrome, *Am J Ophthalmol* 64:587, 1967.

77. Wedemeyer LL et al: Fibrous histiocytoid leprosy of the cornea, *Cornea* 12:532, 1993.

78. Bron AJ, Seal DV: The defenses of the ocular surface, *Trans Ophthalmol Soc UK* 105:18, 1986.

79. Coyle PK, Sibony PA: Tear immunoglobulins measured by ELISA, *Invest Ophthalmol Vis Sci* 27:622, 1986.

80. Fredrickson AB: Behavior of mixed culture of microorganisms, *Annu Rev Microbiol* 31:63, 1977.

81. Locatcher-Khorazo D, Sullivan N, Gutierrez E: *Staphylococcus aureus* isolated from normal and infected eyes: phage types and sensitivity to antibacterial agents, *Arch Ophthalmol* 77:370, 1967.

82. Watt PJ: Pathogenic mechanism of organisms virulent to the eye, *Trans Ophthalmol Soc UK* 105:26, 1986.

83. Wilson LA: *Bacterial conjunctivitis*. In Duane T, Jaeger E, editors: *Clinical ophthalmology*, vol 4, Philadelphia, 1988, Harper & Row.

84. Ostler HB: *Diseases of the external eye and adnexa: a text and atlas*, Baltimore, 1993, Williams & Wilkins.

85. Londer L, Nelson DL: Orbital cellulitis due to *Haemophilus influenzae*, *Arch Ophthalmol* 91:89, 1974.

86. King S et al: Nosocomial *Pseudomonas aeruginosa* conjunctivitis in a pediatric hospital, *Infect Control Hosp Epidemiol* 9:77, 1988.

87. Steere AC et al: Lyme arthritis: an epidemic of oligoarticular arthritis in children and adults in three Connecticut communities, *Arthritis Rheum* 20:7, 1977.

88. Bruhn FW: Lyme disease, *Am J Dis Child* 138:467, 1984.

89. Winward KE, Smith JL: Ocular disease in Caribbean patients with serologic evidence of Lyme borreliosis, *J Clin Neurol Ophthalmol* 9:65, 1989.

90. Blegval O: Tuberculosis of the conjunctiva, *Acta Ophthalmol* 14:200, 1936.

91. Wan WL et al: The clinical characteristics and course of adult gonococcal conjunctivitis, *Am J Ophthalmol* 102:575, 1986.

92. Ullman S et al: *Neisseria gonorrhoeae* keratoconjunctivitis, *Ophthalmology* 94:525, 1987.

93. Thygeson P, Kimura S: Chronic conjunctivitis, *Trans Am Acad Ophthalmol Otolaryngol* 67:494, 1963.

94. Leibowitz HM: Antibacterial effectiveness of ciprofloxacin 0.3% ophthalmic solution in the treatment of bacterial conjunctivitis, *Am J Ophthalmol* 112(suppl):29S, 1991.

95. Jacobson JA et al: Safety and efficacy of topical norfloxacin versus tobramycin in the treatment of external ocular infections, *Antimicrob Agents Chemother* 32:1820, 1988.

96. Miller IM et al: Topically administered norfloxacin compared with topically administered gentamicin for the treatment of external ocular bacterial infections, *Am J Ophthalmol* 113:638, 1992.

97. Gwon A, the Ofloxacin Study Group: Ofloxacin vs tobramycin for the treatment of external ocular infection, *Arch Ophthalmol* 110:1234, 1992.

98. Bron AJ et al: Ofloxacin compared with chloramphenicol in the management of external ocular infection, *Br J Ophthalmol* 75:675, 1991.

99. Rosenthal RL, Blackman A: Bone marrow hypoplasia following use of chloramphenicol eye drops, *JAMA* 191:136, 1965.

100. Duke-Elder S: *Vol VIII-Diseases of the outer eye, part 1.* In Duke-Elder S, editor: *System of opthalmology,* London, 1965, CV Mosby.

101. Arnold R, Whildin J: Rhinosporidiosis of the conjunctiva, *Am J Ophthalmol* 25:1227, 1942.

102. Neumayr TG: Bilateral rhinosporidiosis of the conjunctiva, *Arch Ophthalmol* 71:39, 1964.

103. Gori S, Scasso A: Cytologic and differential diagnosis of rhinosporidiosis, *Acta Cytol* 38:361, 1994.

104. Rodenbiker HT, Ganley JP: Ocular coccidioidomycosis, *Surv Ophthalmol* 24:263, 1980.

105. Slack JW et al: Blastomycosis of the eyelid and conjunctiva, *Ophthalmol Plast Reconstr Surg* 8:143, 1992.

106. Kreibig W: Beiderseitige matastatsche ophthalmis durch Blastomyzeten (Bilateral metastatic ophthalmia from blastomycosis), *Klin Monatsbl Augenheilkd* 104:64, 1940.

107. Duke-Elder S: *Vol VIII-Diseases of the outer eye, part 1.* In Duke-Elder S, editor: *System of ophthalmology,* London, 1965, CV Mosby.

108. Judson FN: Assessing the number of genital chlamydial infections in the United States, *J Reprod Med* 30:269, 1985.

109. Schachter J et al: Are chlamydia infections the most prevalent venereal disease?, *JAMA* 231:1252, 1975.

110. Schachter J: Chlamydial infections, *N Engl J Med* 298:428, 1978.

111. Schachter J, Causse G, Tarizzo ML: Chlamydiae as agents of sexually transmitted diseases, *Bull World Health Organ* 54:245, 1976.

112. Thompson SE, Washington AE: Epidemiology of sexually transmitted *Chlamydia trachomatis* infections, *Epidemiol Rev* 5:96, 1983.

113. Morax V: *Les conjonctivites folliculaires,* Paris, 1933, Masson et Cie.

114. Darougar S, Viswalingam ND: Marginal corneal abscess associated with adult chlamydia ophthalmia, *Br J Ophthalmol* 72:774, 1988.

115. Dawson C et al: Experimental inclusion conjunctivitis in man. III. Keratitis and other complications, *Arch Ophthalmol* 78:341, 1967.

116. Yoneda C et al: Cytology as a guide to the presence of chlamydial inclusions in Giemsa-stained conjunctival smears in severe endemic trachoma, *Br J Ophthalmol* 59:116, 1975.

117. Schachter J et al: Evaluation of laboratory methods for detecting acute TRIC agent infection, *Am J Ophthalmol* 70:377, 1970.

118. Taylor HR, Agarwala N, Johnson SL: Detection of experimental *Chlamydia trachomatis* eye infection in conjunctival smears and in tissue culture by use of fluorescein-conjugated monoclonal antibody, *J Clin Microbiol* 20:391, 1984.

119. Hawkins DA et al: Rapid, reliable diagnosis of chlamydial ophthalmia by means of monoclonal antibodies, *Br J Ophthalmol* 69:640, 1985.

120. Bialasiewicz AA, Jahn GJ: Evaluation of diagnostic tools for adult chlamydial keratoconjunctivitis, *Ophthalmology* 94:532, 1987.

121. Sheppard JD et al: Immunology of adult chlamydial conjunctivitis, *Ophthalmology* 95:434, 1988.

122. Buisman NJF et al: Chlamydia keratoconjunctivitis: determination of *Chlamydia trachomatis* specific secretory immunoglobulin A in tears by enzyme immunoassay, *Graefes Arch Clin Exp Ophthalmol* 230:411, 1992.

123. Darougar S et al: Rapid serological test for diagnosis of chlamydial ocular infections, *Br J Ophthalmol* 62:503, 1978.

124. Wang S, Grayston J: Immunologic relationship between genital TRIC, lymphogranuloma venereum, and related organisms in a new microtiter indirect immunofluorescence test, *Am J Ophthalmol* 70:367, 1970.

125. Arffa RC, Kowalski RP, Springer DS: The value of serology in the diagnosis of adult chlamydial keratoconjunctivitis, *Ophthalmology* 95(suppl):145, 1988.

126. Tabrizi SN, Lees MI, Garland SM: Comparison of polymerase chain reaction and culture techniques for detection of *Chlamydia trachomatis,* *Mol Cell Probes* 7:357, 1993.

127. Talley AR et al: The use of polymerase chain reaction for the detection of chlamydial keratoconjunctivitis, *Am J Ophthalmol* 114:685, 1992.

128. Talley AR, Garcia-Ferrer F, Laycock KA et al: Comparative diagnosis of neonatal chlamydial conjunctivitis by polymerase chain reaction and McCoy cell culture, *Am J Ophthalmol* 117:50, 1994.

129. Martin DH et al: A controlled trial of a single dose of azithromycin for the treatment of chlamydial urethritis and cervicitis, *N Engl J Med* 327:921, 1992.

130. Marx R: Sociomedical aspects of trachoma, *Acta Ophthalmol (Copenh)* 66(suppl 183):1, 1988.

131. Taylor HR et al: Hygiene factors and increased risk of trachoma in central Tanzania, *Arch Ophthalmol* 107:1821, 1989.

132. West SK et al: Facial cleanliness and risk of trachoma in families, *Arch Ophthalmol* 109:855, 1991.

133. Brechner RJ, West S, Lynch M: Trachoma and flies: individual vs environmental risk factors, *Arch Ophthalmol* 110:687, 1992.

134. Whitcher JP: *Chlamydial keratitis and conjunctivitis: clinical disease.* In Smolin G, Thoft RA, editors: *The cornea: scientific foundations and clinical practice,* Boston, 1994, Little, Brown & Co.

135. Jones BR: The prevention of blindness from trachoma, *Trans Ophthalmol Soc UK* 95:19, 1975.

136. Taylor HR et al: An animal model of trachoma II: the importance of repeated infection, *Invest Ophthalmol Vis Sci* 23:507, 1982.

137. Grayston JT et al: Importance of reinfection in

the pathogenesis of trachoma, *Rev Infect Dis* 7:717, 1985.

138. MacCallan A: The epidemiology of trachoma, *Br J Ophthalmol* 15:369, 1931.

139. Dawson C, Jones B, Darougar S: Blinding and non-blinding trachoma: assessment of intensity of upper tarsal inflammatory disease and disabling lesions, *Bull World Health Organ* 52:279, 1975.

140. Darougar S, Jones BR: Trachoma, *Br Med Bull* 39:117, 1983.

141. Reacher MH et al: T cells and trachoma: their role in cicatricial disease, *Ophthalmology* 98:334, 1991.

142. Dawson CR, Jones BR, Tarizzo ML: *Guide to trachoma control,* Geneva, 1981, World Health Organization.

143. Tabbara KF, Babb AA: Lacrimal system complications in trachoma, *Ophthalmology* 87:298, 1980.

144. Taylor PB, Burd EM, Tabbara KF: Comparison of diagnostic laboratory techniques in the various stages of trachoma, *Ophthalmology* 94(suppl):123, 1987.

145. Bettman JW Jr et al: Inclusion conjunctivitis in American Indians of the Southwest, *Am J Ophthalmol* 70:363, 1970.

146. Rapoza PA et al: Direct immunofluorescence monoclonal antibody staining of conjunctival smears for trachoma. Paper presented at the annual meeting of the Ocular Microbiology and Immunology Group, Dallas, November, 1987.

147. Tabbara KF, Rahi A: Enzyme immunoassay in the detection of chlamydial antigens in patients with trachoma, *Ophthalmology* 94(suppl):123, 1987.

148. Bailey RL et al: Polymerase chain reaction for the detection of ocular chlamydial infection in trachoma-endemic communities, *J Infect Dis* 170:709, 1994.

149. Bobo L et al: Diagnosis of *Chlamydia trachomatis* eye infection in Tanzania by polymerase chain reaction/enzyme immunoassay, *Lancet* 338(8771):347, 1991.

150. Dawson CR et al: Intermittent trachoma chemotherapy: a controlled trial of topical tetracycline or erythromycin, *Bull World Health Organ* 59:91, 1981.

151. Dawson CR, Jones BR, Tarisso ML: *Guide to trachoma control.* In: *Programmes for the Prevention of Blindness,* Geneva, 1981, World Health Organization.

152. Bailey RL et al: Randomised controlled trial of single-dose azithromycin in treatment of trachoma, *Lancet* 342:453, 1993.

153. Dawson CR, Schachter J: Strategies for treatment and control of blinding trachoma: cost-effectiveness of topical or systemic antibiotics, *Rev Infect Dis* 7:768, 1985.

154. Ostler B, Schachter J, Dawson C: Acute follicular conjunctivitis of epizootic origin, *Arch Ophthalmol* 82:587, 1969.

155. Viswalingam ND, Wishart MS, Woodland RM: Adult chlamydial ophthalmia (paratrachoma), *Br Med Bull* 39:123, 1983.

156. Duke-Elder S, Leigh AG: *System of ophthalmology,* vol 8, *Diseases of the outer eye,* St Louis, 1965, Mosby–Year Book.

157. Buus DR et al: Lymphogranuloma venereum conjunctivitis with a marginal corneal perforation, *Ophthalmology* 95:792, 1988.

158. Meyer GP, Reber J: A case of corneal ulcer associated with lymphogranuloma venereum, *Am J Ophthalmol* 24:161, 1941.

159. Scheie HG, Crandall AS, Henle W: Keratitis associated with lymphogranuloma venereum, *JAMA* 135:333, 1947.

160. Endicott JN, Kirconnel WS, Beam D: Granuloma inguinale of the orbit with bony involvement, *Arch Otolaryngol* 96:457, 1972.

Eight

Noninfectious Causes of Conjunctival Inflammation

A number of noninfectious disorders can cause conjunctival inflammation, and these should be considered in the differential diagnosis, particularly in chronic or recurrent disease. A partial list is given in Table 8-1. Some specific entities are discussed below.

ALLERGIC CONJUNCTIVITIS

Each of the following diseases appears to be related, at least in part, to an immediate-type hypersensitivity reaction, which is also called an *anaphylactic reaction*. Antigen (allergen) reacts with IgE (or IgG) antibody bound to mast cells or circulating basophils, causing release of pharmacologic mediators. It is essential that two adjacent antibodies attached to the same mast cell bind an antigen. This results in the activation of serine esterase at the outer membrane, which in turn initiates a chain of reactions that results in an increase in the mast cells' permeability to calcium ions. The influx of calcium ions activates enzymes that release energy and cause fusion of intracellular granules with the cell membrane, releasing pharmacologic mediators. The mediators include histamine, serotonin, heparin, eosinophil chemotactic factors of anaphylaxis, leukotrienes (C, D, and E), prostaglandins, platelet-activating factor, bradykinin, lysosomal hydrolases, and pro-

Table 8-1	Noninfectious Causes of Conjunctival Inflammation and Injection

Atopic
  Allergic conjunctivitis
  Vernal catarrh
  Atopic keratoconjunctivitis
  Contact dermatoconjunctivitis

Other primary conjunctival diseases
  Superior limbic keratoconjunctivitis
  Masquerade syndrome (carcinoma)
  Floppy eyelid syndrome
  Lid imbrication
  Limbal dyskeratosis

Ocular disease
  Blepharitis
  Meibomitis
  Episcleritis*
  Scleritis*
  Intraocular inflammation*
  Angle-closure glaucoma*

Medications—toxic effects of many drugs, particularly:
  Gentamicin
  Idoxuridine
  Neomycin
  Preservatives

Dermatologic disorders (in part)
  Acne rosacea
  Psoriasis
  Atopic dermatitis
  Discoid lupus erythematosus
  Cicatricial pemphigoid
  Erythema multiforme
  Other mucous membrane diseases

Other systemic diseases
  Gout* (see Fig. 21-35)
  Thyroid disease*
  Kawasaki disease
  Scleroderma
  Dermatomyositis
  Polyarteritis nodosa*
  Relapsing polychondritis*
  Reiter's syndrome
  Behçet's disease
  Toxic shock syndrome*
  Ataxia telangiectasia*
  Paget's disease*
  Arteriovenous fistulae (Fig. 8-1)*
  Blood dyscrasis: polycythemia, leukemia, multiple myeloma, dysproteinemia*

Environmental and irritative
  Ultraviolet radiation
  Therapeutic radiation
  Foreign particles (e.g., fiberglass)
  Ophthalmia nodosa (caterpillar hairs)
  Burdock (thistle)
  Diffenbachia plant

*These conditions cause conjunctival hypermia but not conjunctival inflammation.

teases. These mediators cause increased vascular permeability, mucosal edema, mucus secretion, and chemotaxis.

The levels of intracellular cyclic adenosine monophosphate (cAMP) and cyclic guanine monophosphate (cGMP) influence the release of these mediators from the mast cells and basophils. Elevation of intracellular cAMP inhibits the release of mediators, whereas elevation of cGMP enhances their release. Prostaglandins E_1 and E_2 and stimulation of β_2-adrenergic receptors (e.g., with epinephrine or norepinephrine) increase the level of cAMP, while stimulation of α_2-adrenergic receptors (e.g., with phenylephrine) reduces the cAMP level. Stimulation of cholinergic receptors (e.g., by acetylcholine or carbachol), serotonin, and ascorbate leads to increased intracellular levels of cGMP. Phosphodiesterase inhibitors (e.g., aminophylline and caffeine) decrease the breakdown of cAMP. Allergy symptoms can be alleviated by drugs that increase the level of cAMP or decrease the level of cGMP. The mechanism of action of disodium chromoglycate, lodoxamide, and other "mast cell stabilizers" is unclear. They may prevent calcium influx.

Patients with allergic conjunctivitis have elevated levels of IgE in their tears and serum. Tear IgE and IgG specific to inciting allergens are produced in the eye.[1,2]

The diagnosis can be inferred from a history of atopy, development of reactions after contact with an allergen, and itching. Further evidence can be obtained by observation of eosinophils in conjunctival scrapings, conjunctival challenge with dilute preparation of an allergen,[3-5] measurement of tear IgE levels,[6] reaction to intradermal challenge with the allergen, or detection of specific IgE in serum (radioallergosorbent technique [RAST] or enzyme-linked immunoadsorbent assay [ELISA]).

A number of conditions are considered atopic: asthma, allergic rhinitis and conjunctivitis, urticaria, and atopic dermatitis. They tend to occur together in the same family and in the same individual. The tendency toward atopy is inherited, probably on a multifactorial basis. Between 10% and 20% of the population are affected by atopy.

Conjunctivitis Due to Airborne Allergens

This common condition results from a type I immediate hypersensitivity reaction to an airborne allergen. The most common allergen is ragweed (hay fever), but a wide variety of antigens can be responsible, including other plant pollens, dust, animal danders, and mold spores. Shortly after exposure, the patient develops

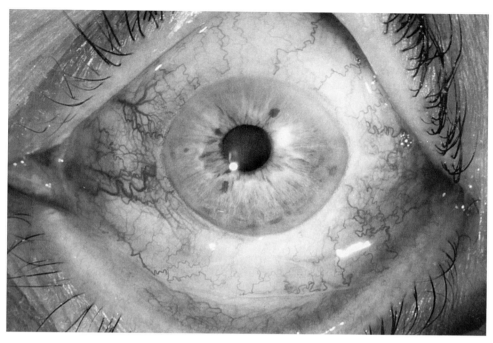

Figure 8-1
Conjunctival injection (due to increased venous pressure) and chemosis associated with a dural-cavernous fistula. (Courtesy of Diane Curtin, Pittsburgh, PA.)

itching, burning, and tearing. Rhinitis or sinusitis is commonly present. Many of these patients manifest other forms of immediate hypersensitivity, such as asthma, atopic dermatitis, food and drug allergies, and urticaria-angioedema. The symptoms are often seasonal, related to the amount of allergen present in the air. The peak months for grass pollen allergy are May and June, whereas ragweed pollen allergy peaks in late summer and early autumn.

Signs include conjunctival hyperemia, edema, and chemosis (Fig. 8-2), a mild papillary response, lid edema, and mucoid discharge. The edema can give the conjunctiva a milky appearance. Mild lid and periorbital edema can be seen. Venous dilation can cause the lower lids to appear darker than normal. The conjunctivitis is usually bilateral and symmetric.

The diagnosis can usually be made on the basis of history and examination. Conjunctival scrapings often demonstrate eosinophils; however, their absence does not exclude the diagnosis.[7,8] Tear IgE levels can be measured and may be helpful in diagnosis and in monitoring response to treatment.[9] A rapid response to appropriate therapy, such as antihistamines or corticosteroids, is also suggestive. Some special tests are particularly useful for identifying the specific allergen(s): intradermal skin testing and

identification of specific serum IgE (RAST, ELISA). A diluted preparation of an allergen can be instilled in the conjunctival sac and the reaction observed, although this method is seldom practical.[10-12]

Treatment

Exposure to the allergen(s) should be reduced as much as possible. Cool compresses and topical vasoconstrictors, such as naphazoline or tetrahydrozoline up to five times daily, provide some symptomatic relief. However, tolerance may develop and rebound exacerbation of symptoms may occur after discontinuing vasoconstrictors. They can also cause severe hypertensive crises in patients on monoamine oxidase inhibitors.

Oral and topical antihistamines are often useful. Most topical antihistamines are commercially available only in combination with a vasoconstrictor. In one study the combination of a vasoconstrictor and a topical antihistamine (antazoline) was superior to either treatment alone.[13] A new long-acting H_1 antihistamine, levocabastine 0.05%, was recently approved for topical ophthalmic use and has been demonstrated to be effective in relieving the symptoms of allergic conjunctivitis.[14-18] In one study it was significantly more effective than 4% cro-

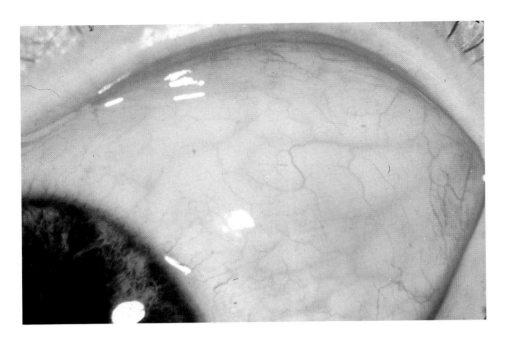

Figure 8-2
Hay fever reaction in conjunctiva with large conjunctival wheal.

molyn in inhibiting allergic conjunctivitis after administration of a topical allergen.[19] The recommended dose is four times daily.

The mast cell stabilizers disodium cromoglycate (cromolyn sodium) 4% (Crolom; Bausch & Lomb Pharmaceuticals, Tampa, FL)[20,21] and lodoxamide 0.1% (Alomide; Alcon Laboratories, Fort Worth, TX) can be effective in patients with chronic disease. These are given four times daily, and their effect is not evident until 2 to 3 weeks of treatment.

Topical corticosteroids are very effective in relieving symptoms, but the risks of chronic treatment usually outweigh the benefits. Desensitizing immunotherapy may be a useful approach to patients with severe disease, particularly if it is accompanied by rhinitis or sinusitis. Desensitizing immunotherapy involves repeated injections or oral doses of allergen extracts in slowly increasing amounts. Its mechanism of action is uncertain, but it is associated with increased blocking IgG antibody titers, generation of specific suppressor T cells, and nonspecific target cell desensitization.[22] Oral immunotherapy was reported to be effective in alleviating the symptoms of hay fever conjunctivitis.[23]

Vernal Keratoconjunctivitis

Vernal keratoconjunctivitis (VKC) is a bilateral, seasonal inflammation caused by allergy that is usually seen in young patients.[24,25-27] It occurs most often between 6 years of age and puberty.[28] Before puberty boys are affected two to three times as often as girls, but because the prevalence in girls rises after puberty, by the age of 20 the sexes are affected almost equally. The disease usually diminishes in severity during the teen years and disappears in the early twenties, but it can persist for decades in some individuals.

Vernal keratoconjunctivitis affects all races and occurs in all parts of the world. The limbal form appears to be more common in blacks and American Indians. The disease is more common in dry, warm climates, such as the Middle East, the Mediterranean basin, and Central America. In more temperate climates, VKC tends to be seasonal, occurring with the onset of spring and decreasing in the fall. During the colder months the symptoms decrease, but the conjunctival changes usually persist with only slight regression. The signs of the limbal form of the disease are more likely to regress, and in mild cases they can resolve completely. In tropical climates the seasonal variation is often less marked.

Clinical Manifestations

Itching, the most outstanding symptom of VKC, is usually the earliest symptom and may precede all conjunctival signs of disease. Photo-

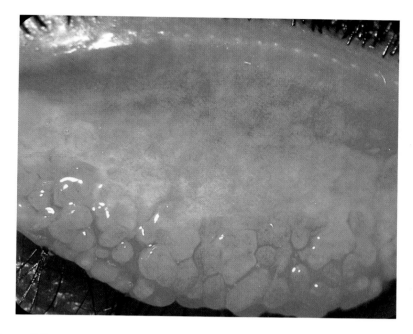

Figure 8-3
Giant papillary hypertrophy (cobblestone appearance) of upper tarsal conjunctiva.

phobia is also often prominent, and the child responds by continually keeping his or her face turned toward the ground. Other symptoms include burning, lacrimation, and foreign body sensation. These symptoms are often associated with a thick, sticky, mucoid discharge.

The earliest sign of VKC may be a simple hyperemia, which is quickly followed by a more marked response characterized by conjunctival thickening or hyperplasia. Hyperplasia can be most prominent either in the superior tarsal conjunctiva (palpebral form) or around the limbus (limbal form). In the palpebral form, the tarsal conjunctiva initially appears dull and pale and may have a milky-blue hue. Later, papillae are the most prominent finding. They can be small and few in number early; but with progression they become larger, more elevated, polygonal, and flat-topped (Fig. 8-3). When they are numerous and tightly packed, the tarsal conjunctiva can have the classic cobblestone appearance. The weight of the papillae can cause a mechanical ptosis. The lower tarsal conjunctiva can also demonstrate papillary hypertrophy, but it is less severely affected, and giant papillae are rarely seen. (Giant papillae are more often seen in this location in atopic keratoconjunctivitis [AKC]).

Limbal involvement appears as semitransparent, smooth, gelatinous elevations (Fig. 8-4), which may be broad and uniform or may form distinct nodules. Their corneal edges are sharp, but they blend gradually into the conjunctiva. They can involve any portion of the limbus or its entire circumference; some authors say that the interpalpebral limbus is most commonly affected, whereas others implicate the superior limbus. The limbal elevations can extend onto the peripheral cornea, often leaving focal areas of opacity and micropannus after their regression. Small epithelial cysts and marginal pits can occur. The pits are translucent, round, nondepressed areas within the opaque limbus and represent localized resolution of limbal infiltration.

Small, flat or mildly elevated, grayish-white to yellow dots, called *Trantas' dots,* can be present on the limbal elevations (Fig. 8-5). These structures are usually seen only at the upper limbus, but they can appear on the bulbar conjunctiva, semilunar folds, and very rarely on the tarsal conjunctiva or cornea. The dots consist of degenerating eosinophils and epithelial cells. They are transient, usually not lasting longer than a week. The dots may be seen in the deep layers of the epithelium; however, they gradually become more superficial and break through to the surface. (Trantas' dots also can occur in chronic AKC and with soft contact lens wear.)

Corneal involvement in VKC can take several forms. As mentioned previously, a micro-

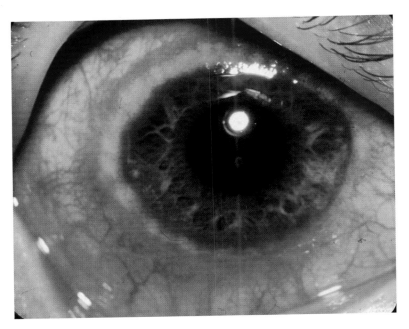

Figure 8-4
Limbal vernal catarrh exhibiting gelatinous elevations.

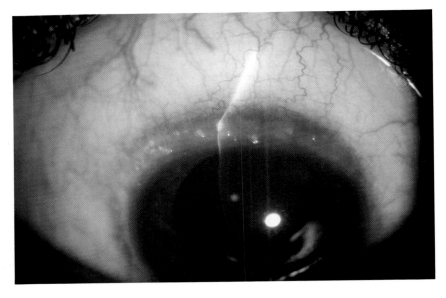

Figure 8-5
Gelatinous superior limbal elevations, with overlying fine white plaques (Trantas' dots) in limbal vernal.

pannus can occur. Another form is a farina-ceous epitheliopathy (keratitis epithelialis ver-nalis of Tobgy), which consists of tiny, gray-white, intraepithelial corneal opacities, like a dusting of flour.[29,30] The opacities are most prominent in the superior cornea, with relative sparing of the periphery, and they stain with fluorescein and rose bengal red. A more intense form of farinaceous keratitis can occur, produc-ing the appearance of a cobweb or syncytium (Fig. 8-6). This form is more common in pa-tients with palpebral vernal keratitis and tends to be transient, lasting days to weeks.

Characteristic corneal ulcers also can occur (in about 3% to 4% of patients).[25] These are horizontally oval or shield-shaped and are usu-

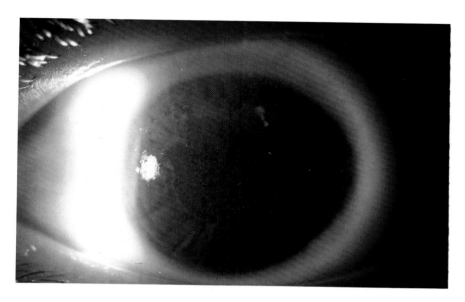

Figure 8-6
Farinaceous epithelial keratopathy in vernal keratoconjunctivitis.

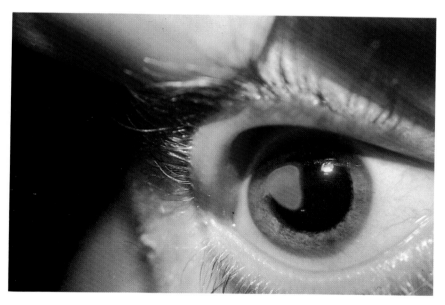

Figure 8-7
Shieldlike ulcer of cornea occasionally seen in vernal catarrh. (From Grayson M, Keates RH: *Manual of diseases of the cornea,* Boston, 1969, Little, Brown & Co.)

ally located in the superior half of the cornea (Fig. 8-7), but inferior ulcers can also be seen.[31,32] These ulcers are shallow and have thickened opaque edges. The base can be transparent or gray, or yellow inflammatory deposits can be present. The deposits can be elevated above the level of the surrounding epithelium. They often heal slowly but do not vascularize.

As they heal a gray plaque can form in the bed, which gradually shrinks, leaving an oval or ring opacity in the superficial stroma. Bacterial infection or sterile ulceration and perforation can occur before healing is completed.[27,32]

Shield ulcers are most common in very young patients, particularly those with large papillae. The ulcers and the other epithelial findings may result from mechanical irritation of the corneal surface by the abnormal palpebral conjunctiva[30] or the toxicity of the inflammatory mediators.[33]

Less often, a deep, fascicular keratitis can be seen. An arc-like or annular opacity can be seen in the peripheral stroma, separated by a clear zone from the limbus (vernal pseudogerontoxon). There appears to be a higher incidence of keratoconus in patients with VKC,[34] although the reason for this relationship is not clear. Corneal involvement appears to be less common in patients with purely limbal VKC.[35]

The most characteristic feature of conjunctival scrapings in VKC is the presence of eosinophils and free eosinophilic granules. In addition, fibrin, mucus, epithelial cells, polymorphonuclear leukocytes, and basophils may be present.

Vernal keratoconjunctivitis generally abates in the teens and disappears in the twenties. Eventually there is complete resolution of all conjunctival signs; there is no residual scarring unless it has been inappropriately treated by radiation or surgery. The corneal involvement usually does not result in changes that reduce vision; however, myopic astigmatism or keratoconus may require optical correction. Excessive steroid treatment can lead to cataract formation or secondary infection.

Histopathology
In early VKC new vessels and cellular infiltration are seen in the conjunctival substantia propria (see Fig. 3-6). Large numbers of eosinophils are accompanied by polymorphonuclear leukocytes, basophils, and mast cells and in later stages by lymphocytes and macrophages.[24,36-38] An increased amount of connective tissue is seen in the substantia propria; it becomes hyalinized and forms the fibrous core of the papillae. The overlying conjunctival epithelium becomes thickened, increasing from the normal two layers to 5 to 10 layers of irregular, edematous cells. Mast cells, eosinophils, and basophils also are present in the epithelium. In advanced cases the epithelium atrophies to one cell layer and can become keratinized.

Eosinophil granule major basic protein was identified in the beds of corneal ulcers associated with VKC.[39] Eosinophil granule major basic protein can inhibit epithelial migration and protein synthesis.

Pathogenesis
Strong evidence suggests a role for type I hypersensitivity, but type IV hypersensitivity may also be involved. Evidence for the role of type I hypersensitivity includes a frequent personal or family history of allergies and other forms of atopy; a high concentration of eosinophils and mast cells in the conjunctiva; a relatively high incidence of systemic eosinophilia[40]; elevated tear IgE and IgG antibodies, including specific antibodies to allergens such as grass and ragweed[27,41-44]; elevated tear histamine[45] and complement[46]; and response to agents that inhibit mast cell degranulation. In patients with specific IgE antibodies against house dust mites, symptoms of VKC correlated well with the quantity of dust mites in their homes.[47]

Several other findings, however, are not explained by this mechanism. Some patients do not have elevated tear IgE[30,35] (although at least some of these patients have elevated IgG$_4$ antibody, which may also participate in type I reactions). There is proliferation of connective tissue and mixed cellular infiltrate. Occasionally there is no association with other atopic diseases, and high numbers of basophils are present in the conjunctiva. The latter situation suggests that cutaneous basophil hypersensitivity, a type IV reaction, may play a role.[48,49]

Differential Diagnosis
The keratoconjunctivitis associated with atopic dermatitis, atopic keratoconjunctivitis (AKC), can be confused with VKC (Table 8-2). Both occur in atopic individuals, are associated with itching, and may be exacerbated by warm weather. Patients with VKC may have atopic dermatitis, and certainly both VKC and AKC can occur simultaneously. The papillae associated with AKC are usually small and involve the lower tarsal conjunctiva. The discharge is meager and watery, and there are few eosinophils and minimal or no free eosinophilic granules in scrapings. Conjunctival scarring and shrinkage of the inferior fornix are common in AKC but do not occur in VKC.

Trachoma should also be considered in the differential diagnosis. Trachoma produces round, translucent limbal follicles of uniform size; however, they may be accompanied by true pits (Herbert's pits), tarsal follicles, or conjunctival scarring. Conjunctival scrapings in trachoma may contain polymorphonuclear cells, plasma cells, lymphocytes, Leber cells, and epithelial inclusions, but no eosinophils.

Treatment
Fortunately, VKC is self-limiting and only rarely causes a permanent decrease in vision. Nevertheless, it can be quite disabling. The objective of treatment is to reduce symptoms to permit

Table 8-2	Diseases of Immediate-Type Hypersensitivity			
	Allergic Conjunctivitis (Hay Fever)	Vernal Kerato-conjunctivitis	Atopic Kerato-conjunctivitis	Giant Papillary Conjunctivitis
Hypersensitivity type	I	I, ?IV	I, ?IV	?I, IV
Conjunctiva				
Scarring	–	–	Inferior fornix and papillae	–
Chemosis	+	+	+ (acute)	–
Papillae	Mild diffuse	Medium-giant upper lid	Usually small lower lid	Medium-giant upper lid
Limbus	Normal	Gelatinous elevations Trantas' dots Cysts Marginal pits Pseudogerontoxon	Gelatinous elevations Trantas' dots Cysts	Contact lens–induced keratoconjunctivitis Superior injection Gelatinous elevations Trantas' dots
Cornea		Micropannus Epitheliopathy "Shield" ulcer	Punctate keratitis Vascularization Opacification Marginal ulceration	Micropannus Superior keratopathy Filaments
Conjunctival scrapings	Eosinophils	Eosinophils Free eosinophilic granules Basophils	Eosinophils Basophils	Eosinophils

the child to function as normally as possible, while avoiding iatrogenic complications.

A number of general measures can improve symptoms and may be sufficient in mild cases. Moving to a cooler climate is the most effective form of management, but it clearly is not often practical. Attempts should be made to identify and limit exposure to allergens. Air-conditioning is helpful because it decreases room temperature and filters out airborne allergens. Cool compresses, irrigation with cold saline, and patching provide immediate but transient relief. Densensitization has not proved beneficial.

Topical vasoconstrictors, such as naphazoline, can be applied up to four times daily and are helpful in some cases. A mucolytic agent (e.g., acetylcysteine 10% four times daily) is often beneficial when mucous discharge is prominent. Systemic and topical antihistamines are not useful.

If these measures are not sufficient, a mast cell stabilizer such as cromolyn sodium 4% (Crolom)[50-54] or lodoxamide 0.1%[55,56] (Alomide)

is given four times daily. These agents are beneficial in most cases, but 2 to 3 weeks of treatment may be necessary before their effect is evident. Patients with a history of atopic disease have a greater response. The mast cell stabilizers must be used continuously, at least during the appropriate seasons; they are not effective when applied only during exacerbations. If the eye solution is not available, the 4% nasal solution of cromolyn sodium (Nasalcrom; Fisons Corporation, Rochester, NY) can be used as an eyedrop.[57]

Topical corticosteroids can provide dramatic relief, but because of the chronic nature of the disease and the risks of prolonged steroid use, steroid treatment is kept to a minimum. In most cases intermittent pulse therapy is sufficient. During severe exacerbations, prednisolone acetate 1% or dexamethasone phosphate 0.1% is given every 2 hours during the day, for 4 days, and then tapered over 1 to 2 weeks. This regimen may need to be repeated three to four times per year. If necessary, oral steroids can also be given in a 1- to 2-week pulse. In the

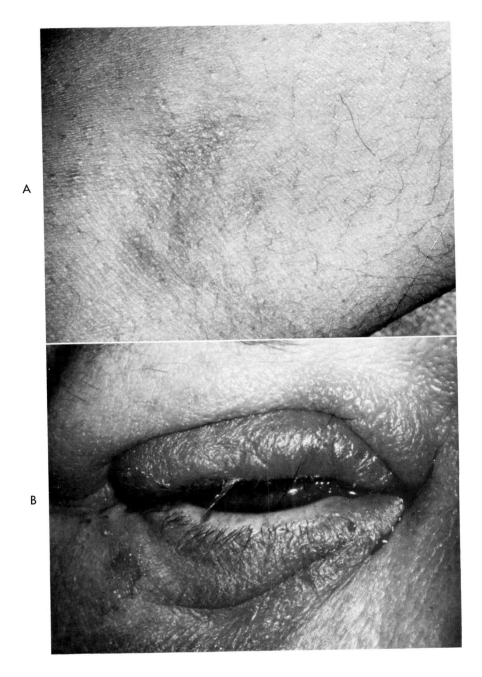

Figure 8-8
A, Antecubital skin lesions in atopic dermatitis. Skin in eczema can be weeping and crusting or dry and lichenified. **B,** Eyelids may be thick and lichenified in atopic dermatitis with keratoconjunctivitis.

most persistent cases, daily doses of dilute steroid may be necessary. Topical cyclosporine 2% has been reported to improve signs and symptoms during use, but further evaluation is required.[58,59] Cryotherapy of the superior tarsal conjunctiva can provide short-term relief, possibly by degranulating large numbers of mast cells.[60] Superior tarsal excision and replacement with mucous membrane was helpful in some severe cases, but large papillae sometimes formed at the superior edge of the graft.[61]

Corneal ulcers are treated by optimizing medical therapy of the VKC, with a mast cell stabilizing drug given four times daily and topi-

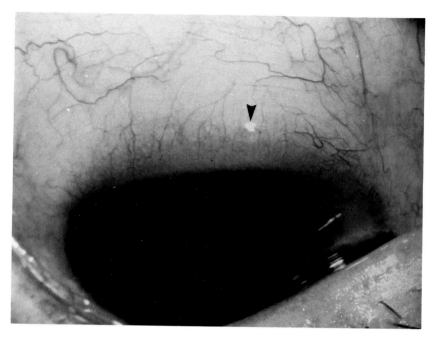

Figure 8-9
Limbal bleb may be seen in atopic conjunctival keratitis (*arrow*).

cal corticosteroid drops every 2 hours while the patient is awake. A broad-spectrum topical antibiotic drop can be used to help prevent infection. If the patient is cooperative, inflammatory deposits should be scraped from the bed of the ulcer. If there is no significant epithelialization in 1 week, a bandage contact lens can be placed. If inflammatory deposits are present and the epithelium is not healing, the deposits should be removed.[32] It may be necessary to perform this procedure in the operating room, particularly in young children.

Atopic Dermatitis with Keratoconjunctivitis

Atopic dermatitis is an inflammatory skin disease usually found in patients with other forms of atopy. It appears to have a genetic basis, probably via multifactorial inheritance. Atopic dermatitis also can be seen in some immuno-deficiency disorders, such as Wiskott-Aldrich syndrome and ataxia-telangiectasia.

Clinical Manifestations

Atopic dermatitis can begin at any age, but onset during infancy is most common. The duration and severity are quite variable; after infantile onset it can resolve by 2 years of age or can persist into adulthood. The skin lesions are dry, erythematous, vesicular, and pruritic. Scratching leads to excoriations, weeping, scal-ing, and crusting. In infants the forehead, cheeks, and extensor surfaces of the extremities are most involved, and in older patients the antecubital and popliteal areas, neck, wrists, and ankles are more likely to be affected (Fig. 8-8A). The face and eyelids are often affected in the more severe cases. The lids can become thickened, indurated, and lichenified (Fig. 8-8B). Weeping fissures often occur at the lateral canthi, and punctal eversion or stenosis can occur. Staphylococcal superinfections are common.[62]

Conjunctival involvement occurred in 16% of patients in one series from the Mayo Clinic.[63] The conjunctival inflammation is accompanied by itching, burning, tearing, photophobia, and mucoid discharge. The disease usually affects both eyes. Seasonal exacerbations and precipitation of symptoms by antigens, such as animal dander, dust, and certain foods, can occur in some patients.[64] The conjunctiva often appears hyperemic and chemotic during active disease. In chronic cases it is pale and congested, with a papillary response. Medium or giant papillae can be present, usually inferiorly; the upper tarsal conjunctiva often appears milky, without formation of large papillae. Gelatinous elevations, thick broad opacifications (usually superior), epithelial cysts (Fig. 8-9), and Trantas' dots can be seen at the limbus. Scarring can occur and tends to be focal and develop in the

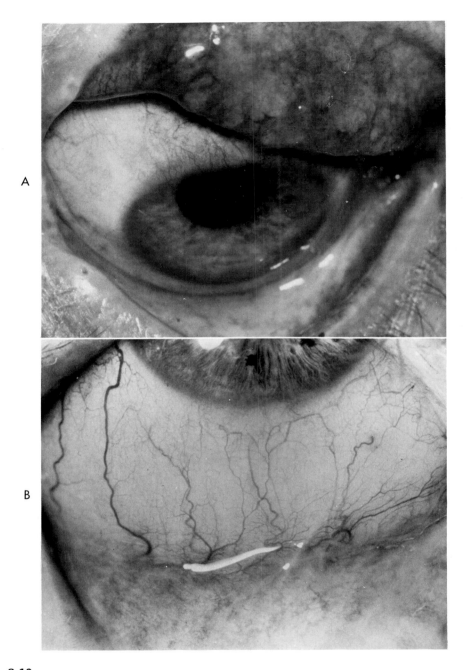

Figure 8-10
A, Papillary hypertrophy of conjunctiva in case of atopic keratoconjunctivitis. **B,** Atopic keratoconjunctivitis with cicatrization of cul-de-sac.

centers of the papillae (Fig. 8-10*A*) and in the inferior fornix (Fig. 8-10*B*). It can be severe enough to cause symblepharon, entropion, and trichiasis.

The most common corneal finding is punctate keratitis, which is most prominent inferiorly. Marginal ulceration, vascularization, and stromal opacification can occur (Fig. 8-11). In one series subepithelial fibrosis was present in 58% of patients and corneal neovascularization in 38%.[65] Secondary infection with bacteria or herpes simplex[64,66] (Fig. 8-12) is common. Keratoconus is also more common in these patients.[64,66,67]

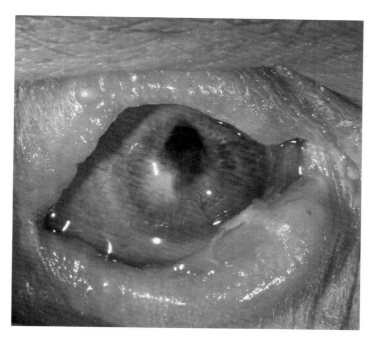

Figure 8-11
Extensive corneal thinning, scarring, and vascularization in atopic keratoconjunctivitis.

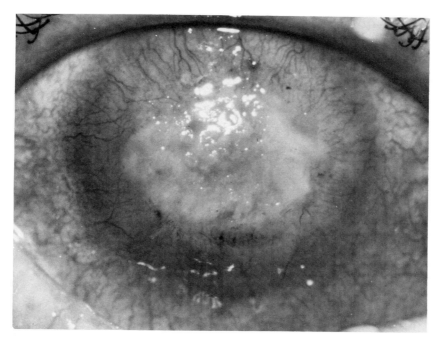

Figure 8-12
Herpes simplex infection of cornea in patient with atopic dermatoconjunctivitis.

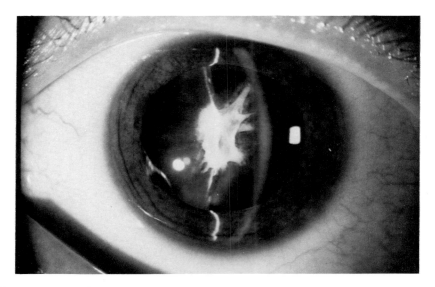

Figure 8-13
Anterior subcapsular cataract of atopic keratoconjunctivitis. (From Wiley L, Arffa R, Fireman P: *Allergic and immunologic ocular diseases.* In Fireman P, Slavin R, editors: *Atlas of allergic and immunologic diseases,* New York, 1991, Gower.)

Anterior and posterior subcapsular cataracts (Fig. 8-13) occur in approximately 8% of patients.[64,67-69] The opacities usually begin between 16 and 18 years of age and can progress rapidly.

Histopathology
The conjunctivae of patients with AKC have increased numbers of B cells, macrophages, Langerhans cells, and activated T cells and lower numbers of suppressor T cells.[70] Mast cell density is increased.[71]

Pathogenesis
The pathogenesis is unknown, but patients have evidence of both immediate-type hypersensitivity and abnormal cell-mediated immunity. The role of immediate-type hypersensitivity is suggested by a frequent family history of atopy, a high incidence of positive immediate skin test reactions, elevated serum levels in more than 80% of patients, elevated tear IgE levels,[64,65] and frequent eosinophilia.[72] However, there is little correlation between allergic disease or serum IgE and clinical findings.

Impaired cell-mediated immunity is suggested by the increased susceptibility of these patients to skin infections by viruses, bacteria, and fungi and decreased delayed-type skin test reactivity.[54,73] The number of circulating T cells, particularly suppressor T cells, is decreased in patients with active disease,[74] and in vitro studies have demonstrated decreased suppression of IgE synthesis by T cells from patients with atopic dermatitis.[75] Therefore, an impairment of suppressor T-cell function may lead to the elevation of IgE production.

Treatment
The treatment of AKC is similar to that of VKC, but patients with AKC can develop scarring and are more susceptible to superinfection, particularly with herpes simplex, and cataract formation. Symptomatic treatment with cool compresses, topical vasoconstrictors, and antihistamines may be helpful. A mast cell stabilizer (cromolyn sodium 4% or lodoxamide 0.1% four times daily) is often effective in severe cases.[76-78]

Topical corticosteroids are very effective for decreasing inflammation and relieving symptoms, but their use increases the risk of superinfection and cataract. They are certainly indicated when inflammation is producing ectropion, symblepharon, or corneal scarring, but even in these cases the lowest possible dose should be used for the shortest possible time. Systemic corticosteroids may be necessary in some cases but are particularly dangerous in these patients with defective cell-mediated immunity and a high incidence of fungal, staphylococcal, and herpetic infections.

Some patients with atopic dermatitis have the hyper-IgE syndrome. This syndrome includes chronic atopic dermatitis, recurrent pyogenic skin and lung infection, markedly elevated serum IgE, and sometimes defective neutrophil chemotaxis. In some of these patients eye disease was markedly improved by plasmapheresis.[79]

GIANT PAPILLARY CONJUNCTIVITIS

Giant papillary conjunctivitis (GPC), a condition initially described in contact lens wearers, is characterized by increased mucus, mild itching, and the development of giant papillae in the upper tarsal conjunctiva.[80,81] A spectrum of clinical findings is associated with this disease; giant papillae are present only in the more advanced cases. Identical findings can be found in association with ocular prostheses,[82,83] corneal shells, exposed nylon sutures,[84,85] cyanoacrylate glue,[86] extruded scleral buckles,[87] filtering blebs,[88] and elevated calcific plaques.

Clinical Manifestations

The earliest symptoms of GPC associated with contact lens wear are itching after removal of the lens and mild mucoid discharge, which is most evident the following morning. With progression, itching and then pain occur while the lens is in the eye. Mucous discharge increases, and this can coat the lens rapidly after insertion and decrease vision or cause the lids to stick together in the morning. The conjunctival findings often lag behind the symptoms.[89]

Enlarged papillae (>0.3 mm) develop on the upper tarsal surface, and the conjunctiva loses its transparency (Fig. 8-14). In soft contact lens wearers, the papillae tend to affect the middle and superior portions of the tarsus most. They gradually enlarge (to >1 mm) and can become flat-topped and densely packed, creating a cobblestone appearance. It may be easier to visualize the papillae with fluorescein instillation. In hard contact lens wearers, the papillae tend to be smaller, more widely separated, and concentrated in the middle or inferior tarsal conjunctiva.

Fluorescein staining of the tops of the papillae can be seen and is a sign of disease activity.[90] Coating of the contact lens surface is often noted and can become quite heavy. Mucous globs or strands may be found on the conjunctival surface or at the canthi. Advanced cases are characterized by gelatinous limbal nodules and Trantas' dots.[91]

Histopathology

Histopathologically, GPC appears similar to VKC, except that there are fewer eosinophils and basophils in GPC.[81] The papillae represent thickened substantia propria, filled with a normal density of lymphocytes and plasma cells. The overlying epithelium is thickened and irregular. In addition, mast cells are often found in the epithelium, and eosinophils or basophils can be present in the epithelium or the substantia propria. Patients with GPC were found to have meibomian gland dropout, and the meibomian gland excreta had greater viscosity than in contact lens wearers without GPC.[92]

Pathogenesis

That this condition can result from chronic trauma by prostheses, sutures, or scleral buckles indicates that trauma alone can be a sufficient stimulus. However, most contact lens wearers do not develop GPC, suggesting that some additional mechanism is usually involved. The lens coating appears to play a role: Increased coatings on lenses exacerbate GPC,[89] and when lenses from patients with GPC were placed in eyes of monkeys they induced a GPC-like reaction, whereas virgin lenses did not.[93]

Elevated levels of IgG, IgE, IgM, C3, and neutrophil chemotactic factor have been found in the tears of patients with GPC.[94-96] Neutrophil chemotactic factor is produced by injured conjunctival epithelial cells and can cause an inflammatory reaction similar to GPC.[96] Many authors have concluded that there is a humeral or cell-mediated immunologic reaction to antigens present on the lens, and that trauma may facilitate the exposure of the conjunctival lymphoid system to the antigens. To date, however, specific sensitivity to any of the antigens on these lenses has not been demonstrated.

Treatment

Although cessation of exposure to the foreign body is the most effective treatment, patients are often unwilling to discontinue contact lens wear. In these cases it is frequently possible to continue contact lens wear if certain measures are taken. First, lens wear should be discontinued until the eye is quiet; symptoms such as hyperemia and discharge should resolve, but conjunctival papillae resolve very slowly or not at all. Mild topical steroids can be given to speed this process. If the patient was wearing a hydrogel lens, switching to a gas-permeable lens often increases lens tolerance. However, continued hydrogel lens wear is sometimes achieved through the following steps:

1. Reduce lens coatings as much as possible through good lens hygiene, regular enzymatic cleaning (weekly or biweekly), and frequent replacement of lenses (including disposable lenses).
2. Avoid the use of sensitizing chemicals (e.g., thimerosal).
3. Switch to a smaller-diameter, thinner-edged lens.
4. Use cromolyn sodium 4% or lodoxamide 0.1% four times daily to reduce or prevent exacerbation of the disease.[97] (The package inserts state that these medications should not be given while the lens is in the eye,

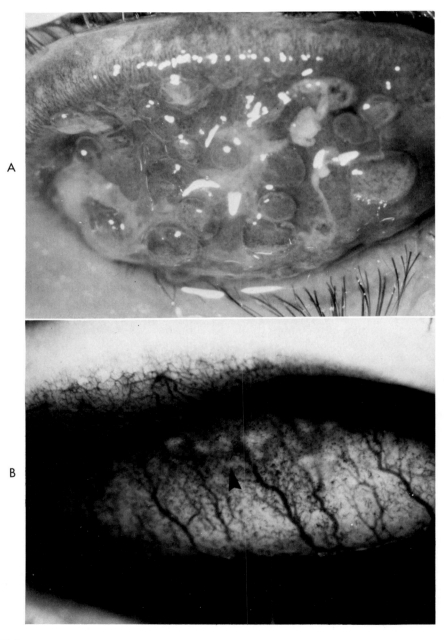

Figure 8-14
A, Giant papillary reaction of upper tarsal plate in soft contact lens wearer. **B,** Milder reaction in wearer of soft contact lens (*arrow*).

but I am not aware of any ill effects from this practice.)

FLOPPY EYELID SYNDROME

Floppy eyelid syndrome, which is a noninfectious cause of chronic conjunctivitis, is characterized by the presence of a lax, easily everted upper lid. The syndrome was first described by Culbertson and Ostler in 1981,[98] and many other cases have been described since,[99-106] indicating that this is a relatively common disorder. It is more common in men, but also affects women and children.[107]

Clinical Manifestations

Patients complain of redness, irritation, foreign body sensation, and mucoid discharge. The symptoms usually are worse in the morning and improve over the course of the day. Intermittent blurring of vision and mild itching may also be present.

One or both eyes can be affected, and this appears to relate to which side the patient sleeps on; if he or she consistently sleeps on one side, the ipsilateral eye is the one affected; otherwise both lids are affected. Many patients with this disorder are obese, but obesity is not necessarily present.

On examination, the most prominent feature is laxity of the upper lid, which must be tested for to be appreciated. By pulling the lid skin upward, the lid everts (Fig. 8-15). Spontaneous eversion can also occur by squeezing the lids closed (Fig. 8-16). When pulling upward on the lashes, as in standard lid eversion, the lid rolls upward, with no resistance from the tarsus. The tarsus feels soft and rubbery and is easily folded.

A papillary response is evident in the superior tarsal conjunctiva, and mucus strands can be seen. A coarse punctate keratopathy, which can be diffuse or primarily superior, superior corneal pannus,[98,104] filaments,[104] and mild ptosis may also be present. Schirmer's test has indicated decreased tear flow in some patients.

Punctate epithelial keratopathy and keratoconus are commonly associated with floppy eyelid syndrome.[99,108] In one review, they were found in 45% and 10% of cases, respectively.[106] Bilateral corneal neovascularization was observed in one case.[109]

Associated Findings

Scrapings have yielded primarily polymorphonuclear leukocytes with some lymphocytes. In rare cases eosinophils also are present.[100] Histologic specimens of the superior tarsus show a dense chronic inflammatory infiltrate in the substantia propria, with a normal-appearing tarsus.[98,100,102,103] Immunohistochemical analysis demonstrated markedly reduced tarsal elastin in four patients.[110] Occasionally keratinization of the surface epithelium[1] and subepithelial scarring[3] are present.

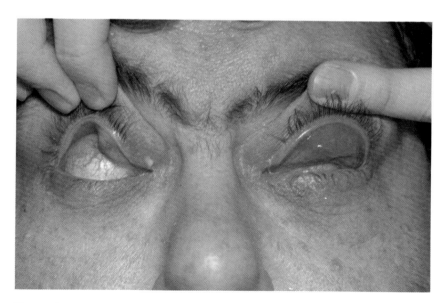

Figure 8-15
Eversion of the upper lids with superior traction in floppy eyelid syndrome.

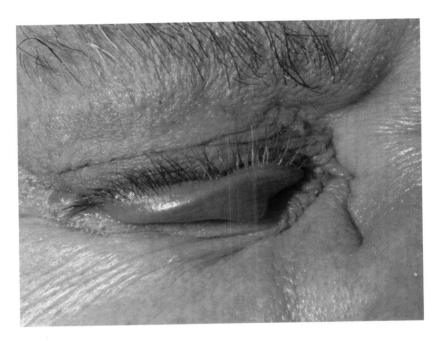

Figure 8-16
Spontaneous eversion of upper lid with forced closure in floppy eyelid syndrome.

Floppy eyelid syndrome has been noted in association with several diseases, including sleep apnea,[40,111] hyperglycinemia,[101] blepharochalasis,[103] and keratotorus,[105] but in none is there a clear relationship.

Etiology

The cause of floppy eyelid syndrome is unknown, except that it is often related to obesity. However, no endocrinologic abnormalities have been identified in these patients.[98,99] Culbertson and Ostler[98] proposed that lid eversion occurred during sleep, resulting in contact of the upper lid and cornea with the pillow, and this has been reported by some of the patients' spouses. Although this may often be the case, the underlying cause for the laxity of the upper lids is unknown.

Treatment

Treatment is aimed at eliminating lid eversion or contact with bedclothes. The simplest methods are taping the lids shut at night and using an eye shield. These measures provide at least temporary relief in most patients and can be used to confirm the diagnosis. Permanent relief can be obtained with horizontal lid shortening procedures.[101,102,104] Lubricants, cromolyn sodium, and contact lenses have not been found to be very useful.

LID IMBRICATION SYNDROME

Chronic overriding or imbrication of a lax upper lid on the lower lid can cause conjunctival inflammation. The lower lid lashes rub the tarsal surface of the upper lid, causing papillary conjunctivitis and occasionally tarsal ulcers.[112] Patients complain of irritation, tearing, and foreign body sensation. The superior tarsal conjunctiva stains with rose bengal (Fig. 8-17), and the amount of staining correlates with the severity of the disease.[113] Persistent epithelial defects can occur, and floppy eyelid syndrome may be present. In some cases lubrication is sufficient treatment, but in most cases surgical intervention, such as eyelid shortening or lateral canthal tendon plication, is necessary.

MUCUS FISHING SYNDROME

Mucus fishing is a behavior that contributes to inflammation and mucus production in some patients with conjunctivitis. Described by McCulley, Moore, and Matoba in 1985,[114] this syndrome is brought about by self-induced mechanical trauma to the conjunctiva during removal of mucus filaments from the eye. The patients have underlying conditions that cause mucus production, most commonly keratoconjunctivitis sicca, but they induce further irrita-

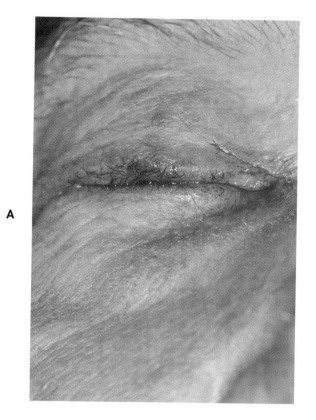

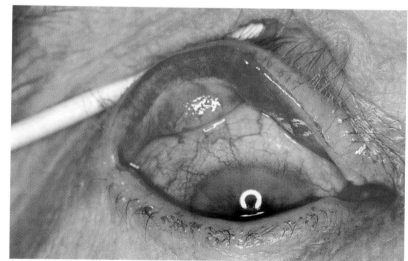

Figure 8-17
A, Imbrication of the lower lid beneath the upper lid. **B,** Rose bengal staining and papillary response on the superior tarsal conjunctiva. (Courtesy of Eric Donnenfeld, Rockville Center, NY.)

tion and mucus production by using their fingers, cotton swabs, tissues, cotton balls, or washcloths to remove the mucus. When patients are asked to demonstrate this behavior, it is evident that conjunctival contact occurs, most commonly in the medial interpalpebral conjunctiva. Rose bengal staining is usually present in the traumatized area.

Once the diagnosis is made, the patient can be educated about avoiding contact with the eye. Cessation of mucus fishing, combined with treatment of the underlying disorder, leads to resolution of signs and symptoms.

MASQUERADE SYNDROME

Occasionally conjunctival tumors grow in a diffuse, minimally elevated manner and appear as a chronic conjunctivitis.[115-118] Squamous cell carcinoma is the most common type to manifest itself in this manner, but sebaceous carcinoma may also do so.[116,119,120] The conjunctivitis is unilateral and may have persisted for years. The involved conjunctiva is diffusely inflamed, mildly thickened, and may contain vascular tufts or subepithelial scarring (Fig. 8-18). A mucoid discharge may be present. The cornea frequently displays a diffuse, nonspecific, punctate keratitis. Cytologic examination of conjunctival scrapings may suggest malignancy by the presence of atypical and pleomorphic cells and multinucleated cells. A biopsy should be performed whenever the disease is suspected and probably in all cases of idiopathic chronic conjunctivitis unresponsive to therapy. It is important to obtain specimens from several sites and to take a wedge specimen from the lid if sebaceous carcinoma is suspected.

REITER'S SYNDROME

Reiter's syndrome consists of conjunctivitis, urethritis, arthritis, circinate balanitis, shallow ulcerations of the buccal mucosa, and a characteristic dermatitis, keratoderma blennorrhagicum. Young men are primarily affected. It is seen worldwide and is the most common cause of arthritis in young men. It is strongly correlated with HLA-B27; more than 76% of patients with Reiter's syndrome have HLA-B27 versus an incidence of less than 10% in the general population. Infectious origins have been proposed, but the evidence is contradictory and inconclusive. Some cases occur after diarrheal illness, including epidemics of bacillary dysentery,[121] *Campylobacter jejuni*,[122] and *Salmonella* enteritis.[123] Other cases appear to relate to venereal disease, particularly nongonococcal urethritis, which is most commonly caused by chlamydial infection[124,125] or *Mycoplasma (Ureaplasma urealyticum)*. Therefore, in at least some patients the disease appears to be triggered by an infectious

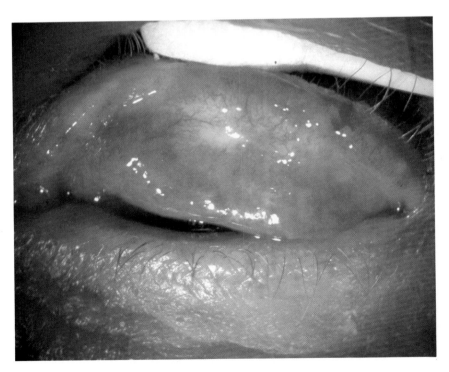

Figure 8-18
Masquerade syndrome. Note abnormal surface and scarring of superior tarsus caused by superficially spreading sebaceous cell carcinoma.

process in the urogenital tract or gut coupled with a specific genetic background.[126]

The gastrointestinal or genitourinary symptoms usually precede the onset of other symptoms by days to weeks. The most common manifestation of Reiter's syndrome is arthritis, which occurs in more than 90% of patients. It is typically an acute, oligoarticular, and asymmetric arthritis most frequently affecting the lower extremities. Mucocutaneous lesions, mainly oral and genital, are also seen in a high percentage of patients. These lesions are painless red macules that can be easily overlooked. The lesions of keratoderma blennorrhagicum consist of painless hyperkeratotic papules that occur most often on the palms and soles but may also appear elsewhere. Some individuals have pleuritis, pericarditis, aortic insufficiency, or neurologic manifestations.

The diagnosis is made clinically, because no specific laboratory findings are present. The presence of oligoarticular, seronegative, asymmetric arthritis lasting longer than 1 month and found in association with urethritis or cervicitis is sufficient for diagnosis of Reiter's syndrome.[127-129]

Reiter's syndrome is usually self-limited, subsiding in 6 weeks to 6 months, and complete remission with full recovery of the joints is the rule. However, relapses can occur and may be precipitated by sexual exposure. Skin and mucous membrane lesions heal without a trace. In a minority of patients the arthritis persists and can be disabling. In rare cases, patients with clinical features of Reiter's syndrome develop typical psoriatic arthritis.

Ocular Manifestations

Ocular involvement can occur at any time during the course of the disease. Conjunctivitis is the most common ophthalmic manifestation of Reiter's syndrome.[130] Iridocyclitis, episcleritis, scleritis, and keratitis may also be seen.[131,132] The conjunctivitis is papillary in nature, usually bilateral, with mucopurulent discharge. It is occasionally recurrent. Conjunctival scarring occurs in rare cases.[130] The iridocyclitis is nongranulomatous, and posterior synechiae are rare. The corneal complications consist of punctate epithelial lesions, central erosive corneal lesions, and peripheral subepithelial opacities (Fig. 8-19).[130,132]

As with the systemic disease, ocular involvement is usually self-limited. Topical corticosteroids may be necessary for keratitis or iritis. Systemic steroids should be avoided because they can aggravate the skin disease. Patients should be tested for chlamydial infection, which, if present, should be treated with systemic tetracycline or erythromycin.

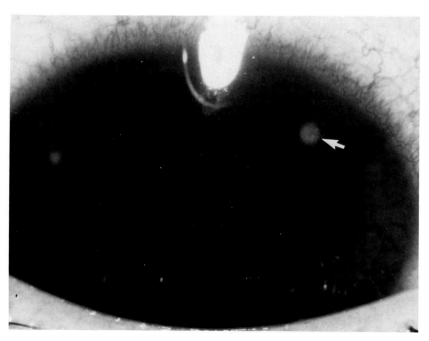

Figure 8-19
Subepithelial lesions (*arrow*) of the cornea in Reiter's syndrome.

KAWASAKI DISEASE (MUCOCUTANEOUS LYMPH NODE SYNDROME)

Kawasaki disease is an acute multisystem disease of children consisting of fever, characteristic mucous membrane and skin findings, and lymphadenopathy. A widespread arteritis is present that can affect the coronary arteries. There is reddening of the palms and soles, membranous fingertip desquamation, a polymorphous exanthem of the trunk without crust or vesicles, and reddening of the lips, tongue, and oral mucosae.

Most affected children have bilateral conjunctival injection.[133] Exudative conjunctivitis,[134] subconjunctival hemorrhage, superficial punctate keratopathy, and anterior uveitis[135] can also be seen.[136]

SUPERIOR LIMBAL KERATOCONJUNCTIVITIS

Superior limbal keratoconjunctivitis (SLK) is a frequently unrecognized cause of chronic, recurrent keratoconjunctivitis. Because it is a distinct clinical entity, SLK can usually be diagnosed readily if the clinician is familiar with the condition. Accurate diagnosis, in turn, enables initiation of the proper therapy and avoidance of harmful or ineffective measures. Often the patient has been using topical antibiotic, antiviral, or corticosteroid medications, which achieve little or no response. In fact, such medications are likely to produce toxic or allergic reactions that can obscure the signs of the original disease. Therefore, a high index of suspicion must be maintained by the ophthalmologist to diagnose all cases of SLK.

Since the disorder was first recognized in the early 1960s by Theodore[137,138] and Thygeson,[139-141] little has been added to the description. SLK is a chronic, inflammatory condition of the eye that can cause considerable ocular irritation.[142] SLK most commonly is bilateral, but often one eye is more severely involved. Exacerbations may affect one eye first and then the other. It occurs most commonly between 20 and 60 years of age.[143] Cases have been reported in patients from 4 to 81 years of age, with a mean age of 49 years. At least 75% of the cases occur in females,[143-145] and there appears to be no racial predilection. The disease occurs nationwide in the United States; the cases occur sporadically and are nonfamilial. There is no seasonal variation. Abnormal thyroid function, most commonly hypothyroidism, has been reported in 26% to 50% of patients with SLK.[144,146-149]

The disease is quite unpredictable in duration and recurrence. Periods of remission and exacerbation occur, with individual attacks lasting for a few days to longer than a year. The disease may persist for several weeks to 10 years or perhaps even longer, but most cases eventually resolve spontaneously. Visual loss does not occur except through inappropriate treatment.

Clinical Manifestations

The symptoms of SLK are usually more severe than objective findings would suggest. One of the foremost complaints is a burning sensation. In addition, patients may experience irritation, foreign body sensation, pain, photophobia, ptosis, and blepharospasm. Visual impairment, discharge, and itching of the eyes are not usually encountered.

Papillary hypertrophy and marked inflammation occur on the superior tarsal conjunctiva. In severe cases this area may have a diffuse velvety appearance, but medium or giant papillae do not form. The severity of disease on the superior tarsus usually parallels that of the superior limbus. In extremely severe cases, a membrane can be seen on the superior tarsus.[143] The conjunctiva of the lower lid is not involved.

The superior limbus is almost always involved by papillary hypertrophy and hyperemia. A fleshy, gray thickening of epithelium occurs in the superior limbal area (Fig. 8-20). A boggy apron of conjunctiva, folding over the superior limbus, is occasionally seen. Fine epithelial keratitis is often present in the upper fifth of the cornea. In severe cases edema or even bullous keratopathy can affect the superior cornea. A micropannus occasionally is noted.

Filaments in the area of the superior limbus are present in a third of the cases (Fig. 8-21) and may also occur on the bulbar and tarsal conjunctiva.[138] The appearance of filaments usually is accompanied by an acute worsening of the symptoms; desquamation of filaments can lead to epithelial loss. When filaments occur, they may overshadow the picture of the underlying disease, and the condition may be misdiagnosed simply as filamentary keratitis.

Hyperemia of the superior bulbar conjunctiva arranged in a "corridor" fashion is a constant finding and is most evident when the patient's gaze is directed downward (Fig. 8-22). This injection is most intense at the limbal area and fades as it approaches the superior fornix. The conjunctiva is thickened and often luster-

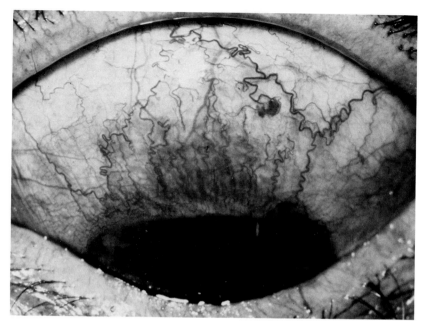

Figure 8-20
Superior limbal keratoconjunctivitis. Note thickening and graying of epithelium in superior limbal area, associated with characteristic vascular injection of bulbar conjunctiva. (From Grayson M: *Perspectives in ophthalmology,* vol 1, Hagerstown, MD, 1976, Ankho International Co.)

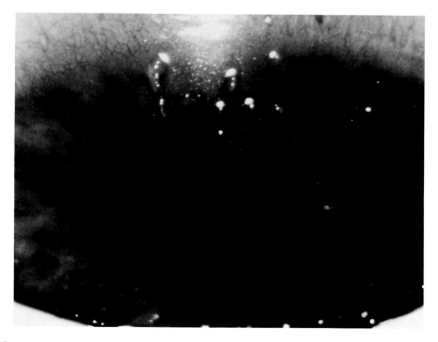

Figure 8-21
Filaments on the superior limbal cornea in superior limbal keratoconjunctivitis. (From Grayson M: *Perspectives in ophthalmology,* vol 1, Hagerstown, MD, 1976, Ankho International Co.)

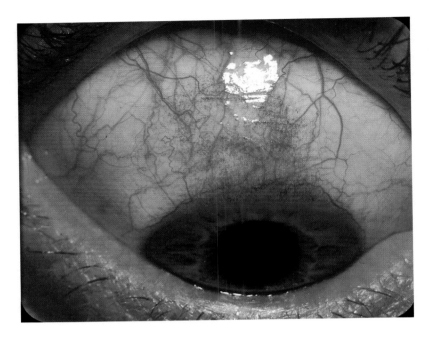

Figure 8-22
Superior bulbar conjunctiva in superior limbal keratoconjunctivitis showing a corridor of injection and staining with rose bengal red.

less because of keratinization of the surface. The remaining conjunctiva exhibits a mild hyperemia.

Other possible findings include increased mucus, pseudoptosis, and edema of the superior bulbar conjunctiva. Decreased corneal sensation and decreased vision caused by induced astigmatism occur in rare cases.[144]

The instillation of rose bengal reveals rather characteristic involvement of the cornea, limbus, and conjunctiva.[150] Fine and uniform areas of epithelial staining are found immediately above and below the superior limbus. Superficial, punctate staining of the bulbar conjunctiva usually involves the 10:30 to 1:30 area and extends about 4 to 5 mm above the limbus (Fig. 8-22). Corneal staining is often seen extending 1 to 2 mm centrally from the limbus. Similar but less extensive staining may be seen with fluorescein.

Areas of localized dryness of the involved superior bulbar conjunctiva may be present, but tear production is usually normal. However, in cases with decreased tear production, inferior filaments and interpalpebral conjunctival staining may be present along with the typical superior changes. It is best to treat the dry eye state first (e.g., with lubricants, punctal occlusion) before treating the SLK.

Laboratory Evaluation

Giemsa-stained scrapings from the superior bulbar conjunctiva show keratinization of the epithelial cells (see Fig. 4-7).[151] The keratinized epithelial cells contain keratohyalin granules. With further keratinization the cytoplasm decreases in volume and takes on a purplish hue. Some epithelial cells may demonstrate degenerated nuclei that appear pyknotic and shrunken. Scrapings of the palpebral conjunctiva may be normal or may reveal similar changes. A mild inflammatory reaction, with polymorphonuclear cells predominating, may be present. It has been reported that in Papanicolaou-stained scrapings of the superior bulbar conjunctiva, the nuclear chromatin may be condensed into unusual figures such as an **S** shape, bar, or coil.[152] The significance of these findings is not clear.

Biopsy specimens of the bulbar conjunctival epithelium exhibit keratinization, acanthosis, and mild dyskeratosis. Cytoplasmic edema, nuclear pyknosis, and intracellular accumulation of glycogen are seen.[144,151,153,154] Electron microscopy shows that the keratinization characteristics of the conjunctival epithelium are similar to those occurring in normal skin.[153] In addition, nuclear changes similar to those reported in conjunctival scraping specimens were observed: an abnormal aggregation of the nuclear chromatin, with formation of multilobed nuclei and multinucleated cells.[152,155]

Biopsy specimens of the epithelium and stroma of the palpebral conjunctiva demonstrate an inflammatory infiltration consisting of neutrophils, lymphocytes, and plasma cells with a preponderance of neutrophils. An inflammatory exudate of similar cellular makeup may be present overlying the thickened conjunctiva.[151] Staining with the periodic acid-Schiff or alcian blue does not occur. The laboratory test of consistent value seems to be the finding of keratinized cells.

Differential Diagnosis

Differential diagnosis can be approached by considering the following conditions with or without filaments:

Conditions without filaments
  Trachoma
  Marginal infiltrates in the superior cornea
  Limbal vernal keratoconjunctivitis
  Phlyctenulosis
  Giant papillary conjunctivitis
  Contact lens–induced keratoconjunctivitis

Conditions with filaments
  Keratoconjunctivitis sicca
  Masquerade syndrome

In none of the nonfilamentous conditions listed is there significant bulbar conjunctival staining. Corneal staining, follicles, and scarring on the upper tarsal conjunctiva, Herbert's pits, and gross pannus help differentiate trachoma. The presence of basophilic intracytoplasmic inclusions and response to specific treatment for trachoma aid in the differentiation. Limbal vernal disease may be differentiated by the presence of fragmented eosinophils on scrapings, the gelatinous appearance of the limbal lesions, with overlying Trantas' dots, and giant papillae on the upper tarsal plate. In addition, the seasonal nature and response of vernal disease to steroids and cromolyn sodium are important clues. The limbal phlyctenule has a characteristic clinical picture. This raised, yellow-white, self-limited conjunctival limbal lesion is primarily associated with a sensitivity to staphylococci.

The corneal and conjunctival staining of keratoconjunctivitis sicca is mainly in the interpalpebral zone. If the eye is dry enough to cause filament formation, Schirmer's test is usually markedly abnormal, and the precorneal tear film is filled with debris. A loss of luster occurs on the corneal surface. Scrapings may reveal goblet cells.

The differentiation of contact lens–induced keratoconjunctivitis (CLIK) and SLK may be difficult in contact lens wearers. This is discussed in the section on CLIK. As with any case of chronic conjunctivitis, masquerade syndrome should be suspected, and if the conjunctiva appears dysplastic, a biopsy should be performed. Misdiagnosis of sebaceous cell carcinoma as SLK was reported in one case.[120]

Etiology

The cause of SLK is unknown. Viral and fungal cultures have been negative. Bacterial cultures have yielded normal flora, including *Staphylococcus epidermidis* and diphtheroids. Eosinophils, basophils, and inclusions have not been found. The frequent association with thyroid disease may suggest some immunologic connection, but no evidence exists that the disease occurs on an immunologic basis.[156]

Wright[149] has suggested that the initial pathologic process occurs in the superior tarsal conjunctiva, with development of chronic inflammation and tightness of the lid against the globe. He proposed that this interfered with the normal removal of surface cells from the epithelium of the bulbar conjunctiva.

The hypothesis proposed by Wilson and Ostler[157,158] best explains all the findings in this disease. According to this hypothesis, SLK results from a combination of increased tension of the upper lid against the globe and increased mobility of the upper bulbar conjunctiva. The increased tension of the upper lid may be caused by edema or exophthalmos, which may be related to thyroid disease or to chronic inflammation from other causes. Laxity or edema of the superior bulbar conjunctiva may arise from hypothyroidism or aging or may be congenital. The movement of the lid against the conjunctiva and of the conjunctiva against the globe results in chronic mechanical irritation. The response of the eye to this is injection, papillary hypertrophy, cellular infiltration, and abnormal epithelial maturation, with surface keratinization.

Silver nitrate treatment removes the abnormal conjunctival epithelium and temporarily improves symptoms until the process again results in an abnormal surface. Scarring of the bulbar conjunctiva to the globe, which may occur with prolonged inflammation, multiple silver nitrate treatments, or cautery or conjunctival resection, prevents the abnormal movement of the conjunctiva.

It is interesting to note that SLK occurred in the superior temporal conjunctiva in a patient with esotropia[157] and that thyroid patients with lid retraction seem not to develop SLK.[149]

Treatment

Topical application of silver nitrate solution improves the condition in most patients, and in some cases complete remission is achieved.[138,143] Filaments often disappear, and the symptoms and clinical findings usually are reduced by the next day. Limbal staining is most resistant to treatment and may take several weeks to disappear. Two or three treatments at least 2 days apart may be required before relief is obtained. As mentioned, however, recurrences are frequent after 4 to 6 weeks, and retreatment is required.

A cotton-tipped applicator that has been impregnated with a 0.5% to 1% solution of silver nitrate is used. Ampules marketed for Credé prophylaxis contain 1% silver nitrate and may be diluted with sterile water (not sodium chloride) for use. My practice has been to treat both the upper tarsal and bulbar conjunctiva. The silver nitrate–moistened applicator is rubbed vigorously over both surfaces. Afterward the eye is irrigated with normal saline.

Strong concentrations of silver nitrate cause chemical burns and silver staining of the cornea. Solid-tipped silver nitrate applicators must be avoided, because their use may result in a severe burn and opacification of the cornea that may necessitate penetrating keratoplasty.[159,160]

Simple mechanical scraping of the involved conjunctiva with a platinum spatula may be effective.[149,161] Pressure patching and bandage soft contact lens wear provide relief in some patients.[149,154,161] Cromolyn sodium was found to be effective by some researchers[162] but not by others.[149] Lodoxamide tromethamine 0.1% four times daily was reported to be effective in three patients.[154] In a few cases topical decongestants, zinc salts, and artificial tears may bring about temporary, symptomatic relief but will have no effect on the progression of the disease. Cryotherapy also has been advocated but does not appear to be as effective as silver nitrate treatment.

Thermocauterization of the superior bulbar conjunctiva often is effective, even in cases that do not respond to silver nitrate.[163] I recommend this procedure over silver nitrate cauterization in most cases. To perform the procedure, the superior bulbar conjunctiva is ballooned up with an injection of local anesthetic, and small burns are created in an even distribution throughout the affected area.

Recession or resection of the superior bulbar conjunctiva usually is effective in cases that do not respond to other treatments.[154,164,165] The superior conjunctiva and Tenon's membrane is dissected off the limbus and sclera from the 10:30 to 1:30 positions and for 5 to 8 mm posteriorly. The conjunctiva may be excised or recessed with the edges sutured to the globe with 7-0 chromic sutures. In the rare case that symptoms recur after this procedure, silver nitrate treatment or repeat resection are still effective.[165] In one study, botulinum toxin administration to the orbital portions of the obicularis muscles improved or eliminated symptoms in 76% of patients.[166]

CONTACT LENS–INDUCED KERATOCONJUNCTIVITIS

In 1981, Wilson[167] became the first to recognize that contact lens wear could cause a condition simulating SLK. Since then several authors have reported series of patients with this syndrome, which has come to be called *CLIK*.[168-171]

Clinical Manifestations

The symptoms of CLIK include redness, irritation, burning, itching, photophobia, crusting, and tearing. Vision is often mildly reduced, and wearing contact lenses may exacerbate the symptoms.

Superior conjunctival injection and limbal papillary hypertrophy usually are present. The superior corneal epithelium usually is irregular, thickened, and gray with punctate fluorescein staining. This may extend down from the limbus in a **V** pattern toward the visual axis (Fig. 8-23). Subepithelial opacities often are present. Pannus may be present beneath the abnormal epithelium and may extend several millimeters onto the cornea. The superior tarsal conjunctiva may be normal or may display a mild to moderate papillary response. Filaments are present in a minority of cases. A summary of the differentiating features of CLIK and SLK is given in Table 8-3.

If untreated, progressive corneal involvement occurs (Fig. 8-24).[172] The epithelium becomes thicker and grayer and a greater area is involved. The pannus progresses centrally, and deep stromal vascularization can occur. Resolution may not occur after the patient stops wearing contact lenses. In severe cases the entire cornea can be covered by thickened, hazy epi-

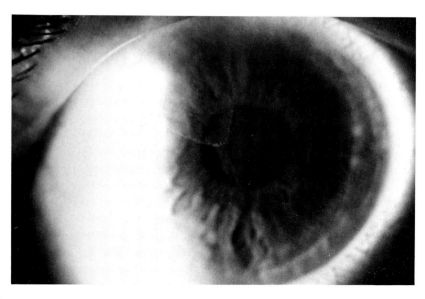

Figure 8-23
Contact lens–induced keratoconjunctivitis. Note the irregular, thickened, and gray epithelium extending down from the superior limbus toward the visual axis.

Table 8-3	Differentiating Features of Contact Lens–Induced Keratoconjunctivitis (CLIK) and Superior Limbic Keratoconjunctivitis (SLK)	
Clinical Features	**CLIK**	**SLK**
Age (most common)	15 to 35 yrs	40 to 60 yrs
Decreased vision (from keratopathy)	Common	No
Exacerbations and remissions unrelated to contact lens wear	No	Yes
Thyroid disease	No	Common
Response to contact lens wear	Worsens	Can improve
Itching	Common	No
More than minimal hyperemia of nasal temporal and inferior bulbar conjunctiva	Common	No
Keratopathy extending >3 mm below upper limbus	Common	No
Gelatinous papillary hypertrophy of limbus	Common	No
Gross pannus (>2 mm)	Occasionally	No
Subepithelial opacification	Common	No
Corneal filaments	Occasionally	Common
Eosinophils in conjunctival scrapings	Occasionally	No
Response to cessation of contact lens wear	Yes	No

Adapted from Wilson FM II: *Differential diagnosis of superior limbic keratoconjunctivitis and papillary keratoconjunctivitis associated with contact lenses.* In Hughes WF, editor: *The year book of ophthalmology 1981,* Chicago, 1981, Mosby–Year Book.

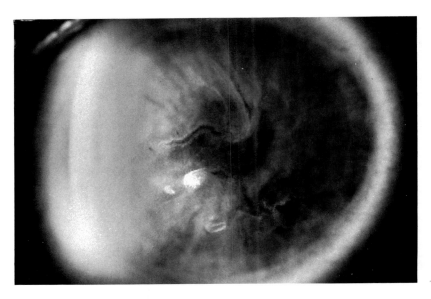

Figure 8-24
Diffuse irregularity, opacification, and thickening of corneal epithelium related to contact lens wear (contact lens–induced keratoconjunctivitis). (Courtesy of Richard A. Thoft, Pittsburgh, PA.)

thelium, superficial stromal scarring can be present, and recurrent ulceration can occur.

In conjunctival scrapings, early keratinization of the epithelium, a moderate polymorphonuclear response, and occasional lymphocytes are seen.[169,170] Eosinophils may be present in some patients. Biopsy specimens exhibit keratinization, acanthosis, and intracellular edema of the epithelium.[171] A chronic inflammatory infiltrate is present in the conjunctival stroma, with polymorphonuclear cells, plasma cells, and mononuclear cells.

Etiology

In many cases CLIK appears to be related to thimerosal exposure. Thimerosal was present in lens care solutions in most of the reported cases, but only a small minority of patients exhibited reactions to thimerosal on patch testing.[168,170,171] The incidence of CLIK appears to be decreasing because most contact lens solutions no longer contain thimerosal. Mechanical factors have also been implicated.[173]

Most likely several factors can play a role: mechanical irritation of the superior limbus; exposure to preservatives and other chemicals in lens solutions; proteins, organisms, and other materials deposited on contact lenses; and hypoxia of the epithelium beneath the lens, which would be expected to be greatest under the superior lid.

Treatment

Cessation of lens wear is the main treatment. Resolution of signs and symptoms occurs in most cases and takes several weeks to more than a year. Silver nitrate treatment or conjunctival resection, as used for SLK, may be helpful.[170] Lens wear often can be reinstituted, with refitting, switching to gas-permeable hard contact lenses, or avoidance of thimerosal-containing solutions.[169,171]

If corneal epitheial changes do not resolve with cessation of lens wear, surgical treatment may be necessary. Limbal[174,175] or conjunctival[176] autografts have restored the corneal surface in some cases. Experimental work in rabbits suggests that limbal autografts are superior to conjunctival autografts.[177]

LIGNEOUS CONJUNCTIVITIS

Ligneous conjunctivitis is a chronic membranous conjunctivitis seen in childhood.[178-183] It is most common in children but can occur at any age, even at birth. It is more frequent in females and is equally likely to be bilateral or unilateral. In several reports, two siblings have developed ligneous conjunctivitis, and in one case two generations were affected.

Immediately preceding or concomitant with the development of conjunctivitis, many pa-

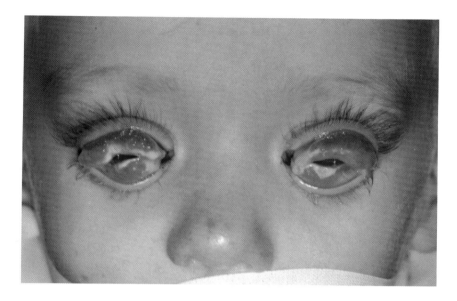

Figure 8-25
Ligneous conjunctivitis involving all four lids. (Courtesy of Eugene Helveston and Forrest D. Ellis, Indianapolis, IN.)

tients have signs and symptoms of acute systemic disease, including upper respiratory infections, tonsillitis, otitis media, sinusitis, vulvovaginitis, cervicitis, and fever. In some cases family members or other close contacts developed a conjunctivitis at the same time that cleared rapidly.[184] In one such case both parents had a streptococcal conjunctivitis. Cases have occurred following excision of a pinguecula[185] and strabismus surgery.[186]

The eyes are often injected, and mucoid discharge may be present. The membranes are thick, yellow-white or red, and exhibit a hard, boardlike appearance (Fig. 8-25). They may be sessile or pedunculated and arise from the tarsal or bulbar conjunctiva. If the membranes are removed, the area beneath bleeds and the membrane regrows, usually in a few days. Corneal involvement occurs occasionally, and it can lead to perforation and loss of the globe. The course is usually chronic, lasting 4 to 44 years. Spontaneous resolution may occur after many recurrences.

Ligneous conjunctivitis may be associated with similar lesions affecting other mucous membranes[180] or the middle ear.[187] Tracheal involvement may be life threatening.[188,189]

Histopathologic sections of the membrane have revealed subepithelial deposits of eosinophilic amorphous material, granulation tissue, and chronic inflammatory cells. The amorphous material is composed of fibrin, albumin, and immunoglobulins.[180,185,187,190] Eosinophils, mononuclear cells, neutrophils, and mast cells may be present.

The cause of ligneous conjunctivitis is unclear. Hidayat and Riddle[180] suggested that the disorder was related to an abnormal hyperpermeability of blood vessels, but this may be a secondary phenomenon. Bateman et al.[191] believe that ligneous conjunctivitis is genetic and most likely inherited in an autosomal recessive pattern.

Ligneous conjunctivitis has generally been resistant to treatment. Numerous treatments have been proposed, with case reports illustrating success in some patients and failures in others. Hyaluronidase,[178,192] fibrinolysin,[193] alphachymotrypsin,[185] cryotherapy,[193] and cromolyn sodium[188] have all been recommended. Azathioprine was effective in one case.[180] Topical cyclosporine was effective in three cases,[190,194] but failed in two others.[195] Total excision of the membrane, combined with excision of the tarsus and conjunctiva, and replacement with donor sclera was effective in another case.[196] Antibiotics, steroids, antiviral agents, cautery, and beta and x-ray irradiation have been ineffective.[188] In the largest series, 17 patients were treated with excision combined with meticulous cautery and perioperative topical treatment, and control was obtained in 76%.[197] Topical heparin, 1000 or 5000 IU/ml, topical corticosteroid (e.g., 1% prednisolone), and in 12 patients alpha-chymotrypsin, 2500 or 5000 IU/ml, were administered intensively until the conjunctival surface re-epithelialized and slowly tapered thereafter.

REFERENCES

1. Ballow M et al: IgG specific antibodies to rye grass and ragweed pollen antigens in the tear secretions of patients with vernal conjunctivitis, *Am J Ophthalmol* 95:161, 1983.
2. Dart JKG et al: Perennial allergic conjunctivitis: definition, clinical characteristics and prevalence, *Trans Ophthalmol Soc UK* 105:513, 1986.
3. Moller C et al: The precision of the conjunctival provocation test, *Allergy* 39:37, 1984.
4. Giovannini M, Spada E, Broccoli MP: Conjunctival provocation tests in suspected allergic conjunctivitis: a clinical study, *Ophthalmologica* 201:1, 1990.
5. Leonardi A et al: Correlation between conjunctival provocation test (CPT) and systemic allergometric tests in allergic conjunctivitis, *Eye* 4:760, 1990.
6. Baratz KH, Foulks GN: Rapid tear IgE analysis in ocular diseases using the touch tear system, *Invest Ophthalmol Vis Sci* 4:198, 1992.
7. Abelson MB, Madiwale N, Weston JF: Conjunctival eosinophils in allergic ocular disease, *Arch Ophthalmol* 101:631, 1983.
8. Theodore FH: The significance of conjunctival eosinophilia in the diagnosis of allergic conjunctivitis, *Ear Nose Throat J* 30:653, 1951.
9. Baratz KH, Foulks GN: Rapid tear IgE analysis in ocular diseases using the touch tear system, *Invest Ophthalmol Vis Sci* 4:198, 1992.
10. Moller C et al: The precision of the conjunctival provocation test, *Allergy* 39:37, 1984.
11. Giovannini M, Spada E, Broccoli MP: Conjunctival provocation tests in suspected allergic conjunctivitis: a clinical study, *Ophthalmologica* 201:1, 1990.
12. Leonardi A et al: Correlation between conjunctival provocation test (CPT) and systemic allergometric tests in allergic conjunctivitis, *Eye* 4:760, 1990.
13. Abelson MB et al: Effects of Vasocon-A in the allergen challenge model of acute allergic conjunctivitis, *Arch Ophthalmol* 108:520, 1990.
14. Abelson MB, Smith LM: Levocabastine: evaluation of histamine and compound 48/80 models of ocular allergy in humans, *Ophthalmology* 95:1494, 1988.
15. Pipkorn U et al: A double-blind evaluation of topical levocabastine, a new specific H1 antagonist, in patients with allergic conjunctivitis, *Allergy* 40:491, 1985.
16. Rimas M et al: Topical levocabastine protects better than sodium cromoglycate and placebo in the conjunctival provocation test, *Allergy* 45:18, 1990.
17. Wihl JA et al: Levocabastine eyedrops vs. sodium cromoglycate in seasonal allergic conjunctivitis, *Clin Exp Allergy* 21:37, 1991.
18. Abelson MB et al: Evaluation of the new ophthalmic antihistamine, 0.05% levocabastine, in the clinical allergen challenge model of allergic conjunctivitis, *Clin Immunol* 94:458, 1994.
19. Abelson MB, George MA, Smith LM: Evaluation of 0.05% levocabastine versus 4% sodium cromolyn in the allergen challenge model, *Ophthalmology* 102:310, 1995.
20. Kray KT et al: Cromolyn sodium in seasonal allergic conjunctivitis, *J Allergy Clin Immunol* 76:623, 1986.
21. Allansmith MR, Ross RN: Ocular allergy and mast cell stabilizers, *Surv Ophthalmol* 30:229, 1986.
22. Norman PS, Lichtenstein LM: *Allergic rhinitis.* In Samter M, editor: *Immunological diseases,* ed 4, Boston, 1988, Little, Brown & Co.
23. Taudorf E et al: Oral immunotherapy in birch pollen hayfever, *J Allergy Clin Immunol* 80:153, 1987.
24. Smolin G, O'Connor GR: *Ocular immunology,* Philadelphia, 1981, Lea & Febiger.
25. Neumann E et al: A review of 400 cases of vernal conjunctivitis, *Am J Ophthalmol* 74:166, 1959.
26. Allansmith MR: *Vernal conjunctivitis.* In Duane TD, editor: *Clinical ophthalmology,* vol 5, Philadelphia, 1988, Harper & Row.
27. Buckley RJ: Vernal keratoconjunctivitis, *Int Ophthalmol Clin* 28:303, 1988.
28. Rice NSC, Jones BR: Vernal keratoconjunctivitis: an allergic disease of the eyes of children, *Clin Allergy* 3:629, 1973.
29. Togby AF: Keratitis epithelial vernalis, *Bull Ophthalmol Soc Egypt* 28:104, 1935.
30. Jones BR: Vernal keratitis, *Trans Ophthalmol Soc UK* 81:215, 1961.
31. Shuler JD, Levenson J, Mondino BJ: Inferior corneal ulcers associated with palpebral vernal conjunctivitis, *Am J Ophthalmol* 106:106, 1988.
32. Cameron JA: Shield ulcers and plaques of the cornea in vernal keratoconjunctivitis, *Ophthalmology* 102:985, 1995.
33. Udell IJ et al: Eosinophil granule major basic protein and Charcot-Leyden crystal protein in human tears, *Am J Ophthalmol* 92:824, 1981.
34. Khan MD et al: Incidence of keratoconus in spring catarrh, *Br J Ophthalmol* 72:41, 1988.
35. Tuft SJ, Dart JKG, Kemeny M: Limbal vernal keratoconjunctivitis: clinical characteristics and immunoglobulin E expression compared with palpebral vernal, *Eye* 3:420, 1989.
36. Collin HB, Allansmith MR: Basophils in vernal conjunctivitis in humans: an electron microscopic study, *Invest Ophthalmol Vis Sci* 16:858, 1977.
37. Easty DL et al: Immunological investigations in vernal eye disease, *Trans Ophthalmol Soc UK* 100:98, 1980.
38. Morgan G: The pathology of vernal conjunctivitis, *Trans Ophthalmol Soc UK* 91:467, 1971.

39. Trocme SD et al: Eosinophil granule major basic protein deposition in corneal ulcers associated with vernal keratoconjunctivitis, *Am J Ophthalmol* 115:640, 1993.
40. Alimuddin M: Vernal conjunctivitis, *Br J Ophthalmol* 39:160, 1955.
41. Samra Z et al: Vernal keratoconjunctivitis: the significance of immunoglobulin E levels in tears and serum, *Int Arch Allergy Appl Immunol* 74:158, 1984.
42. Ballow M, Mendelson L: Specific immunoglobulin E antibodies in tear secretions of patients with vernal conjunctivitis, *J Allergy Clin Immunol* 66:112, 1980.
43. Allansmith MR, Hahn GS, Simon MA: Tissue, tear and serum IgE concentrations in vernal conjunctivitis, *Am J Ophthalmol* 81:506, 1976.
44. Ballow M et al: IgG specific antibodies to rye grass and ragweed pollen antigens in the tear secretions of patients with vernal conjunctivitis, *Am J Ophthalmol* 95:161, 1983.
45. Abelson MB, Baird RS, Allansmith MR: Tear histamine levels in vernal conjunctivitis and other ocular inflammations, *Ophthalmology* 87:812, 1980.
46. Ballow M, Donshik PC, Mendelson L: Complement proteins and C3 anaphylatoxin in tears of patients with conjunctivitis, *J Allergy Clin Immunol* 76:473, 1985.
47. Mumcuoglu YK et al: House dust mites and vernal keratoconjunctivitis, *Ophthalmologica* 196:175, 1988.
48. Allansmith MR et al: Conjunctival basophil hypersensitivity in the guinea pig, *J Allergy Clin Immunol* 78:919, 1986.
49. Friedlander MG, Cyr R: Ocular findings in systemic cutaneous basophil hypersensitivity, *Invest Ophthalmol Vis Sci* 18:964, 1979.
50. Easty DL, Rice NSC, Jones BR: Disodium cromoglycate (Intal) in the treatment of keratoconjunctivitis, *Trans Ophthalmol Soc UK* 91:491, 1971.
51. Easty DL, Rice NSC, Jones BR: Clinical trial of topical disodium cromoglycate in vernal keratoconjunctivitis, *Clin Allergy* 2:99, 1972.
52. Kazdan JJ et al: Sodium cromoglycate (Intal) in the treatment of vernal keratoconjunctivitis and allergic conjunctivitis, *Can J Ophthalmol* 11:300, 1976.
53. Foster CS: The cromolyn sodium collaborative study group: evaluation of topical cromolyn sodium in the treatment of vernal keratoconjunctivitis, *Ophthalmology* 95:194, 1988.
54. Baryishak YR et al: Vernal keratoconjunctivitis in an Israeli group of patients and its treatment with sodium cromoglycate, *Br J Ophthalmol* 66:118, 1982.
55. Caldwell DR et al: Efficacy and safety of lodoxamide 0.1% vs. cromolyn sodium 4% in patients with vernal keratoconjunctivitis, *Am J Ophthalmol* 113:632, 1992.
56. Santos CI et al: Efficacy of lodoxamide 0.1% ophthalmic solution in resolving corneal epitheliopathy associated with vernal keratoconjunctivitis, *Am J Ophthalmol* 117:488, 1994.
57. Fiscella RG, Siegel FP, Weisbecker C: Alternative solution for Optocrom, *Am J Hosp Pharm* 49:70, 1992.
58. Ben Ezra D et al: Cyclosporine eyedrops for the treatment of severe vernal keratoconjunctivitis, *Am J Ophthalmol* 101:278, 1986.
59. Holland EJ, Olsen TW, Ketcham JM et al: Topical cyclosporine A in the treatment of anterior segment inflammatory disease, *Cornea* 12:413, 1993.
60. Singh G: Cryosurgery in palpebral vernal catarrh, *Ann Ophthalmol* 14:252, 1982.
61. Tse DT et al: Mucous membrane grafting for severe palpebral vernal conjunctivitis, *Arch Ophthalmol* 101:1879, 1983.
62. Rich LF, Hanifin JM: Ocular complications of atopic dermatitis and other eczemas, *Int Ophthalmol Clin* 25:61, 1985.
63. Garrity JA, Liesegang TJ: Ocular complications of atopic dermatitis, *Can J Ophthalmol* 19:21, 1984.
64. Tuft SJ et al: Clinical features of atopic keratoconjunctivitis, *Ophthalmology* 98:150, 1991.
65. Foster CS, Calonge M: Atopic keratoconjunctivitis, *Ophthalmology* 97:992, 1990.
66. Easty D et al: Herpes simplex keratitis and keratoconus in the atopic patients. A clinical and immunological study, *Trans Ophthalmol Soc UK* 95:267, 1975.
67. Brunsting LA, Reed WB, Bair HL: Occurrence of cataracts and keratoconus with atopic dermatitis, *Arch Dermatol* 72:237, 1955.
68. Cowan A, Klauder JV: Frequency of occurrence of cataracts in atopic dermatitis, *Arch Ophthalmol* 43:759, 1950.
69. Amemiya T, Matsuda H, Vehara M: Ocular findings in atopic dermatitis with special reference to the clinical features of atopic cataract, *Ophthalmologica* 180:129, 1980.
70. Foster CS, Rice BA, Dutt JE: Immunopathology of atopic keratoconjunctivitis, *Ophthalmology* 98:1190, 1991.
71. Morgan SJ et al: Mast cell hyperplasia in atopic keratoconjunctivitis: an immunohistochemical study, *Eye* 5:729, 1991.
72. Rocklin RE, Pincus S: *Atopic dermatitis.* In Samter M, editor: *Immunological diseases,* ed 4, Boston, 1988, Little, Brown & Co.
73. Palacios J, Fuller EW, Blaylock WK: Immunological capabilities of patients with atopic dermatitis, *J Invest Dermatol* 47:484, 1966.
74. Leung DYM, Rhodes AR, Geha RS: Enumeration of T cell subsets in atopic dermatitis using monoclonal antibodies, *J Allergy Clin Immunol* 67:450, 1981.
75. Hemady Z et al: Abnormal regulation of in vitro IgE synthesis by T cells obtained from patients with atopic dermatitis, *Clin Immunol Immunopathol* 35:156, 1985.
76. Ostler HB: Acute chemotic reaction to cromolyn, *Arch Ophthalmol* 100:412, 1982.

77. Jay JL: Clinical features and diagnosis of adult atopic keratoconjunctivitis and the effect of treatment with sodium cromoglycate, *Br J Ophthalmol* 65:335, 1981.

78. Ariyanayagam M et al: Topical sodium cromoglycate in the management of atopic eczema, *Br J Dermatol* 112:343, 1985.

79. Aswad MI, Tauber J, Baum J: Plasmapheresis treatment in patients with severe atopic keratoconjunctivitis, *Ophthalmology* 95:444, 1988.

80. Spring TF: Reaction to hydrophilic lenses, *Med J Aust* 1:499, 1974.

81. Allansmith MR, Korb DR, Greiner JV: Giant papillary conjunctivitis induced by hard or soft contact lens wear: quantitative histology, *Ophthalmology* 85:766, 1978.

82. Srinivasan DB et al: Giant papillary conjunctivitis with ocular prosthesis, *Arch Ophthalmol* 97:892, 1979.

83. Meisler DM, Krachmer JH, Goeken JA: An immunopathologic study of giant papillary conjunctivitis associated with an ocular prosthesis, *Am J Ophthalmol* 92:368, 1981.

84. Jolson AS, Jolson SC: Suture barb giant papillary conjunctivitis, *Ophthalmic Surg* 15:139, 1984.

85. Sugar A, Meyer RF: Giant papillary conjunctivitis after keratoplasty, *Am J Ophthalmol* 91:239, 1981.

86. Carlson AN, Wilhelmus KR: Giant papillary conjunctivitis associated with cyanoacrylate glue, *Am J Ophthalmol* 104:437, 1987.

87. Robin JB et al: Giant papillary conjunctivitis associated with an extruded scleral buckle, *Arch Ophthalmol* 105:619, 1987.

88. Heidemann DG, Dunn SP, Siegal MJ: Unusual causes of giant papillary conjunctivitis, *Cornea* 12:78, 1993.

89. Allansmith MR, Ross RN: Giant papillary conjunctivitis, *Int Ophthalmol Clin* 28:309, 1988.

90. Abelson MB, Allansmith MR: Ocular allergies. In Smolin G, Thoft RA, editors: *The cornea: scientific foundations and clinical practice,* Boston, 1983, Little, Brown & Co.

91. Meisler DM, Zaret CR, Stock EL: Trantas' dots and limbal inflammation associated with soft contact lens wear, *Am J Ophthalmol* 89:66, 1980.

92. Mathers WD, Billborough M: Meibomian gland function and giant papillary conjunctivitis, *Am J Ophthalmol* 114:188, 1992.

93. Ballow M et al: An animal model for contact lens-induced giant papillary conjunctivitis, *Invest Ophthalmol Vis Sci* 28:39, 1987.

94. Donshik PC, Ballow M: Tear immunoglobulins in giant papillary conjunctivitis, *Am J Ophthalmol* 96:460, 1983.

95. Ballow M, Donshik PC, Mendelson L: Complement proteins and C3 anaphylatoxin in tears of patients with conjunctivitis, *J Allergy Clin Immunol* 76:473, 1985.

96. Elgebaly SA et al: Neutrophil chemotactic factor in the tears of giant papillary conjunctivitis

97. Kruger CJ et al: Treatment of giant papillary conjunctivitis with cromolyn sodium, *CLAO J* 18:46, 1992.

98. Culbertson WW, Ostler HB: The floppy lid syndrome, *Am J Ophthalmol* 92:568, 1981.

99. Parunovic A: Floppy eyelid syndrome, *Br J Ophthalmol* 67:264, 1983.

100. Schwartz LK, Gelender H, Forster RK: Chronic conjunctivitis associated with "floppy eyelids," *Arch Ophthalmol* 101:1884, 1983.

101. Gerner EW, Hughes SM: Floppy eyelid with hyperglycinemia, *Am J Ophthalmol* 98:614, 1984.

102. Dutton JJ: Surgical management of floppy eyelid syndrome, *Am J Ophthalmol* 99:557, 1985.

103. Goldberg R et al: Floppy eyelid syndrome and blepharochalasis, *Am J Ophthalmol* 102:376, 1986.

104. Moore MB, Harrington J, McCulley JP: Floppy eyelid syndrome: management including surgery, *Ophthalmology* 93:184, 1986.

105. Parunovic A, Bozidar I: Floppy eyelid syndrome associated with keratotorus, *Br J Ophthalmol* 72:634, 1988.

106. Culbertson WW, Tseng SC: Corneal disorders in floppy eyelid syndrome, *Cornea* 13:33, 1994.

107. Eiferman RA et al: Floppy eyelid syndrome in a child, *Am J Ophthalmol* 109:356, 1990.

108. Donnenfeld ED et al: Keratoconus associated with floppy eyelid syndrome, *Ophthalmology* 98:1674, 1991.

109. Imbert P et al: Bilateral corneal neovascularization and floppy eyelid syndrome: a case report, *J Fr Ophthalmol* 13:223, 1990.

110. Netland PA et al: Histopathologic features of the floppy eyelid syndrome: involvement of tarsal elastin, *Ophthalmology* 101:174, 1994.

111. Woog JJ: Obstructive sleep apnea and the floppy eyelid syndrome, *Am J Ophthalmol* 110:314, 1990.

112. Karesh JW, Nirankari VS, Hameroff SR: Eyelid imbrication: an unrecognized cause of chronic ocular irritation, *Ophthalmology* 100:883, 1993.

113. Donnenfeld ED et al: Lid imbrication syndrome: diagnosis with rose bengal staining, *Ophthalmology* 101:763, 1994.

114. McCulley JP, Moore MB, Matoba AY: Mucus fishing syndrome, *Ophthalmology* 92:1262, 1985.

115. Theodore FH: Conjunctival carcinoma masquerading as chronic conjunctivitis, *Eye Ear Nose Throat Monthly* 46:1419, 1967.

116. Brownstein S, Codere F, Jackson WB: Masquerade syndrome, *Ophthalmology* 87:259, 1980.

117. Irvine AR: Diffuse epibulbar squamous cell epithelioma, *Am J Ophthalmol* 64:550, 1967.

118. Wolfe JT et al: Sebaceous carcinoma of the eyelid: errors in clinical and pathologic diagnosis, *Am J Surg Pathol* 8:597, 1984.

119. Foster CD, Allansmith MR: Chronic unilateral

blepharoconjunctivitis caused by sebaceous carcinoma, *Am J Ophthalmol* 86:218, 1978.

120. Condon GP, Brownstein S, Codere F: Sebaceous cell carcinoma of the eyelid masquerading as superior limbal keratoconjunctivitis, *Arch Ophthalmol* 103:1525, 1985.
121. Paronia I: Reiter's disease, *Acta Med Scand* 131(suppl 213):1, 1948.
122. Saari KM, Kaurenen O: Ocular inflammation in Reiter's syndrome associated with *Campylobacter jejuni* enteritis, *Am J Ophthalmol* 90:572, 1980.
123. Saari KM et al: Ocular inflammation in Reiter's disease after *Salmonella* enteritis, *Am J Ophthalmol* 90:63, 1980.
124. Week LA et al: Urethritis associated with *Chlamydia*: clinical and laboratory diagnosis, *Minn Med* 59:288, 1976.
125. Martin DH et al: *Chlamydia trachomatis* infections in men with Reiter's syndrome, *Ann Intern Med* 100:207, 1984.
126. Calin A, Fries JF: An "experimental" epidemic of Reiter's syndrome revisited: follow-up evidence of genetic and environmental factors, *Arthritis Rheum* 84:564, 1976.
127. Willkens RF et al: Reiter's syndrome: evaluation of preliminary criteria for definite disease, *Arthritis Rheum* 24:844, 1981.
128. Keat A: Reiter's syndrome and reactive arthritis in perspective, *N Engl J Med* 309:1606, 1983.
129. Lee DA et al: The clinical diagnosis of Reiter's syndrome: ophthalmic and nonophthalmic aspects, *Ophthalmology* 93:350, 1986.
130. Ostler HB et al: Reiter's syndrome, *Am J Ophthalmol* 71:986, 1971.
131. Mills RP, Kalina RE: Reiter's keratitis, *Arch Ophthalmol* 87:447, 1972.
132. Wiggins RE, Steinkuller PG, Hamill MB: Reiter's keratoconjunctivitis, *Arch Ophthalmol* 108:280, 1990.
133. Meade R, Brandt L: Manifestations of Kawasaki disease in New England outbreak of 1980, *J Pediatr* 100:558, 1982.
134. Ammerman S et al: Diagnostic uncertainty in atypical Kawasaki disease and a new finding: exudative conjunctivitis, *Pediatr Infect Dis* 4:210, 1985.
135. Burns J et al: Anterior uveitis associated with Kawasaki syndrome, *Pediatr Infect Dis* 4:258, 1985.
136. Ohno S et al: Ocular manifestations of Kawasaki's disease (mucocutaneous lymph node syndrome), *Am J Ophthalmol* 93:713, 1982.
137. Theodore FH: The collected letters of the International Correspondence Society of Ophthalmologists and Otolaryngologists, Series 6, June 30, 1961, p. 89.
138. Theodore FH: Superior limbal keratoconjunctivitis, *Eye Ear Nose Throat Monthly* 442:25, 1963.
139. Thygeson P: Further observations on superficial punctate keratitis, *Arch Ophthalmol* 66:158, 1961.
140. Thygeson P: Observations of filamentary keratitis. Transactions of the 102nd annual meeting of the American Medical Association, Section of Ophthalmology, 1963.
141. Thygeson P, Kimura SJ: Chronic conjunctivitis, *Trans Am Acad Ophthalmol Otolaryngol* 67:494, 1963.
142. Grayson M, Wilson FM II: Superior limbal keratoconjunctivitis, *Perspect Ophthalmol* 1:234, 1977.
143. Theodore FH: Further observations on superior limbal keratoconjunctivitis, *Trans Am Acad Ophthalmol Otolaryngol* 71:341, 1967.
144. Cher I: Clinical features of superior limbal keratoconjunctivitis in Australia: a probable association with thyrotoxicosis, *Arch Ophthalmol* 82:580, 1969.
145. Corwin ME: Superior limbal keratoconjunctivitis, *Am J Ophthalmol* 66:338, 1968.
146. Sutherland AL: Superior limbal keratoconjunctivitis, *Trans Ophthalmol Soc N Z* 21:89, 1969.
147. Tenzel RR: Comments on superior limbal filamentous keratitis, *Arch Ophthalmol* 79:508, 1968.
148. Theodore FH: Comments on findings of elevated protein bound iodine in superior limbal keratoconjunctivitis, *Arch Ophthalmol* 79:508, 1968.
149. Wright P: Superior limbal keratoconjunctivitis, *Trans Ophthalmol Soc UK* 92:555, 1972.
150. Theodore FH: *Diagnostic dyes in superior limbal keratoconjunctivitis and other superficial entities.* In Turtz AI, editor: Proceedings of the Centennial Symposium: Manhattan Eye, Ear and Throat Hospital, vol 1: *Ophthalmology,* St Louis, 1969, Mosby–Year Book.
151. Theodore FH, Ferry AP: Superior limbal keratoconjunctivitis: clinical and pathological correlations, *Arch Ophthalmol* 84:481, 1970.
152. Wander AH, Musukawa T: Unusual appearance of condensed chromatin in conjunctival cells in superior limbal keratoconjunctivitis, *Lancet* 2:42, 1981.
153. Collin HB et al: Keratinization of the bulbar conjunctival epithelium in superior limbal keratoconjunctivitis: an electron microscopic study, *Acta Ophthalmol (Copenh)* 56:531, 1978.
154. Donshik PC et al: Conjunctival resection treatment and ultrastructural histopathology of superior limbal keratoconjunctivitis, *Am J Ophthalmol* 85:101, 1978.
155. Collin HB et al: The fine structure of nuclear changes in superior limbal keratoconjunctivitis, *Invest Ophthalmol Vis Sci* 17:79, 1978.
156. Eiferman RA, Wilkins EL: Immunologic aspects of superior limbal keratoconjunctivitis, *Can J Ophthalmol* 14:85, 1979.
157. Wilson FM, Ostler HB: Superior limbal keratoconjunctivitis, *Int Ophthalmol Clin* 26:99, 1986.
158. Ostler HB: *Superior limbal keratoconjunctivitis.* In Smolin G, Thoft RA, editors: *The cornea: scientific foundations and clinical practice,* Boston, 1987, Little, Brown & Co.
159. Grayson M, Pieroni D: Severe silver nitrate

injury to the eye, *Am J Ophthalmol* 70:227, 1970.

160. Laughrea PA, Arentsen JJ, Laibson PR: Iatrogenic ocular silver nitrate burn, *Cornea* 4:47, 1985.

161. Mondino BJ, Zaidman GW, Salamon SW: Use of pressure patching and soft contact lenses in superior limbal keratoconjunctivitis, *Arch Ophthalmol* 100:1932, 1982.

162. Confino J, Brown SI: Treatment of superior limbal keratoconjunctivitis with topical cromolyn sodium, *Ann Ophthalmol* 19:129, 1987.

163. Udell IJ et al: Treatment of superior limbal keratoconjunctivitis by thermocauterization of the superior bulbar conjunctiva, *Ophthalmology* 93:162, 1986.

164. Tenzel K: Resistant superior limbal keratoconjunctivitis, *Arch Ophthalmol* 89:439, 1973.

165. Passons GA, Wood TO: Conjunctival resection for superior limbal keratoconjunctivitis, *Ophthalmology* 91:966, 1984.

166. Mackie IA: Botulinum toxin in the management of theodore's superior limbal keratoconjunctivitis, presented at the Ocular Microbiology and Immunology Group meeting, Atlanta, October, 1995.

167. Wilson FM: *Differential diagnosis of superior limbal keratoconjunctivitis and papillary keratoconjunctivitis associated with contact lenses.* In Hughes WF, editor: *Year Book of Ophthalmology 1981,* Chicago, 1981, Mosby–Year Book.

168. Miller RA, Brightbill FS, Slama SL: Superior limbal keratoconjunctivitis in soft contact lens wearers, *Cornea* 1:293, 1982.

169. Stenson S: Superior limbal keratoconjunctivitis associated with soft contact lens wear, *Arch Ophthalmol* 101:402, 1983.

170. Fuerst DJ, Sugar J, Worobec S: Superior limbal keratoconjunctivitis associated with cosmetic soft contact lens wear, *Arch Ophthalmol* 101:1214, 1983.

171. Sendele DD et al: Superior limbal keratoconjunctivitis in contact lens wearers, *Ophthalmology* 90:616, 1983.

172. Bloomfield SE, Jakobiec FA, Theodore FH: Contact lens induced keratopathy: a severe complication extending the spectrum of keratoconjunctivitis in contact lens wearers, *Ophthalmology* 91:290, 1984.

173. Carpel EF: Superior limbal conjunctivitis, *Arch Ophthalmol* 102:662, 1984 (letter).

174. Kenyon KR, Tseng SC: Limbal autograft transplantation for ocular surface disorders, *Ophthalmology* 96:709, 1989.

175. Jenkins C et al: Limbal transplantation in the management of chronic contact-lens-associated epitheliopathy, *Eye* 7:629, 1993.

176. Clinch TF, Goins KM, Cobo LM: Treatment of contact lens-related ocular surface disorders with autologous conjunctival transplantation, *Ophthalmology* 99:634, 1992.

177. Tsae RJ, Sun TT, Tseng SC: Comparison of limbal and conjunctival autograft transplantation in corneal surface reconstruction in rabbits, *Ophthalmology* 97:446, 1990.

178. Firat T: Ligneous conjunctivitis, *Am J Ophthalmol* 78:679, 1974.

179. Firat T, Tinaztepe B: Histochemical investigations on ligneous conjunctivitis and a new method of treatment, *Acta Ophthalmol (Copenh)* 48:3, 1970.

180. Hidayat AA, Riddle PJ: Ligneous conjunctivitis: a clinicopathologic study of 17 cases, *Ophthalmology* 94:949, 1987.

181. McGrand JC, Rees DM, Garry J: Ligneous conjunctivitis, *Br J Ophthalmol* 53:373, 1969.

182. Spaeth GL: Chronic membranous conjunctivitis: a persisting problem, *Am J Ophthalmol* 64:300, 1967.

183. Spencer LM, Straatsma BR, Foos RY: Ligneous conjunctivitis, *Am J Ophthalmol* 80:365, 1968.

184. Ostler HB: *Diseases of the external eye and adnexa: a text and atlas,* Baltimore, 1993, Williams & Wilkins.

185. Girard LJ, Veselinovic A, Font RL: Ligneous conjunctivitis after pingueculae removal in an adult, *Cornea* 8:7, 1989.

186. Bierly JR et al: Ligneous conjunctivitis as a complication following strabismus surgery, *J Pediatr Ophthalmol Strabismus* 31:99, 1994.

187. Marcus DM et al: Ligneous conjunctivitis with ear involvement, *Arch Ophthalmol* 108:514, 1990.

188. Cooper TJ, Kazdan JJ, Cutz E: Ligneous conjunctivitis with tracheal obstruction: a case report, with electron microscopy findings, *Can J Ophthalmol* 14:57, 1979.

189. Cohen SR: Ligneous conjunctivitis: an ophthalmic disease with potentially fatal tracheobronchial obstruction. Laryngeal and tracheobronchial features, *Ann Otol Rhinol Laryngol* 99:509, 1990.

190. Holland EJ et al: Immunohistochemical findings and results of treatment with cyclosporine in ligneous conjunctivitis, *Am J Ophthalmol* 107:160, 1989.

191. Bateman JB et al: Ligneous conjunctivitis: an autosomal recessive disorder, *J Pediatr Ophthalmol Strabismus* 23:137, 1986.

192. Francois J, Victoria-Troncoso V: Treatment of ligneous conjunctivitis, *Am J Ophthalmol* 65:674, 1968.

193. Melikian HE: Treatment of ligneous conjunctivitis, *Ann Ophthalmol* 17:763, 1985.

194. Rubin BI et al: Response of reactivated ligneous conjunctivitis to topical cyclosporine, *Am J Ophthalmol* 112:95, 1991.

195. Kaan G, Ozden O: Therapeutic use of topical cyclosporine, *Ann Ophthalmol* 25:182, 1993.

196. Berlin AJ et al: Scleral grafting in the management of ligneous conjunctivitis, *Ophthalmic Surg* 13:288, 1982.

197. De Cock R et al: Topical heparin in the treatment of ligneous conjunctivitis, *Ophthalmology* 102:1654, 1995.

Nine

Approach to Diseases of the Cornea

To aid the diagnosis of corneal disease it is useful to categorize diseases according to clinical findings, as was done for conjunctival disease in Chapter 6 (Table 9-1). The differential diagnosis can be greatly reduced using even a limited number of characteristics. The presence or absence of each of the following are useful in categorization: epithelial ulceration (not punctate or focal fluorescein staining), vascularization, thinning, inflammatory cell infiltration, accumulation of noninflammatory material, and suppuration (liquid pus and tissue necrosis). The location of the disease, whether central, diffuse, or marginal (within 3 mm of the limbus), and the layer(s) involved are clearly important. Whether or not vision is decreased and whether the disease is unilateral or bilateral can also be useful.

ULCERATIVE KERATITIS

Infiltrative Ulcerative Keratitis
Infiltrative ulcerative keratitis is usually caused by infection. Bacterial infection is most common, but fungal, parasitic, and viral infections also occur (Table 9-2). These infections most commonly involve the central cornea, but marginal or ring infections can occur. Noninfectious infiltrative ulcerative keratitis is more common in the peripheral cornea. Immunologic infiltrates associated with lid disease (catarrhal infiltrates) and sterile contact lens–related infiltrates are the most common types of marginal infiltrative ulcerative keratitis, but many systemic inflammatory diseases (e.g., collagen vascular diseases) can also cause infiltrative ulcerative marginal keratitis.

Central
A central corneal infection is a threat to vision and to the eye itself; it is a true ocular emergency. Therefore, it is important to learn to diagnose and treat corneal infectious infiltrates and ulcers. Clues to the cause of the infiltration

Table 9-1 Clinical Classification of Corneal Diseases

ULCERATIVE
  Infiltrative (suppurative)
    Central
    Marginal
  Noninfiltrative
    Central
    Marginal

EPITHELIAL
  Staining
  Filaments
  Vascularization
  Accumulations
  Thickening and opacification
  Intraepithelial cysts

SUBEPITHELIAL
  Infiltrative
  Accumulations

STROMAL
  Inflammatory
    Noninfiltrative edema (disciform keratitis)
    Infiltrative (interstitial keratitis)
      Suppurative
  Noninflammatory
    Central/diffuse
      Edema
      Accumulations
      Thinning
    Localized
    Marginal
      Edema
      Accumulations
      Thinning

POSTERIOR STROMAL
  Accumulations

DESCEMET'S/ENDOTHELIUM
  Accumulation
  Inflammation
  Endothelial cell abnormalities

Table 9-2 Central Infiltrative Ulcerative Keratitis

INFECTIOUS
  Bacteria
    Nearly all bacterial pathogens. Most common:
      Staphylococci
      Streptococci
      Pseudomonas spp.
      Serratia spp.
      Escherichia coli
      Moraxella spp.
  Fungi
    Candida
    Fusarium
    Aspergillus
    Penicillium
    Cephalosporium
    Others
  Viruses
    Herpes simplex
    Varicella
    Mumps
    Cytomegalovirus (in newborns)
    Measles (in kwashiorkor syndrome or vitamin A deficiency)
  Parasites
    Acanthamoeba spp.
    Nosema spp.

STERILE
  Contact lens–related infiltrates
  Catarrhal infiltrates
  Persistent epithelial defects

can be derived from a history and clinical examination, but in most cases laboratory testing is necessary. Some diagnostic points are provided here. The initial laboratory evaluation and treatment are discussed in the next sections.

Bacterial ulcers are usually accompanied by conjunctival infection and chemosis, lid edema, decreased vision, pain, tearing, photophobia, and purulent discharge. The corneal epithelium is ulcerated and there is gray-white to yellow stromal infiltration, sometimes with necrosis and stromal loss. The surrounding cornea is often edematous. Anterior chamber cells,

inflammatory endothelial plaques, and hypopyon can be present.

Fungal ulcerative keratitis can be indistinguishable from bacterial keratitis, but in some cases differentiating characteristics are present. A history of trauma with plant matter is suggestive of fungal infection. In some fungal infections, particularly those caused by filamentous fungi, the infiltrate margins are feathery, with irregular extensions into the adjacent stroma (see Fig. 11-5). The surface of the infiltrate can be elevated above the plane of the uninvolved cornea (see Fig. 11-4). Satellite lesions, foci of infiltration up to several millimeters away from the main area of infiltrate, as well as ring infiltrates surrounding the main infiltrate can be present (see Fig. 11-6). The course is often one of slow progression.

Herpes simplex infection is seen most commonly as an epithelial dendrite, subepithelial scarring, or disciform edema, and these are usually relatively easy to differentiate from bacterial keratitis. Less often a necrotizing, infiltrative keratitis occurs (see Fig. 12-13), probably caused by active viral proliferation in the stroma, and this presents more of a diagnostic dilemma. A history of previous herpetic keratitis or of recurrent ocular disease may be elicited. In herpetic infection corneal sensitivity is usually decreased, and this can be a helpful feature. However, bacterial and herpetic ulcers can be indistinguishable clinically, and bacterial infection often occurs in patients with corneas scarred by previous herpetic infection. Therefore, laboratory diagnosis often is required. In herpetic keratitis scrapings may contain multinucleated giant cells, and viral culture or immunologic tests can confirm the diagnosis.

Central stromal infiltration and ulceration rarely occur in varicella (chickenpox), mumps, measles, and cytomegalovirus infection. The systemic disease is clearly evident, but whether the corneal disease is caused by viral infection or secondary bacterial infection cannot be determined without laboratory examination. Corneal ulceration in measles occurs mainly in the setting of kwashiorkor syndrome or vitamin A deficiency. Cytomegalovirus corneal ulceration affects newborn infants with disseminated disease and immunosuppressed hosts.

Acanthamoeba corneal infections occur in contact lens wearers or after trauma in non–contact lens wearers. These patients usually exhibit a slowly progressive course, with exacerbations and remissions. The amount of pain is often greater than would be expected from the appearance. Radial perineural infiltrates (diagnostic), decreased sensation, an adjacent scleritis, and surrounding ring infiltrates are common (see Figs. 11-12 to 11-16). The diagnosis can often be made clinically. Scrapings, culture, and, in some cases biopsy, should be performed if acanthamoeba infection is suspected.

Sterile infiltrates often occur in contact lens wearers, and it can be very difficult to differentiate these from infectious infiltrates. Sterile infiltrates tend to be smaller (<1 mm), multiple, or arcuate in shape, and tend not to be associated with significant pain, discharge, epithelial defect, or anterior chamber reaction (Fig. 9-1).[1] In some cases these infiltrates appear to be reactions to thimerosal use (Fig. 9-2). However, it is not possible to be certain that any infiltrate is sterile. Therefore for any infiltrate associated with lens wear, it is best to discontinue lens wear, scrape and culture, forgo patching the eye, and follow up with the patient closely. Depending on the degree of suspicion of infection and the severity of the infiltrate, regular-strength or fortified antibiotics are administered.

Catarrhal ulcers are an immunologic reaction to organisms on the lid margin, most commonly staphylococci. They usually affect the marginal cornea, but can occur centrally, particularly if previous inflammation has caused superficial vascularization to extend to the central cornea. The ulcers are usually small (<1 mm), and more than one may be present (see Fig. 19-27).

Noninfectious infiltration can affect a preexistent epithelial defect. Typically, multiple small infiltrates occur at the margin of the defect.

Laboratory Evaluation. Scrapings and bacterial, fungal, and viral cultures should be obtained in nearly all cases. Only if the infiltrate and epithelial defect are less than 1 mm in diameter, the patient is not immunocompromised, and there is no marked anterior chamber reaction can empiric broad-spectrum antibacterial therapy be given without obtaining cultures. Every ophthalmologist should be equipped to take adequate scrapings of the ulcer and should know how to interpret the findings. The techniques of obtaining corneal specimens, staining, and culture media are discussed in detail in Chapter 4. Briefly, corneal smears should be obtained for Gram's and Giemsa staining, and specimens should be inoculated onto blood agar, chocolate agar, and thioglycolate broth. If fungal infection is suspected, a smear should be examined with a fungal stain (e.g., periodic acid–Schiff or Gomori methenamine-silver), and a fungal medium such as Sabouraud's dextrose agar should be inoculated.

If the patient has been wearing contact lenses, the lens case and lens care solutions should be cultured. In some cases these will indicate the causative organism(s) when corneal cultures do not. Similarly, if a patient has been taking ocular medications, specimens from each should be taken for culture.

Initial Antibiotic Therapy. Initial treatment is based on the interpretation of the corneal smears and a clinical assessment of the severity of the keratitis. If bacteria, fungi, amoeba, or other agents are identified in the smear, and the history and examination are consistent with infection caused by the identified agent, specific treatment for that agent is instituted. If a causative agent is not identified, bacterial keratitis should be suspected and antibiotic treatment should be given until a more definitive diagnosis can be made.

The therapy given depends on the severity of the keratitis, the presence of other ocular disease, and the immunologic status of the host.

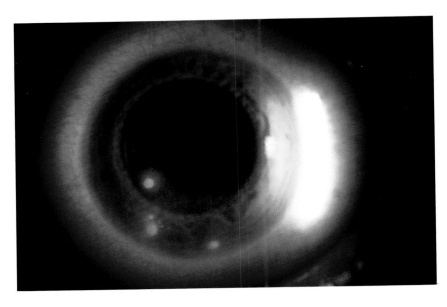

Figure 9-1
Sterile corneal infiltrates associated with contact lens wear.

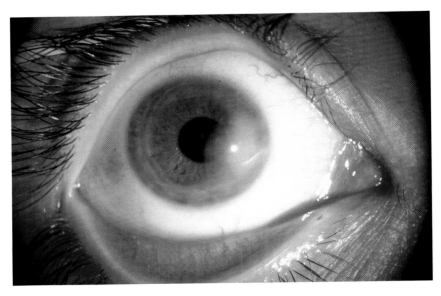

Figure 9-2
Sterile corneal infiltrates associated with contact lens wear. This patient exhibited a reaction to thimerosal on patch testing. (Courtesy of Diane Curtin, Pittsburgh, PA.)

This is a situation in which the experience and clinical judgement of the physician has a strong influence on the decisions made. If there is any question about the course to take it is usually safer to use more aggressive antibiotic treatment. Broad-spectrum antibiotic treatment can be obtained with ciprofloxacin, ofloxacin, or a combination of fortified agents, such as cefazolin, 50 mg/ml, and tobramycin, 14 mg/ml. These antibiotics should be administered every 30 minutes to every 3 hours. Antibiotic treatment is discussed further in Chapter 10.

Marginal

Both infectious and immunologic infiltrates can occur in the limbal cornea (Table 9-3). Catarrhal infiltrates related to staphylococcal

Table 9-3	Marginal Infiltrative Ulcerative Keratitis

INFECTIOUS
  Bacteria
    Neisseria spp.
    Staphylococcus spp.
    Streptococcus pyogenes
    Haemophilus spp.
    Moraxella lacunata
    Actinomyces
    Clostridium diphtheriae
    Coliforms
    Syphilis
    Pseudomonas spp.
  Fungi
    Candida
  Viruses
    Herpes simplex
    Influenza
    Varicella

STERILE
  Catarrhal infiltrates
  Phlyctenulosis
  Acne rosacea
  Psoriasis
  Systemic inflammatory diseases
    Rheumatoid arthritis
    Systemic lupus erythematosus
    Discoid lupus erythematosus
    Progressive systemic sclerosis
    Relapsing polychondritis
    Inflammatory bowel disease
    Polyarteritis nodosa
    Wegener's granulomatosis

blepharitis are probably most common. These are typically 0.5 to 2 mm long, located approximately 1 mm central to the limbal vessels, and are associated with an epithelial defect (see Fig. 19-28). However, infectious infiltrates can have the same appearance. One helpful differentiating feature is that catarrhal infiltrates are often multiple, while infectious ulcers are rarely so. The presence of blepharitis or meibomitis and evidence of previous marginal inflammation suggests catarrhal ulceration.

Virtually any organism that can infect the central cornea can also produce an infection that primarily involves the marginal cornea. Marginal corneal ulcers can also occur as a complication of bacterial conjunctivitis. *Neisseria* spp., *Staphylococcus* spp., *Streptococcus pyogenes*, *Haemophilus aegyptius*, *Haemophilus influenzae*, *Moraxella lacunata*, *Actinomyces*, *Clostridium diphtheriae*, coliforms, and syphilis infections can be associated with marginal corneal infiltrates.[2] Marginal infiltrates can also be associated with food allergies, influenza, and bacillary dysentery.

Occasionally, catarrhal infiltrates and infiltrates associated with bacterial conjunctivitis will coalesce to form a ring ulcer (see Fig. 10-4). More commonly, ring ulcers occur after penetrating trauma. *Pseudomonas aeruginosa, Proteus* spp., *Staphylococcus aureus, Escherichia coli, Bacillus* spp.,[3] *Actinomyces* spp., and *Streptococcus* spp.[4] can cause ring ulcers.

Blood-borne organisms can also cause a marginal corneal infection. This type of infection (called *metastatic*) begins in the limbal stroma as a yellowish infiltrate. It progresses rapidly to form an abscess, and spreads circumferentially as well as anteriorly and posteriorly. If not treated, it breaks through to the surface and produces a ring ulcer.

Phlyctenulosis is an inflammation of the conjunctiva or cornea that appears to be a cell-mediated hypersensitivity to a topical infectious antigen (see Chapter 19). Small marginal ulcers occur central to areas of superficial vascularization (see Figs. 19-27 and 19-28). Multiple ulcers, evidence of previous episodes, triangular corneal scars (with their base at the limbus), and lid inflammation may be present. Associated infections include *S. aureus, Mycobacterium tuberculosis, Coccidioides immitis,* and *Candida* spp. Similar appearing lesions can occur in acne rosacea and psoriasis (see Chapter 22).

Peripheral corneal ulceration can occur in autoimmune diseases, particularly rheumatoid arthritis, or in Mooren's ulceration. These ulcers typically develop in a concentric shape near the limbus and may be associated with adjacent scleritis (see Figs. 19-3, 19-11, and 19-18). Cellular infiltration is usually minimal or absent, but marked infiltration can occur. Necrotizing scleritis of any etiology can be associated with infiltrated marginal ulceration.

Laboratory Evaluation. Scrapings and cultures (bacterial, fungal, and viral) should be obtained from most marginal infiltrated ulcers, and certainly all those greater than 1 mm in diameter. If bacteria are seen on Gram's stain or if the etiology of the ulcer is unclear, broad-spectrum antibiotic therapy should be administered (see previous section). Cultures should also be taken from the lid margin if the infiltrates appear to be catarrhal or phlyctenular. Lid hygiene should be initiated and an antibiotic ointment applied to the lid margin four times daily.

Differentiation of marginal ulceration related to systemic inflammatory disease from infectious ulceration can be difficult. Often, cultures need to be taken and antibiotic treatment initiated because the possibility of infection cannot be eliminated. If these diseases are suspected, systemic evaluation should be performed. Systemic and local treatment is necessary (see Chapter 19).

Noninfiltrative Ulcerative Keratitis

Central

Central epithelial defects can develop from many causes. The most common causes are probably trauma and recurrent erosions, and these are associated with mild ocular inflammation. Central epithelial defects also develop in eyes with severe conjunctivitis, such as epidemic keratoconjunctivitis and gonorrhea. Other causes include dry eye, exposure, and neurotrophic keratitis. Stromal ulceration can occur with any epithelial defect, with or without infection. Sometimes an infection is present without infiltration. This occurs occasionally with bacterial infection, usually at an early stage, and is often associated with contact lens wear. Acanthamoeba, herpes simplex, and nonvirulent fungi can also cause an ulcerative noninfiltrative keratitis.

More often, the stromal ulceration is noninfectious. This can occur in the presence of any chronic epithelial defect but is especially likely when keratitis sicca is present or topical corticosteroids are administered. Stromal lysis and even perforation can occur. These ulcers are usually located in the interpalpebral space, where the cornea is more prone to the effects of drying.

Scrapings and bacterial and viral cultures should be obtained from any ulcer with a persistent epithelial defect or stromal loss. If infection is not present, treatment is directed at determining the cause of the ulceration and promoting epithelial healing (see Chapter 15).

Marginal

Most cases of noninfiltrative marginal ulceration are noninfectious (Table 9-4). Many systemic inflammatory diseases can be associated with marginal corneal ulceration. In many of these cases adjacent scleral inflammation is also present; however, symptoms are often mild (see Fig. 19-2). The ulcers usually progress circumferentially more than centrally. Superficial vascularization often accompanies epithelialization.

Serious ocular and systemic complications can occur in these diseases, so their presence must be recognized. All patients with marginal noninfiltrative keratitis should be questioned about the presence of these diseases, and a "re-

Table 9-4	Causes of Noninfiltrative Marginal Ulceration
Systemic inflammatory diseases	
Rheumatoid arthritis	
Systemic lupus erythematosus	
Relapsing polychondritis	
Inflammatory bowel disease	
Polyarteritis nodosa	
Wegener's granulomatosis	
Mooren's ulcer	
Herpes simplex	
Exposure	
Psoriasis	
Necrotizing scleritis	
Posttrauma	
Postsurgery	

view of symptoms" is a specific part of patient history. Referral to an internist or rheumatologist for further investigation is often appropriate. If systemic inflammatory disease is present, systemic therapy must be initiated or, or if already administered, altered. These diseases are covered in more detail in Chapter 19.

Clinically identical ulceration occurs in many patients without systemic inflammatory disease, and is called Mooren's ulcer (see Figs. 19-33 to 19-35). Usually seen in the elderly, Mooren's ulcer is usually painful and unilateral. Similar ulceration can also occur after trauma or surgery (e.g., cataract extraction, penetrating keratoplasty). Some of these cases are associated with systemic inflammatory disease, dry eyes, or steroid treatment. Necrotizing scleritis of any cause can be associated with marginal corneal ulceration.

Limbal herpes simplex is usually associated with infiltration, but in some cases ulceration can occur without an infiltrate. The ulcers are usually small and are often associated with decreased corneal sensation, superficial vascularization, and anterior chamber reaction.

NONULCERATIVE INFLAMMATORY KERATITIS

Epithelial Disease
Epithelial Staining

Punctate epithelial keratitis can result from any disease of the corneal epithelium. It accompanies many forms of lid and conjunctival inflammation as well as corneal disease. This is discussed in Chapter 3.

Focal epithelial keratitis is a term that can be

Condition	Usual Location and Number of Filaments
Herpes simplex (transitory)	Usually single filament
Sutures/wound	One to a few near suture or wound
After corneal abrasion and erosion (transitory)	Usually at the site of erosion or abrasion
Occlusion (including ptosis)	Diffuse
Keratoconjunctivitis sicca Psoriasis (rare)	Interpalpebral
Superior limbal keratoconjunctivitis	Upper third of cornea
Neurotrophic keratopathy	Interpalpebral
Toxicity from topical ophthalmic medications	Lower third of cornea
Bullous keratopathy	Diffuse

Table 9-5   Filaments

used to describe the coarser or grouped epithelial lesions, which may be seen in a number of diseases (see Fig. 3-12). These lesions appear like the cytopathologic effect caused by some viruses in culture, and in many cases represent a similar process occurring in the corneal epithelium. They may contain white flecks, and stain irregularly with fluorescein, with areas of dye uptake and negative staining due to elevation. Inflammatory cells may be present within the epithelial lesions. The following diseases cause these lesions:

1. Adenoviral keratoconjunctivitis
2. Thygeson's superficial punctate keratitis
3. Herpes simplex
4. Herpes zoster
5. Adult inclusion conjunctivitis
6. Drug toxicity
7. Vaccinia
8. Measles
9. Mumps
10. Varicella

A distinct type of epithelial disease occurs in vernal conjunctivitis. *Farinaceous epitheliopathy* consists of tiny, gray-white, intraepithelial opacities, which appear like a dusting of flour and stain with fluorescein and rose bengal. They are most prominent in the superior cornea, and there is relative sparing of the periphery. In severe disease the epithelium can take on the appearance of a cobweb or syncytium (see Fig. 8-8).

Epithelial dendrites occur only in herpes simplex, varicella, and herpes zoster viruses. However, other lesions can be dendritic in shape: mucoid plaque, healing epithelial defect, acanthamoeba infection, and tyrosinosis. Early herpes lesions can be stellate rather than dendritic.

Filaments

The presence of filaments is a nonspecific clinical sign, but the etiology can usually be determined by examination (Table 9-5). Epithelial filaments appear as small mucoid deposits adherent to the corneal surface (see Fig. 3-11). They stain with fluorescein and rose bengal. The mechanism of their formation is controversial. Filaments consist of a coil of epithelial cells attached to the cornea at one end, with adherent mucus and other debris. They are associated with irritation and foreign body sensation. Following is a list of the conditions that should be considered when filamentary keratitis is observed:

1. Superior limbic keratoconjunctivitis
2. Ptosis or lid occlusion in adults
3. Keratoconjunctivitis sicca
4. Neuroparalytic keratopathy
5. Recurrent erosions
6. Corneal trauma
7. Neurotrophic keratopathy
8. Herpes simplex keratitis
9. Chronic bullous keratopathy
10. Toxicity from topical ophthalmic medications
11. Corneal surgery/sutures
12. Brain stem injury
13. Atopic dermatitis

Filaments are often transient, related to an acute temporary condition, such as patching or a healing dendrite. In these cases simple removal of the filament is often sufficient treatment. When filaments are chronic or recurrent, measures must be taken to reduce or prevent filament formation. If possible the underlying condition should be treated: artificial tears or punctal occlusion for dry eye; surgical correction for ptosis; silver nitrate or conjunctival cautery for superior limbic keratoconjunctivitis. Hypertonic drops and ointment (5% NaCl) four times daily often reduce filament formation. Application of a bandage contact lens can be effective in severe cases. The lens can often be removed after several weeks without recurrence of filaments.

Superficial Vascularization

Superficial corneal vascularization can occur with chronic or recurrent corneal inflamma-

Table 9-6	Causes of Superficial Corneal Vascularization

ULCERATIVE KERATITIS
Any bacterial, fungal, viral, or parasitic infection
Herpes simplex (most common)
Persistent epithelial defects
Marginal ulceration due to systemic inflammatory disease

CONJUNCTIVITIS
Trachoma
Adult inclusion conjunctivitis
Atopic keratoconjunctivitis
Vernal keratoconjunctivitis
Superior limbal keratoconjunctivitis
Conjunctival scarring

SKIN DISEASE
Acne rosacea
Cicatricial pemphigoid
Erythema multiforme
Toxic epidermal necrolysis
Epidermolysis bullosa
Psoriasis
Keratosis follicularis spinulosa decalvans
Hydroa vacciniforme
Keratitis-ichthyosis-deafness syndrome
Xeroderma pigmentosum
Acanthosis nigricans

PHLYCTENULOSIS
LID DISEASE
Staphylococcal blepharitis
Trichiasis
Entropion
Exposure

TRAUMA
Lacerations
Chemical
Thermal
Radiation

LIMBAL TUMORS
PRIMARY CORNEAL AMYLOIDOSIS
CONTACT LENS WEAR
SCLERITIS
PORPHYRIA
ANIRIDIA
TERRIEN'S MARGINAL DEGENERATION
PTERYGIUM
ONCHOCERCIASIS

Table 9-7	Patterns of Vascularization

SUPERIOR VASCULARIZATION WITHOUT STROMAL DISEASE
Superior limbal keratoconjunctivitis
Adult inclusion conjunctivitis
Trachoma
Vernal keratoconjunctivitis
Contact lens wear

INFERIOR VASCULARIZATION MOST PROMINENT
Staphylococcal blepharitis
Cicatricial pemphigoid
Entropion
Psoriasis

ARCUATE-SHAPED MARGINAL VASCULARIZATION WITH STROMAL THINNING AND OPACIFICATION
Systemic inflammatory diseases
Mooren's ulcer
Scleritis
Terrien's marginal degeneration

SPECIFIC TYPES OF VASCULARIZATION
Phlyctenulosis
Pterygium
Aniridia

tion, severe acute inflammation, or ulcerative keratitis (Table 9-6). Evidence of skin disease, lid position abnormalities, blepharitis, meibomitis, and chronic conjunctival inflammation should be sought.

In many cases with longstanding vascularization the cause of the vascularization cannot be determined from examination, and the history provided by the patient will be more elucidating. However, some clues can be gleaned from the location of vascularization and the presence or absence of stromal thinning and opacification (Table 9-7). For example, scars left by phlyctenulosis are typically triangular, with the base at the limbus. Stromal thinning can occur with repeated attacks. Progressive corneal vascularization occurs in patients with aniridia, eventually leading to vascularization and superficial opacification of the entire corneal surface.

Accumulations

Substances can accumulate in the corneal epithelium in a vortex (whorllike) pattern (see Fig. 24-11) (Table 9-8). The pattern reflects the growth pattern of the epithelial cells. Cells move centrally from the limbus, and the greatest desquamation occurs slightly below the center of the cornea. Therefore, materials that accumulate progressively in epithelial cells are seen in highest concentration centrally and least near the limbus. Many of the drugs associated with this picture exhibit cationic amphiphilia, and it has been hypothesized that these drugs may penetrate lysosomes and form complexes with polar lipids, and that these complexes are unable to pass from the lysosomes or

Table 9-8 Cornea Verticillata

DISORDERS OF METABOLISM
Fabry's disease (see Figs. 21-12 and 21-13)
Tangier disease
Mucolipidosis type IV
Sialidosis

DRUGS
Amiodarone[8,9] (see Fig. 27-11)
Tilorone[7,10]
Naproxen[11]
Suramin[12]
Clofazimine[13]
Chloroquine and related drugs (hydroquinone, monobenzone) (see Fig. 24-10)
Chlorpromazine
Indomethacin[14]
Meperidine hydrochloride
Quinacrine
Tamoxifen

PIGMENT
Striate melanokeratosis
Iron

Table 9-9 Conditions Associated with Thickening and Opacification of the Corneal Epithelium

Chemical burns
Contact lens wear
Surgery
Aniridia (see Fig. 5-15)
Primary corneal epithelial dysplasia
Melkersson-Rosenthal syndrome
Tyrosinemia type II
Keratosis follicularis spinulosa decalvans
Refsum disease
Ichthyosis vulgaris
Pityriasis rubra pilaris
Keratosis follicularis

be degraded, resulting in progressive accumulation.[5-7] Usually no treatment is required, but in some cases the deposits are severe enough to interfere with vision. In this case epithelial debridement can be performed.

Iron deposition in the corneal epithelium occurs with aging and with conditions that disturb the normal pattern of epithelial migration over the cornea. The most common form of iron deposition is the *Hudson-Stähli line,* which is seen as a brown, green, yellow, or white irregular horizontal line in the deep central epithelium. Seen mainly in patients over 50 years of age, it may have a verticillate pattern. Epithelial iron deposition occurs adjacent to any elevation of the corneal surface, such as filtering blebs, pterygia, Salzmann's nodular degeneration, and corneal ectasia (e.g., keratoconus) (see Chapter 24).

Thickening and Opacification

Thickening and opacification of the epithelium occurs with chronic inflammation and vascularization. It is usually localized, and by itself not of diagnostic value. However, when epithelial thickening and opacification persist in the absence of inflammatory disease, several diagnoses must be considered. Conditions that disturb epithelial maturation and replenishment can cause peripheral or diffuse epithelial thickening and opacification (Table 9-9). Limbal epithelial stem cell injury can result from chemical burns, contact lens wear, and surgery. Sectoral,

wedge-shaped abnormalities or diffuse epithelial thickening and opacification can result. There may be a congenital abnormality of the limbal epithelium in aniridia.

In primary corneal epithelial dysplasia areas of frosted or opalescent epithelium, with smooth or fringelike (fimbriated) edges, are seen. They can be multiple, extend from the limbus or lie free in the cornea, and can be unilateral or bilateral. No limbal mass is present, and vascularization usually does not occur. They progress slowly, waxing and waning in their extent (see Chapter 27).

Amorphous gray-white epithelial and subepithelial deposits that can extend like fingers from the superior cornea can be seen in multiple myeloma (see Fig. 19-22). Corneal epithelial and stromal crystals can also be seen (see Fig. 19-21).

Thickening and opacification of the corneal epithelium occurs in Melkersson-Rosenthal syndrome, tyrosinemia type II, keratosis follicularis spinulosa decalvans, Refsum disease, ichthyosis, and pityriasis rubra pilaris. Thickening and opacification of Bowman's layer with overlying focal epithelial thickening and opacification occurs in Melkersson-Rosenthal syndrome (see Chapter 22). On retroillumination the lesions appear as a dense central horizontal core with graceful swirling rods resembling horse hair (see Fig. 22-58).

Bilateral central intraepithelial and subepithelial opacification occurs in tyrosinemia type II (Richner-Hanhart syndrome). The lesions are thick and plaquelike and may have a dendritic or sunburst configuration (see Fig. 21-31). Erosions and ulcerations can occur, but vascularization usually does not develop. Corneal involvement occurs in most cases and usually precedes the skin lesions. Circumferential pannus with diffuse, superficial, farinaceous opacities and thickening and irregularity of the epithelium is rarely seen in keratosis follicularis spinulosa decalvans (see Fig. 22-51*A*). Female carriers may show recurrent erosions, epithelial or subepithelial opacities, and prominent corneal nerves. Keratinization of the corneal epithelium can be seen in ichthyosis (see Figs. 22-42 and 25-43) and pityriasis rubra pilaris.

Epithelial biopsy should be performed if the diagnosis is unclear. Limbal epithelial transplantation may be helpful in some cases with limbal corneal injury.

Intraepithelial Cysts

Intraepithelial cysts are most commonly seen in epithelial basement membrane dystrophy (see Fig. 17-7). They can be unilateral or bilateral, localized or diffuse. Other signs of basement membrane abnormalities, such as fingerprints or geographic areas of opacification and elevation, can be present. Intraepithelial cysts can also be seen in contact lens wear, related to hypoxia, Meesmann's dystrophy (see Fig. 17-2), cytosine arabinoside treatment (see Fig. 24-12), and corneal edema. Meesmann's is an autosomal dominant condition in which bilateral central epithelial cysts are seen (see Chapter 17).

Subepithelial Disease
Subepithelial Infiltrates

Subepithelial infiltrates can follow active epithelial lesions, or they may occur without clinical epithelial involvement. Most cases occur concomitant with or subsequent to conjunctivitis (Table 9-10). Active subepithelial keratitis is associated with light sensitivity and in some cases decreased vision. The overlying epithelium can exhibit punctate fluorescein staining.

Irregular, dendritic, or relatively round subepithelial infiltrates can develop in herpes simplex and zoster infections. They usually develop as the epithelial lesions heal. Corneal sensation is often decreased. Stromal edema, stromal loss (thinning), and anterior chamber reaction are often present. In herpes zoster typical skin lesions are present.

Round subepithelial infiltrates often develop 8 to 15 days after the onset of epidemic keratoconjunctivitis (see Fig. 12-39). Multiple infiltrates are present, primarily affecting the central cornea. They can last for months or years and exhibit exacerbations. Similar, usually smaller and less persistent lesions can occur in pharyngoconjunctival fever, adult inclusion conjunctivitis (see Fig. 7-13), and trachoma. In trachoma, a gross pannus and conjunctival scarring can be present. The subepithelial le-

Table 9-10	Causes of Subepithelial Infiltration

ROUND (NUMMULAR), MULTIPLE
Viral
　Herpes simplex
　Herpes zoster
　Adenovirus (epidemic keratoconjunctivitis, pharyngoconjunctival fever)
　Acute hemorrhagic conjunctivitis
　Newcastle disease
　Infectious mononucleosis (peripheral)
Chlamydial
　Trachoma
　Adult inclusion conjunctivitis
Sterile contact lens–related infiltrates
Nummular keratitis (Dimmer's)
Cogan's interstitial keratitis (early)
Reiter's syndrome (peripheral)
Acanthamoeba (often fine)
Leprosy
Onchocerciasis
Corneal transplant rejection
?Lyme disease (usually multiple levels)

DENDRITIC, SINGLE
Herpes simplex
Herpes zoster
Varicella

IRREGULAR
Herpes simplex
Acanthamoeba
Healing phase of ulcerative keratitis (bacterial, fungal, or viral)
Posttrauma

sions may be as large as 2 mm and may scar. They are usually superficial and affect the superior cornea. In adult chlamydial keratoconjunctivitis subepithelial infiltrates can affect any portion of the cornea and can appear identical to those seen in adenoviral infection, although they are usually smaller. In each of these diseases there is a clear history of conjunctivitis preceding development of the lesions.

Brucellosis has also been reported as a cause of nummular keratitis.[15] In syphilis, subepithelial opacities can precede the interstitial keratitis and may be deep, round, and scattered. Early in the course of Cogan's interstitial keratitis the only sign may be peripheral subepithelial nummular infiltrates (see Fig. 19-32). Vestibuloauditory symptoms are usually present.

Fine (punctate) white opacities can affect the epithelium and subepithelial or anterior stroma in lepromatous leprosy (see Chapter 10). They do not stain with fluorescein, and may be surrounded by a gray, milky stromal opacity. The superior temporal cornea is most frequently affected. The *punctate keratitis* begins at the limbus and gradually extends centrally and deeper into the stroma. This results in a wedge-shaped affected area, deeper peripherally and more superficial centrally. Occasionally coalescence of the lesions or superficial or stromal vascularization develop. The punctate lesions regress with antileprotic therapy.

Dimmer's nummular keratitis develops without conjunctivitis. It usually occurs unilaterally in agricultural workers with exposure to irrigation water, and is rare in this country (see Figs. 12-43 and 12-44). Infiltrates may also be present at deeper levels.

Subepithelial infiltrates can develop in onchocerciasis. Microfilariae, 0.3 mm in length, can invade the cornea. There is little reaction to the live organisms, but dead microfilariae elicit an infiltrative reaction consisting of lymphocytes and eosinophils. The infiltrates are approximately 0.5 mm in diameter, and can be found anywhere in the stroma, although they are more common peripherally. The disease is bilateral. The disease should be suspected in people in endemic ares, such as sub-Saharan Africa, Central America, and northern South America. Live organisms can frequently be seen in the cornea and anterior chamber. Skin infection has usually been present for many years. Definitive diagnosis is made by skin biopsy.

Sterile subepithelial infiltrates commonly develop in contact lens wearers. They may be single or multiple, are usually less than 1 mm in diameter, and are most common in the midperiphery (Fig. 9-1). Peripheral nummular infiltrates occasionally occur in infectious mononucleosis. Often they are seen at all levels of the stroma but sometimes may be limited to the subepithelial stroma (see Fig. 12-41). The lesions can coalesce and vascularize. There is usually a recent history of systemic illness. Serologic testing can be diagnostic. Peripheral nummular subepithelial infiltrates can also develop in Reiter's syndrome and can persist for months.

Patchy anterior stromal infiltrates can occur early in *Acanthamoeba* keratitis. The overlying epithelium is usually irregular, with fine opacities (see Fig. 11-13). Fine opacities may also be seen in the anterior stroma. Other characteristic symptoms and signs, such as severe pain, radial perineural infiltrates, and ring infiltrates may be present.

Noninfiltrative Deposits

Interpalpebral subepithelial deposits can be seen in calcific band keratopathy, hyperuricemia, spheroidal degeneration, and rarely gelatinous droplike dystrophy. Band keratopathy often affects eyes with chronic intraocular inflammation, but it can also be related to hypercalcemia (see Chapter 16). The calcium deposits are gray to white and subepithelial, with distinct borders (see Figs. 16-17 and 16-18). They can be central, limbal, or can form a band across the entire interpalpebral cornea. Similar deposits can be seen with hyperuricemia, but they may be browner in color and painful (see Fig. 21-36), and after topical use of phenylmercuric nitrate (see Fig. 24-2).

Spheroidal degeneration, also known as labrador keratopathy, and climatic droplet degeneration begin as small subepithelial golden droplets near the 3 o'clock and 9 o'clock limbus. They may progress centrally, darken, opacify, and coalesce. In severe cases the deposits can extend in a plaquelike fashion across the central cornea, reducing vision (see Fig. 16-20), and can become nodular, elevating the epithelium.

Nodular subepithelial deposits elevating the corneal epithelium are also seen in Salzmann's nodular degeneration and gelatinous droplike dystrophy. The elevations in Salzmann's nodular degeneration are bluish white or sometimes yellow-white, and are usually arranged in a circular fashion around the pupillary area (see Figs. 16-24 and 16-25). These nodules often appear within or adjacent to an area of previous scarring or at the edge of a longstanding pannus, but they can occur in any area of the cornea. They can decrease vision if they occur in the visual axis, and can cause recurrent erosions. Salzmann's degeneration occurs in adults of any age and is most commonly bilateral. A history of previous corneal inflammation is common, particularly of phlyctenular and trachomatous disease.

In gelatinous droplike dystrophy, bilateral, central, raised, multinodular, subepithelial mounds of amyloid are seen (see Fig. 17-28). These are white on direct illumination and transparent on retroillumination but can become yellow and milky with time. Flat subepithelial opacities can be seen surrounding the mounds. Early in the dystrophy the deposits are fairly flat and can resemble bandshaped keratopathy. In the late stages the cornea can have a diffuse, mulberry-like appearance, and neovascularization can occur.

As mentioned earlier, amorphous gray-white epithelial and subepithelial deposits can develop in the superior corneal periphery in multiple myeloma. Superficial punctate lesions and linear subepithelial corneal opacities, mainly located in the upper paralimbal region, can be seen in acrodermatitis enteropathica. These are radiating, white to light brown, slightly whorllike opacities passing from the limbus about two thirds of the distance to the corneal center (see Fig. 22-56). Unique minute, yellow-brown, subepithelial opacities are seen in Kyrle's disease (see Fig. 22-52). Their greatest density and deepest penetration occur at the limbus, the least at the corneal center. In dermochondral dystrophy of Francois, white or brownish, irregular subepithelial opacities are seen. Deformities of the hands and feet and xanthomalike skin nodules are present. These skin conditions are discussed further in Chapter 22.

Reis-Bücklers' dystrophy is an autosmal dominant dystrophy that presents as subepithelial opacification. The earliest finding, seen in early childhood, is a fine reticular opacification at the level of Bowman's layer. With time the cornea becomes progressively more clouded by superficial, gray-white opacities that may be linear, geographic, honeycombed, or ringlike (see Figs. 17-11 and 17-12). The opacities are most dense in the central or midperipheral cornea. The deposits elevate the corneal surface producing irregular astigmatism. Decreased vision and recurrent erosions develop.

Anterior stromal scarring can be seen after many corneal diseases. It is characterized by hard, noninfiltrative opacities, which may be associated with vascularization and elevation or depression of the corneal surface.

Inflammatory Stromal Disease

Nonulcerative stromal inflammation can take several forms. Disciform keratitis is a disk-shaped area of stromal edema of variable size that may be central or peripheral. Signs of endothelial inflammation such as keratitic precipitates and mild cellular infiltration are sometimes present. Interstitial keratitis is defined by more severe stromal inflammation, with marked infiltration and rapid development of vascularization. Ringshaped infiltrates are donutshaped areas of stromal infiltration with inflammatory cells. Partial rings can also be seen. Within the center of the ring is an antigen, such as a foreign body or infectious agent, which may not be visible.

Disciform Keratitis

The clinical appearance of disciform keratitis varies little between infectious agents. However, most of the diseases can be diagnosed by their systemic manifestations (Table 9-11). Herpes simplex, the most common cause of disciform keratitis, and *Acanthamoeba* infections are

Table 9-11   Causes of Disciform Keratitis

Herpes simplex (see Figs. 12-11 and 12-12)
Herpes zoster (see Fig. 12-31)
Varicella
Mumps (see Fig. 12-46)
Epstein-Barr virus
Variola
Vaccinia
Acanthamoeba (see Fig. 11-13)
Kawasaki disease
Adenovirus

the only types without systemic disease. Distinguishing between these can be difficult. Corneal sensation is frequently reduced in both. However, in *Acanthamoeba* keratitis there is a history of contact lens wear or trauma in all cases, pain is often more prominent, typical epithelial changes are often present, and topical steroid treatment is less effective. Radial perineural infiltrates (see Fig. 11-15) and nodular scleritis (see Fig. 11-16) can be present. If a disciform keratitis that is presumed to be herpetic is not responding to topical corticosteroids as expected, a corneal biopsy should be performed to look for *Acanthamoeba* cysts.

Interstitial Keratitis

Intersitial keratitis is caused by a wide range of diseases (Table 9-12). In most cases it is an inflammatory reaction to infectious organisms that pass into the corneal stroma from the limbal circulation (Table 9-13). Theoretically, the type of reaction depends on the number of organisms in the circulation, their size, how well they penetrate the stroma, and their antigenicity. The interstitial keratitis usually involves all layers of the stroma. The disease may be limited to the periphery or may affect the entire width. Depending on the number of organisms and the intensity of the reaction the infiltrates can be nummular or confluent.

Blood-borne Organisms. The classic interstitial keratitis of this type is that caused by congenital syphilis. In the past, syphilis has accounted for over 90% of cases of interstitial keratitis.[16] Although no survey has been performed recently, active interstitial keratitis due to congenital or acquired syphilis is now uncommon. Most often, patients have quiescent scarring and vascularization that have been present for decades. The interstitial keratitis of congenital syphilis usually begins between 5 and 20 years of age. Other stigmata of congenital syphilis, such as dental abnormalities, deafness, and

Table 9-12	Causes of Interstitial Keratitis

BACTERIAL
  Syphilis
  Tuberculosis
  Leprosy
  Relapsing fever
  ?Post streptococcal
  Lyme disease

VIRAL
  Herpes simplex
  Herpes zoster
  Variola
  Varicella
  Rubeola
  Mumps
  Epstein-Barr

PARASITIC
  Onchocerciasis
  Leishmaniasis
  Schistosomiasis
  Trypanosomiasis

SYSTEMIC INFLAMMATORY DISEASE
  Systemic lupus erythematosus
  Wegener's granulomatosis
  Rheumatoid arthritis
  Progressive systemic sclerosis
  Relapsing polychondritis
  Inflammatory bowel disease
  Polyarteritis nodosa
  Discoid lupus erythematosus
  Cogan's syndrome

SARCOID
LYMPHOGRANULOMA VENEREUM
KAPOSI'S SARCOMA
DRUG TOXICITY (E.G., GOLD, ARSENICALS)

Table 9-13	Classification of Interstitial Keratitis

CIRCULATING ORGANISMS
  Bacteria
    Syphilis
    Tuberculosis
    Leprosy
    Lyme disease
    ?Relapsing fever
  Viral
    Epstein-Barr
    Mumps
    Rubeola
    Vaccinia
    Variola
    Varicella
  Parasitic
    Onchocerciasis
    Trypanosomiasis

EXTENSION OF LIMBAL DISEASE
  Lymphogranuloma venerum
  Scleritis
  Systemic inflammatory diseases
    Wegener's granulomatosis
    Systemic lupus erythematosus
  ?Leishmaniasis
  Leprosy

SPREAD FROM CORNEAL NERVES
  Herpes simplex
  Herpes zoster
  ?Leprosy

UNKNOWN
  Cogan's syndrome

saddle nose, are usually present. The intersitial keratitis is typically bilateral, affects mainly the posterior stroma, proceeds from the periphery to the center, and is associated with significant anterior chamber reaction.

The interstitial keratitis in tuberculosis is usually unilateral, deep, and limited to one sector of the cornea, usually inferior (see Fig. 10-17). Interstitial keratitis occurs in about 6% of patients with leprosy. It occurs late in the disease, so the diagnosis is not in question. Bilateral deep infiltration begins peripherally and extends centrally (see Fig. 10-18). Unlike luetic interstitial keratitis, vascularization is minimal and late.

Interstitial keratitis frequently occurs in onchocerciasis. The subepithelial infiltrates and other manifestations of punctate keratitis in onchocerciasis were discussed previously. Num-

mular infiltrates can occur throughout the stroma, and can coalesce. A diffuse infiltrating and vascularizing process, called *sclerosing keratitis,* can also be seen. It begins in the nasal and temporal periphery and extends centrally. In all these conditions live microfilariae can usually be seen in the corneal stroma as well as the anterior chamber. The patient has been in an endemic region, and skin disease has been present for many years.

Relapsing fevers are a group of acute infections caused by louse-borne or tick-borne spirochetes of the genus *Borrelia.* They are characterized by recurrent cycles of fever, headache, myalgia, and weakness lasting several days, separated by periods of apparent recovery. Superficial, mild, interstitial keratitis, associated with mild neovascularization, can occur. During febrile episodes the organism can be seen in blood smears examined with Giemsa or Wright's stains.

Trypanosomiasis is a rare cause of bilateral interstitial keratitis, but is important to diagnose because the keratitis responds to antitrypanosomal therapy. Interstitial keratitis occurs in the African form (sleeping sickness), which is manifested by fever, transient circinate rashes, hepatosplenomegaly, central nervous system changes, and areas of nonpitting edema. The corneal signs are not distinctive.

Typical systemic manifestations are present in most of the other infectious causes of this type of interstitial keratitis, such as mumps, rubeola, and leprosy. Lyme disease and Epstein-Barr virus infection (see Fig. 12-41) can be exceptions. Lyme disease is caused by infection with the spirochete *Borrelia burgdorferi,* acquired by tick bite. The systemic disease may not be apparent. Multiple infiltrates are present at all levels of the stroma. The disease can be unilateral or bilateral. The diagnosis can be made by determination of serum IgG antibody titer to *B. burgdorferi.* Infection with Epstein-Barr virus (infectious mononucleosis) is typically associated with fever, malaise, sore throat, and lymphadenopathy. However, in some cases it can be associated with minimal or no symptoms. It is most common between 10 and 35 years of age. The diagnosis is made by the mononuclear spot test, the heterophil test, and detection of antibodies to Epstein-Barr virus antigens.

Extensions of Limbal Disease. The interstitial keratitis in lymphogranuloma venereum is part of a sclerokeratitis. The scleritis is the most prominent feature, but corneal involvement can be severe. The superior cornea is usually affected, but the entire cornea can become opaque. Parinaud's oculoglandular syndrome, regional adenopathy, lymphedema of the lids, and proctitis are suggestive of the diagnosis. Staining and culture of scrapings and biopsy specimens are necessary to identify the organism.

Stromal infiltration and vascularization can occur adjacent to scleritis of any etiology. They may be accompanied by stromal edema, lipid deposition, and thinning. Many systemic inflammatory diseases can be associated with scleritis and peripheral interstitial keratitis (Table 9-12). Rare cases of interstitial keratitis have been reported in association with leishmaniasis. These patients have involvement of the eyelids and conjunctiva as well.

Spread from Corneal Nerves. Interstitial keratitis occasionally occurs in herpes simplex and herpes zoster infections. It is not clear whether live virus is present or only viral and altered host antigens. The virus may enter the stroma directly by release from corneal nerves or by extension from epithelial infection. The diagnosis of herpes zoster is usually not difficult because of the typical rash, but keratitis can occur months or years after the rash subsides. Decreased sensation, a history of recurrent attacks, and a previous dendrite can suggest the diagnosis of herpes simplex. Culture is rarely helpful in herpetic interstitial keratitis.

Unknown Origins. The initial signs of interstitial keratitis in Cogan's syndrome are faint subepithelial infiltrates in the periphery. Later, deep yellow, nodular opacities develop. Mild vascularization and anterior chamber reaction may be seen. Vestibuloauditory symptoms are usually present. It is important not to miss this diagnosis, because delay in treatment can result in permanent loss of hearing.

Evaluation. In most cases systemic treatment has no effect on interstitial keratitis; topical corticosteroids are the only treatment of benefit. However, it may be important to recognize and treat the systemic disease in order to prevent other complications. Conditions in which systemic treatment improves the keratitis are the systemic inflammatory diseases, trypanosomiasis, and drug toxicity. Conditions that are important to recognize and treat to prevent systemic complications include Cogan's syndrome, syphilis, tuberculosis, Lyme disease, systemic inflammatory diseases, and onchocerciasis.

In many cases the cause of the interstitial keratitis can be determined from history and physical examination. In the absence of evident systemic disease, laboratory testing should be performed for syphilis, tuberculosis, and Lyme disease. Epstein-Barr virus titers can be performed to make the diagnosis, but the results do not affect treatment.

Ring Infiltrates

Partial or complete ringshaped stromal infiltrates can develop in a number of conditions. They probably result from antigen-antibody complex formation, with infiltration of polymorphonuclear lymphocytes. The ring surrounds an area containing antigen, which can be a foreign body, infectious agent, or chemical. Ring infiltrates can be seen in bacterial infections, especially *Pseudomonas* (see Fig. 10-11), herpes simplex (see Fig. 12-14), *Acanthamoeba* (see Fig. 11-14), fungal keratitis, corneal burns, and with abuse of topical anesthetic agents (see Fig. 25-8). Usually the rings are central or midperipheral, but occasionally they can be marginal. Topical corticosteroids can be used to reduce the infiltration if any infection present has been appropriately treated.

Marginal ring infiltrates can occur in a number of infectious and inflammatory diseases. Most of these were discussed in the section on marginal infiltrative ulcerative keratitis. Marginal staphylococcal catarrhal infiltrates can coalesce to form a partial ring. Marginal infiltration occurs in hyperacute conjunctivitis, scleritis, influenza, gram-negative bacillary dysentery, and systemic inflammatory diseases such as rheumatoid arthritis, polyarteritis nodosa, Wegener's granulomatosis, and systemic lupus erythematosus.

Stromal Abscesses

Stromal abscesses can develop below intact epithelium. They are most common after surgery or trauma, when the organism becomes implanted in deep tissue or enters through a wound or suture tract. Stromal abscesses can also develop from metastatic blood-borne infection. They arise near the limbus as intrastromal infiltrates and progress to abscess formation. They extend circumferentially and centrally, and usually eventually break through to the surface.

Noninflammatory Stromal Disease
Central/Diffuse

Edema. Noninflammatory stromal edema usually occurs from endothelial pump failure. This can be caused by trauma, Fuchs' dystrophy, ocular ischemia, posterior polymorphous dystrophy, graft rejection or failure, and iridocorneal endothelial syndrome. Corneal edema can also occur from Descemet's membrane detachment and corneal hydrops in keratoconus. The edema is greatest centrally, or in an area of previous injury (e.g., superiorly after cataract surgery). There is no infiltration or vascularization.

Fuchs' dystrophy is progressive, bilateral, and fairly symmetric. It may be familial. Endothelial abnormalities, such as guttae, fine pigment deposition, and a diffuse beaten-metal appearance are usually present. Posterior polymorphous dystrophy can also present as bilateral corneal edema. It is usually transmitted as a dominant trait. Most cases are nonprogressive, but endothelial decompensation can develop in some patients. Characteristic endothelial lesions, such as vesicles, blisters, and bands, or signs of anterior segment dysgenesis may be present. (Both of these diseases are discussed in more detail below and in Chapter 18.)

Unilateral corneal edema can occur in the iridocorneal endothelial syndrome. Other ante-

Table 9-14   Diffuse Corneal Accumulations
DISORDERS OF LIPID METABOLISM
Metachromatic leukodystrophy (congenital and infantile forms)
GM_1 gangliosidosis
Niemann-Pick disease
Sandhoff disease (rare)
Apoprotein A-1 deficiency
Lecithin-cholesterol-acyltransferase deficiency
Tangier disease
Fish eye disease
DISORDERS OF CARBOHYDRATE METABOLISM
Mucopolysaccharidosis (see Fig. 21-19)
Macular corneal dystrophy
Sialidosis
OTHERS
Mucolipidoses (types II, III, IV)
Zellweger syndrome

rior segment abnormalities, including peripheral anterior synechiae, ectropion uveae, iris atrophy, iris nodules, and glaucoma usually permit diagnosis (see Chapter 18). Unilateral diffuse corneal edema can also be seen in ocular ischemia. Intraocular inflammation, cataract, retinal, and iris neovascularization may also be present. Patients with corneal hydrops present with an acute onset of central stromal edema, with pain and reduced vision (see Fig. 17-45). Most will have a history of keratoconus and signs of keratoconus in the fellow eye. Corneal graft failure and rejection can present with graft edema without signs of inflammation.

Congenital diffuse corneal edema can be seen in congenital hereditary endothelial dystrophy (see Fig. 18-11), posterior polymorphous dystrophy, and congenital glaucoma. Congenital glaucoma can be differentiated by the elevated intraocular pressure. It is not possible to clinically differentiate the other two conditions. They can both be inherited in autosomal dominant or autosomal recessive patterns. See Chapter 5 for the causes of cloudy corneas in infants.

Accumulations. Diffuse clouding occurs in many metabolic diseases. In most of these the pattern of corneal clouding is nonspecific (Table 9-14). Gray-white-yellow dots progressively accumulate in the stroma and can become confluent (see Fig. 21-19). Differentiation of the diseases is based on the systemic manifestations. In other conditions a specific pattern of stromal corneal deposits is seen. These are described in Table 9-15.

Table 9-15 Specific Patterns of Stromal Accumulations	
Disease	**Pattern**
Mannosidosis	Superficial corneal opacities
Fucosidosis	Central anterior corneal opacification
Cystinosis	Crystals, peripheral > central, anterior > posterior (see Fig. 21-26)
Gold	Dustlike, yellow-brown to purple-violet granules, mainly posterior, denser inferiorly
STROMAL CORNEAL DYSTROPHIES	
Granular	Discrete gray-white, irregularly shaped, in the central anterior stroma (see Figs. 17-17 and 17-18)
Lattice	Fine lines, some bifurcating, and dots, irregular opacities, central > peripheral, anterior > posterior (see Figs. 17-22 and 17-23)
Macular	Diffuse clouding with poorly demarcated, dense gray-white opacities (see Fig. 17-29)
Schnyder's crystalline	Ringshaped or disciform opacities in the central cornea, sometimes crystals evident (see Fig. 17-36)
Fleck	Small discrete opacities, widely scattered in stroma (see Figs. 17-34 and 17-35)
Mosaic (crocodile) shagreen	Grayish-white polygonal opacities, separated by clear spaces (see Fig. 16-8)

Thinning. Central corneal thinning unrelated to anterior stromal ulceration occurs in keratoconus, keratoglobus, and posterior keratoconus. Keratoconus is characterized by thinning and ectasia of the central cornea (see Figs. 17-41 to 17-50). It is usually bilateral, but can be highly asymmetric. Vision is reduced by irregular astigmatism. Corneal topography analysis is the most sensitive means of diagnosis, but characteristic findings are present on examination in more advanced cases (see Chapter 17). Keratoglobus is a rare, bilateral, globular corneal ectasia. The stroma is diffusely thinned and ectatic, often producing high myopia and irregular astigmatism (see Figs. 17-52 to 17-55). Generalized posterior keratoconus is a rare congenital condition in which the entire posterior surface of the cornea is more curved than normal. Central corneal thinning can be present, but the anterior corneal curvature is normal. It is not progressive. Localized posterior keratoconus can also occur.

Localized

Lipid accumulations in the cornea appear as dense, yellow-white opacities that may fan out with feathery edges (see Fig. 16-37). They can affect any part of the cornea. Multicolored crystals may be seen, usually at the edge of the opacity, and blood vessels may extend from the limbus to the affected area. Lipid deposition usually occurs in corneas with vascularized stromal scars, but in some cases there is no history of corneal disease (see Chapter 16).

Infectious crystalline keratopathy is an uncommon form of corneal infection. A crystalline stromal opacity develops without infiltration, ulceration, or other signs of inflammation (see Fig. 10-5). It most commonly affects corneal grafts. Relatively nonvirulent bacteria and fungi can be responsible.

Stromal scarring can be seen after any form of ulcerative or interstitial keratitis. The scarring is white-gray and may be associated with thinning, edema, or vascularization. The pattern of scarring may be suggestive of the process that produced it, but in most cases is not.

Marginal

Edema. Marginal noninflammatory corneal edema occurs as a result of trauma. Sectoral edema occurs adjacent to previous surgical incisions or lacerations and in areas of chronic or recurrent endothelial injury, such as from contact by intraocular lens implants, drainage valves, epithelial downgrowth, or an intact vitreous face. Circumferential peripheral edema can be seen after cataract extraction, usually intracapsular. This is called *Brown-McLean* syndrome. The peripheral 1 to 3 mm of the cornea is involved. The endothelium may have an orange, punctate pigmentation. The edema is usually stable but can progress to involve the central cornea.

Accumulations. The most common accumulation in the marginal corneal stroma is *corneal arcus,* which is a bilateral hazy ring of yellow-white deposits separated from the limbus by a lucid interval (see Figs. 16-3 and 16-4). The deposits affect the superior and inferior cornea first, but eventually spread to affect the entire circumference. The posterior and anterior stroma are affected more than the midstroma. Numerous crisscrossing lines of relative clarity can be seen throughout the arcus.

Yellow-white infiltrations of the peripheral stroma can be seen in Langerhans cell granulomatosis (see Fig. 19-24). Crystalline material in the paralimbal superficial stroma in association with fundus albipunctatus is the rare marginal crystalline dystrophy of Bietti (see Chapter 17). In Lowe's syndrome, which includes congenital cataracts, glaucoma, Fanconi's syndrome, mental retardation, and ocular automanipulation, a mild haze can affect the peripheral stroma. A faint brown peripheral corneal clouding can be seen in Von Gierke's disease, an autosomal recessive disorder of glucose metabolism (see Chapter 20).

Thinning. Furrow degeneration or senile marginal degeneration is characterized by thinning of the stroma in the lucid interval between an arcus and the limbus (see Fig. 16-9). It almost always occurs in elderly patients with prominent arcus. There is no inflammation or vascularization.

Terrien's marginal degeneration is characterized by progressive marginal corneal thinning with vascularization and lipid deposition at the central edge (see Figs. 16-26 to 16-28). It most commonly begins in the superonasal quadrant and progresses circumferentially, and rarely centrally as well. It is usually asymptomatic and bilateral, and can occur at any age (see Chapter 16). In some cases it is difficult to distinguish these from the scars following marginal ulcerative keratitis, such as in rheumatoid arthritis, Mooren's ulcer, and staphylococcal marginal keratitis.

Pellucid marginal degeneration is characterized by a narrow band of stromal thinning between 4 o'clock and 8 o'clock that is 1 to 2 mm in width and separated from the limbus by 1 to 2 mm of clear cornea (see Fig. 16-32). There is no stromal opacification or vascularization. It is usually diagnosed between 20 and 40 years of age. Patients present with decreased vision due to astigmatism.

A *delle* is a localized thinning of the cornea that occurs adjacent to corneal or conjunctival elevation (see Fig. 14-7). They are caused by localized dehydration of the stroma due to a lack of wetting by the lid. They are covered by epithelium, and there is no infiltration. Most will improve 1 to 2 hours after taping the lids.

Posterior Stromal Disease
Opacities

A variety of posterior opacities have been described in older patients and probably represent degenerative changes. The presence of tiny, punctate, gray opacities immediately anterior to Descemet's membrane is called *cornea farinata* (see Chapter 16). Larger dendritic, stellate, boomerang, circular, dot, linear, or filiform opacities are seen in pre-Descemet's dystrophy (see Fig. 17-40). The deposits can be central, peripheral, or diffuse (see Chapter 17). Punctate, linear, branching, or filiform deep stromal deposits, which are gray-white on direct illumination and transparent on retroillumination (see Fig. 16-16), are called *polymorphic amyloid degeneration* or *parenchymatous dystrophy of Pillat*. None of these affects vision.

Similar pre-Descemet's opacities can be seen in X-linked ichthyosis (see Fig. 22-41) Larger white or gray deep stromal opacities can also be seen.

Irregular sheetlike stromal opacities can occur as a congenital abnormality. This has been called *posterior amorphous corneal dystrophy*. The opacities can affect the central or peripheral cornea, can involve any portion of the stroma but are most prominent posteriorly, and can be associated with other congenital anterior segment abnormalities.

Old syphilitic interstitial keratitis can also present as deep stromal opacification. It is typically bilateral, affects the central cornea, and vascularization is evident (see Fig. 10-13).

Endothelial Disease
Inflammatory Disease

The most common form of endothelial inflammation is allogeneic graft rejection. This may be seen as a line of keratic precipitates, extending from limbus to limbus, which marches across the cornea, leaving opacified endothelium and stromal edema in its wake (Khodadoust line). Randomly distributed keratic precipitates or anterior chamber cells are other presentations. In some cases increased corneal thickness is the only sign.

A linear pattern of endothelial inflammation and destruction can occur in nongrafted corneas. The appearance and process appear to be similar to those of corneal graft rejection. A line of keratic precipitates progresses across the cornea, destroying the endothelieum and leaving stromal edema in its wake. Herpes simplex can cause such a picture unilaterally (see Chapter 12).[17,18] It can also be seen as a recurrent, bilaterally symmetric process in otherwise healthy eyes,[19,20] or associated with active pars planitis.[21] The etiology is unknown, but an autoimmune process has been proposed.[19] Single or multiple inflammatory endothelial plaques are another form of endothelial inflammation seen with herpes simplex.

One pedigree has been described in which there appeared to be a dominantly inherited form of recurrent keratoendotheliitis.[22] Attacks usually began around 10 years of age and recurred two to three times per year, lasting days to weeks. Corneal edema, guttae, and mild anterior chamber reaction were noted during attacks, and some patients developed stromal opacities after multiple attacks.

Accumulations

Yellow-brown, red, blue, or green coloration of peripheral Descemet's membrane (see Fig. 21-34) occurs from copper deposition in Wilson's disease and other liver diseases with elevated liver copper, in exogenous chalcosis, and with copper-containing intraocular foreign bodies (see Chapter 24). Pigmentation of the iris and anterior lens capsule (sunflower cataract) can also be present.

Fine yellow-brown-white deposits can be seen near Descemet's membrane in the interpalpebral cornea in patients on phenothiazines, most commonly chlorpromazine. Similar deposits are seen in the central lens, beneath the anterior capsule.

Endothelial Cell Abnormalities

Corneal Guttae. *Corneal guttae* are fine droplike dimples in the corneal endothelium (see Fig. 18-1). With direct illumination they appear as refractile circular excavations in the endothelial surface. On specular reflection they are black holes in the endothelial mosaic. They affect primarily the central cornea, and can be associated with fine pigment deposition. They are seen in a majority of patients over 40 years of age, in Fuchs' dystrophy, as a congenital anomaly, and in association with corneal trauma and inflammation.

In Fuchs' dystrophy the guttae are bilateral and progressive. They can become confluent, giving Descemet's membrane a beaten-metal appearance. Stromal and epithelial edema can occur. The disease can be familial.

Congenital cornea guttata is also bilateral but is not progressive. It can be also be familial, and can be associated with other congenital malformations, including anterior polar cataract and mandibulofacial dysostosis.

Posterior Polymorphous Dystrophy. Posterior polymorphous dystrophy is a hereditary condi-

tion, usually transmitted as a dominant trait. Nodular, grouped vesicular, and blisterlike lesions are seen most commonly. Flat gray-white opacities, gray thickenings of Descemet's membrane, and sinuous broad or clear bands with white scalloped margins can also be seen (see Figs. 18-12 to 18-15). Occasionally it presents as a cloudy cornea at birth. Posterior polymorphous dystrophy can be associated with anterior segment dysgenesis and glaucoma. It is usually nonprogressive or very slowly progressive, but endothelial decompensation develops in some patients.

Iridocorneal Endothelial Syndrome. The iridocorneal endothelial syndrome encompasses a spectrum of iris and corneal endothelial abnormalities occurring unilaterally, and is usually diagnosed between 30 and 50 years of age. The most common endothelial abnormality is a fine hammered-metal appearance of the endothelium, which can be focal or diffuse. Stromal and epithelial edema commonly develops. Associated iris abnormalities include progressive atrophy of the iris stroma, peripheral anterior synechiae, corectopia, ectopion uvea, iris hole formation, and iris nodules. Increased intraocular pressure is common.

Epithelial Ingrowth. Epithelial ingrowth is a rare complication of penetrating corneal incisions or lacerations. The epithelium may be seen on the posterior corneal surface. It is translucent and thicker than endothelium, usually with a whitish leading edge. A similar membrane may be seen on the iris.

REFERENCES

1. Stein RM et al: Infected vs sterile corneal infiltrates in contact lens wearers, *Am J Ophthalmol* 105:632, 1988.
2. Duke-Elder S, Leigh AG: *Diseases of the outer eye, part 2*, St Louis, 1965, Mosby–Year Book.
3. O'Day DM et al: The problem of *Bacillus* species infection with special emphasis on the virulence of *Bacillus cereus*, *Ophthalmology* 88:833, 1981.
4. Liesegang TJ, Samples JR, Waller RW: Suppurative interstitial ring keratitis due to *Streptococcus*, *Ann Ophthalmol* 16:392, 1984.
5. Lullman H, Lullman-Rauch R, Wassermann O: Lipidosis induced by amphiphilic cationic drugs, *Biochem Pharmacol* 27:1103, 1978.
6. D'Amico DJ, Kenyon KR: Drug-induced lipidoses of the cornea and conjunctiva, *Int Ophthalmol* 4:67, 1981.
7. Lullman-Rauch R: Mucopolysaccharidosis (MPS) in ocular tissues as induced by amphi-

philic di-cationic drugs, *Lens Eye Toxic Res* 7:263, 1990.

8. Wilson FM, Schmitt TE, Grayson M: Amiodarone-induced cornea verticillata, *Ann Ophthalmol* 12:657, 1980.

9. Kaplan LJ, Cappaert WE: Amiodarone keratopathy, *Arch Ophthalmol* 100:601, 1982.

10. Weiss JN, Weinberg RS, Regelson W: Keratopathy after oral administration of tilorone hydrochloride, *Am J Ophthalmol* 89:46, 1980.

11. Szmyd L, Perry HD: Keratopathy associated with the use of naproxen, *Am J Ophthalmol* 99:598, 1985.

12. Teich SA et al: Toxic keratopathy associated with suramin therapy, *N Engl J Med* 314:1455, 1986.

13. Walinder PE, Gip L, Stempa M: Corneal changes in patients treated with clofazimine, *Br J Ophthalmol* 60:526, 1976.

14. Burns DA: Indomethacin, reduced retinal sensitivity, and corneal deposits, *Am J Ophthalmol* 66:825, 1968.

15. Woods AC: Nummular keratitis and ocular brucellosis, *Arch Ophthalmol* 34:490, 1946.

16. Duke-Elder S, Leigh AG: *Diseases of the outer eye, part 2*, St Louis, 1965, Mosby–Year Book.

17. Vannas A, Ahonen R: Herpetic endothelial keratitis: a case report, *Acta Ophthalmol (Copenh)* 59:296, 1981.

18. Robin JB, Steigner JB, Kaufman HE: Progressive herpetic corneal endotheliitis, *Am J Ophthalmol* 100:336, 1985.

19. Khodadoust AA, Attarzadeh A: Presumed autoimmune corneal endotheliopathy, *Am J Ophthalmol* 93:718, 1982.

20. Ohashi Y et al: Idiopathic corneal endotheliopathy, *Arch Ophthalmol* 103:1666, 1985.

21. Khodadoust AA et al: Pars planitis and autoimmune endotheliopathy, *Am J Ophthalmol* 102:633, 1986.

22. Ruusuvaara P, Setäläka K: Keratoendotheliitis fugax hereditaria: a clinical and specular microscopic study of a family with dominant inflammatory corneal disease, *Acta Ophthalmol (Copenh)* 65:159, 1987.

Ten

Infectious Keratitis: Bacterial

ULCERATIVE BACTERIAL KERATITIS

Infectious corneal ulcers can be caused by viruses, bacteria, fungi, or parasites. In the developed countries of the world herpes simplex is by far the most common cause of corneal infection. Bacteria are next in frequency, followed by fungi and parasites. Bacterial keratitis will be discussed in this chapter, fungal and parasitic infections are discussed in Chapter 11. Herpes simplex and other viral infections are discussed in Chapter 12. The differential diagnosis of infiltrative ulcerative keratitis was discussed in Chapter 9.

Pathogenesis
Several mechanisms protect the surface of the eye from infectious agents, some of which were discussed in Chapter 7. The lids physically block organisms from entering the eye and remove them from the corneal surface. The mechanical flushing action of the tears is important as a defense against infection, as is the presence of lysozyme, lactoferrin, beta-lysin, and natural antibodies (principally IgA) in the tears. Mucus can trap and remove organisms.[1] Intact epithelial surfaces are an important line of defense against infection. The adherent glycocalyx and mucin layers on the corneal surface may inhibit microbial attachment and penetration. The normal flora of the ocular surface helps prevent overgrowth of indigenous organisms or invasion by pathogens.

The eye's acute, nonspecific inflammatory reaction to injury, through phagocytosis of the invaders by neutrophils and, later, macrophages, helps the immunocompetent host control or destroy invading organisms. Specific humoral and cellular reactions also counteract opportunists, but require 5 to 8 days to develop unless there has been previous exposure to the invading agent. The nonspecific inflammatory reaction ordinarily takes care of all opportunists that have breached the conjunctival epithelium; in the uncompromised host the specific humoral and cellular reactions are needed only if the microbic inoculum is overwhelming.

Interference with any of these defense mechanisms predisposes the host to corneal infection. Lid abnormalities such as exposure, trichiasis, entropion, or lagophthalmos are frequently associated with infection. Dry eyes and lacrimal drainage obstruction reduce the flushing of organisms from the surface and the availability of antibacterial proteins. Antibiotics often play a role in the development of opportunistic infections of the cornea by inhibiting the normal, relatively benign flora of the conjunctival sac to allow growth of more pathogenic bacteria.

Contact lenses have become increasingly associated with corneal infections.[2] In one study there was a 435% increase in the incidence of ulcerative keratitis from the 1950s to the 1980s, and contact lens wear was determined to be the primary risk factor.[3] Soft lenses, particularly those worn on an extended basis (overnight wear), are associated with the highest risk.[4-6] The risk of ulcerative keratitis increases over eightfold with overnight wear.[7] Use of disposable extended-wear lenses appears to increase, rather than reduce the risk.[4,8,9] However, daily wear of disposable contact lenses was associated with a significantly lower risk of severe keratitis.[4] The rates of ulcerative keratitis in aphakic persons wearing contact lenses are much higher than rates among cosmetic wearers of the same lens type.[10]

Contact lenses deprive the cornea of oxygen, serve as a source of microbes, damage the corneal epithelium, and interfere with protective tear flow. Patients who do not care for their lenses properly are more likely to develop an infection, but infections also occur in people without obvious breaks in technique.[11] In rabbits, the presence of organisms in the contact lens is not sufficient to cause ulcerative keratitis. The addition of significant hypoxia often leads to ulceration.[12] Other conditions that reduce the integrity of the corneal epithelium include bullous keratopathy, dry eyes, medication toxicity, corneal anesthesia, recurrent erosions, chemical or physical injury, and viral infection.

Localized or systemic impairment of immune response frequently contributes to corneal infections. The use of topical corticosteroids is the most common cause of localized immunosuppression. The following systemic conditions can result in a compromised host and thus facilitate the development of corneal infection: immunosuppressive drugs, extensive body burns, pregnancy (last trimester), chronic alcoholism, severe malnutrition, infancy, old age, immunodeficiency syndromes such as Wiskott-Alrich syndrome and AIDS, drug addictions,[13,14] malignancy, and diabetes.

The most common precipitating event in microbial keratitis is the development of an epithelial defect. Thus, an abrasion, foreign body, erosion, or rupture of an epithelial bulla often precedes a central corneal ulcer. In individuals with decreased systemic resistance, such as those listed above, or in patients with decreased local defenses, such as those with keratoconjunctivitis sicca, organisms normally present in the tear film can produce infections. Alternatively, pathogenic bacteria can be introduced in foreign bodies, through poor hygiene, in contact lenses, or in topical medications.[15] Gram-negative bacteria, including *Pseudomonas, Serratia,* and *Proteus,* have been isolated from ocular medications used by patients who developed infectious keratitis.[16]

Only a few organisms can penetrate intact epithelium: *Neisseria gonorrhoeae, Corynebacterium diphtheriae, Haemophilus aegyptius,* and *Listeria.* In rare cases organisms reach the corneal stroma through hematogenous spread; in such cases the organisms typically cause perilimbal infection.

The physician should recognize the eye's natural defense mechanisms, using them to advantage and refraining from thwarting them. It is also important to diagnose underlying conditions that may have led to the infection and to correct or ameliorate them if possible.

Organisms

Bacteria that cause keratitis may be classified according to type, Gram's stain, and desire for oxygen, as outlined below.

I. Gram-positive organisms
   A. Aerobes
      1. Micrococci
         a. *Staphylococcus aureus*
         b. *Staphylococcus epidermidis*
      2. Streptococci
         a. Alpha-hemolytic streptococci
         b. Beta-hemolytic streptococci
         c. Nonhemolytic streptococci
         d. *Streptococcus pneumoniae*

3. Bacilli
  a. Spore-forming
     (1) *Bacillus*
     (2) *Clostridium*
  b. Non–spore-forming
     (1) *Corynebacterium*
     (2) *Listeria*
  B. Anaerobes
    1. Cocci
       a. *Peptostreptococcus*
       b. *Peptococcus*
    2. Bacilli
       a. Spore-forming: *Clostridium*
       b. Non–spore-forming
          (1) *Actinomyces*
          (2) Propionibacterium
  C. Acid-fast bacilli
    1. *Mycobacterium*
    2. *Nocardia*
II. Gram-negative organisms
  A. Aerobes
    1. Diplococci: *Neisseria*
    2. Rods
       a. Enterobacteriaceae
          (1) *Escherichia*
          (2) *Klebsiella*
          (3) *Enterobacter*
          (4) *Proteus*
          (5) *Serratia*
          (6) *Citrobacter*
       b. Others
          (1) *Pseudomonas*
          (2) *Azotobacter*
          (3) *Acinetobacter*
    3. Diplobacillus: *Moraxella*
    4. Coccobacillus: *Haemophilus*
  B. Anaerobes
    1. Rods (non–spore-forming)
       a. *Fusobacterium*
       b. *Bacteroides*

The relative frequency of different bacterial ulcers differs geographically within the United States. It appears that staphylococcal infections are seen more frequently in the eastern and northeastern regions of the United States, whereas *Pseudomonas* infections are found more often in the more temperate climates of the country. *S. pneumoniae* was previously the most common corneal pathogen, particularly in the eastern and western regions of the country, but its relative incidence has declined.[17,18] Now *Pseudomonas* and staphylococcal infections are more common.

As with any bacterial disease, the manifestations and severity of corneal infections depend on the organism and the host's response.[19] The virulence of an organism is determined by its ability to adhere to the corneal surface, to penetrate the epithelium, to multiply and spread within the corneal tissue, and to resist the host's defenses, as well as its elaboration of toxins. Less virulent organisms can cause disease only in compromised corneas, whereas the most virulent organisms can cause severe disease in relatively intact corneas.

Following are the bacteria that most commonly cause corneal ulcers in an uncompromised cornea:

1. *Pseudomonas aeruginosa*
2. *S. pneumoniae*
3. *Moraxella*
4. Beta-hemolytic streptococcus
5. *Klebsiella pneumoniae*

Many other organisms are less frequently seen (e.g., *Escherichia coli, Proteus, Mycobacterium fortuitum,* and *Nocardia*).

Opportunistic pathogens are microbic agents that have been regarded as contaminants or harmless inhabitants but that, in the compromised host, can multiply and produce corneal disease. In the compromised cornea, *S. aureus* is the most common cause of central corneal ulcers; however, a wide range of microorganisms can produce serious disease:

1. *S. aureus*
2. *S. epidermidis*
3. Alpha-hemolytic streptococci
4. Beta-hemolytic streptococci
5. *P. aeruginosa*
6. *Proteus*
7. *Enterobacter aerogenes*
8. Others (e.g., *Escherichia* and *Nocardia*)

The following organisms are particularly frequent in contact lens wearers:

1. *P. aeruginosa*
2. *Serratia marcescens*
3. *S. aureus*
4. *S. epidermidis*
5. Other Enterobacteriaceae: *E. coli, Klebsiella, Proteus*

In children the organisms that cause keratitis are similar to those seen in adults.[20-22] In two studies, *P. aeruginosa* was the most common cause of infection in children under 3 years of age,[20,22] but in another study no cases of *P. aeruginosa* were seen in this age range.[21] The risk factors for corneal infection are similar to those in adults: trauma, corneal surgery, contact lens wear, and systemic illness.

Clinical Manifestations

When a bacterial corneal ulcer develops, conjunctival injection and chemosis, lid edema, decreased vision, pain, tearing, photophobia, and purulent discharge are usually present. The tear film contains numerous cells and debris. The conjunctival reaction is usually nonspecific, with a mainly papillary response and injection, which is greatest near the limbus. In some cases, particularly gonococcal, pneumococcal, and *Haemophilus* infections, corneal ulceration occurs in the setting of a bacterial conjunctivitis, and conjunctival inflammation can be more prominent. Marked discharge, chemosis, and membranes may be present.

The corneal epithelium becomes ulcerated, and the stroma exhibits infiltration and may be gray-white and necrotic. Infiltration and edema of the cornea may even be observed in areas away from the site of the ulcer. Stromal abscesses may be evident as small, deep infiltrates beneath relatively clear stroma and intact epithelium. An anterior chamber reaction is often present, and in more severe cases fibrin plaques may be observed on the endothelium, and a fibrinoid aqueous or hypopyon may be seen.

The hypopyon results from an outpouring of fibrin and polymorphonuclear leukocytes from the vessels of the iris and ciliary body. Usually the hypopyon is sterile as long as Descemet's membrane is intact. A hypopyon can be seen with any bacterial infection (Fig. 10-1) but it is relatively more common in ulcers caused by *S. pneumoniae* (Fig. 10-2) and *Pseudomonas* (Fig. 10-3). It should be remembered that hypopyons are also seen with viral and fungal corneal ulcers. Noninfectious causes of hypopyon include Behçet's syndrome, abuse of topical anesthetic agents, severe alkali burns, and therapeutic contact lenses (particularly in anesthetic corneas).

The clinical signs and symptoms of bacterial corneal ulcers vary with the virulence of the organism, the previous status of the cornea, the duration of infection, the immune status of the host, and previous antibiotic and corticosteroid use. More virulent organisms cause greater stromal destruction and elicit a more marked host response, hence the sign and symptoms of infection are more pronounced. In immunosuppressed patients, or with corticosteroid use, the signs of inflammation, including redness, pain, infiltration, and anterior chamber reaction, are relatively reduced, and greater ulceration and extension of infection can occur before presentation.

The use of hydrophilic contact lenses can alter the presentation of bacterial ulcers. Infections associated with contact lenses are often multifocal, and the epithelial and stromal infiltration is more diffuse. Contact lens wearers who present with corneal abrasions may have early bacterial infections. Often a patient whose eye is patched for a contact lens–associated

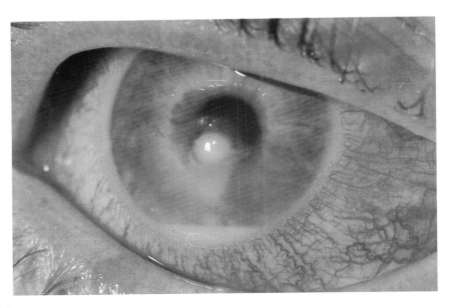

Figure 10-1
Hypopyon ulcer resulting from staphylococcal infection. The infiltrate is round and localized, with more or less distinct borders.

abrasion without any sign of infiltration returns with a well-developed corneal ulcer the following day.[23] It probably is best not to use an eye patch on contact lens wearers with abrasions, but rather to take cultures, begin antibiotic therapy, and reevaluate the patient's condition the following day.

Specific Bacterial Ulcers

In some cases the appearance of an ulcer can suggest a particular bacterial agent or group of agents. The characteristic features of infections produced by some agents are discussed below. However, it should be kept in mind that the clinical appearance is never diagnostic, isola-

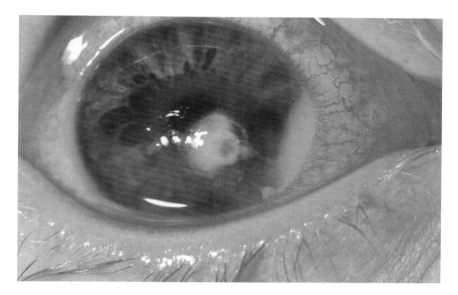

Figure 10-2
Central corneal ulcer caused by *Streptococcus pneumoniae*. The eccentric location of the hypopyon was caused by the patient lying on his side.

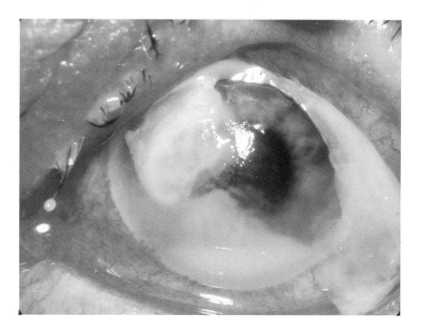

Figure 10-3
Hypopyon ulcer caused by *Pseudomonas aeruginosa* infection. Note extensive lysis of the collagen structure.

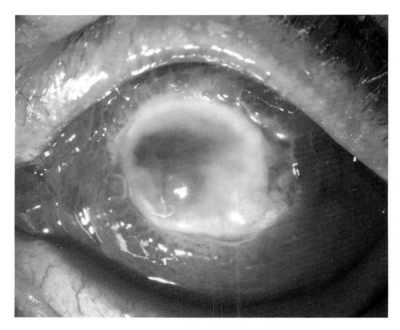

Figure 10-4
Ring ulcer caused by *Pseudomonas*. (Courtesy of Diane Curtin, Pittsburgh, PA.)

tion and identification of the causative organism or organisms are essential in all cases.

Ring Ulcers

Ring ulcer of the cornea is an uncommon finding in ocular infectious disease. Its occurrence is an indication of the devastating nature of the inflammatory reaction and usually foretells a grave prognosis for the eye. This condition can result from hematogenous spread of the bacteria or penetrating injury at the limbus. A variety of microorganisms can cause ring ulcers, including *Bacillus* spp. (most frequent), *P. aeruginosa* (Fig. 10-4), *Streptococcus, Listeria,* and *Proteus* spp.[24]

Infectious Crystalline Keratopathy

Infectious crystalline keratopathy is an uncommon form of corneal bacterial infection.[25,26] The stromal opacity is crystalline in appearance, resembling a snowflake, and is not associated with a cellular infiltrate or other signs of ocular inflammation. The infection usually occurs within a corneal graft, lying within the midstroma with clear stroma superficial to it. The epithelium often is intact (Fig. 10-5). Most cases have been caused by alpha-hemolytic streptococci, but *S. pneumoniae,*[27] *S. epidermidis,*[28] *Haemophilus aphrophilus, Peptostrepto-*

coccus, Candida[29] and other fungi[30] have also been reported. In one case only calcium was seen.[30] The organisms are difficult to culture and a biopsy is often necessary for diagnosis. Antibiotic treatment often has been unsuccessful, and keratoplasty has been required.

The reasons for the lack of inflammatory response and the crystalline appearance are unclear. When one isolate was injected into rabbit corneas, crystalline keratitis developed only if periocular corticosteroids were administered.[31] However, crystalline opacities developed after inoculation of certain strains of *S. pneumoniae*[27] and *Streptococcus sanguis*[32] without corticosteroid treatment. The authors proposed that the nature of the capsular polysaccharide influenced the host inflammatory response in these cases.

Staphylococci

S. aureus is often found on normal skin and mucous membranes, including conjunctiva, and is an opportunistic corneal pathogen. Staphylococci produce many enzymes, including lipases, nucleases, fibrinolysin, hyaluronidase, protease, and lysozyme, and toxins, such as hemolytic toxins and toxic shock syndrome toxin.

The corneal ulcer resulting from *S. aureus*

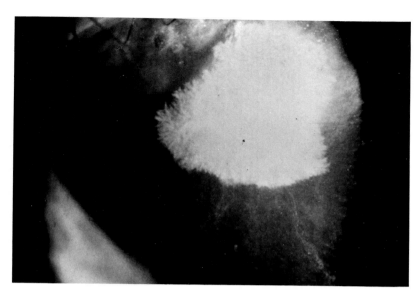

Figure 10-5
Infectious crystalline keratopathy caused by *Streptococcus sanguis* in a graft. (Courtesy of Massimo Busin, Bonn, Germany.)

tends to be round or oval and often remains localized with distinct borders (see Fig. 10-1); however, on occasion the ulcer may be diffuse, demonstrating microabscesses in the anterior stroma that are connected by stromal infiltrates. *S. aureus* ulcers tend to develop more in depth than in width and often are associated with hypopyon and endothelial plaques. Staphylococcal blepharitis often is present.

Non-*aureus* staphylococci, such as *S. epidermidis*, can be isolated from most normal eyes and are an equally frequent cause of keratitis. These staphylococci are also opportunists, affecting primarily compromised corneas. Although *S. aureus* is more virulent, antibiotic resistance is more common among non-*aureus* strains.[33] The corneal ulcers are usually superficial and slow growing.

Corneal ulcers produced by non-*aureus* staphylococci appear similar to those caused by *S. aureus,* except they tend to be more indolent, with less infiltration and anterior chamber reaction. However, severe ulcers can occur.

Streptococci

S. pneumoniae is found in the upper respiratory tract in half of the population; its proximity to the eye may account for the frequency of problems associated with it. Pneumococcal ulcers frequently occur after corneal trauma and often have been associated with chronic dacryocys-

titis. Most pneumococci are surrounded by a polysaccharide capsule, which protects them against phagocytosis, but encapsulation is not necessary to produce keratitis.[34] The cytolytic toxin pneumolysin is important in the ocular virulence of this bacteria.[35]

S. pneumoniae tend to produce acute, purulent infections. Severe pain, photophobia, and decreased vision are seen early in the infection. The keratitis may be localized or may have a tendency to spread in one direction, usually centrally. The edge may be undermined and covered by overhanging tissue. Pneumococcal ulcers have a tendency to be accompanied by a marked anterior chamber reaction, including hypopyon (see Fig. 10-2), and perforation is more common (Fig. 10-6).[34]

Alpha-hemolytic streptococci are present in the upper respiratory tract and the mouth. This organism is relatively nonvirulent and causes infections mainly in corneas with chronic disease. They commonly occur following prolonged use of topical corticosteroids or complicate herpetic infection or keratoconjunctivitis sicca. The ulcer bed is often elevated and moderately to markedly opaque.[36] Infectious crystalline keratopathy (discussed above) is most commonly caused by alpha-hemolytic streptococci.

S. pyogenes (beta-hemolytic streptococcus) is an infrequent cause of corneal infections, and the ulcers tend to be severe. Marginal corneal

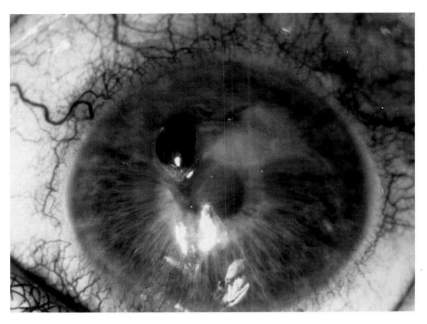

Figure 10-6
Perforated corneal ulcer with iris prolapse.

ulcers resulting from this organism may also be associated with dacryocystitis.[37] *S. faecalis* can cause an ulcer of the cornea in the presence of severely impaired host resistance or after epithelial injury.

Other Gram-Positive Organisms

Gram-positive rods, an infrequent cause of keratitis, usually involve the cornea only when host resistance is impaired. *Bacillus cereus* has emerged as an important ocular pathogen, possibly one of the most destructive organisms to affect the eye.[24] Most cases of *B. cereus* infection have occurred as a result of hematogenous dissemination, usually in intravenous drug abusers. Cases have also occurred after penetrating injury, particularly with soil-contaminated foreign bodies. Characteristically severe pain develops within 24 hours of the injury and is followed rapidly by chemosis, periorbital swelling, and extreme proptosis. Shortly thereafter, low-grade fever may occur, accompanied by a moderate leukocytosis. Invariably a ring of edema forms in the peripheral cornea followed by the rapid development of a circumferential corneal abscess.

Listeria[38-40] and *Corynebacteria* are uncommon causes of corneal infection. Anaerobic gram-positive bacteria often reside in the skin and mucous membranes and are seen in the fecal flora. In rare cases peptostreptococci, *Propi-*onibacterium acnes,[41] *Clostridium*,[42] and other gram-positive species have been recovered from corneal ulcers.[43,44] *Clostridium* can produce gas that can be seen in the anterior chamber, stroma, or under the epithelium.[42]

Corneal ulcers caused by the gram-positive filamentous bacteria *Nocardia* and *Actinomyces* are usually indolent and may simulate the indolent ulcers caused by *Moraxella* and *M. fortuitum*. *Nocardia* is present in soil, and corneal infection usually follows trauma, particularly with soil contamination. *Nocardia* and *Actinomyces* ulcers also may simulate mycotic corneal ulcers because of the presence of "hyphate edges" and satellite lesions, and they may be elevated (Fig. 10-7)[45,46] The base of a *Nocardia* ulcer can have a "cracked windshield" appearance, which can also occur with atypical mycobacteria. Anterior chamber reaction is usually minimal. One case presented as chronic epithelial defect with "calcareous" bodies at the epithelial edge.[47] Sulfonamides, including trimethoprim-sulfamethoxazole,[47,48] and ampicillin are recommended for treatment of *Nocardia* keratitis. Polyhexamethylene biguanide (see Chapter 11) was effective in one case.[49] Penicillin is recommended for *Actinomyces* infections.

Pseudomonas aeruginosa

P. aeruginosa is one of the most important corneal pathogens and is the most common gram-

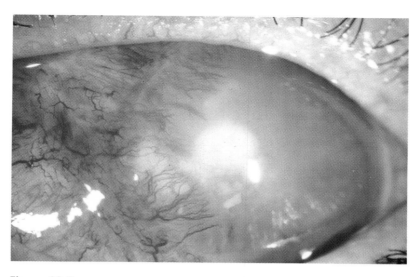

Figure 10-7
Nocardia corneal ulcer.

negative organism causing corneal ulcers.[50] *P. aeruginosa* is found on skin, in saliva, and in the gastrointestinal tract and occurs ubiquitously in the environment. It has been found as a contaminant in hospitals, in fluorescein solutions,[51] eye mascara,[52] and poorly cared for contact lens cases. *Pseudomonas* and *Serratia* are the most common causes of corneal infection in contact lens wearers.[2,53] *Pseudomonas* also frequently causes keratitis in comatose patients[54] and is frequently cultured from patients with tracheostomies.

Surface tissue damage must be present for *Pseudomonas* adherence and infection.[55,56] The virulence of *Pseudomonas* organisms is related to their elaboration of lipases, hemolysins, proteases, and exotoxins and the presence of a surface glycocalyx.[57] The surface glycocalyx allows the organisms to adhere to host cells and to each other and enhances resistance to phagocytosis and antibody-mediated complement killing; exotoxin A, similar to diphtheria toxin, inhibits protein synthesis in human cells, particularly macrophages; lipases attack cell membranes; and proteases digest the proteoglycan ground substance and can destroy small blood vessels. Some clues to which of these factors are most responsible for the severity of these ulcers has been obtained from studies of keratitis in laboratory animals. Immunization against endotoxin,[58] slime capsule,[59] outer membrane proteins,[60] or elatase[61] significantly decreased the severity of *Pseudomonas* ulcers, but immunization against proteases and exotoxin A did not.[61,62] Injection of endotoxin or elastase was

not sufficient to induce formation of a ring infiltrate.[61]

Host enzymes, released in response to *Pseudomonas* infection, also appear to play a large role in the destructive effect.[63] Significantly less corneal and anterior chamber inflammation was seen after *Pseudomonas* injection into the corneas of leukopenic rabbits than in normal animals.[64] The relative importance of bacterial and host factors in the destructiveness of *Pseudomonas* corneal infections is unclear.

Clinically, *P. aeruginosa* often causes a rapidly spreading ulcer, which can extend to twice its size in 24 hours (see Fig. 10-3), and perforation can occur in 2 to 5 days. The ulcer is most commonly central or paracentral. Dense stroma infiltrates and necrosis are characteristic and are often accompanied by edema of the surrounding cornea, posterior corneal stromal folds, endothelial plaques, and hypopyon. Diffuse epithelial graying, or a "ground glass" appearance, is often noted in the nonulcerated portion of the cornea. A copious mucopurulent discharge that may have a greenish color often adheres to the ulcer surface. The greenish color is caused by a fluorescent pigment produced by some strains, and it causes the exudate to fluoresce when exposed to ultraviolet light.

Early descemetocele formation, melting, and perforation are not infrequent. Circumferential progression of paracentral and marginal ulceration is common, and a ring ulcer can form (see Fig. 10-4). *Pseudomonas* corneal infection can extend into the sclera, worsening the prognosis (Fig. 10-8).[65] The corneal infection can smolder

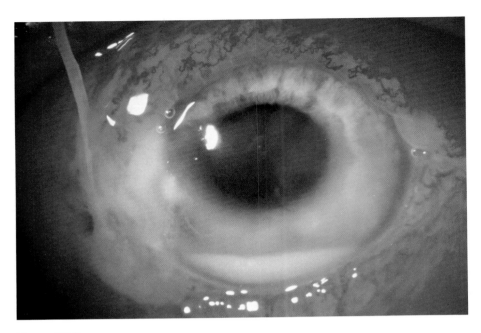

Figure 10-8
Pseudomonas corneoscleritis. (Courtesy of Edward Alfonso, Miami, FL.)

for a long time after treatment is initiated and can recur many days after therapy has been discontinued, particularly if steroids are administered.[66,67] Thus therapy should be continued for several weeks after apparent clinical cure, and steroids should be used cautiously.

Contact lens–associated *Pseudomonas* infections can also manifest themselves as several elevated granular opacities.[68] Less virulent *Pseudomonas* strains can produce more indolent infections, similar to those caused by other bacteria. These strains may lack the enzymes or toxins found in more virulent strains.

Moraxella

Moraxella organisms are commonly found in the nasopharynx and genitourinary tract. They can cause corneal infection in compromised hosts, particularly alcoholics, diabetics, and malnourished and other debilitated patients. The corneal ulcer is an indolent paracentral or peripheral (most commonly inferior) one that usually is oval in shape and localized with an undermined necrotic edge. It progresses deep into the stroma over days or weeks, and untreated ulcers may perforate. Hypopyon may or may not be present. The organism is present in the depths of the crater. The anterior segment is highly inflamed, and the host's resistance usually is low.

Enterobacteriaceae

Enterobacteriaceae spp. such as *E. coli, Serratia, Klebsiella,* and *Proteus* used to be relatively uncommon causes of bacterial keratitis, but such infections are becoming more frequent, particularly in association with contact lens wear. Otherwise, they are seen primarily in compromised eyes. *S. marcescens* appear to the member of this group most commonly involved in contact lens–related infections. It contains an endotoxin and protease and can cause a severe ulcer resulting in perforation.[69,70] Peripheral infiltrates and paracentral ulcers can also occur. In compromised eyes *Proteus vulgaris* is probably most common. *Proteus* spp. can cause a severe keratitis, similar to *Pseudomonas* (Fig. 10-9), and perforation and ring ulcer have been seen.

Neisseria

The gram-negative cocci *N. gonorrhoeae* and *Neisseria meningitidis* can invade the cornea after conjunctivitis through an intact epithelium and cause an ulcer. These ulcers are extremely dangerous, particularly in newborns, because they can lead rapidly to corneal perforation (see Fig. 7-8). Marked purulent discharge, injection, and chemosis usually are present. Systemic treatment is required. Further discussion of gonococcal infection and the current treatment recommendations can be found in Chapter 7.

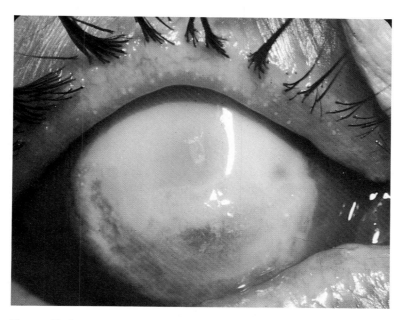

Figure 10-9
Severe keratitis caused by *Proteus mirabilis.*

Atypical Mycobacteria

Atypical mycobacteria are acid-fast organisms that are harbored in soil. *M. fortuitum,*[71-73] *M. chelonei,*[74-76] *M. avium-intracellulare,*[77] and *M. gordonae*[78,79] produce corneal ulcers, most commonly after trauma. The corneal ulcers are similar to those produced by *Moraxella* and *Nocardia* in that they are indolent, progressing slowly over weeks or months.[74] The bed of the ulcer can have a "cracked windshield" appearance. Anterior chamber reaction is often minimal. Any recalcitrant ulcer should prompt suspicion of a *Mycobacterium* spp., and an acid-fast stain and culture on Löwenstein-Jensen medium should be obtained. Topical amikacin is the most frequently used agent. In one study the combination of amikacin and erythromycin was most effective in vitro against *Mycobacterium chelonei* isolates.[80] However, medical treatment often is unsuccessful, and the lesion may need to be removed surgically. Lamellar keratectomy can debulk or eradicate the infection and may avoid penetrating keratoplasty.[81]

Laboratory Work

An etiologic diagnosis is important in dealing with bacterial keratitis to guide antibiotic therapy.[82] The mere clinical appearance of the ulcer is not enough to warrant a specific etiologic diagnosis, and "shotgun" therapy often is ineffective. Every ophthalmologist should be equipped to take adequate scrapings of the ulcer and should know how to interpret the findings. The techniques of obtaining corneal specimens, staining, and culture media are discussed in Chapter 4. Briefly, corneal smears should be obtained from Gram's and Giemsa staining, and specimens should be inoculated onto blood agar, chocolate agar, and thioglycolate broth. If fungal infection is suspected, a smear should be examined with a fungal stain (e.g., periodic acid–Schiff or Gomori methenamine-silver), and a fungal medium such as Sabouraud's dextrose agar should be inoculated. If inflammation worsens or persists despite treatment, reculturing and, in many cases, corneal biopsy are indicated.

If the patient has been wearing contact lenses, the lens case and lens care solutions should be cultured. In some cases these will indicate the causative organism or organisms when corneal cultures do not. Similarly, if a patient has been taking ocular medications, specimens from each should be taken for culture.

Rapid detection tests are becoming available for some bacteria. The limulus lysate test uses horseshoe crab cells to detect endotoxin-producing gram-negative bacteria (see Chapter 4). An enzyme immunoassay for detecting group A streptococci is available and appears to be useful in corneal infections.[83]

Treatment
Initial Antibiotic Therapy

In any case in which a bacterial keratitis is suspected, antibiotic treatment should be given until a more definitive diagnosis can be made. The initial treatment is based on the interpretation of the corneal smears and a clinical assessment of the severity of the keratitis. There is disagreement over whether to begin with broad-spectrum coverage or to tailor initial therapy based on the smear morphology. In previous editions of this text, Jones' method of specifically tailored initial therapy was recommended.[84,85] However, most cornea specialists, including myself, now prefer to use broad-spectrum therapy in most cases. Gram's stain results do not correlate that highly with culture results, particularly if the observer is inexperienced or if a number of organisms or no organisms are seen. In the best of circumstances, in experienced hands and if a single organism is seen in the Gram's stain, the culture results are consistent approximately 70% to 80% of the time.[84-86] Because the consequences of not covering for the causative organism can be very serious and smears are often inaccurate, most now recommend administering broad-spectrum antibiotics.[87-89] The objection to broad-spectrum coverage is that it increases the risk of antibiotic side effects and antagonism and that no broad-spectrum coverage can treat all possible organisms.[85]

Broad-spectrum coverage can be obtained with combined therapy with an aminoglycoside and a cephalosporin or with a fluoroquinolone, either ciprofloxacin or ofloxacin (Table 10-1). Cefazolin is more active in vitro against penicillinase-producing staphylococci and streptococci than bacitracin and erythromycin, is less toxic topically than bacitracin, and is less irritating than methicillin and other semisynthetic penicillins. It also provides coverage against some gram-negative rods, including *E. coli* and *Klebsiella*. Vancomycin has increased gram-positive coverage, particularly against staphylococci and enterococci, but is more irritating.

Gentamicin and tobramycin have been the initial antibiotics of choice for coverage against gram-negative rods. This is based on their sta-

Table 10-1 Broad-spectrum Initial Antibiotic Therapy		
	Selection of Agents	
Results of Smears	**Topical**	**Intravenous**
One bacterium 2 types of bacteria No microorganisms	Cefazolin (50 mg/ml) and tobramycin (14 mg/ml) (vancomycin [50 mg/ml] or bacitracin [10,000 U/ml] instead of cefazolin in penicillin allergic patients) or Ciprofloxacin (3 mg/ml) or ofloxacin (3 mg/ml)	
Exceptions		
Hyperacute conjunctivitis with gram-negative cocci on smear	Penicillin G or bacitracin	Ceftriaxone, or ciprofloxacin (see Chapter 7)
Severe keratitis with gram-negative rods, consider adding	Piperacillin, ciprofloxacin or polymyxin B	
Hyphae	Natamycin*	
Yeasts	Amphotericin B*	
Acid-fast bacilli	Amikacin	
Scleral extension, add		Cefazolin and gentamicin or ciprofloxacin (oral)

*See Table 11-6.

bility, good corneal and intraocular penetration, and broad bactericidal activity, which includes *Pseudomonas, Enterobacter, Klebsiella,* and other aerobic gram-negative organisms. Tobramycin is two to four times more active by weight than gentamicin against *Klebsiella, Enterobacter, Serratia,* and *Proteus.* In addition, in our laboratory, tobramycin has been active against a significantly higher percentage of *Pseudomonas* isolates (84% vs. 60%).

The combination of cefazolin and tobramycin is effective against approximately 95% of all ocular bacterial isolates and all common bacteria. Their main disadvantage is that they are not commercially available as fortified solutions and must be prepared for topical use. Tobramycin is also irritating and toxic to the epithelium.

Single-agent therapy with ciprofloxacin also appears to be effective for about 95% of cases of bacterial keratitis.[90] In a multicenter, randomized study ciprofloxacin was as effective as fortified tobramycin/cefazolin therapy.[91] It is commercially available and is well tolerated. However, the effectiveness of ciprofloxacin in the treatment of streptococcal keratitis is unclear. In one study, only approximately 50% of streptococci isolated from bacterial keratitis were sensitive to ciprofloxacin in vitro.[92] However, many ulcers with streptococci that are resistant in vitro clinically respond to treatment,[91] and cases with streptococci that are sensitive in vitro may not respond.[93] It appears that ciprofloxacin resistance can develop during ocular use.[94]

In vitro, ofloxacin has better gram-positive coverage; in the same study 73% of isolates were sensitive to ofloxacin.[92] It has similar gram-negative activity, except ofloxacin is at least four times less active against *P. aeruginosa.* In a recent multicenter, randomized study of bacterial keratitis, topical ofloxacin 0.3% was as effective as fortified cefazolin and tobramycin and was better tolerated.[95] Ofloxacin was effective against organisms believed to be resistant, such as *Streptococcus* spp. and *P. acnes.* A combination of either ciprofloxacin or ofloxacin plus cefazolin was effective in vitro against all ocular isolates.[92]

Because of the increased convenience and tolerance of ciprofloxacin and ofloxacin, I use these agents in many cases. Combination drug therapy, such as cefazolin or vancomycin plus tobramycin or ciprofloxacin, theoretically covers a broader spectrum of bacteria and may be preferable in some cases, such as large or central ulcers, ulcers associated with hypopyon, or in eyes worsening despite antibiotic treatment. Many rarer bacterial causes of keratitis are not adequately treated by any of these regimens. The most important of these rarer causes is *Neisseria.* If keratitis is associated with a hyperpurulent conjunctivitis and if gram-negative cocci are present in smears, topical bacitracin or penicillin, saline lavage, and intravenous penicillin G or ceftriaxone should be administered (see Chapter 7). In those unusual cases in which acid-fast mycobacteria, fungi, or *Acanthamoeba* are seen in smears, specific therapy for these agents is administered.

Treatment should also be modified in severe keratitis when smears contain gram-negative rods, causing suspicion of *Pseudomonas* involvement. Using two effective agents is often advantageous in cases of *Pseudomonas* infection, particularly before sensitivity is determined. This is because the need for treatment is urgent, because no one agent is effective against all isolates, and because experimentally using two agents appears to be more effective than using only one.[96] I use a combination of tobramycin and either polymyxin B or ciprofloxacin in

Table 10-2 Severity Grade of Microbial Keratitis		
	Severity Grade	
Feature	**Nonsevere**	**Severe***
Rate of progression	Slow, moderate	Rapid
Suppuration		
Area	< 6 mm diameter	> 6 mm diameter
Depth	Superficial two thirds	Inner one third
Depth of ulceration	Superficial one third	Inner one third
Perforation	Unlikely to occur	Present, imminent
Scleral suppuration	Absent	Present

From Jones DB: *Ophthalmology* 88:814, 1981.
*An ulcer is considered severe if it meets three or more of these criteria.

these cases, but ticarcillin, piperacillin, and carbenicillin are also good choices.

Grading the severity of infection is useful in estimating the urgency of appropriate treatment and the risk of perforation and in predicting the causative organism or organisms (Table 10-2). If an infection is judged to be mild, standard-strength topical antibiotics will probably be effective, and the risk of initially ineffective therapy is reduced. In some mild cases, when the patient has already received antibiotics, corneal scrapings can be delayed for 12 to 24 hours to increase the likelihood of isolating the responsible organism.

Routes of Antibiotic Therapy

Topical. For many antibiotics animal studies have demonstrated that concentrations higher than those in the commercially available solutions are more effective in killing bacteria[96-98]; however, clinically the advantage is less evident.[99] Because there does not appear to be an increase in the adverse effects of these medications when the fortified doses are used, it is probably best to use the higher concentrations. Exceptions to this are the fluoroquinolones, ciprofloxacin and ofloxacin, and polymixin B, where the concentration recommended for bacterial keratitis is available commercially. (Polymyxin B [10,000 U/ml] is available in combination with trimethoprim in Polytrim [Allergan, Irvine, CA].) Many other antibiotics are not available commercially as ophthalmic solutions and must be prepared from intravenous solutions.

The methods of preparation of fortified antibiotic solutions are given in Table 10-3. Two antibiotics should not be mixed together in the same container, and the antibiotic solution should be replaced every 5 to 7 days. The antibiotic remains effective for at least 4 weeks,[100,101] but the preservative concentration is reduced, and contamination can occur.

Increasing the frequency of antibiotic drop administration, up to every 30 minutes, has been demonstrated to increase stromal concentrations and bacterial eradication.[96] Part of the benefit of frequent administration of drops may be by washing away bacteria and inflammatory products from the ocular surface. An initial loading dose can achieve peak corneal concentrations more quickly.[102] If a single agent is being used, it can be given every 5 minutes for five applications. Two agents can be alternated every 5 minutes until each has been given five times. If a commercial preparation is available it can be given in this manner until the fortified solution is available. Thereafter doses can be given every 15 minutes to 1 hour over the first day. Some authors recommend administering drops every 15 minutes around the clock in every case, but this appears to be excessive. Even in the worst cases, administration every 30 minutes is sufficient, and in many cases hourly medication is used. If two antibiotics are used, they can be alternated (e.g., every 30 minutes) or given together (5 minutes apart) every hour.

Subconjunctival. The use of subconjunctival antibiotics is controversial. They can rapidly produce high corneal drug levels, but this is short lasting, with subtherapeutic levels reached by 9 hours.[98] In animal models, fortified topical antibiotics are equally as effective as subconjunctival injections,[96-98,103,104] and subconjunctival injections do not provide additional effect when fortified antibiotic solutions are administered.[50,104] Because similarly high concentrations of antibiotics can be obtained in the infected eye by the less traumatic means of frequent topical drops, topical medication seems more logical and just as effective a form of therapy as subconjunctival antibiotics. This is important, especially because subconjunctival antibiotic therapy has certain disadvantages, including patient apprehension, more ocular inflammation, more pain than topical therapy, and a risk of intraocular administration.

Therefore, I recommend subconjunctival antibiotics in only a few situations: when frequent topical administration is not possible, when fortified antibiotic solutions are not available, or to initiate treatment when topical administration will be delayed. In children, topical administration may be limited, so it may be necessary to perform subconjunctival injections every 12 to 24 hours. Chloral hydrate sedation, 100 mg/kg, topical anesthesia, and physical restraint often are sufficient and are preferable to general anesthesia.[20] The antibiotic injection should be placed adjacent to the site of infection, and if two different antibiotics are given, they should be injected at different sites. The methods of preparation of subconjunctival antibiotic injections are given in Table 10-4.

Other Routes. Systemic antibiotics are not routinely recommended for treating infected corneal ulcers. Even in inflamed eyes, only low concentrations of antibiotics usually can be achieved in the cornea and aqueous humor after systemic administration, and using these systemic drugs does not appear to add to the effect of topical or subconjunctival antibiotics. Systemic antibiotics have been recommended for cases with corneal perforation or endophthalmitis. However, recently the Endophthalmitis Vitrectomy Study found that systemic antibiotics were not useful in the treatment of endophthalmitis.[104a] Systemic antibiotics may be useful in eyes with scleral infiltration and for infections in which extraocular tissues are frequently involved, such as infection caused by *Neisseria,* infants with *Pseudomonas* keratitis, or when *Haemophilus* keratitis is accompanied by cellulitis.

Other techniques of antibiotic administration have been proposed. Continuous irrigation can be achieved through a small plastic catheter passed through the lid[105] or by means of a cannulated contact lens, such as the Morgan Therapeutic lens (Wilson Ophthalmic Corporation, Mustang, OK). These devices require partial patient immobilization and are relatively impractical. Hydrophilic contact lenses, made of plastic polymer or collagen, can serve as a reservoir of antibiotic and produce high corneal concentrations.[106,107] These can reduce the necessity for frequent administration of drops; however, they also reduce removal of mucopurulent material and accompanying destructive enzymes from the corneal surface.

Temporary canalicular occlusion is another method of increasing the efficacy of topical antibiotics. Intracanalicular collagen implants in rabbits prolonged the retention of antibiotic in tears, increased stromal concentration, and increased bacterial killing.[108] Iontophoresis can deliver high doses of antibiotics to the corneal stroma,[109] but this has not been tested clinically.

Antibiotic treatment is given at home if the patient is able to comply with the taxing regimen and can return for daily examinations.[110] Certainly any outpatient who is not responding to treatment should be admitted to the hospital, and incorrect technique or poor compliance with treatment should be suspected.

Specific Antibiotics

The following section contains information about antibiotics used to treat corneal ulcers. Tables 10-5 and 10-6 provide a general survey of microbial organisms and antibiotic agents suitable for treatment. Table 10-7 compiles facts concerning the most-used antibiotic agents and classifies them according to their effectiveness and penetration into the eye. As mentioned before, Tables 10-3 and 10-4 list the dosages and

methods of preparation for fortified topical and subconjunctival antibiotics commonly used to treat bacterial keratitis, and the dosages are summarized in Table 10-8.

Penicillins. Penicillins are bactericidal antibiotics that inhibit the biosynthesis of cell wall mucopeptides by sensitive bacteria. All of the penicillins contain a 6-aminopenicillanic acid nucleus, which consists of a β-lactam ring and a thiazolidine ring and differ in the side chains attached to this nucleus.

The major adverse effects of penicillins are hypersensitivity reactions, which occur in approximately 10% of patients, and range from minor skin rash or urticaria to an anaphylactic reaction that may be fatal. Drug-induced fevers are common. Other reactions are enterocolitis, neutropenia, platelet dysfunction, elevated serum glutamic oxaloacetic transaminase, renal toxicity, and hemolytic anemia. Penicillin sensitivity can be determined using an intradermal injection of penicilloyl-polylysine prior to therapy.

Penicillin G. Penicillin G (benzylpenicillin), one of the first penicillins, is effective against gram-positive cocci and *Neisseria, Moraxella,* and many *Klebsiella pneumoniae* isolates. It is not effective against most staphylococci, because they produce a penicillinase, which breaks down the β-lactam ring. Penicillin G is the most active agent against most gram-positive and gram-negative anaerobes, except for *Bacteroides fragilis.*[84]

When given systemically, penicillin penetrates fairly well into the aqueous humor of the normal eye. Intraocular inflammation reduces the effect of the blood–aqueous humor barrier; thus high levels of penicillin are found in the intraocular fluids of inflamed eyes. Penicillin G is absorbed poorly from the gastrointestinal tract, so it must be given intravenously or intramuscularly.

Ampicillin. Ampicillin is effective against a wider spectrum of gram-negative organisms than is penicillin G but is less active against streptococci, staphylococci, and pneumococci. Like penicillin G, it is destroyed by bacterial penicillinase. The spectrum of action against gram-negative organisms includes *Haemophilus influenzae, Proteus mirabilis,* and many strains of *E. coli, Salmonella, Shigella,* and *Moraxella.* Ampicillin is not effective against *P. aeruginosa.*[84]

Penicillinase-resistant Penicillins. This group of semisynthetic penicillins includes oxacillin, cloxacillin, dicloxacillin, methicillin, and nafcillin. These drugs are strongly resistant

Text continued on p. 230

Table 10-3 Preparation of Topical Antibiotics Commonly Used for Treatment of Bacterial Corneal Ulcers

Antibiotic	Remove	Add	Place	Content	Final Concentration
Ampicillin	7 ml from 15-ml tear bottle	3.4 ml to 1-g vial of ampicillin	2 ml from vial in tear bottle	2 ml ampicillin and 8 ml tears	50 mg/ml
Bacitracin	9 ml from 15-ml tear substitute bottle	3 ml tears to each of three vials	All 3 ml from each of three vials (total 9 ml) in original tear substitute bottle	9 ml reconstituted bacitracin and 6 ml tears	10,000 U/ml
Erythromycin lactobionate	7 ml from 15-ml tear bottle	10 ml to 500-mg vial	2 ml from vial in tear bottle	2 ml reconstituted erythromycin and 8 ml tears	10 mg/ml
Neomycin	1 ml from 15-ml tear substitute bottle	1 ml tears to one vial neomycin (500 mg)	1 ml reconstituted neomycin into tear substitute bottle	1 ml neomycin and 14 ml tears	8 mg/ml
Kanamycin		1 vial (500 mg in 2 ml) kanamycin to 15-ml tear bottle		2 ml kanamycin and 15 ml tears	30 mg/ml
Penicillin G	3 ml tears from 15-ml tear substitute bottle	3 ml tears to one vial penicillin G (5 megaunits)	3 ml reconstituted penicillin in tear substitute bottle	3 ml penicillin G and 12 ml tears	110,000 U/ml
Carbenicillin		1 ml carbenicillin (100 mg) to 15-ml tear bottle		1 ml carbenicillin and 15 ml tears	6 mg/ml

Antibiotic					Concentration
Vancomycin	2 ml tears from 15-ml tear substitute bottle	2 ml tears to one vial vancomycin (500 mg)	2 ml reconstituted vancomycin in tear bottle	2 ml vancomycin and 13 ml tears	33 mg/ml
Gentamicin		2 ml parenteral solution (40 mg/ml) to 5-ml bottle ophthalmic gentamicin			14 mg/ml
Cefazolin		5 ml of sterile water to 1-g vial of cefazolin	5 ml cefazolin in 15-ml tear bottle	5 ml cefazolin and 15 ml artificial tears	50 mg/ml
Tobramycin		2 ml of tobramycin (40 mg/ml) to 5-ml bottle ophthalmic preparation		2 ml tobramycin parenteral and 5 ml tobramycin ophthalmic	14 mg/ml
Methicillin	6 ml from 15-ml tear bottle	1.5 ml to 1-g vial of methicillin	1 ml methicillin in tear bottle	1 ml methicillin and 9 ml tears	50 mg/ml
Amikacin	7 ml tears from 15-ml tear substitute bottle	2 ml of amikacin (250 mg/ml) to tear bottle		2 ml amikacin and 8 ml artificial tears	50 mg/ml
Ticarcillin		1 ml ticarcillin (100 mg/ml) to 15-ml tear substitute		1 ml ticarcillin and 15 ml tears	7 mg/ml
Piperacillin	5.3 ml from 15-ml tear substitute	9 ml of sterile saline to 2-gm vial of piperacillin	0.3 ml reconstituted piperacillin in tear bottle	0.3 ml piperacillin (66.7 mg/ml) and 9.7 ml tears	7 mg/ml
Polymyxin B	6 ml from 15-ml tear substitute	5 ml to polymyxin B (500,000 U/vial)	1 ml reconstituted polymyxin in tear bottle	1 ml polymyxin (100,000 U/ml) and 9 ml tears	10,000 U/ml

Table 10-4   Subconjunctival Antibiotic Preparation and Dosage of Commonly Used Drugs for Treatment of Bacterial Corneal Ulcers

Antibiotic	Dose per Vial	Diluent Volume	Concentration	Injection Volume	Total Dose
Amikacin	100 mg	—	50 mg/ml	0.5 ml	25 mg
Ampicillin	1 g	5 ml	200 mg/ml	0.5 ml	100 mg
Bacitracin	50,000 U	2.5 ml	20,000 U/ml	0.5 ml	10,000 units
Carbenicillin	1 g	5 ml	200 mg/ml	0.5 ml	100 mg
Cefazolin	500 mg	2.5 ml	200 mg/ml	0.5 ml	100 mg
Cephaloridine	500 mg	2.5 ml	200 mg/ml	0.5 ml	100 mg
Clindamycin	600 mg/4 ml	4 ml	75 mg/ml	0.5 ml	38 mg
Colistin*	150 mg	2 ml	75 mg/ml	0.3 ml	25 mg
Erythromycin	1 g	5 ml	200 mg/ml	0.5 ml	100 mg
Gentamicin	80 mg	—	40 mg/ml	0.5–1.0 ml	20–40 mg
Methicillin	1 g	5 ml	200 mg/ml	0.5 ml	100 mg
Neomycin	500 mg	1 ml	500 mg/ml	0.5–1.0 ml	250 to 500 mg
Penicillin G*	5 megaunits	2.5 ml	2 megaunits/ml	0.25–0.5 ml	0.5 to 1 megaunit
Piperacillin	2 g	10 ml	200 mg/ml	0.5 ml	100 mg
Polymyxin B	50 mg	5 ml	10 mg/ml	0.5 ml	5 mg
Ticarcillin	—	—	100 mg/ml	1.0 ml	100 mg
Tobramycin	80 g	—	20 mg/ml	0.25 ml	20 mg
Vancomycin	500 mg	5 ml	100 mg/ml	0.25 ml	25 mg

*Painful subconjunctival infection can be avoided if tetracaine is applied topically before injection. To re-enforce this, 4% cocaine may be applied with a cotton-tipped applicator to the area of the intended injection. Use a tuberculin syringe with a 27-gauge needle, and inject 0.5 ml of 1% lidocaine. This may be given before the injection of the drug or with the drug. Parenteral colistimethate sodium is the generic name for colistin to be used for subconjunctival injection.

Table 10-5 General Survey of Antimicrobial Coverage*

Organism	First Choice	Alternative Agents
GRAM-POSITIVE COCCI		
Staphylococcus aureus or *S. epidermidis*		
Non–penicillinase-producing	Penicillin	Cefazolin, vancomycin, ciprofloxacin, ofloxacin, imipenem
Penicillinase-producing	Methicillin (topically); oxacillin or nafcillin (systemically)	Cefazolin, vancomycin, ciprofloxacin, ofloxacin, imipenem
Methicillin-resistant	Vancomycin	Trimethoprim/sulfamethoxazole, minocycline
Streptococci		
Group A (*Streptococcus pyogenes*)	Penicillin	Cefazolin, vancomycin, erythromycin, azithromycin
Group B (*Streptococcus agalactiae*)	Penicillin	Ampicillin, cefazolin, vancomycin, erythromycin
Group D (*Enterococcus, Streptococcus bovis*)	Penicillin	Vancomycin, ciprofloxacin, ofloxacin
Viridans group	Penicillin	Cefazolin, vancomycin
Streptococcus pneumoniae	Penicillin	Cefazolin, erythromycin, vancomycin, chloramphenicol
GRAM-NEGATIVE COCCI		
Neisseria gonorrhoeae	Ceftriaxone	Ciprofloxacin, ofloxacin, cefixime, cefoxitin, cefotaxime, cefuroxime
Neisseria meningitidis	Penicillin	Third-generation cephalosporins, chloramphenicol
Branhamella catarrhalis	Gentamicin	Cefazolin, penicillin, ampicillin, erythromycin, chloramphenicol
Moraxella	Gentamicin	Fluoroquinolones, tobramycin, erythromycin, chloramphenicol, ?cefazolin, ampicillin-sulbactam
GRAM-POSITIVE BACILLI		
Clostridium spp.	Penicillin	Chloramphenicol, metronidazole, clindamycin, vancomycin
Bacillus spp.	Gentamicin	Gentimicin, vancomycin, clindamycin, fluoroquinolone, chloramphenicol, imipenem, erythromycin
Corynebacterium diphtheriae	Bacitracin	Penicillin, erythromycin, clindamycin, rifampin, tetracycline, vancomycin
Listeria monocytogenes	Ampicillin	Penicillin, chloramphenicol, erythromycin, tetracycline, vancomycin, cefazolin
GRAM-NEGATIVE BACILLI		
Acinetobacter	Imipenem	Tobramycin, gentamicin, or amikacin, usually with ticarcillin or piperacillin
Aeromonas	Trimethoprim/ sulfamethoxazole	Gentamicin, tobramycin, ciprofloxacin, ofloxacin, imipenem
Bacteroides fragilis	Clindamycin	Chloramphenicol, imipenem, cefoxitin, piperacillin
Bacteroides spp.	Penicillin	Clindamycin, cefoxitin, chloramphenicol, metronidazole
Enterobacter	Imipenem	Fluoroquinolone, ceftriaxone, ceftazidime, an aminoglycoside plus piperacillin or ticarcillin

Continued

Table 10-5	General Survey of Antimicrobial Coverage—cont'd	
Organism	**First Choice**	**Alternative Agents**
GRAM-NEGATIVE BACILLI—cont'd		
Escherichia coli	Aminoglycoside	Fluoroquinolone, third-generation cephalosporin
Haemophilus influenzae	Cefotaxime or ceftriaxone	Cefuroxime, fluoroquinolone, ampicillin, chloramphenicol
Klebsiella pneumoniae	Aminoglycoside	Cephalosporin, fluoroquinolone
Proteus mirabilis	Fluoroquinolone	Aminoglycoside, third-generation cephalosporin
Pseudomonas aeruginosa	Tobramycin	Ceftazidime, ciprofloxacin, piperacillin, imipenem, aztreonam
Serratia marcescens	Aminoglycoside	Third-generation cephalosporin, fluoroquinolone, piperacillin, ticarcillin, imipenem, aztreonam
Shigella	Fluoroquinolone	Ceftriaxone, ampicillin, chloramphenicol, ?piperacillin, ?polymyxin B
MISCELLANEOUS ORGANISMS		
Actinomyces israelii	Penicillin	Chloramphenicol, tetracycline, ?ampicillin, bacitracin, clindamycin, vancomycin
Nocardia spp.	Trimethoprim/ sulfamethoxazole	Amikacin, minocycline, clofazimine, erythromycin, sulfonamides, minocycline
Atypical mycobacteria	Amikacin plus erythromycin	Rifampin, clofazimine, streptomycin, imipenem, fluoroquinolone

*Modified from Reese RE, Betts RF, editors: *Handbook of antibiotics*, Boston, 1993, Little, Brown & Co.

to destruction by bacterial penicillinase. (Bacterial penicillinase is also called β-lactamase, and drugs resistant to it are called β-lactams.) The semisynthetic penicillins are less effective against nonpenicillinase-producing gram-positive microorganisms than is penicillin G. They should be reserved to treat infections known to be caused by penicillinase-producing staphylococci.[84]

S. aureus isolates resistant to all β-lactams are referred to as *methicillin resistant*. They have an altered penicillin-binding protein as the basis of their resistance and are resistant to all penicillins and cephalosporins. Vancomycin, trimethoprim/sulfamethoxazole, and minocycline may inhibit methicillin-resistant staphylococci.

Other Penicillins. Carbenicillin and ticarcillin are carboxy penicillins with decreased activity against gram-positive organisms but a wider spectrum of activity against gram-negative organisms.[82,84,111] They are useful against *P. aeruginosa*, indole-positive *Proteus*, *Enterobacter* and non–β-lactamase-producing *Haemophilus*, *N.*

meningitidis, and *N. gonorrhoeae*. They are not penicillinase resistant. Some evidence suggests that carbenicillin and ticarcillin are synergistic with gentamicin against *Pseudomonas* organisms, but there is also evidence that they antagonize the effect of gentamicin.[112] Ticarcillin is four times more active than carbenicillin.

Carbenicillin is not available for intravenous use. The main indication for parenteral administration would be in combination with gentamicin or tobramycin in keratitis caused by *Pseudomonas*. Use for other gram-negative infections is guided by sensitivity testing.

Piperacillin is a ureido penicillin, which is a derivative of ampicillin. It has even greater activity against *P. aeruginosa* and the Enterobacteriaceae than ticarcillin and carbenicillin. It also has excellent activity against *Neisseria*, *Haemophilus*, and streptococcal species. It is destroyed by β-lactamases.

Peptide Antibiotics.

Bacitracin. Bacitracin acts similarly to penicillin G by interfering with cell wall synthesis and binding to cell membranes to produce false pores and flux of ions. It is a peptide antibiotic, composed of peptide-linked amino acids. Bacitracin is bactericidal and is effective against *Neisseria,* gram-positive cocci, *H. influenzae,* and some gram-positive bacilli, including *C. diphtheriae, Clostridium,* and *Actinomyces.* Bacitracin is effective against penicillinase-producing staphylococci.[84]

The use of bacitracin in ophthalmology should be restricted to topical administration and subconjunctival injection; it is too toxic for systemic use. Fortified bacitracin is irritating to the ocular surface and can cause a keratopathy. Allergic sensitization is rare.

Polymyxin B. Polymyxin is another peptide antibiotic that alters cell membrane permeability. It is active against many gram-negative organisms, including *Pseudomonas, Salmonella, Shigella, Klebsiella* and *E. coli.* It is not effective against *Proteus* or *Serratia.* Like bacitracin, it is limited to topical use.

Aminoglycosides. Aminoglycoside antibiotics are bactericidal, achieving this by binding to bacterial ribosomes and blocking protein synthesis. They are active against the Enterobacteriaceae (e.g., *E. coli, Serratia, Enterobacter,* and *Klebsiella*) and against *Pseudomonas* and most *S. aureus,* but not streptococci.

All aminoglycosides can cause ototoxicity and nephrotoxicity. Excretion is primarily by glomerular filtration, so extremely high concentrations are present in renal cortical tissue, and serum levels are dependent on glomerular function. If aminoglycosides are given systemically, renal function should be tested so that the dose can be adjusted if renal function is reduced and to monitor for renal toxicity. The renal toxicity is usually mild and reversible; however, it can result in renal failure.

Ototoxicity occurs in 2% to 12% of patients receiving systemic treatment, is dose- and duration-related, and is permanent in approximately 50% of these patients. Aminoglycosides should not be given concurrently with other ototoxic agents.[84] Commercial gentamicin and tobramycin eyedrops inhibit epithelial wound healing.[113] However, it is not clear whether this is due to the drug or to other ingredients, such as preservatives and vehicles. A tissue culture study did not observe inhibition of epithelial healing by tobramycin.[114] Aminoglycosides can cause punctate keratopathy or pseudomembranous conjunctivitis.

Gentamicin. Gentamicin is effective against most gram-negative bacteria, including *P. aeruginosa, E. coli, S. marcescens, Proteus, Klebsiella,* and *Moraxella.* Gentamicin is active against staphylococci and some streptococci but not against pneumococci. As mentioned previously, although carbenicillin may act synergistically with gentamicin in vitro, there is also some evidence that in vivo the combination may be antagonistic.

Tobramycin. Tobramycin is similar to gentamicin in antimicrobial activity and toxicity, but it is reported to be two to four times more active in vitro, by weight, against *P. aeruginosa.*[115] It is also effective against many gentamicin-resistant strains. In our laboratory, 84% of *P. aeruginosa* isolates were sensitive to tobramycin and only 62% were sensitive to gentamicin. However, gentamicin was effective against a greater percentage of streptococcal isolates, and more effective against *Serratia.* For keratitis caused by sensitive organisms, there has been no evidence to date that tobramycin is superior clinically to gentamicin. The toxicity of the two drugs is similar. The doses for tobramycin are the same as for gentamicin.

Amikacin. Many strains of *Pseudomonas* resistant to gentamicin and tobramycin are sensitive to amikacin, a semisynthetic aminoglycoside. Most acquired resistance to aminoglycosides involves microbial enzymatic inactivation of the drugs in the bacterial membrane or near the site of drug transport. Amikacin is resistant to inactivation by most bacterial enzymes. Fluoroquinolones, carboxy penicillins, piperacillin, and polymyxin B are other therapeutic alternatives. Amikacin is also active against some atypical mycobacteria.

Neomycin. Neomycin is effective against a wide spectrum of gram-negative bacteria as well as staphylococci. Neomycin may be given topically or subconjunctivally (Table 10-8). Commercially, it is most commonly available in combination with polymyxin B and bacitracin. Hypersensitivity reactions and punctate keratitis occasionally occur. Neomycin does not inhibit epithelial healing.[113] Because subconjunctival injections may be quite painful, it is advisable to instill a topical anesthetic agent, followed by an injection of 0.5 ml of 1% lidocaine. The lidocaine should be allowed to diffuse; then the neomycin should be injected slowly and carefully.

Erythromycin. Erythromycin is a macrolide antibiotic that is bacteriostatic in low concentrations and bactericidal in high concentrations. It is effective against gram-positive cocci, gram-positive bacilli, *Neisseria,* and *Moraxella.* It is also effective against chlamydia and mycoplasma. The drug is used frequently when a pa-

Table 10-6 Antibiotic Sensitivities of Common Bacteria

	Amikacin	Ampicillin	Bacitracin*	Cefazolin*	Ceftazidime	Cefuroxime	Chloramphenicol*	Ciprofloxacin*	Erythromycin*	Gentamicin*	Methicillin	Neomycin	Ofloxacin*	Penicillin G*	Piperacillin	Polymyxin B*	Sulfonamides*	Tetracyclines*	Tobramycin*	Trimethoprim-Sulfamethoxazole	Vancomycin
GRAM-POSITIVE COCCI																					
Staphylococcus coagulase negative	+	±	+	⊕	+	+	+	±	±	+	+	+	+	−	±	−	+	±	+	+	+
*Staphyloccus aureus**	+	−	+	⊕	+	+	+	±	+	+	+	+	+	−	±	−	+	+	+	+	+
Methicillin-resistant staphylococci	−	−	⊕	−	−	−	+	+	−	±	+	−	+	−	−	−	+	±	±	+	+
alpha-Hemolytic streptococci*	−	+	+	+	+	+	+	±	+	±	+	−	±	⊕	+	−	+	±	±	+	+
beta-Hemolytic streptococci*	−	+	±	⊕	+	+	±	+	+	±	+	−	±	⊕	+	−	±	±	±	±	+
Enterococci	−	⊕	+	−	−	−	+	±	±	−	+	−	±	±	+	−	±	+	±	±	+
*Streptococcus pneumoniae**	−	+	+	⊕	+	+	+	±	+	−	±	−	+	⊕	+	−	+	±	+	+	+
Anaerobic *Streptococcus* spp.	−	±	+	+		+	+	±	+	−	±	−	+	⊕	+	−		±	±		
GRAM-POSITIVE BACILLI																					
Bacillus spp.*			−	−		±	+	+	±	⊕	−	+	+	−		−	+	±	+		+
Clostridium spp.			±	±		+	±	−	±	−		−	+	⊕	+	−		±	−		+
Corynebacterium spp.*		±	⊕	±	−		+	±	±	±	±	+	±	±		+	±	+	±	+	
Listeria monocytogenes		⊕					+	±	+	±			+	±		−		+			
GRAM-NEGATIVE COCCI																					
*Branhamella cotarrhalis**			+	+	+	±	+	+	+	+	±	+	+		+	+	+	+	+	+	−
Neisseria spp.*		⊕	+	+	+	±	±	+	+	+	±	±	+	⊕	+	±	+	±	+		

GRAM-NEGATIVE BACILLI

- Acinetobacter spp.*
- Bacteroides fragilis
- Bacteroides spp.
- Citrobacter spp.
- Enterobacter spp.*
- Escherichia coli
- Haemophilus influenzae*
- Klebsiella spp.*
- Moraxella spp.*
- Proteus mirabilis
- Proteus spp. (indole positive)
- Pseudomonas aeruginosa
- Pseudomonas spp.*
- Salmonella spp.
- Serratia spp.*
- Shigella spp.

OTHERS

- Actinomyces spp.*

Organism	Susceptibility pattern (across drug columns)
Acinetobacter spp.*	− + + + + + − − + ⊕ − ⊕ − + − − + ⊕
Bacteroides fragilis	− − − − + − − − ⊕ − − ⊕
Bacteroides spp.	− − − ⊕ ⊕ − + ⊕ + ⊕ − ⊕ + ⊕
Citrobacter spp.	− + +± +± +± + +± +± +± +± +± +± + +± +± +±
Enterobacter spp.*	− ⊕ ⊕ + ⊕ +± + ⊕ + + +± ⊕ ⊕ +± +±
Escherichia coli	− + + +± + ⊕ +± + + + ⊕ +± +
Haemophilus influenzae*	− + + + + + + +± ⊕ + +± + + ⊕
Klebsiella spp.*	− + + +± + +± +± +± + + + + ⊕ + +±
Moraxella spp.*	− + + ⊕ + + + + + + +± + + +
Proteus mirabilis	− + + + + + + + + ⊕ +± ⊕ + +± +±
Proteus spp. (indole positive)	− + + + +± + + + + + + +± +
Pseudomonas aeruginosa	− − − − +± + + − − − − + ⊕ +±
Pseudomonas spp.*	− − − − +± +± − − − − − + ⊕ −
Salmonella spp.	− + + + + + + + + ⊕ + + ⊕
Serratia spp.*	− + ⊕ + + + ⊕ + + + + + + ⊕
Shigella spp.	− + + + + + + + ⊕ + + + ⊕

OTHERS

Organism	Susceptibility pattern
Actinomyces spp.*	+ + + +± + +| + ⊕ − + +| +| +| + + +

*Data from Campbell Laboratory, Pittsburgh, PA.

+ = 80% to 100% of isolates sensitive.

± = 40% to 79% of isolates sensitive.

− = less than 40% of isolates sensitive.

⊕ Drug of choice or commonly used drug.

Table 10-7   Spectrum, Penetration, and Action of Principal Antibiotics Used to Treat Bacterial Corneal Ulcers

Drug	Spectrum		Penetration	Action	Important Facts
	Gram-positive organisms	Gram-negative organisms			
Amikacin	−	+		Bactericidal	Active against large number of gram-negative bacteria resistant to gentamicin, kanamycin, and tobramycin Active against mycobacteria Cochlear toxicity
Ampicillin	+	±	Good	Bactericidal	Not effective against penicillinase-producing staphylococci, indole-positive *Proteus* or *Pseudomonas*
Bacitracin	+	−		Bactericidal	Allergy is rare; not to be given systemically because of toxicity
Carbenicillin	+	+	Fair	Bactericidal	May be synergistic with gentamicin in severe *Pseudomonas, Proteus*, and *Escherichia coli* infections; not effective against penicillinase producing staphylococci, *Klebsiella*, or *Serratia*
Cephalosporins (similar in action to penicillins)	+	±	Good	Bactericidal	Effective against penicillinase-producing staphylococci and streptococci (except enterococci) and isolates of *E. coli, Klebsiella*, and *Proteus mirabilis;* not good against *Pseudomonas* indole-positive *Proteus*, or *Haemophilus influenzae*
Chloramphenicol	+	+	Good	Bacteriostatic	Serious blood dyscrasias
Cloxacillin	+	−		Bactericidal	Penicillinase resistant
Dicloxacillin	+	−	Good	Bactericidal	Penicillinase resistant
Erythromycin	+	−		Bacteriostatic	Topical ointment is used, subconjunctival injection is also given; may be employed when patient is allergic to penicillin
Fluoroquinolones	+	+	Good	Bactericidal	Variable activity against streptococci; resistance can develop rapidly
Gentamicin	±	+	Poor	Bactericidal	Effective against *Pseudomonas* and some staphylococci Nephrotoxic, ototoxic

| Table 10-7 | | Spectrum, Penetration, and Action of Principal Antibiotics Used to Treat Bacterial Corneal Ulcers—cont'd | | | |

Drug	Spectrum Gram-positive organisms	Gram-negative organisms	Penetration	Action	Important Facts
Methicillin	+	−	Poor	Bactericidal	Effective against penicillinase-producing staphylococci Nephrotoxic; depresses bone marrow
Neomycin	±	+	?Good	Bactericidal	For topical and subconjunctival use only Hypersensitivity
Oxacillin	+	−	Poor	Bactericidal	Penicillinase resistant
Penicillin G	+	−	Good in inflamed eye	Bactericidal	Hypersensitivity
Piperacillin	+	+		Bactericidal	Particularly useful against *Pseudomonas*
Polymyxin B	−	+	Poor	Bactericidal	Effective against *Pseudomonas* but not against *Proteus vulgaris* Nephrotoxic
Sulfonamides	+	+	Good	Bacteriostatic	Hypersensitivity
Tetracyclines	+	+		Bacteriostatic	Effective against *Chlamydia;* not for pregnant women or children under 8 years of age, take on an empty stomach
Tobramycin	±	+		Bactericidal	Effective against most penicillinase-producing staphylococci, as well as *Pseudomonas, Enterobacter, Klebsiella, Serratia,* and *E. coli* Ototoxic and nephrotoxic, with some neuromuscular toxicity

tient is allergic to the penicillins or cephalosporins. Erythromycin is used as either a topical solution or an ointment in a concentration of 5 mg/ml. It is well tolerated but penetrates the cornea poorly. Subconjunctival injections of 5 to 10 mg in a small volume of distilled water may be used. Erythromycin can be given orally, at a dose of 1 to 2 g per day in four divided doses, but it commonly causes gastrointestinal symptoms. When used concurrently with oral theophylline, blood levels of theophylline can be increased, sometimes to toxic levels.

Cephalosporins. The cephalosporins are semisynthetic compounds, similar to penicillin, derived from a naturally occurring antibiotic produced by the fungus *Cephalosporium.*[116] Like penicillin, they are bactericidal and exert their effect by interfering with cell wall synthesis. All of these drugs are effective against nonpenicillinase-producing staphylococci, pneumococci, and streptococci and some strains of gram-negative bacilli, particularly *E. coli, P. mirabilis,* and *Klebsiella.* The first-generation cephalosporins (e.g., cephalothin, cephaloridine, cefazolin, and cephalexin) are effective against most penicillinase-producing staphylococci. The second-generation cephalosporins (e.g., cefamandole, cefoxitin, and cefuroxime) have a wider gram-negative spectrum than the first-

Table 10-8 Dosages for Principal Antibiotics Used to Treat Bacterial Keratitis

Drug	Topical	Subconjunctival	Systemic
Amikacin	50 mg/ml	25 mg	15 mg/kg/day IM or slow IV in two or three divided doses*
Ampicillin	—	100 mg	2–4 g every 4 hours IV*
Amoxicillin	—	—	500 mg–1 g every 8 hours orally*
Bacitracin	10,000 U/ml	—	—
Carbenicillin	4 mg/ml	100 mg	—
Cefazolin	50 mg/ml	100 mg	0.5–1.5 g every 6 hours IV*
Cefotaxime	?	?	1–2 g every 8 hours IV*
Cefoxitin	?	?	2 g every 6 to 8 hours IV*
Ceftazidime	?	?	1–2 g every 8 hours IV*
Cefuroxime	?	?	750 mg–1.5 g every 8 hours IV*
Chloramphenicol	5 mg/ml	100 mg	—
Ciprofloxacin	3 mg/ml	?	500–750 mg orally every 12 hours*
Clindamycin	—	40 mg	600 mg every 8 hours IV
Erythromycin	5 mg/g ointment	100 mg	2–4 g daily orally in four divided doses or 1 g every 6 hours IV
Gentamicin	14 mg/ml	20–40 mg	3–5 mg/kg/day IM or IV in 8-hour doses*
Imipenem	?	?	500 mg–1 g every 6 hours*
Methicillin	—	75–100 mg	—
Nafcillin	—	75–100 mg	2–2.5 g every 4 hours IV with 0.5 g probenecid orally four times daily
Neomycin	5 mg/g 3.5 mg/ml solution	250–500 mg	—
Ofloxacin	3 mg/ml	?	300–400 mg orally every 12 hours*
Oxacillin	—	75–100 mg	2–2.5 g every 4 hours IV with 0.5 g probenecid orally four times daily
Penicillin G	100,000 U/ml	0.5–1 million U (300–600 mg)	2–4 megaunits every 4 hours IV with 0.5 g probenecid orally four times daily*
Polymyxin B	10,000 U	10 g	—
Piperacillin	6.7 mg/ml	100 mg	3–4 g every 4 to 6 hours IV*
Sulfacetamide	30%	—	—
Ticarcillin	6.7 mg/ml	100 mg	200–300 mg/kg/day IV into 4 hour doses
Tobramycin	14 mg/ml	20 to 40 mg	3–5 mg/kg/day IM or IV into 8 hour doses
Vancomycin	50 mg/ml	25 mg	1 g every 12 hours IV

*Doses must be modified in renal failure.

generation cephalosporins, but none of these are effective against *Pseudomonas*. Some of the third-generation drugs, particularly ceftazidime and cefoperazone, have some activity against *Pseudomonas,* but the minimum inhibitory concentrations are fairly high, so single-agent treatment with these agents is not recommended.

None of the cephalosporins are very effective against methicillin-resistant staphylococci or enterococcal streptococci.[117]

Cephalosporins have been proposed as an alternative antibiotic for use when a patient is known to be allergic to penicillin. Approximately 1% to 8% of patients known to be sensitive to penicillin will have a reaction to a cephalosporin, so the drug should be administered with caution.[118]

Cefazolin is a first-generation cephalosporin that is commonly used to treat bacterial keratitis. It often is used with an aminoglycoside in initial broad-spectrum antibiotic treatment. It can be given topically (50 mg/ml) or subconjunctivally (100 mg/ml). It is relatively nontoxic to the corneal epithelium.

Cefuroxime, a commonly used second-generation cephalosporin, has increased activity against *H. influenzae* and other gram-negative bacilli, while maintaining good activity against *S. aureus, S. pneumonia,* and group A and group B streptococci. The usual systemic dose is 750 mg to 1.5 g every 8 hours.

Third-generation cephalosporins (cefotaxime, cefoperazone, moxalactam, ceftriaxone, ceftazidime, cefixime) are less active than first-generation cephalosporins against *S. aureus* but are very active against streptococci, *H. influenzae, Neisseria,* and most Enterobacteriaceae.[119] Ceftazidime is the best cephalosporin for *P. aeruginosa.* In one rabbit study it was very effective against *P. aeruginosa* keratitis.[120] Ceftriaxone and cefotaxime are recommended in the treatment of *Neisseria* (see Chapter 7). Experience with the newer generation cephalosporins in keratitis is limited.

Fluoroquinolones. Fluoroquinolones are a new class of antibiotics that inhibit DNA replication. They are bactericidal, binding to DNA gyrase (bacterial topoisomerase II) and inhibiting superhelical coiling of DNA during replication. Ciprofloxacin has a broad spectrum of activity that includes *Pseudomonas,* gram-positive cocci, anaerobes, chlamydia, and mycobacteria. The combination of ciprofloxacin and an antipseudomonal penicillin (e.g., ticarcillin, piperacillin) is synergistic for about 20% to 50% of isolates of *P. aeruginosa.*[121] Ciprofloxacin penetrates the cornea relatively well.[122] In animal models of infectious keratitis a topical solution of 3 mg/ml was found to be as or more effective than fortified cefazolin and vancomycin against methicillin-sensitive *S. aureus,*[123,124] more effective than fortified cefazolin or tobramycin and equally as effective as vancomycin against methicillin-resistant *S. epidermidis,* and as effective as fortified tobramycin against *Pseudomonas.*[124] In another animal study of *S. aureus* keratitis, ciprofloxacin was not as effective as fortified tobramycin against a methicillin-sensitive strain, and only effective against a methicillin-resistant strain if given very early in infection.[125]

In one clinical study topical ciprofloxacin 0.3% was effective in 92% of 148 culture-positive cases of bacterial keratitis.[90] In another study, a ciprofloxacin-treated group was compared with a retrospective control group treated with fortified cefazolin and gentamicin, and no significant differences were observed.[126] Clinical resistance to ciprofloxacin treatment has been observed with some infections, including cases caused by *S. pneumoniae, S. epidermidis,* and *Xanthomonas maltophila.*[127]

Ciprofloxacin 0.3% is well tolerated topically, with no significant epithelial toxicity.[128] However, a high concentration (100 μg/ml) was found to inhibit corneal epithelial cell growth in tissue culture.[114] It commonly forms a white precipitate, usually in the area of the epithelial defect.[90] This can decrease visualization of the infiltrate and may inhibit epithelial healing. The precipitate can resolve despite continued treatment or can persist despite cessation of treatment. An ointment form of ciprofloxacin is under investigation and appears to be well tolerated and effective.[129] Systemic administration of ciprofloxacin results in intraocular levels approximately 10% of those achieved in serum, and reaches the minimum inhibitory concentration[90] of many bacterial species, including *S. epidermidis* and *Bacillus* spp.[130,131] Fluoroquinolones are not recommended for use in children or pregnant women, because they have been found to produce cartilage erosions in young animals. Antacids containing magnesium or aluminum, and sucralfate can impair absorption.

Norfloxacin has a spectrum of antimicrobial activity similar to ciprofloxacin, but is less active against *P. aeruginosa, Streptococcus* spp., *Chlamydia trachomatis,* and most anaerobic bacteria.[132-134] It was not as effective as ciprofloxacin against an aminoglycoside-resistant strain of *P. aeruginosa* in an experimental model of keratitis.[135] In one study it had epithelial toxicity comparable with that of an aminoglycoside,[128] while another study found epithelial toxicity only at a very high concentration (100 μg/ml).[114] A topical ophthalmic preparation is commercially available but has been approved in the United States only for treatment of bacterial conjunctivitis.

Ofloxacin has a spectrum of activity similar to that of ciprofloxacin. Ofloxacin appears to have better coverage for gram-positive ocular pathogens,[92] but is four times less active against *P. aeruginosa.* In a recent multicenter, randomized study of bacterial keratitis topical ofloxacin 0.3% was as effective as fortified cefazolin and tobramycin and was better tolerated.[136] A combination of either ciprofloxacin or ofloxacin plus cefazolin was effective in vitro against all ocular isolates.[92] Ofloxacin penetrates well into the aqueous after topical or oral administration, which indicates that it penetrates well into the stroma.[137] The oral dose of ofloxacin is 300 to 400 mg every 12 hours.

Chloramphenicol. Chloramphenicol is bacteriostatic and acts by inhibiting protein synthesis. It is active against a wide range of gram-positive and gram-negative organisms (see Table 10-6) and is most useful against ampicillin-resistant *H. influenzae*. Chloramphenicol penetrates well into aqueous and vitreous humor after parenteral or oral administration. Its wide spectrum, excellent penetration, and convenience of use should have made this a desirable drug; however, its adverse effects limit its use.

The most serious adverse reaction is bone marrow suppression, which can be severe and irreversible.[82,84] Other adverse reactions include skin rash, optic neuritis, "gray" illness, and gastrointestinal inflammation. The reactions may be idiosyncratic and not dose related, or toxic and dose related. Systemic administration of chloramphenicol should be reserved for severe infections in which the causative organism is known to be sensitive to chloramphenicol and to no other drug.

Only one well-documented case of bone marrow suppression has been reported after topical use of chloramphenicol, and prolonged treatment with large doses was given.[138] However, it is probably wise to avoid topical use of this drug unless it is absolutely necessary, mainly for medicolegal reasons.

Tetracyclines. Tetracyclines are bacteriostatic antibiotics that interfere with bacterial protein synthesis by blocking attachment of transfer RNA to ribosomes. Tetracyclines are effective against a broad spectrum of gram-positive and gram-negative bacteria, as well as *Chlamydia, Mycoplasma,* and Rickettsiae. They inhibit *Actinomyces*, mycobacteria, *Borrelia*, and *Treponema pallidum*. However, many bacterial isolates are resistant, so its use should be guided by sensitivity testing. Tetracyclines are indicated in the treatment of rickettsial infections, sexually transmitted chlamydial infections, *Mycoplasma*, Lyme disease, brucellosis, and relapsing fever. Oral tetracycline has also been shown to reduce corneal ulceration after alkali burns in experimental animals.[139]

Topically, tetracycline has good corneal penetration and rarely causes adverse reactions. Gastrointestinal absorption of orally administered tetracyclines is inhibited by iron, antacids, dairy products, and other calcium-containing products. Absorption is best if tetracyclines are taken on an empty stomach. Doxycline and minocycline are more expensive than tetracycline, but they can be given every 12 to 24 hours, which may improve compliance. Systemic side effects include gastrointestinal upset, phototoxicity, pseudotumor cerebri, renal toxicity, and hepatic dysfunction. Tetracyclines cause bone and tooth discoloration and enamel hypoplasia and should not be given to pregnant women or to children under 8 years of age.

Sulfonamides. The sulfonamides are bacteriostatic agents that inhibit bacterial synthesis of folic acid. They are active against a variety of gram-positive and gram-negative bacteria, as well as chlamydia. They are not first-line drugs for most causes of keratitis but are the treatment of choice for *Nocardia*. Penetration of topical preparations is good, and these drugs are well tolerated, including fortified solutions (30%). After systemic administration, allergic reactions, even Stevens-Johnson syndrome, can occur, as well as blood dyscrasias and gastrointestinal upset.

Trimethoprim. Trimethoprim is a diaminopyrimidine that also inhibits bacterial folic acid synthesis. It is active against most gram-positive aerobic cocci and gram-negative rods, with the exception of *P. aeruginosa* and *Bacteroides*. It is not an effective agent for *Neisseria*. Systemically, it is usually used in combination with sulfamethoxazole. The ophthalmic preparation Polytrim (Allergan, Irvine, CA) contains trimethoprim, 1 mg/ml, and polymyxin B, 10,000 U/ml. It is approved for the treatment of conjunctivitis. It is generally well tolerated but can cause stinging and burning on administration, and, rarely, hypersensitivity.

Vancomycin. Vancomycin is a glycopeptide antibiotic that has been used with increasing frequency because many staphylococci are resistant to other antibiotics. Vancomycin is bactericidal and acts by inhibiting cell wall synthesis. It is effective against most gram-positive bacteria, including methicillin-resistant staphylococci and hemolytic and nonhemolytic streptococci. It can be used in combination with an aminoglycoside or fluoroquinolone to achieve broad-spectrum antibacterial coverage. For systemic use vancomycin must be administered intravenously. Vancomycin is ototoxic and mildly nephrotoxic and can increase the nephrotoxicity and ototoxicity of an aminoglycoside. Subconjunctival injections (25 mg) can cause sloughing, and it can be irritating topically (50 mg/ml). Intravitreal use appears to be well tolerated.

Rifampin. Rifampin is effective against mycobacteria, chlamydia, and some gram-positive and gram-negative bacteria.[140] Rifampin inhibits bacterial growth by blocking RNA-polymerase activity. Clinically, it is used in the treatment of mycobacterial infections. It is used orally in the treatment of tuberculosis and topically in the treatment of atypical mycobacteria.

Others. Imipenem is a member of the carbapenem class of β-lactam antibiotics, which are resistant to bacterial β-lactamase. It has the widest spectrum of any β-lactam antibiotic. Imipenem is active against most bacteria, including *Pseudomonas*, streptococci, and staphylococci, except for methicillin-resistant strains. It appears to exhibit synergism with aminoglycosides against many strains of *Pseudomonas* but may exhibit antagonism with cephalosporins and expanded penicillins.[141] A 5-mg/ml topical solution was found to be effective against an aminoglycoside-resistant *Pseudomonas* strain in a rabbit model.[142] Aztreonam, another new β-lactam antibiotic also has broad gram-negative aerobe activity but is not active against gram-positive organisms. It is a rational alternative for gram-negative bacillary infections in the penicillin-allergic patient.

Fusidic acid has been used since the 1960s to treat severe systemic staphylococcal infections, but it recently became available in Europe commercially as a topical ophthalmic preparation. It is a bactericidal drug with good corneal penetration even when the epithelium is intact, and it is effective against β-lactamase–producing and methicillin-resistant staphylococci, *Branhamella,* and *Neisseria.* In one clinical study, fusidic acid was proven save and effective in the treatment of staphylococcal keratitis.[143]

Adjunctive Therapy

Cycloplegics should be used to increase comfort and decrease formation of posterior synechiae. Mucopurulent and necrotic debris should be removed daily. Factors that contributed to the development of the infection or that could impair healing should be eliminated, if possible. Entropion, trichiasis, or lagophthalmos should be corrected. Punctal occlusion or lateral tarsorrhaphy should be considered in patients with keratitis sicca.

Collagenase inhibitors such as ethylenedi-aminetetraacetic acid, acetylcysteine, or heparin have been proposed, on a theoretic basis, to decrease stromal ulceration by bacterial and host enzymes. However, such agents have not been found beneficial clinically. Tuftsin, a naturally occurring protein that enhances the phagocytic and bactericidal activity of polymorphonuclear leukocytes, potentiated the effect of gentamicin against *Pseudomonas* keratitis in rabbits,[144] but it has not been tested clinically.

Corticosteroids

The use of corticosteroids in the management of microbial keratitis is controversial. Corticosteroids are effective agents for suppression of the harmful effects of the host inflammatory response, but they also impair the phagocytosis and intracellular killing of bacteria by host effector cells. In experimental studies of *S. aureus* and *P. aeruginosa* keratitis, topical corticosteroids have not interfered with bacterial killing by appropriate antibiotics.[145-148] The course was no different from that seen when the antibiotics were used alone. Clinically, corticosteroid use has appeared to promote recurrence of *Pseudomonas* keratitis.[66]

In summary, the safety or efficacy of corticosteroids in human microbial keratitis has not been established.[41] I recommend that corticosteroids not be used in most cases of bacterial keratitis. They may be used to decrease scarring under certain conditions: after at least 4 to 5 days of antibiotic therapy, if the infectious process appears to be resolving, if concurrent bactericidal antibiotic treatment is given, and if reduction of scarring will improve visual outcome. In addition, it is preferable that the epithelium be intact and that the infection not be caused by *Pseudomonas*.

Course

It is essential to follow carefully the progress of the corneal ulcer.[84] At each examination the area and density of infiltration, the size and depth of ulceration, the size of the epithelial defect, the amount of stromal edema, the extent of scleral involvement, and the anterior chamber reaction should be recorded. Measurements can be made with the continuous beam adjustment on a Haag-Streit slit-lamp microscope.

Untreated corneal ulcers, whether peripheral or paracentral at the onset, tend to progress toward the central cornea away from the vascularized limbus. Early signs of improvement include a decrease in the infiltrate's "fluffiness," a blunting of the perimeter, decreased discharge,

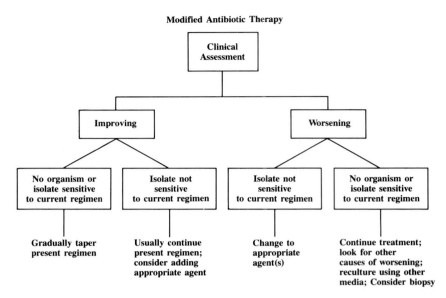

Figure 10-10
Modification of initial antibiotic therapy.

increased comfort, and decreased anterior chamber reaction. Later, a decrease in density and size of the infiltrate, reepithelialization, and vascularization are seen. The most helpful signs of improvement are the blunting of the perimeter of the stromal suppuration, reduction in the cellular infiltrate, reduction of the edema in the adjacent stroma, and progressive epithelialization. Fibrin exudate on the endothelium and hypopyon may resolve slowly and do not necessarily reflect the degree of improvement of the corneal process. In general, during the first 24 to 48 hours a lack of progression indicates that the treatment is effective. However, early progression of the keratitis can occur despite appropriate antibiotic treatment, particularly in *Pseudomonas* infections.

Many danger signs point to further trouble, such as increases in pain, the surface area of the ulcer, cellular stromal infiltration, suppuration, or anterior chamber reaction; or lysis of corneal stroma (see Fig. 10-3) or, at times, sclera.

Modification of therapy after 24 to 48 hours depends on the progress of the keratitis and culture results (Fig. 10-10). If the keratitis is improving, usually the initial regimen should be continued regardless of culture results. Often organisms that are not sensitive to an agent in vitro are sensitive at the high stromal levels achieved with topical administration of fortified antibiotics. If two agents were initiated and the isolate is sensitive to only one of them, the second agent can be discontinued or replaced

with a more appropriate antibiotic.

If the keratitis is worsening and preliminary identification suggests that the initial antibiotic regimen is ineffective, a more appropriate antibiotic should be given. Tables 10-5, 10-6, and 10-9 can be used as guides for modified antibiotic therapy. More definitive identification and sensitivity determination can be used to further refine therapy when this information becomes available.

If no organism is isolated or if the isolated organism is sensitive to the current regimen and the keratitis continues to worsen beyond 1 or 2 days, other infectious and noninfectious causes for the keratitis must be considered. The patient should be examined for keratitis sicca, trichiasis, entropion, or other conditions that could contribute to the keratitis. Noninfectious causes of infiltrative ulcerative keratitis should also be considered, such as those discussed in Chapter 9.

Tissue may be destroyed through mechanisms other than replication of microorganisms. For example, if extensive tissue damage has occurred, corneal ulceration will progress despite elimination of viable bacteria because of white cell infiltration and dissolution of necrotic stroma. The objectives at this stage of management are to halt additional structural alteration, promote stromal healing and reepithelialization, and prevent drug toxicity.[43] Corneal ringshaped infiltrates can occur with infections caused by gram-negative bacteria, particu-

Organism	Antibiotic*		
	Topical	Subconjunctival	Intravenous†
Gram-positive cocci, no further identification	Cefazolin	Cefazolin	Nafcillin
Staphylococcus	Cefazolin	Cefazolin	Nafcillin
Streptococcus	Penicillin G	Penicillin G	Penicillin G
Anaerobic gram-positive cocci	Penicillin G	Penicillin G	Penicillin G
Gram-negative cocci, hyperpurulent conjunctivitis (*Neisseria* spp.)	Ciprofloxacin	Penicillin G	Ceftriaxone (see Chapter 7)
Gram-negative cocci, no hyperpurulent conjunctivitis	Gentamicin	Gentamicin	Gentamicin
Branhamella spp.	Gentamicin	Gentamicin	?Gentamicin
Moraxella spp.	Gentamicin	Gentamicin	?Gentamicin or ciprofloxacin
Gram-positive rods, no further identification	Vancomycin	Vancomycin	?Vancomycin
Bacillus spp.	?Gentamicin vs ciprofloxacin	Gentamicin	?Gentamicin
Corynebacterium spp.	Bacitracin	Penicillin G	Penicillin G
Listeria spp.	Ampicillin	Ampicillin	Ampicillin
Gram-positive filamentous rods	Trimethoprim and sulfamethoxasole	Amikacin	Trimethoprim and sulfamethoxasole
Gram-negative rods, no further identification	Tobramycin and piperacillin	Tobramycin	Tobramycin
Coliforms‡	Gentamicin	Gentamicin	Gentamicin
Pseudomonas spp.	Tobramycin and piperacillin	Tobramycin	Tobramycin
Haemophilus influenzae	Ciprofloxacin	?Chloramphenicol	?Cefotaxime
Anaerobic gram-negative rods, no further identification	Chloramphenicol	Clindamycin	Clindamycin
Acid-fast bacilli	Amikacin and erythromycin	Amikacin	Amikacin

Table 10-9   Modified Antibiotic Therapy Based on Preliminary Identification of Selected Organisms

*See Table 10-7 for doses.

†Reserve intravenous antibiotics for scleral suppuration.

‡Includes *Escherichia coli, Enterobacter* spp., *Citrobacter* spp., *Klebsiella* spp., *Serratia* spp., and *Shigella* spp.

larly *Pseudomonas* (Fig. 10-11). These infiltrates appear to be an immunologic reaction to bacterial endotoxin,[149,150] and respond to corticosteroids. They generally are seen 10 to 14 days after the onset of the infection. It is important to differentiate these infiltrates from worsening or recurrence of infection.

Herpetic keratitis, atypical bacteria, fungi, and parasites may be present, and repeat corneal specimens should be obtained and examined for these agents. If the keratitis is indolent, antibiotic therapy can be discontinued for 1 to 2 days before reculture. A corneal biopsy should also be considered, because it is more likely to be diagnostic than a scraping.

Strict guidelines cannot be provided for the reduction or termination of antibiotics in kera-

titis that is improving with therapy. The duration of viable organisms in the cornea can vary according to the responsible bacteria, duration of infection, severity of the suppuration, depth of involvement, and other factors. Repeat corneal cultures during therapy are not reliable. Epithelialization alone cannot be used to indicate the resolution of infection, because any of these antibiotics can deter epithelial healing and produce other toxic and allergic reactions.

In general, if clinical improvement is seen, antibiotic drops can be reduced in frequency after 48 to 72 hours of therapy. Usually the interval between drops is doubled every 3 to 4 days. During tapering of fortified drops treatment can be switched to commercial-strength drops after the frequency of administration has

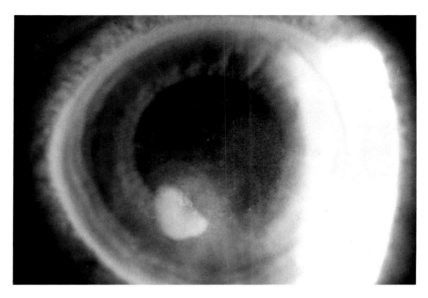

Figure 10-11
Immunologic ring infiltrate around bacterial keratitis.

been decreased to four to six times per day. Treatment usually is continued at least until the epithelium is healed and, particularly for *Pseudomonas* infections, often is continued for 1 to 2 weeks longer. If the patient has been hospitalized, he or she can be discharged once the keratitis is improving and the regimen is reduced to one that the individual can follow without assistance. The patient should be alert to the danger signs of resurgent keratitis and should promptly report increased pain, decreased vision, or purulent discharge.

The severe inflammatory reaction from virulent bacterial ulcers of the cornea can lead to permanent changes such as anterior polar cataracts, posterior and anterior synechiae, increased intraocular pressure, descemetocele or perforation, stromal scars, and edema of the cornea.

Surgical Treatment

Tissue adhesive (cyanoacrylate) is useful in treating or preventing corneal perforation (see Fig. 19-10). With progressive stromal necrosis or descemetocele formation, applying tissue adhesive can reduce the likelihood of perforation. The adhesive is also bacteriostatic.[151] Perforations of up to 2 mm in diameter can be sealed with tissue adhesive, restoring integrity to the globe. Iris can be left in the wound, or the anterior chamber can be restored with air or viscoelastic material. A stromal or scleral plug can be used in conjunction with adhesive to close larger perforations. Necrotic stroma, epithelium, and other debris must be removed from the ulcer bed before the adhesive is applied. Usually a bandage contact lens must be put in place afterward. The adhesive is left in place until it loosens spontaneously, the bed becomes vascularized, or keratoplasty is performed.

A patch graft or penetrating keratoplasty are other alternatives for corneal perforation. Conjunctival flaps can be used to treat ulcers that are unresponsive to medical therapy.[152,153] The flap brings blood vessels to the infected area to facilitate removal of bacteria, to promote healing, and to provide a stable surface. Conjunctival flaps are particularly useful in peripheral keratitis, where a partial flap can be placed without compromising vision. All necrotic material should be removed before placement of the flap, or the flap itself may necrose. Also, a flap alone is not sufficient treatment for a perforation.

Keratoplasty can also be considered when ulceration and necrosis progress despite medical treatment, particularly if all the involved tissue can be removed. The results of keratoplasty in acutely infected or inflamed eyes vary; the surgery is more complicated, intraocular inflammation and scarring are increased, and the risk of rejection and glaucoma are greater, especially in larger grafts.[154,155] The chance of a clear graft is fairly good if the graft's diameter is 8 mm or less, and in one report the results were equal to those cases in which surgery was delayed until the keratitis had resolved.[155] Certainly the globe and the potential for vision can be preserved by this type of surgery, even if the risk for rejection is high. It is best to treat with antibiotics for 24 to 36 hours before surgery, even if perforation is present, and to remove all the infected tissue. Culture and histologic examination of the removed tissue should be performed.

Various other treatments have been used to kill bacteria or remove infected stroma. Because *Pseudomonas* organisms seem to be susceptible to cryotherapy in vivo, this may be considered as an adjunct to medical and surgical treatment of severe *Pseudomonas* infections.[156] *Pseudomonas* corneal ulcers with scleral extension have been treated successfully with combined keratoplasty and cryotherapy.[157] Carbon dioxide[158] and excimer lasers[159] have proved capable of removing infected stroma.

NONULCERATIVE BACTERIAL KERATITIS

Syphilis

In older literature, approximately 90% of interstitial keratitis is caused by syphilis, with 87% resulting from congenital lues and 3% from acquired lues. However, the incidence of congenital syphilis declined, and currently active syphilitic interstitial keratitis is uncommon. At the University of Minnesota, syphilis caused only 3.6% of the cases of active interstitial keratitis seen from 1985 to 1994.[160] Between 1941 and 1983, the national incidence of congenital syphilis declined by 98%, only 239 cases of congenital syphilis were reported in 1983.[161] Since then the incidence increased to 2841 in 1990, and then declined.[162] European countries did not see this recent increase in cases. The incidence of infectious syphilis has increased since the late 1970s, but interstitial keratitis is uncommon in these cases.

Children are more likely to develop syphilis if their mothers had untreated syphilis of short duration, (e.g., less than 1 year) rather than longer duration. The risk of infection of the fetus during untreated early maternal syphilis is estimated to be 75% to 95%, decreasing to approximately 35% for untreated maternal syphilis of greater than 2 years' duration.[161] Approximately 50% of fetuses infected prenatally are born dead or die soon after birth. Forty percent of children who survive through infancy develop symptomatic syphilis.

Clinical Manifestations

The manifestations of prenatally acquired syphilis can be divided into those that appear early, usually between 2 and 10 weeks of age, and those that appear late (i.e., after 2 years of age). Early signs include rhinitis, mucocutaneous lesions, hepatosplenomegaly, lymphadenopathy, anemia, and jaundice. Late manifestations can result from active disease that remains untreated or from injuries to anlage during gestation. These include interstitial keratitis, nerve deafness, dental and skeletal abnormalities, arthropathy, and neurosyphilis.

Residual stigmata of congenital syphilis include scaphoid scapulae, high palatine arch, epiphyseal enlargement, rhagades, and perforation of the palate or nasal septum. Hutchinson's teeth are small, widely spaced, barrel-shaped upper central permanent incisors, frequently with a central notch in the thickened biting edge. Mulberry molars are 6th-year molars with multiple, poorly developed cusps rather than the usual four. Hutchinson's triad is classic: characteristic appearance of the teeth, deafness, and interstitial keratitis. Rhagades are linear scars at the angles of the mouth and nose caused by secondary bacterial infection of the early perioral lesions.

In early congenital syphilis mucocutaneous lesions can affect the lid and conjunctiva. A papular eruption can occur on the lids, leading to ulceration, punctal stenosis, lash loss, andlid margin deformity. Lesions similar to rhagades of the mouth can occur at the lateral canthus. Mucous patches can occur on the conjunctiva. They can manifest as dull erythematous patches, as a gray exudate overlying an erosion, like a conjunctival phlyctenule, or as an exuberant, fleshy mass. Like other lesions in early congenital syphilis, these are infectious, and spirochetes can be demonstrated in the tissue.

In late congenital syphilis, lid gummas, scleritis, and dacryoadenitis can be seen. Interstitial keratitis occurs in about one third of patients with late congenital syphilis. Interstitial keratitis seems to have a higher incidence in females.[163] About two thirds of the cases resulting from congenital syphilis occur when patients are between 5 years of age and the late teens; cases after age 30 are rare. The congenital form of disease is usually bilateral (80%), with the second eye becoming involved within a year in 75% of cases. As time passes, the second eye has a lesser tendency to be affected, being involved after 5 years in only 2% of cases.

The first signs of interstitial keratitis, which may precede symptoms by as much as several

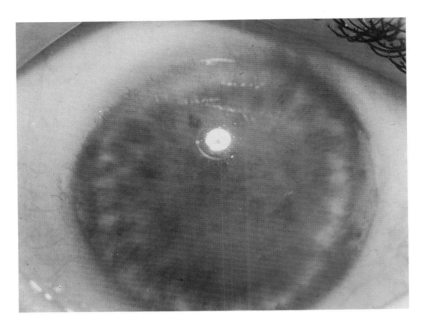

Figure 10-12
Diffuse opacity of the cornea from luetic interstitial keratitis.

weeks, consist of an indistinct cellular infiltrate and edema in the endothelium followed by keratic precipitates and tiny opacities of the stroma. If untreated, the disease then passes through progressive, florid, and retrogressive stages.

The progressive stage, which usually lasts 1 to 2 weeks, begins with severe symptoms of pain, lacrimation, photophobia, and blepharospasm and is accompanied by circumcorneal vascular injection. The cornea becomes rapidly and extensively cloudy over a period of a few days. Blood vessels begin to enter the peripheral cornea. Iridocyclitis and anterior choroiditis occur during this stage.

In the florid stage the changes that began in the progressive stage become more evident. The infiltration becomes more dense and vascular ingrowth progresses. The acute inflammation of the eye and heavy deep vascularization of the cornea persist for about 2 to 4 months.

The corneal cloudiness is a result of changes in all corneal layers. Stromal cellular infiltration usually appears as faint gray, soft-edged opacities that increase in number and coalesce to form a general haze. In other cases the process is generalized from the start, or clouding begins centrally. It imparts to the cornea a ground-glass appearance and can reduce vision to light perception. Epithelial edema occurs and may progress to vesicle and bullae formation.

Vascular invasion occurs in areas with stro-mal infiltration and starts from the periphery. Both superficial and deep vascularization can be seen. Superficial vessels, which can extend several millimeters onto the cornea, produce a crescentic elevation, which has been called an "epaulet" of vascularization. Deeper vessels run between the stromal lamellae in long, wavy, parallel lines. The extent of vascular invasion can vary widely, but usually the whole cornea becomes vascularized. If the opacities begin in one sector, the vascularization is also sectoral. Extensive invasion of the deeper cornea by vessels can cause the cornea to appear a dull reddish pink, the so-called "salmon patch." Vascular invasion continues for 4 to 5 weeks.

A wrinkling or folding of Descemet's membrane usually occurs. Linear formations of corneal guttae, dense endothelial opacities, and clumped keratic precipitates can be seen.

Next, the retrogressive stage begins, the inflammation and symptoms begin to subside, and clearing starts. This stage lasts from 1 to 2 years. In most cases, clearing begins peripherally, proceeds centrally, and is accompanied by thinning of the cornea. The amount of clearing is remarkable, especially in young people; however, usually some opacity is left centrally as a diffuse haze (Fig. 10-12). These changes are usually most prominent posteriorly and in some cases are limited to the pre-Descemet's area (Fig. 10-13). The blood vessels, which tend to persist as fine opaque lines, are not obliterated, al-

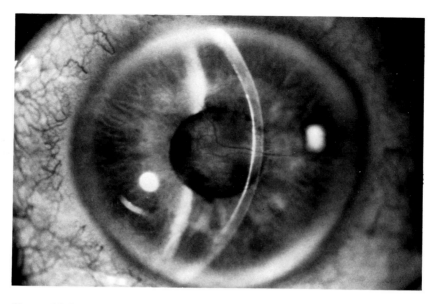

Figure 10-13
Pre-Descemet's scarring from old luetic interstitial keratitis.

though thinner branches of larger vessels might become closed. In some the lumen is so small that a red blood cell is able only occasionally to pass through. These vessels were called "ghost vessels" in the past because they persisted but were not thought to carry blood. In severe cases the corneal endothelium can be destroyed or damaged, resulting in permanent corneal edema. There may be splits in Descemet's membrane,[164] hyaline ridges, and networks attached to the endothelium.

Band keratopathy, corneal thinning, lipid keratopathy, and Salzmann's degeneration can also be seen.[165] Astigmatism can occur because of corneal irregularity and thinning. Late glaucoma may occur[166,167] as a result of hypertrophy of Descemet's membrane over the chamber angle,[164] inflammatory injury to the meshwork, synechiae, or narrow anterior chamber angles. The presentation may be acute or chronic.

There are many variations from the typical course of the disease. The disease may remain in the periphery of the cornea, be confined to one sector only, and be of short duration, or it may have more than one separate center of inflammation with its own vascular invasion existing simultaneously. It can involve the central cornea primarily or exclusively. In these cases there is often a ringshaped stromal infiltrate and a ringlike pattern of exudates in Descemet's membrane. Posterior corneal abscesses, marginal corneal ulceration, and rarely central ulceration can occur.

Generally, recurrences are transient and mild; they occur in about 9% of cases and may be associated with mild trauma (Fig. 10-14), laceration, or impairment of general health.

Acquired Syphilis. The interstitial keratitis in acquired syphilis may occur within months after the onset of the infection but generally occurs 10 years later. The clinical course closely resembles that in congenital syphilis except that interstitial keratitis in acquired syphilis is usually uniocular (60% of cases), frequently milder, limited to a sector of cornea, and occasionally more amenable to treatment (Fig. 10-15).

Pathogenesis
Based on the following indirect evidence, it appears that the host's immune response to the infection, rather than active bacterial proliferation, is responsible for the clinical disease:

1. Interstitial keratitis rarely develops in early congenital syphilis when *T. pallidum* abounds; it usually is delayed by many years.
2. Treponemes are rarely found in the corneas of patients with active interstitial keratitis.
3. Interstitial keratitis does not respond to penicillin or other antitreponemal agents and may actually worsen.
4. The cornea often shows prompt clinical improvement with corticosteroids.

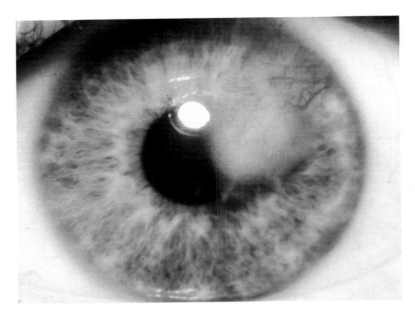

Figure 10-14
Recurrence of interstitial keratitis because of trauma. Note the sectoral response. (Courtesy of F. Wilson II, Indianapolis, IN.)

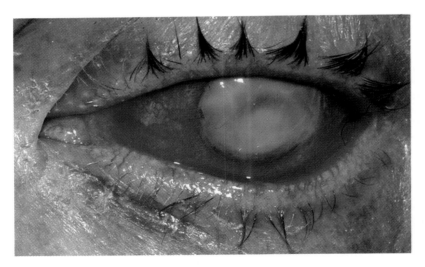

Figure 10-15
Diffuse keratitis in acquired syphilis. (Courtesy of Eric Donnenfeld, Rockville Center, NY.)

Diagnosis

The diagnosis of interstitial keratitis at any stage is predominantly clinical. Bilateral extensive edema and cellular infiltration of the stroma with deep vascularization should be considered as lues until proved otherwise. The presence of iridocyclitis, chorioretinitis, optic neuritis, or sclerokeratitis is also suggestive of syphilis.

However, to see an acute attack today is rare; most cases now seen are in adults with residua of previous disease, which can be diagnosed by a careful history and examination. The hallmark is stromal scarring, opacification, and residual deep vascularization. Deep stromal opacities, usually with a metallic sheen reflex in front of Descemet's membrane, and stromal "ghost" vessels, which can be identified on di-

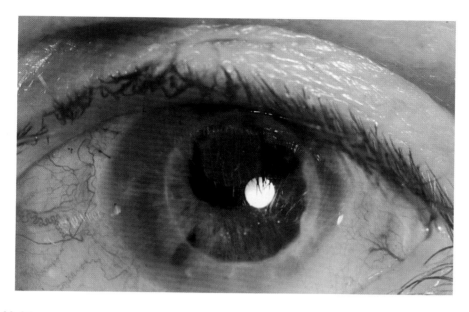

Figure 10-16
When scarring from interstitial keratitis sufficiently impairs vision, good results are obtained with penetrating keratoplasty.

rect illumination or retroillumination, are seen. Findings of uveal involvement include atrophy of the iris stroma, posterior synechia, salt-pepper fundus, large patches of depigmentation and pigment proliferation, and a picture resembling retinitis pigmentosa, with vascular attenuation.

The patient's history is often helpful. A patient with corneal scarring from congenital syphilis usually reports the occurrence of an ocular inflammation in childhood that lasted several months to years. There may be a previous history of a positive serologic test or treatment for venereal disease or a family history of positive serology, venereal disease, abortions, or stillbirths.

Examination should be performed for other physical evidence of congenital lues, including frontal bossing, overgrowth of maxillary bones, Hutchinson's teeth, early loss of teeth, saddle nose, rhagades, and saber shins.[168]

Serologic testing is often useful. Reagin tests, such as the Venereal Disease Research Laboratory (VDRL) or rapid plasma reagin, are indicators of recent or active disease but may also be elevated in certain other diseases, such as lupus erythematosus, malaria, and heroin addiction. The fluorescent treponemal antibody absorption test (FTA-ABS) and microhemagglutination assay test (MHA-TP) detect patient serum antibodies against treponemes. The FTA-ABS and MHA-TP are more sensitive and specific and will remain positive even after treatment.[169,170]

The differential diagnosis of interstitial keratitis is discussed in more detail in Chapter 9. Any patient with interstitial keratitis should also be questioned about vestibuloauditory symptoms and exposure to or history of tuberculosis.

Treatment

Late burned-out interstitial keratitis needs no local treatment other than keratoplasty when indicated for decreased vision (Fig. 10-16).[171] In general, results are good.

During the active disease topical steroids can be used to suppress inflammation. Although some ophthalmologists believed that interstitial keratitis should run its course without steroid treatment, it appears that the end result is better when steroids are administered; however, the disease may be prolonged. Without treatment or with heavy metal treatment, 25% to 50% of eyes recover to 20/30 or better vision, and 70% recover to 20/60 or better; with steroid treatment, 85% to 90% recover to 20/30 vision or better. Topical steroid drops are initially administered eight times a day and then gradually tapered after the acute process is controlled. Treatment may have to be continued for 18 months to 2 years. Cycloplegia is also of benefit. If possible, the pupil should be kept moving,

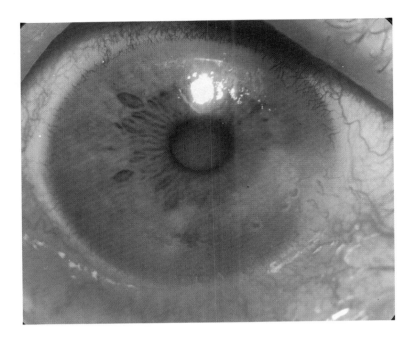

Figure 10-17
Sectoral interstitial keratitis caused by tuberculosis.

but symptoms may necessitate the use of atropine during the active stages of the disease.

Treatment of the systemic disease does not seem to have any dramatic effect on the course of interstitial keratitis except that it may cause a flare-up, probably from liberation of antigen as in systemic Herxheimer's reaction. In addition, treatment of congenital syphilis does not prevent the onset of keratitis later, and penicillin treatment during the first attack of keratitis does not prevent subsequent involvement of the other eye.

Antimicrobial therapy should be given not for the eyes but for the presence of active systemic disease. If the patient has not received adequate systemic treatment in the past, if the treatment status is unknown, or if there are any signs or symptoms of neurosyphilis, the cerebrospinal fluid should be examined. Signs of neurosyphilis are pleocytosis, increased protein concentration, and VDRL reactivity. In primary, secondary, or early latent lues benzathine penicillin G (1.2 million U in each buttock) is sufficient. In late congenital syphilis, 2.4 million U of aqueous procaine penicillin intramuscularly or intravenously is given daily for 10 days to prevent or treat cardiovascular, central nervous system, visceral, and osseous lesions.[169] If neurosyphilis is present, aqueous procaine penicillin is administered as described earlier, with

probenecid, 500 mg, by mouth, four times daily during the first 10 days, followed by benzathine penicillin G 2.4 million U intramuscularly weekly for three doses.

Tuberculosis

Tuberculosis interstitial keratitis is a rare disease in developed countries; even in the 1920s, when tuberculosis was much more prevalent than today, it accounted for less than 2.0% of cases of interstitial keratitis.[172] The keratitis may appear similar to luetic interstitial keratitis, but it is more often unilateral and sectoral. In tuberculosis the cornea is often involved in the peripheral inferior sector only (Fig. 10-17), where it forms a dense, abscesslike, nodular opacity shaped like a ring. The infiltration is greatest in the middle and deeper layers of the cornea, and vascular ingrowth is mainly anterior; the central cornea is relatively spared. A sector-shaped sclerokeratitis or phlyctenulosis may also be seen. The clearing is less rapid and less complete than that of the syphilitic variety, leaving a dense, sectorlike scar. As in syphilitic interstitial keratitis, the host's response to bacterial antigens, and not active corneal infection, is probably responsible for the clinical disease. A focus of tuberculous disease lies elsewhere in the body. A positive tuberculin skin test and a negative FTA-ABS test aid in diagno-

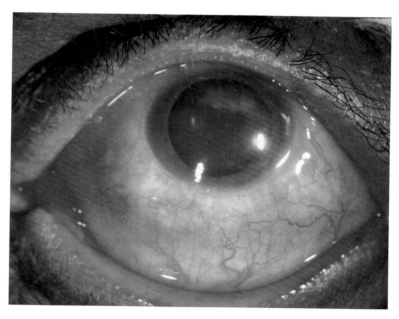

Figure 10-18
Interstitial keratitis and punctate keratitis in leprosy.

sis. There may be a history of tuberculous disease or evidence of disease elsewhere in the body.

The systemic infection should be treated with antituberculous drugs such as isoniazid, streptomycin, or rifampin.[173] Topical steroids and cycloplegics are used for the corneal disease, as for syphilitic interstitial keratitis.

Leprosy

Most of the estimated 15 million worldwide cases of leprosy are seen in developing countries, particularly those in tropical and subtropical regions. Most cases in the United States are seen in immigrants from endemic areas. Leprosy is divided clinically into tubercluloid and lepromatous types. Lepromatous leprosy is characterized by limited immunity, with large numbers of organisms present in the body and tissue damage related mainly to infiltration and destruction by the organisms. Tuberculous leprosy occurs in the presence of a high degree of immune resistance, with a relatively small number of organisms eliciting a strong cell-mediated response. Leprosy affects mainly the nerves, skin, and eyes.

Ocular Manifestations

Ocular involvement is more common and more severe in the lepromatous type. Corneal disease can take several forms. The most common finding is decreased sensation due to fifth nerve involvement. The severity of the hyposensitivity is related to the duration of the disease.[174,175] Superficial punctate keratopathy, mainly interpalpebral, is also commonly seen and can be caused by corneal anesthesia, seventh nerve palsy, trichiasis, entropion, ectropion, or lagophthalmos.

Corneal inflammation occurs in three forms: superficial punctate keratitis, leprotic pannus, and interstitial keratitis[176-178] (Fig. 10-18). The superficial punctate keratitis begins in the superior temporal quadrant as discrete white superficial opacities near the limbus. These opacities resemble grains of chalk and lie in the epithelium and subepithelial stroma. They do not stain with fluorescein and are asymptomatic. They can spread inferiorly and centrally and with time can coalesce, resulting in a diffuse haze. More rarely they can become vascularized or lead to deeper stromal inflammation. Iritis frequently accompanies the keratitis. The chalk-dust opacities are composed of lepra bacilli surrounded by a polymorphonuclear infiltrate.

Nodular lepromata are frequently seen subconjunctivally, particularly at the temporal limbus (see Fig. 7-6). Superficial vessels may grow out from them over the peripheral cornea, producing leprotic pannus. They are frequently associated with similar nodules of the iris.

Interstitial keratitis occurs in approximately 6% of cases and is seen late in the disease. Deep infiltration and vascularization begin in the periphery and move centrally, sometimes involving the visual axis. It is commonly bilateral, and most frequently affects the superotemporal quadrant. In contrast to luetic interstitial keratitis, vascularization is scant and late.

Multiple small, creamy-white pearls may be present on the surface of the iris. These are clumps of active and degenerative bacilli. Exposure keratitis, glaucoma, chronic conjunctivitis, lid nodules, thickened corneal nerves—sometimes with beading (beads on a string)—loss of eyebrows and eyelashes, distortion of the lids, and seventh nerve palsy can also occur. Scleritis can occur by direct infiltration of organisms, often by extension from the uvea or lid, or as part of erythema nodosum leprosum, an immunologic reaction with characteristic skin lesions.

Pathogenesis

Lepromatous leprosy appears to develop in patients with reduced cell-mediated immunity and produces more severe clinical manifestations. Numerous nodular skin lesions and progressive thickening of the skin, particularly on the face and extensor surfaces of the extremities, produce the characteristic leonine facies. Diffuse involvement of peripheral nerves and lymph nodes occurs.

Primary leprous keratitis results from invasion of the cornea by lepra bacilli, via the corneal nerves, the limbal vessels, or by direct extension. Granulomatous inflammation occurs in the form of giant cells that contain the *Mycobacterium leprae* bacilli (lepra cells), large lipid-laden (foamy) macrophages, lymphocytes, and plasma cells. There is a predilection for involvement of nerve bundles, with such granulomatous lesions in and around the nerves. The predilection of leprosy for involvement of the anterior segment of the eye may be the result of its relatively low temperature.[179]

Diagnosis and Treatment

The clinical appearance is often sufficient to make the diagnosis. The conjunctiva can be scraped and an acid-fast stain performed, but the yield is relatively low. Biopsies of conjunctival or cutaneous lesions are more likely to demonstrate the pleomorphic acid-fast bacilli as well as the typical inflammatory lesions. The organism cannot be grown in vitro.

Systemic treatment involves long-term use of clofazimine, rifampin, and dapsone. Topical steroids are used to treat active keratitis or iritis.

Lyme Disease

Lyme disease is a multisystem disorder caused by infection with *Borrelia burgdorferi*, acquired through tick bites. The diagnosis is often difficult because signs and symptoms can be intermittent and vague. A characteristic rash, erythema chronicum migrans usually develops 4 to 20 days after the tick bite. It begins as a red macule or papule that expands to form a large annular red lesion with a relatively clear center. A flu-like illness is often present. Weeks to months later neurologic manifestations, cardiac disease, and arthritis can develop.

Conjunctivitis is probably the most common ocular manifestation. In one study it was seen in 11% of patients.[180] Periorbital edema, iritis, episcleritis, ischemic optic neuropathy, optic disc edema, and cranial neuropathies have also been seen. Several cases of keratitis have been reported in patients with Lyme disease.[181-184] Multiple infiltrates were present at all levels of the stroma. Unilateral and bilateral cases occurred, and keratic precipitates were present in some cases. The infiltrates responded to topical steroid treatment.

The diagnosis is made on the basis of medical history, clinical findings, and serologic tests. Antibodies to *B. burgdorferi* are usually measured by enzyme-linked immunosorbent assay (ELISA); however, serology testing is not well standardized. In one recent study four patients with ocular disease had borderline or negative ELISA serology but were positive by western blot analysis.[185]

Relapsing Fever

Relapsing fever is the name given to a group of acute infections caused by spirochetes of the genus *Borrelia*. In the United States the infections are mainly tick-borne and occur most often in the mountainous areas of the west. Clinically the disease is manifested by an abrupt onset of fever and headache, sometimes accompanied by neurologic symptoms, rash, jaundice, hepatosplenomegaly, and eye pain. The first attack usually lasts about 1 week, and then after an interval of 1 to 2 weeks symptoms return. Relapses become shorter and milder with time.

Iritis is the most frequent ocular complication.[186,187] Interstitial keratitis can also occur. It is usually superficial and mild and occurs in the late stages of infection.[188]

Stromal Abscesses

Stromal abscesses can develop below intact epithelium. They are most common after surgery or trauma, where the organism becomes implanted in deep tissue or enters through a wound or suture tract. Stromal abscesses can also develop from metastatic blood-borne infection. They arise near the limbus as intrastromal infiltrates, and progress to abscess formation. They extend circumferentially and centrally and usually eventually break through to the surface.

REFERENCES

1. Fleiszig SM et al: Modulation of *Pseudomonas aeruginosa* adherence to the corneal surface by mucus, *Infect Immun* 62:1799, 1994.
2. Wilhelmus KR: Review of clinical experience with microbial keratitis associated with contact lenses, *CLAO J* 13:211, 1987.
3. Erie JC et al: Incidence of ulcerative keratitis in a defined population from 1950 through 1988, *Arch Ophthalmol* 111:1665, 1993.
4. Nilsson SE, Montan PG: The hospitalized cases of contact lens induced keratitis in Sweden and their relation to lens type and wear schedule: results of a three-year retrospective study, *CLAO J* 20:97, 1994.
5. Schein OD et al: The relative risk of ulcerative keratitis among users of daily-wear and extended-wear soft contact lenses, *N Engl J Med* 321:773, 1989.
6. Poggio EC et al: The incidence of ulcerative keratitis among users of daily-wear and extended wear soft contact lenses, *N Engl J Med* 321:779, 1989.
7. Schein OD et al: The impact of overnight wear on the risk of contact lens-associated ulcerative keratitis, *Arch Ophthalmol* 112:186, 1994.
8. Buehler PO et al: The increased risk of ulcerative keratitis among disposable soft contact lens users, *Arch Ophthalmol* 110:1555, 1992.
9. Matthews TD et al: Risks of keratitis and patterns of use with disposable contact lenses, *Arch Ophthalmol* 110:1559, 1992.
10. Glynn RJ et al: The incidence of ulcerative keratitis among aphakic contact lens wearers in New England, *Arch Ophthalmol* 109:10, 1991.
11. Bowden FW et al: Patterns of lens care practices and lens product contamination in contact lens associated microbial keratitis, *CLAO J* 15:49, 1989.
12. Solomon OD et al: Testing hypotheses for risk factors for contact lens-associated infectious keratitis in an animal model, *CLAO J* 20:109, 1994.
13. Sachs R, Zagelbaum BM, Hersh PS: Corneal complications associated with the use of crack cocaine, *Ophthalmology* 100:187, 1993.
14. Aristimuno B et al: Spontaneous ulcerative keratitis in immunocompromised patients, *Am J Ophthalmol* 115:202, 1993.
15. Schein OD et al: Microbial contamination of in-use ocular medications, *Arch Ophthalmol* 110:82, 1992.
16. Schein OD et al: Microbial keratitis associated with contaminated ocular medications, *Am J Ophthalmol* 105:361, 1988.
17. Ostler HB, Okumoto M, Wilkey C: The changing pattern of the etiology of central bacterial corneal (hypopyon) ulcer, *Trans Pacific Coast Ophthalmol Soc* 55:237, 1974.
18. Asbell P, Stenson S: Ulcerative keratitis: survey of 30 years' laboratory experience, *Arch Ophthalmol* 100:77, 1982.
19. Jones DB: Pathogenesis of bacterial and fungal keratitis, *Trans Ophthalmol Soc UK* 98:367, 1978.
20. Ormerod LD et al: Microbial keratitis in children, *Ophthalmology* 93:449, 1986.
21. Clinch TE et al: Microbial keratitis in children, *Am J Ophthalmol* 117:65, 1994.
22. Cruz OA et al: Microbial keratitis in childhood, *Ophthalmology* 100:192, 1992.
23. Clemons CS et al: *Pseudomonas* ulcers following patching of corneal abrasions associated with contact lens wear, *CLAO J* 13:161, 1987.
24. O'Day DM et al: The problem of *Bacillus species* infection with special emphasis on the virulence of *Bacillus cereus*, *Ophthalmology* 88:833, 1981.
25. Meisler DM et al: Infectious crystalline keratopathy, *Am J Ophthalmol* 97:337, 1984.
26. Reiss GR, Campbell RJ, Bourne WM: Infectious crystalline keratopathy, *Surv Ophthalmol* 31:69, 1986.
27. Matoba A et al: Infectious crystalline keratopathy due to *Streptococcus pneumoniae*: possible association with serotype, *Ophthalmology* 101:1000, 1994.
28. Lubniewski AJ et al: Posterior infectious crystalline keratopathy with *Staphylococcus epidermidis*, *Ophthalmology* 97:1454, 1990.
29. Wilhelmus KR, Robinson NM: Infectious crystalline keratopathy caused by *Candida albicans*, *Am J Ophthalmol* 112:322, 1991.
30. Weisenthal RW et al: Postkeratoplasty crystalline deposits mimicking bacterial infectious crystalline keratopathy, *Am J Ophthalmol* 105:70, 1988.
31. McDonnell PJ et al: Characterization of infectious crystalline keratitis caused by a human isolate of *Streptococcus mitis*, *Arch Ophthalmol* 109:1147, 1991.
32. Hunts JH et al: Infectious crystalline keratopathy; the role of bacterial exopolysaccharide, *Arch Ophthalmol* 111:528, 1993.
33. Bowers R et al: Non-aureus staphylococcus in corneal disease, *Invest Ophthalmol Vis Sci* 30(suppl):380, 1989.
34. Okumoto M, Smolin G: Pneumococcal infections of the eye, *Am J Ophthalmol* 77:346, 1974.
35. Johnson MK et al: Confirmation of the role of pneumolysin in ocular infections with *Streptococcus pneumoniae*, *Curr Eye Res* 11:1221, 1992.
36. Ostler HB: *Diseases of the external eye and adnexa: a text and atlas*, Baltimore, 1993, Williams & Wilkins.

37. Kim HB, Ostler HB: Marginal corneal ulcer due to beta-streptococcus, *Arch Ophthalmol* 95:454, 1977.

38. Holland S et al: Corneal ulcer due to *Listeria monocytogenes, Cornea* 6:144, 1987.

39. Holbach LM, Bialasiewicz AA, Boltze HJ: Necrotizing ring ulcer of the cornea caused by exogenous *Listeria monocytogenes* serotype IVb infection, *Am J Ophthalmol* 106:105, 1988.

40. Zaidman GW, Coudron P, Piros J: *Listeria monocytogenes* keratitis, *Am J Ophthalmol* 109:334, 1990.

41. Jones DB: Decision-making in the management of microbial keratitis, *Ophthalmology* 88:814, 1981.

42. Stern GA, Hodes BL, Stock EL: *Clostridium perfringens* corneal ulcer, *Arch Ophthalmol* 97:661, 1979.

43. Jones DB, Robinson NM: Anaerobic ocular infections, *Trans Am Acad Ophthalmol Otolaryngol* 83:309, 1977.

44. Coster DJ, Badenoch PR: Host, microbial and pharmacological factors affecting the outcome of suppurative keratitis, *Br J Ophthalmol* 71:96, 1987.

45. Srinivasan M, Sharma S: *Nocardia asteroides* as a cause of corneal ulcer: case report, *Arch Ophthalmol* 105:464, 1987.

46. Hirst LW, Merz WC, Green WR: *Nocardia asteroides* corneal ulcer, *Am J Ophthalmol* 94:123, 1982.

47. Perry HD, Nauheim JS, Donnenfeld ED: *Nocardia asteroides* keratitis presenting as a persistent epithelial defect, *Cornea* 8:41, 1989.

48. Donnenfeld ED et al: Treatment of *Nocardia* keratitis with topical trimethoprim-sulfamethoxazole, *Am J Ophthalmol* 99:601, 1985.

49. Lin JC et al: Treatment of *Nocardia asteroides* keratitis with polyhexamethylene biguanide (PHMB), *Ophthalmology* 102(suppl):153, 1995.

50. Hyndiuk RA: Experimental *Pseudomonas* keratitis, *Trans Am Ophthalmol Soc* 79:541, 1981.

51. Vaughan DG: Contamination of fluorescein solutions, *Am J Ophthalmol* 39:55, 1955.

52. Wilson LA, Ahearn DC: *Pseudomonas*-induced corneal ulcers associated with contaminated eye mascara, *Am J Ophthalmol* 84:112, 1977.

53. Golden B, Fingerman L, Allen HF: *Pseudomonas* corneal ulcers in contact lens wearers: epidemiology and treatment, *Arch Ophthalmol* 85:543, 1971.

54. Hutton WL, Sexton RR: Atypical *Pseudomonas* corneal ulcers in semicomatose patients, *Am J Ophthalmol* 73:37, 1972.

55. Stern GA, Weitzenkorn D, Valenti J: Adherence of *Pseudomonas aeruginosa* to the mouse cornea: epithelial versus stromal adherence, *Arch Ophthalmol* 100:1956, 1982.

56. Stern GA, Lubniewski A, Allen C: The interaction between *P. aeruginosa* and the corneal epithelium, *Arch Ophthalmol* 103:1221, 1985.

57. Dart JKG, Seal DV: Pathogenesis and therapy of *Pseudomonas aeruginosa* keratitis, *Eye* 2(suppl):S46, 1988.

58. Kreger AS et al: Immunization against experimental *Pseudomonas aeruginosa* and *Serratia marcescens* keratitis: vaccination with lipopolysaccharide endotoxins and proteases, *Invest Ophthalmol Vis Sci* 27:932, 1986.

59. Maresz-Babczyszyn J, Sokalska M: Immunity to *Pseudomonas* keratitis in rabbits vaccinated with extracellular slime from mucoid *Pseudomonas aeruginosa* strains producing proteases, *Arch Immunol Ther Exp (Warsz)* 29:653, 1981.

60. Moon MM et al: Monoclonal antibodies provide protection against ocular *Pseudomonas aeruginosa* infection, *Invest Ophthalmol Vis Sci* 29:1277, 1988.

61. Ijiri Y et al: The role of *Pseudomonas aeruginosa* elastase in corneal ring abscess formation in pseudomonal keratitis, *Graefes Arch Clin Exp Ophthalmol* 231:521, 1993.

62. Steuhl KP et al: Relevance of host-derived and bacterial factors in *Pseudomonas aeruginosa* corneal infections, *Invest Ophthalmol Vis Sci* 28:1559, 1987.

63. Kessler E, Mondino B, Brown SI: The corneal response to *Pseudomonas aeruginosa*: histopathological and enzymatic characterization, *Invest Ophthalmol Vis Sci* 16:116, 1977.

64. Hobden JA et al: *Pseudomonas aeruginosa* keratitis in leukopenic rabbits, *Curr Eye Res* 12:461, 1993.

65. Raber IM et al: *Pseudomonas* corneal-scleral ulcers. Paper presented at the annual meeting of the Ocular Microbiology and Immunology Group, San Francisco, Nov 3, 1970.

66. Harbin T: Recurrence of a corneal *Pseudomonas* infection after topical steroid therapy: report of a case, *Am J Ophthalmol* 58:670, 1964.

67. Alfonso E et al: *Pseudomonas* corneoscleritis, *Am J Ophthalmol* 103:90, 1987.

68. Rosenfeld SI et al: Granular epithelial keratopathy as an unusual manifestation of *Pseudomonas* keratitis associated with extended-wear soft contact lenses, *Am J Ophthalmol* 109:17, 1990.

69. Kreger AS, Griffin QK: Corneal damaging proteases of *Serratia marcescens, Invest Ophthalmol Vis Sci* 14:190, 1975.

70. Lass JF et al: Visual outcome in eight cases of *Serratia marcescens* keratitis, *Am J Ophthalmol* 92:384, 1981.

71. Zimmerman LE, Turner, L, McTigue JW: *Mycobacterium fortuitum* infection of the cornea: a report of two cases, *Arch Ophthalmol* 82:596, 1969.

72. Hu F-R: Infectious crystalline keratopathy caused by *Mycobacterium fortuitum* and *Pseudomonas aeruginosa, Am J Ophthalmol* 109:738, 1990.

73. Dugel PU et al: *Mycobacterium fortuitum* keratitis, *Am J Ophthalmol* 105:661, 1988.

74. Newman PE et al: A cluster of cases of *Mycobacterium chelonei* keratitis associated with outpatient office procedures, *Am J Ophthalmol* 97:344, 1984.

75. Bullington RH, Lanier JD, Font RI: Nontuberculous mycobacterial keratitis: report of two cases and review of the literature, *Arch Ophthalmol* 110:519, 1992.

76. Crane TB et al: *Mycobacterium chelonei* keratopathy and visual rehabilitation by a triple procedure, *Ophthalmic Surg* 21:802, 1990.

77. Knapp A, Stern GA, Hood CI: *Mycobacterium avium-intracellulare* corneal ulcer, *Cornea* 6:175, 1987.

78. Moore MB, Newton C, Kaufman HE: Chronic keratitis caused by *Mycobacterium gordonae, Am J Ophthalmol* 102:516, 1986.

79. Telahun A, Waring GO, Grossniklaus HE: *Mycobacterium gordonae* keratitis, *Cornea* 11:77, 1992.

80. Matoba A et al: Combination drug testing of *Mycobacterium chelonae, Invest Ophthalmol Vis Sci* 34:2786, 1993.

81. Hu F-R: Extensive lamellar keratectomy for treatment of nontuberculous mycobacterial keratitis, *Am J Ophthalmology* 120:47, 1995.

82. Herman PE: General principles of antimicrobial therapy, *Mayo Clin Proc* 52:603, 1977.

83. Sobol WM et al: Rapid streptococcal antigen detection in experimental keratitis, *Am J Ophthalmol* 107:60, 1989.

84. Jones DB: A plan for antimicrobial therapy in bacterial keratitis, *Trans Am Acad Ophthalmol Otolaryngol* 79:95, 1975.

85. Jones DB: Initial therapy of suspected microbial corneal ulcers. II: Specific antibiotic therapy based on corneal smears, *Surv Ophthalmol* 24:97, 1979.

86. Asbell P, Stenson S: Ulcerative keratitis. Survey of 30 years' laboratory experience, *Arch Ophthalmol* 100:77, 1982.

87. Baum J: Initial therapy of suspected microbial corneal ulcers. I: Broad spectrum antibiotic therapy based on prevalence of organisms, *Surv Ophthalmol* 24:97, 1979.

88. Baum J: Therapy for ocular bacterial infection, *Trans Ophthalmol Soc UK* 105:69, 1986.

89. Limberg ML: A review of bacterial keratitis and bacterial conjunctivitis, *Am J Ophthalmol* 112(suppl):2S, 1991.

90. Leibowitz HM: Clinical evaluation of ciprofloxacin 0.3% ophthalmic solution for treatment of bacterial keratitis, *Am J Ophthalmol* 112(suppl):34S, 1991.

91. Hyndiuk RA et al: Comparison of ciprofloxacin ophthalmic solution 0.3% to fortified tobramycin/cefazolin in the treatment of bacterial corneal ulcers, *Ophthalmology* 102(suppl):101, 1995.

92. Bower KS, Kowalski RP, Gordon YJ: Which quinolone when combined with fortified cefazolin would be best for the treatment of bacterial keratitis?, *Invest Ophthalmol Vis Sci* 35(suppl):1674, 1994.

93. Hwang DG et al: Clinical failures associated with ciprofloxacin monotherapy of streptococcal keratitis, *Ophthalmology* 102(suppl):101, 1995.

94. Hwang D et al: Frequent recovery of fluoroquinolone-resistant and methicillin-resistant staphylococci following topical ciprofloxacin use, paper presented at the Ocular Microbiology and Immunology Group Meeting, Atlanta, October, 1995.

95. O'Brien TP et al: Efficacy of ofloxacin vs cefazolin and tobramycin in the therapy for bacterial keratitis: report from the bacterial keratitis study reserach group, *Arch Ophthalmol* 113:1257, 1995.

96. Davis SD, Sarff LD, Hyndiuk RA: Antibiotic therapy of experimental *Pseudomonas* in guinea pigs, *Arch Ophthalmol* 95:1638, 1977.

97. Davis SD, Sarff LD, Hyndiuk RA: Topical tobramycin therapy of experimental *Pseudomonas* keratitis: an evaluation of some factors that potentially enhance efficacy, *Arch Ophthalmol* 96:123, 1978.

98. Baum J, Barza M: Topical vs subconjunctival treatment of bacterial corneal ulcers, *Ophthalmology* 90:162, 1983.

99. Stern GA, Driebe WT: The effect of fortified antibiotic therapy on the visual outcome of severe bacterial corneal ulcers, *Cornea* 1:341, 1982.

100. Osborn E et al: The stability of 10 antibiotics in artificial tears, *Am J Ophthalmol* 82:775, 1976.

101. Bowe BE, Snyder JW, Eiferman RA: Fortified ophthalmic antibiotic preparations: an in-vitro study of potency and storage mechanisms, *Invest Ophthalmol Vis Sci* 30(suppl):199, 1989.

102. Glasser DB et al: Loading doses and extended dosing intervals in topical gentamicin therapy, *Am J Ophthalmol* 99:329, 1985.

103. Davis SD, Sarff LD, Hyndiuk RA: Comparison of therapeutic routes in experimental *Pseudomonas* keratitis, *Am J Ophthalmol* 87:710, 1979.

104. Leibowitz HM, Ryan WJ, Kupferman A: Route of antibiotic administration in bacterial keratitis, *Arch Ophthalmol* 99:1420, 1981.

104a. Results of the Endophthalmitis Vitrectomy Study. Randomized trial of immediate vitrectomy and of intravenous antibiotics for the treatment of postoperative bacterial endophthalmitis, *Arch Ophthalmol* 113:1479, 1995.

105. Burris TE, Newsome DI, Rowsey JJ: Hessburg subpalpebral antibiotic lavage of *Pseudomonas* corneal and corneoscleral ulcers, *Cornea* 1:347, 1982.

106. Matoba AY, McCulley JP: The effect of therapeutic soft contact lenses on antibiotic delivery to the cornea, *Ophthalmology* 92:97, 1985.

107. O'Brien TP et al: Use of collagen corneal shields versus soft contact lenses to enhance penetration of topical tobramycin, *J Cataract Refract Surg* 14:505, 1988.

108. Gilbert ML, Wilhelmus KR, Osato MS: Intracanalicular collagen implants enhance topical antibiotic bioavailability, *Cornea* 5:167, 1986.

109. Rootman DS et al: Iontophoresis of tobramycin for the treatment of experimental *Pseu-*

domonas keratitis in the rabbit, *Am J Ophthalmol* 106:262, 1988.

110. Groden LR, Brinser JH: Outpatient treatment of microbial corneal ulcers, *Arch Ophthalmol* 104:84, 1986.

111. Bodey GP et al: Carbenicillin therapy for *Pseudomonas* infection, *JAMA* 218:62, 1971.

112. McLoughlin JE, Reeves DS: Clinical and laboratory evidence for inactivations of gentamicin by carbenicillin, *Lancet* 1:261, 1971.

113. Stern GA et al: Effect of topical antibiotic solutions on corneal epithelial wound healing, *Arch Ophthalmol* 101:644, 1983.

114. Nakamura M et al: Effects of antimicrobials on corneal epithelial migration, *Curr Eye Res* 12:733, 1993.

115. Neu HC: Tobramycin: an overview, *J Infect Dis* 134(suppl):1, 1976.

116. Thompson RL: The cephalosporins, *Mayo Clin Proc* 52:625, 1977.

117. Thornsberry C: Review of in vitro activity of third-generation cephalosporins and other newer beta-lactam antibiotics against clinically important bacteria, *Am J Med* 79(suppl 2A):14, 1985.

118. Donowitz GR: Third-generation cephalosporins, *Infect Dis Clin North Am* 3:595, 1989.

119. Neu H: Pathophysiologic basis for the use of third-generation cephalosporins, *Am J Med* 88(suppl 4A):3S, 1990.

120. Kremer I et al: The effect of topical ceftazidime on *Pseudomonas* keratitis in rabbits, *Cornea* 13:360, 1994.

121. Neu HC: Synergy and antagonism of antimicrobial combinations with quinolones, *Eur J Clin Microbiol Infect Dis* 10:255, 1991.

122. McDermott JL et al: Corneal stromal penetration of topical ciprofloxacin in humans, *Ophthalmology* 100:197, 1993.

123. Callegan MC et al: Topical antibiotic therapy for the treatment of experimental *Staphylococcus aureus* keratitis. *Invest Ophthalmol Vis Sci* 33:3017, 1992.

124. Lauffenburger MD, Cohen KL: Topical ciprofloxacin versus topical fortified antibiotics in rabbit models of *Staphylococcus* and *Pseudomonas* keratitis, *Cornea* 12:517, 1993.

125. Callegan MC et al: Ciprofloxacin versus tobramycin for the treatment of staphylococcal keratitis, *Invest Ophthalmol Vis Sci* 35:1033, 1994.

126. Parks DJ et al: Comparison of topical ciprofloxacin to conventional antibiotic therapy in the treatment of ulcerative keratitis, *Am J Ophthalmol* 115:471, 1993.

127. Snyder ME, Katz HR: Ciprofloxacin-resistant bacterial keratitis, *Am J Ophthalmol* 114:336, 1992.

128. Cutarelli PE et al: Topical fluoroquinolones: antimicrobial activity and in vitro corneal epithelial toxicity, *Curr Eye Res* 10:557, 1991.

129. Wilhelmus KR et al: Keratitis Study Group: treatment of keratitis with ciprofloxacin ointment, *Arch Ophthalmol* 111:1210, 1993.

130. Sweeney GJ et al: Penetration of ciprofloxacin into the aqueous humor of the uninflamed human eye after oral administration, *J Antimicrob Chemother* 26:99, 1990.

131. Baba FZ et al: Intravitreal penetration of oral ciprofloxacin in humans, *Ophthalmology* 99:483, 1992.

132. Heessen TW, Muytjens HL: In vitro activities of ciprofloxacin, norfloxacin, pipemidic acid, cinoxacin, and nalidixic acid against *Chlamydia trachomatis, Antimicrob Agents Chemother* 25:123, 1984.

133. King A, Phillips I: The comparative in vitro activity of eight newer quinolones and nalidixic acid, *J Antimicrob Chemother* 18(suppl):1, 1986.

134. Wolfson JS, Hooper DC: The fluoroquinolones: structures, mechanisms of action and resistance, and spectra of activity in vitro, *Antimicrob Agents Chemother* 28:581, 1985.

135. Reidy JJ et al: The efficacy of topical ciprofloxacin and norfloxacin in the treatment of experimental *Pseudomonas* keratitis, *Cornea* 10:25, 1991.

136. O'Brien TP, Bacterial Keratitis Study Group: Comparative clinical efficacy of topical ofloxacin vs. combined fortified cefazolin plus tobramycin in therapy of acute bacterial keratitis, *Invest Ophthalmol Vis Sci* 36(suppl):862, 1995.

137. von Gunten S et al: Aqueous humor penetration of ofloxacin given by various routes, *Ophthalmology* 117:87, 1994.

138. Rosenthal RL, Blackman A: Bone marrow hypoplasia following use of chloramphenicol eye drops, *JAMA* 191:136, 1965.

139. Seedor JA et al: Systemic tetracycline treatment of alkali-induced corneal ulceration in rabbits, *Arch Ophthalmol* 105:268, 1987.

140. Wilkie J, Smolin G, Okumoto M: The effect of rifampicin on *Pseudomonas* keratitis, *Can J Ophthalmol* 7:309, 1972.

141. Wade JC et al: Potential of imipenem as single-agent empiric antibiotic therapy of febrile neutropenic patients with cancer, *Am J Med* 78:62, 1985.

142. Sawusch MR et al: Topical imipenem therapy of aminoglycoside-resistant *Pseudomonas* keratitis in rabbits, *Am J Ophthalmol* 106:77, 1988.

143. Tabbara K, Antonios S, Alvarez H: Effects of fusidic acid on staphylococcal keratitis, *Br J Ophthalmol* 73:136, 1989.

144. Smith PC, Zam S, Stern GA: The effect of tuftsin in the treatment of experimental *Pseudomonas* keratitis, *Cornea* 5:181, 1986.

145. Leibowitz HM, Kupferman A: Topically administered corticosteroids: effect on antibiotic-treated bacterial keratitis, *Arch Ophthalmol* 98:1287, 1980.

146. Davis SD, Sarff LD, Hyndiuk RA: Corticosteroid in experimentally induced *Pseudomonas* keratitis: failure of prednisolone to impair the efficacy of tobramycin and carbenicillin therapy, *Arch Ophthalmol* 96:126, 1978.

147. Smolin G, Okumoto M, Leong-Sit L: Combined gentamicin-tobramycin-corticosteroid treatment. II: Effect on gentamicin-resistant *Pseu-*

domonas keratitis, *Arch Ophthalmol* 98:473, 1980.

148. Hobden JA et al: Prednisolone acetate or prednisolone phosphate concurrently administered with ciprofloxacin for the therapy of experimental *Pseudomonas aeruginosa* keratitis, *Curr Eye Res* 12:469, 1993.

149. Mondino BJ et al: Corneal rings with gram-negative bacteria, *Arch Ophthalmol* 95:2222, 1977.

150. Belmont JB et al: Noninfectious ring-shaped keratitis associated with *Pseudomonas aeruginosa, Am J Ophthalmol* 93:338, 1982.

151. Eiferman RA, Snyder JW: Antibacterial effect of cyanoacrylate glue, *Arch Ophthalmol* 101:958, 1983.

152. Gundersen T: Conjunctival flaps in the treatment of corneal disease with reference to a new technique of application, *Arch Ophthalmol* 60:880, 1958.

153. Buxton JN, Fox ML: Conjunctival flaps in the treatment of refractory *Pseudomonas* corneal abscess, *Ann Ophthalmol* 18:315, 1986.

154. Zu DN et al: Therapeutic keratoplasty in the management of purulent corneal ulceration: report of 100 cases, *Jpn J Ophthalmol* 23:412, 1979.

155. Hill JC: Use of penetrating keratoplasty in acute bacterial keratitis, *Br J Ophthalmol* 70:502, 1986.

156. Codere F, Brownstein S, Jackson B: *Pseudomonas aeruginosa* scleritis, *Am J Ophthalmol* 91:706, 1981.

157. Eiferman RA: Cryotherapy of *Pseudomonas* keratitis and scleritis, *Arch Ophthalmol* 97:1637, 1979.

158. Sarno EM et al: Carbon dioxide laser therapy of *Pseudomonas aeruginosa* keratitis, *Am J Ophthalmol* 97:791, 1984.

159. Serdarevic O et al: Excimer laser therapy for experimental *Candida* keratitis, *Am J Ophthalmol* 99:534, 1985.

160. Harrison AR, Chen K, Holland EJ: Etiologies of interstitial keratitis, Paper presented at the Ocular Microbiology and Immunology Group meeting, Atlanta, October 1995.

161. Holmes KK, Likehart SA: *Syphilis,* In Braunwald E et al, editors: *Harrison's principles of internal medicine,* ed 11, New York, 1987, McGraw-Hill.

162. Dunn RA et al: Surveillance for geographic and secular trends in congenital syphilis—United States, 1983-1991, *MMWR CDC Surveill Summ* 42 (SS-6):59, 1993.

163. Duke-Elder S, Leigh AG: *System of ophthalmology,* vol VIII, *Diseases of the outer eye,* St. Louis, 1965, Mosby–Year Book.

164. Waring GO et al: Alterations of Descemet's membrane in interstitial keratitis, *Am J Ophthalmol* 81:773, 1976.

165. Vannas A, Hogan MH, Wood I: Salzmann's nodular degeneration of the cornea, *Am J Ophthalmol* 79:211, 1975.

166. Grant MW: Late glaucoma with interstitial keratitis, *Am J Ophthalmol* 79:87, 1975.

167. Lichter PR, Shaffer RN: Interstitial keratitis and glaucoma, *Am J Ophthalmol* 68:241, 1969.

168. Duke-Elder S, Leigh AG: *System of ophthalmology,* vol VIII, *Diseases of the outer eye,* St. Louis, 1965, Mosby–Year Book.

169. Ryan SJ et al: Persistence of virulent *Treponema pallidum* despite penicillin therapy in congenital syphilis, *Am J Ophthalmol* 73:258, 1972.

170. Smith JL: Testing for congenital syphilis in interstitial keratitis, *Am J Ophthalmol* 72:816, 1971.

171. Rabb MF, Fine M: Penetrating keratoplasty in interstitial keratitis, *Am J Ophthalmol* 67:907, 1969.

172. Duke-Elder S, Leigh AG: *System of ophthalmology,* vol VIII: *Diseases of the outer eye,* St. Louis, 1965, Mosby–Year Book.

173. Treatment of tuberculosis, *Am Rev Respir Dis* 127:790, 1983.

174. Karacorlu MA, Cakiner T, Saylan T: Corneal sensitivity and correlations between decreased sensibility and anterior segment pathology in ocular leprosy, *Br J Ophthalmol* 75:117, 1991.

175. Dana MR et al: Ocular manifestations of leprosy in a noninstitutionalized community in the United States, *Arch Ophthalmol* 112:626, 1994.

176. Duke-Elder S, Leigh AG: *System of ophthalmology,* vol VIII: *Diseases of the outer eye,* St. Louis, 1965, Mosby–Year Book.

177. Spaide R et al: Ocular findings in leprosy in the United States, *Am J Ophthalmol* 100:411, 1985.

178. Shields JA, Waring GO, Monte LG: Oclar findings in leprosy, *Am J Ophthalmol* 77:880, 1974.

179. Hobbs HE et al: Ocular histopathology in animals experimentally infected with *Mycobacterium leprae* and *M. lepraemurium, Br J Ophthalmol* 62:516, 1978.

180. Steere AC et al: The early clinical manifestations of Lyme disease, *Ann Intern Med* 99:76, 1983.

181. Baum J et al: Bilateral keratitis as a manifestation of Lyme disease, *Am J Ophthalmol* 105:75, 1988.

182. Bertuch AW, Rocco E, Schwartz WG: Lyme disease: ocular manifestations, *Ann Ophthalmol* 20:376, 1988.

183. Kornmehl EW et al: Bilateral keratitis in Lyme disease, *Ophthalmology* 96:1194, 1989.

184. Flach AJ, LaVoie PE: Episcleritis, conjunctivitis, and keratitis and ocular manifestations of Lyme disease, *Ophthalmology* 97:973, 1990.

185. Karma A et al: Diagnosis and clinical characteristics of ocular Lyme borreliosis, *Am J Ophthalmol* 119:127, 1995.

186. Southern PM Jr, Sanford JP: Relapsing fever: a clinical and microbiological review, *Medicine* 48:129, 1969.

187. Hamilton JB: Ocular complication in relapsing fever, *Br J Ophthalmol* 27:68, 1943.

188. Duke-Elder S, Leigh AG: *Diseases of the outer eye, part 2,* In Duke-Elder S, editors: *System of ophthalmology,* St. Louis, 1966, Mosby–Year Book.

Eleven

Infectious Keratitis: Fungal and Parasitic

FUNGAL KERATITIS

Although fungal infection in the cornea is relatively rare in temperate climates, it is common in tropical climates. Overall, the number of cases of fungal keratitis has increased over the past 20 to 30 years because of improved diagnosis in addition to an increased incidence.[1-5] Fungi are ubiquitous, but infection occurs when they accidentally penetrate normal barriers, such as with penetrating trauma, or when normal host defenses are impaired. Despite advances in both diagnostic techniques and antifungal agents, diagnosis and management continue to be a challenge for the ophthalmologist. Morbidity in fungal infections tends to be greater than that in bacterial keratitis because the diagnosis is often delayed and because available drugs are not as effective. It is necessary, therefore, to be aware of the clinical presentation of fungal keratitis, to promptly suspect its presence, and to implement proper laboratory investigation to establish the diagnosis. Both medical and surgical management are not as well defined as in bacterial keratitis and depend more on clinical judgment. An informed, reasoned approach is essential.

Classification of Fungi

Almost any species of fungus is capable of causing corneal infection, but relatively few are seen with any regularity.[4,6] These fungi can be divided into filamentous, yeast, and dimorphic forms.[7] All fungi digest their food externally, by releasing hydrolytic enzymes into their immediate surrounding and absorbing the digested products. Fungal pathogens rely on these digestive enzymes to penetrate host tissues. Fungi also produce substances to inhibit the growth of other microbes, which often inhabit the same ecosystem and thus compete for the same food supply. Many of these substances have been developed as pharmacologic antibiotics (e.g., penicillin, nystatin, and amphotericin B).

Most fungi can reproduce sexually or asexually, by formation of conidia or by budding.

Filamentous Fungi

Filamentous fungi are also known as *molds*. These fungi occur as long filaments, called *hyphae*, which grow by apical extension. The hyphae of these multicellular fungi branch, forming a tangled mass on the culture medium called a *mycelium* (Fig. 11-1). Hyphae have rigid cell walls that typically contain chitin, glucan, and mannan (Fig. 11-2). The hyphae may be divided into compartments by cell walls, called *septae*. One or more nuclei can be present in each compartment; the septae can be regular or sparse.

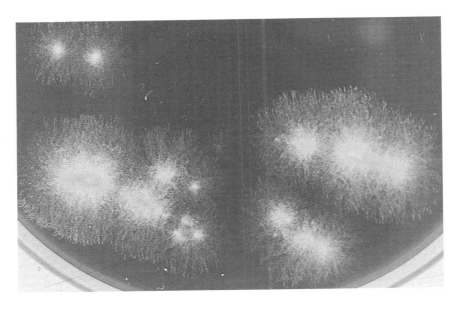

Figure 11-1
Blood agar plate incubated at room temperature showing *Aspergillus fumigatus* mycelia.

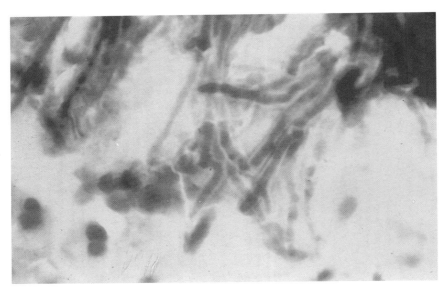

Figure 11-2
Giemsa-stained scraping from corneal ulcer exhibiting nonseptate hyphae.

Septate Organisms. The following septate filamentous fungi are most often associated with ocular disease: *Fusarium, Aspergillus, Acremonium (Cephalosporium), Penicillium, Cladosporium, Curvularia, Alternaria,* and *Paecilomyces.*

These filamentous organisms predominantly affect normal eyes after corneal abrasion or trauma involving some kind of vegetable matter. The fungi are ubiquitous and are found both outside and inside the home, mainly on organic matter. *Fusarium* spp., most commonly *Fusarium solani,* are the most common corneal fungal pathogens in the southern United States,[7] and probably in the Western hemisphere. They are primarily plant pathogens, and *Fusarium* keratitis often occurs in agricultural workers. *Aspergillus* infection is nearly as common. *Aspergillus fumigatus* is the most common species. *Aspergillus* generally can be found in decaying vegetation and soil.

Nonseptate Organisms. There is no regular division of the hyphae by septae; the filaments exist as long tubes with numerous nuclei scattered throughout. The fungi in this group rarely cause corneal disease but can cause hematogenous endophthalmitis and sinus and orbital infections. The most common pathogens are *Mucor, Rhizopus, Absidia,* and yeasts.

Yeasts are fungi with usual and dominant growth as unicellular organisms. They often produce pseudohyphae and buds, and occasionally true hyphae depending on the environment. The following organisms are most significant: *Candida, Cryptococcus,* and *Torulopsis.*

Candida spp. are opportunistic pathogens that are part of the normal flora of the skin; respiratory, gastrointestinal, and vaginal musoca; and occasionally conjunctiva. Corneal ulcers caused by *Candida* usually occur in eyes in which there is some predisposing factor. Agricultural exposure and trauma occurring outdoors are not usually factors in the pathogenesis of yeast keratitis. Infections can also occur in the lacrimal passages, lids, and conjunctiva. In tissues, *Candida* commonly form hyphae.

Yeasts do not form a mycelium in culture. On Sabouraud media they form white, opaque, smooth colonies, which may be mistaken for staphylococcal colonies (Fig. 11-3).

Dimorphic Fungi

Dimorphic fungi possess two distinct morphologic forms: the yeast phase, which occurs in tissues; and a mycelial phase, which occurs on media and natural surfaces. Dimorphic fungi

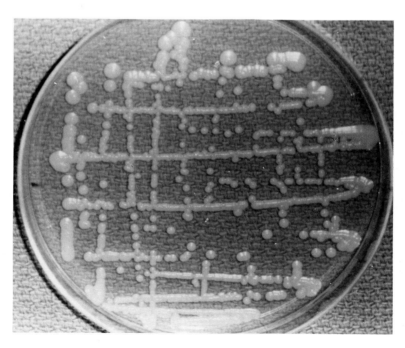

Figure 11-3
Colonies of *Candida albicans* growing on Sabouraud medium can be mistaken for colonies of staphylococci.

rarely cause keratitis but are important pathogens. The following are the most commonly seen dimorphic fungi: *Blastomyces,*[8] *Coccidioides, Histoplasma,* and *Sporothrix.*

Pathogenesis

In general, fungal keratitis is more prevalent in warmer climates, such as the southern and southwestern regions of the United States. In these areas there is a marked seasonal variation in the incidence of fungal keratitis, particularly the forms caused by filamentous fungi. For instance, in Florida the incidence of fungal keratitis is highest between November and March, when the climate is cool, dry, and windy[7]; in India the incidence is greatest in September and October during harvesting.[9] In cooler climates, infection with yeasts is more common than infection with filamentous fungi, and there is less seasonal variation.

Many corneal ulcers are caused by fungi that are commonly considered to be saprophytes (i.e., fungi that live on dead or decaying organic matter). About 7% of normal healthy eyes have fungi on the lids or conjunctiva at one time or other, probably as transient inhabitants.[10,11] The most common species are *Candida, Penicillium, Aspergillus, Rhodotorula, Cladosporium,* and *Alternaria.*

The most virulent fungal infections occur in persons with no apparent deficiency in resistance. These cases usually are associated with injury to the cornea from twigs and other plant matter. Nylon line lawn trimmers are a source of such injury.[12] Less virulent organisms, such as *Candida albicans,* are seen more in compromised hosts, such as those with Sjögren's syndrome, erythema multiforme, endocrinopathy, immunodeficiency, diabetes, alcoholism, or hypovitaminosis A. Corneal disease, such as persistent epithelial defect, stromal ulceration, herpes simplex infection, topical steroid use, and contact lens wear, also appears to predispose an eye to fungal infection, particularly yeast infection.

Corneal infections are relatively difficult to establish in experimental animals, even after intrastromal injection, and the mechanisms underlying the development of human disease are unclear. These fungi do elaborate proteases and toxins, such as the trichothenes, cytotoxins produced by some species of *Fusarium* and *Acremonium,* and aflatoxin, a liver carcinogen, as well as serine proteases produced by *Aspergillus.*[13-15] Gliotoxins produced by *Penicillium, Aspergillus,* and *Gliocladium* have antibacterial, antiviral, and antiphagocytic properties. However, the role of these substances in corneal disease is unknown. In one study of 18 *Fusarium* isolates, neither sterol content nor toxin production by the isolates correlated with the severity of the clinical infections.[16] Some filamentous fungi appear to be relatively nonimmunogenic; they can proliferate extensively in the cornea without eliciting much inflammatory response. In addition, their large size inhibits phagocytosis. Topical steroids may enhance their replication.

A number of *Candida* virulence factors have been identified. The ability to produce hyphae by some strains is associated with increased virulence.[17] Hyphal and pseudohyphal mannoproteins inhibit attachment and digestion by neutrophils.[17] Hyphal forms also appear to be capable of invading epithelial cells and leukocytes.[18] The large size of the hyphae and pseudohyphae also inhibits phagocytosis. *Candida* spp. produce proteolytic enzymes and lipases, which aid host invasion, and a surface protein aids epithelial adherence.[18,19] Resistance to *Candida* infection appears to depend on the location: Resistance to mucocutaneous infection is mainly T-cell dependent, but resistance to disseminated disease depends more on other innate defenses, such as neutrophils.[20]

Fungi can contaminate contact lens solutions, as well as the lenses themselves.[21,22] In rare cases, fungi can lead to keratitis. Filamentous fungi are more likely to cause keratitis in cosmetic or aphakic soft contact lens wearers, and yeasts more likely in therapeutic lens wearers.[23] Good contact lens hygiene and heat disinfection are the best methods for preventing fungal contamination.

Clinical Manifestations

In most infections, symptoms and signs occur within 1 to 2 days. Symptoms are similar to those caused by bacterial ulcers, except that fungal ulcers are more often indolent. In some cases days or weeks may elapse before the patient seeks medical care.

Corneal ulcers caused by filamentous fungi often have grayish white infiltration, with rough-textured surface areas elevated above the plane of the uninvolved cornea (Fig. 11-4). The margins, which are irregular and extend into the adjacent stroma, may exhibit a feathery outline. Foci of infiltration can be seen several millimeters away from the main area of involvement (Fig. 11-5); these are called *satellite lesions.* The epithelium can be intact over the infiltrate. An endothelial plaque may be seen parallel to the ulcer. A ring infiltrate may sur-

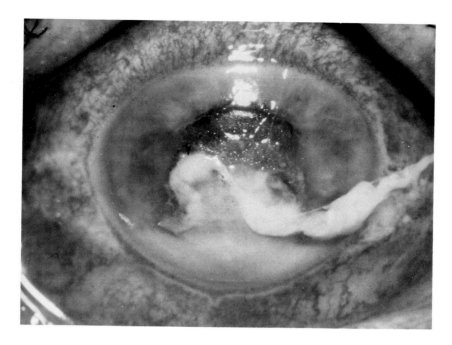

Figure 11-4
Fungal keratitis with stromal infiltration and hypopyon. Note the raised edge and extensive purulent discharge.

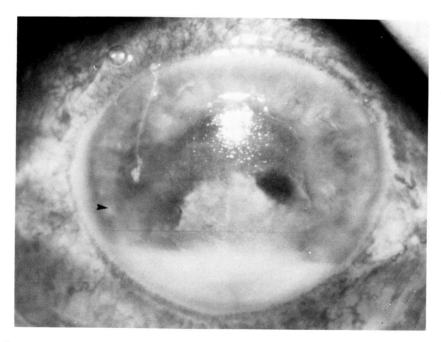

Figure 11-5
Satellite lesion (*arrow*) in fungal ulcer with large hypopyon and extensive stromal necrosis.

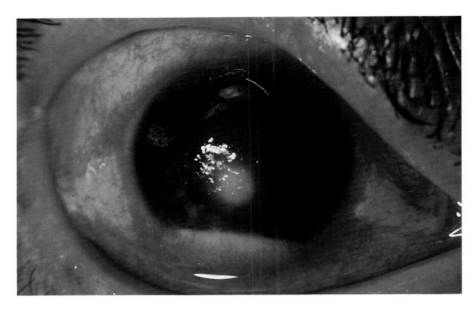

Figure 11-6
Candida albicans corneal infection.

round the primary lesion, most likely representing an antibody response to fungal antigen.
In addition, a hypopyon and purulent discharge may occur, even when the infiltrate appears minimal (Fig. 11-4). Conjunctival injection and anterior chamber reaction may be
quite severe.

The clinical appearance of filamentous fungal keratitis is quite variable and often indistinguishable from bacterial, viral, or parasitic infection. Early infections may resemble staphylococcal infection, especially if they are near
the limbus, or herpes simplex keratitis. *Nocardia, Actinomyces, Streptomyces,* mycobacteria,
and other bacteria can present similarly. Infection that occurs beneath an intact epithelium
can also occur with herpes viruses, *Acanthamoeba,* and some avirulent bacteria (e.g., *Streptococcus viridans*). Ring infiltrates also occur
with keratitis that is caused by herpes viruses,
Acanthamoeba, and gram-negative rods.

A history of trauma with organic matter
should suggest the possibility of fungal infection. The presence of infiltrates with feathery
edges and infiltration that is dry, gray, and elevated above the epithelial surface are also suggestive of fungal infection.

Yeast infections tend to present a slightly different picture. They usually appear as an oval,
plaquelike, elevated lesion that is reasonably
well outlined and often widely surrounded by
stromal edema. These more closely resemble a

Table 11-1	Comparison of Fungal Keratitis Caused by Filamentous Fungi vs. Yeasts

FILAMENTOUS FUNGI
Occurs more frequently in young people (occupational and outdoor activity)
Signs may be present 24 to 48 hours after
injury
Usually no predisposing factor
Involved area can be localized and is often elevated; epithelial defect may or may not be
present; often has feathery edges and satellite lesions
Inflammation can be mild or severe, with hypopyon and endothelial plaque

YEASTS
Usually occur in a compromised host; preexisting corneal disease or steroid treatment
Usually more focal and suppurative, resembling bacterial keratitis
Edges not feathery, and satellitism not usually
seen; often elevated

bacterial keratitis (Fig. 11-6). The differences between filamentous and yeast fungal keratitis is
listed in Table 11-1.

Histopathology

Severe inflammation of the cornea can result
from fungal infection caused by replicating and

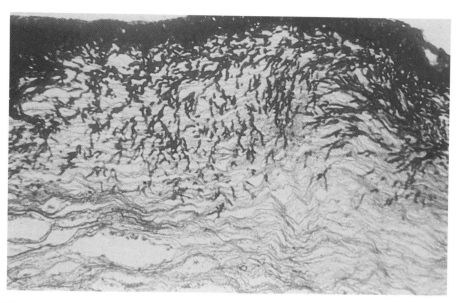

Figure 11-7
Fungus makes its way through corneal lamellae and may penetrate Descemet's membrane (periodic acid–Schiff stain).

nonreplicating fungi, mycotoxins, proteolytic enzymes, and soluble fungal antigens.[24] These agents can result in necrosis of the corneal lamellae, acute inflammation, antigenic response with immune ring formation, hypopyon, and severe uveitis.[25,26] In general, the virulence of the filamentous fungi ranges from the more destructive *Fusarium solanae* through many species, including those of *Cephalosporium, Aspergillus,* and *Penicillium,* to the more leisurely pathogens, such as *Phialophora,* which may grow indolently in the cornea over a period of months.

The inflammatory response tends to be less marked than in bacterial keratitis, and the epithelium is frequently intact over the infection. Multiple microabscesses may surround the main lesion of central ulceration and infiltration. Limbal infiltration with lymphocytes and plasma cells increases with progressive keratitis and can result in a ring abscess. The infection tends to become deeper with time. In more advanced disease, fungi may be absent from the surface and the superficial stroma, which may explain the difficulty in recovering the organisms in scrapings. The hyphae can penetrate through the stromal lamellae (Fig. 11-7) and Descemet's membrane and spread into the anterior chamber. When this occurs, it is usually seen as a retrocorneal or anterior chamber inflammatory mass adjacent to an area of deep

keratitis.[27] Some *Fusarium* spp. appear to have a predilection for infecting the posterior chamber, where their accumulation can cause severe glaucoma.[28]

Diagnosis
Although the clinical history and appearance may be suggestive of fungal keratitis, definite diagnosis requires laboratory confirmation. As discussed earlier, infection with herpes simplex, *Nocardia, Actinomyces, Streptomyces,* mycobacteria, other bacteria, and *Acanthamoeba* can result in a similar picture.

Three to four scrapings should be taken from the ulcer under slit-lamp microscope magnification and examined. The smears are air-dried or fixed with methanol and stained with Giemsa stain, Gram's stain, and with one or two special fungal stains (see Chapter 4).[29,30] All staining material and all media should be fresh. Gram's stain will darken the fungus walls; Giemsa stain will highlight the cytoplasm, but the walls are seen only by contrast (Fig. 11-2). Probably the best stain for fungi is Gomori's methenamine silver technique; however, it is relatively difficult and time consuming to perform. Periodic acid–Schiff stain, calcofluor, potassium hydroxide (ink–KOH), or acridine orange are other options. The next step is to inoculate the proper media. At least one medium appropriate for fungi should be inoculated

Table 11-2   Activity of Antifungal Agents*

	Amphotericin B	Natamycin	Miconazole	Clotrimazole	Ketoconazole	Flucytosine	Nystatin
YEASTS							
Candida	+	±	±	+	+	+	+
Torulopsis	+	+	−	+	−	+	
FILAMENTOUS FUNGI							
Fusarium	±	+	−	±	±	−	
Aspergillus	+	+	+	+	−		±
Paecilomyces	−	−	+	±	+		−
Curvularia	+	+	+		+		
Cladosporium	+	+	+	±		+	
Penicillium	+	+					±

*Based on limited experimental and human data. Susceptibility in individual cases can vary greatly.

whenever fungal keratitis is a possibility, such as one of the following:

1. Blood agar plate incubated at room temperature and 37°C (*Fusarium* grows well at 37°C)
2. Sabouraud medium (gentamicin added) incubated at room temperature (probably the most sensitive)
3. Beef heart infusion broth (gentamicin added) at room temperature kept on a platform shaker

Most fungal isolates grow out within 2 to 3 days, but some can take 3 weeks or more. The frequency of identification of fungal elements in smears depends on the quality of the specimen, the experience of the observer, the stain, and the duration of infection. Even with experienced observers, Gram's- and Giemsa-stained smears are positive in one third to three fourths of cases.[7,31-33] Nevertheless, it is important to examine smears because they often contain fungi even though no growth is obtained in culture.[34] In one series of 171 ulcers clinically suspected to be fungal, cultures were positive in 51% of eyes, and KOH wet-mount preparation was positive in 94%.[35] In another study, calcofluor white was significantly more sensitive than KOH wet-mount in demonstrating fungal pathogens.[36] Specific fungal identification is not possible, but yeasts and filamentous fungi usually can be differentiated. Biopsy may be necessary for diagnosis, particularly in longstanding infection.[37]

Treatment

Antimicrobial therapy for fungal keratitis is currently not as well developed as therapy for bacterial keratitis. No ideal agent—one that would be fungicidal and lack toxicity and that could penetrate the cornea well—is available. The available agents tend only to inhibit growth and allow the host to eradicate the infection. Penetration of most agents is limited, and many are irritating or toxic to the ocular surface.

Antifungal Agents

The main drugs used for treatment of filamentous and yeast infection of the cornea are amphotericin B, natamycin, nystatin, imidazole compounds (clotrimazole, miconazole, and ketoconazole), and flucytosine.

Tables 11-2 through 11-5 summarize the spectrum of activity, dosages, and other characteristics of these drugs.

Amphotericin B. Amphotericin B is a heptaene polyene. Polyenes work by binding to ergosterols in fungal cell membranes. To a lesser extent, they also binds sterols (e.g., cholesterol) present in human cell membranes, which is one of the reasons for their toxicity. The bound amphotericin forms channels in the cellular membrane that allow passage of ions, leading to electrolyte imbalance and death of the cells.

Amphotericin B is consistently active against *Candida*, *Cryptococcus*, and *Aspergillus* spp., but is variably active against *Fusarium* spp. In one animal study, amphotericin B was found to be the most effective agent against two strains of *C. albicans*.[38] It was the most frequently used agent before the development of natamycin and was effective in many cases, but resistance was common and toxicity limited its use.[1,39]

Amphotericin B is fungistatic, insoluble, and relatively toxic, and it cannot penetrate intact epithelium.[40,41] Stromal penetration of denuded, inflamed stroma is better, but only a small percentage of the drug present is active.[42]

Table 11-3	Review of Antifungal Agents				
Drug	**Type**	**Routes**	**Topical Penetration***	**Topical Toxicity**	**Comments**
Amphotericin B	Polyene	Topical Systemic†	Poor	+	Unstable in light, water, heat, and pH extremes Systemic use causes damage to erythrocytes and renal tubules
Natamycin	Polyene	Topical	Fair	+	Insoluble and unstable
Miconazole	Imidazole	Topical Subconjunctival Systemic (intravenously)	Good	−	Unstable in solution; must be reformed weekly
Clotrimazole	Imidazole	Topical Subconjunctival	?	+ (especially commercial preparations)	
Ketoconazole	Imidazole	Topical Systemic (oral)	Good	−	Systemic administration generally well tolerated, but hepatotoxicity can occur
Flucytosine	Pyrimidine	Topical Systemic (oral)	Good	−	Best used in combination with amphotericin B Systemic administration is generally well tolerated but bone marrow and liver toxicity can occur
Nystatin	Polyene	Topical	?		

*De-epithelialized cornea.
†Not effective for keratitis and very toxic.

It is unstable in light, water, heat, and pH extremes.[43]

The adverse effects of topical amphotericin include burning, chemosis, epithelial clouding, greenish discoloration, and punctate keratopathy. These effects are partly caused by the bile salt used to stabilize the drug in solution. Dilute preparations (0.05% to 0.15%) are less toxic and appear to be as effective.[44] Systemic administration is toxic and ineffective for keratitis. The toxicity is related to membrane damage in erythrocytes and renal tubular cells.[45]

Current recommendations are to use a concentration of 0.05%, with an initial application every 5 minutes for 1 hour and then one drop hourly. Amphotericin B should be prepared in distilled water for eye drops because it precipitates in sodium chloride solution. Amphotericin B should not be given as a subconjunctival injection because it is painful and can lead to local necrosis. Amphotericin B–soaked collagen shields appear to be as effective as frequently instilled amphotericin B drops in experimental fungal keratitis.[46]

Natamycin. Natamycin (pimaricin 5%), a tetraene polyene antibiotic, is the only antifungal agent commercially available for ophthalmic use. Like amphotericin B, it alters the permeability of fungal cell membranes by binding to sterols. Instead of forming ionic channels, natamycin accumulates in the membranes, disrupting their integrity.

Like amphotericin B, natamycin is insoluble and lacks stability, but it is less toxic.[47] It penetrates the de-epithelialized cornea well, and to a much lesser extent also penetrates intact epithelium.[42] As with amphotericin B, only a small

Table 11-4   Dosages of Antifungal Agents

Drug	Topical	Initial Topical Frequency	Subconjunctival	Systemic
Amphotericin B	0.05% (0.5 mg/ml)	Every 5 minutes for 1 hour, then hourly	750 mg	*
Natamycin	5% (50 mg/ml)	Every 30 minutes for the first 3 to 4 days, then six to eight times daily	—	—
Miconazole	1% (10 mg/ml)	Hourly	5–10 mg	30 mg/kg/day intravenously
Clotrimazole	1% (10 mg/ml)	?Hourly	5–10 mg	—
Ketoconazole	1%–2% (10–20 mg/ml)	?Hourly	—	200–400 mg/day orally in one dose
Flucytosine	1% (10 mg/ml)	?Hourly	—	150 mg/kg/day orally in four divided doses
Nystatin	50,000 to 100,000 U/ml	Every 2 hours	—	—

*Not effective in keratitis. If contemplated, obtain infectious disease consultation.

Table 11-5   Initial Therapy of Fungal Keratitis

Fungus	Topical	Subconjunctival*	Systemic*
Filamentous	Natamycin	Miconazole	Miconazole
Yeast	Amphotericin B	Miconazole	Flucytosine

*May be added to topical use, depending on severity of keratitis.

percentage of the intrastromal drug is bioactive.[48] It appears to be effective only against relatively superficial infections. Natamycin has a broad spectrum of activity against filamentous fungi and is the drug of choice for these organisms.[3,48-50] It is also effective against yeasts, including *C. albicans*. In South Florida, Forster and Rebell[51] found natamycin to be effective in 85% of *Fusarium solani* infections, 60% of infections caused by other nonpigmented filamentous fungi, 90% of those caused by pigmented filamentous fungi, and 75% of yeast infections.

A 5% suspension is applied topically, and it usually "adheres" to the ulcer site. It also forms a ropelike strand in the inferior fornix, which may serve as a reservoir for the drug. For the first 3 to 4 days, drops should be given every half hour,[52] and then decreased to six to eight times per day. With frequent or prolonged use, it can cause epithelial toxicity.

Nystatin. Nystatin is another polyene antifungal agent that is used commonly as a dermatologic ointment for yeast infections. A solution (50 to 100,000 U/ml) can be formulated for treatment of superficial *Candida* keratitis. The dermatologic cream can also be used for ocular infections. Nystatin is administered every 2 hours initially.[53] If the ointment form is used, any excess should be wiped from the lid margin after each instillation.

Imidazole Compounds. The imidazole compounds inhibit synthesis of ergosterol, which is needed for fungal cell membranes, and at higher concentrations can directly damage the fungal cell wall.[54] In vitro they are fungistatic at low concentrations and fungicidal at high concentrations, but it is unlikely that these higher concentrations can be achieved in the cornea. In vitro the minimum inhibitory concentrations for human isolates are higher for imidazole agents than for the polyenes.[50,55] Subconjunctival injection of miconazole, fluconazole, saperconazole, and ketoconazole in rabbits resulted in measurable stomal levels for 4 to 8 hours.[56] Itraconazole persisted in the cornea for at least 24 hours.

Miconazole can be used topically, subconjunctivally, or systemically. Good stromal levels occur after subconjunctival injection and after topical administration if the epithelium is removed.[57] Aqueous levels are high after intravenous administration. Miconazole is relatively unstable in solution and must be reformulated weekly. Miconazole is active against most yeasts and many filamentous fungi but is variably active against *Fusarium* and *Aspergillus* spp.[58] With limited experience, topical,[59,60] combined topical and subconjunctival (with oral ketoconazole),[61] and intravenous miconazole[62] have been effective in most human cases. Both topical and subconjunctival administration have been well tolerated. However, in one case vesicular epithelial elevations with surrounding superficial punctate keratitis were noted, and resolved with discontinuation of the drug.[63]

Ketoconazole is more water soluble and is better absorbed after systemic administration than other imidazoles. Good corneal levels are obtained after topical, subconjunctival, or oral administration.[64] In both experimental models and limited human trials, oral or topical ketoconazole has been effective in every case,[65-67] except in one animal study in which neither oral nor topical ketoconazole was effective against one strain of *A. fumigatus*.[68] Topical preparations (1% to 2%) have been well tolerated, as has systemic administration, although hepatotoxicity can occur. Terfenadine and astemizole are contraindicated in patients taking ketoconazole.

Clotrimazole also has broad antifungal activity and appears to be of most value in treatment of infection with *Aspergillus*.[69] Too toxic for systemic use, it is well tolerated when given topically in a 1% concentration. Oral fluconazole had a significant therapeutic effect on experimental *A. fumigatus* and *C. albicans* ulcers in one study.[70]

Flucytosine. Flucytosine[71,72] (5-fluorocytosine, or Ancobon, Roche Laboratories, Nutley, NJ) is a fluorinated pyrimidine and is fungistatic.[73,74] Flucytosine is selectively taken up by susceptible fungi and deaminated to fluorouracil, which blocks thymidine synthesis.[48] It is not metabolized by human cells; up to 95% of the dose is excreted. However, gastrointestinal flora can convert flucytosine to fluorouracil, which is then absorbed. Flucytosine is effective against *Candida* and *Cryptococcus* and certain strains of *Aspergillus, Penicillium,* and *Cladosporium,* but is not effective against *Fusarium* or *Cephalosporium.* Some yeast strains are resistant, and resistance can develop during therapy, both of

which reduce its usefulness. In general, the results have been disappointing when flucytosine is used alone. Combined treatment, particularly with amphotericin B, is probably best because the combination appears to be more effective and the chance for resistance is reduced.

Topically, flucytosine is used as drops in a 1% solution (10 mg/ml) every hour and appears to be well tolerated. It appears to penetrate the corneal well when administered topically and penetrates both the cornea and anterior chamber well when administered orally.[50] The combinations of flucytosine and miconazole or natamycin were found to be synergistic in vitro against *Aspergillus* spp. keratitis.[75] The combination of flucytosine and amphotericin B may be particularly valuable in systemic candidiasis. The suggested oral dose is 50 to 150 mg/kg/day in four divided doses. Systemic administration is relatively risk-free, but bone marrow and liver toxicity can occur. These complications are dose-related and reversible if the drug is withdrawn. Therefore, regular hematologic and liver function evaluation should be performed. Gastrointestinal upset and skin rashes can also occur.

Selection of Therapy

Several factors limit the determination of efficacy of antifungal agents: (1) the number of cases of fungal keratitis is small; (2) in vitro susceptibility testing has not been standardized and has not correlated well with clinical results; and (3) testing in laboratory animals has been limited. Therefore, precise guidelines for drug therapy cannot be given. Because the greatest cumulative experience has been with natamycin and has shown it to be relatively effective and nontoxic, there is some bias toward its continued use. However, the newer agents have some potential benefits, and as more experience is accumulated they may supplant natamycin as the drug of choice.

Antifungal therapy should not be initiated without laboratory evidence of fungal keratitis because the clinical history and appearance are not diagnostic; prolonged therapy is required; the response is slow and easily confused with the normal resolution of many nonfungal processes; and the agents are often toxic. If necessary, repeated scrapings and cultures or biopsy should be performed to make the diagnosis.

In fungal keratitis, selection of the proper antifungal agent is based mainly on clinical response. Identification of the fungus in smears or culture media may be useful in the initial selection, but the susceptibility of different strains of the same species can vary greatly. Sensitivity determinations can be useful, but they are not performed by many laboratories and are unreliable even when available.[76] If testing is performed, broth dilution appears to be the most reliable method. Certainly, if the patient is doing well on one drug, treatment should not be changed unless toxicity to the drug develops. Tables 11-2 through 11-5 summarize the selection of antifungal agents for treatment.

The response to treatment is usually extremely slow. Improvement is often not seen until an effective agent has been given for weeks. Signs of improvement of a fungal ulcer are decreased size of the central corneal infiltrate, disappearance of the satellite lesions, and rounding out of the feathery margins. Persistent epithelial staining may be noticed, but this often indicates toxicity from medications. Conjunctival injection and chemosis often result from antifungal agents, so their presence or absence cannot be used as an indication of the success of therapy.

Severe corneal damage can occur rapidly as a result of replicating fungi, mycotoxins, and enzymes, and the battle may be lost, particularly if treatment is delayed or if a more virulent fungus is present. If there is no response to medication, the corneal infiltration and ulceration expand and a descemetocele or perforation can occur. This may happen despite effective microbial therapy; the host response to the infection, including difficulty with phagocytosis and removal of nonviable fungi, may itself cause progressive inflammation and ulceration.

As in bacterial keratitis, whenever the keratitis appears to be worsening despite therapy, repeat scrapings and cultures should be obtained. Another pathogen may be present, the initial diagnosis may have been incorrect, or there may be toxicity from medications. Reinfection from contaminated ocular medications or intravenous drug abuse should also be considered. If, in fact, the fungus appears to be resistant to the current regimen, another agent should be selected (Table 11-2).

Treatment should be continued long enough to allow the normal body defenses to cope with the remaining organisms. Long-term therapy (at least 6 weeks) should be anticipated. Negative scrapings or cultures during treatment are not sufficient to indicate eradication of the fungal agent, and great care should be exercised in discontinuing treatment. After medication is discontinued, the patient should be followed up closely for evidence of recrudescence.

When infection extends into the anterior chamber, intraocular antifungal therapy is required. Often, keratoplasty, lensectomy, excision of the involved iris, and vitrectomy are also necessary.[27] Amphotericin B (10 μg) appears to be the best intraocular agent; miconazole (40 μg) also may be effective and appears to be well tolerated.[77]

Corticosteroids

In fungal infections, invasion of the cornea is aided by alteration of the host. One of the ways to impair host defenses at the time of inoculation of the fungal organism is through steroid use. Steroids aid growth of many fungi in the cornea and impair their elimination by the host.

The aim of giving corticosteroids in conjunction with the proper antifungal agent[78,79] is the control of active inflammation to minimize or eliminate structural alteration. If steroids are given for this reason, they should be given only after antifungal treatment has resulted in clinical improvement. Systemic steroids should not be given, effective antifungal agents should be given before topical steroids are introduced, and the patient must be immunologically competent and should be followed up carefully. One must be prepared for the possibility of rapid worsening, including ulceration and perforation.

If fungal infection is diagnosed in a patient who has been treated with topical corticosteroids, the medication should be decreased gradually. Corticosteroids reduce inflammatory cell response to the infection, and when treatment is stopped, an exuberant response, with great release of destructive enzymes, can occur. Under these circumstances the cornea can perforate.

Surgical Treatment

Regular debridement of the base of the ulcer is useful to remove organisms, necrotic stroma, and other inflammatory debris. This procedure can be performed with a scalpel blade or Kimura spatula. If the infection is superficial and localized, lamellar keratectomy can be useful.[80] However, this procedure usually is mainly a "debulking" of the infection; the infection often extends farther than it appears clinically, so such surgery results in incomplete removal. Treatment should be continued and the patient monitored carefully.

A conjunctival flap, the main treatment before development of antifungal agents, can still be useful in unresponsive cases. Bringing host vessels to the site of infection often improves killing and removal of the fungi and can prevent perforation. A lamellar keratectomy

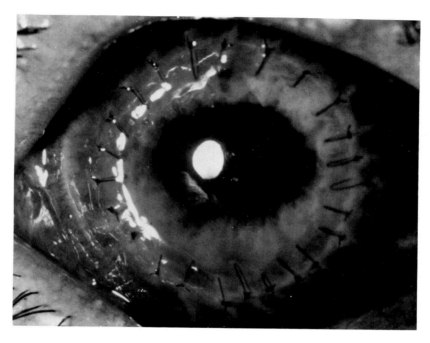

Figure 11-8
Penetrating keratoplasty, 8.5 mm, for the perforated fungal ulcer in Figure 11-5.

should be performed first and all necrotic stroma removed. Conjunctival flaps are particularly useful in localized peripheral infections; a partial inlay flap can treat the infection, greatly shortening the course and reducing morbidity while preserving vision.

If perforation occurs, tissue adhesive can be used to restore integrity. Penetrating keratoplasty can be useful if progressive ulceration or perforation occurs or if the infection does not respond to medical treatment[33,81-86] (Fig. 11-8). Lamellar grafts should be avoided because of the frequent presence of fungi in the residual cornea, which can lead to recurrence of infection even if the cornea is clear clinically. The graft should encompass all clinically involved cornea, but incomplete removal should be expected. Antifungal therapy should be continued and steroid use minimized. Despite the likelihood that fungi are already present in the anterior chamber or are introduced during surgery, endophthalmitis rarely occurs.[27,87] Medical therapy is successful in the majority of cases and usually should be exhausted before resorting to keratoplasty. If a large residual corneal scar results from the ravages of the disease, a corneal transplant can be performed at a later date, with a better prognosis. Forster and Rebell[51] reported that some form of early therapeutic surgery was required in 11 of 61 cases of fungal keratitis at their institution, with penetrating keratoplasty being performed in nine cases. Patients most likely to require keratoplasty were those with deep-seated infections and those who received corticosteroids before diagnosis.

PARASITIC KERATITIS

Parasitic infections of the cornea are rare in the United States but are a major cause of morbidity and blindness in other parts of the world. Onchocerciasis is one of the four leading causes of blindness worldwide, affecting 40 to 50 million people in Africa and Central America, approximately 1 million of whom develop blindness.[88] Interest in parasitic infections in the United States has increased recently because of the emergence of *Acanthamoeba* as an important pathogen. Although still rare, it has been recognized with increased frequency, and treatment options are limited, often inadequate, and controversial.

Acanthamoeba
Acanthamoeba is a genus of free-living protozoa of the subphyla Sarcodina. Like other protozoa, they are unicellular and can exist in two forms—active trophozoite and dormant cyst.

The trophozoite form (16 to 47 μm long) is motile, proliferates, and feeds on bacteria, fungi, and other unicellular organisms. In adverse conditions the trophozoites encyst, forming a double wall containing cellulose. The cyst form (10 to 25 μm in diameter) is much more resistant to extreme environments, as well as to chlorine and other antimicrobial agents.

Acanthamoeba are ubiquitous, having been found in all types of liquid media, including tap water, bottled water, swimming pools, hot tubs, and contact lens solutions, as well as soil and air.[89] Their prevalence appears to peak during warmer weather. *Acanthamoeba* can be isolated from the mouth and pharynx of some asymptomatic adults and children,[90,91] and humoral immunity appears to be common in the general population.[92] Thus, although we are probably constantly exposed to these organisms, clinical infections rarely result. The reasons for the development of clinical infections are not known. It is likely that a break in the epithelial surface is necessary for entry of the organism, and repeated exposure or inoculation into an immunoprivileged site, such as the cornea, may also be required. Concomitant infection with bacteria, fungi, or viruses may be necessary initially to provide the *Acanthamoeba* organism with food.[93,94] Like fungi, *Acanthamoeba* can be relatively nonimmunogenic; they often exist in the cornea without surrounding inflammatory cell infiltration. They release enzymes, including phospholipases, lysozyme, and cellulase. Some species are more pathogenic than others, but the factors that determine virulence have not been identified.

The first case report of *Acanthamoeba* keratitis appeared in 1974.[95] Few additional cases were reported until the mid-1980s, when numerous cases were diagnosed.[96-102] It appeared that cases are not just more likely to be recognized, but that the incidence of the disease increased rapidly. Since then the incidence appears to have stabilized. Although patients of any age can be affected, *Acanthamoeba* keratitis is most common in young adults who are usually in good health and are immunocompetent.

The majority of cases have been related to contact lens wear, most commonly soft contact lenses, and the use of contaminated solutions, including tap water, well water, homemade saline solutions, and saliva. *Acanthamoeba* is usually isolated from one or more of these sources. In a study of the water taps of 50 contact lens wearers in England, *Acanthamoeba* spp. were isolated from 6.[103] *Acanthamoeba* cysts and trophozoites are capable of adhering to soft contact lenses.[104] However, at least in a hamster

model, keratitis does not develop unless the contaminated lens is placed in an eye with an epithelial abrasion.[105] Bacteria and fungi are also present in the lens cases and solutions in many cases, and may serve as a food source for the *Acanthamoeba*.[106] Many bacteria and fungi, including common external ocular flora, such as *Staphylococcus epidermidis* and *Corynebacterium*, support *Acanthamoeba* growth.[107]

Cases not associated with contact lens wear have followed corneal trauma, but the source of the *Acanthamoeba* is often unclear.[108] Cases have also occurred after penetrating keratoplasty.[109]

Once in the cornea, *Acanthamoeba* can grow on epithelial cells and keratocytes.[110] They elaborate collagenase, neuraminidase, and other proteolytic enzymes that may play a role in invasion and destruction of the cornea.[111]

Clinical Manifestations

The clinical features of *Acanthamoeba* keratitis are given in Table 11-6.[112] Symptoms include pain, photophobia, irritation, foreign body sensation, tearing, and decreased vision. The pain is often severe and out of proportion to the signs of inflammation. In the earliest stages of infection, signs may be limited to the epithelium. Epithelial defects, pseudodendrites (Fig. 11-9), punctate staining, haze, granularity, elevated epithelial lines, and microcysts may be

Table 11-6	Clinical Features of *Acanthamoeba* Keratitis	
Feature	**Frequency**	**When Present**
Pain	++++	E,L*
Ring infiltrate	+++	L
Central stromal infiltrate	+++	L
Epithelial haze, punctate staining, pseudodendrites, elevated lines	++	E,L
Recurrent epithelial breakdown	++	E,L
Decreased corneal sensation	++	E,L
Radial keratoneuritis	+	E
Scleritis	+	L
Adenopathy	+	
Hypopyon	+	L
Increased intraocular pressure	+	L

*E, Early; L, late.

present. In early stromal involvement, edema is more prominent than infiltration (Fig. 11-10). The pattern of stromal infiltration varies, but it is generally most dense in the midperiphery, sometimes forming a complete ring (Fig. 11-11). There is usually a central infiltrate, but the cornea within the ring can be relatively clear. A double ring, or a central infiltrate alone, can also be observed. Satellite infiltrates, which

may appear granular, may be present outside the ring. The epithelium overlying the infiltrates can be intact, but recurrent epithelial breakdown is common.

Radial keratoneuritis occurs in a minority of cases but is relatively specific, because it occurs rarely in other conditions (Fig. 11-12). (Radial keratoneuritis was reported in one case of *Pseudomonas aeruginosa* keratitis.[113]) Fluffy infiltrates

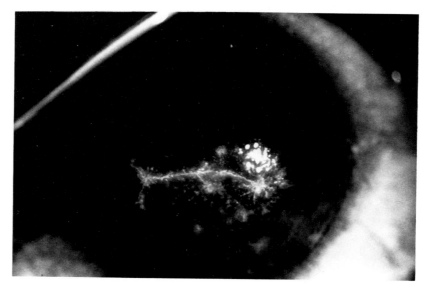

Figure 11-9
Pseudodendritic epithelial staining in *Acanthamoeba* keratitis.

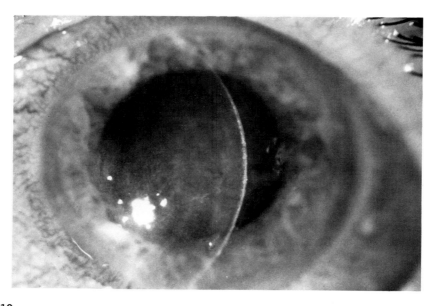

Figure 11-10
Stromal edema and epitheliopathy, resembling herpetic disciform keratitis, in *Acanthamoeba* infection.

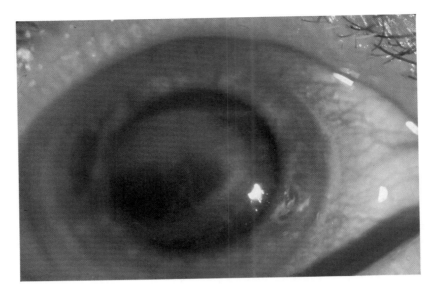

Figure 11-11
Ring infiltrate in *Acanthamoeba* keratitis. (Courtesy of Diane Curtin, Pittsburgh, PA.)

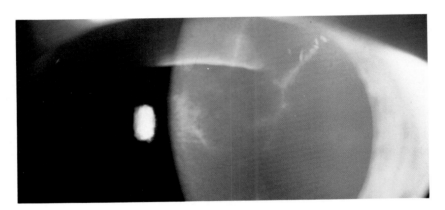

Figure 11-12
Radial keratoneuritis in *Acanthamoeba* keratitis. (Courtesy of Scott Portnoy, Pittsburgh, PA.)

are observed along the course of one or more corneal nerves. These infiltrates may involve the central or peripheral portions of the nerves; they are often transient and can precede other forms of stromal infiltration.[100] Neural inflammation may be responsible for the unusually intense pain that many of these patients experience. It can also explain why decreased corneal sensation is frequently observed.

Nodular or diffuse scleritis may be associated with the keratitis, usually adjacent to the limbus (Fig. 11-13). Anterior chamber reaction is usually present and can be severe enough to produce a hypopyon or increased intraocular pressure. Adenopathy has been present in some cases. Secondary bacterial infection, most often due to streptococci, has occurred in some patients.

Diagnosis

As can be inferred from the previous description, the clinical presentation of *Acanthamoeba* keratitis is rarely diagnostic. However, some features should make one suspect *Acanthamoeba,* and this suspicion is most important in making the diagnosis. Specimens should be inoculated into nonnutrient agar, which has been overlayed with *Escherichia coli* or *Enterobacter aerogenes,* although growth on blood agar, chocolate agar, Sabouraud agar, or Löwenstein-

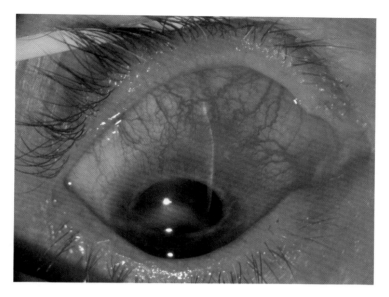

Figure 11-13
Nodular scleritis in *Acanthamoeba* keratitis. (Courtesy of Diane Curtin, Pittsburgh, PA.)

Jensen agar has occurred in some cases. Most standard stains, including Gram's, Giemsa, or Wright's, will indicate the organism when it is present in smears, but often a careful search by an experienced observer is required. Calcofluor white and acridine orange can facilitate detection.

These tests are often unsuccessful, however, particularly early in the course of infection. Removal and examination of intact but abnormal epithelium may be helpful, but corneal biopsy is often required for diagnosis. If the patient has worn contact lenses, the lenses and all solutions should be cultured. Isolation of the organisms is suggestive and may be sufficient to initiate therapy, provided the clinical presentation is consistent.

Treatment

Overall, the treatment for *Acanthamoeba* keratitis has been disappointing, to some extent because the infection was usually well advanced before diagnosis; however, available treatment options are suboptimal. A few drugs kill trophozoites in vitro, but is unclear whether any are cysticidal. Improvement is slow with any of these agents, and unless medical treatment is initiated very early in the course of an infection, prolonged therapy is necessary. It is likely that excystation or host removal of remaining organisms is required to eliminate the infection.

Early penetrating keratoplasty has been advocated by some to remove or debulk the resistant infection. Although this procedure can be successful, in many cases the organism is present in the remaining tissue, and infection recurs in the graft. *Acanthamoeba* infection frequently extends into apparently clear stroma, and its limits cannot be appreciated without tissue examination. Recurrent infections in the corneal graft tend to be even more difficult to treat than primary infections.

In general, medical therapy should be pursued if the condition is responsive. Penetrating keratoplasty is best performed after prolonged medical treatment; in reported cases, recurrences were less common if medical treatment had been given for at least 4 months before surgery.[112] Penetrating keratoplasty can be considered earlier, however, if the diagnosis is made early in the course of infection and it is felt that all involved tissue can be excised. Certainly, if perforation occurs, keratoplasty may be necessary to preserve the globe.

Diamidines. To date the experience with propamidine has been the most extensive, and some medical cures have been achieved, mainly in combined use with polymyxin B–neomycin–gramicidin drops.[114-116] Propamidine has antibacterial and antifungal activity and is sold over the counter in Britain but is not available in the United States. The recommended treatment regimen is as follows: Initially, propamidine and polymyxin B–neomycin–gramicidin drops are alternated every 30 to 60 minutes for 3 days around the clock. For the remainder of the first week, drops are given hourly during the day and every 2 hours at night. Administration is then gradually tapered to four times a day. Dibromopropamidine ointment can be given at bedtime. Treatment should be continued for at least 1 year in most cases. Propamidine is toxic to the epithelial surface, often causing conjunctival injection and chemosis, corneal epithelial microcysts, and punctate keratopathy.[117] Resistance can develop during therapy.[118]

Imidazoles. Miconazole, clotrimazole, and ketoconazole were effective in vitro against some strains of *Acanthamoeba.* Topical miconazole, topical clotrimazole 1% to 2%, and oral ketoconazole (200 to 400 mg/day) were effective in some patients but not in others.[116,119] Probably the most effective imidazole is clotrimazole, which has been used successfully in several cases in conjunction with propamidine or after unsuccessful treatment with propamidine.[120] In some of these cases, clotrimazole was the most effective agent in vitro. In some patients, the 1% dermatologic cream (commercially available) is tolerated, but in others clotrimazole powder must be obtained from Schering Laboratories (Kenilworth, NJ) and a 1% to 2% suspension formulated in artificial tears. Miconazole may be effective, but also can be irritating, and must be reformulated weekly because it is unstable in solution. Although oral ketoconazole may be useful, it carries a small risk of hepatotoxicity.

Polymeric biguanides. Polyhexamethylene biguanide (PHMB) is a disinfectant used commonly in swimming pools and occasionally in contact lens solutions.[121] It damages cytoplasmic membranes and inhibits essential respiratory enzymes in susceptible organisms. It is effective against trophozoites and cysts.[122,123] In one in vitro study it was more effective than propamidine, paramomycin, and imidazoles against 23 clinical isolates.[124] A 0.02% solution is effective in many cases of *Acanthamoeba* keratitis, including many that do not respond to treatment with propamidine and neomycin.[123,125] However, some patients do not respond, even when the isolate is found to be sensitive in vitro. Combination therapy with PHMB, propamidine, and neomycin was effective in all five patients in one study.[124]

Others. The aminoglycosides neomycin and paromomycin appear to be less effective than the previous two groups, but they may be useful in combination with other agents. Neomy-

cin is somewhat toxic and can induce hypersensitivity reactions. Clinical experience with other agents, such as natamycin and ciproxolamine, is limited.

Other Treatment. In *Acanthamoeba* keratitis, as in other forms of infectious keratitis, the use of corticosteroids is controversial. Corticosteroids reduce inflammation and increase comfort but also reduce the host's capacity to eradicate the infection. In *Acanthamoeba* keratitis, the currently available antimicrobial agents cannot kill all the organisms in the cornea, particularly the cyst forms, and the host response appears to be particularly important. In addition, corticosteroids inhibit excystation of the organism into the more susceptible trophozoite form, at least in vitro.[126] Clinically, the effect of corticosteroids on outcome is not clear, but results seem to be better if corticosteroid use is avoided or kept to a minimum and only used during effective antiamebic therapy.

Epithelial debridement can reduce or eliminate the infective load in early disease. Dimethylsulfoxide was found to enhance the effectiveness of propamidine isethionate against *Acanthamoeba* cysts in vitro.[127] The usefulness of cryotherapy of infected corneas is not clear. It did not prevent recurrence of *Acanthamoeba* after keratoplasty in one case,[128] but it did appear to be useful in five others.[129] In two in vitro studies, the cysts were resistant to cryotherapy in one[130] and sensitive to it in another[131]; the combination of cryotherapy and antibiotics was more effective than antibiotics alone.

Relief of the pain associated with these infections can be difficult. Success with sulindac, a nonsteroidal antiinflammatory agent, has been reported in some patients. In resistant cases retrobulbar injections of alcohol may be used. A 1-ml injection, consisting of 1/3 ml absolute alcohol and 2/3 ml 2% lidocaine, will provide anesthesia for 2 to 4 weeks, with full recovery. Temporary ptosis and other nerve palsies can also occur.

Recommendations. Treatment should be initiated with a combination of PHMB and propamidine. Propamidine and PHMB drops are alternated every 30 to 60 minutes for 3 days around the clock. For the remainder of the first week, drops are given hourly during the day and every 2 hours at night. Administration is then gradually tapered to four times a day. I recommend that corticosteroids be avoided if possible. They can be used to reduce inflammation, particularly if there is marked anterior chamber reaction or secondary glaucoma, if effective

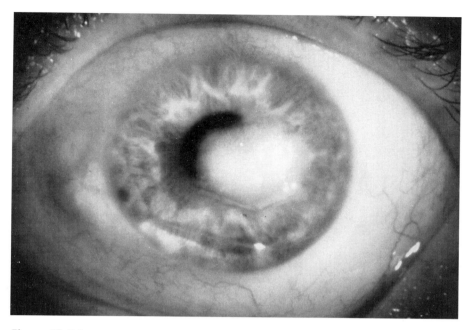

Figure 11-14
Microsporidial stromal keratitis. (Courtesy of Richard Davis, Columbia, SC)

amebicidal therapy is being administered. Prolonged amebicidal treatment is required in most cases, but the duration of treatment is unclear. I recommend treatment for 1 year in most cases. Subepithelial infiltrates can develop late in the course of the disease, sometimes when antibiotics or corticosteroids are tapered.[132] The infiltrates respond to topical corticosteroids and in some cases to antibiotic therapy. Whether these infiltrates are immunologic or infectious is unknown.

Prevention

Proper contact lens hygiene can probably prevent the development of *Acanthamoeba* keratitis. Homemade saline solutions, tap water, and saliva should be avoided. Patients should not swim while wearing their lenses. Avoidance of bacterial and fungal contamination of lenses, lens cases, and solutions will probably also help prevent *Acanthamoeba* infection. Heat disinfection is effective in killing *Acanthamoeba* cysts and trophozoites. Hydrogen peroxide disinfection systems were effective if they did not contain a metal catalyst and exposure was for at least 2 hours.[133] Chlorhexidine and benzalkonium have variable effect: They appear to kill both trophozoites and cysts of some isolates, but in other cases they were not effective against either.[133-136] Thimerosal, sorbic acid, ethylenediaminetetraacetic acid, and quaternary ammonium compounds are generally ineffective.

Microsporidia

Microsporidia are small obligate intracellular protozoa. Two types of ocular infections have been observed—stromal keratitis and infections of the corneal and conjunctival epithelium. The organisms responsible for these two types of infections appear to be different. Stromal keratitis cases appear to be caused by a binucleated oval spore that is *Nosema*-like, while infection of the corneal and conjunctival epithelium is caused by a spore containing a single nucleus that is a member of the genus *Encephalitozoon*.[137] The latter appears to be a newly identified species, called *Encephalitozoon hellem*.[138] The keratitis can be suppurative and ulcerative (Fig. 11-14) and is seen in healthy individuals.[139-141]

Microsporidial infection of the corneal and conjunctival epithelium is commonly seen in patients with AIDS.[138,142-144] Dryness, pain, foreign body sensation, light sensitivity, and decreased vision may be present. Vision can be normal or markedly reduced. A mild hyperemia of the inferior fornix can be seen, but conjunctival inflammation is usually not present. The corneal epithelium has numerous fine opacities, many of which stain with fluorescein (Fig. 11-15). The lesions tend to be denser in the in-

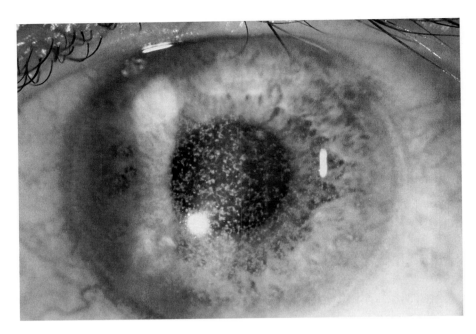

Figure 11-15
Superficial microsporidial keratitis in a patient with AIDS. (Courtesy of Diane Curtin, Pittsburgh, PA.)

terpalpebral area, where the epithelium can be raised. A mild iritis can be present, but corneal infiltrates or stromal extension have not been observed.

The diagnosis can be made by microscopic examination of conjunctival scrapings or debrided corneal epithelium. The organisms are ovoid, approximately 2 by 3 μm. They are seen in the cytoplasm of epithelial cells. They stain purple-blue with Giemsa stain, and are gram-positive. Microsporidia can also be identified by staining with calcofluor, trichrome blue,[145] and fluorescence with Uvitex 2B.[146] Definitive identification requires electron microscopy. Epithelial disease that appears similar to microsporidial infection can be seen in patients with AIDS who are being treated with ganciclovir.[147] The keratopathy resolves 1 to 3 months after discontinuation of ganciclovir.

The epithelial infection tends to be chronic, without spontaneous resolution. Debridement of infected epithelium can be helpful. Topical propamidine isethionate (0.1%) and fumagillin have been effective in some cases. Fumagillin appears to be more effective and is minimally toxic to the ocular surface.[148] Systemic itraconazole was effective in one case.[144] Gastrointestinal microsporidial infections are also commonly seen in AIDS patients and often respond to albendazole or metronidazole.[149]

Leishmania

Leishmania are flagellated obligate intracellular protozoa that are members of the subphylum Mastigophora. They are found in Africa, Central America, the Middle East, India, and South America. The reservoir of the organisms is in rodents and dogs, and infection is transmitted to humans by infected sandflies. Lid infection is common. Involvement of the conjunctiva or cornea is seen more commonly in the Americas and usually occurs by autoinoculation from a nearby infection or direct extension. Large ulcerating granulomas can occur. Trachoma-like follicles and avascular nodules can be seen on the palpebral conjunctiva. Corneal involvement begins as a phlyctenule-like process but quickly progresses to deep infiltration and abscess formation.[150] Perforation can occur after 3 to 4 weeks. In one patient, diffuse cellular infiltration and vascularization of the superficial stroma was seen in both eyes.[151] Treatment is with meglumine antimoniate and stibogluconate sodium, either intravenously or intramuscularly.

Onchocerciasis

Onchocerca volvulus is a filarial nematode (threadworm) that is an endemic cause of infection (river blindness) in Central and Western Africa, Central America, and the northernmost por-

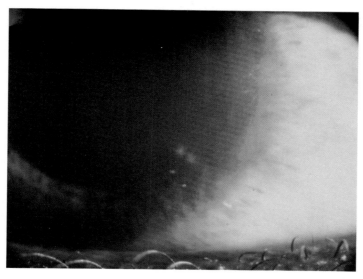

Figure 11-16
Nummular corneal infiltrates caused by *Loa loa*. (Courtesy of Massimo Busin, Bonn, Germany.)

tions of South America. Larvae are transmitted to humans via the *Simulium* black fly. These develop into adults in the subcutaneous tissue, and the females release microfilaria that migrate through the skin and subcutaneous tissue. The microfilaria are 0.22 to 0.36 mm long and 5 to 10 μm in diameter. They can migrate into any portion of the globe, including the conjunctiva, cornea, and anterior chamber, either by direct invasion or via the blood.

In endemic areas most individuals are infected in the first few years of life. The living organism tends to be well tolerated, but a reaction ensues following its death. The more severe complications usually occur after many years of chronic infestation or with microfilaricidal treatment.

Ocular findings generally develop 1.5 to 5 years after skin involvement. The earliest evidence of ocular involvement is the presence of live organisms. The living microfilaria are easily seen in the anterior chamber, and this is facilitated by having the patient sit with his or her head between the knees for 2 minutes before examination to concentrate the organisms in the central anterior aqueous. Detection of live microfilaria in the corneal stroma is more difficult because they are transparent, immobile, and often coiled.

Signs of conjunctival involvement include injection, chemosis, swelling of the lids, limbitis, and phlyctenules.[152] The conjunctival inflammation is often chronic. *Limbitis* is seen as small, pale, yellow globules at the limbus, which often form acutely, either spontaneously or after initiation of antifilarial treatment. The lesions are thought to represent eosinophilic granuloma formation around dead microfilaria.

The earliest corneal inflammatory lesions occur near the limbus as a localized transient reaction around a dead worm. The cellular infiltrate consists of lymphocytes and eosinophils.[153] Later, other "snowflake" or nummular infiltrates can occur throughout the stroma and are also transient. All of these localized infiltrates are referred to as *punctate keratitis*.[154] In severe cases the nummular opacities can coalesce. A more severe reaction, *sclerosing keratitis*, often causes blindness. It is a diffuse infiltrative process that begins at 4 and 8 o'clock and extends inferiorly and centrally. It can progress upward to involve the entire cornea, leaving permanent scarring and vascularization in its wake.[155,156] The worms are usually visible above the infiltration. In a murine model of sclerosing keratitis the infiltrate is composed primarily of CD4+ T cells.[157]

In addition to the aforementioned findings, anterior uveitis, optic neuritis, optic atrophy, and chorioretinitis may occur in onchocerciasis. Ivermectin, 150 mg/kg orally, repeated every 6 months appears to be the most effective treatment and is less likely than diethylcarbamazine to cause exacerbation of ocular inflammation.[158-160] Treatment lowers the number of microfilaria in the anterior chamber and cornea and the incidence of punctate keratitis, but the effect on the long-term incidence of sclerosing keratitis, chorioretinitis, and blindness is less clear.[161,162]

Trypanosomiasis

Trypanosomiasis occurs in both African and American variants and is caused by different species of *Trypanosoma*, a hemoflagellate. A bilateral interstitial keratitis, similar to luetic keratitis, can occur in the African type.[163,164] Conjunctivitis, palpebral and periorbital edema, and preauricular adenopathy may also be present. In contrast to most other causes of interstitial keratitis, in trypanosomiasis the corneal inflammation responds to systemic antibiotic therapy. If appropriate anti-trypanosomal treatment is begun early in the course of the interstitial keratitis, the inflammation clears without significant scarring. Suramin and pentamidine are the drugs of choice for trypanosomiasis. Melarsoprol is added if central nervous system involvement is present.

Other Parasites

A number of other parasites can cause corneal inflammation, including *Loa loa* (Fig. 11-16) and *Multiceps*.[165,166] Larvae have also been observed in the corneal stroma or adherent to the corneal endothelium.[167-169] In each case the larvae appeared to be dead. In two cases there was an inflammatory reaction.

REFERENCES

1. Jones DB, Sexton RR, Rebell G: Mycotic keratitis in South Florida: a review of thirty-eight cases, *Trans Ophthalmol Soc UK* 89:781, 1969.
2. Forster RK, Rebell G: The diagnosis and management of keratomycoses: I. Cause and diagnosis, *Arch Ophthalmol* 93:975, 1975.
3. Jones BR: Principles in the management of oculomycosis: XXXI Edward Jackson Memorial Lecture, *Am J Ophthalmol* 79:15, 1975.
4. Jones BR, Richards AB, Morgan G: Direct fungal infection of the eye in Britain, *Trans Ophthalmol Soc UK* 89:727, 1969.
5. Doughman DJ et al: Fungal keratitis at the University of Minnesota 1971-1981, *Trans Am Ophthalmol Soc* 80:235, 1982.
6. O'Day DM: Selection of appropriate antifungal therapy, *Cornea* 6:238, 1987.
7. Liesegang TJ, Forster RF: Spectrum of microbial keratitis in South Florida, *Am J Ophthalmol* 90:38, 1980.
8. Rodrigues MM, Laibson P: Exogenous mycotic keratitis caused by *Blastomyces dermatitidis*, *Am J Ophthalmol* 75:782, 1973.
9. Poria VC et al: Study of mycotic keratitis, *Indian J Ophthalmol* 33:229, 1985.
10. Ando N, Takatori K: Fungal flora of the conjunctival sac, *Am J Ophthalmol* 94:67, 1982.
11. Wilson LA et al: Fungi from the normal outer eye, *Am J Ophthalmol* 67:52, 1969.
12. Clinch TE et al: Fungal keratitis from nylon line lawn trimmers, *Am J Ophthalmol* 114:437, 1992.
13. Burda CD, Fisher E: Corneal destruction by extracts of *Cephalosporium mycelium*, *Am J Ophthalmol* 50:926, 1960.
14. Wogan GN: Mycotoxins, *Annu Rev Pharmacol* 15:437, 1975.
15. Zhu WS et al: Extracellular proteases of *Aspergillus flavus*: fungal keratitis, proteases and pathogenesis, *Diagn Microbiol Infect Dis* 13:491, 1990.
16. Raza SK et al: An in-vitro study of the sterol content and toxin production of Fusarium isolates from mycotic keratitis, *J Med Microbiol* 41:204, 1994.
17. Nelson RD et al: Candida mannan: chemistry, suppression of cell-mediated immunity and possible mechanisms of action, *Clin Microbiol Rev* 4:1, 1991.
18. Cutler JE: Putative virulence factors of *Candida albicans*, *Annu Rev Microbiol* 45:187, 1991.
19. Ghannoum MA, Abu-Elteen KH: Pathogenicity determinants of *Candida*, *Mycoses* 33:265, 1990.
20. Rogers TJ, Balish E: Immunity to *Candida albicans*, *Microbiol Rev* 44:660, 1980.
21. Donzis PB et al: Microbial contamination of contact lens care systems, *Am J Ophthalmol* 104:325, 1987.
22. Simmons RB et al: Morphology and ultrastructure of fungi in extended-wear soft contact lenses, *J Clin Microbiol* 24:21, 1986.
23. Wilhelmus KR et al: Fungal keratitis in contact lens wearers, *Am J Ophthalmol* 106:708, 1988.
24. Aronson SB, Elliot JH: *Ocular inflammation*, St Louis, 1972, Mosby–Year Book.
25. Dudley MA, Chick EW: Corneal lesions produced in rabbits by an extract of *Fusarium moniliforme*, *Arch Ophthalmol* 72:346, 1964.
26. Arora R, Venkateswamy K, Mahajan VM: Keratomycosis: a retrospective histopathologic and microbiologic analysis, *Ann Ophthalmol* 20:306, 1988.
27. Pflugfelder SC et al: Exogenous fungal endophthalmitis, *Ophthalmology* 95:19, 1988.
28. Jones BR et al: Corneal and intraocular infection due to *Fusarium solani*, *Trans Ophthalmol Soc UK* 89:757, 1969.
29. Jones DB et al: Early diagnosis of mycotic keratitis, *Trans Ophthalmol Soc UK* 89:805, 1969.
30. Wilson LA, Sexton RR: *Laboratory aids in diagnosis*. In Duane T, Jaeger E, editors: *Clinical ophthalmology*, vol 4, Philadelphia, 1988, Harper & Row.
31. Jones DB: *Strategy for the initial management of suspected microbial keratitis*. In New Orleans Academy of Ophthalmology: symposium on medical and surgical diseases of the cornea, St Louis, 1980, Mosby–Year Book.
32. Rosa H, Miller D, Alfonso EC: The changing

spectrum of fungal keratitis in South Florida, *Ophthalmology* 101:1005, 1994.

33. Dunlop AA et al: Suppurative corneal ulceration in Bangladesh: a study of 142 cases examining the microbiological diagnosis, clinical and epidemiological features of bacterial and fungal keratitis, *Aust NZ J Ophthalmol* 22:105, 1994.

34. Ishibashi Y, Hommura S, Matsumoto Y: Direct examination vs culture of biopsy specimens for the diagnosis of keratomycosis, *Am J Ophthalmol* 103:636, 1987.

35. Vajpayee RB et al: Laboratory diagnosis of keratomycosis: comparative evaluation of direct microscopy and culture results, *Ann Ophthalmol* 25:68, 1993.

36. Chander J et al: Evaluation of calcofluor staining in the diagnosis of fungal corneal ulcer, *Mycoses* 36:243, 1993.

37. Ishibashi Y, Kaufman HE: Corneal biopsy in the diagnosis of keratomycosis, *Am J Ophthalmol* 101:288, 1986.

38. O'Day DN, Robinson RD, Head WS: Efficacy of antifungal agents in the cornea: I. A comparative study, *Invest Ophthalmol Vis Sci* 24:1098, 1983.

39. Anderson B, Chick EW: Treatment of corneal fungal ulcers with amphotericin B and mechanical debridement, *South Med J* 56:270, 1963.

40. Green WR, Bennett JE, Goos RD: Ocular penetration of amphotericin B, *Arch Ophthalmol* 73:769, 1965.

41. O'Day DM et al: Corneal penetration of amphotericin B and natamycin, *Curr Eye Res* 5:877, 1986.

42. O'Day DM et al: Bioavailability and penetration of topical amphotericin B in the anterior segment of the rabbit eye, *J Ocul Pharmacol* 2:371, 1986.

43. Bindschadler DO, Bennett JE: A pharmacologic guide to the clinical use of amphotericin B, *J Infect Dis* 170:427, 1969.

44. Wood TO, Tuberville AW, Monnett R: Keratomycosis and amphotericin B, *Trans Am Ophthalmol Soc* 83:397, 1985.

45. Medoff G, Kobayaski GS: Strategies in the treatment of systemic fungal infections, *N Engl J Med* 302:145, 1980.

46. Pleyer Uwe et al: Use of collagen shields containing amphotericin B in the treatment of experimental *Candida albicans*-induced keratomycosis in rabbits, *Am J Ophthalmol* 113:303, 1992.

47. Raab WP: *Natamycin (pimaricin): its properties and possibilities in medicine,* Stuttgart, 1972, Georg Thieme Verlag.

48. Johns KJ, O'Day DM: Pharmacologic management of keratomycoses, *Surv Ophthalmol* 33:178, 1988.

49. Jones DB, Forster RL, Rebell G: *Fusarium solani* keratitis treated with natamycin (pimaricin): 18 consecutive cases, *Arch Ophthalmol* 88:147, 1972.

50. Forster RK: *Fungal keratitis and conjunctivitis:* *clinical disease.* In Smolin G, Thoft RA, editors: *The cornea: scientific foundations and clinical practice,* Boston, 1994, Little, Brown & Co.

51. Forster RK, Rebell G: The diagnosis and management of keratomycoses: II. Medical and surgical management, *Arch Ophthalmol* 93:1134, 1975.

52. O'Day DM et al: In vitro and in vivo susceptibility of *Candida* keratitis to topical polyenes, *Curr Eye Res* 6:363, 1987.

53. Ostler HB: *Diseases of the external eye and adnexa: a text and atlas,* Baltimore, 1993, Williams & Wilkins.

54. Bodey GP: Azole antifungal agents, *Clin Infect Dis* 14(suppl 1):S161, 1992.

55. Robinson N, Penland R, Osato M: Comparative efficacy of new azole antifungal agents against human ocular isolates, *Invest Ophthalmol Vis Sci* 31(suppl):451, 1990.

56. Klippenstein K et al: The qualitative evaluation of the pharmacokinetics of subconjunctivally injected antifungal agents in rabbits, *Cornea* 12:512, 1993.

57. Foster CS, Stefanyszyn M: Intraocular penetration of miconazole in rabbits, *Arch Ophthalmol* 97:1703, 1979.

58. Stevens DA, Levine HB, Deresinski SC: Miconazole in coccidioidomycosis: II. Therapeutic and pharmacologic studies in man, *Am J Ophthalmol* 80:191, 1976.

59. Foster CS: Miconazole therapy of keratomycosis, *Am J Ophthalmol* 91:622, 1981.

60. Mohan M, Panda A, Gupta SK: Management of human keratomycosis with miconazole, *Aust NZ J Ophthalmol* 17:295, 1989.

61. Fitzsimons R, Peters AL: Miconazole and ketoconazole as a satisfactory first-line treatment for keratomycosis, *Am J Ophthalmol* 101:605, 1986.

62. Ishibashi Y, Matsumoto Y, Takei K: The effects of intravenous miconazole on fungal keratitis, *Am J Ophthalmol* 98:433, 1984.

63. Zaidman GW: Miconazole corneal toxicity, *Cornea* 10:90, 1991.

64. Hemady RK, Chu W, Foster CS: Intraocular penetration of ketoconazole in rabbits, *Cornea* 11:329, 1992.

65. Torres MA et al: Topical ketoconazole for fungal keratitis, *Am J Ophthalmol* 100:293, 1985.

66. Ishibashi Y, Kaufman HE: Topical ketoconazole for experimental *Candida* keratitis in rabbits, *Am J Ophthalmol* 102:522, 1986.

67. Ishibashi Y: Oral ketoconazole therapy for keratomycosis, *Am J Ophthalmol* 95:342, 1983.

68. Komadina TG et al: Treatment of *Aspergillus fumigatus* keratitis in rabbits with oral and topical ketoconazole, *Am J Ophthalmol* 99:476, 1985.

69. Jones DB, Jones BR, Robinson NM: Clotrimazole (Canesten) therapy of fungal keratitis, *Chemotherapy* 6:189, 1975.

70. O'Day DM: Orally administered antifungal therapy for experimental keratomycosis, *Trans Am Ophthalmol Soc* 88:685, 1990.

71. Steer PL et al: 5-Fluorocytosine, an oral antifungal compound: a report on clinical and laboratory experience, *Ann Intern Med* 76:15, 1972.

72. Symoens J: Clinical and experimental evidence on miconazole for the treatment of systemic mycoses: a review, *Proc R Soc Med* 70:4, 1977.

73. Block E, Bennett J: Pharmacologic studies with 5-fluorocytosine, *Antimicrob Agents Chemother* 1:476, 1972.

74. Bennett JE: Flucytosine, *Ann Intern Med* 86:319, 1977.

75. Searl SS et al: Aspergillus keratitis with intraocular invasion, *Ophthalmology* 88:1244, 1981.

76. O'Day DM et al: In vitro and in vivo susceptibility of *Candida* keratitis to topical polyenes, *Invest Ophthalmol Vis Sci* 28:874, 1987.

77. Tolentino FI et al: Toxicity of intravitreous miconazole, *Arch Ophthalmol* 100:1504, 1982.

78. Newmark E, Ellison AC, Kaufman HE: Combined pimaricin and dexamethasone therapy of keratomycosis, *Am J Ophthalmol* 71:718, 1971.

79. O'Day DM, Moore T, Aronson S: Deep fungal corneal abscess: combined corticosteroid therapy, *Arch Ophthalmol* 86:414, 1971.

80. Sanitato JJ, Kelly CG, Kaufman HE: Surgical management of peripheral fungal keratitis, *Arch Ophthalmol* 102:1507, 1984.

81. Polack FM, Kaufman HE, Newmark E: Keratomycosis, medical and surgical treatment, *Arch Ophthalmol* 85:410, 1971.

82. Singh G, Malik SR: Therapeutic keratoplasty in fungal corneal ulcers, *Br J Ophthalmol* 56:41, 1972.

83. Forster RK, Rebell G: Therapeutic surgery in failures of medical treatment of fungal keratitis, *Br J Ophthalmol* 59:366, 1975.

84. Sanders N: Penetrating keratoplasty in treatment of fungus keratitis, *Am J Ophthalmol* 70:24, 1970.

85. Jones BR, Jones DB, Richards AB: Surgery in the management of keratomycosis, *Trans Ophthalmol Soc UK* 89:887, 1976.

86. Hill JC: Use of penetrating keratoplasty in acute bacterial keratitis, *Br J Ophthalmol* 70:502, 1986.

87. Wilson LA, Cavanagh HD: Penetrating keratoplasty for exogenous *Paecilomyces* keratitis followed by postoperative endophthalmitis, *Am J Ophthalmol* 98:552, 1984.

88. O'Day J, Mackenzie CD: Ocular onchocerciasis: diagnosis and current clinical approaches, *Trop Doct* 15:87, 1985.

89. Warhurst DC: Pathogenic free-living amoebae, *Parasitol Today* 1:24, 1985.

90. Wang SS, Feldman HA: Isolation of *Hartmanella* species from human throats, *N Engl J Med* 277:1174, 1967.

91. Rivera F et al: Pathogenic and free-living protozoa cultured from the nasopharyngeal and oral regions of dental patients, *Environ Res* 33:428, 1984.

92. Cursons RTM, Brown TJ, Keys EA: Immunity to pathogenic free-living amoebae, *Lancet* 1:877, 1977.

93. Martinez AJ, Janitschke K: *Acanthamoeba*, an opportunistic microorganism: a review, *Infection* 13:251, 1985.

94. Jones DB: *Acanthamoeba*—the ultimate opportunist?, *Am J Ophthalmol* 102:527, 1986.

95. Nagington J et al: Amoebic infection of the eye, *Lancet* 2:1547, 1974.

96. Hirst LW et al: Management of *Acanthamoeba* keratitis: a case report and review of the literature, *Ophthalmology* 91:1105, 1984.

97. Cohen EJ et al: Diagnosis and management of *Acanthamoeba* keratitis, *Am J Ophthalmol* 100:389, 1985.

98. Moore MB et al: *Acanthamoeba* keratitis associated with soft contact lenses, *Am J Ophthalmol* 100:396, 1985.

99. Theodore FH et al: The diagnostic value of a ring infiltrate in acanthamoebic keratitis, *Ophthalmology* 92:1471, 1985.

100. Moore MB et al: Radical keratoneuritis as a presenting sign in *Acanthamoeba* keratitis, *Ophthalmology* 93:1310, 1986.

101. Moore MB et al: *Acanthamoeba* keratitis: a growing problem in hard and soft contact lens wearers, *Ophthalmology* 94:1654, 1987.

102. Florakis GJ et al: Elevated epithelial lines in *Acanthamoeba* keratitis, *Arch Ophthalmol* 106:1202, 1988.

103. Seal D, Stapleton F, Dart J: Possible environmental sources of *Acanthamoeba* sp. in contact lens wearers, *Br J Ophthalmol* 76:424, 1992.

104. John T, Desai D, Sahm D: Adherence of *Acanthamoeba castellanii* cysts and trophozoites to unworn soft contact lenses, *Am J Ophthalmol* 108:658, 1989.

105. van Klink F et al: The role of contact lenses, trauma, and Langerhans cells in a Chinese hamster model of *Acanthamoeba* keratitis, *Invest Ophthalmol Vis Sci* 34:1937, 1993.

106. Larkin DFP, Kilvington S, Easty DL: Contamination of contact lens storage cases by *Acanthamoeba* and bacteria, *Br J Ophthalmol* 74:133, 1990.

107. Larkin DFP, Easty DL: External eye flora as a nutrient source for *Acanthamoeba*, *Graefes Arch Clin Exp Ophthalmol* 228:458, 1990.

108. Sharma S, Srinivasan M, George C: *Acanthamoeba* keratitis in non-contact lens wearers, *Arch Ophthalmol* 108:676, 1990.

109. Parrish CM, Head WS, O'Day DM: *Acanthamoeba* keratitis following keratoplasty without other identifiable risk factors, *Arch Ophthalmol* 109:471, 1991.

110. Stopak SS et al: Growth of *Acanthamoeba* on human corneal epithelial cells and keratocytes in vitro, *Invest Ophthalmol Vis Sci* 32:354, 1991.

111. He Y et al: In vivo and in vitro collagenolytic activity of *Acanthamoeba castellanii*, *Invest Ophthalmol Vis Sci* 31:2235, 1990.

112. Auran JD, Starr MB, Jakobiec FA: *Acanthamoeba* keratitis: a review of the literature, *Cornea* 6:2, 1987.

113. Feist RM, Sugar J, Tessler H: Radial keratoneuritis in *Pseudomonas* keratitis, *Arch Ophthalmol* 109:774, 1991.

114. Wright P, Warhurst D, Jones BR: *Acanthamoeba* keratitis successfully treated medically, *Br J Ophthalmol* 69:778, 1985.

115. Moore MB, McCulley JP: *Acanthamoeba* keratitis associated with contact lenses: six cases of successful management, *Br J Ophthalmol* 73:271, 1989.

116. Berger ST et al: Successful medical management of *Acanthamoeba* keratitis, *Am J Ophthalmol* 110:395, 1990.

117. Johns K, Head S, O'Day D: Corneal toxicity of propamidine, *Arch Ophthalmol* 106:68, 1988.

118. Ficker L et al: *Acanthamoeba* keratitis: resistance to medical therapy, *Eye* 4:835, 1990.

119. Ishibashi Y et al: Oral itraconazole and topical miconazole with debridement for *Acanthamoeba* keratitis, *Am J Ophthalmol* 109:121, 1990.

120. Driebe WT et al: *Acanthamoeba* keratitis: potential role for topical clotrimazole in combination chemotherapy, *Arch Ophthalmol* 106:1196, 1988.

121. Silvany RE, Dougherty JM, McCulley J: Effect of contact lens preservative on *Acanthamoeba*, *Ophthalmology* 98:854, 1991.

122. Burger RM, Franco RJ, Drlica K: Killing acanthamoebae with polyaminopropyl biguanide: quantitation and kinetics, *Antimicrob Agents Chemother* 38:886, 1994.

123. Elder MJ, Kilvington S, Dart JK: A clinicopathologic study of in vitro sensitivity testing and *Acanthamoeba* keratitis, *Invest Ophthalmol Vis Sci* 35:1059, 1994.

124. Varga JH et al: Combined treatment of *Acanthamoeba* keratitis with propamidine, neomycin and polyhexamethylene biguanide, *Am J Ophthalmol* 115:466, 1993.

125. Larkin DFP, Kilvington S, Dart JKG: Treatment of *Acanthamoeba* keratitis with polyhexamethylene biguanide, *Ophthalmology* 99:185, 1992.

126. Mathers WD et al: Immunopathology and electron microscopy of *Acanthamoeba* keratitis. Paper presented at Ocular Microbiology and Immunology Group, New Orleans, November, 1986.

127. Saunders PRP et al: Enhanced killing of *Acanthamoeba* cysts in vitro using dimethylsulfoxide, *Ophthalmology* 99:1197, 1992.

128. Samples JR et al: Management of *Acanthamoeba* keratitis possibly acquired from a hot tub, *Arch Ophthalmol* 105:707, 1984.

129. Binder PS: Cryotherapy for medically unresponsive *Acanthamoeba* keratitis, *Cornea* 8:106, 1989.

130. Meisler DM et al: Susceptibility of *Acanthamoeba* to cryotherapeutic method, *Arch Ophthalmol* 104:130, 1986.

131. Matoba AY et al: The effects of freezing and antibiotics on the viability of *Acanthamoeba* cysts, *Arch Ophthalmol* 107:439, 1989.

132. Holland EJ et al: Subepithelial infiltrates in *Acanthamoeba* keratitis, *Am J Ophthalmol* 112:414, 1991.

133. Silvany RE et al: The effect of currently available contact lens disinfection systems on *Acanthamoeba castellanii* and *Acanthamoeba polyphagia*, *Ophthalmology* 97:286, 1990.

134. Ludwig IH et al: Susceptibility of *Acanthamoeba* in soft contact lens disinfecting systems, *Invest Ophthalmol Vis Sci* 27:626, 1986.

135. Penley CA, Willis SW, Sickler SG: Comparative antimicrobial efficacy of soft and rigid gas permeable contact lens solutions against *Acanthamoeba*, *CLAO J* 15:257, 1989.

136. Brockman RJ et al: Survival of *Acanthamoeba* in contact lens rinse solutions, *Invest Ophthalmol Vis Sci* 28(suppl):370, 1987.

137. Cali A et al: Corneal microsporidioses: characterization and identification, *J Protozool* 38(suppl):215S, 1991.

138. Didier ED et al: Isolation and characterization of a new human microsporidial, *Encephalitozoon hellum* from three AIDS patients with keratoconjunctivitis, *J Infect Dis* 163:617, 1991.

139. Pinnolis M et al: Nosematosis of the cornea: case report, including electron microscopic studies, *Arch Ophthalmol* 99:1044, 1981.

140. Ashton N, Wirasinha P: Encephalitozoonosis (nosematosis) of the cornea, *Br J Ophthalmol* 57:669, 1973.

141. Davis RM et al: Corneal microsporidiosis: a case report including ultrastructural observations, *Ophthalmology* 97:953, 1990.

142. McCluskey PJ et al: Microsporidial keratoconjunctivitis in AIDS, *Eye* 7:80, 1993.

143. Schwartz DA et al: Pathologic features and immunofluorescent antibody demonstration of ocular microsporidiosis (*Encephalitozoon hellum*) in seven patients with acquired immunodeficiency syndrome, *Am J Ophthalmol* 115:285, 1993.

144. Yee RW et al: Resolution of microsporidial epithelial keratopathy in a patient with AIDS, *Ophthalmology* 98:196, 1991.

145. Ryan NJ et al: A new trichrome-blue stain for detection of microsporidial species in urine, stool, and nasopharyngeal specimens, *J Clin Microbiol* 31:3264, 1993.

146. van Gool T et al: Diagnosis of intestinal and disseminated microsporidial infections in patients with HIV by a new rapid fluorescence technique, *J Clin Pathol* 46:694, 1993.

147. Wilhelmus KR et al: Drug-induced corneal lipidosis during AIDS: a condition simulating microsporidial keratoconjunctivitis, *Invest Ophthalmol Vis Sci* 35:255, 1994.

148. Diesenhouse MC et al: Treatment of microsporidial keratoconjunctivitis with topical fumagillin, *Am J Ophthalmol* 115:293, 1993.

149. Asmuth DM et al: Clinical features of microsporidiosis in patients with AIDS, *Clin Infect Dis* 18:819, 1994.

150. Duke-Elder S, Leigh AG: *System of ophthalmology*, vol VIII, *Diseases of the outer eye*, St Louis, 1965, Mosby–Year Book.

151. Roizenblatt J: Interstitial keratitis caused by American (mucocutaneous) leishmaniasis, *Am J Ophthalmol* 87:175, 1979.

152. Joyeux C, Sedan J, Esmenard J: Ocular filariasis: conjunctival lesions in a case of onchocerciasis, *Ann d'Ocul* 173:100, 1936.

153. Garner A: Pathology of ocular onchocerciasis: human and experimental, *Trans R Soc Trop Med Hyg* 70:374, 1976.

154. Von Noorden GK, Buck AA: Ocular onchocerciasis: an ophthalmologic and epidemiologic study in an African village, *Arch Ophthalmol* 80:26, 1968.

155. Duke-Elder S, Leigh AG: *System of ophthalmology,* vol VIII, *Diseases of the outer eye,* St Louis, 1965, Mosby–Year Book.

156. O'Day J, Mackenzie CD: Ocular onchocerciasis: diagnosis and current clinical approaches, *Trop Doct* 15:87, 1985.

157. Chakravarti B et al: Infiltration of CD4+ T cells into cornea during development of *Onchocerca volvulus*-induced experimental sclerosing keratitis in mice, *Cell Immunol* 159:306, 1994.

158. Greene BM et al: A comparison of 6-, 12-, and 24-monthly dosing with ivermectin for treatment of onchocerciasis, *J Infect Dis* 163:376, 1991.

159. Dadzie KY et al: Ocular findings in a double-blind study of ivermectin versus diethylcarbamazine versus placebo in the treatment of onchocerciasis, *Br J Ophthalmol* 71:78, 1987.

160. Taylor HR et al: Treatment of onchocerciasis: the ocular effects of ivermectin and diethylcarbamazine, *Arch Ophthalmol* 104:863, 1986.

161. Rothova A et al: Ocular involvement in patients with onchocerciasis after repeated treatment with ivermectin, *Am J Ophthalmol* 110:6, 1990.

162. Whitworth JA et al: Effects of repeated doses of ivermectin on ocular onchocerciasis: community-based trial in Sierra Leone, *Lancet* 338:1100, 1991.

163. Neame H: Parenchymatous keratitis in trypanosomiasis in cattle and in dogs and in man, *Br J Ophthalmol* 11:209, 1927.

164. Scott JG: Eye changes in trypanosomiasis, *J Trop Med Hyg* 47:15, 1944.

165. Moore MB: *Parasitic infections.* In Kaufman HE et al, editors: *The cornea,* New York, 1988, Churchill Livingstone.

166. Duke-Elder S, Leigh AG: *System of ophthalmology,* vol VIII, *Diseases of the outer eye,* St Louis, 1965, Mosby–Year Book, Inc.

167. Newman PE et al: Fly larva adherent to corneal endothelium, *Am J Ophthalmol* 102:211, 1986.

168. Laborde RP, Kaufman HE, Beyer WB: Intracorneal ophthalmomyiasis, *Arch Ophthalmol* 106:880, 1988.

169. Perry HD, Donnenfeld ED, Font RI: Intracorneal ophthalmomyiasis, *Am J Ophthalmol* 109:741, 1990.

Twelve

Viral Diseases

HERPES SIMPLEX

The Virus

Herpes simplex virus (HSV) is a member of the family Herpesviridae, which also includes cytomegalovirus, varicella-zoster virus (VZV; chickenpox), and Epstein-Barr virus (EBV). All members of this virus group appear morphologically identical by electron microscopy. They are composed of a central double-stranded DNA core and a protein capsid with 162 hollow, cylindric capsomers (Table 12-1). This nucleocapsid is surrounded by an envelope of phospholipoprotein derived from the cytoplasmic membrane of the host cell. The envelope contains viral glycoproteins that project from the surface. The glycoproteins and the capsid proteins

Table 12-1   Properties of Herpes Simplex and Varicella-Zoster Virus

Property	Herpes Simplex	Varicella-Zoster
Morphology		
Core	DNA	DNA
Capsid	Icosahedron; 162 hollow cylindric capsomers	Same
Envelope	Glycoprotein, lipid, carbohydrate	Same
Size	Core 75 μm	Same
	Capsid 90–100 μm	
	Enveloped particle 130–180 μm	
Inclusion body	Intranuclear, eosinophilic Cowdry type A	Same
Antigenic types	Type 1: labial herpes	One type only
	Type 2: genital herpes	
Tissue tropism	Pantropic but prefers epithelium and nervous tissue	Pantropic but prefers epidermis, dermis, and nervous tissue
Animal hosts	Most animals susceptible	Humans only
Tissue culture	Grows on a variety of cells	More fastidious; difficult to culture
Behavior in culture	Particles released into medium; produces diffuse CPE*	Extension occurs by direct passage between contiguous cells; CPE focal and slowly developing
Primary attack	Usually in childhood	Usually in childhood
	Stomatitis or keratoconjunctivitis	Varicella
	Often inapparent	Rarely inapparent
Latency	Sensory ganglia, most commonly gasserian and sacral, autonomic ganglia, and brain stem	Dorsal root and trigeminal ganglia
	Possibly ocular sites	
Ganglionic localization	Neurons	Satellite cells
Triggers for recurrences	Fever, stress, ultraviolet light, trauma, menstruation, others	Immunosuppression, radiation, infection, others

*Cytopathic effect.

induce specific antibody responses from the infected host.

Herpesviruses have the rare ability to cause latent infections: EBV and cytomegalovirus become latent in lymphocytes and secretory glands, herpes zoster in dorsal root and trigeminal ganglia, and HSV in sensory (most commonly trigeminal) or autonomic ganglia and the brain stem. After primary HSV infection at a peripheral site, the virus travels to the regional ganglia, where it can survive for decades in a relatively dormant state.[1] Under certain circumstances the state of infection is altered, and viral production and shedding occur. The virus travels down the nerve to the peripheral end organ and is released, where it can cause recurrent disease.

Types

There are two types of HSV: types 1 (HSV-1) and 2 (HSV-2). HSV-2 generally causes infection be-

low the waist, whereas HSV-1 causes infection above the waist. HSV-2 is recovered principally from the genitals but can also cause neonatal systemic infections, localized skin lesions, aseptic meningitis, and chronic neurologic disease; it may be related to the development of cervical cancer. In disseminated neonatal infection, ocular involvement occurs in about 10% of cases (see Chapter 7). Most cases of neonatal herpes keratitis and conjunctivitis are caused by HSV-2; however, HSV-1 can also cause neonatal keratitis.[2] In adults, approximately 85% of ocular isolates are HSV-1.[3] HSV-2 corneal disease tends to be more severe.[3-5]

Viral Replication

The virus interacts with specific receptors on the surface of human cells (adsorption) and then enters the cell by pinocytosis (penetration). The DNA is released into the cell (uncoating) and travels to the nucleus, where it induces production of both host- and virus-specific enzymes, such as thymidine kinase and DNA polymerase. Viral proteins are synthesized in the cytoplasm and transported to the nucleus, where assembly of nucleocapsids takes place. Viral glycoproteins also become inserted into the host cell membrane. The nucleocapsids bud through the nuclear membrane and are released from the cell. Cowdry type A eosinophilic intranuclear inclusion bodies are thought to be viral particles being assembled in the nucleus of an infected cell.

Primary Infection

Primary infection with HSV-1 most often affects the body surface innervated by the trigeminal ganglion. Viral replication occurs first in mucocutaneous tissues. The cells must have an appropriate HSV receptor molecule on their surface. The receptor has not been identified, but there is evidence that it is structurally related to heparan sulfate, which is commonly present in cell membranes. Productive infection in the mucocutaneous cells leads to cell lysis with release of progeny viruses and infection of contiguous cells.

Invasion of sensory nerve endings occurs soon after infection. Once internalized, the viral nucleocapsids are transported along the axon to the cell nucleus. Productive infection or establishment of latency can result. In productive infection, viral replication occurs in the nucleus of the neuron. Viral nucleocapsid progeny are released into the cytoplasm and enveloped in a transport vesicle. The enveloped virus can be transported along the axon to the nerve endings, where the virus particles are released, probably by fusion of the transport vesicles with the plasma membrane. Further infection of the mucocutaneous tissue can then occur.

Virus can also be released in the ganglion nerve root to infect astrocytes, oligodendroglial cells, and other neurons. It is unclear whether neurons are damaged or destroyed by productive infection, as are other cell types.

Immunization develops after the primary infection. Immunoglobulins are created that are directed against many herpesvirus antigens.

Latency and Reactivation

Infection of some neurons results in a persistent latent infection. The factors that determine whether infection leads to latency or production infection are unknown. Latency can only occur in certain cell types, and it occurs in only a few of those cells. It appears that latency is usually established soon after the initial infection, without prior viral replication. The absence of HSV tegument protein Vmw 65, which stimulates transcription of HSV genes during viral replication, results in the establishment of latent infection.[6] No viral antigen can be detected in the cell membranes during latent infection, so an immune response is not elicited.

The site of latency for production of oral and corneal disease continues to be debated, but it is now clearly established that at least one site of latency is the trigeminal ganglion. Using sensitive detection methods, latent infection with HSV had been demonstrated in 50% to 65% of human trigeminal ganglia obtained at autopsy.[1,7] Only between 0.1% and 3% of neurons in the trigeminal ganglia are latently infected with HSV-1.[8] Studies using newer techniques suggest that the actual numbers may be up to three times greater.[9] Latency has also been shown to occur in autonomic ganglia in humans and, in mice, in the brain stem.

The mechanism by which the virus maintains latency and how this is altered to cause recurrent disease is slowly becoming elucidated. HSV does not lie dormant but actively produces viral RNA, latency-associated transcript (LAT), during latent infection.[10,11] LAT is the antisense copy of RNA that codes for a protein produced early in lytic infection (ICP0). The role of LAT is unclear: it is not necessary for latency, but its absence impairs viral reactivation.[12]

Evidence suggests that latent infection can occur at ocular sites, such as in endothelial cells or keratocytes.[13-15] In human, rabbit, and mice corneas, HSV-1 has been recovered by cocultivation, and HSV DNA and RNA have been detected by in situ hybridization, polymerase chain reaction (PCR), or dot blot techniques.[16-18] LATs have been detected in corneal cells in some studies[19,20] but not in others.[16] Regulation of the LAT promoter is similar in corneal and neuronal cells and is different from that seen in nonneuronal cells.[21]

It is unclear whether mouth or nasopharyngeal primary infection can result in recurrent ocular disease, or whether patients with ocular disease were all inoculated in the conjunctiva at the time of primary infection. At least in mice, latency can be established without clinical ocular disease after introduction of a droplet containing virus to the eye. Conversely, it is possible that oral infection alone can result in ocular disease. The virus can spread from oral to ocular neurons within the ganglion and set up latency there. This has been shown in mice and rabbits: Productive viral infection has been demonstrated in neurons within ganglia, with the release of virions capable of infecting other neurons, and virus can be found in the eye after inoculation of the snout.[22-24]

Infection of a ganglion by one HSV strain does not prevent future infection of that ganglion by another strain, at least in mice.[25] Clinically, in most people a single viral strain is responsible for each disease recurrence, but it appears that a patient can rarely harbor two or more different viruses, either of which can cause recurrent disease at the same location.[26,27] It is also possible that a person can harbor multiple strains of virus at different neurologic sites (e.g., HSV-1 causing labial disease and HSV-2 causing genital disease).

A wide variety of stimuli have been found to be able to stimulate recurrence, including febrile illnesses, stress, menstruation, trauma, sunlight, and heat. In general, immune status does not appear to play a significant role in herpetic reactivation or in the severity of herpetic disease when it does occur. However, severe immunodeficiency can worsen the disease, and high doses of cyclophosphamide can stimulate reactivation.[28] Strain variations among HSV also appear to affect reactivation: Certain strains are associated with higher recurrence rates.[29]

It appears that viral shedding usually occurs without resultant clinical disease. Spontaneous asymptomatic shedding has been demonstrated in animal models and in one human study.[30] The virus can even be recovered from the tears of patients with no known history of herpes keratitis.[31] What causes viral replication in host peripheral tissue, and subsequent clinical disease, is unclear. It may depend on the condition of the epithelium or on local immunologic status; however, it is clear that recurrent clinical disease occurs despite systemic humoral and cell-mediated immunity against the virus. Serum antibody titers do not change with recurrent infections.

Virus and Host Factors

Genetic differences among strains appear to affect the manifestations of infection. The pattern of dendritic epithelial ulceration varies among different strains; each strain produces characteristically shaped ulcers.[32,33] Certain strains are more likely to produce stromal disease, and this is correlated with the amount of glycoprotein D they produce during infection[34,35] and the amount of thymidine kinase activity.[36] In addition, whether or not corticosteroids worsen the course of epithelial infection is strain-related.[37]

Host response to the virus certainly plays a role in the disease process, but the relative importance of viral replication and its by-products (and the host response to them) remain to be elucidated. Most stromal disease appears to be largely immunologic in that intact virus usually cannot be isolated from the stroma or found on electron microscopy.[38] The host response may be elicited by viral antigens that remain after epithelial infection or by viral proteins (but not intact virions) produced by persistent viral DNA (e.g., in keratocytes).[39] Cell-mediated immunity is thought to be primarily responsible for disciform keratitis and antigen-antibody-complement to be responsible for interstitial keratitis, immune rings, and limbal vasculitis;[40] but the evidence is not very strong. Live virus appears to be present more often in necrotizing stromal keratitis, but host immune response also plays a large role.

The role of individual host differences in determining the course of infection appears to be relatively limited. For unknown reasons, herpetic infection does appear to be more frequent in patients with atopic disease.

Epidemiology

Humans are the only natural reservoir of HSV, although experimental infection can be produced in rabbits, mice, primates, and other animals. In the United States, 70% of the population has been infected with HSV by 15 to 25 years of age, and 97% has been infected by 60 years of age, as demonstrated by serum-neutralizing antibody titers.[41] The initial infection is subclinical in 85% to 99% of cases,[42] but these patients all become carriers. Approximately 1% of primary infections will lead to a severe acute systemic illness.[43] Approximately one third of the world's population is affected by recurrent herpes labialis or dermatitis.

Herpes simplex infection is the most common cause of corneal blindness in developed countries. Herpetic keratitis affects approximately 0.5 to 1.5 per 1000 population.[44,45] Both eyes are involved in approximately 12% of patients.[46-48] The rate of recurrence depends on the length of follow-up and varies between 24% and 71% in different series.[44,49,50] In one 30-year study, the recurrence rates were 10% at 1 year, 23% at 2 years, and 63% at 20 years.[46] The time between recurrences is quite variable, ranging from a few weeks to decades. In one study of 141 patients, the median time between episodes was 1.5 years.[49] Approximately one in six patients with herpetic keratitis will have a marked reduction in vision, usually after multiple episodes over 3 to 15 years.[51,52]

Primary Ocular Herpes

Systemic infection with HSV-1 usually occurs within the first few years of life, but cases can

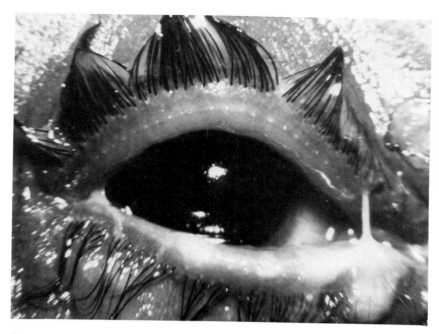

Figure 12-1
Blepharoconjunctivitis of primary herpes simplex.

develop at any age. Young children are typically infected by salivary contamination from an adult with labial herpes; the characteristic clinical disease is an aphthous stomatitis. This primary infection is often unrecognized or entirely subclinical, but it can be severe. Primary infection outside the oral cavity is less common, but it can occur in other mucous membranes (e.g., conjunctiva or skin).

The incubation period is 3 to 12 days. The most common manifestation of primary HSV ocular infection is an acute conjunctivitis with lymphadenopathy, which are usually unilateral, and malaise (Fig. 12-1). The mild cases are follicular in nature; more severe cases are pseudomembranous (50%). Dendrites can occasionally be seen on the bulbar conjunctiva. Keratitis accompanies the conjunctivitis in one third to one half of cases, and there may also be vesicular or ulcerative skin lesions (75%). Corneal involvement usually follows the onset of skin lesions and conjunctivitis by 1 to 2 weeks and can be seen as diffuse superficial punctate keratitis (SPK), focal epithelial lesions, microdendrites, dendrites, or serpiginous ulcers. The skin eruption is similar to that arising elsewhere in the body, with edema and redness followed by vesicles or ulceration (Fig. 12-2). The number and location of vesicles vary, and confusion with herpes zoster can occur. The lesions can be limited to the lid margin, making it appear similar to staphylococcal and *Moraxella* ulcerative blepharitis (Fig. 12-3).

Conjunctivitis usually persists for about 2 weeks, but keratitis can last longer. Preauricular adenopathy, subepithelial scarring, fever, and gastroenteritis can also be seen. Stromal keratitis rarely occurs. A severe vesicular eruption, often referred to as *Kaposi's varicelliform eruption,* can occur and is often seen in patients who have an accompanying immune disease (e.g., atopy). Progression to generalized infection or encephalitis occurs rarely. Involvement of the lacrimal canaliculi can result in permanent strictures and epiphora.

Diagnosis
The diagnosis can be based on history, clinical appearance, cytologic characteristics, virus isolation, and serologic findings. A history of exposure to a parent or relative with labial herpes and a lack of previous herpetic disease are helpful. The clinical appearance can be highly suggestive: A young child with acute follicular or pseudomembranous conjunctivitis probably has primary herpetic disease. However, such a picture can be difficult to differentiate from epidemic keratoconjunctivitis, vaccinia, chlamydia, or zoster. The diagnosis is more likely if vesicles appear on the lids (Fig. 12-2), but vaccinia, herpes zoster, chickenpox, and bacterial blepharitis (*Staphylococcus* or *Moraxella*) also

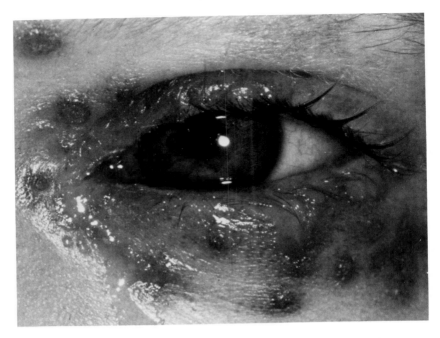

Figure 12-2
Lid vesicles in primary herpes simplex.

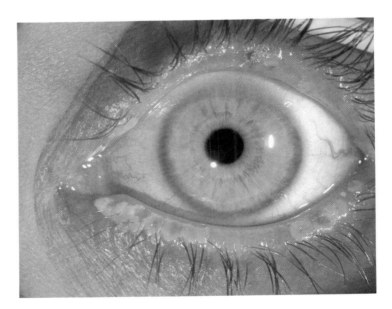

Figure 12-3
Ulcerative blepharitis caused by primary herpes simplex infection.

should be considered. Laboratory methods of diagnosis are discussed in the next section.

Treatment

Primary blepharoconjunctivitis will resolve without treatment. Although it has not been demonstrated, antiviral medication may shorten the course or decrease the risk of corneal complications. Therefore, an antiviral agent should be applied to the eye and skin two to four times a day until the conjunctivitis and skin lesions resolve. Treatment of keratitis is the same as in recurrent disease: debridement and antiviral agents. The child may have to be

Table 12-2 Recurrent Herpes Simplex Type 1		
Characteristics	**Dendritic Keratitis**	**Herpes Labialis**
Latency	Gasserian ganglion	Gasserian ganglion
Trigger mechanisms	Fever most important; also sunburn, stress, menstruation, trauma, depression of cellular immunity by drugs, etc.	Fever most important; also sunburn, stress, menstruation, depression of cellular immunity by drugs, etc.
Premonitory symptoms	Foreign body sensation	Tingling and itching
Number of lesions	Varies from 1 to 10	Varies; often only 1
Intervals between recurrences	Vary with trigger mechanisms, especially with frequency of upper respiratory disease	Vary with trigger mechanisms, especially with frequency of upper respiratory disease
Subepithelial involvement	Varies from none to scar formation	No scarring
Secondary infection	Rare in immunocompetent individuals	Not seen in immunocompetent individuals *Note:* Skin vesicles on face may be superinfected with *Staphylococcus aureus*
Duration (untreated)	50% or more heal within a week; remainder in 2 to 3 weeks	2 days to 3 weeks; average, 9 to 10 days
Disease in patients (immunosuppressed by kidney transplantation, Wiskott-Aldrich syndrome, etc.)	May have severe, chronic stromal disease, keratouveitis, secondary fungal or bacterial infection, perforation	May have deep cutaneous ulceration, dissemination to skin and viscera
Sensitivity	Corneal sensitivity is reduced	Skin area may be sensitive

restrained or anesthetized for debridement, which should be performed gently to prevent injury to Bowman's layer. Cycloplegia may be indicated for symptomatic relief.

Recurrent Herpes

A general classification of recurrent herpes simplex infection with ocular involvement follows:

I. Vesicular eruption of the lids
II. Follicular conjunctivitis
III. Cornea
   A. Epithelial keratitis: active viral replication
      1. Dendritic
      2. Geographic (ameboid)
      3. Marginal (limbal)
   B. Indolent and trophic ulceration (postinfectious herpes): epithelial and stromal ulceration with or without active stromal inflammation
   C. Stromal keratitis
      1. Disciform keratitis
      2. Necrotizing, ulcerative keratitis
      3. Interstitial keratitis
      4. Stromal scarring
   D. Sclerokeratitis
   E. Endotheliitis
   F. Iridocorneal endothelial syndrome
IV. Uveitis
      1. Endotheliitis
      2. Iritis
      3. Multifocal choroiditis

Recurrent lesions generally are localized, superficial, and self-limited (labial fever blister or cold sore) (Table 12-2). Visual loss generally occurs from the cumulative effect of multiple recurrences, with each attack producing additional scarring, vascularization, and thinning. Severe necrotizing stromal disease, interstitial keratitis, or uveitis can occur at any point, with more devastating consequences.

Blepharitis

Eyelid herpes is an uncommon form of recurrent disease. It may appear as isolated vesicles or as a group of vesicles, which can be mistaken for herpes zoster. As in primary disease, ulcerative blepharitis can occur, and herpes simplex should be considered in the differential diagnosis of this condition.[53]

Conjunctivitis

Rarely, recurrent conjunctival herpes can occur without corneal lesions or with only SPK or subepithelial keratitis. The conjunctiva exhibits a moderate to severe papillary and follicular re-

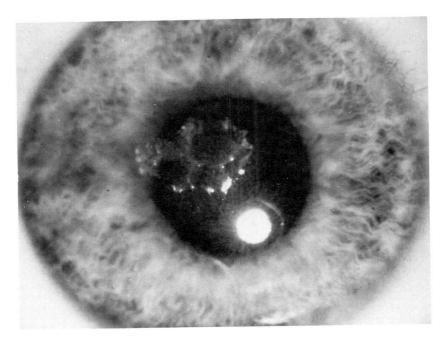

Figure 12-4
Typical dendritic keratitis of herpes simplex.

action and sometimes ulceration. The clinical features can be indistinguishable from those of adenovirus infection.[43,54]

Recurrent Epithelial Infection (Dendritic Keratitis)

Recurrent corneal epithelial disease usually occurs without accompanying conjunctivitis or lid lesions. The infection can appear as SPK, stellate epithelial lesions, dendritic ulcers, or geographic ulcers. The epithelial infection begins as fine punctate lesions that increase in size and later form white plaques of opaque epithelial cells 1 to 2 mm in diameter.[55] There can be a tendency toward palisading of epithelial cells at the periphery of each plaque. These plaques enlarge and develop into an easily recognized dendrite (Figs. 12-4 and 12-5). More than one dendrite can develop. As a dendrite grows, the central epithelium is lost; the peripheral, infected cells stain with rose bengal, and the central area devoid of epithelium stains with fluorescein. The dendritic keratitis can occur at any location on the cornea, but recurrences tend to affect the same area as previous attacks. Stromal infiltration can develop beneath the epithelial lesion. A mild iritis can be present, but keratic precipitates usually do not form.

The epithelial infection usually heals spon-taneously in 5 to 12 days, but it can progress, particularly if topical steroids are administered, to form a geographic (also called *ameboid*) ulcer (Fig. 12-6) or spread to the stroma (3%). Like dendritic ulcers, the geographic ulcers have a margin of opaque, heaped-up cells, which stain with rose bengal. The edges may have a dendritic shape. With time, increasing stromal infiltration and anterior chamber reaction can develop. These ulcers tend to heal slowly, and epithelial ulceration can persist despite resolution of the active viral infection. When this happens the ulcers are called *metaherpetic*, and these are discussed in the next section. During early episodes the loss of corneal sensation is usually confined to the area of the lesion, but with repeated recurrences more generalized anesthesia occurs.

Peripheral, nondendritic herpetic lesions can occur and can resemble staphylococcal marginal keratitis[56] (Fig. 12-7). These lesions tend to respond more slowly to treatment than more central infections and are predisposed to chronic trophic ulceration.[57] Fascicular ulcers resembling a fascicular phlyctenule also can occur (Fig. 12-8). These usually can be differentiated from phlyctenules by their association with dendritic scars and decreased corneal sensation.

In most cases healing occurs with little or no

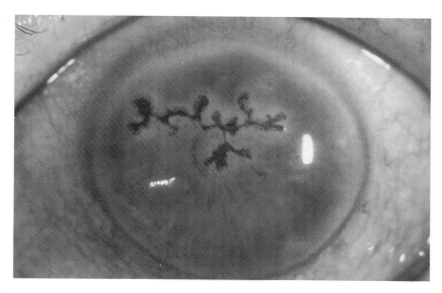

Figure 12-5
Herpes simplex dendrite stained with rose bengal. (Courtesy of Diane Curtin, Pittsburgh, PA.)

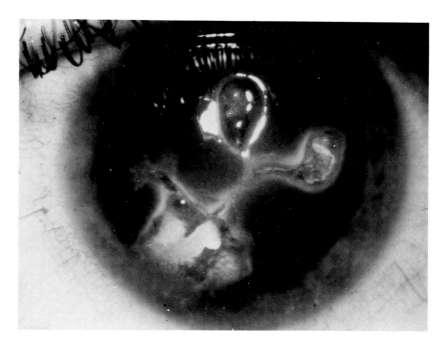

Figure 12-6
Large ameboid dendritic ulcer.

residual scarring. After more severe infections or after multiple attacks, however, superficial stromal scarring, loss of stroma, and vascularization occur. Patients with AIDS are more likely to have peripheral ulcers, have more frequent recurrences, and take longer to heal.[58] The median healing time was 3 weeks in one study.[58]

Postinfectious (Metaherpetic) Ulcers

Sometimes epithelial defects persist or recur after viral epithelial and subepithelial disease. The ulcers can be dendritic, round, or oval, with sinuous or scalloped borders.[59] The edges of the ulcer are gray, appear rolled in, and do not stain with rose bengal.

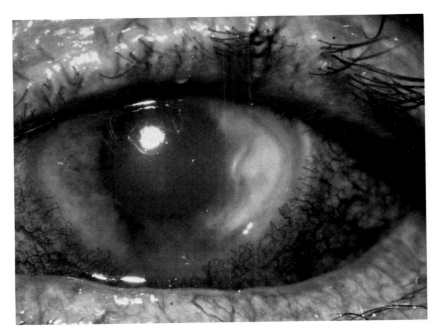

Figure 12-7
Atypical marginal ulcer resulting from herpes simplex virus type 2.

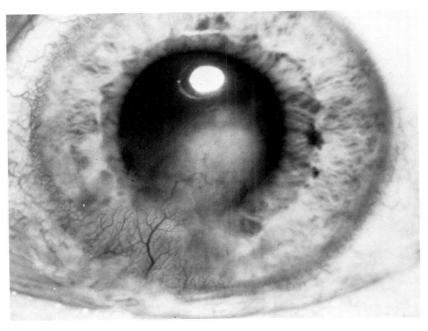

Figure 12-8
Fascicular type of ulcer caused by herpes simplex, resembling a phlyctenular lesion.

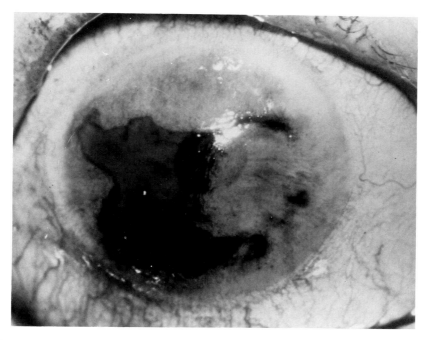

Figure 12-9
Postinfectious herpetic ulcer. The large base stains with rose bengal red. The edges are rolled and heaped up.

By definition, virus cannot be cultured from these lesions. The corneal epithelium fails to cover the defect because of damage to its basement membrane, ongoing stromal inflammation, and the lack of trophic innervation.[60] The edges of the defect consist of piled-up epithelial cells that have failed to cover the ulcer base. The base of this lesion stains with rose bengal red (Fig. 12-9) and fluorescein, in contrast to the active dendritic lesion, in which the base stains only with fluorescein.

It should be noted that live virus can remain in the cornea for a long time. It can be difficult in some cases to distinguish between a recurring erosion or an active viral disease. In these doubtful instances it is advisable to take a viral culture or scraping of the lesion for fluorescent-antibody studies.

Stromal Disease

The patterns of stromal involvement in herpetic keratitis are manifold. Edema, infiltration, vascularization, ulceration, endothelial inflammation, and uveitis can all occur, and their relative contributions vary considerably. However, it is possible to distinguish several common patterns, which can aid in making the diagnosis, guiding treatment, and estimating prognosis. If the stromal reaction is predominantly edema, with mild infiltration and uveitis, it is called *disciform edema;* if infiltration and necrosis dominate, *necrotizing stromal keratitis;* if there is infiltration, edema, and vascularization without ulceration, *interstitial keratitis;* if endothelial inflammation and destruction occur in relative isolation, *endotheliitis;* and if the uveitis is most pronounced, with mild stromal edema, infiltration, or vascularization, *keratouveitis.*

Superficial Stromal Scarring. Residual opacities may be seen in the superficial stroma after epithelial infection, most commonly "ghost" dendrites and small punctate granular lesions. The dendritic opacities are seen as areas of mild subepithelial edema, cellular infiltration, or scarring underlying the site of an epithelial dendrite. Peculiar whitish-yellow subepithelial flecks that appear greasy or granular are frequently seen after herpetic keratitis; the pathogenesis of these particles is uncertain.

Disciform Keratitis. Disciform keratitis is characterized by stromal edema with some cellular infiltration in a circular or oval pattern beneath a dendritic lesion or under intact epithelium. It can occur as a diffuse edematous keratitis (Figs. 12-10 and 12-11) or as an off-visual axis patch of disease. The patient reports photophobia, tearing, mild pain, and if central cornea is involved, reduced vision. There may be a history of previous herpetic disease. Disciform keratitis

can appear as early as 5 to 10 days after the onset of a dendrite. The edema can involve the full thickness of the cornea or may just involve the area beneath the epithelium. Descemet's membrane is often wrinkled, and some degree of uveitis is usually present, especially with

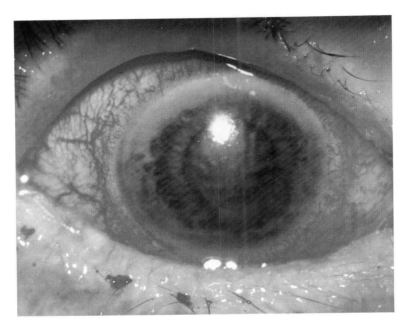

Figure 12-10
Disciform keratitis.

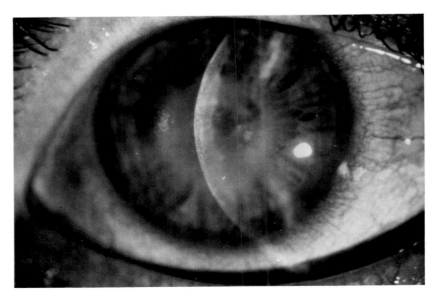

Figure 12-11
Corneal swelling in disciform keratitis as seen with slit-lamp microscope beam. (Courtesy of Diane Curtin, Pittsburgh, PA.)

more severe corneal involvement. The endothelial cells under the disciform area are edematous and can give the appearance of guttae. Fine keratic precipitates may be present posterior to the affected stroma.

Disciform keratitis can heal without complications or can progress to an interstitial keratitis or necrotizing keratitis, with deep scarring.[57,61] Benign cases run a course of several months and heal with minimal scarring. In more severe cases, immune rings, late corneal thinning, scar formation, and neovascularization can occur. Complications of the uveitis, particularly secondary glaucoma, can be seen.[42,62]

The pathogenesis of herpetic disciform keratitis is not known. The disciform lesion may represent an immunologic reaction to herpetic antigen. Cell-mediated immunity is thought to be primarily responsible,[63] but antigen-antibody complexes may also be involved. The antigen may soak into the stroma during epithelial infection or may be produced in the stroma by viral DNA latent in keratocytes or other cells.[39,64] Alternatively, small amounts of live virus may be present, coming from epithelial infection, stromal nerves, or being produced in situ. Others have proposed that the main inflammatory reaction takes place in the endothelium; this reaction may be primarily immunologic or caused by active viral infection.[65-68]

Similar disciform keratitis can be seen with herpes zoster ophthalmicus, vaccinia, mumps, varicella, infectious mononucleosis, *Acanthamoeba*, chemical keratitis (e.g., anesthetic abuse), and corneal trauma (see Chapter 9).

Necrotizing Keratitis. These complicated cases of viral keratitis usually occur in patients who have had previous attacks of herpetic keratitis. In contrast to disciform keratitis, stromal infiltration and necrosis are predominant. In mild cases the infiltrates can be localized and lamellar. In severe cases a stromal abscess can develop, consisting of necrotic cheesy-white infiltration that can occupy the entire thickness of the cornea (Fig. 12-12). The epithelium can be intact, exhibit dendritic ulceration, or break down over stromal infiltration. Edema, ulceration, and vascularization often develop. A ring infiltrate can be seen occasionally surrounding the area of stromal disease (Fig. 12-13). Uveitis is nearly always present and can be severe, with retrocorneal membrane, hypopyon, synechiae formation, secondary cataract, and glaucoma. These cases can be indistinguishable from bacterial, fungal, or *Acanthamoeba* infection.

Severe complications can occur in stromal herpetic keratitis. The stroma can perforate as

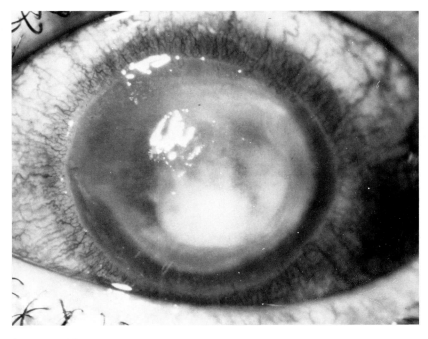

Figure 12-12
Necrotic stromal herpes.

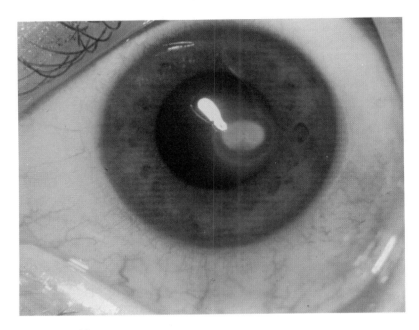

Figure 12-13
Immune ring infiltrate in stromal herpes.

a result of the disease or because of improper treatment. Superinfections with fungi or bacteria can occur.

Necrotizing stromal keratitis is most likely caused by direct viral infection of stroma and a subsequent host immune response. Virus has been observed in pathologic specimens[69] and has been isolated from some of these corneas.[38,66,70] In one study, 20 of 22 keratectomy specimens from patients with ulcerative necrotizing disease displayed HSV antigens versus 4 of 36 specimens from patients with nonulcerative nonnecrotizing keratitis.[71] The relative importance of viral infection and the host's immune response in producing the clinical manifestations, especially the corneal destruction, is not known.

Interstitial Keratitis. The term *interstitial keratitis* is used when infiltration, vascularization, and occasionally necrosis occur beneath intact stroma and epithelium. Single or multiple patches of dense infiltration can form and progress to necrosis and vascularization. They tend to be chronic and indolent, persisting for many months. These cases may result from live virus or from viral proteins produced in the stroma or released from corneal nerves, or as an immunologic response to antigens that have diffused into the stroma after epithelial infection. Herpes is currently one of the most common causes of interstitial keratitis.

Sclerokeratitis
The sclera can become involved when there is peripheral interstitial or ulcerative keratitis. There is often scleral thinning and a great deal of pain, and treatment can be difficult.

Keratouveitis
Herpetic uveitis can be mild and incidental, compared to the corneal disease, or severe and a major source of complications. Disciform keratitis tends to be associated with mild anterior chamber reaction, and necrotizing keratitis with a moderate to severe reaction. A common picture is one of diffuse keratitis with stomal haze, edema, deep and superficial vascularization, and multiple keratic precipitates. In more severe forms, anterior chamber hemorrhage and hypopyon can result (Fig. 12-14). Ovoid sectoral iris atrophy can be seen.

In at least some of these cases, live virus is present in the anterior chamber and possibly in the iris and endothelium as well. HSV has been obtained from the aqueous humor in some cases[62,68,72] and identified histologically in others.[66,73] HSV can infect the superior cervical ganglion of the sympathetic chain, and release of virus from sympathetic nerves in the anterior

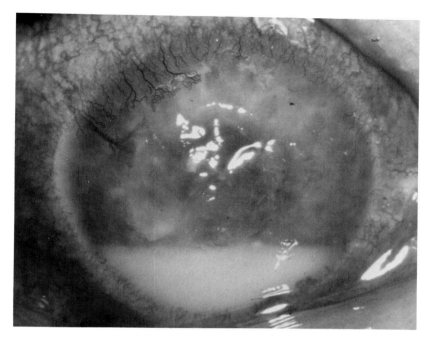

Figure 12-14
Severe herpetic keratouveitis with hypopyon.

segment can result in recurrent keratouveitis. However, in many cases live virus is not present, and the reaction is immunologic. Sundmacher and Neumann-Haefelin[68] found that two types of patients are likely to have live virus in the aqueous: those with serous focal iritis with heavy keratic precipitation and elevated intraocular pressure and those with endotheliitis and elevated pressure. Therefore, these patients are more likely to benefit from antiviral therapy in addition to steroids.

Endotheliitis
In some cases endothelial dysfunction develops peripherally and progresses centrally across the cornea, as in endothelial rejection of a corneal graft.[74,75] In other cases plaques of endothelial inflammation and destruction can be seen.[76] These processes appear to involve active viral replication in the endothelium,[68,74] although subsequent immunologic reaction may also play a role. Some cases develop after epithelial disease.[76]

Iridocorneal Endothelial Syndrome
Herpes simplex viral DNA was present in the endothelium of 16 of 25 specimens from patients with the iridocorneal endothelial syndrome.[77] Herpes infection appears to play a role

in the development of this condition (see Chapter 18).

Diagnosis
The diagnosis of herpes simplex keratitis often can be made clinically. The dendritic epithelial lesions are pathognomonic. A history of recurrent disease, decreased corneal sensation, involvement of multiple corneal layers, and disciform keratitis are all suggestive of herpes simplex.

Cytologic examination typically reveals a mononuclear exudate. Multinucleated giant epithelial cells, typically containing from 2 to 10 nuclei (Fig. 12-15), may be seen in smears of epithelial scrapings and are fairly specific (also seen in varicella and zoster).[78] Intranuclear eosinophilic inclusion bodies, best seen with Papanicolaou stain, are helpful but infrequently found. Viral particles can sometimes be demonstrated with electron microscopy.

Although viral isolation in human cell culture is being performed more often and can provide a definitive diagnosis, it is still unavailable to many and is relatively expensive. Growth is usually observed in 2 to 4 days but can take several weeks. Rose bengal stain should not be applied before obtaining a specimen because it can kill the virus.[79]

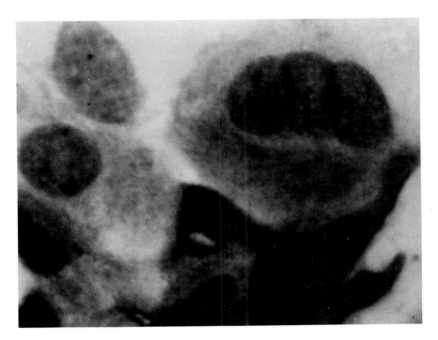

Figure 12-15
Multinucleated epithelial cells seen in scraping of herpes simplex keratitis.

Viral antigens can be detected in specimens fairly rapidly using immunologic tests. Many types are available, including immunofluorescent,[80] immunoperoxidase, enzyme-linked immunosorbent assay (ELISA),[81] and immunofiltration methods.[82] The ELISA and immunofiltration methods appear to be most accurate.[83] Affinity membrane tests have been described, whereby a membrane is touched to the cornea, and viral antigen adherent to the membrane is detected with labeled antibody.[84,85] These tests appear to be simple and sensitive, but more experience is required to assess their usefulness.

Some molecular biology techniques have been used to design potentially more sensitive diagnostic tests. Labeled herpes simplex DNA probes are used to detect viral DNA or RNA in specimens. PCR appears to be as or more sensitive than culture and enzyme immunoassay.[86-88]

Serologic testing may be useful in diagnosing primary infection. A sample should be obtained early in the disease and again after 4 to 6 weeks to document rising titers.

Treatment
Antiherpetic Drugs
Despite the prevalence of viral disease, the availability of antiviral agents has lagged behind that of other microbial agents. The virus usually lies within human cells and utilizes many of the normal human enzymes for repro-

duction. Even after development of specific immunity to HSV, the virus persists in a relatively inaccessible site—central neural tissue—and in a relatively quiescent state.

Drugs marketed for use in herpetic keratitis use inhibition of viral genome synthesis; but in the laboratory, potential agents that act by other mechanisms have been identified. Currently available antiviral agents are listed in Table 12-3.

Idoxuridine. Idoxuridine (IDU), a pyrimidine analog similar to thymidine, was the first clinically effective agent to be approved by the Food and Drug Administration (FDA).[89] It inhibits thymidine kinase, thymidylate kinase, and DNA polymerase and is incorporated into the viral DNA, thus producing a faulty DNA chain. IDU can also affect normal corneal epithelial cells, which also take up the drug[90,91]; however, human thymidine kinase does not use IDU as efficiently as viral thymidine kinase, accounting for the relative selectivity of the agent.

Idoxuridine is useful for epithelial infection[92-95] but not for herpetic uveitis or deep stromal disease. Epithelial keratitis resolves within 10 days with IDU treatment in about 55% to 70% of cases.[96] IDU is relatively unstable, penetrates the stroma poorly, and is quickly metabolized into an inactive form. Resistance to IDU may be encountered.

Table 12-3 Antiviral Agents					
Agent	**Mechanism of Action**	**Administration**	**Topical Penetration**	**Viral Resistance**	**Toxicity**
Idoxuridine (IDU)	Pyrimidine analog Inhibits thymidine kinase, thymidylate kinase, and DNA polymerase Incorporated into viral DNA	Drop 0.1% Ointment 0.5%	Poor	+	+++
Vidarabine (Ara-A)	Pyrimidine analog Inhibits synthesis of viral DNA, mechanism unknown	Ointment 3% Intravenous		Less than IDU	++
Trifluorothymidine	Pyrimidine analog Inhibits thymidylate synthetase Incorporated into viral DNA	Drop 1%	Good	Rare	++
Acyclovir	Purine analog Activated by viral thymidine kinase Inhibits DNA polymerase	Ointment 3% Intravenous Oral	Good	+	+

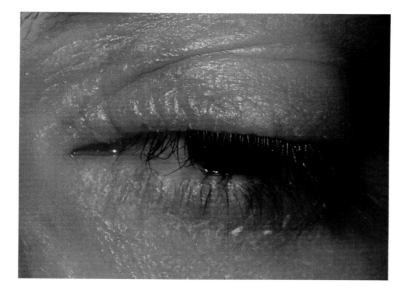

Figure 12-16
Contact dermatitis caused by prolonged use of idoxuridine in treatment of herpes simplex keratitis. (From Wilson FM II: *Surv Ophthalmol* 24:57, 1979.)

Idoxuridine can be toxic in repeated and long-term topical application and is even more toxic in patients with dry eye.[97] In addition, it is topically sensitizing and can cause contact dermatitis (Fig. 12-16). In early toxicity the patient complains of burning or stinging on administration, and a diffuse punctate keratitis is seen. With continued administration, epithelial opacification and irregularity (Fig. 12-17), chronic epithelial defects, subepithelial infiltration, stromal ulceration, narrowing or obliteration of the lacrimal puncta (Fig. 12-18), fol-

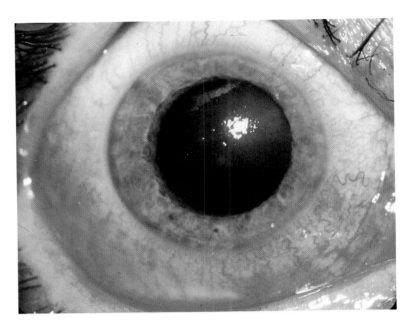

Figure 12-17
Epithelial keratopathy and injection of the inferior conjunctiva in a toxic reaction to idoxuridine used to treat herpes simplex keratitis. (From Wilson FM II: *Surv Ophthalmol* 24:57, 1979.)

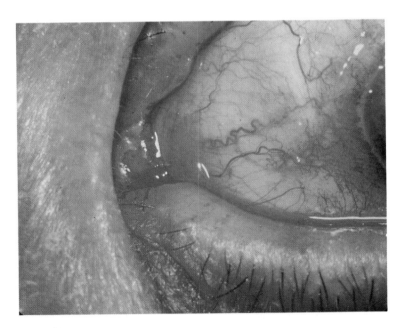

Figure 12-18
Toxic follicular reaction and punctal occlusion secondary to idoxuridine. (From Wilson FM II: *Surv Ophthalmol* 24:57, 1979.)

licular conjunctivitis,[98] cicatricial conjunctivitis, or corneal pannus can develop. Experimentally, IDU inhibits keratocyte mitosis, corneal stromal repair,[99] and epithelial healing,[90] and teratogenicity has been reported in pregnant rabbits.[98] Use of IDU has largely been supplanted by newer agents that require less frequent administration and exhibit less toxicity and better penetration.

Vidarabine (Adenine Arabinoside). Adenine arabinoside (Ara-A) also inhibits synthesis of viral DNA, but the precise mechanism has not been determined. Ara-A is rapidly metabolized to arabinoside hypoxanthine, which, although it is more soluble and enters the stroma and aqueous, has only 20% of the antiviral activity of Ara-A. As a result of its insolubility, Ara-A must be given in ointment form. Ara-A is effective against IDU-resistant strains,[100,101] but Ara-A–resistant strains also exist. Ara-A is as effective as IDU[96,102] and trifluorothymidine (trifluridine; F_3T)[103] in the treatment of epithelial herpes, equal to IDU for stromal disease, but ineffective topically for herpes uveitis. Ara-A is generally better tolerated than IDU, but it can cause similar toxicity, particularly punctate keratopathy,[97,104] and can elicit hypersensitivity reactions. Ara-A impairs stromal healing, comparable with IDU, but was not teratogenic to rabbits in one study.[105] Overall, Ara-A is as effective as IDU in treating epithelial disease and can be used as an alternative in patients unable to use F_3T because of toxicity or allergy.

Trifluridine (Trifluorothymidine). Trifluridine is a halogenated pyrimidine that inhibits thymidylate synthetase and is incorporated into viral DNA, impairing transcription and translation of the viral genome. F_3T is twice as potent and 10 times more soluble than IDU in a 1% solution,[99] which greatly increases its ocular penetration. In the treatment of epithelial disease, F_3T appears to be more effective than IDU[106,107] and about as effective as Ara-A,[103,108] although it appears to be more effective than Ara-A in healing steroid-treated ulcers.[109] F_3T is effective in some IDU- and Ara-A–resistant cases,[106,107,110] and resistance to F_3T is rare. Although as yet unproven, it may be of value for both deep stromal disease and uveitis because therapeutic levels of the drug can be obtained in the iris and anterior chamber.[111]

Toxicity can occur with the use of F_3T drops, especially with more prolonged use (longer than 2 weeks).[97,112] Early signs of toxicity are punctate epithelial erosions and epithelial microcysts. Other complications include filaments, epithelial edema, stromal edema, punctal narrowing, and contact dermatitis. F_3T also tends to impair stromal wound healing. Overall, the toxicity of F_3T appears to be slightly less than that of IDU.

Trifluridine is currently the drug of choice in the United States for topical treatment of ocular herpes. It is equal to or greater than other agents in effectiveness, resistance is rare, and penetration is good. Although acyclovir is of equal or superior value and is widely used in Europe, it is not available in the United States because its superiority to other agents has not been documented sufficiently for FDA approval.

Acyclovir. Acyclovir is an acyclic purine nucleoside analog with highly potent and specific activity against HSV-1 and -2. Noninfected human cells are not affected because viral thymidine kinase is required for activation of the drug (by phosphorylation). Once in its active triphosphate form, it inhibits DNA polymerase. After topical application it penetrates the cornea and reaches the aqueous.[113] It appears to be approximately equal to F_3T and Ara-A in the treatment of epithelial herpes.[114-117] Despite initial optimism, it does not prevent the development of secondary stromal disease.[118] In one study the recurrence rate in patients treated with acyclovir was significantly lower than that in IDU-treated patients.[48]

Acyclovir is less toxic to the ocular surface than are IDU, Ara-A, and F_3T. Experimentally, it has no significant detrimental effect on epithelial or stromal healing.[119] One of the drug's drawbacks is its greater potential for developing resistant strains. In vitro, many mutant herpetic strains have been found that do not produce thymidine kinase at all, or produce an altered thymidine kinase that does not phosphorylate the drug, and are thus resistant.[120] Development of resistance during treatment for keratouveitis has been reported.[121]

Systemic administration of acyclovir has been effective in the treatment of genital herpes simplex[122] and herpes zoster.[123] Use of oral acyclovir in ocular herpes has increased in recent years. It appears to be beneficial in cases in which live virus is suspected to be present in the cornea or anterior chamber, and possibly in reducing recurrence.[124,125] At a dose of 400 mg five times daily, aqueous and tear levels exceed the inhibitory dose$_{50}$ of HSV-1.[126] It is as effective as topical acyclovir for herpes simplex epithelial keratitis[127,128] and is useful in some cases of necrotizing stromal disease, endothelitis, and keratouveitis.[124,125] However, the addition of oral acyclovir to topical corticosteroid and F_3T treatment does not appear to improve the outcome of stromal keratitis.[129]

Oral acyclovir reduces the frequency of genital[130,131] and cutaneous[132] recurrences as long as the drug is continued, and some evidence suggests that it can also reduce ocular recurrences.[125,133] Long-term prophylactic oral acyclovir significantly reduced the recurrence of herpes keratitis and graft failure after penetrating keratoplasty for herpes simplex keratitis.[134]

In cases in which it is likely that virus is present in the anterior chamber—those with focal serous iritis, marked keratic precipitates, and increased pressure and those with endotheliitis—oral acyclovir would probably be effective.

Interferons. Human cells infected with a virus produce interferon, a substance that inhibits viral infection of other cells. A number of different interferons are produced by different cells, but all appear to exert their effect by inhibiting translation of viral genes. Interferons do have an effect on herpetic keratitis; they are less effective than available agents,[135,136] but they do appear to potentiate the effect of other antiviral agents.[137-140] Whether the increase in efficacy is sufficient to warrant the combination of drugs remains to be determined.

Other Agents. 5-[2-Bromovinyl]-2-deoxyuridine (BVDU), like acyclovir, is phosphorylated by viral thymidine kinase into the active form and is therefore relatively selective in its effect. More active against HSV-1 than HSV-2, it has been effective in clinical trials in the treatment of epithelial herpes.[141,142]

(S)-1-(3-hydroxy-2-phosphonylmethoxy-propyl)-cytosine (HPMPC; Cidofovir) is a broad-spectrum DNA polymerase inhibitor that is active against many DNA viruses in vitro. In rabbit models it has been found to be as effective as F_3T in the treatment of HSV-1 dendritic keratitis.[143] It also was effective against adenovirus type 5 in a rabbit model.[144] LAT analogs or other antisense nucleotides may be able to inhibit viral replication and suppress reactivation.

A variety of other agents has been found to be effective in treatment of herpetic keratitis in laboratory animals, including ribavirin and fluoro-deoxy-arabinofuranosyl-iosocytosine (FIAC), but these have not been tested in humans.

Corticosteroids

The use of corticosteroids in herpetic keratitis remains controversial; however, corticosteroids should be used judiciously in treating certain types of herpetic involvement of the cornea. In herpetic keratitis, corticosteroids will reduce the immune response, decreasing edema, infiltration, inflammation, and neovascularization. On the other hand, corticosteroids slow epithelial and stromal healing, enhance collagenolytic enzyme production, increase the risk of microbial superinfection, can induce glaucoma and cataract formation, decrease the host's elimination of viral antigens, and can exacerbate active viral infection. Corticosteroids do not appear to increase the risk of reactivation.[145] They are indicated in the treatment of herpetic diseases caused by the host's immunologic response, but not when there is active viral replication. Once corticosteroids are begun, it is often difficult to discontinue them; a rebound marked inflammatory response can occur.

Unfortunately, in many cases it is not possible to discern whether viral replication or host response is primarily responsible for the clinical disease. In general, corticosteroids are used for disciform keratitis and herpetic uveitis but not for epithelial disease. In two randomized, double-blind, placebo-controlled trials of corticosteroid treatment of stromal keratitis, corticosteroid treatment reduced the duration and severity of stromal inflammation but did not affect the visual outcome.[146,147] Postponing corticosteroid treatment for a few weeks delayed resolution of the stromal keratitis.

In necrotizing stromal keratitis, corticosteroids are sometimes helpful, but the response is unpredictable and caution is indicated. Whenever the epithelium is ulcerated, even if virus is not present, the risk of complications, particularly stromal melting and superinfection, is greater. The risk of complications also seems greater in children. In all cases, the minimum necessary dose should be used, and antiviral medication should be given concomitantly. More specific recommendations are given later.

Specific Treatment
Recurrent Epithelial Keratitis Without Stromal Involvement.
Debridement was the primary treatment for epithelial herpes for many years but has been relatively neglected since the development of antiviral agents. In fact, debridement may be equal or superior to antiviral treatment for epithelial herpes,[148] and the combination of debridement and antiviral treatment is more effective than antiviral treatment

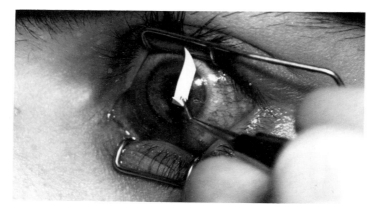

Figure 12-19
Filter paper debridement of herpes simplex virus epithelial keratitis. Dry cellulose acetate filter paper is gently applied to corneal surface.

alone. Reepithelialization may be faster and the incidence of "ghost images" may be lower. Use of a cotton-tipped applicator or cellulose acetate filter paper (Fig. 12-19)[149] is gentler and probably just as effective as scraping. To improve the chances for eliminating the virus, it is best to administer antiviral medication in addition to debridement (Table 12-4).

Trifluridine is administered nine times daily and is continued until at least 3 to 5 days after epithelial healing, for up to 2 weeks. (Antiviral treatment is continued after epithelial healing because of experimental data indicating that virus titers rebound to high levels if antiviral therapy is discontinued too early.[150,151]) One should always be on guard for toxic effects if the drug is continued for more than 2 weeks. Cycloplegia may increase comfort.

A very young child may need to be restrained before debridement is performed. If this is not possible, topical antiviral medication can be used alone or in combination with oral acyclovir.

Limbitis. Limbal inflammation or ulceration caused by HSV can be extremely recalcitrant to treatment. Artificial tears are probably as effective as any other therapy. Fortunately, limbitis tends to resolve spontaneously, over weeks to months, without much residual scarring. Antiviral agents may be useful and are recommended. Corticosteroids should be used only if the visual axis is involved or if symptoms are marked.

Disciform Keratitis. In a randomized, double-blind, placebo-controlled, multicenter clinical trial of corticosteroid treatment of stromal kera-

Table 12-4	Antiviral Treatment of Epithelial Disease[157, 160, 163]
Drug	**Dose**
Trifluridine drops 1% (Viroptic)	Nine times daily
Vidarabine ointment 3% (Vira-A)	Five times daily
Idoxuridine drops 0.1% (Stoxil, Herplex, Dendrid)	Every hour by day
Idoxuridine ointment 0.5% (Stoxil)	Five times daily
Acyclovir, oral (Zovirax)	400 mg five times daily*
Acyclovir ointment 3%†	Five times daily

*Approximate adult dose.
†Available from Burroughs Wellcome, 3030 Cornwallis Rd, Research Triangle Park, NC 27709.

titis, corticosteroid treatment reduced the duration and severity of stromal inflammation but did not affect the visual outcome.[146] Postponing corticosteroid treatment for a few weeks delayed resolution of the stromal keratitis. In another randomized study of the initial episode of disciform keratitis, the addition of topical corticosteroid to topical antiviral treatment significantly reduced the time to resolution but did not affect outcome or recurrence rate.[147] The addition of oral acyclovir does not appear to improve outcome.[129,152]

I use corticosteroids when vision is significantly reduced and in those rare cases when pain is marked. The minimum dose necessary to achieve the desired effect is the best course to follow. Once the keratitis has been treated with steroids, it is difficult to control the recurrent inflammation without again using steroids.[153] One must be certain that steroids are essential to treat the disease because the patient may become committed to steroid use for many months.

Precise guidelines cannot be given, but disciform keratitis tends to be very responsive to steroids, and very dilute doses are often sufficient. Initially, prednisolone acetate 0.125% to 1% can be used two to four times daily; once the desired effect is achieved the dose is gradually tapered. Doses as low as 0.005% daily or 0.125% weekly are often sufficient to prevent a resurgence of the disciform keratitis. It is possible either to increase the interval between drops, from daily to every 2 days up to weekly or to progressively dilute the steroid concentration. (This procedure can be performed by a pharmacist.)

Steroid use is more dangerous if an epithelial defect is present and, in most cases, should be avoided until healing occurs. If necessary, prednisone can be given orally (0.5 to 1.0 mg/kg/day). Cycloplegics are usually beneficial. Concurrent antiviral therapy is also indicated to lessen the risk should viral shedding or reinfection occur. One drop of antiviral medication is given for each steroid drop, up to four times per day.

Persistent Epithelial Defects. Persistent epithelial defects in patients with herpetic keratitis can occur for several reasons, and it is important to determine the exact cause. First, the existence of active viral infection due to antiviral resistance, recurrence, or poor compliance must be determined. Some clinical clues were discussed earlier. More commonly, failure of epithelial healing results from antiviral agent toxicity or persistent anterior stromal inflammation. Basement membrane and anterior stromal injury from repeated herpes attacks can impair the epithelium's ability to cover the corneal surface. Secondary microbial infection is another common cause. Viral, bacterial, and fungal cultures are often useful to rule out active infection. If active viral replication is not present, antiviral medication should be reduced or discontinued. If bacterial infection is not present, antibiotics that interfere with epithelial healing should also be discontinued. Other conditions that impair epithelial healing may be present: dry eye, lagophthalmos, decreased corneal sensation, lid malposition, or trichiasis.

Topical or oral corticosteroids may be helpful in reducing stromal inflammation, but careful monitoring is essential because of the potential for stromal melting. If the surrounding epithelium is hypertrophic or loose it should be removed. Lubricating agents, patching, or a bandage lens will aid reepithelialization. If these measures are not successful a temporary tarsorrhaphy or a conjunctival flap may be necessary.

Stromal Ulceration Without Infiltration. Stromal melting can occur in the presence of a persistent epithelial defect of any cause, even in the absence of active stromal infection. The possible causes and treatment are essentially the same as those discussed in the previous section. If progressive stromal loss is observed, corticosteroids should be avoided, and application of cyanoacrylate glue should be considered.

Stromal Ulceration With Infiltration (Necrotizing Stromal Keratitis). This is the most difficult form of herpes simplex keratitis to manage. Although it appears that active viral infection is present in some cases, the destructive process also can result most often from the host response in the absence of live virus. Viral culture is helpful, and samples should be taken to determine whether bacterial, fungal, or *Acanthamoeba* infection is present.

It is best to begin with antiviral treatment: drops five times daily or ointment three times daily. After several days, if virus is not isolated in culture, topical corticosteroids can be added cautiously to reduce inflammation, infiltration, and patient discomfort. Low doses should be used initially, and the patient must be seen frequently. Oral prednisone (approximately 0.5 to 1.0 mg/kg) is often preferable to topical corticosteroids until the epithelium is healed. If ulceration progresses while the patient is on topical steroids, these drugs should be withheld and oral prednisone administered instead. With progressive stromal loss, cyanoacrylate adhesive application, a conjunctival flap, or therapeutic keratoplasty may be necessary.

In a randomized, double-blind, placebo-controlled multicenter study of the treatment of herpetic stromal keratitis, the addition of oral acyclovir to topical corticosteroid and F_3T treatment affected neither time to resolution nor outcome.[129] I think that a trial of oral acyclovir is warranted when patients are unresponsive to topical antiviral drugs and when steroids are ineffective or contraindicated.

Interstitial Keratitis. If the epithelium is intact, topical corticosteroid use is less risky but should still be prescribed cautiously. Antiviral medication should be given concurrently (matched drop for drop up to four times daily). The treatment is essentially the same as for disciform keratitis, as discussed previously. When corticosteroids are administered, they should be reduced gradually. Cycloplegic agents and topical lubricants are often helpful. Oral acyclovir was not found to be beneficial in patients with stromal keratitis.

Endotheliitis. Virus has been recovered from the anterior chamber in several cases, suggesting that active infection is present. Paracentesis and culture of aqueous humor can be performed to make this determination. Topical F_3T and topical acyclovir have been shown to produce adequate aqueous levels, and they may be effective when used alone; however, I have had success using oral acyclovir in addition. Therefore, I recommend oral acyclovir (400 mg) and F_3T five times daily. Topical corticosteroid, such as 1% prednisolone acetate, can also be given if the epithelium is intact. Acyclovir must be tapered slowly, and prolonged therapy is required in some cases.

Uveitis. In some cases the major site of inflammation is the anterior chamber. Active viral infection is not present in most of these eyes, so corticosteroids are the main treatment. If there is keratitis with a minimal iritis with no hypopyon and no sign of endothelial decompensation, it is best to use a strong cycloplegic agent and antivirals without steroids. In more severe cases, topical corticosteroids are administered (with antiviral prophylaxis), provided the epithelium is intact. If ulceration is present or the response to drops is insufficient, oral corticosteroids are given. As the ulcer epithelializes and stromal inflammation and uveitis improve, use of the systemic steroids should be discontinued and topical steroids initiated, gradually tapering their application.

Oral acyclovir also can be effective, particularly in cases with marked anterior chamber reaction and elevated intraocular pressure, or if virus is isolated from the anterior chamber. If a patient is not responding to steroid and topical antiviral treatment, or if it is not possible to taper oral steroids without reactivation, oral acyclovir (400 mg four or five times a day) should be administered.

Prevention of Recurrence. No treatment can prevent latency or eliminate latent infection. Chronic administration of low doses of antiviral drops does not prevent recurrent ocular infection; however, early treatment of recurrences does seem to lessen the severity and duration of the attack. Thus, it is appropriate for patients to begin antiviral treatment as soon as they sense the onset of an attack. Many patients have prodromal symptoms or clear inciting events, such as fever, extreme stress, or menstruation, and treatment can be initiated at these times.

As was mentioned earlier, chronic administration of oral acyclovir has been clearly demonstrated to reduce the recurrence of genital and cutaneous herpes. There is increasing evidence suggesting that it is also effective for eye disease.[134,154]

Surgical Treatment

Conjunctival Flaps. Conjunctival flaps can provide a stable epithelial surface, stop ulceration, quiet inflammation, and provide comfort. They should be considered in eyes with persistent or recurrent epithelial defects, progressive ulceration, or marked inflammation unresponsive to therapy. They are particularly useful in chronic peripheral ulcers, where a partial flap can be placed without compromising vision.

Penetrating Keratoplasty. If chronic stromal herpes leads to a descemetocele or perforation, keratoplasty may be necessary. A penetrating graft rather than a lamellar graft should be performed, because the incidence of recurrence is much lower.[155,156] If possible, it is better to perform keratoplasty in a quiet eye because the success rate is higher.[157-159]

The extent of vascularization has been inversely related to graft success in some studies[157,158] but not in others.[159-161] The use of intensive postoperative steroid treatment appears to be beneficial.[157] Even in quiet eyes, however, recurrence of herpetic disease in the graft is common (Fig. 12-20), occurring in approximately 15% of eyes within 2 years.* In addition, there is a greater tendency for graft rejection and noninfectious epithelial defects. Oral acyclovir may reduce the risk of recurrence.[134,162]

Approximately 70% to 80% of grafts performed in quiet eyes are clear at 2 years, and 50% to 60% are clear at 5 years.[159,161] If graft failure occurs, the success rate for regrafts is about half that for the primary graft.

Oral corticosteroids are begun 1 to 2 days before keratoplasty, if possible, and are continued for approximately 2 weeks after surgery. Topical corticosteroids are begun the day after surgery and continued as long as necessary to control

---

*References 60a, 111a, 157, 158a, 160, 163.

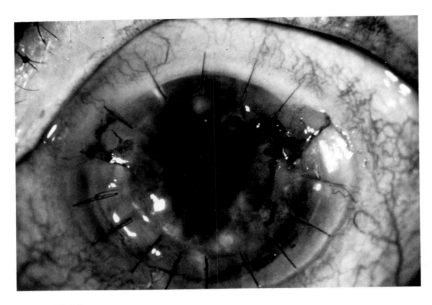

Figure 12-20
Recurrence of herpes simplex virus after penetrating keratoplasty.

inflammation. Topical antiviral prophylaxis does not appear to be beneficial, except during rejection episodes when HSV recurrence is common.[159,163] I use oral acyclovir (400 mg) four or five times daily for 14 days, then twice daily. How long this treatment should be continued is unclear, but effectiveness up to 1 year after surgery has been reported,[134] and indefinite treatment may be advantageous.

Epithelial recurrence is seen most commonly at the graft–host junction as nondendritic epithelial defects. Because it is impossible to differentiate clinically between noninfectious epithelial defects and herpetic recurrence, the index of suspicion must be high and cultures or immunologic testing should be performed. It is often difficult to differentiate between endothelial rejection and herpetic uveitis. If a typical rejection line is present, the diagnosis is clear; if not, the location of keratic precipitates (e.g., graft vs. recipient) is not very helpful. In most cases both corticosteroid and antiviral agents are given.

VARICELLA-ZOSTER

Varicella-Zoster Virus

Varicella-zoster virus is physically similar to the other herpesviruses: It has a DNA core, a protein coat, or capsid, and may have an envelope (Table 12-1). Like HSV, it replicates in the cell nucleus. Humans appear to be the only natural hosts of VZV. Until recently, no animal model of VZV infection was available, limiting research efforts; a guinea pig model of ocular infection has now been developed.[164] The virus can be cultivated in vitro in human cell lines. However, cytopathogenic effects are focal and slow to develop. Extension of individual lesions occurs by direct passage of virus to contiguous cells. Multinucleated giant cells form, and eosinophilic inclusions are seen in the nucleus and occasionally in the cytoplasm of infected cells.

The virus causes both varicella (chickenpox) and herpes zoster (shingles). The initial infection with VZV causes an acute exanthematous disease, chickenpox. The virus spreads from infected skin cells to the sensory nerve endings, with ascent to the ganglia. Acute inflammation is seen in the dorsal root ganglia, with hemorrhagic necrosis. Productive viral infection occurs in neurons and nonneuronal cells. In comparison with HSV-1, the neuron population is far less susceptible to viral-induced damage by VZV.[165]

The virus then becomes latent in the dorsal root ganglia of the spinal cord, or the trigeminal ganglia. VZV DNA and RNA has been detected in some trigeminal, sacral, and thoracic ganglia.[166,167] Latency appears to occur in the satellite cells of the spinal column, not in the neurons.[168] HSV-1 and VZV can be latent in the same trigeminal ganglion. Months to decades after initial infection, these patients can develop zoster by reactivation of endogenous latent virus. The nonneuronal site of latency in the ganglion may explain the clinical features of reactivation.[169,170] Productive replication of virus within the nonneuronal cells results in release of virus particles within the ganglion, with spread to adjacent neurons and nonneuronal cells. Large areas of the ganglion can be affected by inflammation and necrosis, resulting in widespread cutaneous disease in the affected dermatome and chronic neuropathy. Frequent reactivation may occur, but in most cases it is confined by host defenses. When the host is not able to contain the process, extensive multiplication occurs in the ganglion with spread of infection to many neurons. Infectious virus particles then travel down the sensory nerve and infect the skin.

Viral DNA has been found in human corneas up to 8 years after herpes zoster ophthalmicus (HZO).[171] The DNA was found in keratocytes, mononuclear cells, and epithelial cells. This suggests VZV persistence in a latent form in corneal tissue or reactivation of the virus from neural sites without dermal involvement.

Varicella
Epidemiology
Nearly everyone in the United States contracts varicella, usually before the age of 9 years. In less populous areas of the world (such as the tropics), infection is frequently delayed until adulthood. It is an epidemic disease and is highly contagious (80% to 90% of exposed susceptible individuals become infected). Transmission is through contact with respiratory secretions or cutaneous lesions. The incubation period ranges from 10 to 21 days (average, 14 to 17 days).

Clinical Manifestations
The most common initial site of infection is the respiratory mucosa. Replication then occurs in the regional lymph nodes, and viruses are released into the bloodstream. The onset of clinical disease is abrupt, with development of a generalized rash, fever, and malaise. The rash occurs in crops, which appear successively over 2 to 5 days, and follows a characteristic progression from macule to papule and vesicle, encrustation, and healing, usually without scarring. Complete recovery usually occurs in 1 to 2 weeks.

External ocular involvement occurs most commonly as a papillary conjunctivitis, but "pocks" (Fig. 12-21), dendritic keratitis, disciform keratitis, and interstitial keratitis have been reported.[172-174] Pocks can occur in the conjunctiva, appearing as vesicles with inflammatory cell infiltration and surrounding hyperemia and sometimes associated with focal ulceration or hemorrhage.[175] Localized corneal infiltrates, similar to phlyctenules, can also be seen. They usually occur at the time of systemic disease, when they most likely represent active viral infection, but they can also appear months later, possibly as an immunologic response to residual viral antigen. Both corneal and conjunctival lesions resolve spontaneously over 1 to 2 weeks, but the corneal lesions can cause scarring or vascularization (Fig. 12-22).

Punctate epithelial lesions can also occur during the acute systemic disease. Dendritic lesions have been reported several months after the systemic disease, sometimes occurring in eyes with disciform keratitis treated with topical steroids. The dendrites closely resemble zoster lesions.[175-177] The disciform keratitis appears similar to that seen with HSV or zoster.[177-180] It can develop weeks to months after the systemic disease, can last for more than a year, and can recur. The occurrence of dendrites and disciform disease long after the systemic disease suggests local recurrent live viral infection. This may be due to VZV persistence in a latent form in corneal tissue or recurrent viral shedding from neural sites without dermal involvement.

Treatment
The FDA has approved oral acyclovir treatment for cases of chickenpox in children 2 years of age or older. The recommended dose is 800 mg four times daily for 5 days. More prolonged treatment is indicated in immunosuppressed patients. Cool compresses, calamine lotion, and in severe cases oral hydroxyzine hydrochloride (25 mg two to three times daily) can relieve pruritus. Pocks or epithelial lesions may be treated with antiviral medications (e.g., F_3T 0.1% five times daily), although their efficacy has not been determined. Disciform keratitis will respond to corticosteroid treatment, but the same cautions apply as for HSV disciform disease.

Herpes Zoster
Epidemiology
Herpes zoster can occur at any age in anyone who has had varicella. The incidence increases with age: it is five times greater in individuals

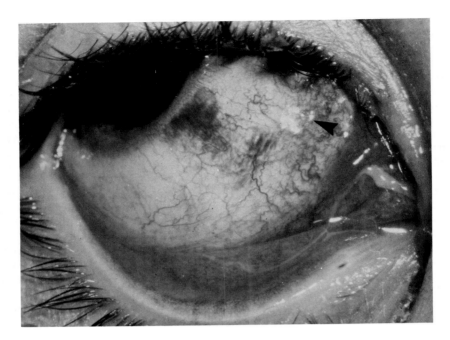

Figure 12-21
Varicella vesicle of conjunctiva (*arrow*).

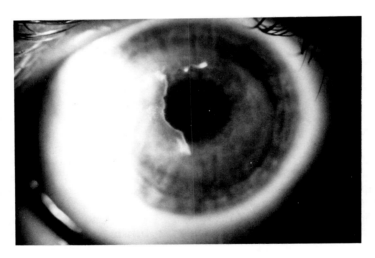

Figure 12-22
Corneal scarring after varicella keratitis. (Courtesy of Diane Curtin, Pittsburgh, PA.)

over 80 years of age than in adults between 20 and 40 years of age. At the other end of the spectrum, herpes zoster can occur in children several months of age.[181,182] Childhood development of zoster is much more likely if the mother has varicella during pregnancy or the child is infected during the first 2 months of life.[183,184] This phenomenon appears to be related to the infant's reduced immunologic reactivity during the primary attack and reduced immunologic memory against the virus. A varicella virus vaccine is now available, and its use may markedly reduce the incidence of herpes zoster in the future.

An increase in the incidence and severity of zoster is seen in patients with impaired immunity, such as those with lymphoma or other malignancies, with AIDS,[185-187] or on immunosuppressive therapy.[188] In most patients, however, no malignancy or immunologic defect can be found.[189,190] Approximately 2% of nonimmunosuppressed patients will develop a second episode of zoster.

Pathogenesis

Herpes zoster seems to be caused by a reactivation of the latent VZV in the dorsal root ganglion or trigeminal ganglion. After reactivation the virus spreads peripherally from the ganglion along the sensory nerve to the skin. The skin eruption is limited to the dermatomes corresponding to the involved sensory ganglion.

In addition to immunosuppression, radiation, syphilis, tuberculosis, malaria, carbon monoxide or arsenic poisoning, and trauma have been implicated in precipitating zoster.[174] Cases also can develop in patients who are exposed to someone with varicella or zoster.[174,191] Neutralizing antibody is present in the serum, but it apparently does not protect against the development of zoster. However, reduction of neutralizing antibody titer below a certain threshold may allow reactivation of the latent virus, and a progressive decrease in titers may occur with age.

Herpes zoster is unusual because ocular disease may become manifest many months after the resolution of the initial illness, with no sign of activity during the interim. For reasons not yet determined, disciform keratitis, iritis, or scleritis often appears 3 to 4 months after the cutaneous eruption, sometimes with minimal early ocular involvement.

The cutaneous lesions of zoster are histopathologically identical to those of varicella. The virus replicates in the strata germinativum and spinosum. Pain may be caused by degeneration of small cutaneous nerve bundles and scarring of the segmental nerve and ganglion. Vasculitis is prominent, with granulomatous or diffusely lymphocytic infiltration.[192,193] Lymphocytic infiltration of nerves (particularly the long ciliary nerve), patchy necrosis of the iris and ciliary body, scleritis, and a granulomatous reaction to Descemet's membrane can also be seen.

Clinical Manifestations

The area supplied by the trigeminal nerve is second only to the thoracic region in frequency of involvement. The first division of the fifth cranial nerve is affected 20 times more than the second and third divisions. When the disease involves the first division of the fifth nerve, it is known as HZO and is of special importance because of the danger to the eye.

The first symptom of herpes zoster is pain, which is accompanied by hyperesthesia of the skin within the distribution of one or more dermatomes. At the onset, a slight elevation of temperature might occur with some evidence of meningeal irritation. A blushing of the skin develops, sometimes simultaneous with the pain, but usually 3 to 4 days later, followed by the appearance of papules that quickly become vesicles. After a few days the clear fluid within the vesicles becomes turbid and yellow; in a short time the vesicles burst and crusts form (Fig. 12-23). If secondary infection does not develop, the crusts disappear rapidly, often leaving white scars in the area. The entire cycle usually takes 3 to 6 weeks. Rarely, infection occurs without development of the typical skin lesions.[194-196]

The most distressing symptom is pain; occasionally it is mild, with a feeling of tingling and numbness, but usually it is throbbing and burning. The pain generally subsides with healing of the eruption but may persist for years. Postherpetic neuralgia (6 months or longer) occurs in less than 4% of patients under 20 years of age, in 30% of patients over 60 years of age, and in 71% of patients 80 years of age and over.[197] The pain may develop several months after the onset of HZO and tends to diminish gradually with time, but in approximately one fourth of cases it persists for more than a year.[198]

In HZO the frontal nerve is involved most often, especially its medial branches (supratrochlear and supraorbital). Hutchinson's rule—that involvement of the eye is likely if the side of the tip of the nose is involved—is essentially true, but there are some exceptions. Eye involvement also occurs in many patients who do not have Hutchinson's sign. A few lesions can develop outside the involved dermatome, past the midline, or even in a remote area of the body, but this usually does not indicate dissemination. The disease is rarely bilateral.[199]

Dissemination of the rash occurs most frequently in debilitated patients, particularly those with lymphomas. Encephalitis and pneumonia (primary varicella pneumonia) are two of the more serious complications that can occur, but even in immunocompromised patients disseminated zoster is rarely fatal.

Ocular Complications

Ocular complications occur in about 50% of cases of HZO, appearing at any time during the eruptive phase or weeks to months after the rash has subsided.[198,200]

Upper Lid. The upper lid generally is affected because of frontal nerve branch involvement. Marked edema of the upper lids with vesicle

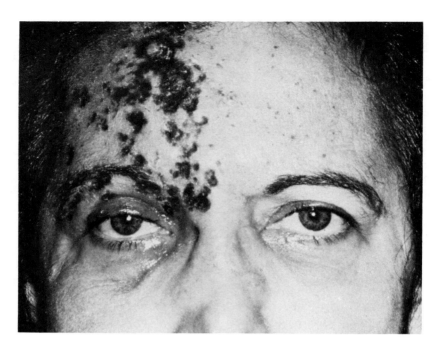

Figure 12-23
Herpes zoster dermatitis with typical lesions along the distribution of the frontal nerve.

formation usually occurs. Lesions on the lid skin most often disappear with little or no scarring, but if scarring occurs, lagophthalmos, entropion, or ectropion of the upper lid may result. Necrosis of the lid and forehead can be seen in the most severe cases. Secondary infection, usually with *Staphylococcus aureus,* streptococci, or canaliculitis, can also develop.

Conjunctiva and Sclera. The conjunctiva is injected, edematous, and may exhibit petechial hemorrhages. Conjunctivitis is usually papillary, but a follicular or membranous form may develop. Occasionally vesicular lesions occur on the palpebral or bulbar conjunctiva and can cause scarring.

Both episcleritis and scleritis can occur. Episcleritis is common, usually develops early, and can last for months.[198] Scleritis may be seen immediately after the skin lesions have waned or 1 to 3 months later.[201] It can be nodular or diffuse and is frequently recurrent. Sclerokeratitis, with peripheral corneal edema, infiltration, and vascularization, may also be seen.

Cornea. Corneal complications occur in approximately 40% of cases of HZO and can take many forms. The most common findings are dendrites and punctate keratitis.[202] The dendritiform figures (Fig. 12-24) are not excavated, but

rather are made up of swollen, heaped-up cells, and have a gray, plaquelike appearance[203-204a] (Table 12-5). The dendrites of zoster stain irregularly with fluorescein but well with rose bengal. Like simplex dendrites, these figures contain live virus. The dendrites are seen most often during the acute disease (4 to 6 days) but can appear many weeks afterward, particularly in patients using topical steroids.[205] They resolve without treatment within 1 month.

Punctate keratitis is seen as multiple, peripheral, focal, raised lesions that stain with rose bengal. These lesions probably contain live virus and may resolve or progress to dendrite formation. Both punctate and dendritic lesions can lead to anterior stromal infiltrates.[202,206] They usually occur 10 days after the onset of the rash and last only a few weeks. They resolve without treatment and appear to respond to topical steroids, but relapse can occur, even as late as 2 years after the onset of the disease.

Disciform keratitis, similar in appearance to that seen in VZV and SV, can occur after HZO (Fig. 12-25). It typically develops 3 to 4 months after the acute disease but can occur at 1 month or after years. The epithelium may not have been involved during the acute attack. Ring infiltrates and necrotizing interstitial keratitis can also occur and are clinically identical to those seen in herpes simplex keratitis. Marginal cor-

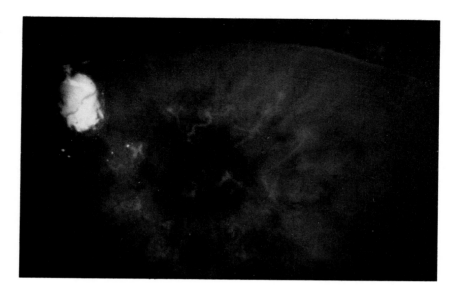

Figure 12-24
Multiple fine dendrites due to herpes zoster. (Courtesy of Massimo Busin, Bonn, Germany.)

neal ulceration can mimic Mooren's ulcer.[207] Corneal vascularization, edema, and scarring are common (Fig. 12-26). The pathogenesis of stromal disease in zoster is presumed to be immunologic, but it is possible that live or latent virus is present. VZV DNA was found in the cornea of a patient with disciform keratitis.[208]

Decreased corneal sensation occurs in approximately 50% of patients, in one third to one half of whom it becomes permanent.[198,202] The complications of neurotrophic keratitis are a major cause of the ocular morbidity of this disease: recurrent epithelial breakdown, persistent epithelial defects, sterile ulceration, vascularization, perforation (Fig. 12-27), and superinfection.

Mucus plaques are seen commonly in zoster keratitis and are often confused with viral dendrites. These plaques are gray, elevated, and linear or branching in shape, and stain well with rose bengal (Fig. 12-28).[204,209] They are usually seen 3 to 4 months after the cutaneous disease and change day to day. They lie over degenerating epithelium and stromal inflammation. Corneal sensation is usually decreased. They can be removed from the surface with gentle scraping, which can be useful in differentiating them from true dendrites.

Iris. Uveitis is seen frequently in HZO; it occurs in most eyes with corneal disease but can be seen in isolation. It usually occurs during the initial attack but can occur months later. The uveitis is most often mild and transient; however, in a considerable number of cases, a severe anterior iridocyclitis develops, which tends to recur. Secondary glaucoma is particularly common.

Single or multiple patches of sectorial iris pigment epithelial loss and atrophy can be seen as a result of an obliterative vasculitis.[210] In extreme cases, anterior segment ischemia and necrosis may develop.[211]

Other Ocular Complications. Herpes zoster rarely affects the retina, but retinal vasculitis, hemorrhagic chorioretinitis, acute retinal necrosis, and nonrhegmatogenous detachments can be seen. Optic neuritis may appear as a retrobulbar neuritis,[212] papillitis, or neuroretinitis. Pupillary abnormalities and cranial nerve palsies also can occur.[213]

Diagnosis

Herpes zoster can usually be diagnosed on clinical grounds, although skin lesions in some cases of herpes simplex can be similar. Laboratory confirmation can be obtained in a number of ways: Vesicular fluid or corneal lesions can be examined with Giemsa or Papanicolaou stain for multinucleated giant epithelial cells and intranuclear eosinophilic inclusion bodies; electron microscopy can demonstrate the virus; and immunologic tests can indicate the presence of VZV antigens.[214] Cultures from early ocular or cutaneous lesions can be inoculated in

Table 12-5 Differentiation of Herpes Zoster and Herpes Simplex Dendrites

Properties	Herpes Zoster Dendrite	Herpes Simplex Dendrite
Appearance	Medusoid "Painted-on" appearance, like plaque heaped on cornea Coarse, swollen epithelial cells reaching in different directions, either from a central focal point or in an elongated branching figure	Delicate, fine, lacy Denuded ulcer
Terminal bulbs	None	May or may not be seen
Staining	Stains poorly with fluorescein	Edges stain with rose bengal red dye; ulcer base stains well with fluorescein, which diffuses into surrounding diseased epithelium
Response to steroid drops	Good	Made worse
Dermatologic findings and distribution	Grouped vesicles with erythematous base; may occur in crops	Grouped vesicles with erythematous base; may occur in crops May be very similar to zoster; therefore what appears to be typical shingles caused by herpes zoster may be caused by simplex virus
	Always in dermatomal distribution	May be in dermatomal distribution, but usually is not
Healing	Heals usually in 2–3 weeks and lasts 5–6 weeks	May heal in 7–10 days, but may persist for 3 weeks
Symptoms	Prodrome of pain and tingling paresthesias or pruritus in two thirds of cases	May have pain and paresthesias
Age incidence	Peak: over 60 years; may occur in children also	1–15 years and 35–50 years
Inflammation	Less in histologic examination	More in skin lesions in pathologic examination
Recurrence	Rare; never in same distribution	Common

human tissue culture. The virus is recoverable only in the early lesions, usually during the first 48 to 72 hours. When ocular disease becomes manifest months after the skin eruption, the diagnosis must be presumptive, based on the history, skin scarring (if present), and consistent clinical picture.

Systemic work-up for malignancy or immunodeficiency disease is generally not indicated; however, a thorough history and review of systems is worthwhile. Herpes zoster is a common presenting manifestation of AIDS, and it is important to question younger patients about their sexual preference, intravenous drug use, or possible exposure by other means and to obtain tests for HIV serum antibodies.[185,186] Medical evaluation is also indicated in patients with cutaneous dissemination or recurrent disease.

Treatment

General. In vitro, VZV is susceptible in IDU, Ara-A, Ara-C, acyclovir, and BVDU; each has been used clinically with some success.[89,123,215-218] Of these, BVDU and acyclovir appear to be the most effective and least toxic.

High doses of oral acyclovir (600 mg five times per day for 10 days) were found to speed resolution of skin lesions, reduce viral shedding, and decrease the incidence of dendritic keratitis, stromal keratitis, and anterior uve-

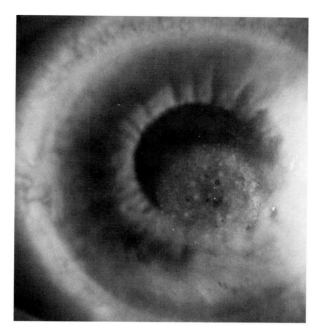

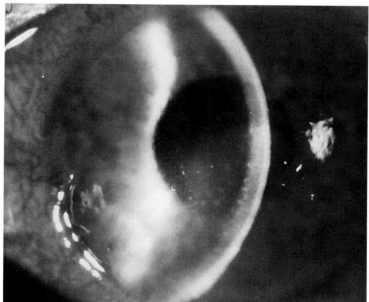

Figure 12-25
Disciform keratitis after herpes zoster. (Courtesy of Diane Curtin, Pittsburgh, PA.)

itis.[123] In this study, treatment was initiated within 7 days of disease onset; when treatment was begun within 72 hours of onset the results were even more marked. There did not appear to be any effect on the incidence or severity of postherpetic neuralgia. The drug was well tolerated. More recently, this group recommended a dose of 800 mg five times daily, and this is now approved by the FDA. Another prospective randomized study comparing oral with topical acyclovir found that institution of oral acyclovir within 3 days of onset of the skin rash significantly reduced ocular complications,[219] while one retrospective study did not observe a

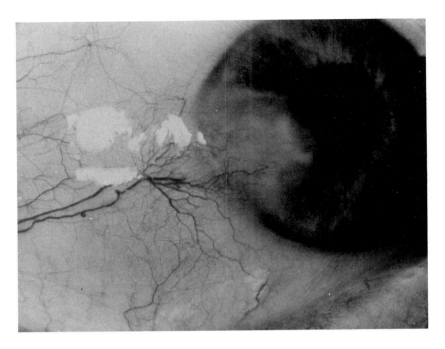

Figure 12-26
Residual scarring after herpes zoster keratitis.

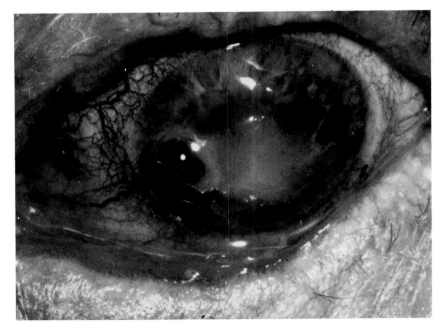

Figure 12-27
Corneal perforation in a case of herpes zoster ophthalmicus.

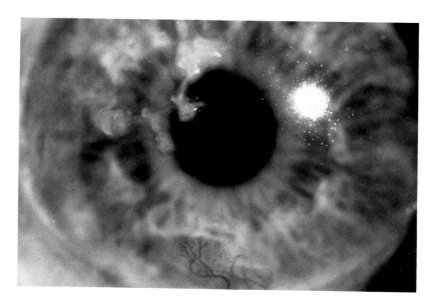

Figure 12-28
Mucus plaque simulating a dendrite.

benefit.[220] Extension of treatment to 21 days or addition of systemic corticosteroids sped healing of the rash and decreased acute pain but conferred little benefit over the standard 10-day acyclovir therapy.[221] Combined topical and oral BVDU also appears to be effective and well tolerated in uncontrolled studies,[215,216] but this medication is not available in the United States.

Administration of oral prednisone to reduce the incidence of postherpetic neuralgia is controversial.[222,223] Most recently, in a large prospective randomized trial the addition of oral corticosteroids to acyclovir had no effect on the frequency of postherpetic neuralgia.[221] On the basis of this study systemic steroids are not recommended for the reduction of postherpetic neuralgia. The current treatment recommendations are summarized in Table 12-6.

In patients with AIDS, herpes zoster can be more severe and less responsive to antiviral therapy. Prolonged intravenous acyclovir may be required. The incidences of corneal involvement, uveitis, and postherpetic neuralgia may be higher than in immunocompetent patients.[187]

Dermal Eruption. When administered alone, topical IDU penetrates the skin poorly, but when combined with dimethyl sulfoxide, its penetration increases. This combination has been effective in reducing symptoms[224] but is not approved for use in the United States. Application of topical acyclovir also may be bene-

Table 12-6	Summary of Recommended Treatment for Acute Herpes Zoster
General*	Acyclovir (800 mg orally five times daily for 10 days)
Skin	Burow's solution, cool compresses, mechanical cleansing
	Topical idoxuridine and dimethyl sulfoxide†
Epithelial keratitis	Debridement or none
Stromal keratitis	Topical corticosteroids
Uveitis	Topical corticosteroids
	Oral corticosteroids, ?oral acyclovir (400 mg four times a day) in severe cases
Corneal mucus plaques	Lubricants, topical corticosteroids, acetylcysteine (10%)

*If less than 7 days after onset.
†Not available in the United States.

ficial, but this has not yet been adequately tested. Burow's solution, cool compresses, and mechanical cleansing are helpful. Some recommend antibiotic ointment to decrease the risk of bacterial superinfection, but this is probably ineffective.

Punctate Epithelial Keratitis and Dendritic Keratitis. These conditions probably result from active viral replication in the epithelium, so it might be expected that antiviral agents would speed their resolution. However, no agent has clearly been demonstrated to be of benefit. One series of studies found that topical acyclovir alone resulted in faster resolution of epithelial disease than topical steroids alone or combined topical acyclovir and steroids,[225,226] but acyclovir was not compared with untreated controls. Another study found no clear benefit of topical acyclovir when used alone, but in combination with a topical corticosteroid inflammation resolved more rapidly.[227] Combined topical and oral BVDU appeared to speed resolution of keratitis, but these studies were uncontrolled.[215,216]

Topical corticosteroids also appear to speed resolution of these lesions,[62,204] but one must be absolutely sure of the diagnosis because such treatment could be disastrous if the dendrite were actually caused by HSV.[228] Debridement may be helpful.[229]

Because no treatment has been clearly demonstrated to be beneficial, and these lesions generally resolve in a few days without treatment, it seems best to withhold both antiviral medication and topical corticosteroids. Systematically administered acyclovir, given for general treatment of herpes zoster, may also treat the epithelial lesions because the drug reaches the tear film.

Stromal Keratitis. Anterior stromal infiltration, disciform keratitis, interstitial keratitis, and sclerokeratitis all respond to topical corticosteroids.[202,230] The risks and benefits of treatment are identical to those for herpes simplex, except that corticosteroids do not appear to exacerbate active viral infection with herpes zoster. The minimum dose necessary to achieve the desired effect should be used. Topical corticosteroids should be used with caution in patients with neurotrophic keratitis, exposure, or epithelial defects because of the increased risk of corneal melting.

Uveitis. Corticosteroids are the mainstay of treatment. Topical treatment is usually sufficient, but in some cases oral prednisone may be necessary. Acyclovir, given systemically or topically, has been reported to be beneficial in some cases,[225] but concurrent corticosteroid treatment was often required.

Nonhealing Epithelial Defects. Most often these defects result from neurotrophic keratitis, but exposure, trichiasis, anterior stromal inflammation, and drug toxicity are also common. Lid position abnormalities should be corrected and unnecessary drugs discontinued. Lubricant drops and ointments and pressure patching are the simplest measures and are usually successful. If not, therapeutic contact lenses, lateral or total tarsorrhaphy, or a conjunctival flap may be necessary.

Corneal Mucus Plaques. Mucus plaques often persist for months but usually resolve without treatment. Topical corticosteroids, lubricants, and mucolytic agents can reduce their formation, but recurrences are frequent.[231]

Pain. Zoster pain can be a serious problem. Administration of levodopa (100 mg three times a day for 10 days) during the acute attack reduced the intensity of pain and appeared to reduce the frequency of postherpetic neuralgia.[232] Cimetidine (300 to 400 mg orally daily for 14 days) has also been reported to relieve pain and itching and speed resolution of vesicles,[233] but the most recent study did not confirm this.[234] Topical capsaicin 0.025% four times daily is effective in relieving pain in approximately three fourths of patients.[235-237] Pain relief is noted after 2 to 6 weeks of treatment. Tricyclic antidepressants, including amitriptyline, imipramine, desipramine, nortriptyline, and doxepin, can alleviate postherpetic neuralgia.[238,239] The recommended dose of amitriptyline and desipramine is 25 to 50 mg orally at bedtime with increasing dosages every 3 to 4 days until a dosage of 75 to 100 mg daily is achieved. Carbamazepine, chlorprothixene, and adenosine monophosphate have all been used but do not appear to be very effective. In intractable cases, stellate ganglion block can provide relief.[240]

Penetrating Keratoplasty. Keratoplasty should be approached with caution. There are no large series of cases, but the success rate is generally poor if there is markedly reduced corneal sensation. However, two centers have recently reported a number of successful outcomes, including some with corneal anesthesia.[241,242] Based on my experience, I would not recommend grafting for patients with markedly reduced cornea sensation. If surgery is contemplated, it is best to wait until at least 1 year after the disease is quiescent. Maintaining epithelial integrity is paramount and should be achieved by obtaining donor tissue with healthy epithelium, protecting this epithelium postoperatively with lubricants, and, in some cases, performing partial or total temporary tarsorrhaphy.

ADENOVIRUS

The Virus

Adenoviruses contain double-stranded DNA surrounded by an icosahedral capsid composed of 252 capsomers. They are not enveloped and measure 1400 Å in diameter. More than 40 immunologically distinct serotypes have been distinguished based on capsomer antigens. As with herpesviruses, viral particle assembly occurs in the nucleus. The virus is relatively easy to isolate in human cell cultures, and recently an animal model of infection has been developed.[243]

Epidemiology

At least 19 serotypes of adenovirus have been associated with ocular infection.[244,245] Certain serotypes (1, 2, 4, 5, and 6) are endemic in the Western world and are mainly associated with respiratory and gastrointestinal infection. These serotypes appear to be a common cause of mild conjunctivitis, often associated with sore throat.[246] Other serotypes (3, 7, 8, 10, 19, 30, and 37) are seen mainly in epidemics where ocular symptoms predominate and tend to be more severe. Antibodies to these serotypes are rare in the normal population of Western countries.[247] The location of the reservoir of these viruses is unclear, but they are much more common in the Orient, and in all geographic locations chronic infections and shedding may occur in some cases.[248,249]

Transmission during epidemics of ocular disease occurs by contamination of fingers, soap, towels, linens, infected surfaces, ophthalmic instruments and solutions,[250] swimming pools,[251] and possibly through sexual contact.[252] One of the most common sites of transmission is the eye clinic. The virus can persist on nonporous surfaces (e.g., tonometer tips) for up to 8 weeks.[253,254] Adequate handwashing and cleansing of ophthalmic instruments are the mainstay of its control. The incubation period is 2 to 14 days, and in epidemic keratoconjunctivitis the person may remain infectious for 10 to 14 days after symptoms develop.

Two distinct clinical forms of epidemic adenoviral conjunctivitis occur—epidemic keratoconjunctivitis (EKC) and pharyngoconjunctival fever (PCF).

Epidemic Keratoconjunctivitis

Epidemic keratoconjunctivitis is most commonly produced by serotypes 8 and 19, but many other serotypes (2, 3, 4, 5, 7, 9, 10, 11, 14, 16, 21, 29, and 37) can produce a similar picture.[255]

Clinical Manifestations

The clinical signs and symptoms of infection vary from minimal or none to severe. Symptoms, which are usually rapid in onset, include watering, soreness, grittiness, and foreign body sensation.[256-259] Most cases are bilateral, with involvement of the second eye frequently occurring 3 to 7 days after involvement of the first. Symptoms and signs in the first eye are usually more severe than in the second. An associated flu-like illness, which may include fever, malaise, respiratory symptoms, nausea, vomiting, diarrhea, and myalgia, is present in some cases. Follicular conjunctivitis is the earliest and most common sign. The follicles are more evident in the inferior fornix. Petechial hemorrhages are often present in the palpebral conjunctiva, and rarely, more extensive hemorrhage is seen. Pseudomembranous or membranous conjunctivitis can occur in more severe cases (Figs. 3-9 and 12-29). Lid edema is common and may be mistaken for cellulitis. Preauricular or submandibular adenopathy develop in the majority of cases, usually within the first few days of symptoms. Conjunctivitis usually resolves in about 2 weeks, but corneal involvement may last much longer.

The characteristic course of the keratitis has been well documented.[260] Approximately 3 to 4 days after the onset of symptoms, a diffuse fine epithelial keratitis appears (Fig. 12-30). Minute white dots, some of which stain with fluorescein or rose bengal, are seen and persist in the majority of cases for 2 to 3 weeks. Approximately 1 week after onset, focal epithelial keratitis develops and persists for 1 to 2 weeks (Fig. 12-31). The focal lesions are similar to those seen in other forms of viral keratitis, with central ulceration and irregular borders with gray-white dots, which may be elevated. Fluorescein stains the central portion of the lesions. Both the diffuse and focal lesions are thought to be caused by active viral infection.

Approximately 2 weeks after onset, subepithelial infiltrates can develop beneath the focal epithelial lesions (Fig. 12-32). The patient then develops increased photophobia and decreased vision. If untreated, these infiltrates gradually fade over weeks or months but can persist for more than 10 years. Histologically, they are composed of lymphocytes and can be associated with overlying defects in Bowman's membrane and epithelial basement membrane.[261] The infiltrates are most likely an immunologic response to viral antigens, which have seeped into the stroma.[262]

Rarely, disciform keratitis, dendritic keratitis, or anterior uveitis can occur.[247,263] In a few cases, chronic or recurrent inflammation has oc-

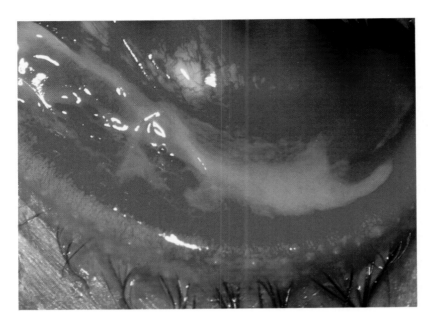

Figure 12-29
Severe conjunctival hyperemia, follicular response, and membrane formation in epithelial kerato-conjunctivitis.

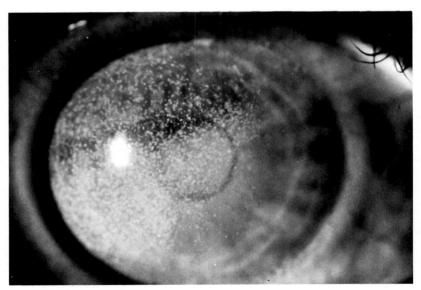

Figure 12-30
Epithelial staining in early epithelial keratoconjunctivitis.

curred after typical EKC, and adenovirus was recovered again many months after the disease onset.[248,249] In some of these cases a chronic papillary conjunctivitis was the only manifestation; in others recurrent focal epithelial keratitis was noted, sometimes over stromal infil-

trates. Chronic steroid use had been present in some cases but not in others.

Pharyngoconjunctival Fever
Pharyngoconjunctival fever is an acute follicular conjunctivitis associated with pharyngitis

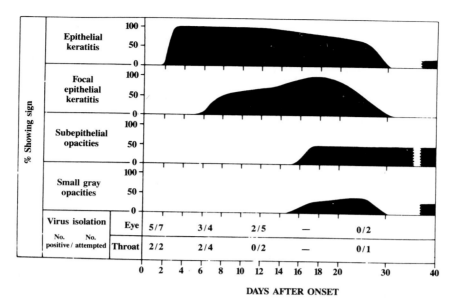

Figure 12-31
Clinical course of keratitis and virus isolations in patients with epidemic keratoconjunctivitis. Diffuse superficial epithelial keratitis is present from the first day in most cases. Focal epithelial lesions (or coarse keratopathy) appear approximately 7 days after onset. Subepithelial opacities form at the site of some of the focal epithelial lesions from the 11th to 15th days. Subepithelial involvement may persist for many months after the epithelium clears. (From Dawson C et al: *Am J Ophthalmol* 69:473, 1970.)

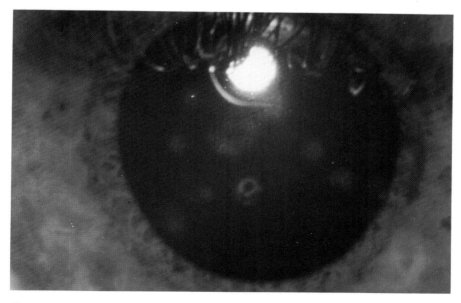

Figure 12-32
Subepithelial corneal infiltrates seen in epithelial keratoconjunctivitis.

and fever that is seen mainly in children[264] (Fig. 12-33). It is most commonly caused by serotypes 3 and 7. PCF is highly contagious and is spread mainly via respiratory secretions but can also be spread through contaminated swimming pools. Tender regional adenopathy is usually present; conjunctival hemorrhage also may occur. A mild diffuse punctate keratitis can be seen; subepithelial infiltrates are rare.

The ocular findings in PCF are similar to those of acute hemorrhagic conjunctivitis and early EKC, but in these diseases patients do not have the systemic symptoms of PCF. There is no specific treatment. Resolution generally occurs in 7 to 14 days.

Diagnosis

In most cases the diagnosis can be made clinically on the basis of history and examination. Differentiation from bacterial infection, especially *Moraxella*, and acute chlamydial infection can be difficult. If bacterial infection is suspected, treatment with a broad-spectrum topical antibiotic (e.g., a fluoroquinolone, polysporin, or polytrim 4 times daily) would be appropriate.

Conjunctival scrapings can be helpful in differentiation. In adenoviral infection they demonstrate a predominantly mononuclear response, and intranuclear inclusions may be seen in the lymphocytes.[265] A mixed polymorphonuclear leukocytic, lymphocytic response is seen in chlamydial infection, and chlamydial inclusions may be present; predominantly polymorphonuclear leukocytes are seen in bacterial infection; and lymphocytes with multinucleated giant cells are seen in herpes simplex.

Immunologic tests, such as Adenoclone,[266] an enzyme immunoassy (Cambridge Bioscience, Worcester, MA), and immunofiltration[267] (V & P Scientific, San Diego, CA) are fairly sensitive (80%) during the first week of infection and are very specific.[268] Adenovirus can be isolated in culture, but it this is not widely available. The PCR technique appears to be applicable in the detection of adenovirus in ocular swabs.[269]

Treatment

The most important measure is prevention of spread of the disease by the patient and physician. The patient should be informed about the length of time the disease is infectious and the types of precautions that are necessary to prevent spread.

No agent has been found to be clinically effective against acute infection. Treatment, therefore, is palliative and can include warm or cold compresses, lubrication, topical vasoconstrictors, and cycloplegic drops. The risk of bacterial superinfection is very low, so prophylactic antibiotic treatment is unnecessary. In one prospective double-blind study, there was no difference between the results of topical treatment with F_3T, dexamethasone, or artificial tears.[270] New agents that have demonstrated antiadenoviral activity in vitro are being investigated. These include S-HPMPC, (S)-1-(3-hydroxy-2-phosphonylmethoxy-propyl)-adenosine (S-HPMPA), ganciclovir, interferons, cyclic GMP, and 3'FLT.[271,272] HPMPC (cidofovir) is effective against adenovirus and HSV in rabbit models.[273]

If membranes form, their removal usually

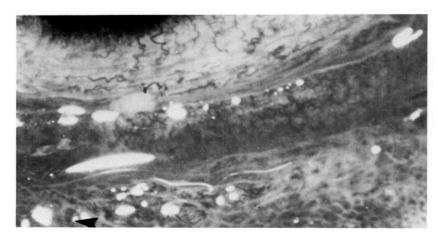

Figure 12-33
Large follicles in the lower tarsal conjunctiva in pharyngoconjunctival fever.

provides some symptomatic relief. Because membranes can result in conjunctival scarring, treatment with a mild steroid, one to two times daily, is recommended. A steroid-sulfacetamide combination drop may be used.

Topical steroids are very effective in relieving the signs and symptoms of subepithelial infiltrates; however, the end result is probably the same, and weaning patients can be very difficult. Steroids are most effective early in the course but also can be beneficial as long as 1 year after onset. In general, their use is indicated if the symptoms are severe or prolonged, if vision is markedly reduced, or if the patient is unable to perform normal activities. The risks and benefits of their use should be discussed with the patient and a mutual decision made. It is probably best to avoid using steroids, if possible, because they are often required for many months, may cause persistent viral infection, and often produce complications.

EPSTEIN-BARR VIRUS

Epstein-Barr virus is a member of the family Herpesviridae. Like other herpesviruses, EBV contains a central double-stranded DNA core, has a protein capsid with 162 hollow, cylindric capsomeres, and the nucleocapsid is surrounded by an envelope. EBV is common worldwide. Infection in children, which is more common in less-developed countries, is usually subclinical. Most teenagers or adults who undergo primary infection develop infectious mononucleosis, which is usually transmitted through saliva by kissing.

Infectious mononucleosis is characterized by fever, lymphadenopathy, and pharyngitis. Headache, malaise, anorexia, and chills are often present. Pharyngitis is maximal for 5 to 7 days then resolves over the next 7 to 10 days. Fever usually persists for 7 to 14 days. Malaise is the most persistent symptom, usually lasting 3 to 4 weeks, but occasionally persists for months.

An acute conjunctivitis can occur during infectious mononucleosis, sometimes with follicles, hemorrhage, chemosis, focal white infiltrates, or membrane development.[274] Conjunctival granulomas have been seen, and these are associated with preauricular adenopathy (see the discussion on Parinaud's oculoglandular syndrome in Chapter 7). In one case a salmon-colored mass was observed on the bulbar conjunctiva.[275] Focal epithelial keratitis can occur during the acute disease, and, in one case, small dendritic lesions were observed from which EBV was isolated.[276]

Interstitial and nummular keratitis can be associated with infectious mononucleosis.[277-279] Most of the opacities are coin-shaped, but they can coalesce to form broader lamellar infiltrates. The opacities are usually multiple and bilateral and are present in all levels of the stroma. They are more common in the peripheral cornea and can become vascularized or develop facets (Fig. 12-34). The epithelium is usually intact, and there is no anterior chamber reaction. Corneal sensation is normal. Other

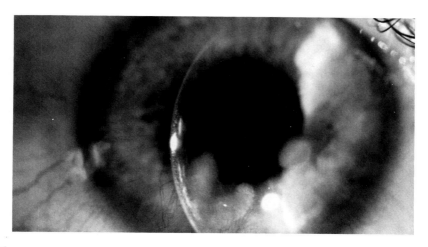

Figure 12-34
Keratitis in Epstein-Barr virus infection consists of nummular infiltrates at multiple levels of the stroma. These infiltrates can become confluent or vascularized.

ocular findings include lid edema (common), dacryoadenitis, episcleritis, uveitis, optic neuritis, retinal edema, and retinal hemorrhages.[174,280,281]

Infectious mononucleosis can be confirmed by a positive heterophil antibody test or serologic evidence of recent EBV infection. In patients with interstitial keratitis, differentiation from herpes simplex and Lyme disease must be made. In most cases rapid improvement in signs and symptoms can be achieved with topical steroids.

NEWCASTLE DISEASE

Newcastle disease is caused by a virus that produces fatal pneumonitis in fowl. Human infections occur in poultry workers and laboratory technicians and are manifested as unilateral, usually follicular, conjunctivitis with scant watery discharge.[282] Preauricular adenopathy is present, and a fine epithelial keratitis and subepithelial infiltrates can be seen. The disease resolves spontaneously without sequelae.

ACUTE HEMORRHAGIC CONJUNCTIVITIS

Acute hemorrhagic conjunctivitis is an acute follicular conjunctivitis that occurs in epidemics. It is caused by enteroviruses, which are members of the family Picornaviridae. Enteroviruses are small, nonenveloped RNA viruses. Polioviruses, echoviruses, and coxsackieviruses are types of enteroviruses. Epidemic conjunctivitis is usually caused by enterovirus type 70 and coxsackievirus type A24.[283] Infection can be transmitted through respiratory, oral, and conjunctival secretions.[284] In contrast to adenovirus, enterovirus 70 survives less than 6 hours on dry, nonporous surfaces such as tonometer tips.[285] Immunity after infection decreases with time, such that most of the patients will not have resistance 7 years after the initial infection, and reinfection can occur.[286,287]

After an incubation period of less than 24 hours, patients develop pain, foreign body sensation, tearing, and photophobia in one eye that rapidly spreads to the other.[288] A mild follicular conjunctivitis is seen, sometimes with subconjunctival hemorrhage and preauricular adenopathy[257,262,289-292] (Fig. 12-35). The frequency of these findings varies considerably in different epidemics. A fine epithelial keratitis and subepithelial infiltrates also can be seen. Nearly all cases resolve without ocular sequelae in 2 to 3 weeks, but neurologic complications, particularly radiculomyelitis, can occur.

OTHER VIRAL INFECTIONS

Viral infection of the external eye can occur in mumps, rubeola, rubella, variola, and vaccinia. The ocular findings in these diseases, as well as a summary of external ocular findings in other viral diseases, are given in Table 12-7. The characteristics of epithelial cell inclusions in viral diseases and chlamydial diseases are listed in Table 4-2.

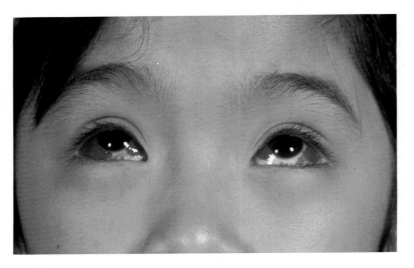

Figure 12-35
Acute hemorrhagic conjunctivitis. (Courtesy of Eric Donnenfeld, Rockville Center, NY.)

DISEASE SUSPECTED TO BE OF VIRAL ORIGIN

Dimmer's Nummular Keratitis

Dimmer's nummular keratitis is a slowly developing, benign keratitis usually occurring unilaterally in young land workers. It is characterized by disc-shaped infiltrates in the superficial stroma that later develop facets, and is not associated with conjunctivitis.[305-307] It was originally described in agricultural workers in Europe, but it appears to be more common in the Far East, where the disease has been called "padi keratitis" because it is usually seen in rice field workers. (*Padi* means "unhusked rice" in the Malayan language.) It also has been reported in South Africa and the United States.

Clinical Manifestations

Dimmer's nummular keratitis presents with foreign body sensation, tearing, photophobia, blurred vision, and some degree of ciliary injection unassociated with any conjunctival discharge. Most patients have a history of trauma and exposure to irrigation water. The onset of symptoms has varied from 1 to 35 days after trauma. The keratitis is characterized by 10 to 50 subepithelial coin-shaped corneal opacities, 0.5 to 1.5 mm in diameter (Figs. 12-36 and 12-37). During the first few weeks of involvement the corneal infiltrates show a nondiscrete, round configuration, and a dull-white opacification that tends to spread and fade off into the surrounding cornea in edematous haze. With time they become more sharply demarcated. These lesions are usually in one plane of the cornea but can be seen at all levels.[307]

During the first 2 to 3 months, some of the nummular lesions may develop central dense nuclei. However, after about the 4th month the nuclei may resorb, resulting in annular forms with much clearer, slightly translucent centers and more opaque, dense rims. In some cases central depressions, or facets, form. Peripheral infiltrates can develop superficial vascularization and, rarely, proceed to ulceration.

The nummular infiltrates gradually resorb and scar, and the central facets become more pronounced. Symptoms typically persist for 9 to 12 months. The infiltrates regress over 6 to 8 years, but some faint scarring and peripheral vascularization can persist indefinitely.

In some cases central lesions coalesce and form a disciform keratitis. Deep stromal involvement with edema and infiltration can also be seen. The deep central stromal infiltrate and edema usually start clearing during the 4th month, although some stromal haze may per-

sist for a couple of years. Epithelial bullae may occur as a result of endothelial injury.

Etiology

The cause of Dimmer's nummular keratitis is unknown, but a viral agent is suspected. Cultures of the corneal lesions and serology have been unfruitful, except in one case in which an unidentified virus was isolated.[307a] It has been suggested that the mechanism is similar to that seen in adenoviral infection.

Treatment

Topical corticosteroids can relieve discomfort and improve vision, but the final outcome appears to be the same. Once begun, treatment usually must be continued for 4 to 8 weeks to prevent recurrence of symptoms.

Thygeson's Superficial Punctate Keratitis

Thygeson's superficial punctate keratitis (TSPK) is characterized by bilateral recurrent focal epithelial keratitis without associated conjunctival or stromal inflammation.[308-312] The etiology is unknown but is suspected to be viral. It can affect all age groups, with the greatest incidence seen in the second and third decades of life. Patients report photophobia, tearing, foreign body sensation, and often a mild decrease in vision. The classic corneal lesion in TSPK is a group of coarse, oval-shaped, slightly raised, white or gray dots that stain with fluorescein (Fig. 12-38). One to 50 of these lesions can be present, with 20 on the average, and they tend to affect the central cornea more than the periphery. This classic picture is seen during active, symptomatic disease; during inactive stages the lesions can disappear; can be flat, gray, intraepithelial dots that do not stain; or can appear stellate. The epithelium is normal between the lesions, and subepithelial opacities do not develop unless toxic drugs, such as IDU, are used. The conjunctiva may be mildly injected; tiny, hairlike filaments may be present; and corneal sensation is normal or only slightly subnormal.

Individual attacks generally last 1 to 2 months, go into remission for 4 to 6 weeks, and then recur; the time course is variable. Usually after 2 to 4 years, the disease resolves without sequelae, but persistence as long as 20 years has been observed, particularly with steroid use.[311]

Symptoms can be relieved and signs suppressed by using soft or hard contact lenses or by applying topical steroids.[313,314] Low concentrations of steroids (e.g., 0.12% prednisolone) two to three times daily, generally only for a

Table 12-7 Summary of Viral External Disease

Virus	Lids	Conjunctivitis	Cornea	Adenopathy	Other Findings	Comments
HERPESVIRUSES						
Herpes simplex (primary)	Vesicles, hyperemia, swelling	Follicular, membranes (50%)	FK*, dendrite	+	Canaliculitis, iritis	
Varicella	Vesicles, hyperemia, swelling	Papillary, pocks	SPK†, dendrites, phlyctenules, disciform keratitis	++	Iritis	
Zoster	Vesicles, marked edema, hyperemia	Usually papillary; can be follicles, membranes, hemorrhages	Dendrites, disciform keratitis	–	Keratouveitis, scleritis, retinitis, others	Typical skin involvement
Epstein-Barr	Mild hyperemia and swelling	Usually papillary, can be follicles, hemorrhages, membranes, infiltrate, granuloma	FK, dendrites, nummular keratitis (late)	+	Infectious mononucleosis, canaliculitis, episcleritis, uveitis, optic neuritis	Usually mild or no conjunctivitis
Cytomegalovirus[293]		Mild follicular		–	Mononucleosis-like illness, chorioretinitis	
ADENOVIRUSES						
Epidemic keratoconjunctivitis	Swelling, hyperemia	Follicles, hemorrhages, membranes	SPK, FK, subepithelial infiltrates	++	Iritis (rare)	Most commonly types 8, 19
Pharyngoconjunctival fever	Swelling, hyperemia	Follicles, hemorrhages, membranes	SPK	++	Pharyngitis, fever	Most commonly types 3, 7
ENTEROVIRUSES						
Acute hemorrhagic conjunctivitis	Mild swelling, hyperemia	Mild follicular response, hemorrhagic	SPK, subepithelial infiltrates	+ (60%)	Radiculomyelitis	Occurs in epidemics, incubation period <24 hrs

	Lid	Conjunctiva	Cornea		Systemic/Other	Comments
PARAMYXOVIRUSES						
Newcastle disease	Mild swelling, hyperemia	Usually follicular	SPK, subepithelial infiltrates	+	Occurs in poultry workers and lab technicians	
Mumps[294–296]	Mild swelling, hyperemia	Catarrhal, occasionally follicular	SPK, disciform keratitis (Fig. 12-39)	−	Episcleritis, scleritis, uveitis, dacryoadenitis, others	
Rubeola (measles)[297–299]	Swelling of plica	Catarrhal, Koplik spots	SPK, rarely interstitial keratitis, corneal ulcers	+	Fever, rash, rarely severe systemic disease, other ocular disease	Severe corneal complications in malnourished children
POXVIRUSES						
Variola (smallpox) (Fig. 12-40)	Swelling, hyperemia	Follicular, can have hemorrhage, pus, pocks	Corneal pocks, disciform keratitis, interstitial keratitis	+	Fever, rash, can be fatal	Now rare
Vaccinia[300–302]	Marked lid swelling, "kissing lesions" (Fig. 12-41)	Catarrhal or purulent, papillary or follicular	SPK, disciform keratitis, interstitial keratitis	++	Malaise, fever	After smallpox vaccination
Molluscum contagiosum	Typical lid lesion(s)	Follicular, rarely primary lesion	SPK, pannus	−		
TOGAVIRUSES						
Rubella[303, 304] (acquired)		Mild catarrhal or follicular	SPK	−	Fever, rash	Conjunctivitis 70%, keratitis 2%
PAPOVAVIRUSES						
Papillomavirus	Warts	Warts, papillae, rarely follicles	SPK	−		
ORTHOMYXOVIRUSES						
Influenza virus		Follicular	−	−	Influenza	

*Focal keratitis.
†Superficial punctate keratitis.

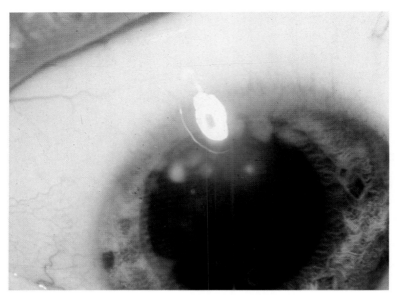

Figure 12-36
Dimmer's nummular keratitis.

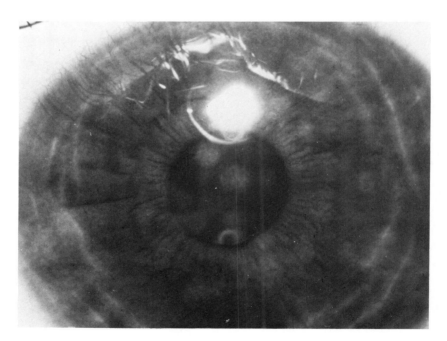

Figure 12-37
Typical coin-shaped lesions in nummular keratitis.

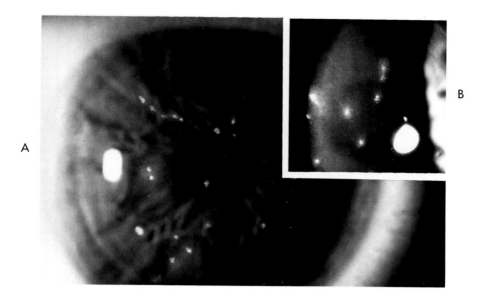

Figure 12-38
Thygeson's superficial punctate keratitis. **A,** Coarse, whitish lesions clustered in central cornea. **B,** More magnified view of the lesions.

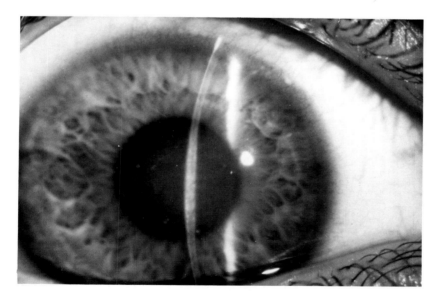

Figure 12-39
Disciform keratitis in mumps. (Courtesy of Eric Donnenfeld, Rockville Center, NY.)

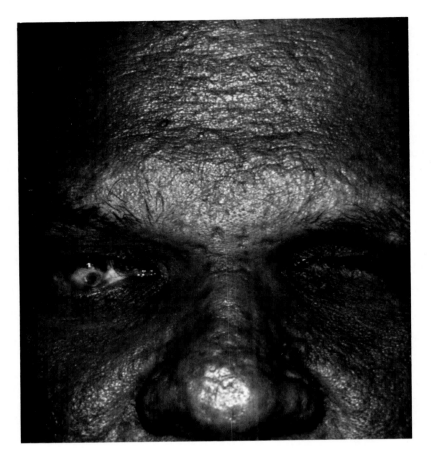

Figure 12-40
Skin and corneal scarring in smallpox. (Courtesy of Eric Donnenfeld, Rockville Center, NY.)

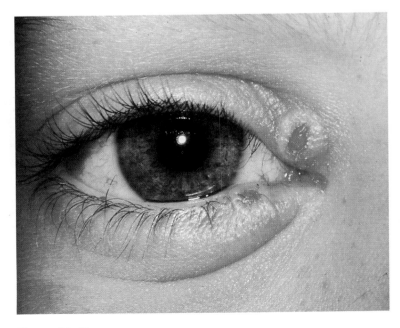

Figure 12-41
Vaccinia of lid.

few days to 2 weeks, are usually sufficient to bring relief. If sufficient response is not obtained or more intensive or prolonged treatment is required, bandage contact lenses can be applied. Antiviral agents do not appear to be beneficial. Removal of the corneal epithelium does not affect the course of the disease.

That TSPK is caused by a virus is supported by the resemblance of the epithelial lesions to those seen in measles, mumps, variola, and adenovirus infection and by electron microscopic evidence of virus particles in epithelial lesions. In two cases a virus was isolated from these lesions: In one case the virus was not identified,[315] and in the other it was identified as VZV.[316] The frequency of HLA-DR3 is significantly increased in patients with TSPK,[312] suggesting an immunologic role.

REFERENCES

1. Baringer JR, Swoveland P: Recovery of herpes simplex virus from human trigeminal ganglions, *N Engl J Med* 288:648, 1973.
2. Pierson RB, Kirkham TH: Neonatal keratitis due to herpesvirus: hominis type 1 infection, *Can J Ophthalmol* 9:429, 1974.
3. Hanna L, Ostler HB, Keshishyan H: Observed relationship between herpetic lesions and antigenic type of *Herpesvirus hominis, Surv Ophthalmol* 21:110, 1976.
4. Oh JO, Stevens TR: Comparison of types 1 and 2 *Herpesvirus hominus* infection of rabbit eyes: I. Clinical manifestations, *Arch Ophthalmol* 90:473, 1973.
5. Stevens TR, Oh JO: Comparison of types 1 and 2 *Herpesvirus hominus* infection of rabbit eyes: II. Histopathologic and virologic studies, *Arch Ophthalmol* 90:477, 1980.
6. Steiner I et al: A herpes simplex virus type I mutant containing a nontransinducing Vmw65 protein establishes latent infection in vivo in the absence of viral replication and reactivates efficiently from explanted trigeminal ganglia, *J Virol* 64:1630, 1990.
7. Efstathiou S et al: Detection of herpes simplex virus-specific DNA sequences in latently infected mice and in humans, *J Virol* 57:446, 1986.
8. Gordon YJ et al: RNA complementary to herpes simplex virus type 1 ICPO gene demonstrated in neurons of human trigeminal ganglia, *J Virol* 62:1832, 1988.
9. Mehta A et al: In situ DNA PCR and RNA hybridization detection of herpes simplex virus sequences in trigeminal ganglia of latently infected mice, *Virology* 206:633, 1995.
10. Gordon YJ et al: RNA complementary to herpes simplex virus type 1 ICPO gene demonstrated in neurons of human trigeminal ganglia, *J Virol* 62:1832, 1988.
11. Rock DDL et al: Detection of latency-related viral RNAs in trigeminal ganglia of rabbits latently infected with herpes simplex virus type 1, *J Virol* 61:3820, 1987.
12. Krause PR et al: Expression of the herpes simplex virus type 2 latency-associated transcript enhances spontaneous reactivation of genital herpes in latently infected guinea pigs, *J Exp Med* 181:297, 1995.
13. Abghare SZ, Stulting RD: Recovery of herpes simplex virus from ocular tissues of latently infected inbred mice, *Invest Ophthalmol Vis Sci* 29:239, 1988.
14. Cook SD, Brown SM: Herpes simplex virus type 1 persistence and latency in cultured rabbit corneal epithelial cells, keratocytes, and endothelial cells, *Br J Ophthalmol* 70:642, 1986.
15. Claoué CMP et al: Does herpes simplex virus establish latency in the eye of the mouse?, *Eye* 1:525, 1987.
16. Laycock KA et al: Herpes simplex virus type 1 transcription is not detectable in quiescent human stromal keratitis by in situ hybridization, *Invest Ophthalmol Vis Sci* 34:285, 1993.
17. Shimomura Y et al: Herpes simplex virus latency in human cornea, *Jpn J Ophthalmol* 37:318, 1993.
18. Cantin E et al: Persistence of herpes simplex virus DNA in rabbit corneal cells, *Invest Ophthalmol Vis Sci* 33:2470, 1992.
19. Rong B-L et al: Detection of herpes simplex virus thymidine kinase and latency-associated transcript gene sequences in human herpetic corneas by polymerase chain reaction amplification, *Invest Ophthalmol Vis Sci* 32:1808, 1991.
20. Cook SD et al: Latency-associated transcripts in corneas and ganglia of HSV-1 infected rabbits, *Br J Ophthalmol* 75:644, 1991.
21. Parng GC et al: Similarities in regulation of the HSV-1 LAT promoter in corneal and neuronal cells, *Invest Ophthalmol Vis Sci* 35:2981, 1994.
22. Easty DL: *Virus disease of the eye,* Chicago, 1985, Mosby–Year Book.
23. Shimeld C et al: *Spread of herpes simplex virus to the eye following cutaneous inoculation in the skin of the snout of the mouse.* In Maudgal JC, Missoten L, editors: *Herpetic eye diseases,* Dordrecht, 1985, D.W. Junk.
24. Claoué C et al: Clinical findings after zosteriform spread of herpes simplex virus to the eye of the mouse, *Curr Eye Res* 6:281, 1987.
25. Gordon Y, Araullo-Cruz T: Herpesvirus inoculation of cornea, *Am J Ophthalmol* 97:482, 1984.
26. Lonsdale DM et al: Variations in herpes simplex virus isolated form human ganglia and a study of clonal variation in HSV-1, *Ann NY Acad Sci* 354:291, 1980.
27. Gerson M: Consecutive infections with herpes simplex virus types 1 and 2 within a three-week period, *J Infect Dis* 149:655, 1984.
28. Openshaw H et al: Acute and latent infection of sensory ganglia with herpes simplex virus: immune control and virus reactivation, *J Gen Virol* 44:205, 1979.

29. Gerdes JC, Smith DS: Recurrence phenotypes and establishment of latency following rabbit keratitis produced by multiple herpes simplex virus strains, *J Gen Virol* 64:2441, 1983.

30. Kaufman HE, Brown DC, Ellison EM: Recurrent herpes in the rabbit and man, *Science* 156:1628, 1967.

31. Kaye S et al: Ocular herpes virus shedding, *Br J Ophthalmol* 74:114, 1990.

32. Centifanto-Fitzgerald YM et al: Ocular disease pattern induced by herpes simplex virus is genetically determined by a specific region of viral DNA, *J Exp Med* 155:475, 1982.

33. Stulting RD, Kindle JC, Nahmias AJ: Patterns of herpes simplex keratitis in inbred mice, *Invest Ophthalmol Vis Sci* 26:1360, 1985.

34. Centifanto-Fitzgerald YM, Fenger T, Kaufman HE: Virus proteins in herpetic keratitis, *Exp Eye Res* 35:425, 1982.

35. Tullo AM et al: Analysis of glycoproteins expressed by isolates of herpes simplex virus causing different forms of keratitis in man, *Curr Eye Res* 6:33, 1987.

36. Gordon YJ, Hilden DM, Becker Y: HSV-1 thymidine kinase promotes virulence and latency in the mouse, *Invest Ophthalmol Vis Sci* 24:599, 1983.

37. Kaufman HE et al: Effect of the herpes simplex virus genome on the response of infection to corticosteroids, *Am J Ophthalmol* 100:114, 1985.

38. Ahonen R, Vannas A, Mäkitie J: Virus particles and leukocytes in herpes simplex keratitis, *Cornea* 3:43, 1984.

39. Gordon YJ: *Herpetic stromal keratitis: a new molecular model and its clinical correlation.* In Cavanagh HD, editor: *The cornea: transactions of the World Congress on the Cornea III,* New York, 1988, Raven Press.

40. Pavan-Langston D: *Viral diseases: herpetic infections.* In Smolin G, Thoft RA, editors: *The cornea: scientific foundations and clinical practice,* Boston, 1983, Little, Brown & Co.

41. Smith J, Pentherer J, MacCallum F: The incidence of herpesvirus hominis antibody in the population, *J Hygiene* 65:396, 1967.

42. Locatcher-Khorazo D, Seegal BC: *Microbiology of the eye,* St Louis, 1972, Mosby–Year Book.

43. Brown DC: Ocular herpes simplex, *Invest Ophthalmol* 10:210, 1971.

44. Norn MS: Dendritic herpetic keratitis: 1. Incidence, seasonal variations, recurrence rate, visual impairment, therapy, *Acta Ophthalmol* 48:91, 1970.

45. Liesegang TJ et al: Epidemiology of ocular herpes simplex: incidence in Rochester, Minn, 1950 through 1982, *Arch Ophthalmol* 107:1155, 1989.

46. Liesegang TJ: Epidemiology of ocular herpes simplex: natural history in Rochester, Minn, 1950 through 1982, *Arch Ophthalmol* 107:1160, 1989.

47. Wilhelmus KR, Falcon MG, Jones BR: Bilateral herpetic keratitis, *Br J Ophthalmol* 65:385, 1981.

48. Uchio E et al: A retrospective study of herpes simplex keratitis over the last 30 years, *Jpn J Ophthalmol* 38:196, 1994.

49. Bell D, Holman R, Pavan-Langston D: Epidemiological aspects of herpes simplex keratitis, *Ann Ophthalmol* 14:421, 1982.

50. Shuster J, Kaufman HE, Nesburn AB: Statistical analysis of the rate of recurrence of herpesvirus ocular epithelial disease, *Am J Ophthalmol* 91:328, 1981.

51. Norn MS: Dendritic (herpetic) keratitis: 2. Follow-up examinations of corneal opacity, *Acta Ophthalmol (Copenh)* 48:214, 1970.

52. Claque CMP, Menage MJ, Easty DL: Severe herpetic keratitis: I. Prevalence of visual impairment in a clinic population, *Br J Ophthalmol* 72:530, 1988.

53. Egerer U, Stary A: Erosive-ulcerative herpes simplex blepharitis, *Arch Ophthalmol* 98:1760, 1980.

54. Darouger S et al: Acute follicular conjunctivitis and keratoconjunctivitis due to herpes simplex virus in London, *Br J Ophthalmol* 62:843, 1978.

55. Jones BR: Differential diagnosis of punctate keratitis, *Int Ophthalmol Clin* 2:291, 1962.

56. Lanier JD: Marginal herpes simplex keratitis, *Ophthalmol Digest* 38:15, 1976.

57. Thygeson P: Marginal herpes simplex keratitis simulating catarrhal ulcer, *Invest Ophthalmol* 10:1006, 1971.

58. Young T et al: Herpes simplex keratitis in patients with acquired immune deficiency syndrome, *Ophthalmology* 96:1476, 1989.

59. Duke-Elder S, Leigh AG: *System of ophthalmology,* vol VIII, *Diseases of the outer eye,* St Louis, 1965, Mosby–Year Book.

60. Kaufman H: Epithelial erosion syndrome: metaherpetic keratitis, *Am J Ophthalmol* 57:984, 1964.

60a. Laibson PR: Surgical approaches to the treatment of active keratitis, *Int Ophthalmol Clin* 13:65, 1973.

61. Pavan-Langston D: Diagnosis and management of herpes simplex ocular infection, *Int Ophthalmol Clin* 15:19, 1975.

62. Pavan-Langston D, Brockhurst RJ: Herpes simplex panuveitis, *Arch Ophthalmol* 81:783, 1969.

63. Hendricks RL, Epstein RJ, Tumpey T: The effect of cellular immune tolerance to HSV-1 antigens on the immunopathology of HSV-1 keratitis, *Invest Ophthalmol Vis Sci* 30:105, 1989.

64. Jones BR: The management of ocular herpes, *Trans Ophthalmol Soc UK* 79:425, 1959.

65. Oh JO: Endothelial lesions of rabbit cornea produced by herpes simplex virus, *Invest Ophthalmol* 9:196, 1970.

66. Collin HB, Abelson MB: Herpes simplex virus in human cornea, retrocorneal fibrous membrane, and vitreous, *Arch Ophthalmol* 94:1726, 1976.

67. Metcalf JF, Reichert RW: Histological and electron microscopic studies of experimental herpetic keratitis in the rabbit, *Invest Ophthalmol Vis Sci* 18:1123, 1979.

68. Sundmacher R, Neumann-Haefelin D: *Herpes simplex virus-positive and virus-negative keratouveitis.* In Silverstein AM, O'Connor GR, editors: *Immunology and immunopathology of the eye,* New York, 1979, Masson Publishing.

69. Dawson CR, Togni B, Moore TE Jr: Structural changes in chronic herpetic keratitis, *Arch Ophthalmol* 79:740, 1968.

70. Shimeld C et al: Isolation of herpes simplex virus from the cornea in chronic stromal keratitis, *Br J Ophthalmol* 66:643, 1982.

71. Holbach L, Foht R, Naumann G: Herpes simplex stromal and endothelial keratitis, *Ophthalmology* 97:722, 1990.

72. Hewson GE: Iritis due to herpes virus, *Ir J Med Sci* 372, 1957.

73. Witmer R, Iwamoto T: Electron microscope observation of herpes-like particles in the iris, *Arch Ophthalmol* 79:331, 1968.

74. Robin JB, Steigner JB, Kaufman HE: Progressive herpetic corneal endotheliitis, *Am J Ophthalmol* 100:336, 1985.

75. Olsen TW et al: Linear endotheliitis, *Am J Ophthalmol* 117:468, 1994.

76. Vannas A, Ahonen R: Herpetic endothelial keratitis: a case report, *Acta Ophthalmol* 59:296, 1981.

77. Alvarado JA et al: Detection of herpes simplex viral DNA in the iridocorneal endothelial syndrome, *Arch Ophthalmol* 112:1601, 1994.

78. Plotkin J, Reynaud A, Olumoto M: Cytologic study of herpetic keratitis, *Arch Ophthalmol* 85:597, 1971.

79. Roat MI et al: Antiviral effects of rose bengal and fluorescein, *Arch Ophthalmol* 105:1415, 1987.

80. Kaufman HE: The diagnosis of corneal herpes simplex infection by fluorescent antibody staining, *Arch Ophthalmol* 64:382, 1960.

81. Dunkel EC et al: Rapid detection of herpes simplex virus (HSV) antigen in human ocular infections, *Curr Eye Res* 7:661, 1988.

82. Cleveland PH, Richman DD: Enzyme immunofiltration staining assay for the immediate diagnosis of herpes simplex virus and varicella zoster virus directly from clinical specimens, *J Clin Microbiol* 25:416, 1987.

83. Kowalski RP, Gordon YJ: Evaluation of immunologic tests for the detection of ocular herpes simplex virus, *Ophthalmology* 96:1583, 1989.

84. Gebhardt BM, Reidy J, Kaufman HE: An affinity membrane test for superficial corneal herpes, *Am J Ophthalmol* 105:686, 1988.

85. Simon MW et al: Comparison of immunocytology to tissue culture for diagnosis of presumed herpesvirus dendritic epithelial keratitis, *Ophthalmology* 99:1408, 1992.

86. Kowalski RP et al: A comparison of enzyme immunoassay and polymerase chain reaction with the clinical examination for diagnosing ocular herpetic disease, *Ophthalmology* 100:530, 1993.

87. Dumas AL, de Ancos E, Herbort CP: Evaluation of the method of DNA amplification (PCR, polymerase chain reaction) for diagnosis of superficial ocular herpes, *Klin Monatsbl Augenheilkd* 200:472, 1992.

88. Yamamoto S et al: Detection of herpes simplex virus DNA in human tear film by the polymerase chain reaction, *Am J Ophthalmol* 117:160, 1994.

89. Kaufman HE, Nesburn AB, Maloney ED: IDU therapy of herpes simplex, *Arch Ophthalmol* 64:382, 1960.

90. Gasset AR, Katzin D: Antiviral drugs and corneal wound healing, *Invest Ophthalmol* 14:628, 1975.

91. Langston RHS, Pavan-Langston D, Dohlman CH: Antiviral medication and corneal wound healing, *Arch Ophthalmol* 92:490, 1974.

92. Kaufman HE, Martola EL, Dohlman CH: Use of 5-iodo-2-deoxyuridine (IDU) in treating herpes simplex keratitis, *Arch Ophthalmol* 68:235, 1962.

93. Laibson PR, Leopold IH: An evaluation of double blind IDU therapy in 100 cases of herpetic keratitis, *Trans Am Acad Ophthalmol Otolaryngol* 68:21, 1964.

94. Patterson A et al: Controlled studies of IDU in the treatment of herpetic keratitis, *Trans Ophthalmol Soc UK* 83:583, 1963.

95. Hart DRL et al: Treatment of human herpes simplex keratitis with idoxuridine, *Arch Ophthalmol* 73:623, 1965.

96. Laibson PR et al: ARA-A and IDU therapy of human superficial herpetic keratitis, *Invest Ophthalmol* 14:762, 1975.

97. Falcon MG et al: *Adverse reactions in the eye from topical therapy with idoxuridine, adenine arabinoside and trifluorothymidine.* In Sundmacher R, editor, *Herpetic eye diseases,* Munich, 1981, Verlag.

98. Itoi M et al: Teratogenicities of ophthalmic drugs: I. Antiviral ophthalmic drugs, *Arch Ophthalmol* 93:46, 1975.

99. Payrau P, Dohlman CH: IDU in corneal wound healing, *Am J Ophthalmol* 57:999, 1964.

100. Pavan-Langston D, Langston RHS, Geary PA: Prophylaxis and therapy of experimental ocular herpes simplex: comparison of idoxuridine adenine arabinoside and hypoxanthine arabinoside, *Arch Ophthalmol* 92:417, 1974.

101. Pavan-Langston D et al: Intravenous and possibly subconjunctival injection of soluble antiviral ARA AMP may be useful in treatment of deep ocular herpetic disease, *Arch Ophthalmol* 94:1585, 1976.

102. Markham RHC et al: Double blind clinical trial of adenine arabinoside and idoxuridine in herpetic corneal ulcers, *Trans Ophthalmol Soc UK* 97:33, 1977.

103. Coster DL et al: Clinical evaluation of adenine arabinoside and trifluorothymidine in the treatment of corneal ulcers caused by herpes simplex virus, *J Infect Dis* 133(suppl A):173, 1976.

104. Pavan-Langston D, Buchanan RA: Vidarabine therapy of herpetic keratitis, *Trans Am Acad Ophthalmol Otolaryngol* 81:813, 1976.

105. Gasset AR, Akaboshi T: Teratogenicity of ade-

nine arabinoside (Ara-A), *Invest Ophthalmol* 15:556, 1976.

106. Pavan-Langston D, Foster CS: Trifluorothymidine and idoxuridine therapy of ocular herpes, *Am J Ophthalmol* 84:818, 1977.

107. Laibson PR et al: Double controlled comparison of IDU and trifluorothymidine in 33 patients with superficial herpetic keratitis, *Trans Am Ophthalmol Soc* 75:316, 1977.

108. Van Bijsterveld OP, Post HJ: *Trifluorothymidine and adenine arabinoside in the treatment of dendritic keratitis.* In Sundmacher R, editor: *Herpetic eye diseases,* Munich, 1981, Verlag.

109. McKinnon JR, McGill JI, Jones BR: *A coded clinical evaluation of adenine arabinoside and trifluorothymidine in the treatment of ulcerative herpetic keratitis.* In Pavan-Langston D, Buchanan RA, Alford CA, editors: *Adenine arabinoside: an antiviral agent,* New York, 1975, Raven Press.

110. Hyndiuk RA et al: Trifluridine in resistant human herpetic keratitis, *Arch Ophthalmol* 96:1839, 1978.

111. Pavan-Langston D, Nelson DJ: Intraocular penetration of trifluridine, *Am J Ophthalmol* 87:814, 1979.

111a. Langston RHS, Pavan-Langston D: Penetrating keratoplasty for herpetic keratitis: decision making and management, *Int Ophthalmol Clin* 15:125, 1975.

112. Wellings PC et al: Clinical evaluation of trifluorothymidine in the treatment of herpes simplex corneal ulcers, *Am J Ophthalmol* 73:932, 1972.

113. Poirier RH et al: Intraocular antiviral penetration, *Arch Ophthalmol* 100:1964, 1982.

114. LaLau C et al: Multicenter trial of acyclovir and trifluorothymidine in herpetic keratitis (acyclovir symposium), *Am J Med* 79:305, 1985.

115. Collum L, Benedict-Smith A, Hillary I: Randomized double-blind trial of acyclovir and idoxuridine in dendritic corneal ulceration, *Br J Ophthalmol* 64:766, 1980.

116. Coster DJ et al: A comparison of acyclovir and idoxuridine as treatment for ulcerative herpetic keratitis, *Br J Ophthalmol* 64:763, 1980.

117. Pavan-Langston D et al: Acyclovir and vidarabine in therapy of ulcerative herpes simplex keratitis: a comparative masked clinical trial, *Am J Ophthalmol* 92:829, 1981.

118. Collum LM et al: Randomized double-blind trial of acyclovir (Zovirax) and adenine arabinoside in herpes simplex amoeboid corneal ulceration, *Br J Ophthalmol* 69:847, 1985.

119. Lass JH, Pavan-Langston D, Park N: Acyclovir and corneal wound healing, *Am J Ophthalmol* 88:102, 1979.

120. Kaufman HE, Rayfield MA: *Viral conjunctivitis and keratitis.* In Kaufman HE et al, editors: *The cornea,* New York, 1988, Churchill Livingstone.

121. Sonkin PL et al: Acyclovir-resistant herpes simplex virus keratouveitis after penetrating keratoplasty, *Ophthalmology* 99:1805, 1992.

122. Nilsen AE et al: Efficacy of oral acyclovir in the treatment of initial and recurrent genital herpes, *Lancet* 2:571, 1982.

123. Cobo LM et al: Oral acyclovir in the treatment of acute herpes zoster ophthalmicus, *Ophthalmology* 93:763, 1986.

124. Bialasiewicz AA, Jahn GJ: Systemic acyclovir therapy in recurrent keratouveitis caused by herpes simplex virus, *Klin Monatsbl Augenheilkd* 185:539, 1984.

125. Schwab I: Oral acyclovir in the management of herpes simplex ocular infections, *Ophthalmology* 95:423, 1988.

126. Collum LMT et al: Oral acyclovir (Zovirax) in herpes simplex dendritic corneal ulceration, *Br J Ophthalmol* 70:435, 1986.

127. Hung SO et al: Oral acyclovir in the management of dendritic herpetic corneal ulceration, *Br J Ophthalmol* 68:398, 1984.

128. Collum LMT, Akhtar J, McGettrick P: Oral acyclovir in herpetic keratitis, *Trans Ophthalmol Soc UK* 104:629, 1985.

129. Barron BA et al: Herpetic eye disease study: a controlled trial of oral acyclovir for herpes simplex stromal keratitis, *Ophthalmology* 101:1871, 1994.

130. Straus SE et al: Suppression of frequently recurring genital herpes: a placebo-controlled double-blind trial of oral acyclovir, *N Engl J Med* 310:1543, 1984.

131. Douglas JM et al: A double-blind study of oral acyclovir for suppression of recurrences of genital herpes simplex virus infection, *N Engl J Med* 310:1551, 1984.

132. Meyrick Thomas RH et al: Oral acyclovir in the suppression of recurrent non-genital herpes simplex virus infection, *Br J Ophthalmol* 113:731, 1985.

133. Pavan-Langston D: *Viral keratitis and conjunctivitis.* In Smolin G, Thoft RA, editors: *The cornea: scientific foundations and clinical practice,* New York, 1994, Little, Brown & Co.

134. Barney NP, Foster CS: A prospective randomized trial of oral acyclovir after penetrating keratoplasty for herpes simplex keratitis, *Cornea* 13:232, 1994.

135. Jones BR et al: Topical therapy of ulcerative herpetic keratitis with human interferon, *Lancet* 2:128, 1976.

136. Sundmacher R, Neumann-Haefelin D, Cantell K: Successful treatment of dendritic keratitis with human leukocyte interferon, *Graefes Arch Clin Exp Ophthalmol* 201:39, 1976.

137. Sundmacher R, Cantell K, Neumann-Haefelin D: Combination therapy of dendritic keratitis with trifluorothymidine and interferon, *Lancet* 2:687, 1978.

138. de Koning EWJ, van Bijsterveld OP, Cantell K: Combination therapy for dendritic keratitis with human leukocyte interferon and trifluorothymidine and interferon, *Br J Ophthalmol* 66:509, 1982.

139. Colin J et al: Combination therapy for dendritic keratitis with human leukocyte interferon and acyclovir, *Am J Ophthalmol* 95:346, 1983.

140. de Koning EWJ, van Bijsterveld OP, Cantell L: Combination therapy for dendritic keratitis with acyclovir and alpha-interferon, *Arch Ophthalmol* 101:1866, 1983.

141. Maudgal P, De Clercq E, Missotten L: Efficacy of bromovinyl-deoxyuridine in the treatment of herpes simplex virus and varicella zoster eye infections, *Antiviral Res* 4:281, 1984.

142. Power WJ et al: Randomised double-blind trial of bromovinyldeoxyuridine (BVDU) and trifluorothymidine (TFT) in dendritic corneal ulceration, *Br J Ophthalmol* 75:649, 1991.

143. Gordon YJ, Romanowski EG, Araullo-Cruz T: HPMPC, a broad-spectrum topical antiviral agent, inhibits herpes simplex virus type 1 replication and promotes healing of dendritic keratitis in the New Zealand rabbit ocular model, *Cornea* 13:516, 1994.

144. Gordon YJ, Romanowski EG, Araullo-Cruz T: Topical HPMPC inhibits adenovirus type 5 in the New Zealand rabbit ocular replication model, *Invest Ophthalmol Vis Sci* 35:4135, 1994.

145. Kibrick S, Takahashi GH, Liebowitz HM: Local corticosteroid therapy and reactivation of herpetic keratitis, *Arch Ophthalmol* 86:694, 1971.

146. Wilhelmus KR et al: Herpetic eye disease study: a controlled trial of topical corticosteroids for herpes simplex stromal keratitis, *Ophthalmology* 101:1883, 1994.

147. Power WJ et al: Acyclovir ointment plus topical betamethasone or placebo in first episode disciform keratitis, *Br J Ophthalmol* 76:711, 1992.

148. Coster DJ, Jones BR, Falson MG: Role of debridement in the treatment of herpetic keratitis, *Trans Ophthalmol Soc UK* 97:314, 1977.

149. Wittpenn JR, Pepose JS: Impression debridement of herpes simplex dendritic keratitis, *Cornea* 5:245, 1986.

150. Jawetz E et al: Studies on herpes simplex: XI. The antivirus dynamics of 5-iodo-2-deoxyuridine in vivo, *J Immunol* 95:635, 1965.

151. Hyndiuk RA, Kaufman HE: Newer compounds in therapy of herpes simplex keratitis, *Arch Ophthalmol* 78:600, 1967.

152. Porter SM, Patterson A, Kho P: A comparison of local and systemic acyclovir in the management of herpetic disciform keratitis, *Br J Ophthalmol* 74:283, 1990.

153. Laibson PR: Current therapy of herpes simplex virus infection of the cornea, *Int Ophthalmol Clin* 13:39, 1973.

154. Colin J, Robinet A, Met F: Preventive treatment of herpetic keratitis with acyclovir tablets, *J Fr Ophthalmol* 16:6, 1993.

155. Rice NSC, Jones BR: Problems of corneal grafting in herpetic keratitis. In Corneal graft failure, Ciba Foundation Symposium 15, Amsterdam, 1973, Elsevier.

156. Witmer R: *Results of keratoplasty in metaherpetic keratitis.* In Sundmacher R, editor: *Herpetic eye diseases,* Munich, 1981, Verlag.

157. Langston R, Pavan-Langston D, Dohlman CH: Penetrating keratoplasty for herpetic keratitis, *Trans Am Acad Ophthalmol Otolaryngol* 79:577, 1975.

158. Foster CS, Duncan J: Penetrating keratoplasty for herpes simplex keratitis, *Am J Ophthalmol* 92:336, 1981.

158a. Polack FM, Kaufman HE: Penetrating keratoplasty in herpetic keratitis, *Am J Ophthalmol* 73:908, 1972.

159. Ficker LA et al: Long-term prognosis for corneal grafting in herpes simplex keratitis, *Eye* 2:400, 1988.

160. Cohen E, Laibson P, Arentsen J: Corneal transplantation for herpes simplex keratitis, *Am J Ophthalmol* 95:645, 1983.

161. Lomholt JA, Baggesen K, Ehlers N: Recurrence and rejection rates following corneal transplantation for herpes simplex keratitis, *Acta Ophthalmol Scand* 73:29, 1995.

162. Beyer CF et al: Oral acyclovir reduces the incidence of recurrent herpes simplex keratitis in rabbits after penetrating keratoplasty, *Arch Ophthalmol* 107:1200, 1989.

163. Cobo LM et al: Prognosis and management of corneal transplantation for herpetic keratitis, *Arch Ophthalmol* 98:1755, 1980.

164. Irvine JA, Dunkel EC, Langston DP: Varicella zoster virus (VZV) induced ocular pathology in guinea pig, *Invest Ophthalmol Vis Sci* 29(suppl): 41, 1988.

165. Wigdahl B, Rong BL, Kinney-Thomas E: Varicella-zoster virus infection of human sensory neurons, *Virology* 152:384, 1986.

166. Vafai A et al: Expression of varicella-zoster virus and herpes simplex virus in normal human trigeminal ganglia, *Proc Natl Acad Sci USA* 85:2362, 1988.

167. Mahalingam R et al: Latent varicella-zoster viral DNA in human trigeminal and thoracic ganglia, *N Engl J Med* 323:627, 1990.

168. Croen KD et al: Patterns of gene expression and sites of latency in human nerve ganglia are different for varicella-zoster and herpes simplex virus, *Proc Natl Acad Sci USA* 85:9773, 1988.

169. Straus SE: Clinical and biological differences between recurrent herpes simplex virus and varicella-zoster virus infections, *JAMA* 262:3455, 1989.

170. Kennedy PG, Steiner I: A molecular and cellular model to explain the differences in reactivation from latency by herpes simplex and varicella-zoster viruses, *Neuropathol Appl Neurobiol* 20:368, 1994.

171. Wenkel H et al: Detection of varicella zoster virus DNA and viral antigen in human cornea after herpes zoster ophthalmicus, *Cornea* 12:131, 1993.

172. Charles NC, Bennett TW, Margolis S: Ocular pathology of the congenital varicella syndrome, *Arch Ophthalmol* 95:2034, 1977.

173. De Luise VP, Wilson FM II: *Varicella and herpes zoster ophthalmicus.* In Duane T, Jaeger E, editors: *Clinical ophthalmology,* vol 5, Philadelphia, 1988, Harper & Row.

174. Ostler HB, Thygeson P: The ocular manifestations of herpes zoster, varicella, infectious mononucleosis and cytomegalovirus disease, *Surv Ophthalmol* 21:148, 1976.

175. Duke-Elder S, Leigh AG: *System of ophthalmology*, vol VIII, *Diseases of the outer eye*, St Louis, 1965, Mosby–Year Book.

176. Nesburn AB et al: Varicella dendritic keratitis, *Invest Ophthalmol* 13:764, 1974.

177. Uchida Y, Kaneko M, Hayashi K: Varicella dendritic keratitis, *Am J Ophthalmol* 89:259, 1980.

178. Awan KJ: Corneal complications of varicella, *Pak J Ophthalmol* 1:147, 1985.

179. Wilhelmus KR, Hamill MB, Jones DB: Varicella disciform stromal keratitis, *Am J Ophthalmol* 111:575, 1991.

180. de Freitas D et al: Delayed onset of varicella keratitis, *Cornea* 11:471, 1992.

181. David TJ, Williams ML: Herpes zoster in infancy, *Scand J Infect Dis* 11:185, 1979.

182. Dworsky M, Whitley R, Alford C: Herpes zoster in early infancy, *Am J Dis Child* 134:618, 1980.

183. Baba K et al: Increased incidence of herpes zoster in normal children infected with varicella zoster virus during infancy: community-based follow-up study, *J Pediatr* 108:372, 1986.

184. Brunell PA, Miller LH, Lovejoy F: Zoster in infancy: failure to maintain virus latency following intrauterine infection, *J Pediatr* 98:71, 1981.

185. Sandor EV et al: Herpes zoster ophthalmicus in patients at risk for the acquired immune deficiency syndrome (AIDS), *Am J Ophthalmol* 101:153, 1986.

186. Cole IL et al: Herpes zoster ophthalmicus and the acquired immune deficiency syndrome, *Ophthalmology* 102:1027, 1984.

187. Kestelyn P et al: Severe herpes zoster ophthalmicus in young African adults: a marker for HTLV-III seropositivity, *Br J Ophthalmol* 71:806, 1987.

188. Dolin R et al: Herpes zoster varicella infections in immunosuppressed patients, *Ann Intern Med* 89:375, 1978.

189. Ragossino MW et al: Population-based study of herpes zoster and its sequelae, *Medicine* 61:310, 1982.

190. Guess HA et al: Epidemiology of herpes zoster in children and adolescents: a population-based study, *Pediatrics* 76:512, 1985.

191. Weller TH: Varicella and herpes zoster, *N Engl J Med* 309:1362, 1983.

192. Hedges TR, Albert DM: The progression of the ocular abnormalities of herpes zoster: histopathologic observations of nine cases, *Ophthalmology* 89:165, 1982.

193. Naumann G, Gass JDM, Font RL: Histopathology of herpes zoster ophthalmicus, *Am J Ophthalmol* 65:533, 1968.

194. Lewis G: Zoster sine herpete, *Br Med J* 2:418, 1958.

195. Uchida Y, Kaneko M, Onishi Y: *Ophthalmic herpes zoster without eruption.* In Henkind P, editor: *Acta XXIV International Congress of Ophthalmology*, vol 2, Philadelphia, 1983, JB Lippincott.

196. Ross JVM: Herpes zoster sine eruptione, *Arch Ophthalmol* 42:808, 1949.

197. Harding SP: Management of ophthalmic zoster, *J Med Virol Suppl* 1:97, 1993.

198. Cobo M et al: Observations on the natural history of herpes zoster ophthalmicus, *Curr Eye Res* 6:195, 1987.

199. Edgarton AE: Herpes zoster ophthalmicus: report of cases and review of literature, *Arch Ophthalmol* 34:40, 114, 1945.

200. Duke-Elder S, Leigh AG: *System of ophthalmology*, vol VIII, *Diseases of the outer eye*, St Louis, 1965, Mosby–Year Book.

201. Dugmore W: Intercalary staphyloma in a case of herpes zoster ophthalmicus, *Br J Ophthalmol* 51:350, 1967.

202. Liesegang TJ: Corneal complications of herpes zoster ophthalmicus, *Ophthalmology* 92:316, 1985.

203. Marsh RJ et al: Herpetic epithelial disease, *Arch Ophthalmol* 94:1899, 1976.

204. Piebenga LW, Laibson PR: Dendritic lesions in herpes zoster ophthalmicus, *Arch Ophthalmol* 90:268, 1973.

204a. Sugar HS: Herpetic keratouveitis: clinical experiences, *Ann Ophthalmol* 3:355, 1971.

205. Jones DB: *Herpes zoster ophthalmicus.* In Golden B, editor: *Ocular inflammatory disease*, Springfield, Ill, 1974, Charles C Thomas.

206. Marsh RJ: Herpes zoster keratitis, *Trans Ophthalmol Soc UK* 93:181, 1973.

207. Mondino BJ, Brown SI, Mondzelewski JP: Peripheral corneal ulcers with herpes zoster ophthalmicus, *Am J Ophthalmol* 86:611, 1978.

208. Yu DD et al: Detection of varicella-zoster virus DNA in disciform keratitis using polymerase chain reaction, *Arch Ophthalmol* 111:167, 1993.

209. Marsh RJ, Fraunfelder FT, McGill JI: Herpetic corneal epithelial disease, *Arch Ophthalmol* 94:1899, 1976.

210. Marsh RJ, Easty DL, Jones BR: Iritis and iris atrophy in herpes zoster ophthalmicus, *Am J Ophthalmol* 78:2, 1974.

211. Crock G: Clinical syndromes of anterior segment ischemia, *Trans Ophthalmol Soc UK* 87:513, 1967.

212. Harrison EQ: Complications of herpes zoster ophthalmicus, *Am J Ophthalmol* 60:1111, 1965.

213. Goldsmith MO: Herpes zoster ophthalmicus with sixth nerve palsy, *Can J Ophthalmol* 3:279, 1968.

214. Liesegang T: Diagnosis and therapy of herpes zoster ophthalmicus, *Ophthalmology* 98:1216, 1991.

215. De Clercq E: Oral (E)-5-(2-Bromovinyl)-2-deoxyuridine in severe herpes zoster, *Br Med J* 281:1, 1980.

216. Maudgal P, De Clercq E, Missotten L: Efficacy of bromovinyl-deoxyuridine in the treatment of herpes simplex virus and varicella zoster eye infections, *Antiviral Res* 4:281, 1984.

217. Balfour H et al: Acyclovir halts progression of herpes zoster in immunocompromised patients, *N Engl J Med* 308:1448, 1983.

218. Bean B, Braum C, Balfour H: Acyclovir therapy for acute herpes zoster, *Lancet* 2:118, 1982.
219. Neoh C et al: Comparison of topical and oral acyclovir in early herpes zoster ophthalmicus, *Eye* 8:688, 1994.
220. Aylward G et al: Influence of oral acyclovir on ocular complications of herpes zoster ophthalmicus, *Eye* 8:70, 1994.
221. Wood MJ et al: A randomized trial of acyclovir for 7 days or 21 days with and without prednisolone for treatment of acute herpes zoster, *N Engl J Med* 330:896, 1994.
222. Esman V et al: Prednisolone does not prevent postherpetic neuralgia, *Lancet* 2:126, 1987.
223. Keckes L, Basheer A: Do corticosteroids prevent postherpetic neuralgia?, *Br J Dermatol* 102:551, 1980.
224. Juel-Jensen BE et al: Treatment of zoster with idoxuridine in dimethyl sulfoxide: results of two double-blind controlled trials, *Br Med J* 4:776, 1970.
225. McGill J, Chapman C: A comparison of topical acyclovir with steroids in the treatment of herpes zoster keratouveitis, *Br J Ophthalmol* 67:746, 1983.
226. McGill J, Chapman C, Mahakasingam M: Acyclovir therapy in herpes zoster infection: a practical guide, *Trans Ophthalmol Soc UK* 103:111, 1983.
227. Marsh R, Cooper M: Double masked trial of topical acyclovir and steroids in the treatment of herpes zoster ocular inflammation, *Br J Ophthalmol* 75:542, 1991.
228. Forrest WM, Kaufman HE: Zosteriform herpes simplex, *Am J Ophthalmol* 81:86, 1976.
229. Wilson FM II: *Varicella and herpes zoster ophthalmicus.* In Tabbara KF, Hyndiuk RA, editors: *Infections of the eye,* Boston, 1986, Little, Brown & Co.
230. Berghaust G, Westerby R: Zoster ophthalmicus: local treatment with cortisone, *Acta Ophthalmol* 45:787, 1967.
231. March RJ: Current management of ophthalmic herpes zoster, *Trans Ophthalmol Soc UK* 96:334, 1976.
232. Kernbaum S, Hauchecome J: Administration of levodopa for relief of herpes zoster pain, *JAMA* 246:132, 1981.
233. Mavligit GM, Talpaz M: Cimetidine for herpes zoster, *N Engl J Med* 310:318, 1984.
234. Levy DW, Banerje AK, Glenny HP: Cimetidine in the treatment of herpes zoster, *J Coll Physicians Lond* 19:96, 1985.
235. Bernstein JE et al: Treatment of chronic postherpetic neuralgia with topical capsaicin, *Am Acad Dermatol* 17:93, 1987.
236. Bucci FA, Gabriels CF, Krohel GB: Successful treatment of postherpetic neuralgia with capsaicin, *Am J Ophthalmol* 106:758, 1988.
237. Watson P et al: Therapeutic advances in the management of post-herpetic neuralgia, *Geriatr Med Today* 7:20, 1988.
238. Watson C et al: Amitriptyline vs placebo in post-herpetic neuralgia, *Neurology* 32:671, 1982.
239. Satterwaite J, Tollison C, Kriegel M: Use of tricyclic antidepressants for the treatment of intractable pain, *Compr Ther* 16:10, 1990.
240. Olson ER, Ivy HB: Stellate block for trigeminal zoster, *J Clin Neurol Ophthalmol* 1:53, 1981.
241. Reed JW, Joyner SJ, Knauer WJ: Penetrating keratoplasty for herpes zoster keratopathy, *Am J Ophthalmol* 107:257, 1989.
242. Marsh RJ, Cooper M: Ocular surgery in ophthalmic zoster, *Eye* 3:313, 1989.
243. Gordon YJ, Romanowski E, Araullo-Cruz T: An ocular model of adenovirus type 5 infection in the NZ rabbit, *Invest Ophthalmol Vis Sci* 33:574, 1992.
244. Adenovirus keratoconjunctivitis, *Br J Ophthalmol* 61:73, 1977 (editorial).
245. Ford E, Nelson KE, Warren D: Epidemiology of epidemic keratoconjunctivitis, *Epidemiol Rev* 9:244, 1987.
246. Gigliotti F et al: Etiology of acute conjunctivitis in children, *J Pediatr* 98:531, 1981.
247. Tullo AB, Higgins PG: An outbreak of adenoviral conjunctivitis in Bristol, *Br J Ophthalmol* 63:621, 1979.
248. Petit TH, Holland GN: Chronic keratoconjunctivitis associated with ocular adenovirus infection, *Am J Ophthalmol* 61:73, 1979.
249. Darougar S et al: Epidemic keratoconjunctivitis and chronic papillary conjunctivitis in London due to adenovirus type 19, *Br J Ophthalmol* 61:76, 1977.
250. Sprague JB et al: Epidemic keratoconjunctivitis: a severe industrial outbreak due to adenovirus type 8, *N Engl J Med* 289:1341, 1973.
251. D'Angelo LJ et al: Pharyngoconjunctival fever caused by adenovirus type 4: report of a swimming pool-related outbreak with recovery of virus from pool water, *J Infect Dis* 140:42, 1979.
252. Harnett GB, Newnhamm WA: Isolation of adenovirus type 19 from the male and female genital tracts, *Br J Vener Dis* 57:55, 1981.
253. Nauheim R et al: Survival of adenovirus on various surfaces, *Invest Ophthalmol Vis Sci* 30(suppl):362, 1989.
254. Gordon R et al: Prolonged recovery of desiccated adenovirus 5, 8, and 19 in vitro may partially explain clinical epidemics, *Ophthalmology* 99(suppl):83, 1992.
255. Tullo A: *The adenoviruses.* In Easty DL, editor: *Virus diseases of the eye,* Chicago, 1985, Mosby–Year Book.
256. Dawson CR, Hanna L, Tagni B: Adenovirus type 8 infections in the United States: ten observations on the pathogenesis of lesions in severe eye disease, *Arch Ophthalmol* 87:258, 1972.
257. Hart JCD et al: Epidemic keratoconjunctivitis: a virological and clinical study, *Trans Ophthalmol Soc UK* 92:795, 1972.
258. Hierholzer JC et al: Adenovirus type 19 keratoconjunctivitis, *N Engl J Med* 290:1436, 1974.
259. O'Day DM et al: Clinical and laboratory evaluation of epidemic keratoconjunctivitis due to adenovirus types 8 and 19, *Am J Ophthalmol* 81:207, 1976.

260. Dawson CR et al: Adenovirus type 8 keratoconjunctivitis in the United States, *Am J Ophthalmol* 69:473, 1970.
261. Lund OE, Stefani JF: Corneal histology after epidemic keratoconjunctivitis, *Arch Ophthalmol* 96:2085, 1978.
262. Jones BR: Epidemic hemorrhagic conjunctivitis in London, 1971, *Trans Ophthalmol Soc UK* 92:625, 1972.
263. Bietti GB, Bruna F: Epidemic keratoconjunctivitis in Italy: some contributions to its clinical aspects, epidemiology and etiology, *Am J Ophthalmol* 43:50, 1957.
264. Kimura SJ et al: Sporadic cases of pharyngoconjunctival fever in northern California, *Am J Ophthalmol* 43:14, 1957.
265. Kobayashi TK et al: Cytological evaluation of adenoviral follicular conjunctivitis by cytobrush, *Ophthalmologica* 202:156, 1991.
266. Kowalski RP, Gordon YJ: Comparison of direct rapid tests for the detection of adenovirus antigen in routine conjunctival specimens, *Ophthalmology* 96:1106, 1989.
267. Cleveland PH, Richman DD: Enzyme immunofiltration staining assay for the immediate diagnosis of herpes simplex virus and varicella-zoster virus directly from clinical specimens, *J Clin Microbiol* 25:416, 1987.
268. Kowalski RP, Gordon YJ: Comparison of direct rapid tests for the detection of adenovirus antigen in routine conjunctival specimens, *Ophthalmology* 96:1106, 1989.
269. Kinchington PR et al: Use of polymerase chain amplification reaction for the detection of adenoviruses in ocular swab specimens, *Invest Ophthalmol Vis Sci* 35:4126, 1994.
270. Ward JB, Siojo LG, Waller SG: A prospective, masked clinical trial of trifluridine, dexamethasone and artificial tears in the treatment of epidemic keratoconjunctivitis, *Cornea* 12:216, 1993.
271. Cook SD: Antiviral agents for ocular adenovirus infections, *Eye* 7(suppl):18, 1993.
272. Gordon YJ: *Adenovirus and other nonherpetic viral diseases.* In Smolin G, Thoft RA, editors: *The cornea: scientific foundations and clinical practice,* Boston, 1994, Little, Brown, & Co.
273. Gordon YJ, Romanowski EG, Araullo-Cruz T: Topical HPMPC inhibits adenovirus type 5 in the New Zealand rabbit ocular replication model, *Invest Ophthalmol Vis Sci* 35:4135, 1994.
274. Librach IM: Ocular symptoms in glandular fever, *Br J Ophthalmol* 40:619, 1956.
275. Gardner BP, Margolis TP, Mondino BJ: Conjunctival lymphocytic nodule associated with the Epstein-Barr virus, *Am J Ophthalmol* 112:567, 1991.
276. Wilhelmus KR: Ocular involvement in infectious mononucleosis, *Am J Ophthalmol* 91:117, 1981.
277. Pinnolis M, McCulley JP, Urman JD: Keratitis associated with infectious mononucleosis, *Am J Ophthalmol* 89:791, 1980.
278. Matoba AY, Wilhelmus KR, Jones DB: Epstein-Barr viral stromal keratitis, *Ophthalmology* 93:746, 1986.
279. Palay DA, Litoff D, Krachmer JH: Stromal keratitis associated with Epstein-Barr virus infection in a young child, *Arch Ophthalmol* 111:1323, 1993.
280. Piel JJ, Thelander HE, Shur EB: Infectious mononucleosis of the central nervous system with bilateral papilledema, *J Pediatr* 37:661, 1950.
281. Tanner OR: Ocular manifestations infectious mononucleosis, *Arch Ophthalmol* 51:229, 1954.
282. Hales RH, Ostler BH: Newcastle disease conjunctivitis with subepithelial infiltrates, *Br J Ophthalmol* 57:694, 1973.
283. Higgins PG: *Acute hemorrhagic conjunctivitis.* In Easty DL, editor: *Virus disease of the eye,* Chicago, 1985, Mosby–Year Book.
284. Yin-Murphy M et al: A recent epidemic of acute hemorrhagic conjunctivitis, *Am J Ophthalmol* 116:212, 1993.
285. Hara E et al: Survival and disinfection of adenovirus type 19 and enterovirus 70 in ophthalmic practice, *Jpn J Ophthalmol* 34:421, 1990.
286. Aoki K, Sawada H: Long-term observation of neutralization antibody after enterovirus 70 infection, *Jpn J Ophthalmol* 36:465, 1992.
287. Bern C et al: Acute hemorrhagic conjunctivitis due to enterovirus 70 in American Samoa: serum-neutralizing antibodies and sex-specific protection, *Am J Epidemiol* 136:1502, 1992.
288. Yang YF et al: Epidemic hemorrhagic keratoconjunctivitis, *Am J Ophthalmol* 80:192, 1975.
289. Kono R et al: Neurologic complications associated with acute hemorrhagic conjunctivitis virus infection and its serologic complication, *J Infect Dis* 129:590, 1974.
290. Whitcher JP et al: Acute hemorrhagic conjunctivitis in Tunisia, *Arch Ophthalmol* 94:51, 1976.
291. Wolken SH: Acute hemorrhagic conjunctivitis, *Surv Ophthalmol* 19:71, 1974.
292. Sklar VEF et al: Clinical findings and results of treatment in an outbreak of acute hemorrhagic conjunctivitis in southern Florida, *Am J Ophthalmol* 95:45, 1983.
293. Garau J et al: Spontaneous cytomegalovirus mononucleosis with conjunctivitis, *Arch Intern Med* 137:1631, 1977.
294. Danielson RW, Long JC: Keratitis due to mumps, *Arch Ophthalmol* 24:655, 1941.
295. Riffenburgh RS: Ocular manifestations of mumps, *Arch Ophthalmol* 66:739, 1961.
296. Mickatavage R, Amadur J: A case report of mumps keratitis, *Arch Ophthalmol* 69:758, 1963.
297. Sandford-Smith JH, Whittle H: Corneal ulceration following measles in Nigerian children, *Br J Ophthalmol* 63:720, 1983.
298. Foster A, Sommer A: Childhood blindness from corneal ulceration in Africa: causes, presentation and treatment, *Bull World Health Organ* 64:619, 1986.

299. Dekkers NWHM: *The cornea in measles*, The Hague, 1981, Dr W Junk Publishers.

300. Ellis P, Winograd LA: Ocular vaccinia: a specific treatment, *Arch Ophthalmol* 68:600, 1962.

301. Petit TH: The poxviruses: vaccinia and variola, *Int Opthalmol Clin* 15:203, 1975.

302. Ruben FL, Lane MJ: Ocular vaccinia: an epidemiologic analysis of 348 cases, *Arch Ophthalmol* 84:45, 1970.

303. Boger WP, Peterson RA, Robb RM: Keratoconus and acute hydrops in mentally retarded patients with congenital rubella syndrome, *Am J Ophthalmol* 91:231, 1981.

304. Hara J et al: Ocular manifestations of the 1976 rubella epidemic in Japan, *Am J Ophthalmol* 87:642, 1979.

305. Dimmer F: A type of corneal inflammation closely related to keratitis nummularis, *Z Augenheilkd* 13:621, 1905.

306. Pillat A: The differential diagnosis of nummular keratitis (Dimmer) and epidemic keratoconjunctivitis, *Am J Ophthalmol* 43:58, 1957.

307. Valenton MJ: Deep stromal involvement in Dimmer's nummular keratitis, *Am J Ophthalmol* 78:897, 1974.

307a. Duke-Elder S, Leigh AG: *System of ophthalmology,* vol VIII, *Diseases of the outer eye,* St Louis, 1965, Mosby–Year Book.

308. Thygeson P: Superficial punctate keratitis, *JAMA* 144:1544, 1950.

309. Thygeson P: Further observations on superficial punctate keratitis, *Arch Ophthalmol* 66:158, 1962.

310. Thygeson P: Clinical and laboratory observation on superficial punctate keratitis, *Am J Ophthalmol* 61:1344, 1966.

311. Tabbara KF et al: Thygeson's superficial punctate keratitis, *Ophthalmology* 88:75, 1981.

312. Darrell RW: Thygeson's superficial punctate keratitis: natural history and association with HLA DR3, *Trans Am Ophthalmol Soc* 79:486, 1981.

313. Forstot SL, Bender PS: Treatment of Thygeson's superficial punctate keratopathy with soft contact lenses, *Am J Ophthalmol* 88:186, 1979.

314. Goldberg DB, Schanzlin DJ, Brown SI: Management of Thygeson's superficial punctate keratitis, *Am J Ophthalmol* 89:22, 1980.

315. Braley AEK, Alexander RC: Superficial punctate keratitis: isolation of a virus, *Arch Ophthalmol* 50:147, 1953.

316. Lemp MA, Chambers RW, Lurdy J: Viral isolation in superficial punctate keratitis, *Arch Ophthalmol* 91:8, 1974.

Thirteen

Blepharitis

The term *blepharitis* encompasses a common yet not well-understood group of diseases. Clinically these diseases have been divided into those that affect mainly the base of the lashes (anterior blepharitis) and those that primarily affect the meibomian glands (posterior blepharitis) (Table 13-1). This division is somewhat artificial in that signs of both types of blepharitis are frequently present, and the nature of their interrelation is obscure.

ANTERIOR LID MARGIN

Anterior blepharitis is a very common disease and often a difficult problem for both the physician and the patient. It is characterized by the accumulation of material around the base of the lashes and erythema of the anterior lid margin. The most common types of anterior blepharitis are the staphylococcal and seborrheic varieties. These are defined clinically; their relationship to staphylococcal infection and seborrhea (overaction of sebaceous glands) is inconsistent.

Staphylococcal Blepharitis
Clinical Manifestations
Patients with staphylococcal blepharitis may be asymptomatic or may report burning, itching, and irritation, which frequently are worse in the morning.[1-3] Hard, brittle, fibrinous scales are commonly seen at the base of the lashes. Scales that encircle the lash are known as *collarettes*. These collarettes are thought to be formed by fibrin exudation from the ulcerated skin at the base of the cilia. As the lash grows, it carries the fibrin out from the lid margin. Less commonly, matted, hard crusts surround the individual cilium (Fig. 13-1). When these crusts are removed, small ulcers of the hair follicles can be seen, and bleeding may occur. Blood vessels on the lid margins may be dilated, and there may be thinning or loss of the lashes (*madarosis*) (Fig. 13-2), white lashes (*poliosis*), misdirected lashes (*trichiasis*), broken lashes, or irregularity of the lid margin (*tylosis*). Folliculitis can be seen as a small pustule surrounding an eyelash.

Seborrheic blepharitis, which is described later in this chapter, is often present, but mei-

Table 13-1 Common Types of Blepharitis				
Feature	Staphylococcal	Seborrheic	Meibomitis	Moraxella
Scales	Hard, brittle tenacious	Greasy, easily removed	Greasy	Macerated epithelium, minimal scaling
Meibomian glands	—	Meibomian abnormalities common	Inspissated plugs, pouting orifices	—
Associated forms of blepharitis	Seborrheic common	Staphylococcal and meibomitis	Seborrheic common	—
Associated skin disease	Seborrheic dermatitis (10%)	Seborrheic dermatitis (100%)	Acne rosacea (two thirds), seborrheic dermatitis (one third)	Occasionally
Bilateral or unilateral	May be unilateral, especially early	Bilateral	Bilateral	Often unilateral
Ulceration	Yes	No	No	No
Keratitis	SPK* (most); marginal infiltrates, phlyctenules	SPK (occasional)	SPK (common), rapid tear breakup time	Marginal infiltrates, occasionally ulcers
Keratitis sicca	50%	33%	33%	—
Hordeola	Frequent	Rare	Common	No
Lash abnormalities	Madarosis, poliosis	No	No	No
Conjunctivitis (injection, papillary response)	Common	Occasional	Common	Always, may be follicular
Treatment	Lid hygiene, topical antibiotics	Lid hygiene, treat dermatitis	Lid hygiene, expression, systemic antibiotics	Topical antibiotics

*Superficial punctate keratopathy.

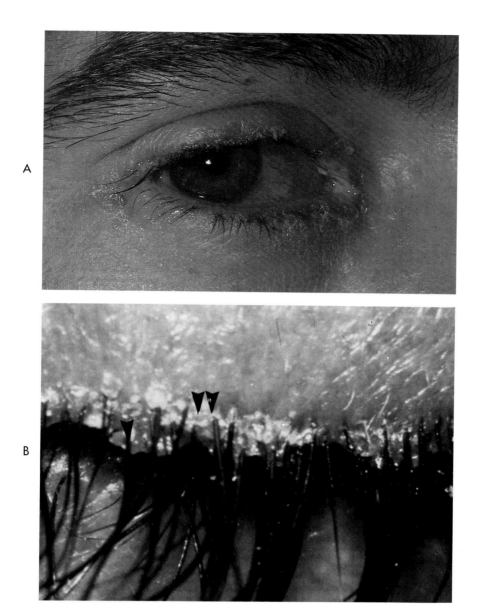

Figure 13-1
A, Ulcerative blepharitis with conspicuous crusting of the lid margin. **B,** When the crust was removed, a bleeding area was visible (*double arrow*). Collarette formation (*single arrow*) can be seen around a cilium.

bomian gland dysfunction is not usually seen. A chronic papillary conjunctivitis also is often present, and this may be accompanied by mucopurulent (predominantly polymorphonuclear) exudate. The conjunctivitis is typically worse in the morning. Hordeola, both external and internal, can accompany the blepharitis. Corneal complications are common, including punctate keratopathy, catarrhal infiltrates, phlyctenules, ulceration, and pannus forma-

tion. The punctate keratopathy predominantly affects the inferior third of the cornea and consists of fine, flat lesions that are regular in shape and may stain with fluorescein or rose bengal. Catarrhal infiltrates and phlyctenules are discussed in Chapter 19.

Pathogenesis
The relationship between staphylococcal blepharitis and *Staphylococcus aureus* infection

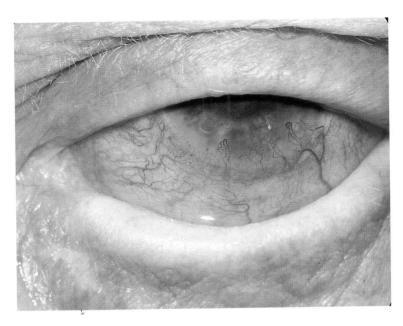

Figure 13-2
Loss of cilia after staphylococcal blepharitis.

is unclear. Staphylococci are common on unaffected lids; non-*aureus* staphylococci can be isolated from 90% to 95% of normal lids, and *S. aureus* from 10% to 35%.[4-6] In patients with signs of staphylococcal blepharitis, *S. aureus* is isolated from the lid margin significantly more often, but still only half of the time or less. Non-*aureus* staphylococci and *Propionibacterium acnes* are isolated in nearly all cases, significantly more often than in patients without blepharitis, and the quantity of bacteria present is greater than in control patients.[4,7,8] *Staphylococcus epidermidis* or other non-*aureus* species may be able to produce the same clinical disease as *S. aureus*. Some researchers have attempted to differentiate the *S. epidermidis* strains found on the lids of patients with blepharitis from those strains found on unaffected lids, but the results have not been very illuminating.[9,10]

The role of staphylococci is suggested by several findings: In 1937 both Allen[11] and Thygeson[12] demonstrated that topical application of a filtrate prepared from a culture of *S. aureus* produced a toxic type of conjunctivitis and keratitis in human volunteers. Later, a filtrate prepared from *S. epidermidis* was also found capable of producing toxic conjunctivitis.[13] Staphylococci produce many enzymes and toxins that may injure the ocular surface. Alpha-toxin, also known as dermonecrotic factor, was suggested by Thygeson to be the one most responsible for such injury. Alpha-toxin appears to increase cell membrane permeability, and it may be responsible for the inferior punctate keratitis seen in affected eyes. Alpha-toxin is produced only by *S. aureus*. Other toxins such as beta-toxin (beta-hemolysin), gamma-toxin, delta-toxin, exfoliative toxin (responsible for signs of toxic epidermal necrolysis), and toxic shock syndrome toxin-1 are elaborated by some staphylococcal strains, and these may play a role in blepharoconjunctivitis.[14] In addition, enzymes such as lysozyme, lipase, fatty wax esterase, and cholesterol esterase can be produced by both *S. aureus* and *S. epidermidis*; these enzymes may alter the ocular flora and meibomian secretions.

In the past, *Pityrosporum ovale* and *Demodex folliculorum* were thought to play a role in staphylococcal blepharitis, but this now seems not to be true. *D. folliculorum* is a microscopic, eight-legged, transparent mite (Fig. 13-3) that commonly infests humans and lives in sebaceous follicles. It covers the base of the lash with a tubular sleeve (Fig. 13-4), and waxy debris forms cuffs around the lashes. Because bacteria are found on *D. folliculorum* bodies, it is possible that the mite serves as a vector for staphylococcal infection.[15-17] The diagnosis of *D. folliculorum* infection can be made by extracting the lash and suspending it in viscous fluid; examination of the base will reveal the mite clinging to the lash. McCulley et al.[7] ex-

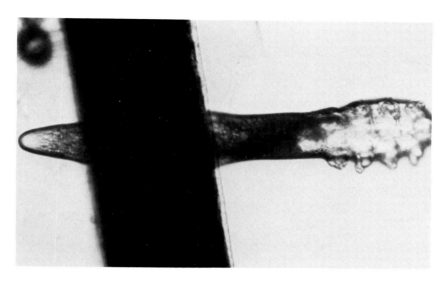

Figure 13-3
Demodex folliculorum.

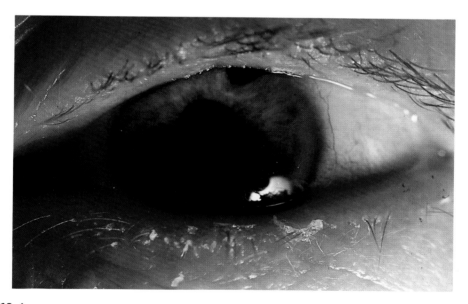

Figure 13-4
Cuffing of the base of a cilium, as seen in an infection of the lid margin caused by *Demodex folliculorum.*

amined lashes from patients in this manner and found *Demodex* in approximately equal frequency in controls and in patients with blepharitis. However, in another study facial mite counts were significantly greater in patients with rosacea than in controls.[18]

Differential Diagnosis

One of the complications of chronic blepharitis is poliosis, a sign also seen in Vogt-Koyanagi-Harada, Waardenburg's, and Behçet's syndromes. Loss of lashes is also seen in trichotillomania (a compulsion to pull out one's own hair) (Fig. 13-5). Patients will often report pull-

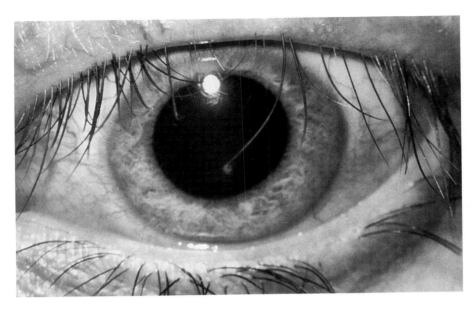

Figure 13-5
Loss of central lashes from trichotillomania. (Courtesy of Robert D. Deitch Jr., Indianapolis, IN.)

ing of lashes, but in many cases the act is unconscious. A combination of behavior therapy and treatment with clomipramine has been reported to be effective.[19]

Staphylococcal blepharitis must be differentiated from dry eyes, although the two conditions frequently occur in the same eye. The corneal staining in staphylococcal blepharitis usually involves the lower third of the cornea, but keratitis sicca is associated with diffuse stain in the interpalpebral zone. Filaments are not usually seen in staphylococcal blepharitis, but they may be seen in dry eye. If the diagnosis is uncertain, Schirmer's testing should be performed.

Treatment

Blepharitis can be very difficult to eradicate; often the disease persists throughout the patient's life. The patient's understanding of the chronic nature of the disease is crucial to its management. However, blepharitis can usually be controlled with a combination of lid hygiene and antibiotic application. The lids can be washed with diluted baby shampoo (one-half or one-third strength) for approximately 1 minute using a cotton swab, cottonball, washcloth, or the tip of the finger. Recently, commercially prepared kits (such as EV Care and EV Lid Cleanser II, Eagle Vision, Memphis, TN; OCuSOFT Lid Scrub, OCuSOFT, Richmond, TX) have become available for this purpose, and they may be superior. Initially the routine is performed twice

daily; after 1 month the frequency is decreased to once daily and continued indefinitely.

Antibiotic ointments also seem to be helpful and can be applied up to four times daily. Erythromycin and bacitracin are the most commonly used antibiotics, but gentamicin can also be used. (Approximately 50% of *S. aureus* isolated from the lids of patients with staphylococcal blepharitis are resistant to sulfonamides, so those drugs should not be used unless sensitivity testing has been performed.) Infection of the meibomian, sweat, and sebaceous glands of the cilia follicles may play a role in the resistance to therapy, because it is difficult or impossible to obtain a therapeutic concentration of any antibiotic in these structures. In resistant cases or cases associated with catarrhal infiltrates or phlyctenulosis, cultures of the lid margin should be performed to direct antibiotic treatment and monitor staphylococcal colonization. I usually instruct patients to apply the antibiotic ointment twice daily, after scrubbing, for 1 month, then to decrease applications to once daily for another month. In most cases this is sufficient. If exacerbations occur, repeat cultures might be advisable to detect colonization by new bacteria.

If lid and conjunctival redness or keratitis persist despite these measures, topical steroids can be used. These can relieve the signs and symptoms of inflammation but should be used cautiously. Applying the ointment to the lids twice daily for 1 to 2 weeks is usually sufficient.

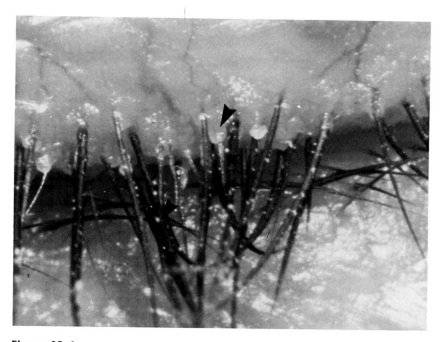

Figure 13-6
Sebaceous blepharitis (*single arrow*). Scales adhere to the side of a cilium (*double arrow*).

When treating pediculi, the nits should be removed manually and the adult organism should be suffocated by applying petroleum jelly. The treatment of catarrhal ulcers and phlyctenules is discussed in Chapter 19.

It is important to realize the difficulties in treating staphylococcal blepharokeratoconjunctivitis. Treatment may have to be continued for a long period, and the patient must understand the chronic nature of the disease. In addition, the physician must recognize the atypical forms of the disease, the different types of corneal involvement, and how tear dysfunction and immunologic complications influence the disease.

Seborrheic Blepharitis

Patients with seborrheic blepharitis complain mainly of burning and itching in the eye. They tend to be older than patients with staphylococcal blepharitis and often have had symptoms for many years.

Large, yellow, greasy scales are seen loosely attached to the side of the cilia (Fig. 13-6). Crusting is present on the lashes and lids (*scurf*), and the lid margins are often red. Staphylococcal blepharitis, meibomian seborrhea, and meibomitis also may be present.[7] Approximately 15% of patients also have corneal involvement, a punctate keratopathy that is found either in the interpalpebral space or over the lower third of the cornea.

Nearly all patients have seborrheic dermatitis, but it is usually mild and is easily overlooked.[5,20] Seborrheic dermatitis is seen as greasy scales over an erythematous patch of skin. The scalp, eyebrows, eyelids, nasolabial folds, and retroauricular or sternal skin may be involved.

Dysfunction of the sebaceous glands is thought to be the cause of seborrheic blepharitis, but the pathogenesis of the clinical findings is unclear. *P. ovale*, a yeast, is seen frequently on scrapings, but its significance is unknown.

This disease also tends to be chronic and incurable, and it is important for the patient to understand this. Treatment consists mainly of lid hygiene, as described for staphylococcal blepharitis. If meibomitis is present, warm compresses, expression of meibomian glands, and oral antibiotics may be helpful. Associated dermatologic abnormalities should be recognized and treated in conjunction with a dermatologist.

Symptoms usually improve over 1 to 2 months, and they then can be controlled with daily scrubs. However, prolonged use of hot compresses, lid massage, and oral antibiotics may be necessary.

POSTERIOR LID MARGIN

The role of meibomian gland dysfunction in blepharitis and blepharoconjunctivitis has not been sufficiently appreciated in the past. McCulley et al., who helped draw attention to meibomian gland dysfunction, has divided the disorder into several types: meibomian seborrhea, primary meibomitis, and secondary meibomitis associated with seborrheic blepharitis.[7,20]

Clinical Manifestations

Meibomian seborrhea is excessive meibomian secretion in the absence of inflammatory signs. The symptoms, mainly a burning feeling in the eye, tend to be more prominent than the signs. The meibomian glands are dilated and easily expressed, releasing large amounts of clear fluid. Excessive foam is often present in the tear film. The orifices are not plugged with inspissated secretions. Meibomian seborrhea is usually seen in conjunction with mild seborrheic blepharitis.

Primary meibomitis is characterized by inflammation around the meibomian gland orifices, pouting of the gland orifices, and solidification of meibomian secretions (Fig. 13-7). The symptoms include burning, tearing, itching, dryness, irritation, and photophobia. The most prominent feature is stagnation of the meibomian gland secretions. This is manifest as dilation of the glands and inspissation of the secretions. The dilated glands can be seen through the tarsal conjunctiva with the aid of a slit-lamp microscope, and the inspissated secretions are oily and often semisolid or yellow. Expression of the secretions is more difficult and often preceded by extrusion of an inspissated plug.

Hyperemia, thickening, and an irregularity of contour (tylosis) may affect the posterior lid margin. Chalazia, tarsitis, or nodules may be seen on the posterior lid; occasionally, the Zeis glands become inflamed. Foamy tears can accumulate in the canthi, or a thick greasy film may be noted. The foam appears to arise from agitation of the oily secretions by blinking. The tear breakup time is reduced. Papillary conjunctivitis and interpalpebral superficial punctate keratopathy are often present.

In the secondary form, which is associated with seborrheic blepharitis, the meibomitis is spotty, with scattered glands or clusters of glands affected. Otherwise the findings are similar.

Virtually all patients with meibomian gland dysfunction have evidence of sebaceous gland dysfunction elsewhere, but it is often subtle. When seborrheic blepharitis is more prominent, seborrheic dermatitis is nearly always present; but when meibomitis is dominant, approximately two thirds of patients have acne rosacea and only one third have seborrheic dermatitis. Acne rosacea may give rise to erythema, telangiectasia, papules, follicular pus-

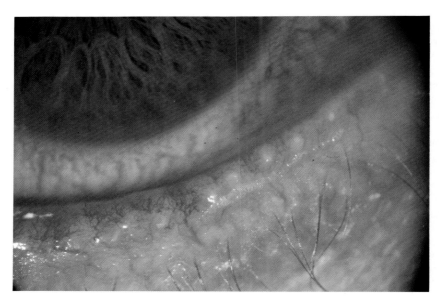

Figure 13-7
Meibomitis, with erythema of the lid margin and inspissation of secretions in the gland orifices.

tules, and hypertrophic sebaceous glands. These signs are found on the forehead, nose, and cheeks (see Chapter 22).

Pathogenesis

Meibomitis does not appear to be related to bacterial infection. No bacteria have been isolated with greater than normal frequency. The role of *Pityrosporum* infection is unclear. Seborrhea responds to antifungal agents, and *P. ovale* in patients with AIDS seborrhea appears to be aggravated by overgrowth of *P. ovale*. However, topical ketoconazole was not significantly more effective than placebo in improving the symptoms and signs of seborrheic blepharitis, despite significantly reducing *Pityrosporum* numbers.[21] The superficial punctate keratopathy looks like that seen in conditions with an unstable tear film, not like that described as secondary to staphylococcus toxin or with anterior blepharitis.[11] An unstable tear film in patients with meibomian keratoconjunctivitis can account for the keratopathy without necessitating the presence of a bacterial exotoxin; however, this may be only one of several pathways involved.

Loss of meibomian glands and stagnation of the gland secretions, which produce the lipid layer of the tear film, may account for the tear film instability.[22] In accordance with this, stabilization of the tear film occurs when fresh secretions from deep within the glands are added by expressing them into the tear film.[23] Also, increased evaporation of tears is seen in patients with meibomian gland dropout.[24]

The observed instability does not appear to be caused by a quantitative decrease in the tear lipid layer, but there may be a qualitative abnormality. Strains of *S. epidermidis* isolated from patients with meibomian gland dysfunction have significantly greater lipase activity than strains from normal eyes,[25] and increased breakdown of lipids into free fatty acids could destabilize the tear film. Previous experiments did not find a biochemical abnormality in secretions from these patients,[26-28] but more recent studies have found significant differences. While normal control subjects may or may not have significant amounts of cholesterol esters in their meibomian gland secretions, all disease groups' secretions contain cholesterol esters.[29] The presence of cholesterol esters stimulates growth of *S. aureus*.[30] Control patients with cholesterol esters and patients with meibomian disease have high levels of unsaturated fatty acids and unsaturated ester fatty alcohols.[31]

The consistent finding of more generalized sebaceous gland dysfunction (the meibomian gland is a specialized sebaceous gland) suggests that these patients have a systemic predisposition to disease in these glands.

Treatment

Like anterior blepharitis, meibomitis is a chronic disease that can be controlled but not cured. Helpful measures include hot compresses, lid massage, lid scrubs, and systemic antibiotics. Hot compresses are applied to the lids for 5 to 10 minutes up to four times daily. Massaging the lids helps express meibomian secretions, relieving stagnation. Systemic tetracycline is usually very effective, both for the meibomitis and for acne rosacea, if present. The initial dose is 250 mg orally four times daily. The drug should be taken on an empty stomach and should not be given to pregnant women or to children under 8 years of age. The mechanism of the beneficial effect is unknown. Most of the staphylococci in patients with chronic blepharitis are resistant to tetracycline. It has been proposed that tetracycline stabilizes the lipid secretions by inhibiting bacterial enzymes.[28] Tetracycline reduces lipase production by *S. epidermidis* and *S. aureus,* including strains resistant to the drug.[32] In a comparison of doxycycline and tetracycline in patients with ocular involvement of acne rosacea, doxycycline (100 mg/day) was significantly less effective than tetracycline in relieving symptoms after 6 weeks of treatment, but after 3 months of treatment there were no significant differences.[33] In patients sensitive to tetracycline, erythromycin, or trimethoprim-sulfamethoxazole can be used.

The value of topical antibiotics is not as clear, but erythromycin, tetracycline, or bacitracin can be used. Topical steroids probably have no benefit.

HORDEOLA

A *hordeolum,* commonly known as a sty, is an acute, suppurative, nodular inflammation of the lid margin. Hordeola may affect primarily the internal (posterior) portion of the lid, when they arise from the meibomian glands, or the external portion (anterior), when they arise from the Zeis glands, sweat glands, or hair follicles (Fig. 13-8). Hordeola often are infectious, most commonly staphylococcal, but they may be sterile acute inflammations in obstructed glands. They often are associated with blepharitis.

Hordeola can rupture spontaneously or resolve slowly. They are treated with hot com-

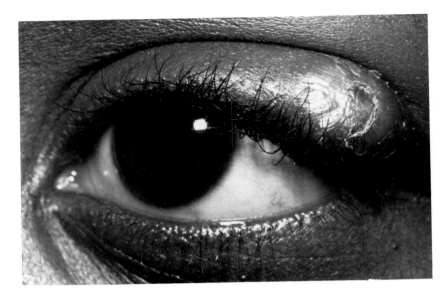

Figure 13-8
External hordeolum (sty).

presses and topical antibiotics. If these measures do not succeed, incision and drainage can be performed. Associated blepharitis should also be treated.

CHALAZIA

A *chalazion* is a sterile, chronic nodular inflammation of a Zeis or meibomian gland. It is a granulomatous reaction to sebaceous material that has been extruded from a plugged gland into the surrounding tissue. It may be insidious in onset or develop acutely and be indistinguishable from a hordeolum. Recently, chronic chalazia were found to be associated with hypercholesterolemia in some patients, and lowering serum cholesterol decreased their occurrence.[34]

Hot compresses may be beneficial. The chalazia can be incised and curetted or left alone. Injection of corticosteroid (approximately 0.1 ml triamcinolone 5 mg/ml) may be of benefit.[35,36]

OTHER CAUSES OF MARGINAL LID INFLAMMATION

Bacterial

Angular blepharitis often is associated with a *Moraxella* infection. The lateral lid margins are wet, macerated, and may be ulcerated (see Fig. 7-10). The blepharitis is usually bilateral, and conjunctivitis is also present. The gram-negative diplobacillus can be identified on smears. *Moraxella* are sensitive to most antibiotics, and the infection responds rapidly to lid scrubs and antibiotic ointment.

Diphtheria blepharitis usually occurs in association with membranous conjunctivitis but can occur as a primary lid infection. It can follow an abrasion, in which case it appears as a moist, eczematoid lesion interspersed with hypertrophic inflammatory areas.[32] It can also begin as a clear vesicle that quickly breaks down to form a central grayish indolent ulcer.

Pseudomonas, coliforms, and *Proteus* are rare causes of blepharitis, mainly in immunosuppressed patients. The eyelids can be involved in both acquired and congenital syphilis. A primary syphilitic lesion (chancre) can occur on the eyelids, usually as a single lesion at the lower lid margin or the inner canthus. A small red papule develops about 3 weeks after inoculation and gradually enlarges and develops central erosion. The edges are rounded and firm, and the base is smooth. If the lid margin is involved, ulceration and tarsal and conjunctival involvement are seen.[38] Painless lymphadenopathy develops 1 to 2 weeks after the chancre appears. Healing occurs over 3 to 6 weeks and can leave scarring, deformity, and madarosis.

In secondary syphilis the lids can be affected by a generalized macular or papular rash, annular skin lesions (syphilids), ulcerative blepharitis, and temporary loss of lashes. Condyloma lata, which are highly infectious lesions, appear

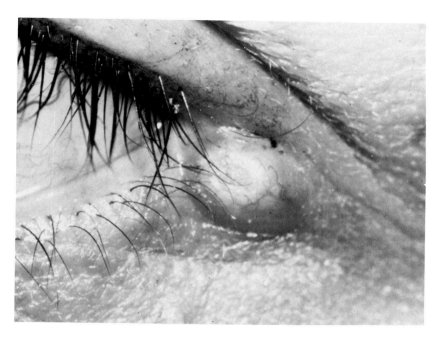

Figure 13-9
Molluscum contagiosum lid lesion.

as flat-topped papules or elevated plaques at the inner canthus. In late benign syphilis gummas can affect the lid. They are usually solitary and are characterized by swelling and infiltration eventually leading to ulceration and local destruction. A papular lid rash, ulceration, lid margin deformity, and lid gummas can also occur in congenital syphilis.

Nodular thickening of the tarsal lid, suggesting multiple chalazia, can occur in lepromatous leprosy.[39] Loss of lashes is common. *Actinomyces,* streptococcal impetigo, and erysipelas can involve the lid by spread of infection from other parts of the face. Other bacteria that can cause lid infection include tuberculosis, psoriasis, yaws, pinta, tetanus, chancroid, glanders, tularemia, anthrax, and *Spirillum minus* (rat-bite fever).

Viral

Marginal lid ulcers may be caused by vaccinia virus and other poxviruses, as well as by herpesvirus. If these viruses are suspected, other skin lesions should be sought and scrapings and cultures of the lid lesions performed.

Herpes simplex can cause a marginal vesicular and ulcerative blepharitis, most commonly in the primary infection. In addition, grouped lesions can occur on the anterior surface of the lids, either in primary or recurrent infection. The lesions begin as clear vesicles on an erythematous base and then open, ulcerate, crust over, and heal, without scarring, over 7 to 14 days (see Fig. 12-3). Scrapings of the base of a lesion may demonstrate multinucleated giant cells or intranuclear inclusions. If there is no associated keratitis, no treatment is necessary, but I commonly prescribe prophylactic antiviral medication (idoxuridine or vidarabine ointment) if the lid margin is involved. Topical acyclovir may speed healing, but it is available only as a dermatologic preparation, and its safety around the eye is unknown. Systemic acyclovir can be considered in severe cases.

Molluscum contagiosum is a poxvirus that commonly infects the lid margins. It occurs most often in adolescents and young adults and is spread by close contact, including sexual contact. In AIDS patients the lesions can be larger and more numerous.[40,41] The molluscum nodule is a pearly white, raised, round, noninflamed lesion with a craterous center. It may be obvious (Fig. 13-9) or subtle (Fig. 13-10). Conjunctival lesions can also occur and are seen as small, white pimples containing caseous material on an erythematous base. Chronic follicular conjunctivitis can occur. In longstanding cases superior micropannus and fine epithelial keratitis can affect the superior cornea, simulating trachoma (Fig. 13-11). A scraping of the conjunctiva reveals mononuclear cells. Molluscum bodies are seen in microscopic sections of the lesion (Figs. 13-12 and 13-13). Treatment is by surgical excision. Hyperfocal cryotherapy

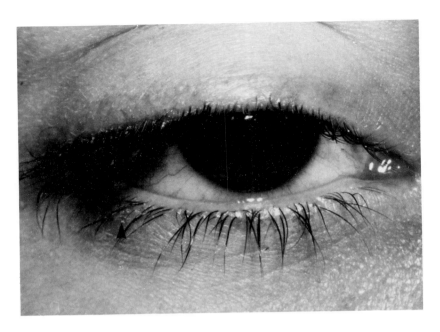

Figure 13-10
Inconspicuous *Molluscum contagiosum* lesion, hidden by cilia (*arrow*), which causes persistent injection of the eye with follicular conjunctivitis.

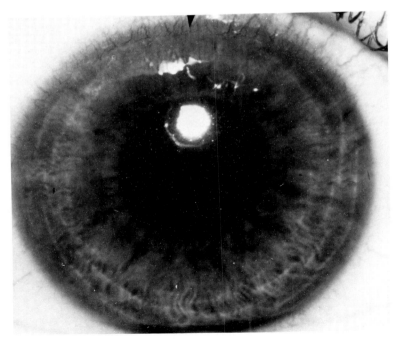

Figure 13-11
Left untreated, a *Molluscum contagiosum* infection can cause pannus (*arrow*).

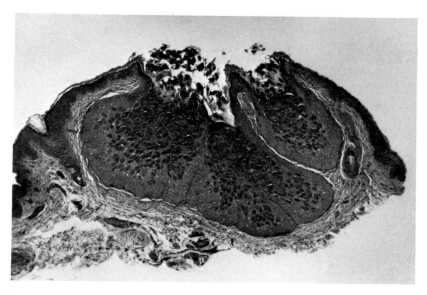

Figure 13-12
A skin lesion caused by *Molluscum contagiosum* with typical cytoplasmic inclusions (H & E, X100) (Courtesy of Bruce L. Johnson, Pittsburgh, PA.)

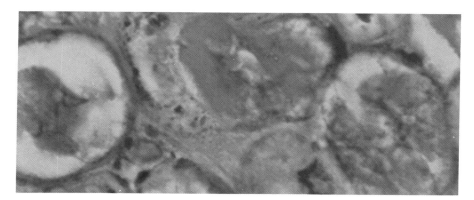

Figure 13-13
Higher magnification of *Molluscum* bodies.

has been reported to be an effective therapy for multiple *Molluscum* lesions in AIDS patients.[42]

Orf, another poxvirus, causes pustular dermatitis in sheep and goats and can cause lid lesions in humans. The lesions begin as an indurated, painless, pruritic dark red papule that gradually enlarges and develops an umbilicated center.[43] Healing with scarring occurs in about 5 weeks.

Verrucae are pedunculated or sessile multilobular lesions caused by papovavirus. When located on the lid margin or conjunctiva, they can cause a mild papillary conjunctivitis or fine epithelial keratitis. A mononuclear response is seen in conjunctival scrapings.

Fungal

Candidal blepharitis resembles staphylococcal blepharitis. Lid erythema, discharge, marginal ulcerations, collarettes, broken lashes, and loss of lashes can be present. Small granulomas can be found near the lash follicle orifices in some patients, and these suggest the diagnosis. Vesicles that progress to pustules and lesions simulating those seen in ringworm infection can be seen.[44] The latter begin as reddish papules that spread peripherally while healing centrally. The central area is scaly, and the margin is sharply defined, slightly elevated, and scaly or vesicular. Many patients with atopic dermatitis and blepharitis have an ulcerative form of blepharitis, and most of these have *Candida* infection.[45]

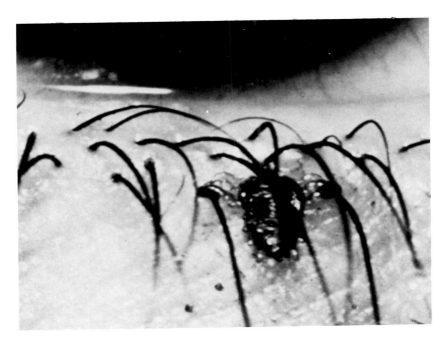

Figure 13-14
Pediculosis (*Phthirus pubis*). The parasite suspends itself between two cilia.

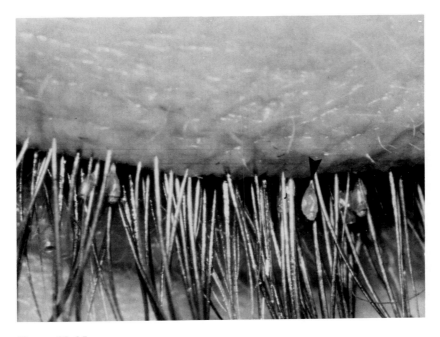

Figure 13-15
Nits (*arrow*).

Other fungi can affect the eyelids, including dermatophytosis, sporotrichosis, blastomycosis, aspergillosis, and rhinosporidiosis.

Others

Phthiriasis palpebrum is an uncommon cause of blepharitis and conjunctivitis and can easily be overlooked.[46] Pubic lice (*Phthirus pubis*) have a predilection for lashes as well pubic hairs because of the appropriate spacing of the cilia (Fig. 13-14). With palpebral phthiriasis, a severe blepharoconjunctivitis can be seen, particularly in children. Symptoms include itching, irritation, and redness of the lid margins as well as conjunctiva. A high index of suspicion and careful examination of the patient's lid margins and eyelashes lead to the proper diagnosis. Nits (louse eggs) are usually seen as small ovoid bodies stuck to the lashes (Fig. 13-15). The adult louse is transparent and can be difficult to see unless it contains blood or other ingested material. The feces of the louse are toxic and cause a follicular conjunctivitis and mild epithelial keratitis.

The condition is best treated by carefully removing the lice and nits from the patient's lashes. Local application of a pediculicide such as yellow mercuric oxide 1% ophthalmic ointment (twice daily for 7 days) or physostigmine ointment (twice daily for 10 days) should be considered when total mechanical removal is impossible. An application of 20% fluorescein has also been found to be effective.[47] Body hair should be examined for infestation with lice, and family members and contacts should also be examined and treated if infected.

Fly larvae can be deposited in the eyelids. Single or multiple lesions can occur and are characterized by itching, pain, and edema. A small sinus tract may be evident, and the larva may be seen in it or expressed from it (see Fig. 7-11). If the larva cannot be expressed, surgical removal is necessary.

Ticks can attach to the eyelids. They should be loosened with a drop of oil, turpentine, or anesthetic prior to removal, so that no body parts are left behind.

Blepharoconjunctivitis can develop in 20% to 45% of patients on oral 13-cis-retinoic acid, which is used to treat basal cell carcinoma, keratinizing dermatoses, and cystic acne.[48] Isotretinoin was found to decrease production of meibomian secretions and increase tear osmolarity in patients.[49] In rabbits given long-term isotretinoin and etretinate, degenerative changes were seen in the meibomian gland acini, leading to cell necrosis and a decrease in the basaloid cells lining the acini walls.[50]

REFERENCES

1. Smolin G, Okumoto M: Staphylococcal blepharitis, *Arch Ophthalmol* 95:812, 1977.
2. Thygeson P: The etiology and treatment of blepharitis: study in military personnel, *Mil Surg* 98:191, 1946.
3. Thygeson P: Complications of staphylococcal blepharitis, *Am J Ophthalmol* 68:446, 1969.
4. Dougherty JM, McCulley JP: Comparative bacteriology of chronic blepharitis, *Br J Ophthalmol* 68:524, 1984.
5. McCulley JP, Sciallis GF: Meibomian keratoconjunctivitis: oculodermal correlates, *CLAO J* 9:130, 1983.
6. Smolin G, Tabbara K, Whitcher J: *Infectious diseases of the eye*, Baltimore, 1984, Williams & Wilkins.
7. McCulley JP, Dougherty JM, Deneau DG: Classification of chronic blepharitis, *Ophthalmology* 89:1173, 1982.
8. Groden LR et al: Lid flora in blepharitis, *Cornea* 10:50, 1991.
9. Dougherty JM, McCulley JP: Bacterial lipases and chronic conjunctivitis, *Invest Ophthalmol Vis Sci* 27:486, 1986.
10. Bowers R et al: Non-*aureus* staphylococcus in corneal disease, *Invest Ophthalmol Vis Sci* 30(suppl):380, 1989.
11. Allen JH: Staphylococcic conjunctivitis, *Am J Ophthalmol* 20:1025, 1937.
12. Thygeson P: Bacterial factors in chronic catarrhal conjunctivitis: role of toxin-forming staphylococci, *Arch Ophthalmol* 18:373, 1937.
13. Valenton M, Okumoto M: Toxin producing strains of *Staphylococcus epidermidis*, *Arch Ophthalmol* 89:186, 1973.
14. Okumoto M: *Infectious agents: bacteria*. In Smolin G, Thoft RA, editors: *The cornea: scientific foundations and clinical practice*, Boston, 1983, Little, Brown & Co.
15. Coston TO: *Demodex folliculorum* blepharitis, *Trans Am Ophthalmol Soc* 65:361, 1967.
16. English FP et al: The vector potential of *Demodex folliculorum*, *Arch Ophthalmol* 84:83, 1970.
17. Jeffery MP: Ocular diseases caused by nematodes, *Am J Ophthalmol* 40:411, 1955.
18. Bonnar E, Eustace P, Powell FC: The *Demodex* mite population in rosacea, *Am Acad Dermatol* 28:443, 1993.
19. Swedo SE, Lenane MC, Leonard HL: Long-term treatment of trichotillomania, *N Engl J Med* 329:141, 1993.
20. McCulley JP, Dougherty JM: Blepharitis associated with acne rosacea and seborrheic dermatitis, *Int Ophthalmol Clin* 25:159, 1985.
21. Nelson ME, Midgley D, Blatchford NR: Ketoconazole in the treatment of blepharitis, *Eye* 4:151, 1990.
22. Mathers WD et al: Meibomian gland dysfunction in chronic blepharitis, *Cornea* 10:277, 1991.
23. McCulley JP, Sciallis GF: Meibomian keratoconjunctivitis, *Am J Ophthalmol* 84:788, 1977.

24. Mathers WD: Ocular evaporation in meibomian gland dysfunction and dry eye, *Ophthalmology* 100:347, 1993.

25. Dougherty JM, McCulley JP: Bacterial lipases and chronic blepharitis, *Invest Ophthalmol Vis Sci* 27:486, 1986.

26. Keith CG: Seborrheic blepharo-kerato-conjunctivitis, *Trans Ophthalmol Soc UK* 87:85, 1967.

27. Cory CC et al: Meibomian gland secretions in the red eyes of rosacea, *Br J Dermatol* 88:25, 1973.

28. McCulley JP: *Meibomitis*. In Kaufman HE et al, editors: *The cornea*, New York, 1988, Churchill Livingstone, Inc.

29. Shine WE, McCulley JP: The role of cholesterol in chronic blepharitis, *Invest Ophthalmol Vis Sci* 32:2272, 1991.

30. Shine WE, Silvany R, McCulley JP: Relation of cholesterol-stimulated *Staphylococcus aureus* growth to chronic blepharitis, *Invest Ophthalmol Vis Sci* 34:2291, 1993.

31. Shine WE, McCulley JP: Role of wax ester fatty alcohols in chronic blepharitis, *Invest Ophthalmol Vis Sci* 34:3515, 1993.

32. Dougherty JM et al: The role of tetracycline in chronic blepharitis. Inhibition of lipase production in staphylococci, *Invest Ophthalmol Vis Sci* 32:2970, 1991.

33. Frucht-Pery J et al: Efficacy of doxycycline and tetracycline in ocular rosacea, *Am J Ophthalmol* 116:88, 1993.

34. Gottsch JD, Greenberg KA: An association of elevated serum cholesterol and multiple recurrent chalazia, *Invest Ophthalmol Vis Sci* 30(suppl):502, 1989.

35. Pizzarello LD et al: Intralesional corticosteroid therapy of chalazia, *Am J Ophthalmol* 85:818, 1978.

36. Sloas HA et al: Treatment of chalazia with injectable triamcinolone, *Ann Ophthalmol* 15:78, 1983.

37. Ostler HB: *Diseases of the external eye and adnexa: a text and atlas,* Baltimore, 1993, Williams & Wilkins.

38. McKee SH: Syphilitic ulcer of the eyelid, *Can Med Assoc J* 35:307, 1936.

39. Holmes WJ: Leprosy of the eye, *Trans Am Ophthalmol Soc* 55:145, 1957.

40. Kohn SR: *Molluscum contagiosum* in patients with acquired immunodeficiency syndrome, *Arch Ophthalmol* 105:458, 1987.

41. Charles NC, Friedberg DN: Epibulbar *Molluscum contagiosum* in acquired immune deficiency syndrome: case report and review of the literature, *Ophthalmology* 99:1123, 1992.

42. Bardenstein DS, Elmets C: Hyperfocal cryotherapy of multiple *Molluscum contagiosum* lesions in patients with the acquired immune deficiency syndrome, *Ophthalmology* 102:1031, 1995.

43. Freeman G, Bron AJ, Juel-Jensen B: Ocular infection with orf virus, *Am J Ophthalmol* 97:601, 1984.

44. Duke-Elder S, MacFaul PA: *The ocular adnexa: Part I. Diseases of the eyelids*. In Duke-Elder S, editor: *System of ophthalmology*, St Louis, 1974, Mosby–Year Book.

45. Huber-Spitzy V et al: Ulcerative blepharitis in atopic patients: is *Candida* species the causative agent?, *Br J Ophthalmol* 76:272, 1992.

46. Couch JM et al: Diagnosing and treating *Phthirus pubis* palpebrarum, *Surv Ophthalmol* 26:219, 1982.

47. Matthew M, D'Souza P, Mehta DK: A new treatment of phthiriasis palpebrarum, *Ann Ophthalmol* 14:439, 1982.

48. Blackman HJ et al: Blepharoconjunctivitis: a side effect of 13-cisretinoic acid therapy for dermatologic diseases, *Ophthalmology* 86:753, 1980.

49. Mathers WD et al: Meibomian gland morphology and tear osmolarity: changes with Accutane therapy, *Cornea* 10:286, 1991.

50. Kremer I et al: Toxic effects of systemic retinoids on meibomian glands, *Ophthalmic Res* 26:124, 1994.

Fourteen

Tear Film Abnormalities

Tear film abnormalities are common and are a great source of irritation both for the patient and the physician. Yet, despite the prevalence of these disorders, our understanding of their cause is poor, diagnostic tests are limited and relatively insensitive, and treatment is inadequate. Classification of tear film abnormalities is limited by this lack of knowledge, but generally the conditions can be divided into those involving an abnormality in the composition of the tear film and those in which the spreading or "surfacing" of the tear film is abnormal. By far the most common abnormality of composition is aqueous tear deficiency, but abnormalities in other tear components, such as lipid and mucin, can also occur. Impaired lid functions, such as lagophthalmos, proptosis, or localized conjunctival elevations are examples of conditions that interfere with tear surfacing.

ABNORMALITIES OF TEAR FILM COMPOSITION

Aqueous
Although aqueous humor deficiency most frequently occurs idiopathically in women in their forties and fifties, it can develop at any age, can affect men, and can be associated with many local and systemic conditions (Table 14-1). The most commonly associated systemic condition is Sjögren's syndrome (SS), which is discussed later in this chapter.

Mucin
The relationship of mucin abnormalities to clinical disease is unclear. It has been proposed that mucin is important in stabilizing the tear film by increasing the wettability of the epithelial surface.[6-9] Wettability is measured clinically by tear film breakup time, and some symptomatic patients are found to have a normal tear volume but rapid tear film breakup. Theoretically, any disease that causes conjunctival scarring will reduce the number of goblet cells and lead to decreased tear mucin. Therefore, a relatively severe mucin deficiency would be expected in cicatricial pemphigoid, erythema

355

Table 14-1	Conditions Associated with Aqueous Tear Deficiency

CONGENITAL CONDITIONS
  Riley-Day syndrome
  Cri-du-chat syndrome
  Multiple endocrine neoplasia
  Lacrimal gland hypoplasia
  Anhidrotic ectodermal dysplasia
  Holmes-Adie syndrome
  Paralytic hyposecretion
  Congenital familial sensory neuropathy with
    anhidrosis

LOCAL CONDITIONS
  Dacryoadenitis (viral or bacterial)
  Irradiation (>30 Gy)[1]
  Trauma
  Benign lymphoepithelial lesion (Mikulicz's
    disease)
  Seventh nerve palsy

AUTOIMMUNE DISEASES
  Rheumatoid arthritis
  Lupus erythematosus
  Polyarteritis nodosa
  Hashimoto's thyroiditis
  Polymyositis
  Others

HEMATOPOIETIC DISEASES
  Lymphoma
  Thrombocytopenic purpura
  Hypergammaglobulinemia
  Waldenström's macroglobulinemia

OTHER SYSTEMIC CONDITIONS
  Celiac disease
  Sarcoidosis
  Graft-versus-host disease
  Pulmonary fibrosis
  Chronic hepatobiliary disease
  Amyloidosis
  HIV infection[2-4]

MEDICATIONS
  Anticholinergic drugs
  Antihistamines
  Tricyclic antidepressants
  Monoamine oxidase inhibitors
  β-blockers
  Hydrochlorothiazide
  ?Oral contraceptives
  Antidiarrheals
  Decongestants
  Thiabendazole
  Antiparkinsonian agents
  Antineoplastic agents
  Retinoids (e.g., etretinate, isotretinoin)
  Many others[5]

multiforme major, vitamin A deficiency, and chemical burns. However, the relationship of mucin deficiency to the changes seen in these conditions has not been well demonstrated.

The correlation between goblet cell density and tear mucin content is poor,[10] and even in cases with severe goblet cell loss, tear mucin content is only moderately reduced.[11] It is possible that a qualitative change in tear mucin occurs, but to date this has not been demonstrated.

Excessive mucin is often noted as mucous strands or plaques. The condition may be caused by increased production or by relative overabundance in aqueous deficiency. Ocular infection, allergies, foreign bodies, and trauma all can stimulate increased production.

Lipid

The only cause of true lipid deficiency is congenital absence of the meibomian glands, a condition that can occur in ectodermal dysplasia. The lack of tear lipids causes increased evaporation of tears, which can lead to corneal thinning.[12] Increased lipid production and abnormal lipid composition may be present in meibomitis, but their role in tear and corneal surface disease remains unclear (see Chapter 13). Staphylococci can produce lipases and other enzymes that alter the lipid composition of the tear film and may affect its stability. Meibomian gland dropout is associated with increased osmolarity of the tear film, probably due to increased evaporation.[13,14]

Clinical Manifestations

The patient complains of burning and irritation, usually in both eyes. Occasionally a foreign body sensation or mucous discharge is also present. The symptoms are exacerbated by reading, watching television, or other tasks involving concentration; drafts or winds; hot, dry environments; and smoke or other particulate matter in the air. The symptoms may be most marked in the morning, on awakening, or in the evening.

Examining the eye with the slit-lamp microscope reveals an increased amount of debris in the tear film, resulting from the poor tear flow. The tear meniscus, or marginal tear strip, may be reduced. Normal meniscus height is 0.2 to 0.3 mm[15]; if it is lower than this, keratoconjunctivitis sicca is likely to be present. Viscous mucous threads may be present in the inferior cul-de-sac. Corneal findings include decreased luster, punctate keratopathy (Fig. 14-1), filaments (Fig. 14-2), mucous plaques, keratinization, band keratopathy,[16] and ulceration.

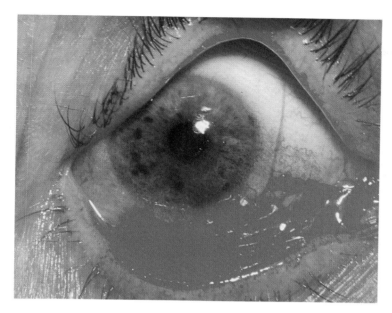

Figure 14-1
Rose bengal red staining of the cornea and conjunctiva in keratoconjunctivitis sicca. Note the extensive amount of stained mucoid material.

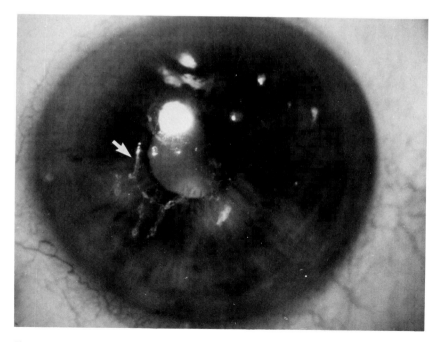

Figure 14-2
Filamentary keratitis (*arrow*) in a patient with Sjögren's syndrome.

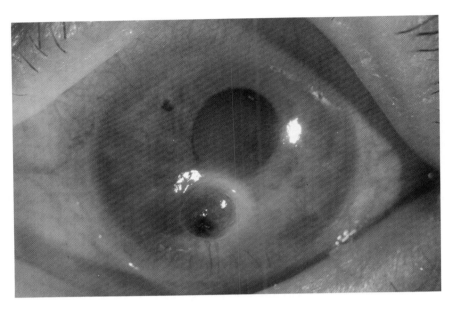

Figure 14-3
Perforation of the cornea with iris prolapse in keratoconjunctivitis sicca.

Dry eyes are prone to infections such as conjunctivitis, blepharitis, and keratitis. Sterile corneal ulceration is also relatively common in patients with dry eyes. Typically the ulcer is round or horizontally oval, noninfiltrated, and located in the interpalpebral cornea. The ulcers tend to progress rapidly, forming deep, steep-walled craters that often perforate (Fig. 14-3). The ulceration usually can be halted with a bandage contact lens or by sealing with cyanoacrylate adhesive, but healing is slow. Penetrating keratoplasty may be required.

Diagnostic Tests
There is no reliable, sensitive test to diagnose dry eyes. If the condition is relatively severe, the diagnosis can be made easily by clinical examination and Schirmer's testing. In milder cases, however, establishing the diagnosis often is difficult or impossible. The three simplest and most common tests are rose bengal staining, Schirmer's test, and tear breakup time.

Rose bengal stain is quite valuable in the diagnosis of keratoconjunctivitis sicca. It stains cells lacking protection by the precorneal tear film and mucus.[17,18] It is the pattern of epithelial injury that suggests dry eyes: interpalpebral cornea and conjunctiva (see Fig. 14-1). In milder cases the staining is limited to the conjunctiva, and in the severest cases most of the cornea also stains. Mucous filaments may be present on the interpalpebral corneal surface.

Schirmer's test is a means of estimating tear production (see the box on page 359). A Schirmer I (unanesthetized) value of less than 5 mm after 5 minutes is considered significant.[19] Test values are reduced in normals after anesthesia, and therefore a reading of 3 mm or less is recommended for this test.[20] Tear production is greatest during the first 1 to 2 minutes after placement of the strip and then slows to a nearly constant rate after 5 minutes.[21] The lower steady rate may be more diagnostic, but this hypothesis has not been tested. Anesthetic-fluorescein solutions such as Fluress (Barnes-Hind, Sunnyvale, CA) and Fluoracaine (Akorn, Abita Springs, LA) contain viscous additives and decrease wetting of Schirmer's strips.[22]

Tear breakup time is the amount of time it takes for a dry spot to appear in the tear film. The test is performed as follows: Fluorescein is instilled in the eye, and the patient is asked to blink several times to distribute the dye. The patient is then asked to look straight ahead (the lids should not be held open), and the examiner observes the tear film with cobalt blue light for development of a black island within the green film. The tear breakup time is the time between the last blink and the appearance of the dry spot. An abnormal tear breakup time is less than 10 seconds. This test is useful in diagnosing tear abnormalities without significant aqueous deficiency. It is not useful if the corneal surface is irregular or if large particles are present in the tear film.

A number of laboratory tests have been used

Tear Function Tests

Schirmer's tests of tear quantity are a measurement of the aqueous layer only. The tests are performed with 5 × 30-mm strips of Whatman filter paper (available commercially from Smith Miller & Patch Laboratories). The paper is folded so that 5 mm of the strip will lie within the lower conjunctival sac, and the remaining 25 mm will project over the lower eyelid. The amount of moistening of the exposed paper is recorded at the end of 5 minutes. It is paramount to remember that these tests are rough measurements only. They are clinically useful as gross indicators of tear function.

Schirmer's Test I (measures total reflex and basic tear secretion)

To minimize reflex tearing, avoid a brightly lit room and instillation of ocular medications before testing. The patient may keep his or her eyes open or closed. If the paper is wetted completely before 5 minutes, note this time; if not, note the amount of wetting at the end of 5 minutes.

Results: Normals will wet approximately 10 to 30 mm at the end of 5 minutes. This amount decreases with age but probably should not be less than 10 mm. If wetting is greater than 30 mm, reflex tearing is intact but not controlled or tear drainage is insufficient. Tear secretion between 5 and 30 mm may be normal, or basal secretion may be low and compensated for by reflex stimulation. A value of less than 5 mm indicates hyposecretion.

Basic Secretion Test (measures basic tear secretion)

Instill topical anesthetic and wait until anesthesia is achieved. The cul-de-sac should be dried before inserting strips. Only basic secretion is being measured. The difference between this test and Schirmer's test I is the amount of reflex secretion. A basic secretion of 3 mm or less after 5 minutes is abnormal.

Schirmer's Test II (measures reflex tear secretion)

Instill topical ocular anesthetic and irritate unanesthesized nasal mucosa by rubbing it with a cotton swab. Measure wetting after 2 minutes. Wetting of less than 15 mm represents failure of reflex secretion. This test is seldom employed, because reflex tearing is usually intact.

---

to detect dry eyes. However, none of these has proved sufficiently sensitive or easy to perform to warrant widespread use.

Tear osmolality appears to be a relatively sensitive laboratory test for dry eyes, but it requires special laboratory equipment to perform.[23] Tear film osmolality presumably is increased because of decreased aqueous flow and increased tear evaporation. This is determined by collecting a tear sample in a glass micropipette and measuring the freezing point in a nanoliter osmometer. An osmolality of more than 312 mOsm/L is considered indicative of dry eyes and in one study was found to have a sensitivity of 76% and specificity of 84%.[24]

Tear lysozyme is decreased in dry eyes. The most common means of measuring tear lysozyme in the laboratory is by an agar diffusion test. Wetted Schirmer's strips are placed on agarose gel containing a suspension of *Micrococcus lysodeikticus,* a bacteria whose cell wall is destroyed by lysozyme. The greater the tear lysozyme concentration, the larger will be the zone of bacterial lysis.[25,19] (The plates are available from the Kallestad Co., Austin, TX.)

In one comparative study tear lysozyme was found to be more accurate than rose bengal staining or Schirmer's testing.[26] However, de-

creased tear lysozyme is not specific for dry eyes; it is also found in herpes simplex infection, bacterial conjunctivitis, smog irritation, and malnutrition.[21] Concentrations also vary with age and with time of day.[27]

Tear lactoferrin, which is also reduced in dry eyes, can be measured using a commercially available antibody assay kit (Lactoplate; Mackeen Consultants, Bethesda, MD). Both basal and reflex tears are measured, and the percent increase in lactoferrin from basal to reflex tears is determined. This test was found to be 96% sensitive in one study[24] but only 35% sensitive and 70% specific in a more recent comparison with tear osmolarity.[28] Danio et al.[29] found that tear lactoferrin level correlated well with the severity of rose bengal staining.

Fluorescein dilution tests measure the decrease in tear fluorescence by the production of new tears. A drop of fluorescein is placed in the eye, and fluorescence is measured over time with a photomultiplier.

Impression cytology can be used to assess goblet cell density and epithelial cell differentiation. Squamous metaplasia and goblet cell loss have been observed in dry eyes (see Chapter 4).[30-35] Impression cytology is useful in diagnosing primary and secondary SS.[36,37]

Sjögren's Syndrome

The classic triad of Sjögren's (pronounced "shurgren's") syndrome consists of dry eyes, dry mouth (xerostomia), and a connective tissue disease, most commonly rheumatoid arthritis.[38-40] However, the syndrome often is incomplete, and its definition has varied; there is still controversy and confusion about its definition. However, it is agreed that the term should not be used to refer to cases of isolated dry eyes, and the syndrome occurs in both a primary and a secondary form. The primary form consists of dry eyes and dry mouth, while the secondary form is dry eyes and/or dry mouth in association with systemic autoimmune disease.

Definition

Because the pathogenesis of SS is unknown, the diagnostic criteria are based on a consensus of opinion rather than on strict scientific data. Several sets of criteria have been proposed over the past decade. Some of the definitions are broader and more inclusive than others.[41] Fox and Saito[42] recommend that the term be reserved for patients who share histologic and serologic features that indicate a systemic autoimmune process in the pathogenesis of the disease. This stricter definition will label a smaller, more homogeneous group with a higher risk of visceral complications. These authors proposed the San Diego Criteria in 1986 (Table 14-2).[42]

The category of probable SS, which does not require a salivary gland biopsy, is most commonly used for routine clinical purposes. Recent reports suggest that gingival impression cytology is nearly as sensitive as minor salivary gland biopsy.[43,44] Patients with dry eye and dry mouth without autoantibodies are labeled with "sicca symptom complex" but not SS. According to these criteria, approximately 22% of patients with dry eyes have SS. However, in one study the incidence of SS-A or SS-B antibodies in patients with dry eye was only 1% to 3%.[45]

Epidemiology

All epidemiologic studies on SS are biased by the criteria used to define the disease, so the prevalence reported varies considerably. Using the above criteria, the prevalence of primary SS is approximately 1 in 1250 individuals.[42] Primary SS usually develops in individuals between 30 and 60 years of age, and women are affected nine times more frequently than men.[25] Secondary SS occurs in 15% to 30% of patients with rheumatoid arthritis,[46,47] in 20% of patients with progressive systemic sclerosis,[48] and in 8% of patients with systemic lupus ery-

Table 14-2	San Diego Criteria for Diagnosis of Sjögren's Syndrome (SS)

I. Primary SS
  A. Symptoms and objective signs of ocular dryness
    1. Schirmer's test less than 8 mm wetting per 5 minutes *and*
    2. Positive rose bengal staining of cornea *or* conjunctiva to demonstrate keratoconjunctivitis sicca
  B. Symptoms and objective signs of dry mouth
    1. Decreased parotid flow rate using Lashley cups or other methods *and*
    2. Abnormal biopsy of minor salivary gland (focus score of ≥2 based on average of four evaluable lobules)*
  C. Evidence of a systemic autoimmune disorder
    1. Elevated rheumatoid factor ≥ 1:320 *or*
    2. Elevated antinuclear antibody ≥ 1:320 *or*
    3. Presence of anti–SS-A (ro) or anti–SS-B (la) antibodies
II. Secondary SS
  Characteristic signs and symptoms of SS (described above) *plus* clinical features sufficient to allow a diagnosis of rheumatoid arthritis, systemic lupus erythematosus, polymyositis, scleroderma, or biliary cirrhosis
III. Exclusions
  Sarcoidosis, preexistent lymphoma, acquired immunodeficiency disease, and other known causes of keratitis sicca or salivary gland enlargement

*Probable SS does not require a minor salivary gland biopsy but can be diagnosed with demonstration salivary function (criteria IA, IB-1, and IC).

thematosus.[49] A few cases of primary and secondary SS have been reported in children.[50-53] There is a higher incidence of other autoimmune diseases in families of patients with primary or secondary SS.[54] SS is associated with certain types of human leukocyte antigen (HLA), and the associations differ among cultures. In whites there is a higher incidence of HLA-DR2, DRw52a, and DQw2.1 in patients with primary SS.[55]

Clinical Manifestations

The same signs and symptoms that are seen in other patients with dry eyes occur in patients with SS. In addition, peripheral corneal infiltration occurs in approximately 10% of patients with SS.[56] Single or multiple marginal subepithelial infiltrates with a lucid interval are seen. The epithelium can break down over the infiltrates, and they can coalesce to form an arcuate infiltrate. They probably are due to deposition of immune complexes. Peripheral corneal ulceration without infiltration can also occur in primary and secondary SS.

Besides the lacrimal and salivary glands, the mucus-secreting glands, respiratory mucosa, and vagina may also be involved in primary SS. Xerostomia may cause difficulty in swallowing and chewing, and ulcers may develop on the tongue and buccal mucous membrane.[39] Other sites of extraglandular involvement include the joints, skin, lungs, kidneys, peripheral and central nervous systems, blood, and muscles. The most common symptoms outside those of dryness are fatigue, myalgias, and arthritis, which are present in approximately 60% of patients.[57] Lymphadenopathy and lung involvement each occur in approximately 14% of patients, and vasculitis occurs in 11%. Autoimmune thyroiditis is relatively common, and some patients require thyroid supplementation. There is a high incidence of serum IgM paraproteins, including cryoglobulins. Lymphoreticular proliferation occurs in 5% to 10% of patients, and there is a 40-fold higher risk of lymphoma, mainly non-Hodgkin's B-cell tumors.[40,58] Central nervous system complications occur in more than 20% of patients with primary SS,[59] and there is a strong association of central nervous system disease with peripheral vasculitis.[60]

Tear and salivary deficiencies are caused by infiltration of the lacrimal and salivary glands with lymphocytes and plasma cells.[61] Infiltrates occur first in the perivascular region of the lobule. Areas of mononuclear cell infiltration are associated with focal degeneration of the glandular acini. Cellular infiltration and glandular atrophy increase, and proliferating ductal epithelial cells form myoepithelial islands. Eventually, the gland tissue is replaced with connective tissue. Biopsy of the more accessible minor glands of the lip and palate demonstrates changes similar to those noted in the lacrimal gland and can facilitate diagnosis.[25] Immunohistochemical studies have shown that most of the lymphocytes in the salivary glands are helper T cells, and that the glandular epithelial cells exhibit high levels of class II HLA molecules (HLA-DR).[62] Helper T cells only interact with antigen presented by HLA-DR molecules. Expression of HLA-DR is probably a result of local production of interferon α by T cells.[63]

Patients with SS have a number of immunologic abnormalities, some of which are helpful in diagnosis. Approximately half of these patients have hypergammaglobulinemia, which usually involves all immunoglobulin classes. Monoclonal gammopathies can also occur, and immune complexes and autoantibodies are common.[64] Rheumatoid factor, antinuclear factor, and antibodies to ribonucleoprotein Ro (SS-A) are seen in most patients. SS-A antibodies are seen in over 90% of patients with primary SS (according to the San Diego criteria) and in approximately 50% of patients with systemic lupus erythematosus, but they are rarely seen in normal adults.[63] SS-A appears to be present in most of the patients with the more serious systemic complications of SS, such as vasculitis, intracranial hemorrhage and infarcts, hyperglobulinemia, and cryoglobulinemia.[57,65] In addition, infants born to women with SS-A antibodies have a greater risk of having cardiac conduction defects.[26] Therefore, detection of SS-A antibodies can be used to identify a subset of SS patients at higher risk for these complications.

Pathogenesis

The pathogenesis of SS is unknown. There appears to be a failure of tolerance mechanisms: T cells that suppress natural and induced "self-reactive" B cells are not functioning properly. This results in the activation of B cells that produce autoantibodies, such as SS-A, SS-B, and rheumatoid factor.

Some researchers have suggested that Epstein-Barr virus (EBV) infection plays a role in the development of SS.[66-68] Primary EBV infection (infectious mononucleosis) usually involves the salivary glands, and the salivary glands are a common site of latent infection. EBV stimulates production of autoantibodies such as rheumatoid factor. Antibodies against EBV nuclear antigen are seen more often in patients with SS.[67,68] Fox et al.[67] found EBV DNA in the saliva and salivary glands of 8 of 20 patients with SS, but not in the saliva of controls or rheumatoid arthritis patients without sicca symptoms.[67] Karameris et al.[69] found EBV DNA in salivary gland epithelial cells from 16 of 23 patients with secondary SS and from 3 of 11 patients with keratoconjunctivitis sicca, but none of 7 controls. Pflugfelder et al.[70] detected EBV DNA in the lacrimal glands and tears of patients with primary SS.[70]

However, EBV reactivation in the salivary glands is also seen in immunosuppressed patients and in those with chronic sialadenitis not associated with SS. Antibody titers against EBV antigens at the onset of disease are comparable with patients with other autoimmune diseases and become progressively elevated only later in the course of SS.[71] EBV reactivation occurs most likely as a consequence of inflammation and immune dysregulation in the salivary and lacrimal glands.[63] Reactivation of EBV may help perpetuate inflammation because EBV is a strong stimulator of T-cell responses.

Diagnosis

Once the diagnosis of dry eyes is made, it is important to consider the possibility of an association with a systemic disease. The patient should be questioned about dryness of the mouth or other mucous membranes, arthritis, and other symptoms of autoimmune disease. The following oral symptoms were found to be most discriminating between SS patients and controls: feeling of dry mouth, difficulty in swallowing dry food, and feeling of dryness when breathing or eating.[72] If these symptoms are present objective testing of parotid flow rate, impression cytology of the buccal mucosa, or biopsy or minor salivary glands should be performed. Parotid flow rate tests include placing a plastic suction cup over the opening of the parotid gland or determining the proportion of a sugarless candy that is dissolved in 3 minutes. If objective signs of dry mouth are present, serum testing for elevated rheumatoid factor, antinuclear antibody, and the presence of anti–SS-A and anti–SS-B antibodies should be performed. The diagnosis of primary SS is made based on the criteria in Table 14-2.

The best means of detecting systemic autoimmune disease in secondary SS is a good review of systems. If suggestive symptoms or signs are present appropriate diagnostic testing should be performed.

Treatment

Artificial Tear Solutions

The mainstay of treatment for dry eyes is artificial tears. Many types of artificial tear solutions are commercially available, and no particular type has been demonstrated to be superior. Most have a polymeric agent such as polyvinyl alcohol, methylcellulose, or dextran to increase viscosity. The solutions with polymeric agents seem to be retained for longer periods, but inspissated material tends to form on the lid margin and in the fornix.[73] Hypotonic solutions have been developed, based on the assumption that reducing the hyperosmolality of the tears in dry eyes will provide more symptomatic relief. Although the effect on osmolality appears to be short-lived,[74] many patients do prefer these drops.

The preservatives in artificial tear solutions, particularly thimerosal and benzalkonium chloride, can elicit contact sensitivity reactions or cause toxicity to the surface epithelium. Nonpreserved solutions are available (e.g., Refresh; Allergan, Irvine, CA; Hypotears PF; Iolab Inc., Claremont, CA; Ocucoat; Storz, St. Louis,

MO) and can be very useful, particularly in patients with severe dryness who must use the drops frequently. A bicarbonate-buffered, preservative-free artificial tear solution was found to be superior to other commercial preservative-free solutions in one animal study.[75] However, all nonpreserved drops are less convenient and must be discarded 24 to 48 hours after opening. The container should not be recapped, because this appears to be associated with increased contamination.[76]

The use of viscoelastic materials, hyaluronic acid, and chondroitin sulfate in artificial tear solutions has been recommended,[77-80] but one double-blind study found no difference in patient preference between these and an artificial tear solution with polyvinyl alcohol.[81]

Autologous serum has been reported to be an effective artificial tear solution,[82] but this has not been tested in a controlled manner. All-trans retinoic acid ointment was initially reported to be very effective,[83] but a subsequent controlled study did not find it to be more effective than a standard artificial tear ointment.[84]

Ointments

Petrolatum-based ointments relieve the symptoms, primarily through lubrication. However, they tend to interfere with vision, so most patients use them only at bedtime. Ointments without preservatives are available and are preferable.

Artificial Tear Inserts

A unique product, Lacrisert (Merck, Sharp & Dome, West Point, PA) is a small pellet of polymer (hydroxypropyl cellulose) that is placed in the inferior fornix. In the presence of tears it slowly dissolves, releasing the polymer into the tear film and retarding its evaporation.[85-88] It is generally used once or twice daily. Lacriserts can be very helpful in some patients with dry eyes, but several problems limit their use. Because many of these patients do not produce enough tears to melt the insert, artificial tear drops must also be used. Some patients have difficulty inserting the pellets in the fornix. Other problems are blurred vision, particularly when looking through the enlarged tear meniscus, and irritation from the presence of the pellet.

Mucolytic Agents

In some patients with marked mucus strands, globs, or filaments, a mucolytic agent will increase comfort. N-acetylcysteine (10% to 20%) can be effective in dissolving excess mucus when given two to four times daily. The Food and Drug Administration has not approved this use of the drug, but it is available and can be formulated by most pharmacists. It burns on instillation and has a distasteful odor. In many patients a course of 3 to 4 weeks of treatment provides prolonged relief; others require chronic treatment.

Punctal Occlusion

Occlusion of the lacrimal puncta can be performed to aid retention of naturally produced and artificial tears.[89,90] The ability of punctal occlusion to improve objective clinical findings has not been well documented,[91] but the procedure is often helpful in patients whose symptoms are not relieved by frequent use of artificial tears. Both the upper and lower puncta should be occluded; occlusion of just one punctum is usually not effective.

The main complication of punctal occlusion is epiphora, which can be prevented by limiting the procedure to patients whose Schirmer's test values are consistently less than 3 mm and by testing with temporary occlusion. Temporary occlusion can be achieved with collagen plugs (Lacrimedics, San Marino, CA), silicone plugs (Eagle Vision, Memphis, TN) (Fig. 14-4), cyanoacrylate adhesive, by suturing the punctum with 10-0 nylon, or by placing a heated spatula on the punctum for 1 second. If symptoms are improved or the frequency of drop use can be reduced, and epiphora does not occur, permanent occlusion may be performed. This is most easily accomplished with cautery, using an electocautery device (Hyfrecator; Birtcher Corp., Los Angeles, CA) or a hand-held cautery. Recanalization can occur, and if several attempts are unsuccessful, the punctum or a portion of the canaliculus can be extirpated.

Moisture Chambers

Evaporation can be retarded by surrounding the eye with a moisture-retaining chamber. Many different types of moisture chambers can be fashioned, including swimming goggles, clear plastic wrap, silicone breast implants, or moist chamber spectacles.[92,93] These are most useful for comatose patients and those with nocturnal lagophthalmos, but they can also aid many severely affected patients. The main drawbacks are their cosmetic unacceptability and their tendency to fog, blurring vision.

Bandage Contact Lenses

Bandage contact lenses are most useful in treating filamentary keratitis. The lens is placed after the filaments are removed from the cornea; the patient experiences immediate symptomatic relief and the filaments usually do not reappear as long as the lens is in place. Bandage lenses are also helpful in cases of recurrent epithelial breakdown or delayed healing, in eyes that are mucin-deficient but have relatively good aqueous flow, and in some cases of exposure keratitis. The lenses can provide some symptomatic relief in patients with marked drying, but other means of treatment should be exhausted first[94] because of the relatively high risk of complications such as infection, vascularization, and chemical reactions.[95] Thicker lenses with a lower water content are preferred to thinner lenses with a higher water content. The former tend not to dehydrate as much, but concomitant artificial tear use is recommended.

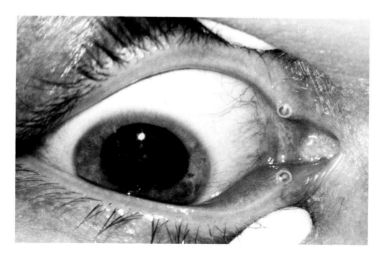

Figure 14-4
Silicone punctal plugs.

Sjögren's Syndrome

Patients with primary SS should be followed up for visceral complications, including lymphoproliferative disease. Thyroid function tests are probably worthwhile. Dry mouth is treated with special toothbrushes that generate peroxide, artificial saliva, and, in some cases, stimulation of secretion with iodides or bromhexine. Patients with dry mouth are prone to dental caries and *Candida* infection. Myalgias and arthalgias are treated with nonsteroidal antiinflammatory agents. Hydroxychloroquine can be added in patients with an elevated sedimentation rate and a positive bone scan. Systemic steroids and other immunosuppressive agents are reserved for life-threatening complications, such as vasculitis, hemolytic anemia, pleuropericarditis, and visceral (such as nervous system, lung, or kidney) manifestations, which are resistant to nonsteroidal antiinflammatory drugs.

Other Treatments

Medications that decrease tear production should be discontinued whenever possible. Using a humidifier in the home is often helpful. Symptomatic improvement and increased tear lysozyme has been reported with oral bromhexine.[15,96] Lateral tarsorrhaphy may be necessary in some patients to help prevent surface breakdown and ulceration. Parotid duct transposition was explored in the past but has been largely abandoned.[97-99] The surgery is tedious, and the secretion is usually excessive and increases during eating.

The effectiveness of topical cyclosporine 2% in secondary SS was evaluated in a randomized, double blind, placebo-controlled trial.[100] Topical cyclosporine significantly decreased rose bengal staining and increased tear breakup time, while Schirmer's test scores were not affected. The authors concluded that topical cyclosporine most likely improved goblet cell function.

Penetrating keratoplasty can be performed for scarring or ulceration caused by dry eyes, but the results usually are poor. Punctal occlusion and temporary tarsorrhaphy are recommended at the time of surgery. Keratoprosthesis can be performed as a last resort.

Psychologic Aspects

The physician's task does not end with prescribing artificial tears. Patients with dry eyes in particular require attention to other psychologic needs. Dry eye conditions are chronic, annoying, and sometimes debilitating. Patients must come to realize not only the limitations of treatment but also that good vision is nearly always maintained. Many patients require reassurance, attention, and compassion from their physician. They also need time to adapt to their condition and adjust their lifestyle, and this usually occurs over several visits. Informational pamphlets, videotaped presentations, and discussions with auxiliary personnel can be very useful. Support groups have been established in many communities to help people with dry eyes deal with their condition, and I have found this to be one of the most effective forms of treatment.

ABNORMALITIES OF TEAR SURFACING

The term *tear surfacing* was introduced by Lemp[101] to refer to the spreading of tears across the corneal and conjunctival surfaces. The lids are primarily responsible for this spreading, and it requires an intact lid margin, contact of the lid with the globe, and complete closure of the lid during blinking. Interference with any of these properties can result in drying of the affected surface areas. Tear surfacing abnormalities are listed in Table 14-3.

Table 14-3 Causes of Tear Surfacing Abnormalities
LID POSITION
Entropion
Ectropion
Tumors
Colobomas and other lid defects
Ptosis surgery
Floppy lid syndrome
LID MOVEMENT (BLINKING)
Seventh nerve palsy
Symblepharon
Severe proptosis
Parkinsonism
Bilateral fifth nerve palsy
Coma
Graves' disease
LOCALIZED SURFACE ELEVATIONS
Pterygium
Limbal tumor
Postsurgical edema
Subconjunctival hemorrhage
Filtering bleb
Many others

Dellen are localized thinnings of the cornea (Fig. 14-5) or sclera (Fig. 14-6) that form adjacent to corneal or conjunctival elevations. They represent localized dehydration caused by lack of wetting by the lid.

Clinical Manifestations

Dellen are differentiated from ulceration by their rapid onset, lack of infiltration, location adjacent to elevations, and coverage by intact epithelium. Their nature can be confirmed by

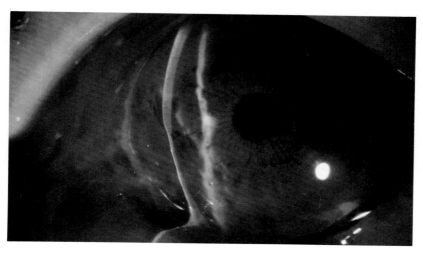

Figure 14-5
Corneal delle adjacent to the area of conjunctival elevation.

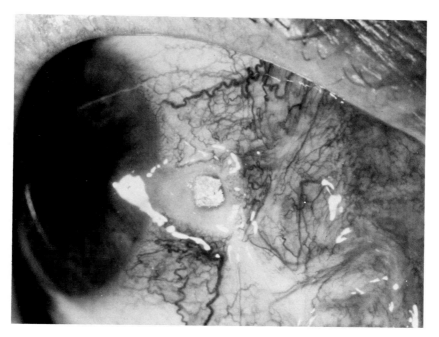

Figure 14-6
Scleral delle.

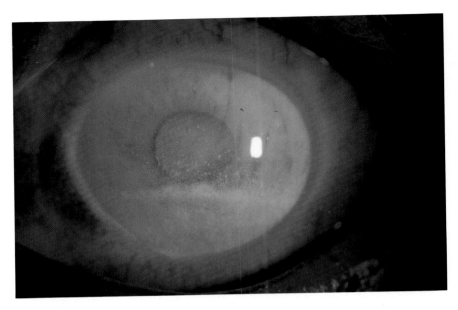

Figure 14-7
Corneal staining in lagophthalmos.

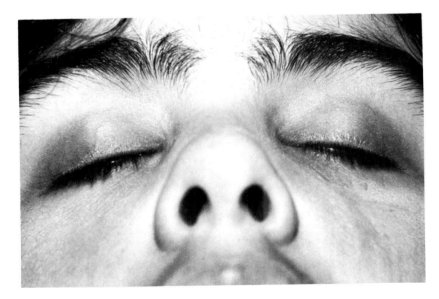

Figure 14-8
Lagophthalmos.

taping the eyelids shut; most will improve in 1 to 2 hours and disappear within 24 to 48 hours.

In most types of tear-surfacing abnormalities, the diagnosis is obvious. However, infrequent or incomplete blinking and lagophthalmos may be difficult to appreciate unless the physician specifically looks for them. The pattern of staining may suggest their presence (see Fig. 3-11); chronic punctate keratopathy of the central or lower cornea usually occurs. Occasionally, the entire lower half of the cornea is involved, or more frequently a horizontal band of keratopathy is seen across the cornea (Fig. 14-7). There is usually a lack of corneal luster as well as diffuse haziness and desiccation of the involved area.

Lagophthalmos is sometimes present only during sleep. The physician should check specifically for this common condition (Fig. 14-8), because otherwise it may be missed. The diagnosis can be made definitely only by the response to nocturnal taping of the lids, because mild surface changes may be present in the morning and then heal later in the day. However, in chronic disease the exposed cornea can develop map-dot-fingerprint lines, spheroidal degeneration, nodules similar to small deposits of Salzmann's nodular dystrophy, and the most common sign, a horizontal brown line of iron deposition, which indicates chronic epithelial damage and irritation.[102]

Treatment

If possible, the primary cause of exposure should be addressed. Abnormalities of lid position can usually be corrected surgically. Most other conditions usually can be adequately treated with artificial tear solutions or ointment. Taping the lids, swimming goggles, or other forms of moisture chambers often are necessary at night. Occasionally, punctal occlusion can be performed to increase the height of the lacrimal lake; in some cases epiphora is preferable to severe drying. If these measures do not provide comfort or maintain epithelial integrity, lateral tarsorrhaphy can be performed. In the most severe cases a total tarsorrhaphy or conjunctival flap can provide comfort and prevent ulceration or perforation.

Corneal dellen and other forms of localized surface drying usually occur adjacent to acute elevations, and tear drops or ointments are sufficient until the elevation subsides. Pterygia and other limbal masses may require surgical excision, and subconjunctival hemorrhages may require drainage.

REFERENCES

1. Parsons JT et al: Severe dry-eye syndrome following external beam irradiation, *Int J Radiat Oncol Biol Phys* 30:775, 1994.
2. Ulirsch RC, Jaffe ES: Sjögren's syndrome-like illness associated with the acquired immunodeficiency syndrome-related complex, *Hum Pathol* 18:1063, 1987.
3. Couderc LJ et al: Sicca complex and infection with human immunodeficiency virus, *Arch Intern Med* 147:898, 1987.
4. Lucca JA et al: Keratoconjunctivitis sicca in male patients infected with human immunodeficiency virus type I, *Ophthalmology* 97:1008, 1990.
5. Fraunfelder FT: *Drug-induced ocular side effects and drug interactions*, ed 3, Philadelphia, 1989, Lea & Febiger.
6. Holly FJ: Formation and rupture of the tear film, *Exp Eye Res* 15:515, 1973.
7. Lemp MA, Dohlman CH, Holly FJ: Corneal desiccation despite normal tear volume, *Ann Ophthalmol* 2:258, 1970.
8. Lemp MA et al: Dry eye secondary to mucus deficiency, *Trans Am Acad Ophthalmol Otolaryngol* 75:1223, 1971.
9. Holly FJ, Lemp MA: Wettability and wetting of corneal epithelium, *Exp Eye Res* 11:239, 1971.
10. Friend J, Kiorpes T, Thoft RA: Conjunctival goblet cell frequency after alkali injury is not accurately reflected by aqueous tear mucin content, *Invest Ophthalmol Vis Sci* 24:612, 1983.
11. Kinoshita S et al: Goblet cell density in ocular surface disease: a better indicator than tear mucin, *Arch Ophthalmol* 101:1284, 1983.
12. Mishima S, Maurice DM: Oily layer of tear film and evaporation from corneal surface, *Exp Eye Res* 1:39, 1961.
13. Gilbard JP et al: Tear film and ocular surface changes after closure of the meibomian gland orifices in the rabbit, *Ophthalmology* 96:1180, 1989.
14. Mathers WD et al: Meibomian gland dysfunction in chronic blepharitis, *Cornea* 10:277, 1991.
15. Scharf JM et al: Influence of bromhexine on tear lysozyme level in keratoconjunctivitis sicca, *Am J Ophthalmol* 92:21, 1981.
16. Lemp MA, Ralph RA: Rapid development of band keratopathy in dry eyes, *Am J Ophthalmol* 83:657, 1977.
17. Feenstra RPG, Tseng SCG: Comparison of fluorescein and rose bengal staining, *Ophthalmology* 99:605, 1992.
18. Feenstra RPG, Tseng SCG: What is actually stained by rose bengal?, *Arch Ophthalmol* 110:984, 1992.
19. van Bijsterveld OP: Diagnostic tests in the sicca syndrome, *Arch Ophthalmol* 82:10, 1969.
20. Lamberts DW, Foster CS, Perry HD: Schirmer test after topical anesthesia and the tear meniscus height in normal eyes, *Arch Ophthalmol* 97:1082, 1979.
21. Lamberts DW: *Keratoconjunctivitis sicca.* In Smolin G, Thoft RA, editors: *The cornea: scientific foundations and clinical practice,* Boston, 1983, Little, Brown & Co.
22. Hodkin MJ, Cartwright MJ, Kurumety UR: In vitro alteration of Schirmer's tear strip wetting by commonly instilled anesthetic agents, *Cornea* 13:141, 1994.
23. Gilbard JP, Farris RL, Santamaria J: Osmolarity of tear microvolumes in keratoconjunctivitis sicca, *Arch Ophthalmol* 96:677, 1978.
24. Farris RL et al: Diagnostic tests in keratoconjunctivitis sicca, *CLAO J* 9:23, 1983.
25. Tabbara KF et al: Sjögren's syndrome: a correlation between ocular findings and labial salivary gland histology, *Trans Am Acad Ophthalmol Otolaryngol* 78:467, 1974.

26. Franco HL et al: Autoantibodies directed against sicca syndrome antigens in the neonatal lupus syndrome, *Am Acad Dermatol* 4:67, 1981.

27. Sen DK, Sarin GS: Biological variations of lysozyme concentration in the tear fluids of healthy persons, *Br J Ophthalmol* 70:246, 1986.

28. Luce A, Farris RL, Nunez JN: A comparison of two diagnostic tests for keratoconjunctivitis sicca: lactoplate and tear osmolarity, *Invest Ophthalmol Vis Sci* 30(suppl):523, 1989.

29. Danio Y et al: Ocular surface damage and tear lactoferrin in dry eye syndrome, *Acta Ophthalmol (Copenh)* 72:433, 1994.

30. Egbert PR, Lauber S, Maurice DM: A simple conjunctival biopsy, *Am J Ophthalmol* 84:793, 1977.

31. Tseng SCG: Staging of conjunctival squamous metaplasia by impression cytology, *Ophthalmology* 92:728, 1985.

32. Nelson JD, Havener VR, Cameron JD: Cellulose acetate impressions of the ocular surface: dry eye states, *Arch Ophthalmol* 101:1869, 1983.

33. Nelson JD, Wright JC: Conjunctival goblet cell densities in ocular surface disease, *Arch Ophthalmol* 102:1049, 1984.

34. Maskin SL et al: Diagnostic impression cytology for external eye disease, *Cornea* 8:270, 1989.

35. Vedreyu VL, Fullard RJ: Enhancements to the conjunctival impression cytology technique and examples of applications in a clinico-biochemical study of dry eye, *CLAO J* 20:59, 1994.

36. Rivas L et al: Correlation between impression cytology and tear function parameters in Sjögren's syndrome, *Acta Ophthalmol (Copenh)* 71:353, 1993.

37. Petroutsos G et al: Diagnostic tests for dry eye disease in normals and dry eye patients with and without Sjögren's syndrome, *Ophthalmic Res* 24:326, 1992.

38. Bloch KJ et al: Sjögren's syndrome: a clinical, pathological and serological study of sixty-two cases, *Medicine (Baltimore)* 44:187, 1965.

39. Sjögren H, Bloch KJ: Keratoconjunctivitis sicca and the Sjögren syndrome, *Surv Ophthalmol* 16:145, 1971.

40. Moustsopoulos HM et al: Sjögren's syndrome (sicca syndrome): current issues, *Ann Intern Med* 92:212, 1980.

41. Vitali C et al: Preliminary criteria for the classification of Sjögren's syndrome: results of a prospective concerted action supported by the European Community, *Arthritis Rheum* 36:340, 1993.

42. Fox RI, Saito I: Criteria for diagnosis of Sjögren's syndrome, *Rheum Dis Clin North Am* 20:391, 1994.

43. Aguilar AJ, Fonseca L, Croxatto JO: Sjögren's syndrome: a comparative study of impression cytology of the conjunctiva and buccal mucosa, and salivary gland biopsy, *Cornea* 10:203, 1991.

44. Liotet S, Konhe O, Wattiaux MI: Sjögren's syndrome diagnosis: a comparison of conjunctival and gingival impressions and salivary gland biopsy, *Adv Exp Med Biol* 350:661, 1994.

45. Farris RL, Stuchell RN, Nisengard R: Sjögren's syndrome and keratoconjunctivitis sicca, *Cornea* 10:207, 1991.

46. Shearn MA: *Sjögren's syndrome.* In Smith LH, editor: *Major problems in internal medicine,* Philadelphia, 1971, Saunders.

47. Andonopoulos AP et al: Secondary Sjögren's syndrome in rheumatoid arthritis, *J Rheumatol* 14:1098, 1987.

48. Drosos A et al: Prevalence of primary Sjögren's syndrome in an elderly population, *Br J Rheumatol* 27:123, 1988.

49. Andonopoulos A et al: Sjögren's syndrome in systemic lupus erythematosus, *J Rheumatol* 17:201, 1990.

50. Mizuno Y et al: Recurrent parotid gland enlargement as an initial manifestation of Sjögren's syndrome, *Eur J Pediatr* 148:414, 1989.

51. Siamopoulou-Mavridou A et al: Sjögren's syndrome in childhood: report of two cases, *Eur J Pediatr* 148:523, 1989.

52. Tomiita M et al: The clinical manifestations of Sjögren's syndrome in children, *Ryumachi* 34:863, 1994.

53. Rocha G, Kavalec C: Sjögren's syndrome in a child, *Can J Ophthalmol* 29:234, 1994.

54. Reveille JD et al: Primary Sjögren's syndrome and other autoimmune diseases in families: prevalence and immunogenetic studies in six kindreds, *Ann Intern Med* 101:748, 1984.

55. Reveille JD, Arnett FC: The immunogenetics of Sjögren's syndrome, *Rheum Dis Clin North Am* 18:539, 1994.

56. Tabbara KF: *Sjögren's syndrome.* In Smolin G, Thoft RA, editors: *The cornea: scientific foundations and clinical practice,* Boston, 1994, Little, Brown & Co.

57. Moutsopoulas HM: *Sjögren's syndrome.* In Braunwald E et al, editors: *Harrison's principles of internal medicine,* ed 14, New York, 1994, McGraw-Hill.

58. Anderson LG, Talal N: The spectrum of benign to malignant lymphoproliferation in Sjögren's syndrome, *Clin Exp Immunol* 9:199, 1971.

59. Alexander EL et al: Neurologic complications of primary Sjögren's syndrome, *Medicine* 61:247, 1982.

60. Molina R, Provost TT, Alexander EL: Peripheral inflammatory vascular disease in Sjögren's syndrome: association with nervous system complications, *Arthritis Rheum* 28:1341, 1985.

61. Williamson J: Keratoconjunctivitis sicca, histology of lacrimal gland, *Br J Ophthalmol* 57:852, 1973.

62. Lindahl G et al: Epithelial HLA-DR expression and T lymphocyte subsets in salivary glands in Sjögren's syndrome, *Clin Exp Immunol* 61:475, 1985.

63. Fos RI, Kang H-I: Pathogenesis of Sjögren's syndrome, *Rheum Dis Clin North Am* 18:517, 1994.

64. Talal N: *Sjögren's syndrome.* In Samter M, editor: *Immunologic diseases,* ed 4, Boston, 1988, Little, Brown & Co.

65. Alexander E: Central nervous system disease in Sjögren's syndrome: new insights into immunopathogenesis, *Rheum Dis Clin North Am* 18:637, 1994.

66. Venables P: *Sjögren's syndrome: differential diagnosis, immunopathology and genetics.* In Scott T et al, editors: *Topical reviews, reports of rheumatic diseases,* London, 1988, ARC Publications.

67. Fox RI, Pearson G, Vaughan JH: Detection of Epstein-Barr virus-associated antigens and DNA in salivary biopsies from patients with Sjögren's syndrome, *J Immunol* 137:3162, 1986.

68. Pflugfelder SC et al: Epstein-Barr virus infection and immunologic dysfunction in patients with aqueous tear deficiency, *Ophthalmology* 97:313, 1990.

69. Karameris A et al: Detection of the Epstein Barr viral genome by an in situ hybridization method in salivary gland biopsies from patients with secondary Sjogren's syndrome, *Clin Exp Rheumatol* 10:327, 1992.

70. Pflugfelder DC et al: Amplification of Epstein-Barr virus genomic sequences in blood cells, lacrimal glands, and tears from primary Sjögren's syndrome patients, *Ophthalmology* 97:976, 1990.

71. Fox RI: Epstein-Barr virus and human autoimmune diseases: possibilities and pitfalls, *J Virol Methods* 241:1218, 1988.

72. Vitali C et al: The European Community Study Group on diagnostic criteria for Sjögren's syndrome: sensitivity and specificity of tests for ocular and oral involvement in Sjögren's syndrome, *Ann Rheum Dis* 53:637, 1994.

73. Swanson A, Jeter D, Tucker P: Ophthalmic vehicles: II. Comparison of ointment and polyvinyl alcohol 1.4%, *Ophthalmologica* 160:265, 1970.

74. Holly FJ, Lamberts DW: Effect of nonisotonic solutions on tear film osmolality, *Invest Ophthalmol Vis Sci* 20:236, 1981.

75. Lopez-Bernal D, Ubels J: Artificial tear composition and promotion of recovery of the damaged corneal epithelium, *Cornea* 12:115, 1993.

76. McCollum CJ et al: Microbial contamination of preservative-free artificial tears with repeated usage, *Ophthalmology* 101(suppl):104, 1994.

77. DeLuise VP, Peterson WS: The use of topical Healon tears in the management of refractory dry-eye syndrome, *Ann Ophthalmol* 16:823, 1984.

78. Polack FM, McNiece MT: The treatment of dry eyes with Na hyaluronate (Healon), *Cornea* 1:133, 1982.

79. Hammer ME, Burch TG: Viscous corneal protection by sodium hyaluronate, chondroitin sulfate, and methylcellulose, *Invest Ophthalmol Vis Sci* 25:1329, 1984.

80. Hamano T et al: Evaluation of the effect of the sodium hyaluronate ophthalmic solution on tear film stability: non-contact specular microscopic evaluation, *Nippon Ganka Gakkai Zasshi* 97:928, 1993.

81. Limberg MB et al: Topical application of hyaluronic acid and chondroitin sulfate in the treatment of dry eyes, *Am J Ophthalmol* 103:194, 1987.

82. Rox RI et al: Beneficial effect of artificial tears made with autologous serum in patients with keratoconjunctivitis sicca, *Arthritis Rheum* 27:459, 1984.

83. Tseng SCG et al: Topical retinoid treatment for various dry-eye disorders, *Ophthalmology* 92:717, 1985.

84. Soong HK et al: Topical retinoid therapy for squamous metaplasia of various ocular surface disorders, *Ophthalmology* 95:1442, 1988.

85. Bloomfield SE et al: Soluble artificial tear inserts, *Arch Ophthalmol* 95:247, 1977.

86. Werblin TP, Rheinstrom SD, Kaufman HE: The use of slow-release artificial tears in the long-term management of keratitis sicca, *Ophthalmology* 88:78, 1981.

87. Guatheron PD, Lotli VJ, LeDouarec JC: Tear film breakup time prolonged with unmedicated cellulose polymer inserts, *Arch Ophthalmol* 97:1944, 1979.

88. Hill JC: Slow-release artificial tear inserts in the treatment of dry eyes in patients with rheumatoid arthritis, *Br J Ophthalmol* 73:151, 1989.

89. Tuberville AW, Frederick WR, Wood TO: Punctal occlusion in tear deficiency syndromes, *Ophthalmology* 89:1170, 1982.

90. Freeman JM: The punctum plug: evaluation of a new treatment for the dry eye, *Trans Am Acad Ophthalmol Otolaryngol* 79:874, 1975.

91. Meyer DR et al: Assessment of tear drainage after canalicular obstruction using fluorescein dye disappearance, *Ophthalmology* 97:1370, 1990.

92. Tsubota K, Yamada M, Urayama K: Spectacle side panels and moist inserts for the treatment of dry-eye patients, *Cornea* 13:197, 1994.

93. Kurihashi K: Moisture aid during sleep for the treatment of dry eye: wet gauze eye mask, *Ophthalmologica* 208:216, 1994.

94. Gassett AR, Kaufman HE: Hydrophilic lens therapy of severe keratoconjunctivitis sicca and conjunctival scarring, *Am J Ophthalmol* 71:1185, 1971.

95. Dohlman CH, Boruchoff SA, Mobilia E: Complications in use of soft contact lenses in corneal disease, *Arch Ophthalmol* 90:367, 1973.

96. Frost-Larsen K et al: Sjögren's syndrome, *Arch Ophthalmol* 98:836, 1980.

97. Katsuelson AB, Zhak EM: Surgical therapy of xerophthalmia by transplantation of parotid duct into conjunctival sac, *Vestn Oftalmol* 30:3, 1951.

98. Bennett JE: The management of total xerophthalmia, *Arch Ophthalmol* 81:667, 1969.

99. Soll DB: Vein grafting in nasolacrimal system reconstruction, *Ophthalmic Surg* 14:696, 1983.

100. Gunduz K, Ozdemir O: Topical cyclosporin

treatment of keratoconjunctivitis sicca in secondary Sjögren's syndrome, *Acta Ophthalmol (Copenh)* 72:438, 1994.

101. Lemp MA et al: The precorneal tear film: I. Factors in spreading and maintaining a continuous tear film over the corneal surface, *Arch Ophthalmol* 3:39, 1970.

102. Katz J, Kaufman HE: Corneal exposure during sleep (nocturnal lagophthalmos), *Arch Ophthalmol* 95:499, 1977.

Fifteen

Epithelial Diseases

NORMAL EPITHELIAL HEALING

Normal epithelial wound healing is a process of cell migration, mitosis, and adhesion. Small defects are covered by migration of adjacent epithelial cells, and this is followed by cell division until the thickness of the epithelium returns to normal.[1,2] The activated, migrating epithelial cells express vimentin[3] and epidermal growth factor (EGF) receptor.[4,5] With larger defects, both migration and mitosis are involved in covering the defect, and more time is required. Cells in the limbal and possibly the extralimbal conjunctiva migrate centripetally during healing of large corneal wounds.[6] If the basement membrane is intact, the epithelial cells attach rapidly, forming hemidesmosomes over the remaining anchoring fibrils (within 24 hours).[7] Healing after injuries that destroy the basement membrane is more complex and can take much longer.

After epithelial wounding, the keratocyte population in the anterior stroma is reduced.[8,9] The reason for this is unclear, but it may be related to osmotic changes. A temporary layer of fibrin and fibronectin forms on the denuded surface and facilitates epithelial migration and attachment.[4, 10-16] The process of cell sliding involves detachment from underlying fibronectin through activation of plasmin, a proteolytic enzyme, and advancement to adjacent fibronectin.[17] The epithelial cells are stimulated by fibrin and fibronectin to release plasminogen activator. Plasminogen activator then causes the conversion of plasminogen into plasmin. The active plasmin decreases epithelial adhesion to the fibrin and fibronectin, allowing advancement of the cell.

Once epithelial integrity is restored, the temporary matrix of fibrin and fibronectin is resorbed. After the epithelial layer is intact, basement membrane and anchoring fibrils are formed. If stroma has been removed, collagen is laid down beneath the epithelium, and new anchoring fibrils may constantly be reformed until normal stromal thickness is achieved.[18]

Table 15-1	Causes of Decreased Corneal Sensation

FIFTH NERVE PALSY
Surgical
Tumors
Aneurysms
Others
CONGENITAL CAUSES
Familial dysautonomia (Riley-Day syndrome)
Goldenhar's syndrome
Möbius' syndrome
Parry-Romberg syndrome
Bassen-Kornzweig syndrome
Isolated congenital trigeminal anesthesia
CORNEAL DYSTROPHIES
Lattice
Granular (rare)
IATROGENIC
Contact lens wear[27]
Trauma to ciliary nerves by laser, cryotherapy, scleral buckling, or diathermy
Corneal incisions: cataract, keratoplasty, epikeratophakia
INFECTION
Herpes simplex
Herpes zoster
Leprosy
SYSTEMIC DISEASE
Diabetes[28, 29]
MEDICATIONS
Topical anesthetic abuse
Atropine[30]
Timolol (usually temporary)[31]
Sulfacetamide 30%[32]
TOXIC CAUSES
Chemical burns
Carbon disulfide exposure
Hydrogen sulfide exposure
FUNCTIONAL CAUSES
Hysteria
MISCELLANEOUS CAUSES
Any condition involving chronic epithelial injury or stromal inflammation

NEUROTROPHIC KERATITIS

Sensory innervation of the cornea can be impaired by many conditions (Table 15-1). Whenever corneal sensation is decreased, epithelial dysfunction occurs. The pathogenesis of the epithelial disease is unclear, but it is believed that the corneal nerves normally provide some type of trophic influence on the epithelium. The nerves may release substances from their sensory endings that are necessary for epithelial cell function. In the absence of innervation, cell metabolism is reduced, permeability is increased,[19] acetylcholine and choline acetyl-

transferase concentrations are reduced,[20,21] and the mitotic rate decreases.[22,23] Epithelial cell attachment is reduced, and fewer desmosomes are observed.[24] Epithelial defects, vascularization, and opacification can occur, even in the absence of injury.[25] These eyes are also prone to infection and trauma, and their ability to heal is markedly reduced.[26] Stromal ulceration often occurs, usually in the presence of persistent epithelial defects.

Corneal Manifestations

Early signs of corneal involvement are the development of a corneal haze and injection of the conjunctiva. These changes may be apparent within 24 hours after section of the trigeminal nerve. Damage and focal loss of epithelial cells lead to punctate keratopathy and decreased corneal luster (Fig. 15-1). In many cases larger erosions develop, and eventually so do broad epithelial defects, most commonly in the interpalpebral cornea. These defects usually are slow to heal, even with treatment. Iritis often accompanies a persistent epithelial defect, and a sterile hypopyon can be seen, usually after placement of a bandage contact lens. Ulceration (Fig. 15-2), perforation, and vascularization often develop before the epithelium heals.

The course of neurotrophic keratitis varies considerably. In many patients with congenital or acquired corneal hypoesthesia, the cornea can appear normal or exhibit only mild punctate staining for years. Then, spontaneously or after minor trauma, an epithelial defect develops; it heals poorly, and infection or sterile ulceration often follow.

Treatment

The only form of treatment available is protecting the corneal surface with lubricants, tarsorrhaphy, or a bandage contact lens. Punctate staining and corneal haziness are treated with artificial tear solutions during the day and ointment at bedtime. If defects develop, patching may result in healing, but often a bandage contact lens or tarsorrhaphy is required. Using bandage contact lenses is more likely to cause complications in these patients. A sterile hypopyon often develops, usually within 1 or 2 days of lens application. For unknown reasons, administration of a cycloplegic agent usually prevents this complication. Both sterile and infectious infiltrates are also common.

A complete tarsorrhaphy usually results in healing of the epithelium and prevents further ulceration. Once the epithelium is intact, the tarsorrhaphy can gradually be opened. Partial

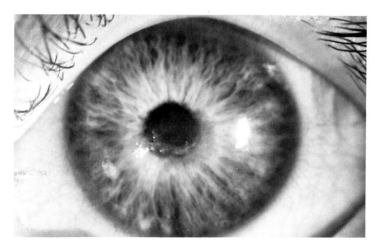

Figure 15-1
Anesthetic cornea with loss of epithelial luster and irregular thickening of the central epithelium.

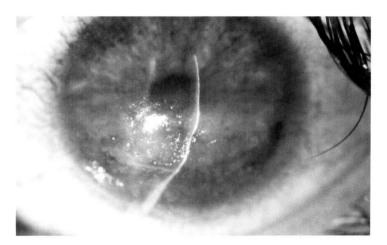

Figure 15-2
Anesthetic cornea with ulceration.

closure may be required permanently, and occasionally total closure must be performed repeatedly or a conjunctival flap must be placed.

RECURRENT EROSIONS

Recurrent erosions are a common problem. Most cases are related to corneal injury, most commonly from fingernails or paper.[33] These erosions may also be seen in patients with diabetes,[34] epithelial basement membrane dystrophy and other corneal dystrophies,[35] other forms of anterior stromal injury, exposure, and Cockayne's syndrome.[36] Causes of recurrent corneal erosions are presented in Table 15-2.

The erosions reflect an abnormality of the epithelial attachment complex, which is comprised of the basement membrane, hemidesmosomes, anchoring fibrils, and anterior stroma.[37-39] After trauma, discontinuities and duplications of attachment complexes are seen for 8 to 12 weeks, and during this period the epithelium is easily removed.[39,40] Damage to Bowman's layer and the anterior stroma or active inflammation in these layers can also prevent adhesion. Primary abnormalities in the attachment complex are seen in epithelial basement membrane (map-dot-fingerprint) dystrophy (see Chapter 17) and diabetes. Thickening of the basement membrane, with reduced penetration of the anchoring fibrils into the

Table 15-2	Causes of Recurrent Corneal Erosions

TRAUMA
Fingernail or paper cuts
Alkali burns
Thermal injury
CORNEAL DYSTROPHIES
Meesmann's
Fuchs'
Reis-Bücklers'
Grayson-Wilbrandt
Epithelial basement membrane
Lattice
Macular
Granular
CORNEAL ANESTHESIA
Herpes simplex
Herpes zoster
Alkali burns
Others
OTHER CORNEAL CONDITIONS
Nontraumatic anterior stromal injury (e.g., infection)
Corneal edema
SYSTEMIC DISEASE
Diabetes
Cockayne's syndrome
Epidermolysis bullosa

stroma, and duplications of anchoring fibrils are seen in the corneas of patients with diabetes.[41] In lattice dystrophy, amyloid deposition occurs between the epithelium and Bowman's layer, disrupting the epithelial attachment complex.[42]

Clinical Manifestations

With recurrent erosions the patient experiences pain, photophobia, tearing, and foreign body sensation.[43] The onset is usually sudden, most often early in the morning (while dreaming), but can occur anytime. The symptoms vary in severity and duration according to the size of the erosion; they can last for minutes to days. The frequency of attacks also varies considerably, and as many as four or five brief attacks may occur each day.

During an acute attack one may see epithelial loss, epithelial microcysts, bullae, loose sheets of epithelium, or epithelial filaments. Visual acuity can be markedly reduced if the visual axis is affected. Between attacks epithelial cysts, surface irregularity, or subepithelial scarring can often be detected.[44,45] The healed epithelial area may even resemble a dendritic figure and may be misdiagnosed as herpetic

keratitis. As with any epithelial defect, bacterial infection can develop.

The physician should look for evidence of abnormal epithelial adhesion in other portions of the cornea and in the fellow eye to detect epithelial basement membrane dystrophy. It has been stated that approximately half of patients with recurrent erosions have evidence of epithelial basement membrane dystrophy.[36]

Treatment

The treatment of recurrent corneal erosion is directed toward reestablishing tight adhesion of the epithelium by a normal epithelial attachment complex. The first goal is healing of the erosion, which can be accomplished with patching or placement of a bandage contact lens. Removal of loose epithelium may facilitate healing.

In many cases little or no treatment is required; the attacks are relatively infrequent and short-lived. Erosions usually abate spontaneously after 1 to 3 years. The simplest method of reducing recurrences is by lubrication, with drops during the day and ointment at bedtime. Although many feel that hypertonic drops and ointment are superior, this was not observed in a randomized trial.[46] Treatment should be continued for at least 3 months.

If further treatment is necessary, several options are available, including anterior stromal puncture, debridement, superficial keratectomy, and bandage contact lens wear. Anterior stromal puncture was introduced by McClean, MaCrea, and Rich[47] to treat recurrent erosions occurring consistently in the same portion of the extraaxial cornea. A 25- or 27-gauge needle is used to create several shallow (less than one fourth depth) punctures in the anterior stroma of the affected area.[48] The needle tip can be bent at 90° to ensure that only the desired depth is achieved. If fine superficial scars are created, the visual axis can be treated without degrading vision. I have found this technique to be very effective. The mechanism of action is unclear, but in rabbits epithelial plugs persist in the wounds for at least 5 months after surgery.[49] In patients with bullous keratopathy anterior stromal puncture stimulated local production of laminin, fibronectin, and type IV collagen.[50] The neodymium:yttrium-aluminum-garnet laser can be used to create localized anterior stromal lesions similar to those produced by needle puncture.[51]

A bandage contact lens can provide comfort and lessen or eliminate erosions. It usually must be worn for at least 3 months and should

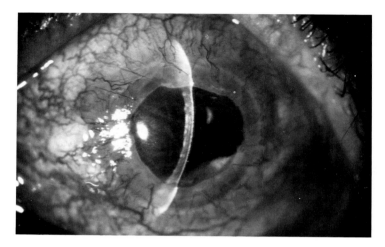

Figure 15-3
Persistent epithelial defect after penetrating keratoplasty. (Courtesy of Diane Curtin, Pittsburgh, PA.)

not be removed until the epithelium appears normal in the affected area.

Scraping of the epithelium and basement membrane can improve adhesion after healing. If the recurrences consistently affect the same portion of the cornea, the epithelium can be removed and the base gently scraped with a blunt instrument, such as a Kimura spatula. If diffuse disease is present, as in epithelial basement membrane dystrophy or in cases that are resistant to other treatment, aggressive debridement of nearly the entire corneal surface (leaving 1 to 2 mm of peripheral epithelium),[52] with gentle burring[53] or superficial keratectomy,[54,55] may be more effective. Burring is performed with a 5-mm fine-grit diamond burr. The epithelium is debrided to within 1 to 2 mm of the limbus, and the exposed Bowman's membrane is polished with the burr. Some eyes experience a myopic shift after this procedure. All these procedures carry a theoretic risk of delayed healing, ulceration, scarring, and infection.

Excimer laser phototherapeutic keratectomy can be performed for refractory recurrent erosions. Symptomatic improvement has been obtained in the majority of patients.[56-58] The affected epithelium is removed and a superficial ablation (4 to 7 μm) of Bowman's membrane is performed. There is no refractive change.

I perform anterior stromal puncture if recurrences consistently affect the same area. If the epithelium is loose, with many cysts or accumulated basement membrane material, localized debridement is also performed, using a Paton or Kimura spatula, and a bandage contact lens is placed. Many patients experience

marked pain after the procedure for 12 to 36 hours. Topical diclofenac four times daily helps relieve pain. Repeat treatments are necessary in some cases, both in previously treated areas and in new areas. Anterior stromal puncture can be performed for diffuse basement membrane disease, but I usually try use of a bandage contact lens first. I also use a bandage contact lens when patients are reluctant to undergo the above procedures. If anterior stromal puncture and debridement are not successful, excimer laser phototherapeutic keratectomy or gentle burring can be performed.

PERSISTENT EPITHELIAL DEFECTS

Nonhealing epithelial defects (Fig. 15-3) are relatively common problems, but a systematic approach to diagnosis and treatment can nearly always lead to resolution. The most common conditions associated with delayed epithelial healing are listed in Table 15-3. A thorough search for these conditions should be performed in any patient with a persistent defect; often a number of conditions are present.

Stromal Ulceration

If epithelial healing is delayed, stromal substance can be lost. This has been hypothesized to result from several mechanisms. With a chronic epithelial defect, polymorphonuclear leukocytes (PMNs) invade the stroma, and excess amounts of the enzymes plasmin and collagenase may be produced. Collagenase can split collagen, making it more vulnerable to de-

Table 15-3	Common Causes of Delayed Epithelial Healing

ABNORMAL LID FUNCTION
Entropion
Ectropion
Lagophthalmos
Trichiasis
MEDICATIONS
Topical antibiotics[60]
  Gentamicin
  Tobramycin
  ?Fluoroquinolones[61]
Topical antivirals
Preservatives
Anesthetic abuse
SYSTEMIC DISEASE
Diabetes mellitus
Severe malnutrition
Vitamin A deficiency
PRIMARY EPITHELIAL DISEASE
Cicatricial pemphigoid
Erythema multiforme major (Stevens-Johnson syndrome)
Atopic keratoconjunctivitis
Other dermatologic conditions
LOCAL CONDITIONS
Corneal anesthesia
Stromal injury: viral (see Fig. 12-10), traumatic, chemical
Keratoconjunctivitis sicca
Active stromal inflammation or infection
Occult foreign body

struction by other proteases. Collagenase has been isolated from ulcerating corneas and is thought to be produced by epithelial cells, PMNs, and keratocytes.[59]

Plasmin can also be secreted by epithelial cells, PMNs, and keratocytes. Plasmin degrades fibrin, fibronectin, and basement membrane components and activates collagenase.[62] Theoretically, excess plasmin production could prevent the formation of an adequate fibrin-fibronectin layer for epithelial attachment and resurfacing. Plasmin also stimulates keratocyte secretion of latent collagenase, converts latent collagenase to active collagenase, and cleaves complement component C3 to produce fragments that are chemotactic for PMNs. In addition to the experimental support for the role of plasmin, elevated tear levels of plasmin have been found in some patients with persistent epithelial defects.[63]

Treatment

If possible, any conditions that impair epithelial healing should be corrected. Dry eyes are treated with lubricants and punctal occlusion, lid position abnormalities are corrected surgically, and unnecessary toxic medications are discontinued.

Progressive measures are then taken, in a stepwise manner, from the least complicated or invasive measure to the most, to obtain healing. Pressure patching, bandage contact lens, or total tarsorrhaphy can be used. If some healing is not obtained within 2 to 3 days, the next measure is taken. Because contact lens wear is usually required for 1 to 3 weeks, hydrophilic polymer contact lenses are preferred to short-lived collagen lenses. It is best to have several types of bandage lenses available because no one type fits all patients. In eyes with marked conjunctival inflammation or elevation, smaller-diameter lenses can be helpful. Pediatric aphakic lenses can be used for this purpose, because they are approximately 12 mm in diameter and are relatively stiff. Larger lenses can be trephined to the correct size. Tarsorrhaphy should be total, or near total, with only a small medial opening for instillation of medications. The tarsorrhaphy should be left in place for at least 10 days. One of the sutures can be tied with a bow knot, over bolsters, allowing loosening for examination and reclosure if healing is incomplete.

Epithelial Transplantation

Transplantation of conjunctival epithelium or limbal corneal epithelium can be used for eyes with recalcitrant epithelial defects.[64-68] The procedure has been used chiefly after chemical or thermal burns but can also be performed in other conditions, such as after penetrating keratoplasty or in cases of herpes simplex keratitis. Transplantation is often successful in cases that are not amenable to other forms of treatment.

Experimental Treatments

Various topical medications have been proposed for enhancing epithelial healing.

Fibronectin and Epidermal Growth Factor. Considerable interest has developed in the use of fibronectin and EGF. As mentioned previously, fibronectin appears to play an important role in epithelial cell migration over a defect. EGF promotes epithelial cell proliferation, another important process in epithelial healing.[16,69,70] Both topical fibronectin[71-73] and EGF[16,69,70,74-76] promote epithelial healing after various types of injury in rabbits. However, in experimental animals the epithelial defects recur, even with continued fibronectin or EGF treatment. The incidence of secondary epithelial breakdown was reduced by combined use of EGF and fibronectin[77] or by adding topical steroid treatment to EGF or fibronectin treatment.[78]

In uncontrolled patient trials, autologous and homologous fibronectin drops appeared to aid in closure of persistent epithelial defects,[79-83] and EGF was reported to promote epithelial healing in patients with corneal disease.[84] In one placebo-controlled study of patients undergoing penetrating keratoplasty, EGF did not promote epithelial healing,[85] but in another controlled study of traumatic corneal epithelial defects EGF significantly enhanced healing.[86] It is possible that more prolonged exposure (more than 2 hours) is necessary to achieve the optimum effect.[87,88] A controlled clinical trial of fibronectin (3.5 mg/ml four times daily) in the treatment of persistent epithelial defects failed to demonstrate efficacy of the medication.[89]

Plasmin Inhibitors. In view of the elevated tear levels of plasmin found in some patients with persistent epithelial defects and the possible role of plasmin in the persistence of epithelial defects and the associated stromal ulceration, the use of plasmin inhibitors has also been investigated recently. Treatment with topical aprotinin, a proteinase inhibitor, appeared to promote epithelial healing.[63] Further studies are needed, and aprotinin currently is not commercially available.

Collagenase Inhibitors. The identification of collagenase in ulcerating corneas caused a great deal of excitement about the possible therapeutic role of collagenase inhibitors. Ethylenediaminetetraacetic acid, cysteine, acetylcysteine, tetracycline, doxycycline,[90] and α- macroglobulin have anticollagenase activity and have been tried. As yet, however, none has been convincingly demonstrated to be of clinical benefit in preventing stromal ulceration.[91]

Others. The topical β-adrenergic receptor blocking agents timolol, levobunolol, betaxolol, and metipranolol were found to accelerate epithelial wound healing in rabbits.[92] Once the epithelial defect is closed, the surface should be protected to facilitate thickening and attachment of the epithelial layer. Lubricants can be continued, a bandage contact lens can be left in place for several weeks, or the tarsorrhaphy can gradually be taken down.

Table 15-4	Corneal Diseases with Limbal Deficiency
Chemical burns
Thermal burns
Contact lens–induced keratoconjunctivitis
Surgical limbal injury (incision, excision, or cryotherapy)
Erythema multiforme major (Stevens-Johnson syndrome)
Severe microbial keratitis
Peripheral inflammatory disorders
Aniridia
Keratitis associated with multiple endocrine deficiencies

LIMBAL STEM CELL DEFICIENCY

Limbal stem cell deficiency can arise in a number of situations (Table 15-4). The corneal epithelium is diffusely thickened, opacified, and often vascularized. Chronic inflammation, photophobia, poor vision, recurrent erosions, and persistent epithelial defects are often seen. Usually the normal limbal palisades of Vogt are absent.[93] There is congenital or acquired loss of limbal epithelial stem cells, resulting in population of the corneal surface with epithelium derived from conjunctiva. Similar corneal changes can be produced experimentally by surgical excision of the limbus.[94] Conditions with conjunctivalization of the corneal epithelium can be differentiated from other corneal diseases resulting in opacification and vascularization by the presence of goblet cells on impression cytology[95] or by staining with monoclonal antibodies.[96,97] Clinical signs of limbal deficiency may not develop for many years after an injury. Neurotrophic keratopathy from diabetes or ischemia is also associated with conjunctivalization of the corneal epithelium, although the mechanism is unclear.[98]

Epithelial transplantation for ocular surface reconstruction was first described by Thoft and others.[64-67,99] Total superficial keratectomy and resection of the perilimbal conjunctiva for 360° were performed. In patients with unilateral disease, conjunctival grafts were then obtained from the unaffected eye and sutured over the limbal cornea. Kenyon and Tseng[68] modified this procedure by using donor limbal epithelium instead of conjunctiva. In a rabbit model, limbal transplantation was more effective than conjunctival transplantation.[100] While there are theoretic advantages to this procedure, it also entails greater risk. In one study of patients with contact lens–induced keratopathy,[101] recurrent epithelial changes were noted in the recipient eyes of patients who had previously worn contact lenses bilaterally. The authors concluded that subclinical limbal disease was present in the donor eyes. In addition, the donor eye appears to be compromised. Experimentally, its capacity to heal large corneal epithelial defects is reduced,[97] and adjacent epithelial haze was reported in one case.[101]

In patients with bilateral disease, Thoft and others obtained peripheral corneal lenticules from fresh donor globes (keratoepithelioplasty).[102,103] This procedure was effective in healing epithelial defects, but rejection usually led to recurrent epithelial opacification. Subsequently, others used limbal allografts to treat patients with bilateral disease or to avoid injury to the fellow eye in unilateral disease.[104,105] Systemic administration of cyclosporine for an average of 3 months after surgery appeared to prevent allograft rejection in one series of 16 patients.[104] Over an average follow-up of 18 months, visual acuity was improved in 13 of 16 eyes. Tsubota et al.[106] achieved similar results using a combination of oral and topical cyclosporine and intravenous dexamethasone. In another series, transplantation of donor conjunctiva from human leukocyte antigen (HLA)–matched relatives (50% or 100% identity) was successful without systemic immunosuppression.[105]

In summary, limbal autograft transplantation is recommended for patients with unilateral limbal deficiency. Where there is a question of bilateral disease, such as in contact lens–induced keratoconjunctivitis or asymmetric alkali burns, it is best to evaluate the donor eye perilimbal epithelium with impression cytology. In patients with bilateral disease, limbal allograft transplantation can be performed. Systemic immunosuppression and/or the use of HLA-matched relatives appears to increase the success rate.

REFERENCES

1. Kuwabara T, Perkins DG, Cogan DG: Sliding of the epithelium in experimental corneal wounds, *Invest Ophthalmol* 15:4, 1976.
2. Pfister RR: The healing of corneal epithelial abrasions in the rabbit: a scanning electron microscopic study, *Invest Ophthalmol* 14:468, 1975.
3. Sundar Raj N et al: Expression of vimentin by rabbit corneal epithelial cells during wound repair, *Cell Tissue Res* 267:347, 1992.
4. Murata T, Ishibashi T, Opomata H: Localizations of epidermal growth factor receptor and proliferating cell nuclear antigen during corneal wound healing, *Graefes Arch Clin Exp Ophthalmol* 231:104, 1993.
5. Beuerman RW, Thompson HW: Molecular and cellular responses of the corneal epithelium to wound healing, *Acta Ophthalmol* 202(suppl):7, 1992.
6. Sandvig KU et al: Cell kinetics of conjunctival and corneal epithelium during regeneration of different-sized corneal epithelial defects, *Acta Ophthalmol* 72:43, 1994.
7. Gipson IK et al: Hemidesmosomal formation in vitro, *J Cell Biol* 97:849, 1983.
8. Szerenyi KD et al: Keratocyte loss and repopulation of anterior corneal stroma after deepithelialization, *Arch Ophthalmol* 112:973, 1994.
9. Campos M et al: Keratocyte loss after corneal deepithelialization in primates and rabbits, *Arch Ophthalmol* 112:254, 1994.
10. Fujikawa LS et al: Fibronectin in healing rabbit corneal wounds, *Lab Invest* 45:120, 1981.
11. Suda T et al: Fibronectin appears at the site of corneal stromal wound in rabbits, *Curr Eye Res* 1:553, 1981.
12. Ohashi Y et al: Appearance of fibronectin in rabbit cornea after thermal burn, *Jpn J Ophthalmol* 27:547, 1983.
13. Fujikawa LS et al: Basement membrane components in healing rabbit corneal epithelial wounds: immunofluorescence and ultrastructural studies, *J Cell Biol* 98:128, 1984.
14. Nishida T et al: Fibronectin promotes epithelial migration of cultured rabbit cornea in situ, *J Cell Biol* 97:1653, 1983.
15. Berman M et al: Ulceration is correlated with degradation of fibrin and fibronectin at the corneal surface, *Invest Ophthalmol Vis Sci* 24:1358, 1983.
16. Watanabe K, Nakagawa S, Nishida T: Stimulatory effects of fibronectin and EGF on migration of corneal epithelial cells, *Invest Ophthalmol Vis Sci* 28:205, 1987.
17. Berman M et al: *The pathogenesis of epithelial defects and stromal ulceration.* In Cavanagh HD, editor: *The cornea: transactions of the World Congress on the Cornea III,* New York, 1988, Raven Press.
18. Goodman WM et al: Unique parameters in the healing of linear partial thickness penetrating corneal incisions in rabbit: immunohistochemical evaluation, *Curr Eye Res* 8:305, 1989.
19. Simone S: de Richerche sul contenuto in acqua totale ed in azoto totale della cornea di coniglio in condizione di cheratite neuroparalytica sperimentale, *Arch Ottalmol* 62:151, 1958.
20. Mittag TW, Mindel JS, Green JP: Trophic functions of the neuron: V. Familial dysautonomia: choline acetyltransferase in familial dysautonomia, *Ann NY Acad Sci* 228:301, 1974.
21. Hallerman W: Zur lakalbehandlung des Auges mit Acetycholin, *Klin Monatsbl Augenheilkd* 121:397, 1952.
22. Sigelman S, Friedenwald JS: Mitotic and wound healing activities of the corneal epithe-

lium: effect of sensory denervation, *Arch Ophthalmol* 52:46, 1954.

23. Mishima S: The effects of the denervation and the stimulation of the sympathetic and the trigeminal nerve on the mitotic rate of the corneal epithelium in the rabbit, *Jpn J Ophthalmol* 1:56, 1957.

24. Araki K et al: Epithelial wound healing in the denervated cornea, *Curr Eye Res* 13:203, 1994.

25. Alper MG: The anesthetic eye: an investigation of changes in the anterior ocular segment of the monkey caused by interrupting the trigeminal nerve at various levels along its course, *Trans Am Ophthalmol Soc* 72:323, 1976.

26. Schimmelpfennig B, Beuerman R: Sensory deprivation of the rabbit cornea affects epithelial properties, *Exp Neurol* 69:169, 1980.

27. Millodot M: Effect of long-term wear of hard contact lenses on corneal sensitivity, *Arch Ophthalmol* 96:1255, 1978.

28. Schwartz DE: Corneal sensitivity in diabetics, *Arch Ophthalmol* 91:174, 1974.

29. Schultz RO et al: Diabetic keratopathy as a manifestation of peripheral neuropathy, *Am J Ophthalmol* 96:368, 1983.

30. Von Oer S: Ueber die Beziehung des Acetylcholine des Hornhautepithels zur Erregungsu: Bertragung von Diesem auf die Sensiblen Nervenenden, *Pflugers Arch* 273:325, 1961.

31. Van Buskirk EM: Corneal anesthesia after timolol maleate therapy, *Am J Ophthalmol* 88:739, 1979.

32. Chang FW, Reinhart S, Fraser NM: Effect of 30% sulfacetamide on corneal sensitivity, *Am J Optom Physiol Opt* 61:318, 1984.

33. Cavanaugh DW et al: Pathogenesis and treatment of persistent epithelial defects, *Trans Am Acad Ophthalmol Otolaryngol* 81:754, 1976.

34. Mandelcorn MS, Blankenship G, Machemer R: Pars plana vitrectomy for management of severe diabetic retinopathy, *Am J Ophthalmol* 81:561, 1976.

35. Akiya S, Brown SI: The ultrastructure of Reis-Bücklers' dystrophy, *Am J Ophthalmol* 72:549, 1971.

36. Brown NA, Bron AJ: Recurrent erosion of the cornea, *Br J Ophthalmol* 60:84, 1976.

37. Goldman JM, Dohlman CH, Kravit RA: The basement membrane of the human cornea in recurrent epithelial erosion syndrome, *Trans Am Acad Ophthalmol Otolaryngol* 73:471, 1969.

38. Kenyon K: The synthesis of basement membrane by epithelium in bullous keratopathy, *Invest Ophthalmol* 8:156, 1969.

39. Khodadoust AA et al: Adhesion of regenerating corneal epithelium: the role of the basement membrane, *Am J Ophthalmol* 65:339, 1968.

40. Kenyon KR et al: Regeneration of corneal epithelial basement membrane following thermal cauterization, *Invest Ophthalmol Vis Sci* 16:292, 1977.

41. Kenyon KR: Recurrent corneal erosion: pathogenesis and therapy, *Int Ophthalmol Clin* 19:169, 1979.

42. Fogle JA et al: Defective epithelial adhesion in anterior corneal dystrophies, *Am J Ophthalmol* 79:925, 1975.

43. Chandler PA: Recurrent erosions of the cornea, *Am J Ophthalmol* 28:355, 1945.

44. Tripathi RG, Bron AJ: Cystic disorders of the corneal epithelium: II. Ultrastructural study of nontraumatic recurrent erosion, *Br J Ophthalmol* 56:73, 1972.

45. Wales HJ: A family history of corneal erosions, *Trans Ophthalmol Soc NZ* 8:77, 1955.

46. Hykin PG et al: The natural history and management of recurrent corneal erosion: a prospective randomised trial, *Eye* 8:35, 1994.

47. McClean EN, MaCrea SM, Rich LF: Recurrent erosion: treatment by anterior stromal puncture, *Ophthalmology* 93:784, 1986.

48. Rubinfeld RS et al: Anterior stromal puncture for recurrent erosion: further experience and new instrumentation, *Ophthalmic Surg* 21:318, 1990.

49. Judge D et al: Anterior stromal micropuncture: electron microscopic changes in the rabbit cornea, *Cornea* 9:152, 1990.

50. Hsu JKW et al: Anterior stromal puncture: immunohistochemical studies in human corneas, *Arch Ophthalmol* 111:1057, 1993.

51. Katz HR et al: Nd:YAG laser photo-induced adhesion of the corneal epithelium, *Am J Ophthalmol* 118:612, 1994.

52. Wood TO, Griffith ME: Surgery for corneal epithelial basement membrane dystrophy, *Ophthalmic Surg* 19:20, 1988.

53. Forstot SL et al: Diamond burr keratectomy for the treatment of recurrent corneal erosion syndrome, *Ophthalmol* 101(suppl):103, 1994.

54. Buxton JN, Constad WH: Superficial epithelial keratectomy in the treatment of epithelial basement membrane dystrophy, *Cornea* 6:292, 1987.

55. Buxton JN, Constad WH: Superficial epithelial keratectomy in the treatment of epithelial basement membrane dystrophy, *Ann Ophthalmol* 19:92, 1987.

56. O'Brart SPS, Kerr Muir MG, Marshall J: Phototherapeutic keratectomy for recurrent corneal erosions, *Eye* 8:378, 1994.

57. Dausch D et al: Phototherapeutic keratectomy in recurrent corneal epithelial erosion, *Refract Corneal Surg* 9:419, 1993.

58. Ohman L, Fagerholm P, Tengroth B: Treatment of recurrent corneal erosions with the excimer laser, *Acta Ophthalmol* 72:461, 1994.

59. Pfister RR et al: Collagenase activity of intact corneal epithelium in peripheral alkaline burns, *Arch Ophthalmol* 86:308, 1971.

60. Stern GA et al: Effect of topical antibiotic solutions on corneal epithelial wound healing, *Arch Opthalmol* 101:644, 1983.

61. Nakamura M et al: Effects of antimicrobials on corneal epithelial migration, *Curr Eye Res* 12:733, 1993.

62. Berman M et al: Plasmin regulates corneal collagenase secretion by degrading fibroblast cell

surface/matrix fibronectin, *Invest Ophthalmol Vis Sci* 25(suppl):6, 1984.

63. Salonen EM et al: Plasmin in tear fluid of patients with corneal ulcers: basis for new therapy, *Acta Ophthalmol (Copenh)* 65:3, 1987.

64. Thoft RA: Conjunctival transplantation, *Arch Ophthalmol* 95:1425, 1977.

65. Thoft RA: Conjunctival transplantation as an alternative to keratoplasty, *Ophthalmology* 86:1084, 1979.

66. Thoft RA: Indications for conjunctival transplantation, *Ophthalmology* 89:335, 1982.

67. Thoft RA: Keratoepithelioplasty, *Am J Ophthalmol* 97:1, 1983.

68. Kenyon KR, Tseng SCG: Limbal autograft transplantation for ocular surface disorders, *Ophthalmology* 96:709, 1989.

69. Frati L et al: Selective binding of the epidermal growth factor and its specific effects on the epithelial cells of the cornea, *Exp Eye Res* 14:135, 1972.

70. Savage CR, Cohen S: Proliferation of corneal epithelium induced by epidermal growth factor, *Exp Eye Res* 15:361, 1973.

71. Nishida T et al: Fibronectin enhancement of corneal epithelial wound healing of rabbits in vivo, *Arch Ophthalmol* 102:455, 1984.

72. Carol LA et al: Topical fibronectin in a rabbit alkali burn model of corneal ulceration, *Invest Ophthalmol Vis Sci* 26(suppl):176, 1985.

73. Tenn PF et al: Fibronectin in alkali burned rabbit cornea: enhancement of epithelial wound healing, *Invest Ophthalmol Vis Sci* 26(suppl):92, 1985.

74. Singh G, Foster CS: Epidermal growth factor in alkali-burned corneal epithelial wound healing, *Am J Ophthalmol* 103:802, 1987.

75. Chung JH, Fagerholm P: Treatment of rabbit corneal alkali wounds with human epidermal growth factor, *Cornea* 8:122, 1989.

76. Reim M et al: Effect on epidermal growth factor in severe experimental alkali burns, *Ophthalmic Res* 20:327, 1988.

77. Singh G, Foster CS: *Treatment of nonhealing corneal ulcers and recurrent corneal erosions.* In Cavanagh HD, editor: *The cornea: transactions of the World Congress on the Cornea III,* New York, 1988, Raven Press.

78. Singh G, Foster CS: Growth factors in treatment of nonhealing corneal ulcers and recurrent erosions, *Cornea* 8:45, 1989.

79. Phan TM et al: Topical fibronectin in the treatment of persistent corneal epithelial defects and trophic ulcers, *Am J Ophthalmol* 104:494, 1987.

80. Nishida T: *Role of fibronectin in corneal epithelial wound healing.* In Cavanagh HD, editor: *The cornea: transactions of the World Congress on the Cornea III,* New York, 1988, Raven Press.

81. Nishida T, Nakagawa S, Manabe R: Clinical evaluation of fibronectin eyedrops on epithelial disorders after herpetic keratitis, *Ophthalmology* 92:213, 1985.

82. Spigelman AV, Deutsch TA, Sugar J: Application of homologous fibronectin to persistent human corneal epithelial defects, *Cornea* 6:128, 1987.

83. Kim KS et al: Clinical efficacy of topical homologous fibronectin in persistent corneal epithelial disorders, *Korean J Ophthalmol* 6:12, 1992.

84. Daniele S et al: The effect of the epidermal growth factor (EGF) on the corneal epithelium in humans, *Graefes Arch Clin Exp Ophthalmol* 210:159, 1979.

85. Kandarakis AS, Page CS, Kaufman HE: The effect of epidermal growth factor on epithelial healing after penetrating keratoplasty in human eyes, *Am J Ophthalmol* 98:411, 1984.

86. Pastor JC, Calonge M: Epidermal growth factor and corneal wound healing: multicenter study, *Cornea* 11:311, 1992.

87. Sheardown H et al: Continuous epidermal growth factor delivery in corneal epithelial wound healing, *Invest Ophthalmol Vis Sci* 34:3593, 1993.

88. Nishida T et al: Differential modes of action of fibronectin and epidermal growth factor on rabbit corneal epithelial migration, *J Cell Physiol* 145:549, 1990.

89. Gordon JF et al: Topical fibronectin ophthalmic solution in the treatment of persistent defects of the corneal epithelium, *Am J Ophthalmol* 119:281, 1995.

90. Perry HD et al: Effect of doxycycline hyclate on corneal epithelial wound healing in the rabbit alkali-burn model: preliminary observations, *Cornea* 12:379, 1993.

91. Berman MB: *Collagenase and corneal ulceration.* In Wolley DR, Evanson JA, editors: *Collagenase in normal and pathological connective tissues,* New York, 1980, John Wiley & Sons, Inc.

92. Reidy JJ et al: Effect of topical β blockers on corneal epithelial wound healing in the rabbit, *Br J Ophthalmol* 78:377, 1994.

93. Kinoshita S et al: Disappearance of palisades of Vogt in ocular surface disease, *Jpn J Clin Ophthalmol* 40:363, 1986.

94. Huang AJW, Tseng SCG: Corneal epithelial wound healing in the absence of limbal epithelium, *Invest Ophthalmol Vis Sci* 32:96, 1991.

95. Tseng SCG et al: Classification of conjunctival surgeries for corneal disease based on stem cell concept, *Ophthalmol Clin North Am* 3:595, 1990.

96. Chen JJY, Tseng SCG: Abnormal corneal epithelial wound healing in partial thickness removal of limbal epithelium, *Invest Ophthalmol Vis Sci* 32:2219, 1991.

97. Chen JJY, Tseng SCG: Corneal epithelial wound healing in partial limbal deficiency, *Invest Ophthalmol Vis Sci* 31:1301, 1990.

98. Puangsricharern V, Tseng SCG: Cytologic evidence of corneal diseases with limbal stem cell deficiency, *Ophthalmology* 102:1476, 1995.

99. Clinch TE, Goins KM, Cobo M: Treatment of contact lens-induced ocular surface disorders

with autologous conjunctival transplantation, *Ophthalmology* 99:634, 1992.

100. Tsai RJF, Sun TT, Tseng SCG: Comparison of limbal and conjunctival autograft transplantation in corneal surface reconstruction in rabbits, *Ophthalmology* 97:446, 1990.

101. Jenkins C et al: Limbal transplantation in the management of chronic contact-lens-associated epitheliopathy, *Eye* 7:629, 1993.

102. Thoft RA: Keratoepithelioplasty, *Am J Ophthalmol* 97:1, 1984.

103. Turgeon PW et al: Indications for keratoepithelioplasty, *Arch Ophthalmol* 108:233, 1990.

104. Tsai RJ-F, Tseng SCG: Human allograft limbal transplantation for corneal surface reconstruction, *Cornea* 13:389, 1994.

105. Kwitko S et al: Allograft conjunctival transplantation for bilateral ocular surface disorders, *Ophthalmology* 102:1020, 1995.

106. Tsubota K et al: Reconstruction of the corneal epithelium by limbal allograft transplantation for severe ocular surface disorders, *Ophthalmology* 102:1486, 1995.

Sixteen

Degenerations

The term *degeneration* is used to describe changes in tissues that cause deterioration and sometimes impair function. Degeneration can either occur as a relatively normal aging process or may be related to a specific disease. It may be unilateral or bilateral; if bilateral, it is often asymmetric. With rare exceptions, there is no family history of or genetic predisposition to degeneration. This condition commonly affects the peripheral cornea, can be accompanied by vascularization, and generally begins in middle or older age.

In contrast, the term *dystrophy* refers to a hereditary, symmetric, bilateral disease that usually affects the central cornea. A dystrophy is avascular, begins early in life, and is unrelated to other systemic or local diseases (Table 16-1).

In many cases, the pathogenesis of the corneal changes is unknown, and classification as degeneration or dystrophy is an estimation. Some diseases have been incorrectly classified in the past, and classification is difficult to change once it is established. For instructional purposes, degenerative conditions can be divided into two types: those that are common and appear to be primarily related to age (involutional) and those that are less common and usually related to specific local and systemic conditions.

INVOLUTIONAL CHANGES

Morphologic Changes
Advancing age frequently brings about minor changes in the gross morphologic characteristics of the cornea, including flattening of the vertical meridian, generalized thinning that is most prominent peripherally, increased stromal relucency, and decreased transparency and luster. In addition, the cornea's refractive index increases slightly, and in some individuals the corneal nerves become more visible. Histopathologically, the epithelial basement membrane and Descemet's membrane show irregular thickening; there is nonspecific degeneration of stromal ground substance and collagen; corneal guttae develop; and endothelial cell density decreases. These changes are usually of little or no clinical importance, except that the vertical flattening of the cornea may alter the refractive

Table 16-1 Differentiation Between Degeneration and Dystrophy

Feature	Degeneration	Dystrophy
Onset	Middle age or older	Usually first decade of life
Laterality	Often unilateral or asymmetric	Bilateral and symmetric
Family history	Uncommon	Common
Vascularization	Common	No
Corneal location	Peripheral	Central

error, requiring relatively more plus cylinder at the 180° axis. Of course, in some cases the decrease in endothelial cell density can lead to corneal edema (Fuchs' dystrophy).

The aging conjunctiva undergoes changes similar to those of the cornea. It becomes thinner, less transparent, and more relucent, mainly because of atrophy of the subepithelial layers. Laxity develops as a result of the loss of elastic tissue, occasionally producing frank redundancy, known as *conjunctivochalasis*. The conjunctival vessels become more prominent, particularly in the interpalpebral area, and tortuosities, varicosities, and small telangiectases may appear.

Pinguecula

A *pinguecula* is a triangular or polygonal, gray-white to yellowish, slightly elevated conjunctival nodule adjacent to the limbus in the horizontal meridian (Fig. 16-1). Pingueculae are seen most commonly on the nasal side and usually occur bilaterally. More densely opacified material can often be seen within the nodule, obscuring the underlying vessels.

Histopathologically, a pinguecula consists of a mass of abnormal subepithelial collagen. The connective tissue is hyalinized, with increased basophilia and curling of the collagen fibrils. The abnormal collagen takes on the staining characteristics of elastic tissue (elastotic degeneration) but is not elastin, because it is resistant to digestion by elastase.[1] The overlying epithelium is usually normal or slightly thinned, but it may be thickened or even mildly dysplastic.

Pingueculae are thought to be caused by the combined effects of age and exposure to sunlight, perhaps with further contribution by exposure to dust and wind or by repeated trauma from lid closure.[2-4] The predilection of pingueculae for the nasal aspect of the interpalpebral conjunctiva is probably related to the fact that this area of the conjunctiva receives the greatest amount of ultraviolet exposure through reflection of sunlight from the side of the nose. Rather than a degeneration of existing collagen, the abnormal material may be abnormal elastic fibers produced by damaged fibroblasts.[5]

Pingueculae have little clinical significance and generally do not require treatment. They can grow in width and height and can extend onto the cornea, at which point they are called *pterygia*. Occasionally, for unknown reasons, they become inflamed and symptomatic (pingueculitis).[6] Pingueculitis can be treated by observation only, with topical steroids, or by excision.

In rare cases, pingueculae have been mistaken for epithelial tumors. The two should be differentiated easily by the subepithelial location of the pingueculae, by the lack of staining of pingueculae with rose bengal, and by the fluorescence of pingueculae in ultraviolet light. Conjunctival scrapings from pingueculae show essentially normal epithelial cells, whereas scrapings from epithelial tumors usually contain cells with neoplastic characteristics. Brown, pinguecula-like lesions have also been noted in patients with Gaucher's disease.[7]

Limbal Girdle
(White Limbal Girdle of Vogt)

Vogt's girdle is a narrow, crescentic, yellow-white line running along the nasal and temporal limbal areas of the cornea in the interpalpebral zone (Fig. 16-2). It is composed of small, irregular, chalklike flecks and opacities lying immediately beneath the epithelium, and it is usually more prominent nasally. Vogt described two types of girdle: type I is now thought to represent early band keratopathy, while type II (Vogt's limbal girdle) appears to represent elastotic degeneration of subepithelial collagen, such as that found in pingueculae. The differentiating characteristics are listed in Table 16-2. Early band keratopathy is separated from the limbus by a narrow lucid interval, while type II extends to the limbus without an intervening clear zone.[8,9] The lucid interval of early band keratopathy can be explained by the fact that calcium deposition ends at the termination of Bowman's membrane, still some distance from the opaque sclerolimbal junction. The elastosis

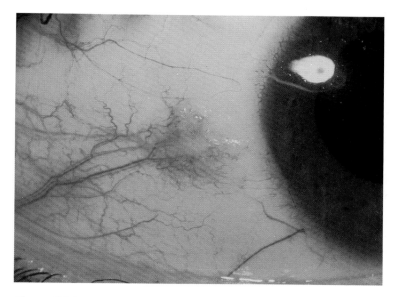

Figure 16-1
Pinguecula.

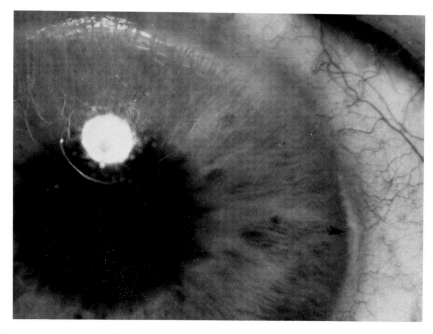

Figure 16-2
Vogt's limbal girdle, type II. No lucid interval is seen; chalklike flecks can be seen in the opacity (*arrow*).

of Vogt's limbal girdle occurs between the end of Bowman's membrane and the sclerolimbal junction so that no lucid interval is seen.

If searched for carefully by indirect lateral illumination, Vogt's limbal girdle can be found in about 60% of patients over 40 years of age

and in all patients over 80 years of age.[9] Its occurrence probably depends largely on exposure to sunlight, as is true of pingueculae. Vogt's girdle has no clinical significance except that it must be distinguished from minimal calcific band keratopathy. Perhaps the severity of the girdle can provide some insight into the degree of actinic radiation to which a patient has been exposed.

Corneal Arcus

Corneal arcus (arcus corneae, gerontoxon, arcus senilis) is a bilateral hazy ring of yellow-white deposits in the peripheral cornea (Fig. 16-3). The deposits appear first in the inferior cornea and then in the superior cornea, eventually encircling the entire cornea. Deposition occurs first in the posterior cornea, initially near Descemet's membrane and then near Bowman's layer. With progression, an anvil- or hourglass-shaped distribution is seen. On slit-lamp examination, numerous criss-crossing lines of relative clarity can be seen throughout the arcus, and in very early cases the posterior corneal haze and lucent lines may simulate a posterior crocodile shagreen.

A lucid interval is present between the peripheral border of the arcus and the limbus. This area is not entirely free of lipid, however, because the deposits extend across the limbus into the adjacent sclera at the level of Descemet's membrane. The central edge of the lucid interval is located at the termination of Bowman's layer, but it is unclear whether the lucid interval is related to the lack of Bowman's layer or to its proximity to the limbal vasculature, because the arcus and its lucid interval can be seen to be displaced centrally in an area of abnormal corneal vascularization. At times the arcus can be wide, extending axially without corneal vascularization, at which time it probably should be classified as a lipid keratopathy (Fig. 16-4).

The incidence of corneal arcus is directly related to age; it is present in 60% of people between 40 and 60 years of age and in nearly ev-

Table 16-2	Differentiation Between Early Band Keratopathy and Limbal Girdle of Vogt	
Early Calcific Band Keratopathy (Type I)	**True Vogt's Girdle (Type II)**
Lucid interval	No lucid interval
Fine crystals	Chalklike flecks
"Swiss cheese holes"	No "holes"
Slightly more superficial	Slightly deeper
Rather smooth central edge	Thornlike extensions from central edge
Calcium	Elastosis
Calcium-adjacent conjunctiva	Pinguecula-adjacent conjunctiva

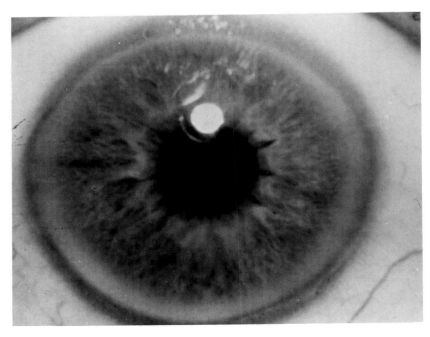

Figure 16-3
Corneal arcus.

eryone over 80.[10] However, arcus is rarely seen in certain populations, such as Canadian Eskimos. It tends to occur earlier in men than in women, and earlier in blacks than in whites.

The arcus is composed of cholesterol esters, cholesterol, and neutral glycerides in the extracellular corneal stroma.[11,12] Its development is related to increasing age, elevation of cholesterol and low-density lipoproteins (LDLs), and increased vascular permeability.[13-18] On average, people 30 to 49 years of age with arcus have higher serum LDL cholesterol concentrations than people without arcus, with an increased likelihood of having markedly elevated values (higher than 5.5 mmol/L).[14,19] The presence of corneal arcus in men 30 to 49 years of age is also a significant risk factor for the development of coronary heart disease and cardiovascular death.[20,21] This remains true even after adjusting for its association with hyperlipidemia. Therefore, patients with arcus should be evaluated by a primary care physician for cardiovascular disease, including a serum lipid profile.

The presence of a unilateral arcus suggests vascular occlusion on the side without arcus.[22] Arcus is rarely a congenital finding (see Chapter 5) and can occur prematurely in lecithin cholesterol acyltransferase (LCAT) deficiency[23] and phytosterolemia.[24]

Cornea Farinata

Cornea farinata is an age-related corneal change comprising innumerable tiny, dustlike gray dots and flecks in the deep corneal stroma (Figs. 16-5 and 16-6). The term "farinata" refers to the farinaceous, or flourlike, appearance of the deposits, which classically are more prominent centrally and best seen with retroillumination. Although the condition is usually bilateral, unilateral cases have been reported. The deposits do not interfere with vision. Cornea farinata sometimes occurs as a familial trait.[25]

The histopathologic characteristics of the cornea from one patient with changes resembling cornea farinata included abnormal keratocytes containing intracytoplasmic vacuoles with lipidlike inclusions.[26] These deposits are probably degenerative.[27] Lipofuscin, a degenerative pigment that accumulates in aged cells, has been found in pre-Descemet's dystrophy, a condition that bears a close clinical resemblance to cornea farinata (see Chapter 17). Cornea farinata is sometimes mistaken for cornea guttata. Careful examination of the posterior surface of the cornea by specular reflection reveals the normal endothelial mosaic pattern underlying the opacities of cornea farinata, which are smaller and more gray-white than those of cornea guttata.

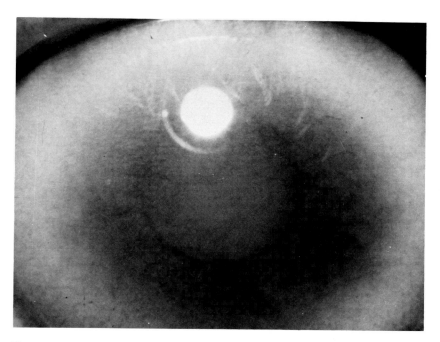

Figure 16-4
Extensive arcus, resulting in lipid deposition in the axial area of the cornea.

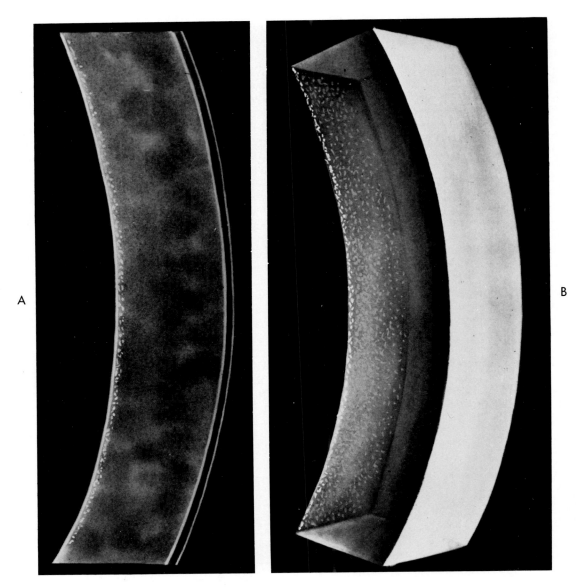

Figure 16-5
A, Cornea farinata consists of punctate opacities in the deep stroma, as seen in this parallel-piped section. These lesions are best seen by retroillumination. **B,** Same lesion and location in optical section.

Descemet's Striae

Small, linear striations in Descemet's membrane are often seen in otherwise normal corneas, perhaps more commonly in older patients.[28] The striae are finer and more subtle than those of striate keratopathy and are not large enough to cause gross irregularities of either Descemet's membrane or the posterior corneal surface. Descemet's striae (also called glass striae) are generally oriented vertically, but they may tilt slightly away from the vertical in either the nasal or temporal direction. They have a double-walled (pipestem) configuration. They have no clinical significance (Fig. 16-7).

Hassall-Henle Bodies

Descemet's membrane normally has a uniform thickness except in the corneal periphery, where localized thickenings are common, particularly with advancing age. These nodular thickenings are called *Hassall-Henle bodies,* or Descemet's "warts." They project toward the

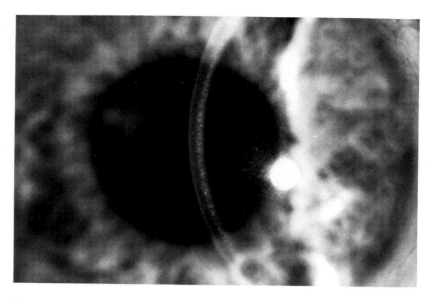

Figure 16-6
Cornea farinata.

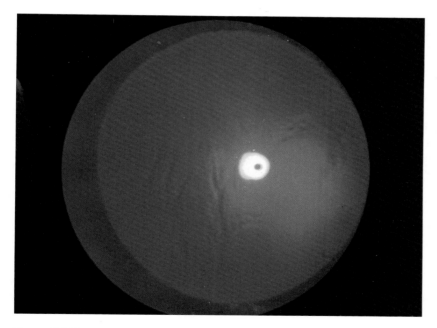

Figure 16-7
Glassy striae, or Descemet's striae, are vertically oriented.

anterior chamber and can be seen in the area of specular reflection as small, circular, dark areas within the normal endothelial mosaic.

Hassall-Henle bodies are histopathologically the same as the excrescences that occur in cornea guttata. They are peripheral, however, and do not indicate corneal disease.

Mosaic (Crocodile) Shagreen

Mosaic shagreen of Vogt consists of grayish white, polygonal opacities separated by relatively clear spaces, creating an appearance likened to crocodile leather (Fig. 16-8).[8] This pattern may be seen in either the anterior or posterior corneal layers, is usually bilateral, and is

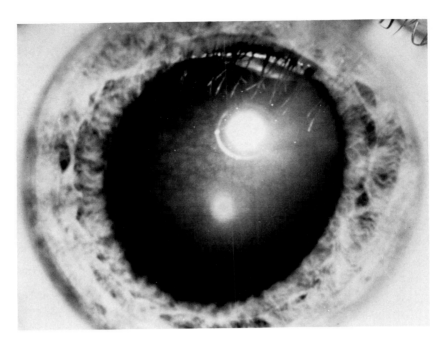

Figure 16-8
Posterior mosaic shagreen. Gray polygonal patches are noted in the deep stroma and Descemet's membrane area.

most prominent centrally. Vascularization does not occur, and only rarely are the opacities dense enough to reduce vision.

Most cases of mosaic shagreen are involutional in origin, but anterior mosaic shagreen has been seen after trauma, in association with band keratopathy, or in a dominantly inherited juvenile form. In one case of posterior crocodile shagreen, an irregular saw-toothed configuration of the collagen lamellae was noted on electron microscopy,[29] but the significance of this finding is unclear.

The cause of both the anterior and posterior forms is unknown, but Bron and Tripathi[30,31] have proposed that anterior mosaic shagreen results from relaxation of the normal tension on Bowman's layer. The collagen lamellae insert obliquely into Bowman's layer and, according to the authors' theory, when tension on Bowman's layer is released, the lamellae support the layer in ridges, which are noted as the clear spaces of the mosaic. A similar pattern can be seen in the fluorescein-stained cornea after applying pressure to the cornea through the lid. It can also be seen in hypotony, or when a hard contact lens flattens a cornea with keratoconus.[32]

Furrow Degeneration

In rare cases thinning can develop in the lucid interval between an arcus and the limbus in elderly persons (Fig. 16-9). This is noninflammatory and asymptomatic. The epithelium is intact, and vascularization and perforation do not occur. More commonly, the false appearance of a furrow can be created by the pattern of lipid deposition, with relative lucency of the anterior lamellae.

Other Involutional Changes

Occasionally, the nerves in an aging cornea may become more visible. A Hudson-Stähli line can also be seen as an involutional change (see Chapter 24).

NONINVOLUTIONAL DEGENERATIONS

Pterygium

Pterygia are fibrovascular overgrowths of the bulbar conjunctiva onto the cornea (Fig. 16-10). They are usually triangular and horizontally oriented, with the base peripheral and the apex central over the cornea. They are located in the palpebral fissure, most commonly on the

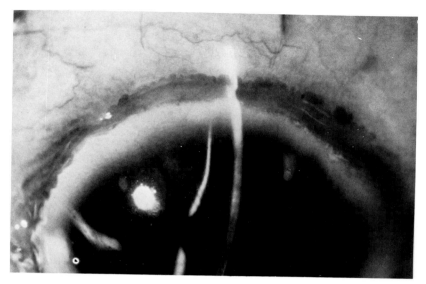

Figure 16-9
Furrow degeneration.

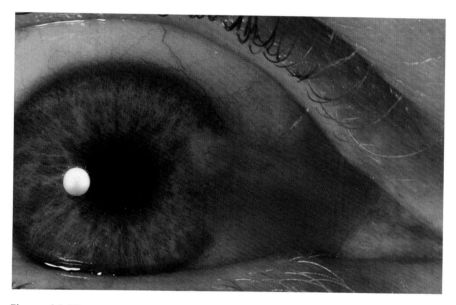

Figure 16-10
Pterygium.

nasal side, but they can occur on the temporal side as well. A grayish, flat, avascular zone usually lies at the apex. An iron line, called *Stocker's line,* may be seen in advance of the pterygium head. Just peripheral to the avascular cap are fine anastomosing and budding vessels, which are particularly present in actively growing pterygia. The body of the pterygium varies in thickness and injection, and these are most prominent during active growth. The vessels are straight and appear to be under tension. Although the head is firmly attached to the cornea, the body can usually be lifted from the globe.

Pseudopterygia must be distinguished from true pterygia. In pseudopterygia the conjunc-

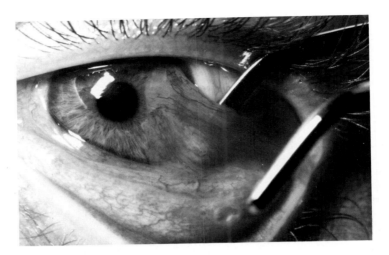

Figure 16-11
Pseudopterygium.

tiva becomes attached to the cornea during peripheral inflammatory disease. A probe can be passed between the conjunctival mass and the globe in pseudopterygia (Fig. 16-11), and this is not possible with true pterygia.

Pterygia most likely are related to ultraviolet radiation and other environmental factors such as heat, wind, dust, and a dry atmosphere.[33,34] The prevalence of pterygia in a population is directly related to the proximity of that population to the equator. In the Western hemisphere, the highest prevalence is seen in Central America and the Caribbean; in the United States the highest rates are seen in the South.[35] Pterygia are more common in men, in people who work outdoors (particularly on sand or concrete), and in people who do not wear spectacles, sunglasses, or a hat while outdoors.[35,36] However, the mechanism of development of the conjunctival lesion and the reason for its growth onto the cornea are unknown. Barraquer[37] has proposed that the limbal elevation produced by the conjunctival lesion causes peripheral corneal drying and microulceration, which induce vascular invasion. However, this is not consistently noted in active pterygia. Kwok and Coroneo[38] proposed that the initial event in pathogenesis was an alteration of limbal stem cells as a result of chronic ultraviolet light exposure, with a resultant breakdown in the normal limbal barrier, allowing conjunctivalization of the corneal epithelium.

Histologically, the conjunctival changes in pterygia are identical to those in pingueculae, with thickening and elastotic degeneration of the subepithelial connective tissue (Fig. 16-12).[4,39] Vascularity is increased, and the overlying epithelium may be mildly dysplastic. Increased numbers of mast cells are present.[40] In primary cases the abnormal material does not extend beneath Tenon's layer and therefore does not become adherent to the sclera. Using immunohistochemical techniques, the cells advancing at the head of the pterygium were found to be cells arisen from the limbal basal epithelium.[41] Fibroblasts are present at the head of the pterygium, advancing between Bowman's layer and the epithelial basement membrane. The fibroblasts exhibit characteristics of transformed cells, with reduced dependence on growth factors for growth and a higher saturation density in culture.[42] Vessels and connective tissue invade this zone, fragmenting and detaching Bowman's layer.

The peak incidence of pterygia is between 20 and 40 years of age. The natural course of pterygia varies considerably. Most commonly they arise from longstanding pingueculae and grow rapidly, over several months, to the limbus.[43] They then progress slowly over the cornea and can take several years to reach the pupil. Growth can stop at any time, and this is indicated by decreased injection, shrinkage of the cap, and regression of the most central vessels. With further involution the head and body flatten and the number of larger vessels decreases.

Pterygia are usually asymptomatic, but they can cause photophobia, tearing, and foreign body sensation. They can also decrease vision by inducing with-the-rule and irregular astigmatism (Fig. 16-13) or by growing across the

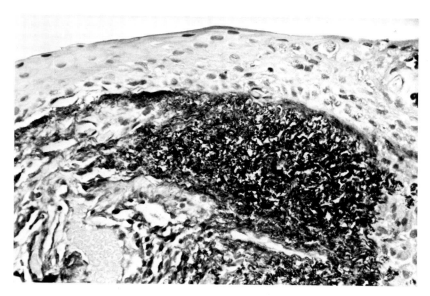

Figure 16-12
Pterygium. Subepithelial curled and fragmented fibers pick up the elastic stain (elastic stain, ×500). (Courtesy of Bruce L. Johnson, Pittsburgh, PA.)

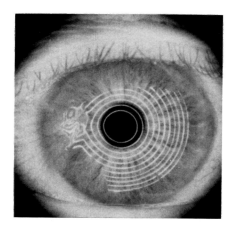

Figure 16-13
Induction of with-the-rule irregular astigmatism by pterygium can be seen with photokeratoscopy.

visual axis. Limited rotation, causing diplopia in peripheral gaze, can be a consequence, usually in recurrent pterygia.

Treatment

Pterygia are usually removed because of the cosmetic blemish, astigmatism, or risk of involvement of the visual axis. Unfortunately, the recurrence rate is high, averaging approximately 40% in various studies.[35,44-46] Recur-

rences generally occur rapidly, arising from the cut conjunctival edge and progressing across the bed of the resection and onto the cornea. Approximately 50% of recurrences are seen within 3 months of surgery, and nearly all are seen by 1 year.[47] The highest rates of recurrence are after surgery on active pterygia; less risk is attached to operating on inactive or atrophic pterygia. The high recurrence rate prompts a conservative approach to pterygia. They should be removed only when necessary because vision has been decreased or because documented recent progression threatens vision.

A number of excision techniques have been described, but none has been clearly demonstrated to be superior. Beta-irradiation,[35,48-57] pedicle or free conjunctival grafts,[58,59-63] and lamellar corneal grafts[64-66] appear to reduce the recurrence rate, but most practitioners reserve these methods to treat recurrent cases. Serious complications, particularly corneoscleral melting and infection, can occur after beta-irradiation.[54,55,57,67,68] In one study, 4.5% of patients had severe scleromalacia after an average dose of 2200 rads.[57] The risk of complications does not appear to be directly related to the total dose of radiation.[55] In a review of infectious complications, the mean latency before infection was over 14 years, so follow-up must be prolonged before safety can be determined.[67]

Postoperative thiotepa (0.5 mg/ml, one drop every 3 hours while awake) for 6 to 8 weeks

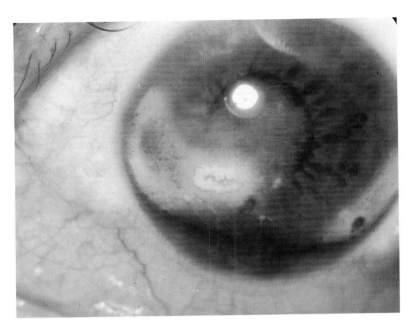

Figure 16-14
Secondary localized amyloid in a patient with interstitial keratitis and band keratopathy. (Courtesy of F. Wilson II, Indianapolis, IN.)

may be beneficial,[69-71] but it also can cause skin and lash depigmentation, conjunctivitis, and scleral ulceration.[71] Townsend[43] presents a more extensive discussion of these techniques.

Topical mitomycin C appears to be very effective in reducing recurrences. In the initial reports mitomycin C was given as a postoperative drop (with a dose of 0.2 mg/ml to 0.4 mg/ml, one drop given twice daily for 5 days to 0.4 mg/ml, one drop every 6 hours for 14 days).[72-75] However, some patients developed corneal or scleral ulceration, secondary glaucoma, iritis, or intractable pain and photophobia.[76-79] A lower dose of 0.01% to 0.02% twice daily for 5 days appeared to be just as effective with a lower risk of complications.[80,81] More recently, an intraoperative dose of mitomycin C (0.2[82,83] or 0.4[84] mg/ml for 3 minutes) appears to be as effective as postoperative drops. It is not clear whether the incidence of serious complications is lower, however. In view of the serious potential complications with mitomycin C, its use should be restricted to those cases in which less risky procedures, such as conjunctival grafting, fail. A single intraoperative dose of 0.2 mg/ml for 2 to 3 minutes appears to be as effective and safer than higher intraoperative or repeated postoperative doses.

For primary pterygia, I recommend a simple excision, leaving bare sclera. The corneal surface should be smoothed as much as possible (a diamond corneal burr can be used for this purpose). If the pterygium recurs, excision is combined with a free or sliding conjunctival flap. If it recurs despite these measures, resection is performed with a single intraoperative dose of mitomycin C.

Amyloid Degeneration

Corneal deposits of amyloid may be seen in primary or secondary localized amyloidosis and in primary systemic amyloidosis. The most common form is secondary localized amyloidosis, which is seen in the cornea (or conjunctiva) after trauma or chronic ocular disease (Figs. 16-14 and 16-15). Some of the problems that cause secondary localized amyloidosis are trachoma, sarcoidosis, lipid proteinosis (Urbach-Wiethe disease), retrolental fibroplasia, phlyctenular disease, interstitial keratitis, uveitis, glaucoma, leprosy, and keratoconus. Secondary amyloidosis associated with climatic droplet keratopathy can appear as multiple lattice lines throughout the stroma.[85]

The amyloid may appear as a small, salmon pink to yellow-white, fleshy, waxy, sometimes nodular mass or masses on the cornea or conjunctiva; as grayish perivascular deposits; as lamellar deposits; or as a subepithelial pannus. The diagnosis usually is made histologically; its

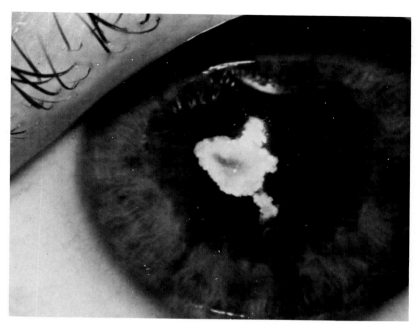

Figure 16-15
Secondary localized amyloidosis of the cornea.

only clinical significance is that it can contribute to decreased vision.

Primary localized amyloidosis occurs as lattice dystrophy, gelatinous droplike dystrophy, or polymorphic amyloid degeneration. The first two conditions are dystrophies and are discussed in Chapter 17. In *polymorphic amyloid degeneration,* punctate, filiform, or linear deposits are seen bilaterally in the stroma of patients over 40 years of age, usually in those in the sixth decade of life (Fig. 16-16). These deposits can be found at all levels, but are most common in the middle and deep stroma. They are gray-white on focal illumination and transparent on retroillumination. The deposits can be central, peripheral, or annular in distribution. The punctate opacities are polymorphic flecklike, stellate, linear, or guttate. The filaments are identical to those seen in lattice dystrophy; they can have beading, striations, or dichotomous branching. There is no progression, vision is not affected, and the cornea remains lustrous. No hereditary pattern has been demonstrated. The amyloid nature of the deposits has been confirmed histologically.[86] This condition most likely is a degenerative disease, and probably is the same condition as parenchymatous dystrophy of Pillat.[87,88] Thomsitt and Bron[89] called it *polymorphic stromal dystrophy.*

The cornea does not become involved in secondary systemic amyloidosis. In primary systemic amyloidosis, purpuric and papillary lesions of the eyelids and conjunctiva may be seen (see Fig. 21-33). Ophthalmoplegias and ptosis can also occur, and in the familial form veillike vitreous opacities or glaucoma are seen.[90] Rarely, families have been reported that exhibit both lattice dystrophy and signs of primary systemic amyloidosis (see Chapter 17).[91,92] Skin changes, cranial nerve palsies, and visceral symptoms have been present. The visual loss is usually milder or delayed, because central deposits are decreased. In contrast to typical lattice dystrophy, however, the deposits extend to the limbus.

Band-Shaped Keratopathy

Band keratopathy of calcific origin usually occurs from drugs, localized ocular inflammatory disease, or systemic disease that causes hypercalcemia. It develops most commonly in eyes with chronic ocular inflammatory disease, particularly uveitis. Children with juvenile rheumatoid arthritis and uveitis are especially prone to the development of band keratopathy. Chronic exposure of the ocular surface to mercury, via eye drops or fumes, can induce calcium deposition. Old interstitial keratitis, corneal edema, glaucoma, trauma, and phthisis are also commonly associated with band keratopathy (Table 16-3).

In rare cases, band keratopathy can occur in

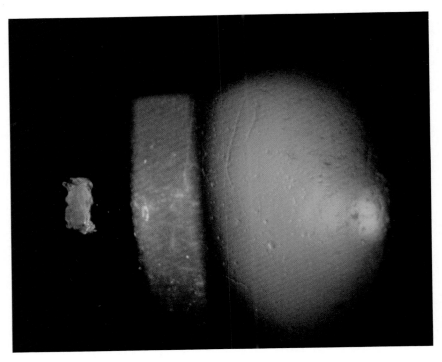

Figure 16-16
Deep stromal punctate and filamentous opacities in polymorphic amyloid degeneration. The opacities appear gray-white on direct illumination and clear on retroillumination. (Courtesy of Robert W. Weisenthal, Syracuse, NY.)

a hereditary form. Calcareous degeneration of the cornea is a similar process that involves all corneal layers. This type of degeneration is seen in phthisis bulbi, necrotic intraocular neoplasm, extensive trauma, and other conditions in which "bone" is formed in other parts of the eye. In many cases band keratopathy occurs in the absence of ocular disease or systemic hypercalcemia.[99] In hyperuricemia, urate crystals can be deposited in the cornea in a band form. In this instance the band keratopathy takes on a brownish color instead of the gray-white opacity seen in calcific band keratopathy. Severe spheroid degeneration can also occur in band form.

Band keratopathy is most often seen in the interpalpebral area. It begins in the periphery (Fig. 16-17) and can extend to involve the visual axis (Fig. 16-18). A lucid interval is seen between the calcific band and the limbus. Small holes in the calcific opacity are noted throughout the band keratopathy, representing areas in which corneal nerves penetrate Bowman's layer. These small holes give a "Swiss cheese" appearance to the layer on slit-lamp examination. The deposits are grayish and flat initially, but with progression they become white and

elevate the overlying epithelium. The band usually develops slowly, over years, but can develop rapidly, particularly in dry eyes.[100]

Histologically, the earliest changes consist of a basophilic staining of the basement membrane of the epithelium. Later, calcium deposits are seen in Bowman's layer (Fig. 16-19) and sometimes in the anterior stroma, and fragmentation and destruction of Bowman's layer occurs.[101,102] The deposition of the calcium in Bowman's layer accounts for the lucid interval, because Bowman's layer does not extend to the absolute limbus. The calcium is deposited extracellularly in local disease, whereas in systemic hypercalcemia the deposits are intracellular.

The mechanism of calcium deposition has not been determined.[101,102] In other tissues, calcium and phosphate concentrations are very close to those that favor precipitation. Mild elevation of either calcium or phosphate levels, elevation of pH, or concentration by evaporation can lead to precipitation. Uveitis may alter corneal metabolism, resulting in a rise in tissue pH and thus favoring precipitation of calcium salts.[103] In experimental animals, however, combined ocular inflammation and hypercal-

Table 16-3   Causes of Band Keratopathy
Hypercalcemia
Sarcoidosis and other granulomatous disease
Renal failure
Hyperparathyroidism
Hematologic malignancies (e.g., multiple myeloma, lymphoma, leukemia)
Acute osteoporosis (including Paget's disease)
Idiopathic hypercalcemia of infancy
Excess vitamin D intake
Bone metastases
Lithium therapy
Milk-alkali syndrome
Thiazides
Gout (urate)
Ocular disease
Chronic nongranulomatous uveitis (juvenile rheumatoid arthritis)
Prolonged glaucoma
Longstanding corneal edema
Phthisis
Spheroid degeneration (can occur in band form)
Norrie's disease
Interstitial keratitis
Idiopathic origin
Mercury
Mercury fumes[93]
Eye drops containing mercury[94]
Chronic irritants (e.g., calomel, calcium bichromate vapor)
Discoid lupus erythematosus
Tuberous sclerosis
Ichthyosis
Rothmund-Thomson syndrome
Progressive facial hemiatrophy (Parry-Romberg syndrome)
Intracameral Viscoat[95-98] (Alcon Pharmaceuticals, Fort Worth, TX)

down over the deposits. The easiest means is by use of ethylenediaminetetraacetic acid (EDTA).*

To apply EDTA, 4% cocaine drops or other topical anesthetic must first be instilled into the cul-de-sac. Cocaine will facilitate removal of the epithelium, which is necessary in order for the EDTA to act. I have found the following to be the most effective method: The epithelium is removed in the area of calcium deposition. A 3-ml plastic syringe is cut approximately 1.5 cm from the handled end; this is inverted and placed firmly against the cornea. The EDTA is dropped into the well thus created and is allowed to react for approximately 2 minutes. The liquid then is absorbed with a cellulose sponge, and the cornea is gently scraped with a Kimura spatula or scalpel blade. The process is repeated until the band is removed. Alternatively, the EDTA can be placed on a small strip of cellulose sponge that is resting on the cornea; the cellulose strip is kept moist by dropping the solution onto the sponge continuously. If necessary, a diamond burr or excimer laser can be used to polish the cornea.[106,107] Removal of calcium with the excimer laser is not recommended, because the calcium is relatively resistant to photoablation. Patching, cycloplegics, and mild antibiotics are employed until reepithelialization has occurred.

If no EDTA is available, anesthetic drops can be instilled, and the cornea can be scraped with a scalpel blade (e.g., no. 15 Bard-Parker).[108] The scraping is continued until all gritty-feeling material is removed.

Spheroid Degeneration

Spheroid degeneration (climatic droplet keratopathy) is one of many names applied to spherical, golden brown, translucent, droplike deposits that may be seen in the subepithelial layers of the cornea and conjunctiva.[108-116] These deposits begin peripherally, most often at the 3 o'clock and 9 o'clock positions, and advance centrally. They may progressively darken, opacify, and coalesce. In severe cases spheroid degeneration can extend in a plaquelike fashion across the central cornea, reducing vision (noncalcific spheroid band keratopathy; Fig. 16-20), and the deposits can become nodular, elevating the epithelium. Clinically (and histopathologically) they fluoresce brightly in ultraviolet light.

cemia did not cause band keratopathy unless the lids were open.[104] Evaporation of tears may favor calcium precipitation by increasing its concentration and making the pH more alkaline. Carbon dioxide is lost from the tears in the palpebral fissure, and this may elevate pH locally. The lack of blood vessels in the cornea may prevent the normal buffering ability of blood serum to inhibit variations in tissue pH.[101] Topical steroid-phosphate preparations may increase the risk of calcium deposition.[105]

Treatment

Band keratopathy can be treated if vision is reduced, if the deposits cause mechanical irritation of the lids, or if the epithelium breaks

---

*The solution is prepared using Endrate (Abbott Laboratories, Birmingham, AL) in a 20-ml ampule containing 150 mg/ml. The ampule is diluted with water to 175 ml. A 0.05 M, 1.7% solution of neutral disodium EDTA is obtained.

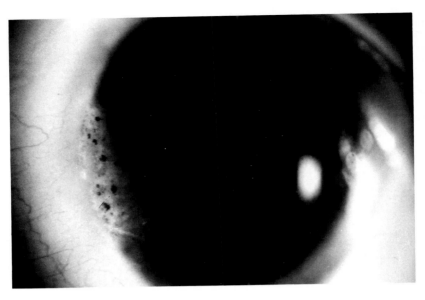

Figure 16-17
Early band keratopathy in a patient with juvenile rheumatoid arthritis. (Courtesy of Diane Curtin, Pittsburgh, PA.)

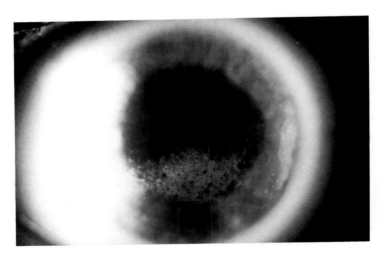

Figure 16-18
More advanced band keratopathy.

Spheroid degeneration occurs almost exclusively in the interpalpebral zones of the cornea and conjunctiva, suggesting that actinic exposure plays a role in its development.[109,117-119] It is more common and more severe in tropical and arid climates with high levels of sunlight. It is more common with increasing age and in those with outdoor occupations.[34,112] Spheroid degeneration is a significant cause of visual impairment in some populations: In a survey in Mongolia it accounted for 7.2% of cases of

blindness and 19.3% of low vision.[120] There is a strong association between conjunctival spheroidal degeneration and pingueculae, and both are probably related to exposure to ultraviolet light.[11,121,122] Chronic mild trauma from wind, sand, or ice; low humidity; and possibly extremes of temperature also may be responsible.

Fraunfelder, Hanna, and Parker[109,123,124] divide spheroid degeneration into three types: the primary corneal type, the secondary corneal type, and the conjunctival type (which can

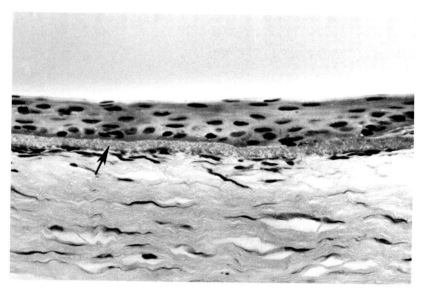

Figure 16-19
Early band keratopathy. Deposition of calcium salts gives Bowman's layer a stippled appearance (*arrow*) (hematoxylin and eosin, ×800). (Courtesy of Bruce L. Johnson, Pittsburgh, PA.)

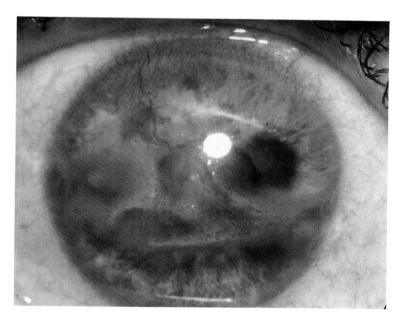

Figure 16-20
Spheroid degeneration in a bandlike distribution.

occur with the primary or secondary corneal types). Primary corneal spheroid degeneration is unrelated to the coexistence of any other ocular disease but is related to advancing age and is usually bilateral. In rare cases, primary band-shaped spheroidal degeneration can develop in childhood. These cases are associated with pho-tophobia, intermittent pain, and slow deterioration in vision.[125] Familial cases have been reported.[126]

The secondary corneal type is a degenerative change that can occur after various longstanding ocular diseases (Fig. 16-21), including glaucoma, herpetic infection, and dystrophies, es-

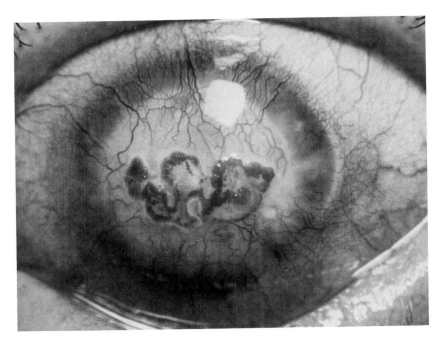

Figure 16-21
Spheroid degeneration occurring secondarily in a failed corneal graft.

pecially Fuchs' endothelial dystrophy and lattice dystrophy. This type can be unilateral or bilateral, central or peripheral, depending on the location of the predisposing disease. The secondary corneal form may also be caused by chronic climatic insults. These cases are usually bilateral, can occur in young people, and are often referred to as tropical or climatic corneal degeneration.

The conjunctival form can occur alone or with either of the corneal types. It is more common in older age groups and may be associated with pinguecula or pterygium. This classification of spheroid degeneration is somewhat arbitrary in that the primary corneal type is probably largely climatic in origin as well, and local corneal inflammation may enhance production of the abnormal material in each type.

The spheroid material is acidophilic and amorphous by light microscopy (Fig. 16-22), finely granular by electron microscopy, extracellular, and proteinaceous.[33,70,71,74,75,80,81] The spheroids are located mainly in the superficial stroma but occasionally may be seen in the deep stroma or within the epithelium.

The composition of spheroid degeneration has long been unclear and to some extent controversial. Different researchers have described the material variously as being colloid, high-tyrosine protein, lipid, keratin-like, a secretory product of abnormal fibrocytes, and elastotic degeneration of collagen. Garner, Morgan, and Tripathi[127] initially believed that the material was a form of keratin and thus originated from the epithelium; however, Garner et al.[112] later concluded that it was more likely collagenous. Hanna and Fraunfelder[124] thought that the substance was of stromal origin, consisting of a fibrocyte-derived granular protein deposited on adjacent collagen fibrils. The composition is not lipid, despite the "oil droplet" clinical appearance. Most researchers now think that the process is basically a stromal one and that epithelial involvement occurs only secondarily after destruction of Bowman's membrane.[4,39,124,127,128] Most likely spheroid degeneration is a type of elastotic degeneration of collagen. The clinically descriptive term of *spheroid degeneration* will be used until the histopathologic nature of the disorder finally is determined.

In most cases the lesions are asymptomatic and require no treatment. If vision is reduced by central involvement, lamellar keratectomy or keratoplasty is indicated. Recurrence is common after conjunctival resection, but the number of lesions is much smaller.[129] Rarely, rapid progression, sterile ulceration, or secondary infection can occur.[130,131]

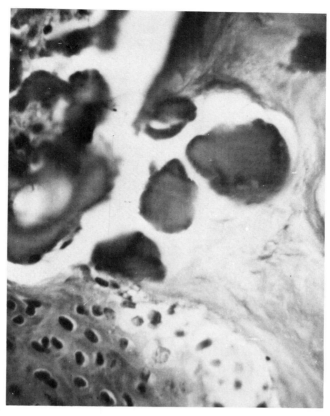

Figure 16-22
Spheroid degeneration. Note the acidophilic amorphous material as seen by light microscopy.

Salzmann's Degeneration

Salzmann's degeneration is a noninflammatory condition comprising elevated, bluish white and sometimes yellow-white subepithelial corneal nodules usually arranged in a circular fashion around the pupillary area (Fig. 16-23). These nodules often appear within or adjacent to an area of previous scarring or at the edge of a longstanding pannus, but they can occur in any area of the cornea. They usually develop slowly and are asymptomatic unless they occur in the visual axis, where they can decrease vision. Occasionally the epithelium can break down over the surface, causing irritation. Salzmann's degeneration occurs in adults of any age and is most commonly bilateral. A history of previous corneal inflammation, particularly of phlyctenular and trachomatous disease, is common.[132,133]

The raised areas consist of hyaline plaques located between the epithelium and Bowman's layer, replacing Bowman's layer in most areas. The nature of the hyaline material is not known, but it does not stain for elastin, amyloid, or reticulin.[133] The epithelium varies in thickness but is usually thinned over the nodules, and the amount of subepithelial basement membrane material is markedly increased.

Treatment is not usually necessary, but surgery may be required if visual acuity is reduced because of involvement of the pupillary area. Excision of the nodules is often sufficient.[134] Sometimes this can be accomplished by simple scraping, but in other cases superficial keratectomy is necessary. Superficial keratectomy can be performed with the excimer laser, but large refractive shifts and increased irregular astigmatism can result.[135] In severe cases, lamellar or penetrating keratoplasty is required.

Terrien's Marginal Degeneration

Terrien's marginal degeneration is an uncommon marginal thinning of the cornea. It occurs more often in males than females, is commonly bilateral, and can occur at any age. It may develop gradually over many years and may be unilateral at first. It is usually asymptomatic unless astigmatism develops.

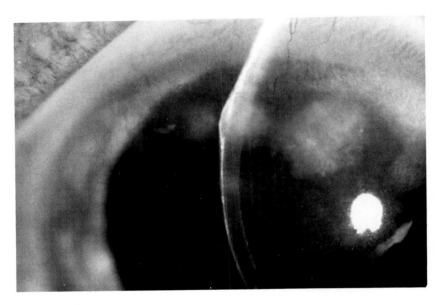

Figure 16-23
Salzmann's degeneration seen by slit illumination.

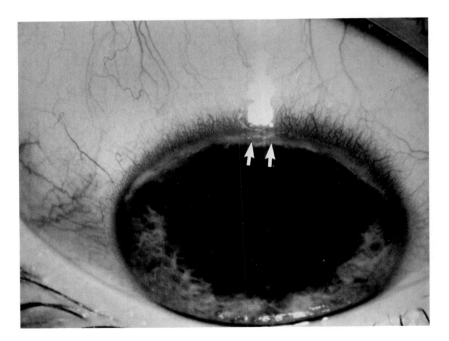

Figure 16-24
Terrien's marginal thinning in the superior aspect of the cornea. A thin lipid line occurs at the central edge of the thinned area (*double arrow*).

Marginal thinning with opacification and superficial vascularization are the dominant features. The degeneration generally begins superonasally, as punctate stromal opacities separated by a lucid zone from the limbus. With time these coalesce, superficial vessels extend over them from the limbus, and the stroma thins. The thinning is in an arcuate shape, without a steep edge, and remains covered by epithelium. A yellow-white line, which appears to be lipid deposition, is seen at the central edge of the thinned area (Fig. 16-24).

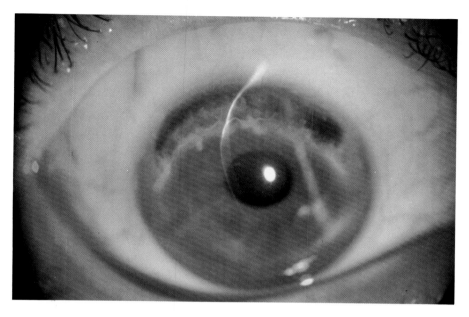

Figure 16-25
Superior corneal thinning and ectasia in Terrien's marginal degeneration. (Courtesy of Diane Curtin, Pittsburgh, PA.)

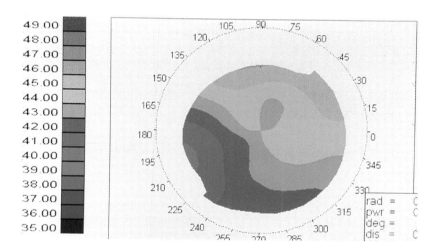

Figure 16-26
Videokeratograph of a patient with Terrien's marginal degeneration, showing superior steepening resulting from superior limbal corneal ectasia.

The thinning can progress circumferentially and in rare cases centrally (Fig. 16-25). Marked thinning can lead to severe astigmatism because of the tilting forward of the central cornea. Corneal topography is characterized by flattening over the areas of peripheral thinning, with relative steepening 90° away (Fig. 16-26).[136] If the area of thinning is small or involves the entire circumference, the central topography can remain relatively spherical. Perforation is uncommon but can occur spontaneously or after minor trauma. Occasionally, the thinning is associated with recurrent inflammation, episcleritis, or scleritis.[137] Breaks in Descemet's membrane can occur, but in contrast to keratoconus, intracorneal pockets of aqueous result, not corneal edema.[138-140] Terrien's marginal degeneration may be confused with

Table 16-4   Comparison of Mooren's Ulcer and Terrien's Marginal Degeneration

Mooren's Ulcer	Terrien's Marginal Degeneration
Unilateral or bilateral	Usually symmetric and bilateral; can be unilateral
Pain and inflammation	Usually painless and not inflamed
Epithelial breakdown at central edge of active ulcers, stains with fluorescein	Epithelium intact, no fluorescein staining
Spreads centrally and circumferentially; slow or rapid progression	Spreads circumferentially; slow progression
Overhanging central edge; can become vascularized with healing; no lipid	Gradual central edge; vascularized base; lipid deposits
Can cause severe corneal melting; corneal destruction	Usually main problem is astigmatism caused by ectasia
Perforation occurs in severe cases	Perforation occurs in 15% of cases as a result of minor trauma

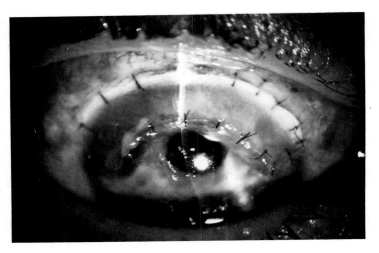

Figure 16-27
Crescentic lamellar graft for Terrien's marginal degeneration.

Mooren's ulcer. The differences between these two conditions are given in Table 16-4.

The cause of Terrien's marginal degeneration is unknown. Histologically, the stromal thinning, vascularization, and lipid deposition are evident, as is local absence of Bowman's membrane, and in some cases healed breaks in Descemet's membrane. Fibrillar degeneration of collagen also is seen.[141,142] An electron microscopic study demonstrated phagocytosis of collagen by histiocytic cells with a high degree of lysosomal activity.[143] Immunohistochemical analysis of one specimen indicated relatively low-grade immune activity: less than 25% of the cells expressed class II histocompatibility antigens; and the ratio of helper/induced to suppressor/cytotoxic T cells was 1:1.[144]

If the thinning becomes so extreme that per-foration is threatened or if astigmatism severely reduces vision, a reconstructive full-thickness or lamellar corneoscleral graft can alleviate the problem.[145-148] These grafts must be hand-fashioned to fit the defect (Fig. 16-27).

Coats' White Ring

Coats' white ring is a small corneal opacity that is the residue of previous injury by a metallic foreign body. On slit-lamp examination the ring is seen as a small, anterior, granular, white, oval ring (Fig. 16-28). Iron deposition is found in Bowman's layer or the anterior stroma.

Pellucid Marginal Degeneration

Pellucid marginal degeneration is an uncommon form of corneal thinning and ectasia. A narrow, arcuate band of corneal thinning is

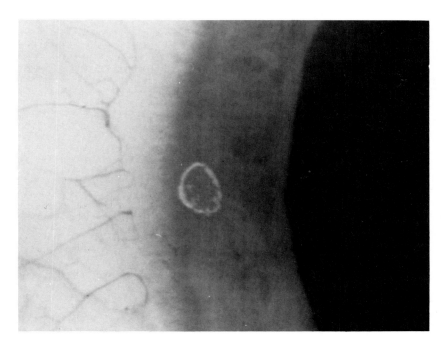

Figure 16-28
Coats' white ring.

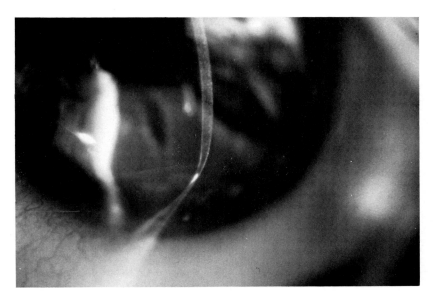

Figure 16-29
Pellucid marginal degeneration. Note the inferior corneal thinning without vascularization or lipid deposition.

seen in the inferior cornea, usually between the 4 o'clock and 8 o'clock positions (Fig. 16-29). The stroma is clear, epithelialized, and nonvascularized. The thinned area usually is 1 to 2 mm in width and is separated from the limbus by 1 to 2 mm of clear cornea. The cornea cen-tral to the thinning is of normal thickness and protrudes forward, creating against-the-rule astigmatism (Figs. 16-30 through 16-32). In contrast to keratoconus, no Fleischer ring, Vogt striae, or conical shape is seen.

Pellucid marginal degeneration usually ap-

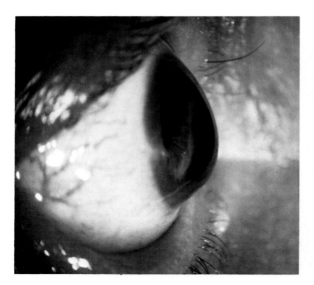

Figure 16-30
Inferior corneal ectasia in pellucid marginal degeneration.

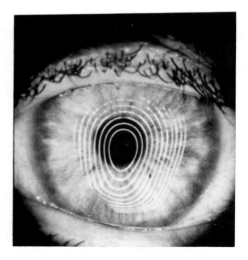

Figure 16-31
Pellucid marginal degeneration. Photo-keratoscopy demonstrates marked central corneal flattening and inferior peripheral steepening in the vertical meridian.

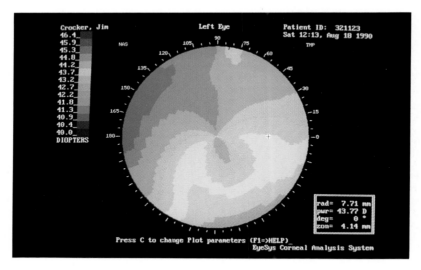

Figure 16-32
Videokeratograph of a patient with pellucid marginal degeneration. Note the typical pattern of oblique inferior peripheral steepening and superior flattening. (Courtesy of Steven E. Wilson, Cleveland, OH.)

pears between 20 and 40 years of age; there is no sexual predilection or family history. However, increased amounts of astigmatism have been reported among families with this type of degeneration.[149] The condition may progress,

usually gradually over several years. Hydrops and corneal scarring can develop, and rupture can occur with trauma.[150-154]

On histologic examination, stromal thinning with localized loss of Bowman's layer has

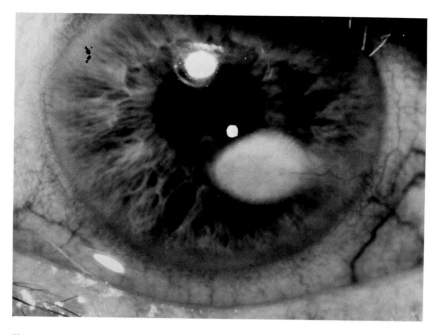

Figure 16-33
Lipid deposit with feathery edges and a central blood vessel.

been noted.[151,155-157] Collagen with 110-nm banding has also been found. Reduced concentration of highly sulfated keratan sulfate epitopes has been observed in corneas with pellucid marginal degeneration and keratoconus.[158]

Pellucid marginal degeneration has features similar to those seen in keratoconus: progressive thinning and ectasia, hydrops, and scarring. It differs, however, in the more peripheral location of the thinning; the lack of a Fleischer ring, Vogt striae, or conical shape; and the slightly older age of affected patients. Some believe that keratoconus and pellucid marginal degeneration are different presentations of the same disease, and this can be determined only by further study of the biochemical processes underlying the diseases.

The major problem for patients with pellucid marginal degeneration is astigmatism caused by protrusion of the central cornea. Usually correction with eyeglasses is inadequate, and contact lens correction is often difficult.[159] When the astigmatism cannot be corrected with either eyeglasses or hard contact lenses, any of several surgical approaches can be tried. Large, inferiorly eccentric penetrating grafts can be performed, but these are prone to vascularization, rejection, and high rates of postoperative astigmatism.[150,160] However, good results were reported in one series.[161] Resection of the thinned cornea,[160,162-164] epikeratopha-

kia,[165] central lamellar keratoplasty, and crescentic peripheral lamellar keratoplasty[166] have also been performed. The best option is unclear at this time.

Lipid Degeneration

Lipid degeneration of the cornea occurs in primary and secondary forms. Secondary lipid deposition is much more common and is usually related to corneal vascularization. It is most commonly associated with trauma, ulceration, hydrops,[167] interstitial keratitis, or herpes zoster keratitis. The pathogenesis of the deposition of lipids is unclear, but it may involve increased vascular permeability, excess production of lipids, or the inability to metabolize lipids.

The lipid is seen as a dense, yellow-white opacity that may fan out with feathery edges from blood vessels (Fig. 16-33).[168] Multicolored crystals (cholesterol) may also be seen at the edge of the opacity, where it is not so dense. The opacity usually develops rapidly, in an area with longstanding vascularization. Histologically, the material consists of neutral fats, phospholipids, and cholesterol, as in corneal arcus.[12,169,170]

Much less frequently, lipid deposits develop in a cornea with no previous history of disease or vascularization.[10,170-175] Serum lipids usually are within normal limits. In one case, histologic examination indicated vascularization, chronic nongranulomatous inflammation, and extracellular lipids, with the same composition as in secondary lipid keratopathy.[174] Therefore, some cases may be secondary, with the original corneal inflammatory disease undiagnosed. In another case no vascularization was observed, and biochemical analysis of the lipid deposits disclosed high concentrations of unesterified cholesterol and sphingomyelin.[176] Penetrating keratoplasty may be required to preserve vision, but deposits can occur in the graft.[172]

In primary lipid degeneration the practitioner should consider some rare causes of serum lipoprotein abnormalities, such as Tangier disease and LCAT deficiency (see Chapter 21). In Tangier disease, visual acuity is good, and hazy stromal infiltrates consisting of fine dots are seen throughout the cornea, densest posteriorly and in the horizontal meridian. A lipid arcus is not present, and vision is not affected. Serum cholesterol is low, high-density lipoproteins (HDLs) are usually markedly deficient, LDLs are low, and very–low-density lipoproteins (VLDLs) are increased. In LCAT deficiency, granular stromal clouding is also seen, but with a peripheral arcus and an outer lucid interval. Vision is not usually affected. LDLs are decreased, and lipoproteins of abnormal structure are seen in the plasma as well as in other tissues of the body, including the cornea.[177] Fish-eye disease is an inherited disorder in which marked corneal clouding can occur, with elevated LDLs and VLDLs and reduced HDLs.[178] Snyder's crystalline dystrophy can present with diffuse corneal clouding, central clouding alone, or central clouding associated with dense arcus.

Laser treatment can reduce the extent or density of the lipid opacities and improve vision in some cases.[179,180] However, several treatments, with thousands of burns, are required, and rapid corneal thinning (leading to keratoplasty) can occur.

Dellen

Dellen (Fuchs' dimples) are areas of localized thinning of the cornea or sclera caused by tear film instability and dryness. The thinning is caused by reversible water loss from the corneal stroma or sclera. Dellen are usually seen in the peripheral cornea adjacent to acute elevations of the conjunctiva (e.g., after surgery or with marked chemosis). Dellen are discussed more fully in Chapter 14 but are mentioned here because they may occur idiopathically in the elderly.

REFERENCES

1. Li ZY et al: Elastic fiber components and protease inhibitors in pinguecula, *Invest Ophthalmol Vis Sci* 32:1573, 1991.
2. Hogan MJ, Alvarado J: Pterygium and pinguecula: electron microscopic study, *Arch Ophthalmol* 78:74, 1967.
3. Sugar S, Kobernick S: The pinguecula, *Am J Ophthalmol* 47:341, 1959.
4. Klintworth GK: Chronic actinic keratopathy: a condition associated with conjunctival elastosis (pingueculae) and typified by characteristic extracellular concretions, *Am J Pathol* 67:327, 1972.
5. Austin P, Jakobiec HA, Iwamoto T: Elastodysplasia and elastodystrophy as pathologic bases of ocular pterygium and pinguecula, *Ophthalmology* 90:96, 1983.
6. Sugar S, Kobernick S: Localized irritative lesions involving pingueculae, *Am J Ophthalmol* 57:94, 1964.
7. Petrohelos M et al: Ocular manifestations of Gaucher's disease, *Am J Ophthalmol* 80:1006, 1975.
8. Vogt A: *Corneal degenerations of various etiology.* In Blodi FC, editor: *Textbook and atlas of slit lamp microscopy of the living eye,* Bonn, 1981, Wayenbargh Editions.
9. Sugar SH, Kobernick S: The white limbal girdle of Vogt, *Am J Ophthalmol* 50:101, 1960.
10. Duke-Elder S, Leigh AG: *System of ophthalmology,* vol 8, Diseases of the outer eye, St Louis, 1965, Mosby–Year Book.
11. Cogan DG, Kuwabara T: Arcus senilis: its pathology and histochemistry, *Arch Ophthalmol* 61:353, 1959.
12. Andrews JS: The lipids of arcus senilis, *Arch Ophthalmol* 68:264, 1962.
13. Walton KW: Studies on the pathogenesis of corneal arcus formation, *J Pathol* 111:263, 1973.
14. Vinger PF, Sachs BA: Ocular manifestations of hyperlipoproteinaemia, *Am J Ophthalmol* 70:563, 1970.
15. Rifkind BM: Corneal arcus and hyperlipoproteinemia, *Surv Ophthalmol* 16:295, 1972.
16. Walton KW, Dunkerley DJ: Studies on the pathogenesis of corneal arcus formation: II. Immunofluorescent studies on lipid deposition in the eye of the lipid-fed rabbit, *J Pathol* 114:217, 1974.
17. Winder AF: Factors influencing the variable expression of xanthelasmata and corneal arcus in familial hypercholesterolemia, *Birth Defects* 18:449, 1982.
18. Pe'er J et al: Association between corneal arcus and some of the risk factors for coronary artery disease, *Br J Ophthalmol* 67:795, 1983.
19. Hughes K et al: Corneal arcus and cardiovascular risk factors in Asians in Singapore, *Int J Epidemiol* 21:473, 1992.
20. Chambless LE et al: The association of corneal arcus with coronary heart disease and cardiovascular disease mortality in the Lipid Re-

search Clinics Mortality Follow-up Study, *Am J Public Health* 80:1200, 1990.

21. Rosenman RH et al: Relation of corneal arcus to cardiovascular risk factors and incidence of coronary disease, *N Engl J Med* 291:1322, 1974.

22. Smith JL, Susac JO: Unilateral arcus senilis: sign of occlusive disease of the carotid artery, *JAMA* 225:676, 1973.

23. Horven I, Effe K, Gjone E: Corneal and fundus changes in familial LCAT deficiency, *Acta Ophthalmol (Copenh)* 52:201, 1974.

24. Björkhem I, Skrede S: *Familial diseases with storage of sterols other than cholesterol: cerebrotendinous xanthomatosis and phytosterolemia.* In Scriver CR et al, editors: *The metabolic basis of inherited disease,* ed 6, New York, 1989, McGraw-Hill.

25. Paufique L, Etienne R: La cornea farinata, *Bull Soc Ophtalmol Fr* 50:522, 1950.

26. Durand I et al: Cornea farinata. Report of a case: clinical, histologic and ultrastructural study, *J Fr Ophtalmol* 13:449, 1990.

27. Curran RE, Kenyon KR, Green WR: Pre-Descemet's membrane corneal dystrophy, *Am J Ophthalmol* 77:711, 1974.

28. Sturrock G: Glassy corneal striae, *Graefes Arch Clin Exp Ophthalmol* 188:245, 1973.

29. Krachmer JH et al: Corneal posterior crocodile shagreen and polymorphic amyloid degeneration, *Arch Ophthalmol* 101:54, 1983.

30. Bron AJ, Tripathi RC: Anterior corneal mosaic: further observations, *Br J Ophthalmol* 53:760, 1969.

31. Tripathi RC, Bron AJ: Secondary anterior crocodile shagreen of Vogt, *Br J Ophthalmol* 59:59, 1975.

32. Dangel ME, Kracher GP, Stark WJ: Anterior corneal mosaic in eye with keratoconus wearing hard contact lenses, *Arch Ophthalmol* 102:888, 1984.

33. Moran DJ, Hollows FC: Pterygium and ultraviolet radiation: a positive correlation, *Br J Ophthalmol* 68:343, 1984.

34. Taylor HR et al: Corneal changes associated with chronic UV irradiation, *Arch Ophthalmol* 107:1481, 1989.

35. Cameron ME: *Pterygium throughout the world,* Springfield, IL, 1965, Charles C Thomas.

36. Mackenzie FD et al: Risk analysis in the development of pterygia, *Ophthalmology* 99:1056, 1992.

37. Barraquer JI: Etiologia y patogenia del pterigiom y de las excavaciones de la cornea de Fuchs, *Arch Soc Am Oftalmol Optom* 5:45, 1964.

38. Kwok LS, Coroneo MT: A model for pterygium formation, *Cornea* 13:219, 1994.

39. Rodrigues MM, Laibson PR, Weinreb S: Corneal elastosis: appearance of band-like keratopathy and spheroidal degeneration, *Arch Ophthalmol* 93:111, 1975.

40. Butrus SI et al: Increased numbers of mast cells in pterygia, *Am J Ophthalmol* 119:236, 1995.

41. Dushku N, Reid TW: Immunohistochemical evidence that human pterygia originate from an invasion of vimentin-expressing altered limbal epithelial basal cells, *Curr Eye Res* 13:473, 1994.

42. Chen JK, Tsai RJ, Lin SS: Fibroblasts isolated from human pterygia exhibit transformed cell characteristics, *In Vitro Cell Dev Biol* 30A:243, 1994.

43. Townsend WM: *Pterygium.* In Kaufman HE et al, editors: *The cornea,* New York, 1988, Churchill Livingstone.

44. Pearlman G et al: Recurrent pterygium and treatment with lamellar keratoplasty with presentation of a technique to limit recurrences, *Ann Ophthalmol* 2:763, 1970.

45. Zauberman H: Pterygium and its recurrence, *Am J Ophthalmol* 63:1780, 1967.

46. Youngson RM: Recurrence of pterygium after excision, *Br J Ophthalmol* 56:120, 1972.

47. Hirst LW, Sebban A, Chant D: Pterygium recurrence time, *Ophthalmology* 101:755, 1994.

48. Alaniz-Cancino F: The use of postoperative beta irradiation in the treatment of pterygium, *Ophthalmic Surg* 13:1022, 1982.

49. Cooper JS, Lerch IA: Postoperative irradiation of pterygia, *Radiology* 135:743, 1980.

50. Hilgers JH: Pterygium, *Am J Ophthalmol* 50:635, 1960.

51. Pico G: *Pterygium: current concept of etiology and management.* In King JH, McTigue JW, editors: *The cornea: World Congress,* Washington, 1965, Butterworth Publishers.

52. Bahrassa F, Datta R: Postoperative beta radiation treatment of pterygium, *Int J Radiat Oncol Biol Phys* 9:679, 1983.

53. Paryani SB et al: Management of pterygium with surgery and radiation therapy: the North Florida Pterygium Study Group, *Int J Radiat Oncol Biol Phys* 28:101, 1994.

54. Wesberry JM Jr, Wesberry JM Sr: Optimal use of beta irradiation in the treatment of pterygia, *South Med J* 86:633, 1993.

55. Dusenbery KE et al: Beta irradiation of recurrent pterygia: results and complications, *Int J Radiat Oncol Biol Phys* 24:315, 1992.

56. Wilder RB et al: Pterygium treated with excision and postoperative beta irradiation, *Int J Radiat Oncol Biol Phys* 23:533, 1992.

57. Mackenzie FD et al: Recurrence rate and complications after beta irradiation for pterygium, *Ophthalmology* 98:1776, 1991.

58. Kenyon KR, Wagoner MD, Hettinger ME: Conjunctival autograft transplantation for advanced and recurrent pterygium, *Ophthalmology* 92:1461, 1985.

59. Hara T et al: Pterygium surgery using the principle of contact inhibition and a limbal transplanted pedicle conjunctival strip, *Ophthalmic Surg* 25:95, 1994.

60. McCoombes JA, Hirst LW, Isbell GP: Sliding conjunctival flap for the treatment of primary pterygium, *Ophthalmology* 101:169, 1994.

61. Riordan-Eva P et al: Conjunctival autografting

in the surgical management of pterygium, *Eye* 7:634, 1993.

62. Allan BD et al: Pterygium excision with conjunctival autografting: an effective and safe technique, *Br J Ophthalmol* 77:698, 1993.

63. Tomas T: Sliding flap of conjunctival limbus to prevent recurrence of pterygium, *Refract Corneal Surg* 8:394, 1992.

64. Poirier RH, Fish JR: Lamellar keratoplasty for recurrent pterygium, *Ophthalmic Surg* 7:38, 1976.

65. Laughrea PA, Arentsen JJ: Lamellar keratoplasty in the management of recurrent pterygium, *Ophthalmic Surg* 17:106, 1986.

66. Busin M et al: Precarved lyophilized tissue for lamellar keratoplasty in recurrent pterygium, *Am J Ophthalmol* 102:222, 1986.

67. Moriarty AP et al: Fungal corneoscleritis complicating beta-irradiation-induced scleral necrosis following pterygium excision, *Eye* 7:525, 1993.

68. Moriarty AP et al: Severe corneoscleral infection: a complication of beta irradiation scleral necrosis following pterygium excision, *Arch Ophthalmol* 111:947, 1993.

69. Meacham CT: Triethylene thiophosphoramide in prevention of pterygium recurrence, *Am J Ophthalmol* 54:751, 1962.

70. Harrison M, Kelly A, Ohlrich J: Pterygium: thio-tepa versus beta radiation, a double-blind trial, *Trans Aust Coll Ophthalmol* 1:64, 1969.

71. Asregadoo ER: Surgery, thio-tepa, and corticosteroid in the treatment of pterygium, *Am J Ophthalmol* 74:960, 1972.

72. Singh G, Wilson MR, Foster CS: Mitomycin eye drops as treatment for pterygium, *Ophthalmology* 95:813, 1988.

73. Hayasaka S et al: Postoperative instillation of low-dose mitomycin C in the treatment of primary pterygium, *Am J Ophthalmol* 106:715, 1988.

74. Singh G, Wilson MR, Foster CS: Long-term follow-up study of mitomycin eye drops as adjunctive treatment of pterygia and its comparison with conjunctival autograft transplantation, *Cornea* 9:331, 1990.

75. Mahar PS, Nwokora GE: Role of mitomycin C in pterygium surgery, *Br J Ophthalmol* 77:433, 1993.

76. Rubinfeld RS et al: Serious complications of topical mitomycin-C after pterygium surgery, *Ophthalmology* 99:1647, 1992.

77. Fujitani A et al: Corneoscleral ulceration and corneal perforation after pterygium excision and topical mitomycin C therapy, *Ophthalmologica* 207:162, 1993.

78. Dunn JP et al: Development of scleral ulceration and calcification after pterygium excision and mitomycin therapy, *Am J Ophthalmol* 112:343, 1991.

79. Ewing-Chow DA et al: Corneal melting after pterygium removal followed by topical mitomycin C therapy, *Can J Ophthalmol* 27:197, 1992.

80. Frucht-Pery J, Ilsar M: The use of low-dose mitomycin C for prevention of recurrent pterygium, *Ophthalmology* 101:759, 1994.

81. Chen PP et al: A randomized trial comparing mitomycin C and conjunctival autograft after excision of primary pterygium, *Am J Ophthalmol* 120:151, 1995.

82. Frucht-Pery J, Ilsar M, Hemo I: Single dosage of mitomycin C for prevention of recurrent pterygium: preliminary report, *Cornea* 13:411, 1994.

83. Cardillo JA et al: Mitomycin administration by single intraoperative application versus postoperative eye drop in pterygium surgery, *Ophthalmology* 102(suppl):131, 1995.

84. Mastropasqua L et al: Effectiveness of intraoperative mitomycin C in the treatment of recurrent pterygium, *Ophthalmologica* 208:247, 1994.

85. Matta CS et al: Climatic droplet keratopathy with corneal amyloidosis, *Ophthalmology* 98:192, 1991.

86. Mannis MJ et al: Polymorphic amyloid degeneration of the cornea, *Arch Ophthalmol* 99:1217, 1981.

87. Pillat A: Zur frage der familíuaren Hornhautentartung: ueber eine einzigartige tiefe scholige und periphere gitterförmige familíre Hornhautdystrophie, *Klin Monatsbl Augenheilkd* 104:571, 1939.

88. Strachan IM: Pre-Descemetic corneal dystrophy, *Br J Ophthalmol* 52:716, 1968.

89. Thomsitt J, Bron AJ: Polymorphic stromal dystrophy, *Br J Ophthalmol* 59:125, 1975.

90. Kaufman HE, Thomas IB: Vitreous opacities diagnostic of familial primary amyloidosis, *N Engl J Med* 261:1267, 1959.

91. Kirk HQ et al: Primary familial amyloidosis of the cornea, *Trans Am Acad Ophthalmol Otolaryngol* 77:411, 1973.

92. Meretoja J: Comparative histopathological and clinical findings in eyes with lattice corneal dystrophy of two different types, *Ophthalmologica* 165:15, 1972.

93. Kennedy RE, Roca PD, Platt DS: Further observations on atypical band keratopathy in glaucomatous patients, *Trans Am Ophthalmol Soc* 72:107, 1974.

94. Kennedy RE, Roca PD, Landers PH: Atypical band keratopathy in glaucomatous patients, *Am J Ophthalmol* 72:917, 1971.

95. Binder PS, Deg JK, Kohl FS: Calcific band keratopathy after intraocular chondroitin sulfate, *Arch Ophthalmol* 105:1243, 1987.

96. Coffman MR, Mann PM: Corneal subepithelial deposits after use of sodium chondroitin, *Am J Ophthalmol* 102:279, 1986.

97. Ullman S, Lichtenstein SB, Heerlein K: Corneal opacities secondary to Viscoat, *J Cataract Refract Surg* 12:489, 1986.

98. Nevyas AS et al: Acute band keratopathy following intracameral Viscoat, *Arch Ophthalmol* 105:958, 1987.

99. Henriksen E: Primary calcareous corneal dystrophy, *Acta Ophthalmol (Copenh)* 60:759, 1982.
100. Lemp MA, Ralph RA: Rapid development of band keratopathy in dry eyes, *Am J Ophthalmol* 83:657, 1977.
101. O'Connor GR: Calcific band keratopathy, *Trans Am Ophthalmol Soc* 70:58, 1972.
102. Pouliquen Y: Ultrastructure of band keratopathy, *Arch Ophthalmol* 27:149, 1967.
103. Doughman DJ et al: Experimental band keratopathy, *Arch Ophthalmol* 81:264, 1969.
104. Economon JW, Silverstein AM, Zimmerman LE: Band keratopathy in a rabbit colony, *Invest Ophthalmol* 2:361, 1963.
105. Taravell MJ et al: Calcific band keratopathy associated with the use of topical steroid-phosphate preparations, *Arch Ophthalmol* 112:608, 1994.
106. Poirier L et al: Results of therapeutic photokeratectomy using the excimer laser: apropos of 12 cases, *J Fr Ophtalmol* 17:262, 1994.
107. O'Brart DP et al: Treatment of band keratopathy by excimer laser phototherapeutic keratectomy: surgical techniques and long term follow up, *Br J Ophthalmol* 77:702, 1993.
108. Young JDH, Finlay RD: Primary spheroidal degenerations of the cornea in Labrador and northern Newfoundland, *Am J Ophthalmol* 79:129, 1975.
109. Fraunfelder F, Hanna C: Spheroid degeneration of the cornea and conjunctiva: III. Incidences, classification and etiology, *Am J Ophthalmol* 76:41, 1973.
110. Freedman A: Climatic droplet keratopathy: I. Clinical aspects, *Arch Ophthalmol* 89:193, 1973.
111. Johnson GJ, Ghosh M: Labrador keratopathy: clinical and pathological findings, *Can J Ophthalmol* 10:119, 1975.
112. Garner A et al: Spheroidal degeneration of cornea and conjunctiva, *Br J Ophthalmol* 60:473, 1976.
113. Ahmad A et al: Climatic droplet keratopathy in a 16-year-old boy, *Arch Ophthalmol* 95:149, 1977.
114. Anderson J, Fuglsang H: Droplet degeneration of the cornea in North Cameroon: prevalence and clinical appearance, *Br J Ophthalmol* 60:256, 1976.
115. Klintworth GK: Chronic actinic keratopathy: a condition associated with conjunctival elastosis (pingueculae) and typified by characteristic extracellular concretions, *Am J Pathol* 67:327, 1972.
116. Gray RH, Johnson GJ, Freedman A: Climatic droplet keratopathy, *Surv Ophthalmol* 36:241, 1992.
117. Taylor HR: Aetiology of climatic droplet keratopathy and pterygium, *Br J Ophthalmol* 64:154, 1980.
118. Taylor HR et al: Corneal changes associated with chronic UV irradiation, *Arch Ophthalmol* 107:1481, 1989.
119. Taylor HR et al: The long-term effects of visible light on the eye, *Arch Ophthalmol* 110:99, 1992.
120. Raasanhu J et al: Prevalence and causes of blindness and visual impairment in Mongolia: a survey of populations aged 40 years and older, *Bull World Health Organ* 72:771, 1994.
121. Norn MS: Prevalence of pinguecula in Greenland and Copenhagen, *Acta Ophthalmol (Copenh)* 57:96, 1979.
122. Norn MS: Spheroid degeneration, pinguecula, and pterygium among Arabs in the Red Sea territory, Jordan, *Acta Ophthalmol (Copenh)* 60:949, 1982.
123. Fraunfelder FT, Hanna C, Parker JM: Spheroid degeneration of the cornea and conjunctiva: I. Clinical course and characteristics, *Am J Ophthalmol* 74:821, 1972.
124. Hanna C, Fraunfelder FT: Spheroid degeneration of the cornea and conjunctiva: II. Pathology, *Am J Ophthalmol* 74:829, 1972.
125. Hida T et al: Primary band-shaped spheroidal degeneration of the cornea: three cases from two consanguineous families, *Br J Ophthalmol* 70:347, 1986.
126. Hida T et al: Familial band-shaped spheroid degeneration of the cornea, *Am J Ophthalmol* 97:651, 1984.
127. Garner A, Morgan G, Tripathi RC: Climatic droplet keratopathy: II. Pathologic findings, *Arch Ophthalmol* 89:198, 1973.
128. Brownstein S et al: The elastotic nature of hyaline corneal deposits: a histochemical, fluorescent, and electron microscopic examination, *Am J Ophthalmol* 75:799, 1973.
129. Norn MS: Conjunctival spheroid degeneration: recurrence after excision, *Acta Ophthalmol (Copenh)* 60:434, 1982.
130. Ormerod LD et al: Serious occurrences in the natural history of advanced climatic keratopathy, *Ophthalmology* 101:448, 1994.
131. Resnikoff S, Filliard G, Dell'Aquila B: Climatic droplet keratopathy, exfoliation syndrome, and cataract, *Br J Ophthalmol* 75:734, 1991.
132. Katz D: Salzmann's nodular corneal dystrophy, *Acta Ophthalmol (Copenh)* 31:377, 1953.
133. Vannas A, Hogan MJ, Wood I: Salzmann's nodular degeneration of the cornea, *Am J Ophthalmol* 79:211, 1975.
134. Wood TO: Salzmann's nodular degeneration, *Cornea* 9:17, 1990.
135. Hersh PS et al: Phototherapeutic keratectomy: strategies and results in 12 eyes, *Refract Corneal Surg* 9(suppl):S90, 1993.
136. Wilson SE et al: Terrien's marginal degeneration: corneal topography, *Refract Corneal Surg* 6:15, 1990.
137. Austin P, Brown SI: Inflammatory Terrien's marginal corneal disease, *Am J Ophthalmol* 98:189, 1981.
138. Soong HK et al: Corneal hydrops in Terrien's marginal degeneration, *Ophthalmology* 93:340, 1986.
139. Ashenhurst M, Slomovic A: Corneal hydrops

in Terrien's marginal degeneration: an unusual complication, *Can J Ophthalmol* 22:328, 1987.

140. Romanchuk KG, Hamilton WK, Braig RF: Terrien's marginal degeneration with corneal cyst, *Cornea* 9:86, 1990.

141. Süveges MD, Levai G, Alberth B: Pathology of Terrien's disease, *Am J Ophthalmol* 74:1191, 1972.

142. Guyer DR et al: Terrien's marginal degeneration: clinicopathologic case reports, *Graefes Arch Clin Exp Ophthalmol* 225:19, 1987.

143. Iwamoto T, DeVoe AG, Farris RL: Electron microscopy in cases of marginal degeneration of the cornea, *Invest Ophthalmol* 11:241, 1972.

144. Lopez JS et al: Immunohistochemistry of Terrien's and Mooren's corneal degeneration, *Arch Ophthalmol* 109:988, 1991.

145. Brown AC, Rao GN, Aquavella JV: Peripheral corneal grafts in Terrien's marginal degeneration, *Ophthalmic Surg* 14:931, 1983.

146. Caldwell DR et al: Primary surgical repair of several peripheral marginal ectasias in Terrien's marginal degeneration, *Am J Ophthalmol* 97:332, 1984.

147. Hahn TW, Kim JH: Two-step annular tectonic lamellar keratoplasty in severe Terrien's marginal degeneration, *Ophthalmic Surg* 24:831, 1993.

148. Pettit TH: Corneoscleral freehand lamellar keratoplasty in Terrien's marginal degeneration of the cornea: long term results, *Refract Corneal Surg* 7:28, 1991.

149. Nagy M, Vigvary L: Beitrage zur atiologie der degeneratio marginalis pellucida corneae, *Klin Monatsbl Augenheilkd* 161:604, 1972.

150. Krachmer J: Pellucid marginal corneal degeneration, *Arch Ophthalmol* 96:1217, 1978.

151. Pouliquen Y et al: Acute corneal edema in pellucid marginal degeneration or acute marginal keratoconus, *Cornea* 6:169, 1987.

152. Golubovíc S, Parunovíc A: Acute pellucid marginal corneal degeneration, *Cornea* 7:290, 1988.

153. Carter JB, Jones DB, Wilhelmus KR: Acute hydrops in pellucid marginal corneal degeneration, *Am J Ophthalmol* 107:167, 1989.

154. Cameron JA: Deep corneal scarring in pellucid marginal degeneration, *Cornea* 11:309, 1992.

155. Francois J, Hassens M, Stockman L: Degeneresence marginale pellucide de la corneé, *Ophthalmologica* 155:337, 1968.

156. Pouliquen Y et al: Degenerescence pellucide marginale de la corneé ou keratocone marginale, *J Fr Ophtalmol* 3:109, 1980.

157. Rodrigues MM et al: Pellucid marginal corneal degeneration: a clinicopathologic study of two cases, *Exp Eye Res* 33:277, 1981.

158. Funderburgh JL et al: Altered antigenicity of keratan sulfate proteoglycan in selected corneal diseases, *Invest Ophthalmol Vis Sci* 31:419, 1990.

159. Astin CL: The long-term use of the SoftPerm lens on pellucid marginal corneal degeneration, *CLAO J* 20:258, 1994.

160. Barraquer JI: Results of the crescent resection in keratotorus, *Dev Ophthalmol* 5:49, 1981.

161. Varley GA, Macsai MS, Krachmer JH: The results of penetrating keratoplasty for pellucid marginal corneal degeneration, *Am J Ophthalmol* 110:149, 1990.

162. Dubroff S: Pellucid marginal corneal degeneration: report on corrective surgery, *J Cataract Refract Surg* 15:89, 1989.

163. Cameron JA: Results of lamellar crescentic resection for pellucid marginal corneal degeneration, *Am J Ophthalmol* 113:296, 1992.

164. Duran JA, Rodriguez-Ares MT, Torres D: Crescentic resection for the treatment of pellucid corneal marginal degeneration, *Ophthalmic Surg* 22:153, 1991.

165. Fronterre A, Portesani GP: Epikeratoplasty for pellucid marginal corneal degeneration, *Cornea* 10:450, 1991.

166. Schanzlin DJ, Samo EM, Robin JB: Crescentic lamellar keratoplasty in pellucid marginal corneal degeneration, *Am J Ophthalmol* 96:253, 1983.

167. Shapiro LA, Farkas TG: Lipid keratopathy following corneal hydrops, *Arch Ophthalmol* 95:456, 1977.

168. Jack RL, Lase SA: Lipid keratopathy: an electron microscopic study, *Arch Ophthalmol* 83:678, 1970.

169. Ciccarelli EC, Kuwabara T: Experimental aberrant lipogenesis, *Arch Ophthalmol* 62:125, 1959.

170. Baum JL: Cholesterol keratopathy, *Am J Ophthalmol* 67:372, 1969.

171. Fine BS, Townsend WM, Zimmerman LE: Primary lipoidal degeneration of the cornea, *Am J Ophthalmol* 78:12, 1974.

172. Friedlander MH et al: Bilateral central lipid infiltrates of the cornea, *Am J Ophthalmol* 84:78, 1977.

173. Savino DF, Fine BS, Alldredge OC: Primary lipidic degeneration of the cornea, *Cornea* 5:191, 1986.

174. Alfonso E et al: Idiopathic bilateral lipid keratopathy, *Br J Ophthalmol* 72:338, 1988.

175. Duran JA, Rodriquez-Ares MT: Idiopathic lipid corneal degeneration, *Cornea* 10:166, 1991.

176. Silva-Araújo A et al: Primary lipid keratopathy: a morphological and biochemical assessment, *Br J Ophthalmol* 77:248, 1993.

177. Gjone E, Bergaust B: Corneal opacity in familial plasma cholesterol ester deficiency, *Acta Ophthalmol (Copenh)* 47:222, 1969.

178. Bron AJ: Corneal changes in the dyslipoproteinemias, *Cornea* 8:135, 1989.

179. Marsh RJ: Argon laser treatment of lipid keratopathy, *Br J Ophthalmol* 72:900, 1988.

180. Baar JC, Foster CS: Corneal laser photocoagulation for treatment of neovascularization: efficacy of 577 nm yellow dye laser, *Ophthalmology* 99:173, 1992.

Seventeen

Dystrophies of the Epithelium, Bowman's Layer, and Stroma

DYSTROPHIES OF THE EPITHELIUM AND BASEMENT MEMBRANE
Meesmann's Dystrophy
Epithelial Basement Membrane Dystrophy

DYSTROPHIES OF BOWMAN'S LAYER
Reis-Bücklers' Dystrophy
Treatment
Anterior Membrane Dystrophy of Grayson-Wilbrandt
Honeycomb Dystrophy of Thiel and Behnke
Inherited Band Keratopathy
Dermochondral Dystrophy of François
Local Anterior Mucopolysaccharide Accumulation

STROMAL DYSTROPHIES
Granular Dystrophy
Lattice Dystrophy
Gelatinous Droplike Dystrophy
Avellino Corneal Dystrophy
Macular Dystrophy
Fleck Dystrophy
Central Crystalline Dystrophy of Schnyder
Marginal Crystalline Dystrophy of Bietti
Central Cloudy Dystrophy of François
Parenchymatous Dystrophy of Pillat
Posterior Amorphous Dystrophy

PRE-DESCEMET'S DYSTROPHIES

ECTATIC DYSTROPHIES
Anterior Keratoconus
Keratoglobus

Posterior Keratoconus
Pellucid Marginal Degeneration

Although a dystrophy may be apparent at birth, it is usually initially seen later in the first or second decade of life. Dystrophies show a hereditary pattern (usually autosomal dominant), are bilateral, symmetric, and may be progressive. They tend to affect the central cornea more than the periphery and to be avascular, and they are usually unrelated to any other local or systemic disease. Of course, there are exceptions to each of these generalizations.

Corneal dystrophies are most easily classified anatomically, because they usually affect only one corneal layer. A pathogenic classification would be preferable, but as yet our understanding of the pathogenesis of corneal dystrophies is limited. Some conditions that have traditionally been classified as dystrophies usually do not show a hereditary pattern and probably are forms of degeneration (e.g., pre-Descemet's dystrophy, epithelial basement membrane dystrophy, and some cases of Fuchs' dystrophy).

DYSTROPHIES OF THE EPITHELIUM AND BASEMENT MEMBRANE

Anterior corneal dystrophies affect the epithelium, basement membrane, and Bowman's layer (Table 17-1). Primary involvement of any one of these layers frequently leads to or is accompanied by changes in the other two layers, so exact classification as to the level of involvement is often difficult and arbitrary. However, Meesmann's dystrophy (juvenile epithelial corneal dystrophy) and epithelial basement membrane dystrophy (Cogan's map-dot-fingerprint dystrophy, bleblike dystrophy, dystrophic re-

Table 17-1	Epithelial and Bowman's Layer Dystrophies			
Dystrophy	Vision	Inheritance	Age at Manifestation	Pathologic Features
Meesmann's	Not usually affected but may decrease	Autosomal dominant	Childhood	Intraepithelial cysts that contain cellular debris PAS*-positive material within epithelial cells and in basement membrane zone
Epithelial basement membrane (map-dot-fingerprint)	Normal or reduced	Usually none; in rare cases autosomal dominant	Adulthood	Debris-containing intraepithelial cysts Insinuation of basement membrane and collagen intraepithelially, accounting for fingerprint and map appearance Recurrent epithelial erosions
Reis-Bücklers'	Reduced	Autosomal dominant	Childhood	?Primary epithelial abnormality Replacement of Bowman's layer with abnormal collagen fibers
Grayson-Wilbrandt	Reduced	Autosomal dominant	Adolescence	PAS-positive material in abnormal amounts in basement membrane zone; extends in undulating fashion into epithelium Infrequent epithelial erosions May be variant of Reis-Bücklers' dystrophy
Honeycomb	Reduced	Autosomal dominant	Childhood	May be variant of Reis-Bücklers' dystrophy
Inherited band keratopathy	Can be reduced	?Autosomal dominant	Adulthood	Calcium deposition in epithelial basement membrane and Bowman's layer
Anterior crocodile shagreen	Not affected	None	Adulthood	Anterior polygonal opacities seen as an involutional change
Local mucopolysaccharide accumulation	May be reduced	None	Infants	Bilateral diffuse clouding caused by acid mucopolysaccharide in Bowman's layer

*Periodic-acid Schiff.

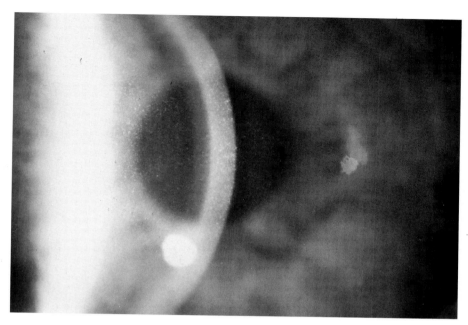

Figure 17-1
Meesmann's dystrophy with fine, intraepithelial opacities. (Courtesy of Diane Curtin, Pittsburgh, PA.)

current erosions) affect primarily the epithelium and basement membrane.

Meesmann's Dystrophy

Meesmann's dystrophy is a rare, bilateral, symmetric, familial corneal disease that begins early in life.[1-4] The major finding is epithelial vesicles, which may be seen as early as 6 months of age and tend to increase in number with age. Meesmann's dystrophy is inherited as an autosomal dominant trait with incomplete penetrance.

This epithelial dystrophy is usually asymptomatic until early adulthood or middle age, when symptoms of lacrimation, photophobia, and irritation may develop. The discomfort is caused by microcysts that rupture onto the epithelial surface. In most instances visual acuity remains good, but irregularity in the corneal surface and mild opacification, which occur in older patients, can impair vision. Families vary widely in the degree of progression over time and in the level of visual impairment.[5]

The bleblike lesions in the epithelium appear on direct illumination as small, white-gray, punctate opacities that are diffusely distributed over the corneal surface but are more pronounced in the interpalpebral zone (Fig. 17-1). On retroillumination, the opacities appear as clear, spherical vesicles that are regular in size and shape (Fig. 17-2). The cysts can coalesce into refractile lines or clusters. In rare cases other forms are seen, such as a whorllike pattern at the level of Bowman's layer, peripheral limbal lesions, or focal wedge-shaped lesions.[1,6] The intervening epithelium is clear. Some of the opacities, presumably those that have ruptured onto the corneal surface, stain with fluorescein and rose bengal. Central corneal thickness is reduced, particularly in younger patients, but increases with worsening epitheliopathy.[5] Corneal sensation may be reduced.

Similar epithelial cysts can be seen in contact lens wearers, epithelial basement membrane dystrophy, and toxicity from local anesthetics; but the uniform size, diffuse distribution, and bilaterality distinguish Meesmann's dystrophy. This condition can also be confused with diffuse marked punctate keratopathy, such as that caused by vernal conjunctivitis, meibomitis, or dry eyes. It is helpful, therefore, to establish the familial nature of the disease.

Histopathologically, the epithelial layer is usually thickened, but it may be thinned. There is disorganization, with poor maturation from the basal layer to the surface. Small debris-containing cysts are found throughout the epithelium; these are the vesicles seen with retroillumination on slit-lamp examination. The cysts are most numerous in the anterior third of the epithelium, and some may open to the

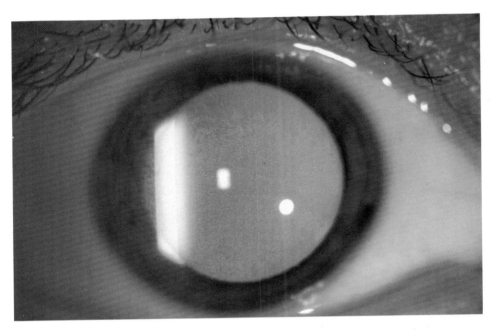

Figure 17-2
Meesmann's dystrophy. On retroillumination, small, clear, vesicles are seen.

corneal surface. The amorphous material within the cysts stains with alcian blue and colloidal iron, indicating the presence of glycosaminoglycans, and with periodic-acid Schiff (PAS). Increased glycogen is seen in the superficial epithelium in some cases and most likely is related to the rapid turnover of cells.[7] The epithelial basement membrane may be abnormally thick and multilaminar and may show fingerlike projections extending into the basal epithelium. Bowman's layer, stroma, endothelium, and Descemet's membrane appear normal.

Electron microscopy reveals an unusual, characteristic material in the epithelial cell cytoplasm called *peculiar substance*.[2-8] This substance is described as a mass of fibrillogranular material intermixed with cytoplasmic filaments. It is seen most prominently in the basal cells and may be the result of degeneration of cytoplasmic filaments.[2] In some cases electron-dense bodies that appear similar to lysosomes have been seen in the basal epithelial cells.[9] The cysts appear to contain degenerated cellular material, such as organelles, and a vacuolated homogenous substance. The walls of the intraepithelial cysts are formed by the cell membranes of adjacent epithelial cells.

Meesmann's dystrophy appears to be caused by an epithelial cell abnormality, which is probably manifested by the development of peculiar substance. This abnormality leads to poor maturation of the epithelial cells and early cell death. The cysts appear to represent pockets of degenerated cells. The other changes, such as increased cell turnover and thickening of the basement membrane, are secondary to the epithelial disease.

Treatment is often unnecessary. However, wearing soft contact lenses has been reported to greatly reduce the number of cysts and the severity of symptoms.[10] The epithelial disease recurs after epithelial debridement and lamellar or penetrating keratoplasty, but it may be delayed or less severe.[3,8] Therefore, if vision is reduced by subepithelial scarring or irregular astigmatism, one of these procedures may be worthwhile. It has been asserted that superficial keratectomy results in reepithelialization without recurrence of epithelial disease.[7]

Epithelial Basement Membrane Dystrophy

Epithelial basement membrane dystrophy (also called Cogan's microcystic epithelial dystrophy or map-dot-fingerprint dystrophy) is a common, bilateral, epithelial dystrophy.[7,11-13] There is usually no hereditary pattern, but some cases show an autosomal dominant inheritance.[14,15] The condition occurs mainly in adults, usually between 40 and 70 years of age, and is slightly more common in women. In familial cases the

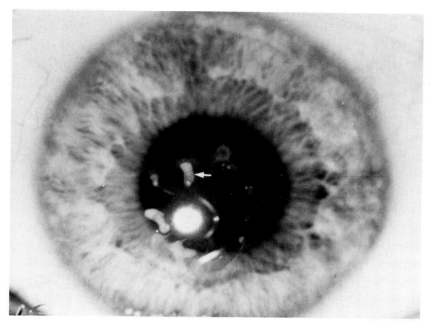

Figure 17-3
Epithelial basement membrane dystrophy. Typical puttylike lesions *(arrow)* and maplike lines can be seen in the epithelium.

onset is between 4 and 8 years of age, and the frequency of attacks decreases gradually with age, being rare after age 50.

Clinical Manifestations

The pattern of epithelial and basement membrane abnormalities varies considerably among patients. It may be seen as dots, maps, fingerprints, blebs, nets, or any combination of these patterns. All types tend to come and go spontaneously and move to affect different portions of the cornea.

Dots are gray-white intraepithelial opacities that vary in size and may be round, oblong, or comma-shaped (Fig. 17-3). With focal illumination, larger dot opacities look like putty. Smaller dots may be closely clustered and clear, and these are best seen on retroillumination. Fluorescein may stain the superficial microcysts or may show negative staining where the epithelium is elevated over cysts.

Fingerprints are clusters of concentric, contoured lines that can occur in any area of the cornea. On direct illumination they are usually seen as white lines, but they are best appreciated by retroillumination, in which they appear refractile (Fig. 17-4). Some lines branch or have club-shaped terminations.

Maps are irregular, geographic-shaped, circumscribed areas that are commonly seen in epithelial basement membrane dystrophy, usually alone or combined with dots (Fig. 17-5). These areas vary in size and have a ground-glass appearance, often with clear lacunae. Maps may be surrounded by gray-white borders or may blend gradually into the normal cornea. They are best seen with broad, oblique illumination.

Blebs are fine, clear, round, and bubblelike and are seen best in retroillumination (Fig. 17-6). They are uniform in size and shape and can be numerous. In the past, cases with only blebs have been called *bleblike dystrophy*.

Nets are refractile lines or rows of blebs that follow the normal anterior corneal mosaic.[16] Nets and blebs do not result in erosions, but they may be associated with maps and fingerprints, which do.

Most patients with anterior basement membrane dystrophy are asymptomatic; however, in many cases epithelial erosions occur or vision is decreased because of surface irregularity. After an erosion occurs, the patient experiences foreign body sensation, pain, photophobia, or tearing. These symptoms develop most commonly early in the morning, while dreaming or upon awakening, but can occur at any time of the day, and they vary considerably in severity and duration. Patients with nonfamilial disease tend to suffer recurrent erosions for no more

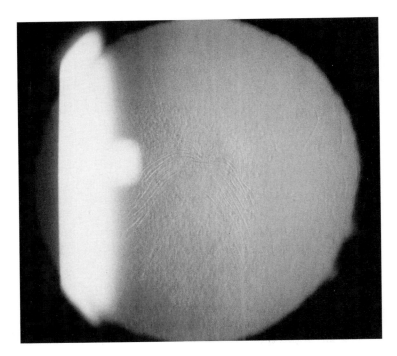

Figure 17-4
Epithelial basement membrane dystrophy. Fingerprint lines often are best appreciated with retro-illumination. (Courtesy of Diane Curtin, Pittsburgh, PA.)

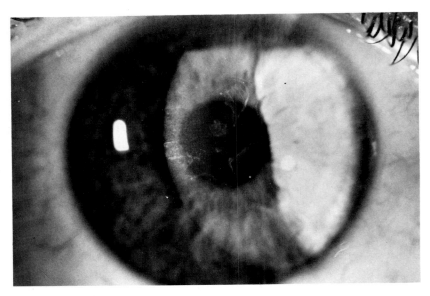

Figure 17-5
Maps of epithelial basement membrane dystrophy.

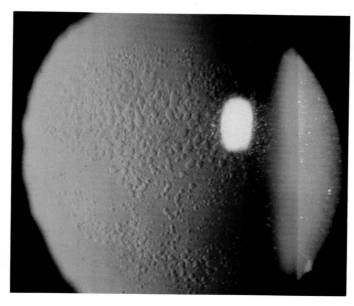

Figure 17-6
Bleb form of epithelial basement membrane dystrophy. (Courtesy of Y. Jerold Gordon, Pittsburgh, PA.)

than a few years, with spontaneous improvement and no significant residual visual loss.[17] A large percentage of patients with recurrent erosions have evidence of epithelial basement membrane dystrophy.[18] Similar changes can be seen after corneal trauma, particularly that caused by fingernails or paper cuts, but they are localized to the traumatized area. These changes have also been noted in patients who have undergone radial keratotomy.[17,19]

Histopathology

In each of these patterns of abnormality, the epithelial basement membrane is abnormal and shows intraepithelial extensions. The map-like changes are related to multilaminar thickening of the basement membrane, with extension of the aberrant membrane into the overlying epithelium. The extensions contain fine fibrillogranular material and are 2 to 6 μm in thickness. Epithelial cells anterior to the abnormal basement membrane do not form hemidesmosomal connections to the membrane, and this probably accounts for their tendency to erode.

The gray-white dot opacities correspond to intraepithelial microcysts (pseudocysts), which contain nuclear debris, cytoplasmic debris, and lipid (Fig. 17-7). There is no visible lining, and the cyst's wall is created by the normal border of the neighboring cell. The cysts form poste-

rior to an intraepithelial extension of aberrant epithelial basement membrane. Epithelial cells beneath the aberrant membrane become vacuolated and liquified, forming the cyst. The cysts may discharge spontaneously onto the corneal surface and thus disappear,[20] producing an erosion in the process.

Fingerprint lines are linear projections of fibrillogranular material into the epithelial layer. The material is covered by a basement membrane, which may be thickened.[21] Blebs are localized mounds of fibrillogranular protein between Bowman's layer and the epithelial basement membrane, indenting the basal epithelium.[22]

Treatment

The treatment of recurrent erosions is discussed in Chapter 15. Corneal topography (Fig. 17-8) and trial of a hard contact lens can document whether a reduction in acuity is related to epithelial irregularity. For these patients, wearing a contact lens improves vision and usually reduces the severity of the basement membrane changes. Debridement of the central epithelium usually reduces surface irregularity and improves vision. I remove the epithelium with a Kimura spatula and place a bandage contact lens. Diclofenac and a broad-spectrum non-toxic antibiotic are administered four times daily until the epithelium heals. It usually takes

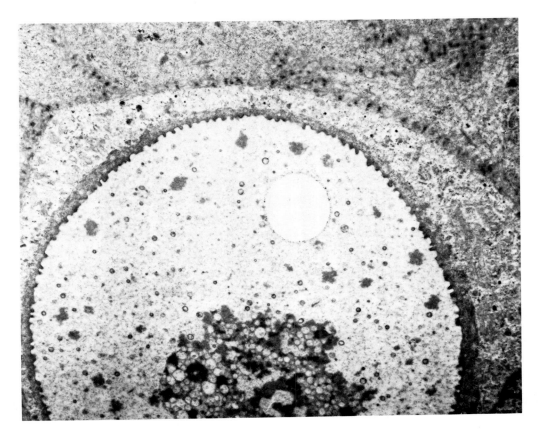

Figure 17-7
Pseudomicrocyst showing a degenerating cell; the pyknotic nucleus and cellular debris can be seen. The cyst's wall is created by the normal border of neighboring cell.

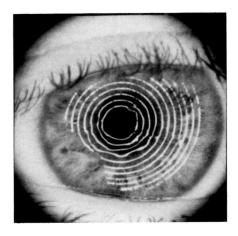

Figure 17-8
Photokeratoscopy demonstrates surface irregularity in epithelial basement membrane dystrophy.

3 weeks before the epithelium becomes uniform and the vision improves. Excimer laser keratectomy may also be useful.

DYSTROPHIES OF BOWMAN'S LAYER

Dystrophies that primarily affect Bowman's layer include Reis-Bücklers' dystrophy, Grayson-Wilbrandt dystrophy, hereditary calcific band keratopathy, and dermochondral dystrophy of François.

Reis-Bücklers' Dystrophy

Reis-Bücklers' dystrophy is transmitted as an autosomal dominant trait with strong penetrance.[23-26] It is bilateral and symmetric. The corneal disease is discernible in early childhood, and symptoms usually begin at about 5 years of age. Recurring attacks of erosion produce photophobia, foreign body sensation, injection, and pain, which can last for several weeks. The erosions recur approximately three to four times a year and gradually decrease in frequency over 5 to 20 years. Vision usually begins to deteriorate when patients are in their twenties.

The earliest finding is a fine reticular opacification at the level of Bowman's layer. With time the cornea becomes progressively more clouded by superficial, gray-white opacities. The opacities may be linear, geographic, honeycombed, or ringlike[23,26] and remain localized to Bowman's layer, except for peaklike projections into the epithelial layer (Figs. 17-9 and 17-10). The opacities are most dense in the central or midperipheral cornea, and the extreme periphery remains transparent. The corneal surface becomes rough and irregularly thickened, producing irregular astigmatism. Corneal sensation decreases with increasing epithelial thickness.[27,28] Hudson-Stähli lines and prominent corneal nerves are often present; vascularization is unusual.[26]

Bowman's layer is absent in many areas and is replaced by fibrocellular connective tissue, which extends into the epithelium in projections (Fig. 17-11).[25-31] The fibrocellular material consists of a mixture of larger collagen fibrils with a diameter of 250 to 400 Å and short, dense, curly fibrils 80 to 120 Å in diameter. In areas where Bowman's layer remains intact, the fibrocellular material accumulates between Bowman's layer and the epithelium. Degenerative changes occur in the basal epithelial cells, and the basement membrane is irregular or absent. The posterior surface of the epithelial

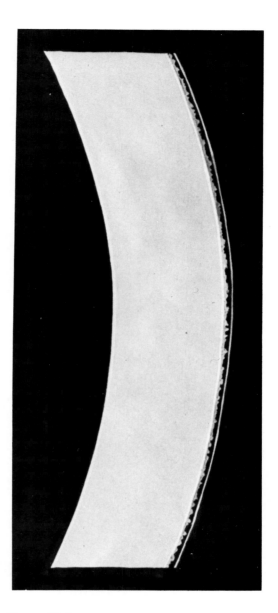

Figure 17-9
Reis-Bücklers' dystrophy. Peaklike projections from the area of Bowman's layer extend into the epithelium.

layer has a saw-toothed configuration. The posterior stroma, Descemet's membrane, and endothelium appear normal.

The nature and location of the primary abnormality in Reis-Bücklers' dystrophy is unclear. Some have proposed that the superficial keratocytes produce abnormal collagen fibrils, damaging Bowman's layer, with secondary epithelial injury.[29,30] Others feel that a primary epithelial cell abnormality leads to the recurrent

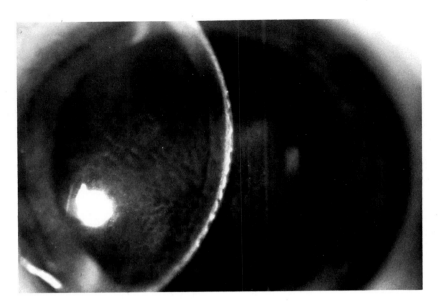

Figure 17-10
Opacities of Reis-Bücklers' dystrophy are interwoven ringlike figures making up a geographic pattern.
(Courtesy of Diane Curtin, Pittsburgh, PA.)

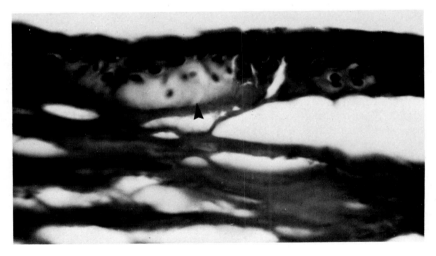

Figure 17-11
In Reis-Bücklers' dystrophy Bowman's layer is absent in some areas and replaced by fibrocellular connective tissue *(arrow)*. (From Grayson M: *Degeneration, dystrophies, and edema of the cornea.* In Duane TD, editor: *Clinical ophthalmology,* vol 4, Hagerstown, MD, 1978, Harper & Row, Publishers. Used with permission of Lippincott-Raven Publishers.)

epithelial erosions, with secondary activation of stromal cells, leading to deposition of the fibrocellular material and absorption of Bowman's layer.[30]

Treatment
The erosions are treated in the same way as erosions of other causes (described in Chapter 15). Surgery is indicated in cases with debilitating recurrent erosions or severe impairment of vision. Lamellar and penetrating keratoplasty have been successful,[25-27,29] but the disease can recur in the graft (Fig. 17-12).[32,33] Superficial keratectomy appears to be equally effective and may eliminate the necessity for a penetrating graft,[29,31,34,35] but the disease can recur after this procedure also. Excimer laser phototherapeutic keratectomy removes the opacity, improving

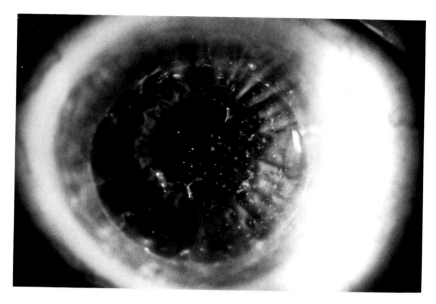

Figure 17-12
Recurrent Reis-Bücklers' dystrophy in a graft. (Courtesy of Diane Curtin, Pittsburgh, PA.)

vision, and reduces erosive episodes.[36,37] However, it can be complicated by a hyperopic refractive shift and irregular astigmatism.

Anterior Membrane Dystrophy of Grayson-Wilbrandt

A dystrophy with a clinical appearance similar to Reis-Bücklers' dystrophy was described by Grayson and Wilbrandt.[38] Two generations of a single family were affected, and the inheritance appeared to be autosomal dominant. The onset of the disease did not occur until 10 or 11 years of age, and erosions were infrequent. Vision was variably affected, with some retaining 20/20 vision and others reduced to 20/200, mainly by epithelial irregularity.

On biomicroscopic examination, moundlike opacities with a gray-white, macular appearance were seen in central Bowman's layer, extending into the epithelium. The lesions varied in size, and the intervening cornea was clear. Corneal sensation was normal.

It is possible that this disorder is an attenuated form of Reis-Bücklers' dystrophy. However, it differs from most cases of Reis-Bücklers' dystrophy in its later onset, infrequency of erosions, variable effect on vision, and normal corneal sensation.

Honeycomb Dystrophy of Thiel and Behnke

Honeycomb dystrophy is a bilateral, subepithelial dystrophy that was described in a single family, transmitted as an autosomal dominant trait.[39] It begins in childhood and runs a progressive course of recurrent erosions and decrease in vision. The vision varies from 20/25 in younger patients to 20/100 in patients 40 to 60 years of age. Corneal erosions cease between the thirties and fifties. A characteristic honeycomb-like opacity is seen at the level of Bowman's layer, with projections into the epithelium. The corneal surface remains smooth, and sensation is not affected.

Honeycomb dystrophy is probably another variant of Reis-Bücklers' dystrophy, especially in view of its occurrence in a pedigree with typical Reis-Bücklers' dystrophy.[40] Other anterior membrane dystrophy variants have been described.[41,42]

Inherited Band Keratopathy

Although band-shaped keratopathy is usually seen as a degeneration in ocular disease or systemic disease, it can occur as an inherited trait. Onset has been described in late adulthood, during puberty, and at birth.[43] In most cases it has been described in siblings of a single generation. Whether this was truly a dystrophy or resulted from undiagnosed ocular or systemic disease is unclear.

Meisler et al.[44] described a family with early onset of yellow-amber–colored anterior stromal globules in a band-shaped distribution.

Dermochondral Dystrophy of François

Dermochondral corneal dystrophy is a rare disorder consisting of a triad of abnormalities: skin

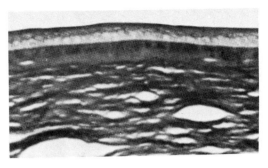

Figure 17-13
Corneal clouding caused by accumulation of acid mucopolysaccharide in Bowman's layer. (From Rodrigues MM, Calhoun J, Harley RD: *Am J Ophthalmol* 79:916, 1975.)

nodules, acquired deformities of the extremities, and a corneal dystrophy.[45,46] The corneal dystrophy is characterized by superficial central white opacities with irregular margins. They can elevate the epithelium. The lesions can develop as early as 3 years of age.[47] On histologic examination the epithelium is abnormal, and Bowman's membrane is poorly defined and contains some keratocytes.

Abnormal ossification of cartilage in the hands and feet leads to abnormal development, subluxations, and tendon retractions. The skin nodules look similar to xanthomas and involve the dorsal surface of joints of fingers, the posterior surface of elbows, and the nose and external ear. They probably represent a proliferation of anomalous fibroblasts.[46]

Local Anterior Mucopolysaccharide Accumulation

Bilateral diffuse corneal clouding with increased acid mucopolysaccharide accumulation in Bowman's layer occurred in two infants without evidence of systemic mucopolysaccharidosis.[48] Bowman's layer was diffusely thickened with abnormal acid mucopolysaccharide (Fig. 17-13). The epithelium, stroma, Descemet's membrane, and endothelium were normal. There were no intracellular vacuoles containing fibrillogranular inclusions or extracellular granular material, which are seen in macular dystrophy.

STROMAL DYSTROPHIES

Stromal dystrophies are hereditary disorders typified by the development of noninflammatory, nonvascularized stromal opacifications of various sizes and shapes. The opacities are bilateral and show specific physical characteristics on biomicroscopic examination. The histologic (Table 17-2) and histochemical (Table 17-3) nature of most of these stromal dystrophies has been identified. Table 17-4 summarizes the features of the stromal dystrophies.

Granular Dystrophy

Granular dystrophy is transmitted as an autosomal dominant trait with complete penetrance. The genetic abnormality has been localized to chromosome 5q.[49] The location is close to that of lattice and Avellino dystrophies, which also map to chromosome 5q.[50] The corneal opacities are usually apparent in the first decade of life as small, discrete, sharply demarcated, grayish white opacities in the anterior axial stroma (Fig. 17-14). At this stage vision is not impaired, and the patient feels no discomfort. As the condition advances, the lesions become larger, increase in number, coalesce, and extend into the deeper stroma. The opacities can vary in shape; they can be round with solid (Fig. 17-14) or relatively clear centers; they can take the form of a "Christmas tree" (Fig. 17-15); or they can resemble snowflakes; sinuous, interlacing tracks; or a sponge imprint (Fig. 17-16). The stroma between the discrete opacities is clear until relatively late in the disease. The opacities can extend toward the periphery of the cornea but never reach the limbus. Corneal sensation is usually normal. In some families recurrent erosions are common, but in most they are unusual.

Atypical forms have been described.[51] Diffuse subepithelial opacification, developing as early as 6 years of age, has been reported in some cases.[52-54] In one type, snowflakelike opacities are seen in the superficial stroma, sometimes extending into the periphery and developing into a diffuse superficial haze by the teen years. In another form, the lesions are small and flecklike, and normal vision is maintained throughout life.[55] Clinical and histologic features of both granular and lattice dystrophies have been observed in families from Avellino, Italy. The condition has been named *Avellino corneal dystrophy,* and is discussed below.

The histopathology of granular dystrophy is characteristic. Eosinophilic hyaline deposits are seen in the stroma and beneath the epithelium. These deposits stain an intense red with Masson trichrome stain (Fig. 17-17) and sometimes stain weakly positive with PAS.[56] The peripheral portions of the deposits may stain with Congo red.[57-59] Deposits that exhibit staining characteristic for amyloid can sometimes be seen sep-

Table 17-2   Stromal Corneal Dystrophies: Histopathologic Features

Dystrophy	Masson Trichrome Stain	Periodic-Acid Schiff Stain	Alcian Blue	Colloid Iron	Congo Red	Oil Red O	Thioflavine T	Birefringence*	Dichroism†
Granular corneal (Groenouw's type I)	+ (red)	± (weak)	–	–	–	–	–	–	–
Macular corneal (Groenouw's type II)	–	+ (pink)	+ (blue)	+	–	–	–	–	–
Lattice	+ (red)	+ (pink)	–	–	+ (orange)	–	+	+	+ (red/green)
Schnyder's crystalline	–	–	–	–	–	+ (red)	–	–	–
Fleck (speckled or mouchetée)	–	–	+ keratocytes (blue)	+	–	+	–	–	–
Pre-Descemet's	–	–	–	–	–	+ (red)	–	–	–

*Birefringence (The linear molecules of the Congo red dye arrange themselves along the axis of the amyloid fibrils; thus dichroism and birefringence can be demonstrated.)

1. Place a polarizing filter in front of the eyepiece lens.
2. Place a polarizing filter between the microscope light and slide.
3. Normally, when perpendicular to each other, no light is seen. However, when the amyloid fibrils stained with Congo red lie in a parallel direction, polarization of the light passing through the first polarizing filter is rotated by the amyloid and passes through the second filter as yellow-green color against a black background.

†Dichroism

1. Place a green filter in front of the microscope light.
2. Place a polarizing filter between the green light and the slide.
3. The parallel-stained Congo red amyloid fibrils absorb green light.
4. If the polarizing is parallel to the fibril axis, the green light is absorbed.
5. If the polarizing plane is at right angles to the fibril, it is not absorbed; thus rotating the polarizing filter will produce red and green colors.

Table 17-3   Abnormal Substances of Stromal Dystrophies

Dystrophy	Abnormal Substance
Granular	Amino acids and phospholipid
Lattice	Amyloid
Gelatinous droplike	Amyloid
Macular	Glycosaminoglycan (?abnormal keratan sulfate)
Central crystalline	Cholesterol
Fleck	Intracellular glycosaminoglycan
Pre-Descemet's	Intracellular lipids
Parenchymatous	?Amyloid

arately from otherwise typical granular deposits.[57,58] Electron microscopy shows electron-dense, trapezoid- or rod-shaped extracellular deposits (Fig. 17-18). These deposits are 100 to 500 μm wide, and their inner structure can display a homogenous, filamentous, or moth-eaten pattern.[17,58-61] The stromal keratocytes in some instances show degenerative changes, with dilation of the endoplasmic reticulum and Golgi apparatus and vacuolization of the cytoplasm.[60] Histochemical studies indicate that the deposits contain tyrosine, tryptophan, and sulfur-containing amino acids, and some contain arginine as well.[62,63] Microfibrillar protein and phospholipid have also been demonstrated.[63] In one study, the deposits were positive for immunoglobulin G and κ and λ immunoglobulin chains.[64]

The exact nature and source of the deposits are not known. Protein and phospholipids, which make up the deposits, are the principal components of cell membranes. It is unclear whether the deposits are produced by epithelium, stromal keratocytes, or both. The characteristic rod-shaped structures have been seen within both epithelial cells and keratocytes.[61] In some recurrences the disease appears to be confined to the epithelium.[65]

Treatment

Most patients with granular dystrophy do not require treatment. Some patients have recurrent erosions, and the treatment of these is discussed in Chapter 15. If vision is markedly reduced, surgery can be performed. If the opacities are largely superficial, epithelial scraping or superficial keratectomy may be sufficient.[54,66] Superficial keratectomy can be performed with an excimer laser.[67,68] For deeper opacities lamellar or penetrating keratoplasty can be performed. Granular dystrophy can appear in the graft as early as 1 year after surgery (Fig. 17-19),[69-72] and is present in nearly all cases by 4 years.[73] Clinically, it usually is noted as a diffuse, subepithelial haze in the peripheral graft or as typical granular lesions in the stroma. The former type represents avascular fibrous tissue between the epithelium and Bowman's layer; it can be removed by superficial keratectomy to restore good vision.[74] The typical electron-dense trapezoid- and rod-shaped deposits can be seen in the stroma and epithelium.[65,70] In view of the near certainty of recurrence, the least invasive surgery necessary to restore vision should be performed. Superficial keratectomy is probably preferable, followed by lamellar and then penetrating keratoplasty. Excimer laser phototherapeutic keratectomy can also be used to treat recurrent granular dystrophy after penetrating keratoplasty.[75]

Lattice Dystrophy

Lattice dystrophy is inherited as an autosomal dominant trait and varies in penetrance and expression.[76] Most cases are bilateral, but unilateral cases have been reported.[77,78] Clinical evidence of corneal disease appears early, usually by 2 to 7 years of age. Visual impairment gradually increases and usually requires keratoplasty by the twenties or thirties. Recurrent erosions are fairly common.

The early corneal lesions typically appear as fine, irregular lines and dots, mainly in the axial cornea and involving the anterior stroma and Bowman's layer.[79] In other cases it appears as discrete round or ovoid nonrefractile subepithelial opacities or as diffuse axial anterior stromal haze.[80] With progression the lesions can appear as small nodules, dots, threadlike spicules (Fig. 17-20), or thicker, radially oriented branching lines. The lines are typically refractile with a double contour and a clear core on retroillumination. With time the lattice lines can extend into the deep stroma and epithelium, and they tend to become opacified. Between the lines refractile dots or small irregular opacities are usually present, but the stroma between these opacities is clear initially. With time the opacities coalesce, and a diffuse ground-glass haze can involve the anterior stroma and midstroma. Anterior involvement leads to recurrent erosions and surface irregularity.

Once the anterior cornea becomes opacified, the appearance can resemble that seen in the later stages of macular and granular dystro-

Dystrophy	Character of Opacity	Clinical Features	Vision	Electron-Microscopic Features	Inheritance	Erosion Symptoms
Granular corneal (Groenouw's type I)	Discrete, gray-white opacities with sharp borders Clear cornea between opacities	Axial region All depths of stroma No involvement of epithelium or Descemet's membrane	Usually good until age 40	Electron-dense, rhomboid-shaped rods Endothelium not affected	Autosomal dominant In rare cases sporadic	–
Lattice	Gray lines resembling pipestemlike threads that are translucent by retroillumination; dot and stromal opacities between these give ground-glass appearance; threadlike opacities may show bulbous areas and dichotomous branching	Scattered latticelike network with bifurcating pipestemlike threads, mainly limited to zone between center of cornea and periphery; seen throughout the stroma and may involve epithelium	Reduced early in life (usually late adolescence)	Nonbranching fibrils (8–10 mm) characteristic of amyloid	Autosomal dominant	+
Gelatinous droplike	Raised multinodular subepithelial mounds	White on direct illumination, transparent on retroillumination Central	Reduced in first decade	Amyloid in and beneath basal epithelium	?Autosomal recessive	+
Macular corneal (Groenouw's type II)	Poorly demarcated, gray-white opacities Diffusely cloudy cornea between large, irregular opaque areas	Entire cornea may be involved, but more dense in axial region Some spots extend to limbus Deep epithelium and endothelium are affected	Affected in late teens	Membrane-bound vacuoles with fibrillogranular material Keratocytes and endothelium affected	Autosomal recessive	+
Schnyder's crystalline	Crystalline deposits, usually	Mostly located in axial area of cornea Hyperlipidemia often present Chondrodystrophy and genu valgum in some families	Usually not markedly disturbed; may be decreased	Notched rectangular crystals	Autosomal dominant	–

Table 17-4 Stromal Corneal Dystrophies

Continued

Table 17-4 Stromal Corneal Dystrophies—cont'd

Dystrophy	Character of Opacity	Clinical Features	Vision	Electron-Microscopic Features	Inheritance	Erosion Symptoms
Fleck (speckled or mouchetée)	Well-demarcated, small, round, doughnutlike opacities	Opacities are located in all levels of stroma	Vision usually is not affected; however, photophobia may be marked	Keratocytes contain cytoplasmic, membrane-bound vacuoles with fibrillogranular material	Autosomal dominant	—
Marginal crystalline (Bietti)	Crystals in cornea	Superficial stromal deposition in paralimbal area	Vision is not affected by crystals Fundus albipunctatus	No studies available	Not definitely established	—
Central cloudy (François)	Diffuse posterior opacity in pupillary zone broken up into segmental areas Seen best via sclerotic scatter In direct illumination opacities are multiple, small, fuzzy-outlined gray areas, polygonal in shape and separated by clearer areas	Opacity densest posteriorly but extends to level of Bowman's layer Does not involve Descemet's membrane May be same as posterior crocodile shagreen	No decrease in vision	No studies available	Autosomal dominant	—
Parenchymatous (Pillat)	Central punctate and filamentous opacities Peripheral ones are also seen but are finer Central opacities affect posterior stroma	Most opacities are larger than those seen in pre-Descemet's dystrophy Appear gray on focal illumination and clear on retroillumination Noted in seventh decade	No decrease in vision	No studies available	?	—
Posterior amorphous	Gray sheets of indistinct corneal opacities	Opacities are at various levels but mostly deep stroma and may involve Descemet's membrane	Vision may be reduced to 20/40	No studies available	Autosomal dominant	—
Pre-Descemet's	Small opacities of varied shapes and sizes: round, comma, dots, dendritic, or linear	Best seen in retroillumination All opacities are in deep stroma	Vision is not affected	Posterior keratocytes contain membrane-bound vacuoles with fibrillogranular material	Autosomal dominant	—

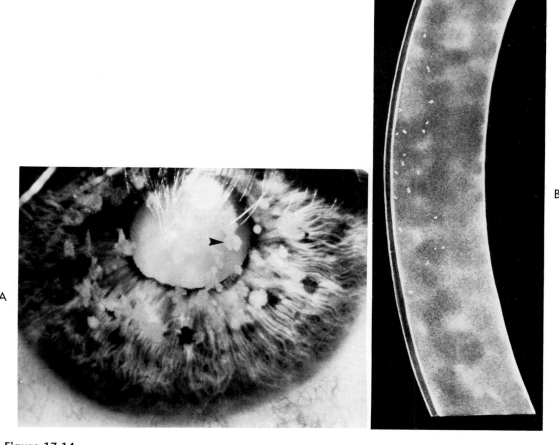

Figure 17-14
A, Lesions in granular dystrophy are discrete, gray-white opacities *(arrow)* with clear corneal stroma between opacities. **B,** Optical section showing the distribution of lesions throughout the stroma.

phies. However, the typical branching lattice lines usually can be seen. Also, refractile opacities can usually be found in lattice dystrophy but not in macular or granular dystrophies.

Other Forms of Lattice Corneal Dystrophy

Other forms of latticelike dystrophy have been described (Table 17-5). In rare cases a similar corneal picture can be seen in association with systemic amyloidosis. This condition was originally described by Meretoja[81-84] and has been called type II lattice dystrophy and familial amyloid polyneuropathy type IV. The latticelike corneal changes usually become manifest between 20 and 35 years of age; in later decades the skin, peripheral nerves, and cranial nerves become involved. In contrast to type I lattice dystrophy, the corneal disease in type II is

milder and later in onset. Vision is good until the seventh decade, and erosive symptoms are less frequent. In type II lattice dystrophy, fewer lattice lines (8 to 20) are present; they are radially oriented, are coarser, and extend to the limbus. There are also fewer amorphous dots.

Another type of latticelike corneal dystrophy (type III) was recently reported in two families in Japan.[85,86] These patients had thick, translucent lattice lines and few amorphous dots. Vision was good until after 40 years of age, and recurrent erosions did not develop. There was no evidence of systemic amyloidosis.

Histopathology

On histologic examination of type I lattice dystrophy, the epithelial layer is irregular, with areas of thickening and thinning.[56,87] The basal

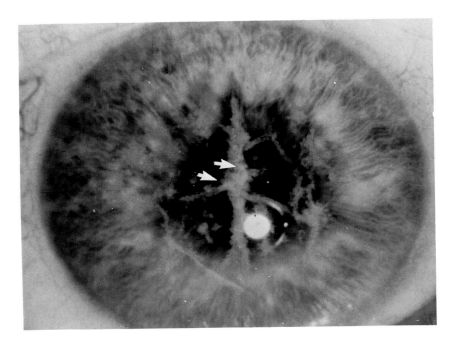

Figure 17-15
Christmas tree opacity (*arrows*) in a case of granular dystrophy. (From Grayson M: *Degeneration, dystrophies, and edema of the cornea.* In Duane TD, editor: *Clinical ophthalmology,* vol 4, Hagerstown, MD, 1978, Harper & Row, Publishers. Used with permission of Lippincott-Raven Publishers.)

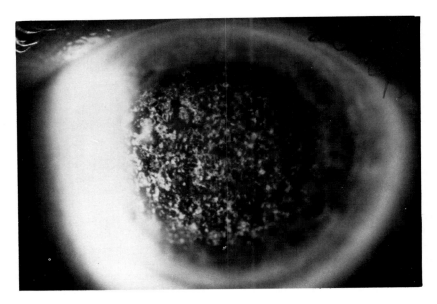

Figure 17-16
Sponge-imprint type of opacities in granular dystrophy.

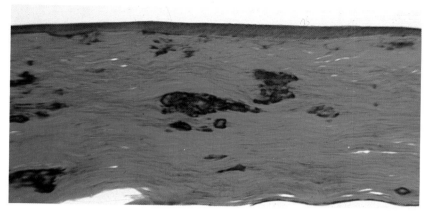

Figure 17-17
Positive Masson's trichrome stain seen in granular dystrophy.

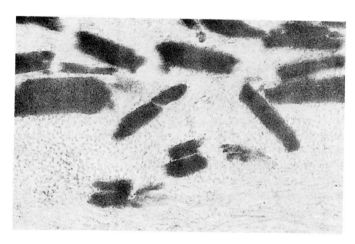

Figure 17-18
Dense, homogeneous, rod-shaped structures characteristic of granular dystrophy as noted with transmission electron microscopy (×36,000). (From Haddad R, Font RL, Fine BS: *Am J Ophthalmol* 83:213, 1977.)

epithelial cells degenerate, and the basement membrane is thickened and discontinuous, without normal hemidesmosomes.[88] Bowman's layer may be absent, thick, or thin in different areas. Deposits of eosinophilic material are seen between the epithelium and Bowman's layer and throughout the stroma (Fig. 17-21). These deposits stain with Congo red (Fig. 17-22), PAS, and thioflavin T; manifest green birefringence when viewed with a polarizing microscope (Fig. 17-23); and exhibit dichroism when viewed with polarization and a green filter.[89,90] These findings are consistent with amyloid, and the amyloid nature has been confirmed by immu-

nofluorescence studies using antisera to human amyloid.[91] In some cases, some of the deposits stain red with Masson's trichrome stain, suggestive of granular dystrophy.[92] In longstanding cases, a degenerative pannus can be seen.[91] Descemet's membrane and the endothelium are essentially normal, although amyloid deposits have been seen rarely in the former.

On electron microscopy, the deposits are composed of fine, electron-dense, nonbranching fibrils 8 to 10 nm in diameter without periodicity.[93-95] Most of the fibrils are highly aligned, which explains the phenomena of dichroism and birefringence. Keratocytes in the

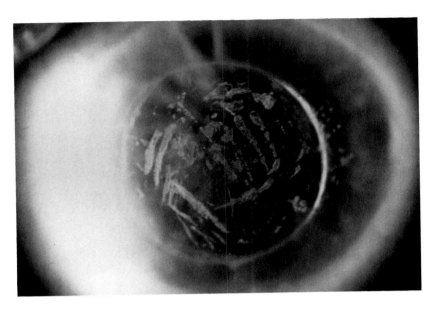

Figure 17-19
Granular dystrophy recurring in a graft. (Courtesy of Diane Curtin, Pittsburgh, PA.)

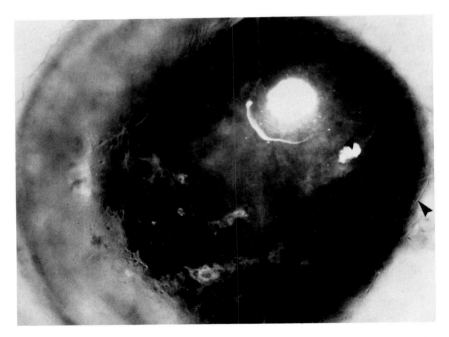

Figure 17-20
Lattice dystrophy. Note the threadlike spicules branching dichotomously (*arrows*).

involved areas are decreased in number; some of them appear quite active, whereas others appear degenerated.[76,89,90,95]

Histologic examination of corneas with type II lattice dystrophy showed a uniform thin layer of amyloid deposits posterior to Bowman's layer.[82] The lattice lines were also composed of amyloid, and they appeared to have replaced corneal nerves. Amyloid was also found beneath the basement membrane of the conjunctival epithelium and in sclera, arteries, skin, peripheral nerves, and other tissues.

Table 17-5 Comparison of Different Types of Lattice Corneal Dystrophy

Characteristic	Type I	Type II (Meretoja)	Type III	Polymorphic Amyloid Degeneration
Inheritance	Autosomal dominant	Autosomal dominant	?Autosomal recessive	None
Onset	Under age 10	20–35 years	Over age 40	Over age 40
Visual acuity	Poor after age 40	Good until age 65	Impaired after age 60	Unaffected
Erosions	Frequent	Infrequent	None	None
Cornea	Numerous, delicate lines; many amorphous deposits; periphery clear	Few thick lines; extend to periphery; few amorphous deposits	Thick lines	Polymorphic punctate opacities, filaments; central, peripheral, or annular distribution
Systemic involvement	None	Amyloidosis involving skin, nerves, arteries, and other organs	None	None
Face	Normal	Facial paresis and blepharochalasis after age 40	Normal	Normal

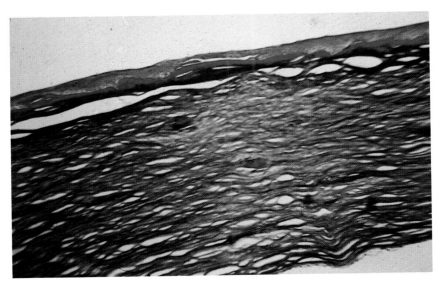

Figure 17-21
Lattice dystrophy. Lesions may be seen subepithelially and in all levels of the stroma.

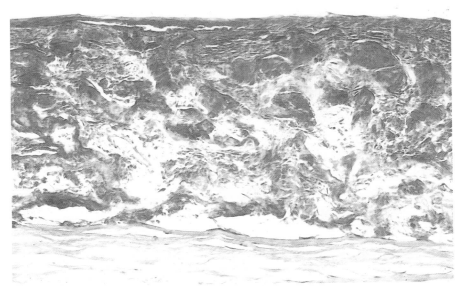

Figure 17-22
Congo red stain of corneal amyloid. (Courtesy of F. Wilson II, Indianapolis, IN.)

Pathogenesis

Amyloid is a noncollagenous, fibrous protein containing 2% to 5% carbohydrate. The structure of the amyloid deposits varies in the different forms of amyloidosis. In immunoglobulin primary systemic amyloidosis, the amyloid contains fragments of immunoglobulin light chains. In hereditary systemic amyloidosis, normal or variant transthyretin, also known as plasma prealbumin, is most frequently accu-

mulated. Many variant transthyretin molecules have been identified.[96] Apolipoprotein A-1, or gelsolin, an actin-severing protein, is found in some kindreds with familial amyloidotic polyneuropathy.

The major component of amyloid deposits associated with secondary systemic amyloidosis is a protein (protein AA) that appears to be a degradation product of a serum acute phase reactant (serum AA) unrelated to immunoglobu-

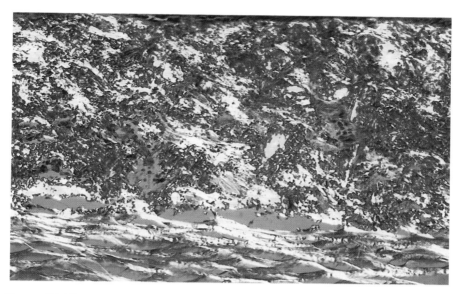

Figure 17-23
Corneal amyloid as seen with polarized light. (Courtesy of F. Wilson II, Indianapolis, IN.)

lins. Both primary and secondary amyloid deposits are associated with a structural protein (protein AP), which is also present in normal serum.

In lattice corneal dystrophy, protein AP is present, but immunoglobulin light chains and protein AA are not.[97,98] In type II, variant gelsolin molecules have been identified, always at nucleotide 654 in the gelsolin gene, which is on chromosome 9q.[99-101] Antibodies to the mutated gelsolin protein and to protein AP bind to amyloid deposits in the cornea and conjunctiva, the perineurium of ciliary nerves, the walls of ciliary vessels, the optic nerve sheaths, the stroma of the ciliary body, and the choriocapillaris.[102]

Mutations in the gelsolin gene are not responsible for type I lattice dystrophy.[103] The gelsolin gene is on chromosome 9q, but type I lattice dystrophy has been localized to 5q. The antibodies to the mutated gelsolin protein found in type II lattice dystrophy do not react with the stromal deposits found in type I.[97] Therefore, it appears that mutations in different genes and on different chromosomes can cause clinically similar forms of lattice dystrophy.

Treatment
If visual acuity is impaired, penetrating keratoplasty can be performed (Fig. 17-24). The likelihood of obtaining a clear graft is high, but the dystrophy can appear in the graft in as little as 3 years.[70,104] Excimer laser phototherapeutic keratectomy can be performed for recurrent erosions or to improve vision. It is indicated in cases in which most of the opacity is less than 100 μm in depth. Lattice dystrophy recurs more frequently than granular or macular dystrophy: In one study 48% of patients had evidence of recurrence from 2 to 26 years after grafting, and 15% required regrafting.[105] Recurrence of lattice lines is unusual; more commonly, dotlike, diffuse, or filamentous subepithelial opacities or diffuse anterior stromal haze are seen.

Gelatinous Droplike Dystrophy
Gelatinous droplike dystrophy is a rare form of primary familial amyloidosis of the cornea.[106-109] It has been seen in Europe and the United States but is much more common in Japan.[110] The pattern of inheritance is unclear but is most likely autosomal recessive. The disorder usually appears in the first decade, with photophobia, lacrimation, and decreased visual acuity. Bilateral, central, raised, multinodular, subepithelial mounds of amyloid are seen (Fig. 17-25). These are white on direct illumination and transparent on retroillumination but can become yellow and milky with time. Flat subepithelial opacities can be seen surrounding the mounds. Early in the dystrophy the deposits are fairly flat and can resemble band-shaped keratopathy.[111] In the late stages the cornea can have a diffuse, mulberry-like appearance, and neovascularization can occur.

The amyloid nature of these deposits has

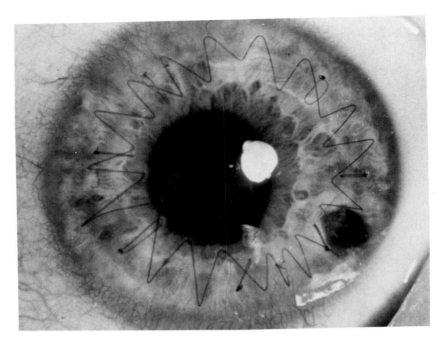

Figure 17-24
Penetrating keratoplasty is used to obtain good vision in patients with lattice dystrophy.

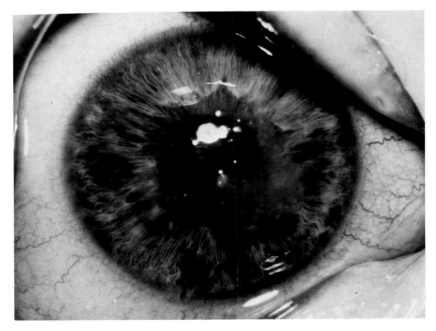

Figure 17-25
Gelatinous droplike dystrophy. Note the raised, multinodular lesions with subepithelial formations of amyloid (*arrow*).

been demonstrated histologically.[106-108] Bowman's layer is usually absent, and amyloid is deposited in the basal epithelial cells, beneath the epithelium, and occasionally in the stroma. The deposits contain protein AP but not protein AA or immunoglobulins.

Penetrating keratoplasty is not very effective.[112] Subepithelial haze develops within 1 year after keratoplasty. Recurrent amyloid deposition, sufficient to decrease vision, typically occurs within 3 years.[107,112] There is also a high incidence of postsurgical complications.[112] Superficial keratectomy, repeated as often as necessary, is probably the best approach,[113] and this can be performed with an excimer laser.

Avellino Corneal Dystrophy

Several pedigrees have been reported that display both clinical and histologic features of both granular and lattice corneal dystrophies.[114-116] Nearly all patients have originated from Avellino, Italy, so the term *Avellino corneal dystrophy* has been proposed. Others have called it granular-lattice dystrophy. The disease is inherited as an autosomal dominant trait with high penetrance. Avellino, granular, and type I lattice dystrophies have each been mapped to chromosome 5q.[50]

These patients have well-circumscribed central anterior stromal opacities and deeper lattice-like lines. A central anterior stromal haze can be seen between the deposits, most often in older individuals. The granular stromal lesions develop early in life and reach their mature quantity relatively early, although they continue to enlarge slowly. The lattice component begins later and progresses for a longer period. The stromal haze is last to develop, usually after the age of 50. The granular lesions are fairly typical, while the lattice deposits tend to be larger and more fusiform than those normally seen in lattice dystrophy. Initially they are found in the mid and deep stroma, but with age they involve the entire thickness. When fully developed they can create the appearance of a snowflake. Recurrent erosions are seen in some patients.

Histologically, superficial granular deposits that appear hyaline with hematoxylin-eosin staining and bright red with Masson-trichrome staining are present. Also seen are numerous fusiform stromal deposits that have the staining characteristics of amyloid. As noted earlier, patients with clinically typical granular dystrophy are often found to have amyloid deposits on histopathology, and patients with typical type I lattice dystrophy have deposits consistent with granular dystrophy. In view of these findings,

and the discovery that Avellino, granular, and type I lattice dystrophies all map to chromosome 5q, some authors have suggested that all three dystrophies result from mutations in the same gene.[117]

Phototherapeutic keratectomy and penetrating keratoplasty have improved vision.[115,118] Granular deposits can recur in the graft.[115]

Macular Dystrophy
Clinical Findings

Macular dystrophy is transmitted as an autosomal recessive trait. Of the three classic stromal dystrophies, macular dystrophy is the most severe. The patient has progressive loss of vision and attacks of irritation and photophobia. In most cases vision is severely impaired by the twenties or thirties. Recurrent erosions are seen, but they are less frequent than in lattice dystrophy. Heterozygous carriers do not manifest any corneal abnormalities.

The corneal changes are first noted usually between 3 and 9 years of age, when a diffuse clouding is seen in the central superficial stroma. With time the clouding extends peripherally and into the deeper stroma. By the teens the opacification involves the entire thickness of the cornea and may extend out to the limbus. Within this sea of haziness are gray-white, denser opacities with indistinct borders (Fig. 17-26). These denser, macular opacities can protrude anteriorly, resulting in irregularity of the epithelial surface (Fig. 17-27), or posteriorly, causing irregularity, grayness, and a guttate appearance of Descemet's membrane (Fig. 17-28). They can enlarge with time and coalesce. The stroma is thinner than normal.[119]

Pathology

Histologically, macular dystrophy is characterized by the accumulation of glycosaminoglycans (acid mucopolysaccharide) between the stromal lamellae, underneath the epithelium, within stromal keratocytes, and within the endothelial cells.[56,57,120] The glycosaminoglycans stain with alcian blue, colloidal iron, and PAS (Figs. 17-27 and 17-28). Degeneration of the basal epithelial cells and focal epithelial thinning are seen over the accumulated material. Bowman's layer is thinned or absent in some areas.

Electron microscopy shows accumulation of mucopolysaccharide within stromal keratocytes.[57,89,121] The keratocytes are distended by numerous intracytoplasmic vacuoles, which appear to be the dilated cisternae of the rough endoplasmic reticulum. Some of these vacuoles are clear, but many contain fibrillar or granular

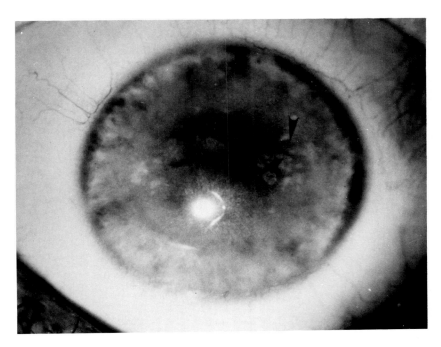

Figure 17-26
Macular dystrophy shows diffuse corneal haze with gray-white dense opacities in the area of haze (*arrows*).

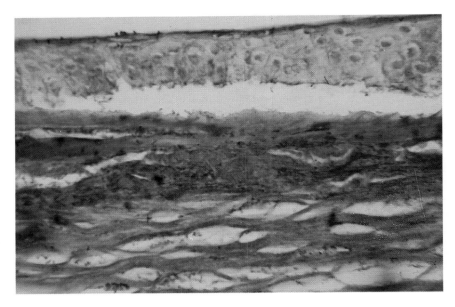

Figure 17-27
Macular dystrophy. Colloidal iron stain indicates accumulation of acid mucopolysaccharide under the epithelium.

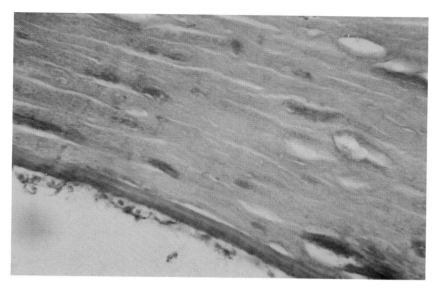

Figure 17-28
Macular dystrophy. Colloidal iron stain shows accumulation of acid mucopolysaccharide in the endothelium.

material, and occasionally membranous lamellar material. The endothelial cells contain material similar to that found in keratocytes. The posterior, nonbanded portion of Descemet's membrane is infiltrated by vesicular and granular material deposited by the abnormal endothelium.

The accumulated material appears to be abnormal keratan sulfate. In culture, the keratocytes produce only glycoprotein precursors of keratan sulfate.[122,123] In one patient there was a defect in a sulfotransferase specific for sulfating lactosaminoglycans.[124] The accumulated material varies; its staining by different anti–keratan sulfate antibodies differs between patients (Fig. 17-29).[125,126] In some patients normal keratan sulfate is also absent from the serum and cartilage.[125,127,128]

The corneal pathology of macular corneal dystrophy differs from that of the systemic mucopolysaccharidoses. There appears to be an abnormality in the synthesis of mucopolysaccharide in macular dystrophy and an abnormality in the breakdown of mucopolysaccharide in the systemic mucopolysaccharidoses. In the systemic mucopolysaccharidoses, the abnormal material accumulates in lysosomal vacuoles, whereas in macular dystrophy it accumulates in endoplasmic reticulum.

Treatment
Good results are obtained from penetrating keratoplasty for macular dystrophy (Fig. 17-30).

Recurrences can be seen in both lamellar and penetrating grafts, but they are usually delayed for many years.[129,130] Host keratocytes invade the graft and produce abnormal glycosaminoglycan. The periphery of the graft is most affected, particularly the superficial and deep layers. Surprisingly, the endothelium and Descemet's membrane also are affected.

Fleck Dystrophy
Fleck dystrophy, which has also been called speckled or mouchetée dystrophy, is rare. It is transmitted as an autosomal dominant trait.[131-134] The condition is usually noted during a routine examination; it is stationary with no loss of visual acuity. Some degree of photophobia may be present.[133] The lesions appear during the first decade of life and are usually bilateral, although they can be asymmetric or unilateral. Small opacities are present in all layers of the corneal stroma except Bowman's layer, and they involve the peripheral as well as central stroma (Figs. 17-31 and 17-32). The lesions are semiopaque, flattened opacities that may be oval, round, comma-shaped, granular, or stellate. Many have a doughnutlike appearance with a relatively clear center. These small opacities are well demarcated, and the intervening stroma is clear. The best way to demonstrate them is on retroillumination. Corneal sensation is normal in most cases, but in some families sensation is decreased.

Fleck dystrophy has been noted in associa-

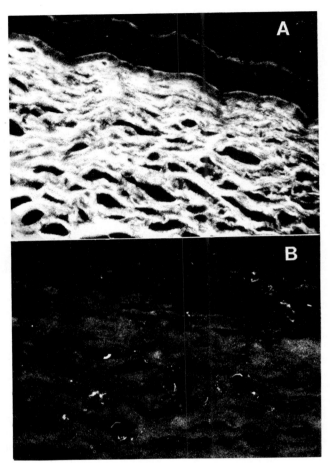

Figure 17-29
Distribution of keratan sulfate in a normal cornea **(A)** and the cornea from a patient with macular corneal dystrophy **(B)**. Cryostat sections of the cornea were reacted with a monoclonal antibody against
keratan sulfate using an indirect immunofluorescence technique. Note the strong staining of keratan sulfate in the normal cornea *(A)* but the absence of staining in the cornea from the patient with macular
corneal dystrophy *(B)*. (Courtesy of Nirmala Sundar-Raj, PhD, Pittsburgh, PA.)

tion with a variety of disorders such as keratoconus, limbal dermoids, central cloudy dystrophy, angioid streaks, papillitis, and punctate
cortical lens opacities.[131,135] It is unclear
whether the relationship is more than coincidental.

Histopathologic studies reveal abnormal,
distended keratocytes throughout the stroma.
The keratocytes stain with oil red O and Sudan
black B, indicating the presence of lipid, and
with alcian blue and colloidal iron, indicating
the presence of mucopolysaccharide.[136,137] On
electron microscopy the keratocytes are seen to
contain varying numbers of membrane-limited
intracytoplasmic vacuoles containing a fibrillogranular material.[136] The vacuoles appear to
arise from the Golgi apparatus and therefore
would be lysosomal vacuoles. Because of this
fleck dystrophy seems to be a storage disorder
of glycosaminoglycans and complex lipids that
is limited to the cornea.

Central Crystalline Dystrophy of Schnyder

Central crystalline dystrophy is transmitted as
an autosomal dominant trait. It is absent at
birth but may be seen as early as 18 months
of age. Visual acuity is not usually affected, but
occasionally it is moderately reduced. The chief
characteristic of the dystrophy is the presence
of bilateral, ring-shaped, or disciform opacities
in the central cornea.[138-141] The opacities often

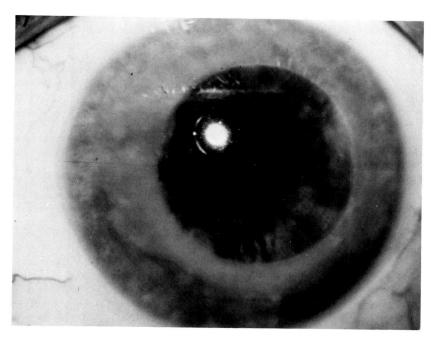

Figure 17-30
Good visual results can be obtained with penetrating keratoplasty in macular dystrophy.

appear to consist of fine, polychromatic, needle-shaped crystals (Fig. 17-33), but in one half of cases a disciform opacity is present without evident crystals.[142] The opacity primarily involves the anterior stroma but may extend into the deeper layers.

Although the opacities usually progress slowly and stabilize in later life, significant progression can occur.[143] A dense corneal arcus frequently develops between 23 and 39 years of age, and after age 40 many patients will have diffuse corneal opacification.[141,144]

A significant number of patients have hyperlipidemia, but the type and severity vary.[139] Within a single family some individuals have only crystalline dystrophy, whereas others have hyperlipidemia and crystalline dystrophy, and still others have only hyperlipidemia. Chondrodystrophy and genu valgum are also present in some families.[139,141,145]

The main histopathologic feature of Schnyder's dystrophy is the presence of cholesterol crystals, noncrystalline cholesterol, cholesterol esters, and neutral fats in the stroma.[139,146-148] The deposits are most numerous in the anterior stroma, but they can extend posteriorly to Descemet's membrane.[149,150] Frozen sections must be performed to avoid dissolution of the crystals during fixation. Destruction of Bowman's layer and the superficial stroma with disorganization of collagen has often been observed. Some keratocytes contain cholesterol crystals, and similar deposits have been noted occasionally in basal epithelial cells.[151]

Schnyder's dystrophy is most likely a localized disorder of cholesterol metabolism, and it may be exacerbated by systemic hyperlipoproteinemia. Burns, Connor, and Gipson[152] administered radiolabeled cholesterol intravenously to a patient with crystalline dystrophy 2 weeks before keratoplasty. The radioactivity in the cornea was higher than in the blood, suggesting active deposition of cholesterol in the cornea.

In most cases of crystalline dystrophy the corneal disease requires no treatment. Serum lipid profiles should be obtained. Penetrating or lamellar keratoplasty can be performed for visual rehabilitation, but the dystrophy can recur.[141] It is important to consider other causes of corneal crystals. (These are discussed in Chapter 3.)

Marginal Crystalline Dystrophy of Bietti

Marginal crystalline dystrophy was described in two brothers who had crystalline material in the superficial stroma of the paralimbal cornea; their vision was not affected[153] (Fig. 17-34).

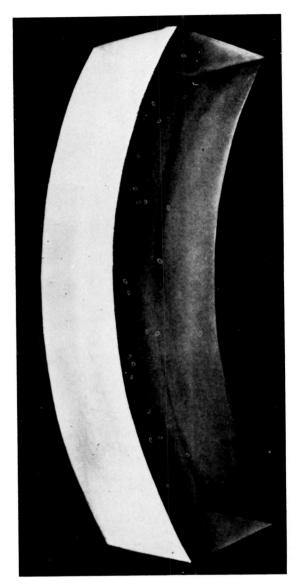

Figure 17-31
Fleck dystrophy. Small, oval, doughnut-shaped, gray-white lesions are seen in the stroma.

Both brothers also had fundus albipunctatus. A few similar cases have been described, and in one case a pathologic examination was performed.[154,155] Cholesterol or cholesterol ester and complex lipid inclusions were seen in corneal fibroblasts and circulating lymphocytes. The retinal crystals diminish with time.[156]

Central Cloudy Dystrophy of François
Central cloudy dystrophy was described as a nonprogressive diffuse clouding of the axial cornea, which is densest posteriorly and fades anteriorly and peripherally (Figs. 17-35 and 17-36).[157-159] The cloud is broken into segments by an interlacing network of clear lines, creating a mosaic pattern. Most likely this condition is the same as posterior mosaic shagreen.

Parenchymatous Dystrophy of Pillat
Parenchymatous dystrophy of the cornea,[160,161] also called polymorphic stromal dystrophy,[162] is most likely the same as polymorphic amyloid degeneration, which is discussed in Chapter 16.[163]

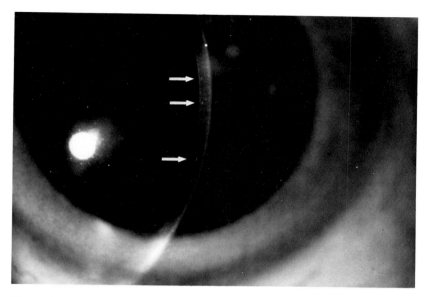

Figure 17-32
Fleck dystrophy.

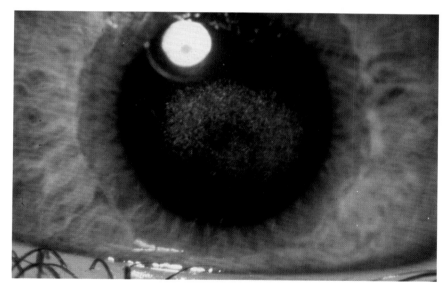

Figure 17-33
Schnyder's crystalline dystrophy. The lesion consists of fine, polychromatic needlelike crystals in the area of Bowman's layer and the anterior stroma.

Posterior Amorphous Dystrophy

Posterior amorphous dystrophy, an autosomal dominant condition, has now been reported in seven families.[164-166] Changes have been noted as early as 16 weeks of age and thus may be present at birth. Progression has not been documented; this condition most likely is a dysgenesis rather than a dystrophy.

Gray, sheetlike opacities can involve any portion of the stroma but are most prominent posteriorly. They can affect any portion of the cornea and are bilaterally symmetric. The haze tends to be denser peripherally and is often interrupted by clear zones. Descemet's membrane may show posterior bowing and distortion of the endothelial mosaic. Generalized corneal

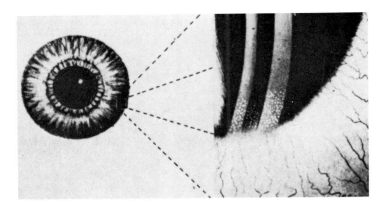

Figure 17-34
Marginal crystalline changes in the cornea. (From Bagolini B, Ioli-Spada G: *Am J Ophthalmol* 65:53, 1968.)

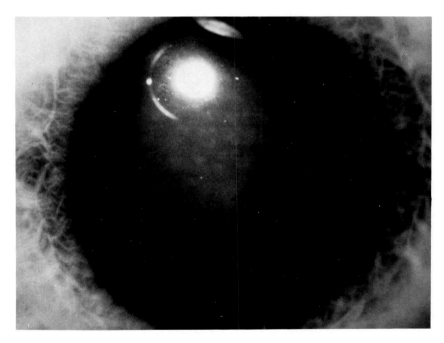

Figure 17-35
Central cloudy dystrophy of François. General clouding of the cornea is broken up into segmental areas of opacity by intervening clear tissue.

thinning, high astigmatism, flattened keratometry, scleralization of the peripheral cornea, and hyperopia may be present.[166] Visual acuity is usually 20/40 or better. Various iris and angle abnormalities have been noted, including a prominent Schwalbe's ring with numerous fine iris processes, pupillary remnants, corectopia, iridocorneal adhesions, and anterior stromal tags.

In one case, collagen fibers in the most posterior stromal lamellae were disorganized. Descemet's layer was interrupted by a band of collagen fibers resembling stroma, and there was loss of endothelial cells.[167] In another case, subepithelial deposits and a thick collagenous layer posterior to Descemet's membrane were seen.[168] The findings in both of these cases suggest abnormalities in development of the posterior cornea. The condition being a dysgenesis rather than a dystrophy is consistent with the early onset, lack of progression, and association with iris abnormalities.[164]

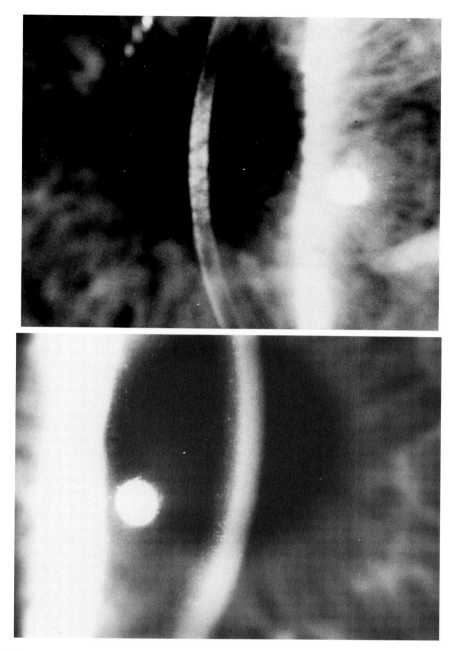

Figure 17-36
Slit-beam microscopy showing distribution of the opacity in central cloudy dystrophy of François.
Inset, Fine dot-, line-, and comma-shaped opacities can be seen adjacent to Descemet's membrane in pre-Descemet's dystrophy. (Courtesy of Robert D. Deitch Jr, Indianapolis, IN.)

PRE-DESCEMET'S DYSTROPHIES

A variety of fine posterior stromal opacities have been described in patients in their fourth decade or older. Most likely these are degenerative diseases rather than dystrophies.[17] However, some of these conditions have been re-

ported in a number of family members, over two to four generations.[169,170] In one family the mother had typical cornea farinata, whereas her daughter had pre-Descemet's dystrophy.

Cornea farinata is sometimes classified with pre-Descemet's dystrophies, but it is more often considered an age-related degeneration. *Cornea*

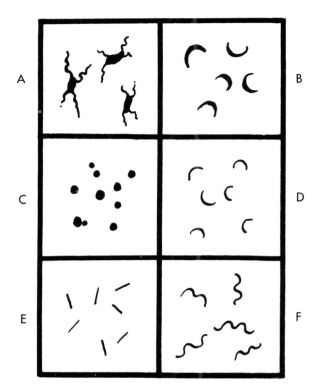

Figure 17-37
Patterns of opacities in the pre-Descemet's dystrophies. **A,** Dendritic. **B,** Boomerang. **C,** Circular.
D, Comma. **E,** Linear. **F,** Filiform.

farinata consists of tiny, punctate, gray opacities in the deep stroma immediately anterior to Descemet's membrane. It is discussed in Chapter 16.

The opacities in pre-Descemet's dystrophy resemble those in cornea farinata, but they are larger and more polymorphous (Fig. 17-36). Grayson and Wilbrandt[171] described primary pre-Descemet's dystrophies that consisted of mixtures of six types of tiny, deep, stromal opacities: (1) dendritic or stellate, (2) boomerang, (3) circular or dot, (4) comma, (5) linear, and (6) filiform (Fig. 17-37). The deposits could be axial, peripheral, or diffuse. The type and location of the opacities showed no correlation with age or with the presence or absence of coexisting ocular or systemic disease.

Histopathologic examination of one case of pre-Descemet's dystrophy demonstrated that the pathologic condition was limited to the keratocytes of the posterior stroma.[172] Within the keratocytes were cytoplasmic vacuoles (secondary lysosomes) that contained lipidlike material, which on electron microscopy consisted of fibrillogranular and electron-dense lamellar inclusions. These findings suggest that the accumulated material most likely was lipofuscin, a degenerative "wear and tear" lipoprotein associated with aging.

Similar opacities have been noted in association with other ocular or systemic abnormalities, and these have been called *secondary pre-Descemet's dystrophies*. Pre-Descemet's dystrophy has been reported in association with keratoconus, epithelial basement membrane dystrophy, posterior polymorphous dystrophy, ichthyosis, central cloudy corneal dystrophy, pseudoxanthoma elasticum, and in female carriers of sex-linked ichthyosis.[170,173-175]

ECTATIC DYSTROPHIES

Anterior Keratoconus

The salient feature of anterior keratoconus is the conical shape of the corneal surface (Fig. 17-38). The incidence has been reported to be 2 in 100,000[176] to 230 in 100,000 population. It may be congenital, but is most commonly diagnosed between 10 and 30 years of age. On aver-

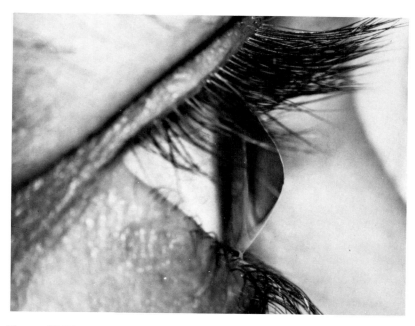

Figure 17-38
Keratoconus.

age it progresses for about 7 to 8 years and then remains stable, but this varies considerably. Progression can be rapid, gradual, or intermittent.

The condition is nearly always bilateral[177] but may be highly asymmetric. Most cases have no familial history of keratoconus, but pedigrees with autosomal dominant and recessive inheritance have been described.[178-180] Photokeratoscopy has shown that apparently unaffected family members have increased central steepening and astigmatism.[181] In familial keratoconus approximately two thirds of affected members have other evidence of connective tissue abnormalities such as syndactyly, Raynaud's phenomenon, and brachydactyly.[182]

Corneal topography analysis, especially computer-assisted videokeratography, is the most sensitive means of diagnosis.[183,184] With photokeratoscopy, the central mires are typically oval, pointing inferonasally, with decreased separation (steepening) of the inferotemporal mires and increased separation (flattening) of the superonasal mires (Fig. 17-39). Most commonly the cone is relatively round and only slightly displaced inferonasally. However, cones can be oval, sagging, small, nipplelike, large, or more peripheral (usually inferior). A central, nipplelike area of ectasia is shown in Figure 17-40.

On computer-assisted videokeratography the majority of patients with keratoconus have peripheral inferior steepening (Fig. 17-41); approximately one fourth have steepening that is confined to the central cornea (Fig. 17-42).[184,185] There is high degree of mirror-image symmetry between the corneas of a patient with keratoconus. While advanced keratoconus is readily identified with these instruments, early forms of the disorder can be difficult to detect. In addition, diagnostic criteria have not been established. It can be difficult to distinguish between early cases of keratoconus, naturally occurring astigmatism, and contact lens–induced corneal warpage. Attempts have been made to determine quantitative characteristics of the topography in keratoconus, which will allow objective differentiation from these other conditions.[186,187] An expert system classifier, based on multiple quantitative topographic indices, was 98% sensitive and 99% specific.[188]

Wearing contact lenses, particularly rigid lenses, can alter the corneal surface, increasing or decreasing curvature and producing regular and irregular astigmatism (corneal warping).[189-191] The cornea usually exhibits relative flattening in the area underneath the lens and steepening elsewhere. Most of the time these changes disappear when the patient stops wearing contact lenses, but in some cases they are permanent.[192] Such corneal warping can appear similar to early keratoconus (Fig. 17-43). In

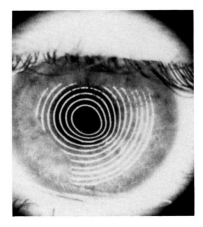

Figure 17-39
Photokeratoscopy in moderate keratoconus demonstrates ovaling of
central mires, with superonasal flattening and inferotemporal steepening.

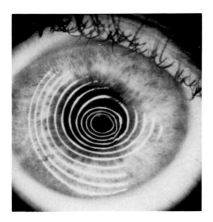

Figure 17-40
Central steep nipplelike cone.

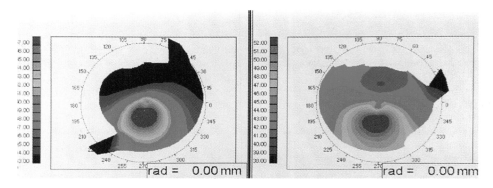

Figure 17-41
Videokeratographs of a patient with bilateral keratoconus, demonstrating inferior corneal steepening.

most cases they can be differentiated, because patients with corneal warping do not have corneal thinning, Descemet's striae, Fleischer rings, or other changes typical of keratoconus. However, in some cases the only way to differentiate is by discontinuing lens wear and obtaining repeated topography measurements. In contact lens–induced corneal warpage, the topography will gradually normalize, although the process can take months.

The conical deformation of the cornea results in a convexity of the lower lid on down gaze, called *Munson's sign.* A *Fleischer ring* is iron deposition in the epithelium around a portion or the entire circumference of the base of the

cone. It is most easily appreciated with oblique cobalt blue illumination (Fig. 17-44). The ring can be useful in determining the size and position of the cone. The cone can also be visualized by retroillumination with the slit-lamp microscope or retinoscope.

The apex of the cornea thins in proportion to the progression of the disease. However, perforation is rare. With ectasia vertical stress lines appear deep in the corneal stroma (*Vogt's striae*) (Fig. 17-45). These lines disappear with gentle pressure on the apex of the cone. Increased visibility of the corneal nerves, posterior crocodile shagreen, and guttae may also be present. Interruptions in Bowman's layer can be seen as clear

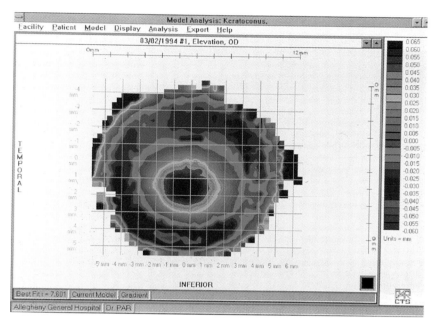

Figure 17-42
Rasterstereography measurement of corneal elevation in a patient with keratoconus. Note the central steepening.

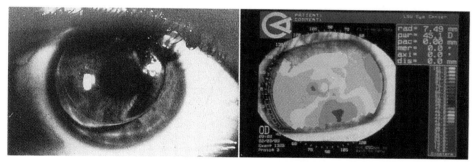

Figure 17-43
Contact lens–induced corneal warpage resembling keratoconus. **Left,** Normal position of a rigid contact lens on the cornea. **Right,** Videokeratograph of the cornea, demonstrating relative flattening of the corneal contour underlying the resting position of the lens and inferior steepening. (From Wilson SE et al: *Ophthalmology* 97:734, 1990.)

spaces in the anterior stroma of the thinned cornea, usually with a vertical orientation.[193] Corneal sensation is reduced, particularly in the inferior cornea.[194] A scissors reflex often is present on retinoscopy.

Fine anterior stromal scars can be seen near the cone apex, caused by ruptures of Bowman's layer. Acute tears in Descemet's membrane can occur in advanced cases, leading to stromal edema in the cone (*corneal hydrops*) (Fig. 17-46).

Hydrops affects approximately 5% of patients with keratoconus.[195] This appears to occur more often in patients with Down syndrome,[196,197] in younger males with advanced corneal ectasia, and in the presence of severe allergic eye disease.[75] It can be precipitated by eye rubbing. The edema can thicken the cornea twofold to threefold but usually resolves in 2 to 3 months, leaving an apical scar (Fig. 17-47). Neovascularization can occur.[198] Sometimes the vision

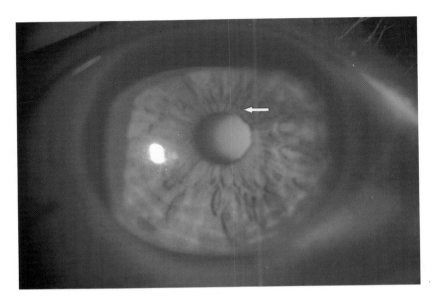

Figure 17-44
Fleischer ring *(arrow).*

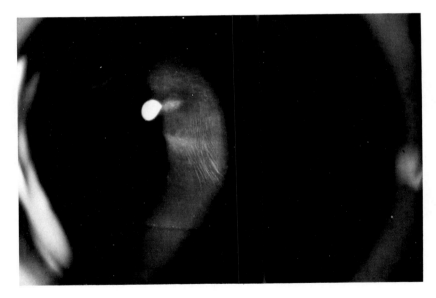

Figure 17-45
Vogt's striae.

is improved or contact lens wear is facilitated by the scarring, as a result of the flattening of the cone, but more often the condition is worsened. A high percentage of these eyes will eventually require keratoplasty.[75]

Associated Conditions
Keratoconus can be associated with a number of conditions (Table 17-6). The association of keratoconus with vernal keratoconjunctivitis,[199,200] atopic dermatitis,[201] and other atopic diseases[202-204] is well documented. The relationship is unclear, but the frequency of their coexistence appears to be significantly greater than expected by chance.[205] Individuals with Down syndrome are significantly more likely to have keratoconus.[194,196,206] Patients with mitral valve prolapse also appear to have a higher incidence

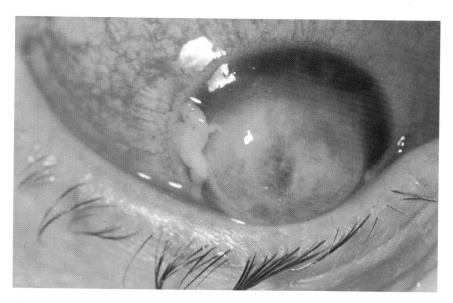

Figure 17-46
Acute corneal hydrops.

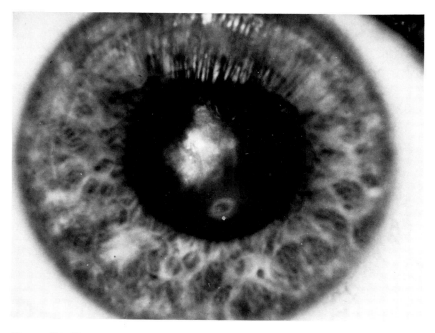

Figure 17-47
Residual scarring from hydrops of the cornea secondary to keratoconus.

of keratoconus.[207] In a series of 50 patients with severe keratoconus, 29 were found to have mitral valve prolapse on echocardiography, compared with 3 of 50 matched controls.[208] Both conditions may result from defects in collagen metabolism.

Histopathology

Fragmentation and fibrillation of Bowman's layer and the epithelial basement membrane are noted in the area of the cone (Fig. 17-48).[209-211] Interruptions of Bowman's layer are common, and scar tissue and activated keratocytes are

Table 17-6	Conditions Associated with Keratoconus

Retinitis pigmentosa
Leber's congenital amaurosis
Ectopia lentis
Congenital cataract
Aniridia
Microcornea
Retinopathy of prematurity
Blue sclera
Vernal keratoconjunctivitis
Atopic dermatitis
Other atopic diseases
Floppy eyelid syndrome[214, 215]
Down syndrome
Mitral valve prolapse[207]
False chordae tendineae
Marfan syndrome
Ehlers-Danlos syndrome
Osteogenesis imperfecta
Apert syndrome
Noonan's syndrome
Crouzon's syndrome
Little disease
Duane's syndrome
Addison's disease
Xeroderma pigmentosa
Laurence-Moon-Bardet-Biedel syndrome

noted in these areas.[212] Electron-dense, PAS-positive material is seen in the stroma and adjacent to the activated keratocytes.[210,211,213] This material is presumed to be an abnormal proteoglycan.

The corneal epithelium may be irregular and thinned over the cone. Fleischer ring is seen as the accumulation of ferritin particles within and between the basal epithelial cells at the base of the cone.[209,216] Corneal hydrops is seen as tears in Descemet's membrane, with extension of adjacent endothelium over the exposed stroma and deposition of new Descemet's material.[217,218]

As the stroma thins, the number of corneal lamellae decreases.[211,219] The diameter of the collagen fibrils increases, as does the interfibrillary distance.[218] However, the hexagonal arrangement of the fibrils is not changed, and the distance does not increase to the point that clarity is lost. The content and distribution of the different collagen types appear to be normal.[220,221]

Biochemical Studies

A variety of biochemical abnormalities have been reported in corneas with keratoconus. Unfortunately, many of these have either not been confirmed or have been contradicted by other studies. Increased reducible collagen cross-

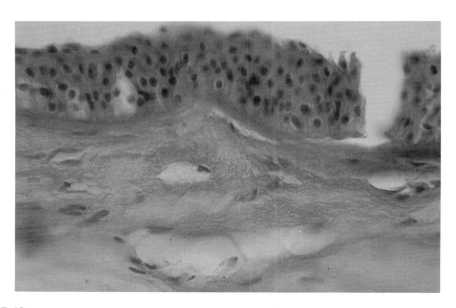

Figure 17-48
Fragmentation and fibrillation of Bowman's layer and basement membrane in keratoconus. (From Grayson M: *Degeneration, dystrophies, and edema of the cornea.* In Duane TD, editor: *Clinical ophthalmology,* vol 4, Hagerstown, MD, 1978, Harper & Row, Publishers. Used with permission of Lippincott-Raven Publishers.)

linking was found in one study,[222] but this was not confirmed in others.[223] In tissue culture, keratocytes from some keratoconus corneas were found to have defects in RNA translation, leading to reduced protein synthesis, but keratocytes from other corneas exhibited normal protein synthesis.[224,225] Collagenolytic activity has been consistently reported to be higher than normal.[219,226,227] The increased collagenolytic activity appears to be related to a decrease in the amount of tissue metalloproteinase inhibitor, rather than an abnormality in the amount of metalloproteinase.[228-230] The levels of lysosomal acid hydrolases were found to be higher in the corneal[231] and conjunctival[232] epithelium of keratoconus patients.

Several studies have suggested that an abnormality in proteoglycans is present. Keratocyte proteoglycan metabolism was found to be abnormal,[233,234] and abnormalities were found in the glycoproteins on the surface of the keratocytes.[235] Total proteoglycan content was found to be increased,[236] and there is a reduction in the amount of highly sulfated keratan sulfate epitopes.[237] Proteoglycan location, in relation to collagen fibrils, was found to be abnormal by electron histochemistry and x-ray diffraction.[238] The interaction between the collagen fibrils and proteoglycans may be important in maintaining normal corneal strength. Therefore, these abnormalities could result in stretching and thinning of the stroma.[239]

Pathogenesis

In view of the diversity of biochemical findings in keratoconus, it has been proposed that keratoconus can be caused by more than one mechanism.[238,240] Collagen may be defective in some patients; for instance, in Ehlers-Danlos syndrome type VI, in which keratoconus can occur, collagen cross-linking is deficient. Supporting this mechanism are studies that show abnormal collagen synthesis by keratocytes, abnormal cross-linking, and increased collagenolytic activity. Other studies have suggested that proteoglycan abnormalities are responsible in some patients.

Wearing hard contact lenses has also been proposed as a cause for keratoconus. Many patients who wear hard contact lenses have developed keratoconus,[241-243] and a relatively high percentage of patients diagnosed as having keratoconus had worn hard contact lenses in the past.[244,245] Certainly, wearing contact lenses, particularly rigid lenses, can cause corneal curvature alterations, which sometimes resemble keratoconus (see above). Most of the time these changes disappear when the patient stops wearing contact lenses, but in some cases they are permanent.[192] Whether the full-blown clinical picture of keratoconus can be induced by wearing contact lenses remains to be determined.

Rubbing the eyes has also been suggested as a cause of keratoconus. The evidence in favor of this is limited; many patients with atopy, Down syndrome, and Leber's tapetoretinal degeneration, which often are associated with keratoconus, rub their eyes excessively.[246-248] Also, in a few cases an initially normal cornea developed keratoconus after intensive massage.[249-251]

Treatment

When eyeglasses are no longer sufficient to correct vision, contact lenses are indicated. Most patients with keratoconus can be fitted successfully with lenses, although it often entails a great deal of time, patience, and trial and error.[252-254] A number of authors have described fitting techniques.[255,256] In some cases this requires use of double posterior curve lenses (Soper),[255] combined soft and hard (piggyback) lenses, or a hard lens with a soft peripheral skirt (e.g., Softperm, Sola/Barnes-Hind, Sunnyvale, CA).

If scarring prevents adequate vision or if the patient cannot wear contact lenses, keratoplasty can be performed. Overall there is a 10% to 20% probability of a patient with keratoconus eventually requiring keratoplasty.[176,257] The risk of progressing to keratoplasty is related to steeper maximum and minimum corneal keratometry, the presence of a corneal cylinder of more than 1.9 mm, reduced best-corrected acuity, younger age (less than 18 years) at presentation, and race (West Indians more than Africans more than Asians more than whites).[84,258,259] The prognosis for a clear graft and visual acuity of 20/40 or better is better than 80%.[260-263] The average astigmatism after surgery is greater than in other keratoplasty patients (approximately 4 to 5 Ds), and one fourth to one fifth of patients will have greater than 6 Ds of astigmatism.[176] Approximately 60% of patients will require contact lens fitting after keratoplasty for correction of myopia, astigmatism, or both.[253] Unfortunately, contact lens wear is associated with endothelial cell injury[264] and probably with an increased risk of infection and rejection. Recurrence of keratoconus in the graft has been reported but is rare.[265,266]

Permanent mydriasis can occur after keratoplasty (Urrets-Zavalia syndrome).[267] The mechanism is unknown, but use of strong mydriatics and iris ischemia caused by pressure of the corneal wound against the iris[268] have been implicated.

Lamellar keratoplasty can also be of value, but it is more difficult and the visual results are not quite as good.[269-271] Still, it may be useful, particularly in patients who cannot cooperate well with postoperative care (e.g., in cases involving Down syndrome or very large or peripheral cones).

Epikeratophakia for keratoconus is a form of onlay lamellar keratoplasty. A lamellar graft lathed to a uniform thickness of 0.3 mm is sutured on top of the cornea to flatten the cone.[272] Only patients without central corneal scarring are candidates. An average of 9 Ds of corneal flattening is obtained, and approximately 80% of patients obtain 20/40 vision or better.[273-275] The rate of visual recovery varies widely but appears to be similar to that after penetrating keratoplasty. If necessary, penetrating keratoplasty can be performed after epikeratophakia, and the results appear similar to those in virgin eyes.[276] The main advantages of epikeratophakia are that it is an extraocular procedure, there is no risk of rejection, and it is technically simpler than lamellar keratoplasty. In general the reported results have been good, but postoperative visual acuity is often not as good as after successful penetrating keratoplasty, and few surgeons perform the procedure today.

Thermokeratoplasty has been used with limited success. Heat is applied to the corneal stroma, shrinking the collagen and flattening the cone.[277,278] The visual results were disappointing, and many complications occurred, including persistent epithelial defects, stromal scarring, instability of the corneal curvature, and aseptic corneal necrosis.[276,279,280]

Elevated apical scars, also called *proud nebulae*, can decrease both contact lens tolerance and vision. In some cases superficial keratectomy will restore the ability to wear a contact lens.[281] This procedure can be performed with an excimer laser.[282,283]

Acute hydrops should be treated conservatively, and the patient should be assured that the condition nearly always improves. Some scarring usually remains, but in some cases the cornea is flattened, and contact lens wear is facilitated. Cycloplegia and hypertonic solutions or ointments may provide some symptomatic relief. The condition usually resolves in 8 to 10 weeks, but some cases take 6 months or more, whereas others never clear. If the condition is not improving after 3 months, keratoplasty is indicated.

Keratoglobus

Keratoglobus is a rare, bilateral, globular corneal ectasia. The stroma is diffusely thinned to one third to one fifth of normal thickness and is often thinnest in the periphery (Figs. 17-49 and 17-50). The cornea is transparent, and its diameter is normal. Intraocular pressure is normal. The corneal ectasia can lead to high myopia and astigmatism (Fig. 17-51). Acute hydrops can occur,[284] and perforation after minimal trauma has occurred in most reported cases.[285-287] Associated ocular conditions include blue sclera, vernal keratoconjunctivitis, and orbital pseudotumor.[288] Pathologic examination has demonstrated focal breaks in or absence of Bowman's layer and stromal thinning to one third to one fifth of normal thickness.[286]

Keratoglobus can be associated with Leber's congenital amaurosis, hyperextensibility of the joints of the hand and ankles, sensorineural hearing defects, and mottling of the teeth (Fig. 17-52).[284-286] Keratoconus and keratoglobus have been observed in different members of the same family; in one family the father had keratoglobus and a son had keratoconus,[289] and in another family a brother had keratoglobus and a sister had keratoconus.[290] Treatment options are limited and not very successful.[288] Contact lens wear is not recommended because of the risk of perforation, but it usually is not possible anyway. Total keratoplasty can be performed, but the sclera is often thin as well, making closure difficult. If surgery is necessary, onlay lamellar keratoplasty (i.e., epikeratophakia) may be preferable.[291] A penetrating graft can be performed later into the thickened bed.

Differential Diagnosis

It is important to differentiate among keratoglobus, keratectasia, and congenital anterior staphyloma. In keratectasia the cornea is bulging, protrudes through the lids, and is opaque, with variable thinning and scarring of the stroma. It usually occurs unilaterally. If the ectatic cornea also contains uveal tissue, the condition is called *congenital anterior staphyloma*. Megalocornea may appear similar to keratoglobus, but the corneal diameter is normal in keratoglobus. The normal diameter and normal intraocular pressure differentiate keratoglobus from congenital glaucoma.

Posterior Keratoconus

Posterior keratoconus is a rare condition characterized by a focal or generalized increase in the curvature of the posterior corneal surface, with normal curvature of the anterior surface. It is more commonly unilateral then bilateral. The

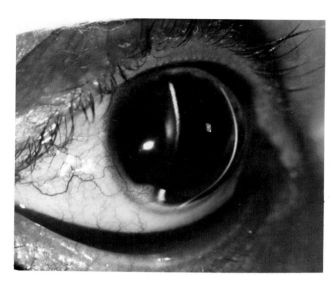

Figure 17-49
Diffusely thin and ectatic cornea in keratoglobus.

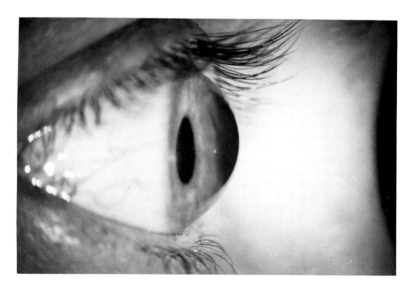

Figure 17-50
Globular cornea in keratoglobus.

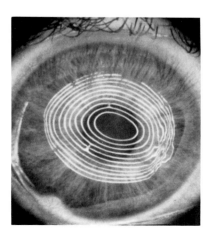

Figure 17-51
Marked astigmatism in keratoglobus.

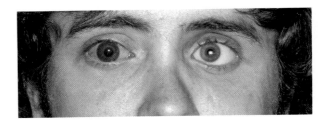

Figure 17-52
Individual with keratoglobus, blue sclera (right eye), and hyperextensible joints. The left eye was enucleated as a result of rupture after minor trauma.

condition is usually present at birth and is non-progressive. It most likely is a form of dysgenesis and thus is discussed in Chapter 5.

Pellucid Marginal Degeneration
Pellucid marginal degeneration is characterized by noninflammatory inferior corneal thinning and ectasia. Some feel that it is a variant of keratoconus. Pellucid marginal degeneration is discussed in Chapter 16.

REFERENCES

1. Meesmann A, Wilke F: Klinische und Anatom-ische Untersuchungen ber eine Bisher Unbe-kannte, Dominant Vererbte Epitheldystrophie der Hornhaut, *Klin Monatsbl Augenheilkd* 103:361, 1939.
2. Kuwabara R, Ciccarelli EC: Meesmann's cor-neal dystrophy, *Arch Ophthalmol* 71:676, 1964.
3. Stocker FW, Holt LB: Rare form of hereditary epithelial dystrophy, *Arch Ophthalmol* 53:536, 1955.
4. Snyder WB: Hereditary epithelial corneal dys-trophy, *Am J Ophthalmol* 55:56, 1963.
5. Wittebol-Post D, van Bijsterveld OP, Delleman JW: Meesmann's epithelial dystrophy of the cornea: biometrics and a hypothesis, *Ophthal-mologica* 194:44, 1987.
6. Tripathi RG, Bron AJ: Cystic disorders of the corneal epithelium: II. Pathogenesis, *Br J Oph-thalmol* 57:375, 1973.
7. Cogan DG et al: Microcystic dystrophy of the corneal epithelium, *Trans Am Ophthalmol Soc* 62:213, 1964.
8. Burns RP: Meesmann's corneal dystrophy, *Trans Am Ophthalmol Soc* 66:531, 1968.
9. Nakaniski I, Brown SI: Ultrastructure of epithe-lial dystrophy of Meesmann, *Arch Ophthalmol* 93:259, 1975.
10. Bourne WM: Soft contact lens wear decreases epithelial microcysts in Meesmann's corneal dystrophy, *Trans Am Ophthalmol Soc* 84:170, 1986.
11. Cogan DG et al: Microcystic dystrophy of the cornea, *Arch Ophthalmol* 92:470, 1974.
12. Trobe JD, Laibson PR: Dystrophic changes in the anterior cornea, *Arch Ophthalmol* 87:378, 1972.
13. Wolter JR, Fralick FB: Microcystic dystrophy of the corneal epithelium, *Arch Ophthalmol* 75:380, 1966.
14. Laibson PR, Krachmer JH: Familial occurrence of dot, map, and fingerprint dystrophy of the cornea, *Invest Ophthalmol* 14:397, 1975.
15. Bron AJ, Burgess SEP: Inherited recurrent cor-neal erosion, *Trans Ophthalmol Soc UK* 101:239, 1981.
16. Bron AJ, Tripathi RC: Anterior corneal mosaic: further observations, *Br J Ophthalmol* 53:760, 1969.
17. Waring GO, Rodriquez MM, Laibson PR: Cor-neal dystrophies: I. Dystrophies of the epithe-lium, Bowman's layer, and stroma, *Surv Oph-thalmol* 23:71, 1978.
18. Brown NA, Bron AJ: Recurrent erosion of the cornea, *Br J Ophthalmol* 60:84, 1976.
19. Nelson JD et al: Map-dot-fingerprint changes in the corneal epithelial basement membrane following radial keratotomy, *Ophthalmology* 92:199, 1985.
20. Polack FM: Contributions of electron micros-copy to the study of corneal pathology, *Surv Ophthalmol* 20:375, 1976.
21. Broderick JD, Dark AJ, Peace GW: Fingerprint dystrophy of the cornea, *Arch Ophthalmol* 92:483, 1974.
22. Dark AJ: Bleb dystrophy of the cornea: histo-chemistry and ultrastructure, *Br J Ophthalmol* 61:65, 1977.
23. Reis W: Familiäre, Fleckige Hornhautentartung, *Dtsch Med Wochenschr* 43:575, 1917.
24. Bücklers M: Ueber eine Weitere Familiäre Horn-hautdystrophie (Reis), *Klin Monatsbl Augen-heilkd* 114:386, 1949.
25. Rice NSC et al: Reis-Bücklers' dystrophy, *Br J Ophthalmol* 52:577, 1968.
26. Jones ST, Stauffer LH: Reis-Bücklers' corneal dystrophy, *Trans Am Acad Ophthalmol Otolaryn-gol* 74:417, 1970.
27. Hall P: Reis-Bücklers' dystrophy, *Arch Ophthal-mol* 91:170, 1974.
28. Wittebol-Post D, van Bijsterveld OP, Delleman JM: The honeycomb type of Reis-Bücklers' dys-

trophy of the cornea: biometrics and interpretation, *Ophthalmologica* 194:65, 1987.

29. Griffith DG, Fine BS: Light and electron microscopic observations in a superficial corneal dystrophy, *Am J Ophthalmol* 63:1659, 1967.

30. Hogan M, Wood I: Reis-Bücklers' corneal dystrophy, *Trans Ophthalmol Soc UK* 91:41, 1971.

31. Kanai A, Kaufman HE, Polack FM: Electron microscopic study of Reis-Bücklers' dystrophy, *Ann Ophthalmol* 5:953, 1973.

32. Olson RJ, Kaufman HE: Recurrence of Reis-Bücklers' corneal dystrophy in a graft, *Am J Ophthalmol* 85:349, 1978.

33. Caldwell DR: Postoperative recurrence of Reis-Bücklers' corneal dystrophy, *Am J Ophthalmol* 85:567, 1978.

34. Wood TO et al: Treatment of Reis-Bücklers' corneal dystrophy by removal of subepithelial fibrous tissue, *Am J Ophthalmol* 85:360, 1978.

35. Schwartz MF, Taylor HR: Surgical management of Reis-Bücklers' corneal dystrophy, *Cornea* 4:100, 1985.

36. McDonnell PJ, Seiler T: Phototherapeutic keratectomy with excimer laser for Reis-Bücklers' corneal dystrophy, *Refract Corneal Surg* 8:306, 1992.

37. Rogers C, Cohen P, Lawless M: Phototherapeutic keratectomy for Reis-Bücklers' corneal dystrophy, *Aust N Z J Ophthalmol* 21:247, 1993.

38. Grayson M, Wilbrandt H: Dystrophy of the anterior limiting membrane of the cornea (Reis-Bücklers' type), *Am J Ophthalmol* 63:345, 1966.

39. Thiel HJ, Behnke H: Eine Bisher Unbekannte Subepitheliale Hereditäre Hornhautdystrophie, *Klin Monatsbl Augenheilkd* 150:862, 1967.

40. Yamaguchi T, Polack FM, Rowsey JJ: Honeycomb-shaped corneal dystrophy: a variation of Reis-Bücklers' dystrophy, *Cornea* 1:71, 1982.

41. Feder RS et al: Subepithelial mucinous corneal dystrophy: clinical and pathological correlations, *Arch Ophthalmol* 111:1106, 1993.

42. Chan CC et al: Anterior corneal dystrophy with dyscollagenosis (Reis-Bücklers type?), *Cornea* 12:451, 1993.

43. Duke-Elder S, Leigh AG: *System of ophthalmology*, vol 8, *Diseases of the outer eye*, St Louis, 1965, Mosby–Year Book.

44. Meisler DM et al: Familial band-shaped nodular keratopathy, *Ophthalmology* 92:217, 1985.

45. Francois J: Dystrophie dermo-chondro-cornéenne familiale, *Ann Oculist* 182:409, 1949.

46. Caputo R et al: Dermochondrocorneal dystrophy (Francois' syndrome): report of a case, *Arch Dermatol* 124:424, 1988.

47. Bierly JR, George SP, Volpicelli M: Dermochondral corneal dystrophy (of Francois), *Br J Ophthalmol* 76:760, 1992.

48. Rodrigues MM, Calhoun J, Harley RD: Corneal clouding with increased acid mucopolysaccharide accumulation in Bowman's membrane, *Am J Ophthalmol* 79:916, 1975.

49. Eiberg H et al: Assignment of granular corneal dystrophy Groenouw type I (CDGG1) to chromosome 5q, *Eur J Hum Genet* 2:132, 1994.

50. Stone EM et al: Three autosomal dominant corneal dystrophies map to chromosome 5q, *Nat Genet* 6:47, 1994.

51. Ruusuvaara P, Setala K, Tarkkanen A: Granular corneal dystrophy with early stromal manifestation: a clinical and electron microscopical study, *Acta Ophthalmol (Copenh)* 68:525, 1990.

52. Haddad R, Font RL, Fine BS: Unusual superficial variant of granular dystrophy of the cornea, *Am J Ophthalmol* 83:213, 1977.

53. Rodrigues MM, Gaster RN, Pratt MV: Unusual superficial confluent form of granular corneal dystrophy, *Ophthalmology* 90:1507, 1983.

54. Sajjadi SH, Javadi MA: Superficial juvenile granular dystrophy, *Ophthalmology* 99:95, 1992.

55. Forsius H et al: Granular corneal dystrophy with late manifestation, *Acta Ophthalmol (Copenh)* 61:514, 1983.

56. Jones ST, Zimmerman LE: Histopathologic differentiation of granular, macular, and lattice dystrophies of the cornea, *Am J Ophthalmol* 51:394, 1961.

57. Garner A: Histochemistry of corneal macular dystrophy, *Invest Ophthalmol* 8:473, 1969.

58. Iwamoto T et al: Ultrastructural variations in granular dystrophy of the cornea, *Graefes Arch Clin Exp Ophthalmol* 194:1, 1975.

59. Smith ME, Zimmerman LE: Amyloid in corneal dystrophies: differentiation of lattice from granular and macular dystrophies, *Arch Ophthalmol* 79:407, 1968.

60. Sornson E: Granular dystrophy of the cornea: an electron microscopic study, *Am J Ophthalmol* 59:1001, 1965.

61. Wittebol-Post D, van der Want JJ, van Bijsterveld OP: Granular dystrophy of the cornea (Groenouw type I): is the keratocyte the primary source after all?, *Ophthalmologica* 195:169, 1987.

62. Garner A: Histochemistry of corneal granular dystrophy, *Br J Ophthalmol* 53:799, 1969.

63. Rodrigues MM et al: Microfibrillar protein and phospholipid in granular corneal dystrophy, *Arch Ophthalmol* 101:802, 1983.

64. Moller HW et al: Immunoglobulins in granular corneal dystrophy Groenouw type I, *Acta Ophthalmol (Copenh)* 71:548, 1993.

65. Johnson BL, Brown SI, Zaidman GW: A light and electron microscopic study of recurrent granular dystrophy of the cornea, *Am J Ophthalmol* 92:49, 1981.

66. Moller HU, Ehlers N: Early treatment of granular dystrophy (Groenouw type I), *Acta Ophthalmol (Copenh)* 63:597, 1985.

67. Hahn TW, Sah WJ, Kim JH: Phototherapeutic keratectomy in nine eyes with superficial corneal diseases, *Refract Corneal Surg* 9(suppl):S115, 1993.

68. Binder PS et al: Human excimer laser keratectomy: clinical and histopathologic correlations, *Ophthalmology* 101:979, 1994.

69. Brownstein S et al: Granular dystrophy of the

cornea: electron microscopic confirmation of recurrence in a graft, *Am J Ophthalmol* 77:701, 1974.

70. Herman SJ, Hughes WF: Recurrence of hereditary corneal dystrophy following keratoplasty, *Am J Ophthalmol* 75:689, 1973.
71. Rodrigues MM, McGavic JS: Recurrent corneal granular dystrophy: a clinicopathologic study, *Trans Am Ophthalmol Soc* 73:306, 1975.
72. Stuart JC, Mund ML: Recurrent granular corneal dystrophy, *Am J Ophthalmol* 79:18, 1975.
73. Lyons CJ et al: Granular corneal dystrophy: visual results and pattern of recurrence after lamellar or penetrating keratoplasty, *Ophthalmology* 101:1812, 1994.
74. Lempert SL et al: A simple technique for removal of recurring granular dystrophy in corneal grafts, *Am J Ophthalmol* 86:89, 1978.
75. John ME et al: Photorefractive keratectomy following penetrating keratoplasty, *J Refract Corneal Surg* 10(suppl):S206, 1994.
76. Klintworth GK: Lattice corneal dystrophy: an inherited variety of amyloidosis restricted to the cornea, *Am J Pathol* 50:371, 1967.
77. Rabb MR, Blodi F, Boniuk M: Unilateral lattice dystrophy of the cornea, *Trans Am Acad Ophthalmol Otolaryngol* 78:440, 1974.
78. Mehta RF: Unilateral lattice dystrophy of the cornea, *Br J Ophthalmol* 64:53, 1980.
79. Stansbury FC: Lattice type of hereditary corneal degeneration: report of five cases, including one of a child of two years, *Arch Ophthalmol* 40:189, 1974.
80. Dubord PF, Krachmer JH: Diagnosis of early lattice corneal dystrophy, *Arch Ophthalmol* 100:788, 1982.
81. Meretoja J: Familial systemic paramyloidosis with lattice dystrophy of the cornea, progressive cranial neuropathy, skin changes and various internal symptoms: a previously unrecognized heritable syndrome, *Ann Clin Res* 1:314, 1969.
82. Meretoja J: Comparative histopathological and clinical findings in eyes with lattice corneal dystrophy of two types, *Ophthalmologica* 165:15, 1972.
83. Purcell JJ et al: Lattice corneal dystrophy associated with familial systemic amyloidosis (Meretoja's syndrome), *Ophthalmology* 90:1512, 1983.
84. Kiuru S: Familial amyloidosis of the Finnish type (FAF): a clinical study of 30 patients, *Acta Neurol Scand* 86:346, 1992.
85. Hida T et al: Clinical features of a newly recognized type of lattice corneal dystrophy, *Am J Ophthalmol* 104:241, 1987.
86. Hida T et al: Histopathologic and immunochemical features of lattice corneal dystrophy type III, *Am J Ophthalmol* 104:249, 1987.
87. Kani A et al: Clinical and histopathological studies of the lattice dystrophy of the cornea, *Act Soc Ophthalmol Jpn* 17:357, 1973.
88. Zechner EM, Croxatto JO, Malbran ES: Superfi-

cial involvement in lattice corneal dystrophy, *Ophthalmologica* 193:193, 1986.
89. François J, Fehér J: Light microscopical and polarization optical study of lattice dystrophy of the cornea, *Ophthalmologica* 164:1, 1972.
90. Hogan M, Alvarado S: Ultrastructure of lattice dystrophy of the cornea: a case report, *Am J Ophthalmol* 64:656, 1967.
91. Bowen RA et al: Lattice dystrophy of the cornea as a variety of amyloidosis, *Am J Ophthalmol* 7:822, 1970.
92. Yanoff M et al: Lattice corneal dystrophy: report of an unusual case, *Arch Ophthalmol* 95:651, 1977.
93. McTigue J: The human cornea: a light and electron microscopic study of the normal cornea and its alterations in various dystrophies, *Trans Am Acad Ophthalmol Otolaryngol* 65:591, 1968.
94. François J, Hanssens M, Teuchy H: Ultrastructural changes in lattice dystrophy of the cornea, *Ophthalmic Res* 7:321, 1975.
95. McTigue JW, Fine BS: The stromal lesion in lattice dystrophy of the cornea: a light and electron microscopic study, *Invest Ophthalmol* 3:355, 1964.
96. Sipe JD: Amyloidosis, *Annu Rev Biochem* 61:947, 1992.
97. Kivela T et al: Immunohistochemical analysis of lattice corneal dystrophies type I and II, *Br J Ophthalmol* 77:799, 1993.
98. Starck T et al: Clinical and histopathologic studies of two families with lattice corneal dystrophy and familial systemic amyloidosis (Meretoja's syndrome), *Ophthalmology* 98:1197, 1991.
99. Gorevic PD et al: Amyloidosis due to a mutation of the gelsolin gene in an American family with lattice corneal dystrophy type II, *N Engl J Med* 325:1780, 1991.
100. Sunada Y et al: Inherited amyloid polyneuropathy type IV (gelsolin variant) in a Japanese family, *Ann Neurol* 33:57, 1993.
101. Maury CP: Gelsolin-related amyloidosis: identification of the amyloid protein in Finnish hereditary amyloidosis as a fragment of variant gelsolin, *J Clin Invest* 87:1195, 1991.
102. Kivela T et al: Ocular amyloid deposition in familial amyloidosis, Finnish: an analysis of native and variant gelsolin in Meretoja's syndrome, *Invest Ophthalmol Vis Sci* 35:3759, 1994.
103. Wiens A et al: Exclusion of the gelsolin gene on 9q32-34 as the cause of familial lattice corneal dystrophy type I, *Am J Hum Genet* 51:156, 1992.
104. Lorenzetti DWC, Kaufman HE: Macular lattice dystrophies and their recurrences after keratoplasty, *Trans Am Acad Ophthalmol Otolaryngol* 71:112, 1967.
105. Meisler DM, Fine M: Recurrence of the clinical signs of lattice corneal dystrophy (type I) in corneal transplants, *Am J Ophthalmol* 97:210, 1984.
106. Akiya S, Ito I, Matsui M: Gelatinous drop-like

dystrophy of the cornea, *Jpn J Clin Ophthalmol* 26:815, 1972.

107. Nagataki S, Tanishima T, Sakomoto T: A case of primary gelatinous drop-like corneal dystrophy, *Jpn J Ophthalmol* 16:107, 1972.

108. Weber FL, Babel J: Gelatinous drop-like dystrophy, *Arch Ophthalmol* 98:144, 1980.

109. Gartry DS, Falcon MG, Cox RW: Primary gelatinous drop-like keratopathy, *Br J Ophthalmol* 73:661, 1989.

110. Ramsey MS, Fine BS: Localized corneal amyloidosis, *Am J Ophthalmol* 75:560, 1972.

111. Kanai A, Kaufman HE: Electron microscopic studies of primary band-shaped keratopathy and gelatinous drop-like corneal dystrophy in two brothers, *Ann Ophthalmol* 14:535, 1982.

112. Shimazaki J et al: Long-term follow-up of patients with familial subepithelial amyloidosis of the cornea, *Ophthalmology* 102:139, 1995.

113. Sugar J: Castroviejo Cornea Society Meeting, Atlanta, October, 1995.

114. Folberg R et al: Clinically atypical granular corneal dystrophy with pathologic features of lattice-like amyloid deposits: a study of three families, *Ophthalmology* 95:46, 1988.

115. Holland EF et al: Avellino corneal dystrophy: clinical manifestations and natural history, *Ophthalmology* 99:1564, 1992.

116. Rosenwasser GOD et al: Phenotypic variation in combined granular-lattice (Avellino) corneal dystrophy, *Arch Ophthalmol* 111:1546, 1993.

117. Folberg R et al: The relationship between granular, lattice type I and Avellino corneal dystrophies: a histopathologic study, *Arch Ophthalmol* 112:1080, 1994.

118. Cennamo G et al: Phototherapeutic keratectomy in the treatment of Avellino dystrophy, *Ophthalmologica* 208:198, 1994.

119. Donnenfeld ED et al: Corneal thinning in macular corneal dystrophy, *Am J Ophthalmol* 101:112, 1986.

120. Snip RC, Kenyon KR, Green RD: Macular corneal dystrophy: ultrastructural pathology of the corneal endothelium and Descemet's membrane, *Invest Ophthalmol* 12:88, 1973.

121. Klintworth GK, Vogel FS: Macular corneal dystrophy: an inherited acid mucopolysaccharide storage disease of corneal fibroblasts, *Am J Pathol* 45:565, 1964.

122. Klintworth GK, Smith CF: Abnormalities of proteoglycans and glycoproteins synthesized by corneal organ cultures derived from patients with macular corneal dystrophy, *Lab Invest* 48:603, 1983.

123. Hassell JR et al: Macular corneal dystrophy: failure to synthesize a mature keratan sulfate proteoglycan, *Proc Natl Acad Sci USA* 77:3705, 1980.

124. Midura RJ et al: Proteoglycan biosynthesis by human corneas from patients with types 1 and 2 macular corneal dystrophy, *J Biol Chem* 265:15947, 1990.

125. Yang CJ et al: Immunohistochemical evidence

of heterogeneity in macular corneal dystrophy, *Am J Ophthalmol* 106:65, 1988.

126. Edward DP et al: Heterogeneity in macular corneal dystrophy, *Arch Ophthalmol* 106:1579, 1988.

127. Thonar EJ et al: Absence of normal keratan sulfate in the blood of patients with macular corneal dystrophy, *Am J Ophthalmol* 102:561, 1986.

128. Edward DP et al: Macular dystrophy of the cornea: a systemic disorder of keratan sulfate metabolism, *Ophthalmology* 97:1194, 1990.

129. Klintworth GK et al: Recurrence of macular corneal dystrophy within grafts, *Am J Ophthalmol* 95:60, 1983.

130. Akova YA et al: Recurrent macular corneal dystrophy following penetrating keratoplasty, *Eye* 4:698, 1990.

131. Streeten BW, Falls HF: Hereditary fleck dystrophy of the cornea, *Am J Ophthalmol* 51:275, 1961.

132. Birndoft LA, Ginsberg SP: Hereditary fleck dystrophy associated with decreased corneal sensitivity, *Am J Ophthalmol* 73:670, 1972.

133. Aracena T: Hereditary fleck dystrophy of the cornea: report of a family, *J Pediatr Ophthalmol* 12:223, 1975.

134. Purcell JJ Jr, Krachmer JH, Weingeist TA: Fleck corneal dystrophy, *Arch Ophthalmol* 95:440, 1977.

135. Gillespie F, Covelli B: Fleck (Mouchetée) dystrophy of the cornea: report of a family, *South Med J* 56:1265, 1963.

136. Nicholson DH, Green WR, Cross HE: A clinical and histopathological study of François-Neetens speckled corneal dystrophy, *Am J Ophthalmol* 83:554, 1977.

137. Kiskaddon BM et al: Fleck dystrophy of the cornea: case report, *Ann Ophthalmol* 12:700, 1980.

138. Luxenburg M: Hereditary crystalline dystrophy of the cornea, *Am J Ophthalmol* 63:507, 1967.

139. Kaseras A, Price A: Central crystalline corneal dystrophy, *Br J Ophthalmol* 54:659, 1970.

140. Bron AJ, Williams HP, Carruthers ME: Hereditary crystalline stromal dystrophy of Schnyder: clinical features of a family with hyperlipoproteinemia, *Br J Ophthalmol* 56:383, 1972.

141. Grop K: Clinical and histologic findings in crystalline corneal dystrophy, *Acta Ophthalmol (Copenh)* 51(suppl 120):52, 1973.

142. Delleman JW, Winkelman JE: Degeneratio corneae cristallinea hereditaria: a clinical, genetical, and histological study, *Ophthalmologica* 155:409, 1968.

143. Ingraham HJ et al: Progressive Schnyder's corneal dystrophy, *Ophthalmology* 100:1824, 1993.

144. Weiss JS: Schnyder's crystalline dystrophy sine crystals: recommendations for a revision of nomenclature. Paper presented at the meeting of the Castroviejo Cornea Society, Atlanta, October, 1995.

145. Fry WE, Pickett WE: Crystalline dystrophy of

the cornea, *Trans Am Ophthalmol Soc* 48:220, 1950.

146. Weller RO, Rodger FC: Crystalline stromal dystrophy: histochemistry and ultrastructure of the cornea, *Br J Ophthalmol* 64:46, 1980.

147. Rodrigues MM et al: Unesterified cholesterol in Schnyder's corneal crystalline dystrophy, *Am J Ophthalmol* 104:157, 1987.

148. McCarthy M et al: Panstromal Schnyder corneal dystrophy: a clinical pathologic report with quantitative analysis of corneal lipid composition, *Ophthalmology* 101:895, 1994.

149. Freddo TF, Polack FM, Leibowitz HM: Ultrastructural changes in the posterior layers of the cornea in Schnyder's crystalline dystrophy, *Cornea* 8:170, 1989.

150. Weiss JS et al: Panstromal Schnyder's corneal dystrophy. Ultrastructural and histochemical studies, *Ophthalmology* 99:1072, 1992.

151. Ghosh M, McCulloch C: Crystalline dystrophy of the cornea: a light and electron microscopic study, *Can J Ophthalmol* 12:321, 1977.

152. Burns RP, Connor W, Gipson I: Cholesterol turnover in hereditary crystalline corneal dystrophy of Schnyder, *Trans Am Ophthalmol Soc* 76:184, 1978.

153. Bagolini B, Ioli-Spada G: Bietti's tapetoretinal degeneration with marginal corneal dystrophy, *Am J Ophthalmol* 65:53, 1968.

154. Harrison RJ, Acheson RR, Dean-Hart JC: Bietti's tapetoretinal degeneration with marginal corneal dystrophy (crystalline retinopathy): case report, *Br J Ophthalmol* 71:220, 1987.

155. Wilson DJ et al: Bietti's crystalline dystrophy: a clinicopathologic correlative study, *Arch Ophthalmol* 107:213, 1989.

156. Bernauer W, Daicker B: Bietti's corneal-retinal dystrophy: a 16-year progression, *Retina* 12:18, 1992.

157. Strachan IM: Central cloudy corneal dystrophy of François: five cases in the same family, *Br J Ophthalmol* 53:192, 1969.

158. Bramsen T, Ehlers N, Baggesen KH: Central cloudy corneal dystrophy of François, *Acta Ophthalmol (Copenh)* 54:221, 1976.

159. Collier MT: Dystrophie moucheté du parenchyme cornéen avec dystrophie nuageuse centrale, *Bull Soc Ophthalmol Fr* 64:608, 1964.

160. Pillat A: Zur frage der familiúaren Hornhautentartung: ueber eine einzigartige tiefe scholige und periphere gitterförmige familíe Hornhautdystrophie, *Klin Monatsbl Augenheilkd* 104:571, 1939.

161. Strachan IM: Pre-Descemetic corneal dystrophy, *Br J Ophthalmol* 52:716, 1968.

162. Thomsitt J, Bron AJ: Polymorphic stromal dystrophy, *Br J Ophthalmol* 59:125, 1975.

163. Mannis MJ et al: Polymorphic amyloid degeneration of the cornea, *Arch Ophthalmol* 99:1217, 1981.

164. Carpel EF, Sigelman RJ, Doughman DJ: Posterior amorphous corneal dystrophy, *Am J Ophthalmol* 83:629, 1977.

165. Dunn SP, Krachmer JH, Ching SS: New findings in posterior amorphous dystrophy, *Arch Ophthalmol* 102:236, 1984.

166. Grimm BB, Waring GO III, Grimm SB: Posterior amorphous corneal dysgenesis, *Am J Ophthalmol* 120:448, 1995.

167. Johnson AT et al: The pathology of posterior amorphous corneal dystrophy, *Ophthalmology* 97:104, 1990.

168. Roth SI, Mittelman D, Stack EL: Posterior amorphous corneal dystrophy: an ultrastructural study of a variant with histopathological features of an endothelial dystrophy, *Cornea* 11:165, 1992.

169. Collier M: Dystrophie nuageuse centrale et dystrophie ponctiforme prédescemétique, *Bull Soc Ophthalmol Fr* 64:1034, 1964.

170. Fernandez-Sasso D, Acosta JEP, Malbran E: Punctiform and polychromatic pre-Descemet's dominant corneal dystrophy, *Br J Ophthalmol* 63:336, 1979.

171. Grayson M, Wilbrandt H: Pre-Descemet dystrophy, *Am J Ophthalmol* 64:276, 1967.

172. Curran RE, Kenyon KR, Green WR: Pre-Descemet's membrane corneal dystrophy, *Am J Ophthalmol* 77:711, 1974.

173. Maeder G, Danis P: Surune nouvelle forme de dystrophie cornéene (dystrophia filiformis profunda corneae) associé à un kératocône, *Ophthalmologica* 114:246, 1947.

174. Franceschetti A, Schlaeppi V: Dégénérescence en bandelettes et dystrophie prédescemétique de la cornée dans un cas d'ichyhyose congénitale, *Dermatologica* 115:217, 1957.

175. Sever RJ, Frost P, Weinstein G: Eye changes in ichthyosis, *JAMA* 206:2283, 1968.

176. Kennedy RH, Bourne WM, Dyer JA: A 48-year clinical and epidemiologic study of keratoconus, *Am J Ophthalmol* 101:267, 1986.

177. Rabinowitz YS, Nesburn AB, McDonnell PJ: Videokeratography of the fellow eye in unilateral keratoconus, *Ophthalmology* 100:181, 1993.

178. Falls HF, Allen AW: Dominantly inherited keratoconus: report of a family, *J Hum Genet* 17:317, 1969.

179. Redmond KB: The role of heredity in keratoconus, *Trans Ophthalmol Soc NZ* 27:52, 1968.

180. Rudemann AD: Clinical course of keratoconus, *Trans Am Acad Ophthalmol Otolaryngol* 74:384, 1970.

181. Rabinowitz YS et al: Corneal topography in family members of patients with keratoconus using computer-assisted corneal topography analysis, *Invest Ophthalmol Vis Sci* 30(suppl): 188, 1989.

182. Ihalainen A: Clinical and epidemiological features of keratoconus: genetic and external factors in the pathogenesis of the disease, *Acta Ophthalmol (Copenh)* 178:1(suppl), 1986.

183. Maguire LJ, Bourne WD: Corneal topography of early keratoconus, *Am J Ophthalmol* 108:107, 1989.

184. Rabinowitz YS, McDonnell PJ: Computer-assisted corneal topography in keratoconus, *J Refract Corneal Surg* 5:400, 1989.

185. Wilson SE, Lin DTC, Klyce SD: Corneal topography of keratoconus, *Cornea* 10:2, 1991.

186. Maeda N et al: Automated keratoconus screening with corneal topography analysis, *Invest Ophthalmol Vis Sci* 35:2749, 1994.

187. Smolek MK, Klyce SD, Maeda N: Keratoconus and contact lens-induced corneal warpage analysis using the keratomorphic diagram, *Invest Ophthalmol Vis Sci* 35:4192, 1994.

188. Maeda N, Klyce SD, Smolek MK: Comparison of methods for detecting keratoconus using videokeratography, *Arch Ophthalmol* 113:870, 1995.

189. Levenson DS: Changes in corneal curvature with long-term PMMA contact lens wear, *CLAO J* 9:121, 1983.

190. Hartstein J: Corneal warping, *Am J Ophthalmol* 60:1103, 1965.

191. Wilson SE et al: Topographic changes in contact lens-induced corneal warpage, *Ophthalmology* 97:734, 1990.

192. Levenson DS, Berry CV: Findings on followup of corneal warpage patients, *CLAO J* 9:126, 1983.

193. Shapiro MB et al: Anterior clear spaces in keratoconus, *Ophthalmology* 93:1316, 1986.

194. Zabala M, Archila EA: Corneal sensitivity and topogometry in keratoconus, *CLAO J* 14:210, 1988.

195. Tuft SJ, Gregory WM, Buckley RJ: Acute corneal hydrops in keratoconus, *Ophthalmology* 101:1738, 1994.

196. Slusher MM, Laibson PR, Mulberger KD: Acute keratoconus in Down's syndrome, *Am J Ophthalmol* 63:1137, 1968.

197. Walsh SZ: Keratoconus and blindness in 469 institutionalized subjects with Down's syndrome and other causes of mental retardation, *J Ment Defic Res* 25:243, 1981.

198. Rowson NJ, Dart JK, Buckley RJ: Corneal neovascularisation in acute hydrops, *Eye* 6:404, 1992.

199. Copeman PWM: Eczema and keratoconus, *Br Med J* 2:977, 1965.

200. Tabbara K, Butrus S: Vernal conjunctivitis and keratoconus, *Am J Ophthalmol* 95:704, 1983.

201. Spencer WH, Fisher JJ: The association of keratoconus with atopic dermatitis, *Am J Ophthalmol* 47:332, 1959.

202. Galin MR, Berger R: Atopy and keratoconus, *Am J Ophthalmol* 45:904, 1958.

203. Sabiston DW: The association of keratoconus, dermatitis, and asthma, *Trans Ophthalmol Soc NZ* 18:66, 1966.

204. Gasset AR, Hison WA, Frias JL: Keratoconus and atopic disease, *Ann Ophthalmol* 10:991, 1978.

205. Rahi A et al: Keratoconus and coexisting atopic disease, *Br J Ophthalmol* 61:761, 1977.

206. Shapiro MB, France T: The ocular features of Down's syndrome, *Am J Ophthalmol* 99:659, 1985.

207. Beardsley SL, Foulks GN: An association of keratoconus and mitral valve prolapse, *Ophthalmology* 89:35, 1982.

208. Sharif KW, Casey TA, Coltart J: Prevalence of mitral valve prolapse in keratoconus patients, *J R Soc Med* 85:446, 1992.

209. Caffi M: Histopathology of keratoconus, *Ann Oftalmol Clin Ocul* 92:429, 1966.

210. McPherson SD, Kiffney GT: Some histologic findings in keratoconus, *Arch Ophthalmol* 79:669, 1968.

211. Pataa C, Joyon L, Roucher RF: Ultra-structure du keratoconus, *Arch Ophthalmol (Paris)* 30:403, 1970.

212. Pouliquen Y: Les fibrocytes dans le keratocone. Aspect morphologique et modification de L'espace extracellulaire: etude en microscopie optique et electronique, *Arch Ophthalmol (Paris)* 32:571, 1972.

213. Teng CC: Electron microscopic study of the pathology of keratoconus: I, *Am J Ophthalmol* 55:18, 1963.

214. Culbertson WW, Tseng SC: Corneal disorders in floppy eyelid syndrome, *Cornea* 13:33, 1994.

215. Donnenfeld ED et al: Keratoconus associated with floppy eyelid syndrome, *Ophthalmology* 98:1674, 1991.

216. Iwamoto R, DeVoe GA: Electron microscopic study of the Fleischer ring, *Arch Ophthalmol* 94:1579, 1976.

217. Stone DK, Kenyon KR, Stark WJ: Ultrastructure of keratoconus with healed hydrops, *Am J Ophthalmol* 82:450, 1976.

218. Waring G, Laibson P, Rodriques M: Clinical and pathologic alterations of Descemet's membrane with emphasis on endothelial metaplasia, *Surv Ophthalmol* 18:325, 1974.

219. Pouliquen Y: Keratoconus: Doyne lecture, *Eye* 1:1, 1987.

220. Nakayasu K et al: Distribution of types I, II, III, IV, and V collagen in normal and keratoconus corneas, *Ophthalmic Res* 18:1, 1986.

221. Zimmerman DR et al: Comparative studies of collagens in normal and keratoconus corneas, *Exp Eye Res* 46:431, 1988.

222. Cannon DT, Foster CS: Collagen cross-linking in keratoconus, *Invest Ophthalmol Vis Sci* 17:63, 1978.

223. Critchfield JW et al: Keratoconus: I. Biochemical studies, *Exp Eye Res* 46:953, 1988.

224. Yue BY, Sugar J, Benveniste K: RNA metabolism in cultures of corneal stromal cells from patients with keratoconus, *Proc Soc Exp Biol Med* 178:126, 1985.

225. Peters DP, Harrison DA, Brandt CR: Heterogeneity of type I collagen expression in human corneal keratoconus fibroblasts, *Ophthalmic Res* 25:273, 1993.

226. Kao WW et al: Increased collagenase and gelatinase activities in keratoconus, *Biochem Biophys Res Commun* 107:929, 1982.

227. Rehany U, Lehay M, Shoshan S: Collagenolytic activity in keratoconus, *Ann Ophthalmol* 14:751, 1982.

228. Brown D et al: Keratoconus corneas: increased gelatinolytic activity appears after modification of inhibitors, *Curr Eye Res* 12:571, 1993.

229. Sawaguchi S et al: Alpha2-macroglobulin levels in normal human and keratoconus corneas, *Invest Ophthalmol Vis Sci* 35:4008, 1994.

230. Kenny MC et al: Increased gelatinolytic activity in keratoconus keratocyte cultures: a correlation to an altered matrix metalloproteinase-2/tissue inhibitor of metalloproteinase ratio, *Cornea* 13:114, 1994.

231. Sawaguchi S et al: Lysosomal enzyme abnormalities in keratoconus, *Arch Ophthalmol* 107:1507, 1989.

232. Fukuchi T et al: Lysosomal enzyme activities in conjunctival tissues of patients with keratoconus, *Arch Ophthalmol* 112:1368, 1994.

233. Robert L et al: Etude morphologique et biochemique du keratocone: II. Etude biochemique, *Arch Ophthalmol (Paris)* 30:589, 1970.

234. Bleckman G, Kresse H: Studies on the glycosaminoglycan metabolism of cultured fibroblasts from human keratoconus corneas, *Exp Eye Res* 30:215, 1980.

235. Yue BY et al: Glycoconjugate abnormalities in cultured keratoconus stromal cells, *Arch Ophthalmol* 106:1709, 1988.

236. Yue BY, Sugar J, Schrode K: Histochemical studies of keratoconus, *Curr Eye Res* 7:81, 1988.

237. Funderburgh JL et al: Altered antigenicity of keratan sulfate proteoglycan in selected corneal diseases, *Invest Ophthalmol Vis Sci* 31:419, 1990.

238. Meek KM et al: The structure of normal and keratoconus human corneas, *Ophthalmic Res* 19:6, 1987.

239. Bron AJ: Keratoconus, *Cornea* 7:163, 1988.

240. Yue BY, Sugar J, Benveniste K: Heterogenicity in keratoconus: possible biochemical basis, *Proc Soc Exp Biol Med* 175:336, 1984.

241. Hartstein J: Keratoconus that developed in patients wearing corneal contact lenses, *Arch Ophthalmol* 80:345, 1968.

242. Hartstein J, Becker B: Research into the pathogenesis of keratoconus. A new syndrome: low ocular rigidity, contact lenses, and keratoconus, *Arch Ophthalmol* 84:728, 1970.

243. Steahly LP: Keratoconus following contact lens wear, *Ann Ophthalmol* 10:1177, 1978.

244. Gasset AR, Houde WL, Garcia-Bengochea M: Hard contact lens wear as an environmental risk in keratoconus, *Am J Ophthalmol* 85:339, 1978.

245. Brightbill FS, Stainer GA: Previous hard contact lens wear in keratoconus, *Contact Intraocular Lens Med J* 5:43, 1979.

246. Ridley F: Eye rubbing and contact lenses, *Br J Ophthalmol* 45:631, 1961.

247. Copeman PW: Eczema and keratoconus, *Br Med J* 2:977, 1965.

248. Karseras AB, Ruben M: Aetiology of keratoconus, *Br J Ophthalmol* 60:522, 1976.

249. Gritz DC, McDonnell PJ: Keratoconus and ocular massage, *Am J Ophthalmol* 106:757, 1988.

250. Coyle JT: Keratoconus and eye rubbing, *Am J Ophthalmol* 97:527, 1984.

251. Koenig SB, Smith RW: Keratoconus and corneal hydrops associated with compulsive eye rubbing, *Refract Corneal Surg* 9:383, 1993.

252. Kastl PR et al: A 20-year retrospective study of the use of contact lenses in keratoconus, *CLAO J* 13:102, 1987.

253. Fowler WC, Belin MW, Chambers WA: Contact lenses in the visual correction of keratoconus, *CLAO J* 14:203, 1988.

254. Smiddy WE et al: Keratoconus: contact lens or keratoplasty, *Ophthalmology* 95:487, 1988.

255. Buxton JN, Keates RH, Hoefle FB: *The contact lens correction of keratoconus.* In Dabezies OH, editor: *Contact lenses: the CLAO guide to basic science and clinical practice,* Orlando, FL, 1984, Grune & Stratton.

256. Soper JW, Jarrett A: Results of a systematic approach to fitting keratoconus and corneal transplants, *Contact Lens J* 9:12, 1975.

257. Tuft SJ et al: Prognostic factors for the progression of keratoconus, *Ophthalmology* 101:439, 1994.

258. Crews MJ, Driebe WT, Stern GA: The clinical management of keratoconus: a 6 year retrospective study, *CLAO J* 20:194, 1994.

259. Dana MR et al: Contact lens failure in keratoconus management, *Ophthalmology* 99:1187, 1992.

260. Payne JW: Primary penetrating keratoplasty for keratoconus: a long-term follow-up, *Cornea* 1:21, 1982.

261. Paglen PG et al: The prognosis for keratoplasty in keratoconus, *Ophthalmology* 89:651, 1982.

262. Girard LJ et al: Allograft rejection after penetrating keratoplasty for keratoconus, *Ophthalmic Surg* 24:40, 1993.

263. Sharif KW, Casey TA: Penetrating keratoplasty for keratoconus: complications and long-term success, *Br J Ophthalmol* 75:142, 1991.

264. Matusda M et al: The effect of hard contact lens wear on the keratoconic corneal endothelium after penetrating keratoplasty, *Am J Ophthalmol* 107:246, 1989.

265. Abelson MB et al: Recurrent keratoconus after keratoplasty, *Am J Ophthalmol* 90:672, 1980.

266. Bechrakis N et al: Recurrent keratoconus, *Cornea* 13:73, 1994.

267. Urrets-Zavalia A: Fixed, dilated pupil, iris atrophy, and secondary glaucoma: a distinct clinical entity following penetrating keratoplasty in keratoconus, *Am J Ophthalmol* 56:257, 1963.

268. Davies PD, Ruben M: The paretic pupil: its incidence and etiology after keratoplasty for keratoconus, *Br J Ophthalmol* 59:223, 1975.

269. Richard J, Paton D, Gasset A: A comparison of penetrating keratoplasty and lamellar keratoplasty in the surgical management of keratoconus, *Am J Ophthalmol* 86:807, 1978.

270. Wood TO: Lamellar transplants in keratoconus, *Am J Ophthalmol* 83:543, 1977.

271. Gasset AR: Lamellar keratoplasty in the treatment of keratoconus: conectomy, *Ophthalmic Surg* 10:26, 1979.
272. Kaufman HE, Werblin TP: Epikeratophakia for the treatment of keratoconus, *Am J Ophthalmol* 93:342, 1982.
273. McDonald MB et al: Epikeratophakia for keratoconus: the nationwide study, *Arch Ophthalmol* 104:1294, 1986.
274. Steinert RF, Wagoner MD: Long-term comparison of epikeratoplasty and penetrating keratoplasty for keratoconus, *Arch Ophthalmol* 106:493, 1988.
275. Benson WH et al: Visual improvement as a function of time after lamellar keratoplasty for keratoconus, *Am J Ophthalmol* 116:207, 1993.
276. Frantz JM, McDonald MB, Kaufman HE: Results of penetrating keratoplasty after epikeratophakia for keratoconus in the nationwide study, *Ophthalmology* 96:1151, 1989.
277. Gasset AR, Kaufman HE: Thermokeratoplasty for keratoconus, *Am J Ophthalmol* 79:226, 1975.
278. Rowsey JJ, Ross JD: Preliminary report of Los Alamos keratoplasty techniques, *Ophthalmology* 88:755, 1981.
279. Aquavella JV, Smith RS, Shaw EL: Alterations in corneal morphology following thermokeratoplasty, *Arch Ophthalmol* 94:2082, 1976.
280. Fogle JA, Kenyon KR, Stark WJ: Damage to epithelial basement membrane by thermokeratoplasty, *Am J Ophthalmol* 83:392, 1977.
281. Moodaley L, Buckley RJ, Woodward EG: Surgery to improve contact lens wear in keratoconus, *CLAO J* 17:129, 1991.
282. Moodaley L et al: Excimer laser superficial keratectomy for proud nebulae in keratoconus, *Br J Ophthalmol* 78:454, 1994.
283. Fagerholm P et al: Nebulae at keratoconus: the result after excimer laser removal, *Acta Ophthalmol (Copenh)* 71:830, 1993.
284. McClellan KA, Billson FA: Acute hydrops in keratoglobus, *Arch Ophthalmol* 105:1432, 1987.
285. Hymas SE, Dar H, Newman E: Blue sclera keratoglobus, *Br J Ophthalmol* 53:53, 1969.
286. Gregoratos N, Bartoscocas C, Papas K: Blue sclera with keratoglobus and brittle cornea, *Br J Ophthalmol* 55:424, 1971.
287. Biglan AW, Brown SI, Johnson BL: Keratoglobus and blue sclera, *Am J Ophthalmol* 83:225, 1977.
288. Cameron JA: Keratoglobus, *Cornea* 12:124, 1993.
289. Cavara V: Keratoglobus and keratoconus: a contribution to nosological interpretation of keratoglobus, *Br J Ophthalmol* 34:621, 1950.
290. Greenfield G et al: Blue sclera and keratoconus: key features of a distinct heritable disorder of connective tissue, *Clin Genet* 4:8, 1973.
291. Cameron JA et al: Epikeratoplasty for keratoglobus associated with blue sclera, *Ophthalmology* 98:446, 1991.

Eighteen

Disorders of the Endothelium

ENDOTHELIAL DYSTROPHIES

Fuchs' Endothelial Dystrophy

Abnormality or loss of endothelial cells occurs with aging and a variety of injuries, such as trauma, inflammation, toxins, and glaucoma. In many cases the manifestations are similar: The earliest sign, corneal guttae, can progress to stromal edema, epithelial edema, and corneal scarring. When these changes are seen in the absence of contributory injury, the condition is called *Fuchs' dystrophy.* Some of these cases may be a result of unrecognized injury; many are related to normal aging or an accelerated aging of the endothelium; and some appear to be true dystrophies, with early onset and hereditary transmission.

Fuchs' dystrophy is a bilateral condition that is usually noted in the elderly and is more common in women.[1,2] Autosomal dominant transmission has been demonstrated in some cases.[3-7] Some reports have suggested an association between Fuchs' dystrophy and open-angle glaucoma,[8] but others have not found this to be the case.[9,10] Two reports noted an association of Fuchs' dystrophy with axial hypermetropia and angle-closure glaucoma.[11,12] Coexistent bilateral Fuchs' dystrophy and keratoconus have also been reported.[13,14]

Clinical Manifestations

Endothelial Changes. Vogt used the term *cornea guttata,* derived from Latin, to describe corneas containing multiple droplike excrescences, or guttae, on the posterior surface. The condition is usually seen in middle-aged or older patients. Corneal guttae have been noted in as many as 70% of patients over 40 years of age.[15,16] In addition to aging, guttae can be associated with corneal trauma and inflammation.[17-19] They do not interfere with vision.

Guttae are seen as dewdroplike, wartlike, endothelial excrescences. On direct illumination they appear as refractile circular excavations on the endothelial surface (Fig. 18-1). They develop first in the central cornea and gradually spread peripherally and become more numerous. Fine pigment deposition is often seen dif-

465

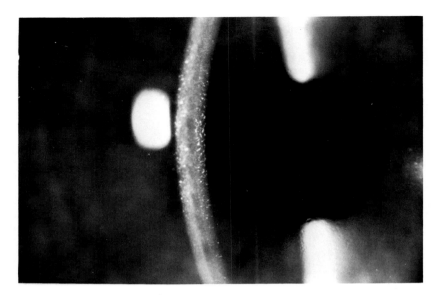

Figure 18-1
Endothelial guttae seen with slit-lamp microscopy.

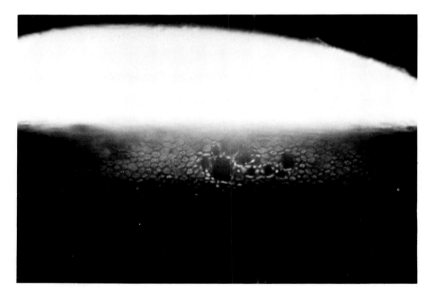

Figure 18-2
Specular micrograph of the endothelium showing guttae (dark holes in endothelial mosaic).

fusely on the posterior corneal surface. With time, Descemet's membrane can develop a beaten-metal appearance. Specular microscopy demonstrates decreased endothelial cell density, polymegathism, and dark holes in the endothelial mosaic (Fig. 18-2), representing guttae.

In some instances the endothelial change is not in guttate form, but rather the endothelium becomes increasingly diffusely relucent, giving the appearance of a grayish membrane.[20,21] Reduced endothelial cell density and cell pleomorphism are seen on specular microscopy.[20] In severe inflammation, edema of the endothelial cells can resemble a guttate cornea, but the condition is transient.[22]

Stromal and Epithelial Edema. If endothelial cell function is sufficiently compromised, stromal edema occurs. Although stromal edema is more likely to occur with decreased endothelial cell density, the density may vary. The number of corneal guttae also does not correlate well: Stromal edema can occur in the absence of guttae.[20] With further impairment of endothelial function, epithelial edema develops. Epithelial edema can occur at different stages depending on the intraocular pressure (IOP). Elevations of IOP cause epithelial edema more readily in a cornea with compromised endothelium and stromal edema.

Some reduction of vision occurs with marked stromal edema (approximately >0.65 mm), but it is usually not until epithelial edema develops that the patient becomes very symptomatic. Epithelial edema causes surface irregularity, haze, photophobia, and recurrent epithelial erosions. At first, epithelial edema occurs only in the morning and clears as the day goes on. This is related to the decreased evaporation of fluid from the surface of the eye during sleep as a result of lid closure. Humid weather can similarly affect vision.

When there is early or moderate stromal edema it is difficult to perceive any changes other than a widening of the slit beam. Therefore, pachometry is useful to detect its presence. In more advanced edema, the stroma can become slightly hazy, the posterior corneal surface is pushed posteriorly, and Descemet's membrane can be thrown into folds. The central cornea can become thicker than the peripheral cornea.

Epithelial edema appears first as fine, clear cysts producing nodular elevations of the surface (bedewing). Topical fluorescein can be helpful in demonstrating bedewing, by producing dark gaps in the fluorescein film ("negative" staining). On retroillumination, the bedewing appears as a fine patina. Fingerprint-like patterns and other linear opacities may be seen in the deep epithelium, probably caused by shifting of the overlying epithelium. With coalescence of the microcysts, epithelial bullae develop. These markedly reduce vision and can rupture, causing pain and foreign body sensation. Subepithelial fibrosis and vascularization can occur in more advanced cases, particularly with recurrent epithelial breakdown (Figs. 18-3 and 18-4).

Histopathology

As noted previously, the main pathologic condition is in the endothelium.[23-25] Guttae are seen as nodular thickenings of Descemet's membrane (Fig. 18-5). They are composed of collagen and most likely are abnormal products of the endothelial cells.[24]

The cell density decreases progressively and cell size increases, with thinning over the Descemet's warts. Some of the endothelial cells take on morphologic features of fibroblasts and produce collagen.[24,25] Other cells show tonofilaments, surface microvilli, and desmosomes, similar to epithelial cells.[26] Descemet's membrane becomes diffusely thickened because of deposition of collagenous basement membrane–like material on the posterior surface (see Fig. 1-25).[24,27-29] The anterior banded portion is relatively normal, but the posterior nonbanded layer is thinned or absent and is replaced by a posterior banded layer.[24,28] The thinness of the posterior nonbanded layer suggests that endothelial cell function becomes abnormal at an early age. The posterior banded layer is probably produced by stressed or abnormal endothelial cells. The sulfur content of Descemet's membrane was found to be decreased and the calcium content increased.[30]

Epithelial edema first appears intracellularly in the basal cells (Fig. 18-6). Later, interepithelial and subepithelial pockets of fluid are seen. Bowman's layer usually remains intact. Subepithelial deposition of collagen and basement membrane–like material can be noted (Fig. 18-7).

Pathogenesis

Although the pathogenesis of Fuchs' dystrophy is not known, several hypotheses have been advanced. One theory is that Fuchs' dystrophy results from an abnormality in the final phases of the differentiation of the corneal endothelium from neural crest cells.[31] Another theory is that corneal inflammation or toxicity plays a role. Endothelial injury from inflammation or toxins can result in reduced cellular density, a thickened abnormal Descemet's membrane, and, in some instance, corneal guttae.[32] A hormonal influence has also been hypothesized, primarily based on the increased incidence and greater severity of disease in women.[2,7,8]

Treatment

Patients with early epithelial edema may benefit from hyperosmotic drops and ointment (Fig. 18-8). Usually 5% NaCl drops are given four to eight times daily and 5% NaCl ointment is given at bedtime. These may reduce epithelial edema and improve both comfort and vision. A hair dryer, held at arm's length or directed across the face, may help "dry out" the corneal surface, and this can be repeated two or three times a day. Lowering of IOP is useful in some cases. Topical corticosteroids are not beneficial.

A bandage contact lens is beneficial in allevi-

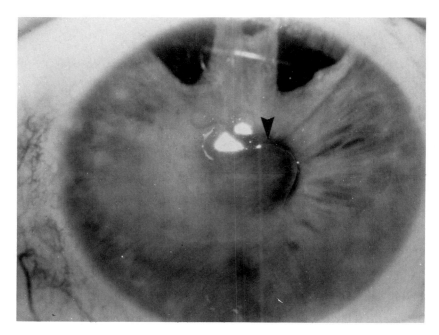

Figure 18-3
Subepithelial fibrosis *(arrow)* can occur in Fuchs' dystrophy.

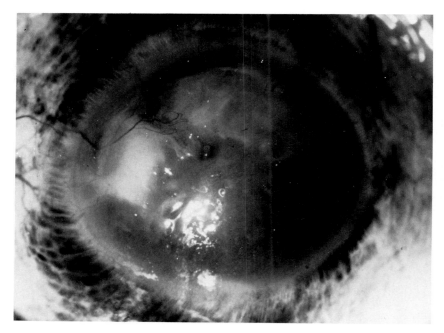

Figure 18-4
Fuchs' dystrophy with epithelial bullae, scarring, and vascularization.

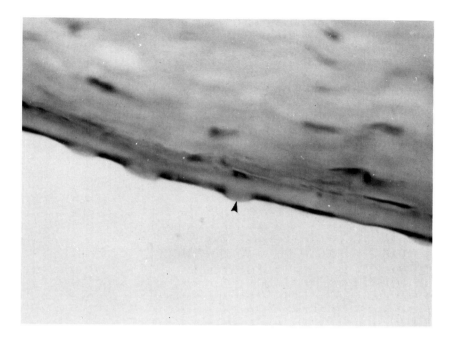

Figure 18-5
Cornea guttata. Descemet's warts are noted with loss of endothelial cells *(arrow).*

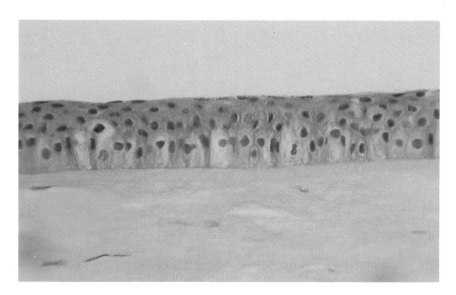

Figure 18-6
Early epithelial edema in Fuchs' dystrophy, clinically seen as bedewing of epithelium. (From Grayson M, Keates RH: *Manual of diseases of the cornea,* Boston, 1969, Little, Brown & Co.)

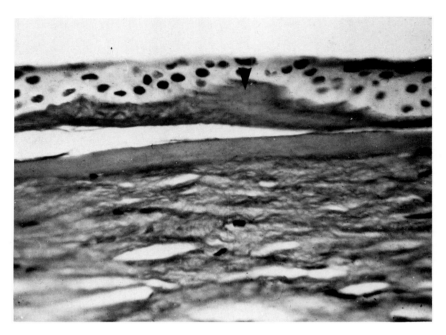

Figure 18-7
In longstanding Fuchs' dystrophy, an increase in basement membrane substance (*arrow*) and alterations in Bowman's layer may be seen.

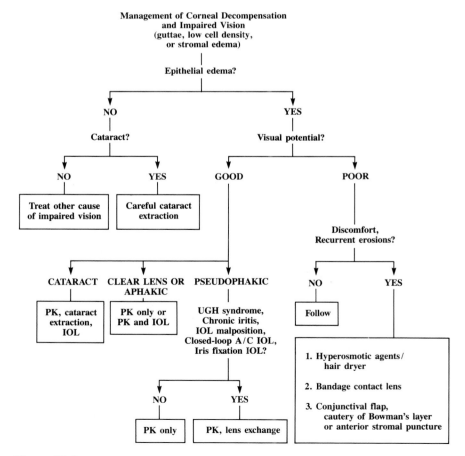

Figure 18-8
Management of corneal decompensation and impaired vision.

ating discomfort resulting from bullae formation and rupture. It is particularly useful in making life more pleasant for patients for whom corneal transplantation is not desired or recommended. Cautery of Bowman's layer, phototherapeutic keratectomy,[33] or a conjunctival flap are other alternatives for these patients.

Penetrating keratoplasty is indicated once visual acuity is decreased to the point of impairing normal activities. The short-term results are quite good (Fig. 18-9),[34,35] but long-term survival of these grafts is questionable. Some studies have found a relatively high incidence of graft failure.[36,37] Cataracts are often present, and combined keratoplasty and cataract extraction can be performed.[38-41] The relative value of separate versus combined procedures has not yet been determined, but most surgeons now perform combined procedures.[42] In the presence of a cataract, the indications for keratoplasty are not well defined. Some have recommended keratoplasty whenever corneal thickness is greater than 0.60 mm,[43] but I usually proceed with cataract extraction alone unless epithelial edema is present. Patients with any lens opacity or those over 60 years of age requiring keratoplasty for Fuchs' dystrophy should have simultaneous cataract extraction. If extraction is not performed, there is a high likelihood of cataract formation that will be sufficient to require surgery within the subsequent 5 years.[44,45]

Congenital Hereditary Endothelial Dystrophy

Congenital hereditary endothelial dystrophy (CHED) can be inherited in both autosomal dominant and autosomal recessive forms. The recessive form is more common and more severe, whereas the dominant form can be associated with deafness.[46-54] The recessive form is present at birth or develops in the neonatal period and is often associated with nystagmus. Patients with dominantly inherited disease have clear corneas early in life, but within a few years they develop slowly progressive opacification.[52,55-57] They do not develop nystagmus.

The essential feature of CHED is bilateral diffuse corneal edema, unrelated to commonly known causes such as congenital glaucoma, intrauterine infections, or mucopolysaccharidosis. The clinical picture can vary from a mild haziness to a moderately severe, diffuse, homogeneous, gray-white, ground-glass appearance of the central cornea that extends to the periphery (Fig. 18-10). The corneal thickness is two to three times greater than normal, but corneal diameter is not enlarged. Macular or dot stromal opacities are sometimes present. Diffuse stromal cloudiness often prevents clinical evaluation of the endothelium and Descemet's membrane, but the latter can sometimes be seen as thickened and gray. Guttae are not pres-

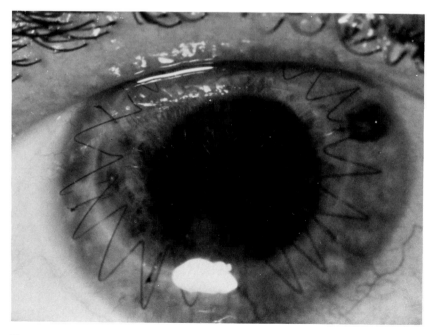

Figure 18-9
Penetrating graft for Fuchs' dystrophy.

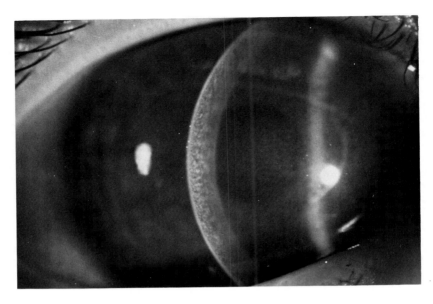

Figure 18-10
Congenital hereditary endothelial dystrophy.

ent, there is no vascularization, and corneal sensation and IOP are normal.

The corneal opacity may either be stationary or show slow progression. Epithelial edema and bedewing can develop, but bullae and discomfort are rarely seen. Visual deprivation–related ocular enlargement was reported in a series of patients with CHED.[58]

This condition appears to result from a degeneration of the endothelium, which may occur in utero or within the first year of life. The anterior banded portion of Descemet's membrane is normal, indicating that the endothelium is functionally normal at least through the 5th month of gestation. However, sometime after the 5th month a defective endothelium secretes abnormal and excessive basement membrane, which accumulates as an aberrant, nonbanded posterior portion of Descemet's membrane.[50,58-64] Endothelial cells are absent or atrophic. Multinucleated endothelial cells may be present.[65] In one study, the endothelial cells did not grow when placed in culture media.[63] Secondary changes related to the stromal and epithelial edema are also noted. Clinically and histologically identical abnormalities have been observed in patients with congenital glaucoma.[66]

Asymptomatic relatives of patients with CHED can manifest corneal changes resembling those of posterior polymorphous dystrophy (PPD).[67] These individuals appear to have a higher risk of producing offspring with CHED.[68]

Differential Diagnosis

Several conditions can present with cloudy corneas at birth, including congenital hereditary stromal dystrophy (CHSD), PPD, congenital glaucoma, Peter's anomaly, birth trauma, intrauterine infection, and sclerocornea. The differential diagnoses of these conditions are discussed in Chapter 5.

Treatment

Keratoplasty in such young children is considerably more difficult to treat than that seen in adults, but good results can be obtained in some cases (see Chapter 5).[69-72]

Posterior Polymorphous Dystrophy

Posterior polymorphous dystrophy is usually transmitted as a dominant trait, but recessive patterns of inheritance have been demonstrated in some pedigrees.[73-75] It is most often bilateral but can be asymmetric and, rarely, unilateral.[76] Some cases are clearly congenital, with cloudy corneas at birth. However, patients with PPD usually demonstrate normal vision and are asymptomatic, so the age of onset can be difficult to determine. Most cases are nonprogressive or very slowly progressive, but in some patients endothelial decompensation can develop, reducing visual acuity.[26]

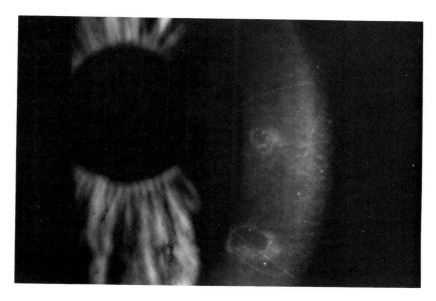

Figure 18-11
Endothelial lesions in posterior polymorphous dystrophy.

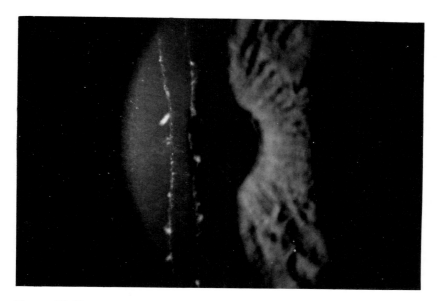

Figure 18-12
Endothelial bands in posterior polymorphous dystrophy.

As indicated by its name, PPD is characterized by deep corneal lesions of various shapes. Nodular, grouped vesicular and blisterlike lesions commonly occur (Fig. 18-11).[77] Gray-white halos often surround the vesicular lesions. Flat gray-white opacities, gray thickenings of Descemet's membrane, sinuous broad bands (Fig. 18-12), or clear bands with white scalloped margins may also be present.[26] The clear bands with scalloped margins can be oriented vertically or horizontally and are often confused with Descemet's tears.[78] The lesions stand out on retroillumination. With specular microscopy the lesions are seen to contain abnormal, pleomorphic cells, with indistinct borders and increased reflective highlights.[79,80] The vesicles and bands appear to be shallow depressions projecting into the posterior cornea.[81]

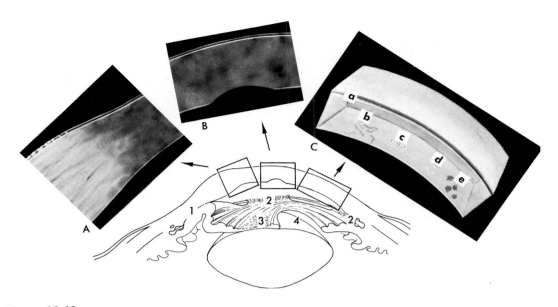

Figure 18-13
A, Posterior polymorphous dystrophy. Diagrammatic representation of biomicroscopic findings: (*1*) iridocorneal adhesions obliterating the trabeculum, (*2*) abnormal iris processes, and (*3*) patchy iris atrophy involving the iris stroma. **B,** Area of circumscribed posterior keratoconus. **C,** En bloc section showing (*a*) calcific deposition in Bowman's membrane, (*b*) "sinuous" opacities, (*c*) vesicular lesions, (*d*) flat, gray-white macular lesions, and (*e*) aggregations of guttae. (From Grayson M: *Trans Am Ophthalmol Soc* 72:516, 1974.)

Specular microscopy can distinguish PPD from Haab's striae[81] and the iridocorneal endothelial (ICE) syndrome.[82]

Posterior polymorphous dystrophy can be associated with anterior segment dysgenesis, prominent Schwalbe's ring, iridocorneal adhesions, abnormal iris processes, iris atrophy, corectopia, and ectropion uveae (Fig. 18-13).[26] IOP elevation occurs in approximately 15% of cases.[26,76,83,84] Band keratopathy,[26] calcium deposition in the deep stroma,[74] and posterior keratoconus[26] may also be seen. In one study in Thailand, 11 of 17 patients with Alport's syndrome had signs of PPD.[85] Renal abnormalities and hearing loss also appeared to be more common in patients with PPD without a history of Alport's syndrome.

Pathogenesis
Electron microscopic studies have revealed the main abnormality to be in the endothelial cell.[26,61,76,86-93] Degeneration of endothelial cells, fibroblast-like cells, and epithelial-like cells are seen. Islands of epithelial-like endothelial cells are found in about two thirds of cases.[93] These cells are larger than normal endothelial cells. They can be multilayered and have extensive microvilli, desmosomal junctions, intracy-

toplasmic filaments, and a decreased number of organelles (Figs. 18-14 and 18-15). The abnormal endothelium can extend across the trabecular meshwork and onto the iris.[87,94] The abnormal endothelial cells can be grown in culture and maintain the abnormal characteristics observed in pathologic specimens.[95] Epithelial-like cells were also observed adjacent to the site of Descemet's rupture in a cornea from a patient with a history of forceps injury at birth.[96] This suggests that the young corneal endothelium can undergo epithelial transformation in response to injury.

In most cases the anterior banded layer of Descemet's membrane is normal, indicating that the abnormality develops late in gestation or shortly after birth. However, in several patients with PPD who developed corneal edema at an early age, the anterior banded layer was thinned and incomplete, indicating onset of the disease before the 12th week of gestation.[97-99] The posterior portion of Descemet's membrane may be thickened by abnormal multilaminate basement membrane material. Corneal guttae and excavations of Descemet's membrane have been described.

The pathogenesis of PPD is unknown, but it has been suggested that the endothelial cells

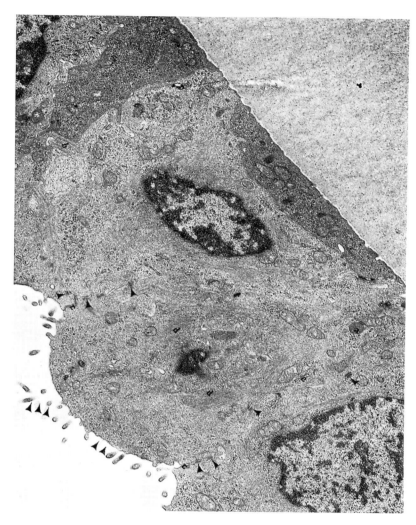

Figure 18-14
Posterior polymorphous dystrophy. Mitochondria are few, and those present are degenerating **(a)**. Desmosomes (*single arrows*) are abundant, and microvilli are numerous (*triple arrow*). Extensive interdigitation between cells **(b)** and zonulae occludens **(c)** is noted. Note extensive intracytoplasmic filaments **(d)** and elongated endoplasmic reticulum **(e)**. *Double arrows* indicate rounded edge or elevated apices of altered cells (×8714.5). (From Grayson M: *Trans Am Ophthalmol Soc* 72:516, 1974.)

undergo transformation into epithelial-like cells, or that their embryonal precursors undergo abnormal differentiation. Epithelial transformation appears to be one of the responses of the young endothelium to disease, as suggested by the finding of epithelial-like cells in a patient with forceps injury.[96] The angle and iris abnormalities may represent spread of these abnormal cells from the cornea, or they may be a broader reflection of the mesenchymal dysgenesis. The percentage of endothelial cells affected and the age at which the cells are affected probably determine the sever-

ity of the clinical disease. In mild cases the remaining intact endothelial cells are able to compensate for the abnormal cells.

Differential Diagnosis
Because PPD can present as a cloudy cornea at birth, it must be differentiated from CHED, CHSD, and other conditions. It is useful to examine the child's parents, because clinical corneal changes consistent with PPD can be present. The differential diagnosis of cloudy corneas at birth is discussed in Chapter 5. Glaucoma, iridocorneal adhesions, and corneal

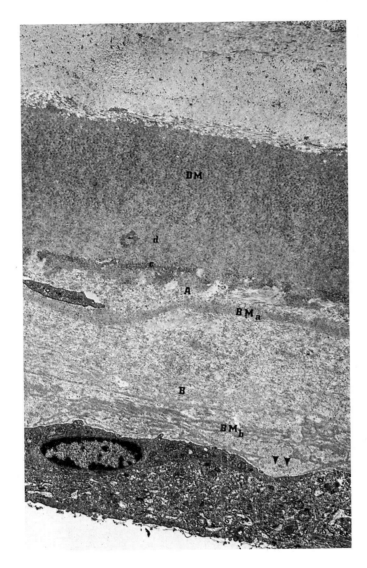

Figure 18-15
Posterior polymorphous dystrophy. An abnormal membrane has been laid down in layers *A* and *B.* The abnormal membrane consists of collagen fibers and laminated areas of basement membrane (*BMa* and *BMb*). A demarcation line (*c*) is visible. *BMa* separates collagen fiber layers *A* and *B. Double arrow* indicates an area in which indentations are made into the posterior cellular layer, possibly representing early guttate lesions. Descemet's membrane (*DM*) shows a narrow nonbanded zone (*d*) (×6394.5). (From Grayson M: *Trans Am Ophthalmol Soc* 72:516, 1974.)

edema can be present in both PPD and Chandler's (ICE) syndrome. The differentiating features are given in Table 18-1. Specular microscopy may also be useful in distinguishing PPD from the ICE syndrome.[82]

Treatment

In most cases no treatment is necessary, but keratoplasty is required occasionally for corneal edema. Early-onset corneal edema has been observed to clear slowly,[97] so observation may be warranted in some cases, particularly in view of the high risk of keratoplasty in infants. In a few cases histologic changes typical of PPD were observed in failed grafts 3 to 9 years after penetrating keratoplasty was performed for PPD.[100,101] These authors hypothesized that abnormal cells from the periphery of the host cornea repopu-

Table 18-1	Comparison of Posterior Polymorphous Dystrophy and Chandler's Syndrome	
Feature	**Posterior Polymorphous Dystrophy**	**Chandler's Syndrome**
Laterality	Bilateral	Unilateral
Heredity	Autosomal dominant	None
Sex distribution	Males = females	Females > males
Onset of symptoms	Any age	Second and third decades
Corneal edema	Occasionally	Usually
Endothelium	Ridges, vesicles, plaques	Fine guttaelike changes
Iridocorneal adhesions	25% (usually microscopic)	100%
Iris stromal atrophy	Absent or minimal	Mild-marked (essential iris atrophy)
Ectropion uveae	Infrequent	Frequent
Glaucoma	Infrequent	100%
Progression	May slowly progress	Fairly rapid

Adapted from Rodrigues MM et al: *Arch Ophthalmol* 98:688, 1980.

lated the posterior graft surface, possibly after destruction of the donor endothelium. In rare instances corneal edema developing in adulthood has improved spontaneously.[73] If extensive angle and iris involvement is present, the resultant glaucoma can be very difficult to manage, and the prognosis for successful keratoplasty is much worse.

IRIDOCORNEAL ENDOTHELIAL SYNDROME

Three different clinical conditions—Chandler's syndrome, essential (or progressive) iris atrophy, and Cogan-Reese iris nevus syndrome—have been grouped together into a single syndrome because their pathologic processes appear to be quite similar.[102] ICE syndrome is a nonfamilial unilateral disease that is more common in women and is usually diagnosed between 30 and 50 years of age.

Clinical Manifestations

The chief characteristics of ICE syndrome are corneal endothelial abnormalities, peripheral anterior synechiae, glaucoma, iris atrophy and hole formation, and iris nodules. The relative prominence of these different features varies widely and is the reason for the original division into three different clinical diseases. In essential iris atrophy, the earliest described condition,[103] the iris features predominate, particularly atrophy, hole formation, and corectopia (Fig. 18-16). In Chandler's syndrome, iris atrophy and corectopia are mild or absent, and corneal endothelial changes and stromal edema are prominent.[104] In the iris nevus syndrome,

nodular, pigmented elevations are present on the surface of the iris (Fig. 18-17).[105] Other corneal and iris abnormalities may or may not be present.

The most common corneal abnormality is a fine hammered-metal appearance of the endothelium.[106] Stromal or epithelial edema commonly develops, with or without an abnormal appearance of the endothelium. Specular examination of the endothelium reveals pleomorphism, polymegathism, and intracellular dark areas.[107-110] Distinct morphologic features have been described that purportedly can be used to distinguish ICE syndrome from PPD.[82] Usually the endothelium is diffusely affected, but in some cases focal areas of normal and abnormal cells are seen.[111] In most of these cases the normal areas disappear with time, but regression of the abnormal endothelium has also been observed.[112]

The fellow eyes are nearly always clinically unaffected, but decreased endothelial cell density and pleomorphism have been noted on specular microscopy.[113] Bilateral clinical disease has also been reported.[114]

In some cases there is progressive atrophy of the iris stroma, peripheral anterior synechiae, and stretching of the iris, with corectopia, ectropion uvea, and hole formation (previously called progressive or essential iris atrophy).[106,115] The peripheral anterior synechiae extend to or beyond Schwalbe's ring and are usually visible without gonioscopy. The pupil is usually eccentric in the direction of the most prominent synechiae, and the majority of iris holes are found in the opposite side. As many as several hundred fine, yellow to brown pedunculated nodules can be present on the iris surface.[105,116] In

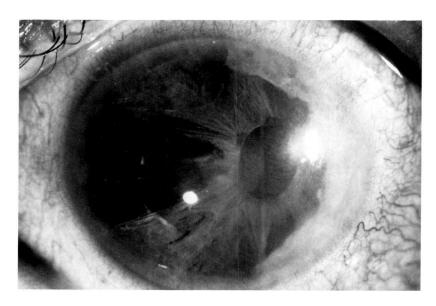

Figure 18-16
Essential iris atrophy with peripheral anterior synechiae and corneal edema.

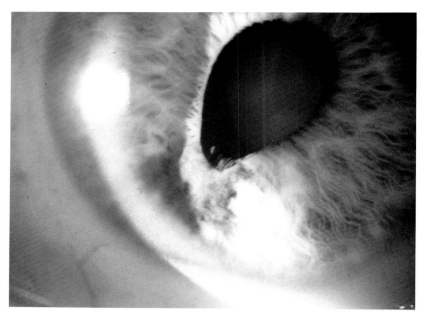

Figure 18-17
Cogan-Reese iris nevus syndrome. (Courtesy of Massimo Busin, Bonn, Germany.)

some cases these iris nodules are the most prominent feature; in others they develop many years after other iris and corneal changes.[117,118] Elevated IOP is common and often requires surgical intervention. Mild signs of intraocular inflammation, such as keratic precipitates, are occasionally seen.

Histopathology

Abnormal endothelial cells are present on the trabecular meshwork, the anterior surface of the iris, and the posterior corneal surface.[112,119-126] The corneal endothelial cells are decreased in number and irregular in shape. They can have epithelial features, including desmosomal junctions, surface microvilli, and increased intracytoplasmic filaments. The endothelial cells express cytokeratins, which are normally present on some epithelial cells but not on endothelium.[127] Descemet's membrane can be thickened or normal but contains an abnormal posterior collagenous layer. Lymphocytes may be seen within the endothelial layer.[122,124-126] The abnormal endothelial cells, together with a basement membrane, extend over the peripheral anterior synechiae and open anterior chamber angle onto the iris surface. Most commonly the membrane covers the iris quadrant toward the pupil that is distorted and not the quadrants containing holes.[102,115] Iris nodules are localized protrusions of normal iris stroma through the cellular sheet that may later become covered by the sheet.[115,122,128,129] Iris ischemia has been noted,[117] but its etiology is unclear.

Pathogenesis

The primary abnormality is most likely a defect in the corneal endothelium.[115] Until recently, the predominant theory was that the endothelium was abnormal congenitally because of an anomalous differentiation of the neural crest mesenchyme, and the abnormal endothelium could not maintain corneal hydration and grew over the angle and iris surface.[130] Currently, ICE syndrome appears to be related to infection with herpes simplex virus (HSV). In one study, 16 of 25 corneas affected by ICE syndrome were positive for HSV DNA, and the DNA was localized within endothelial cells.[131] This theory is supported by the finding of inflammatory cells in some cases, the unilateral occurrence of disease, and the age at onset.

Treatment

Control of IOP can usually be achieved medically. Drugs that lower aqueous production are more effective. Laser trabeculoplasty is not usually effective.[132] Filtering surgery is reasonably successful,[117] but endothelialization of the bleb can occur.

Lowering IOP can reduce corneal edema, but penetrating keratoplasty is often required. Most groups have reported good results with keratoplasty,[133-135] but one observed a high risk of graft reaction and rejection.[136]

OTHER CAUSES OF CORNEAL EDEMA

The differential diagnosis of corneal edema and corneal clouding in infants is discussed in

Table 18-2	Causes of Noninfiltrative Corneal Edema

Dystrophy
    Fuchs' dystrophy
    Posterior polymorphous dystrophy
Corneal hydrops (keratoconus)
Postsurgical causes
    Complicated intraocular surgery
    Lens-implant related
    Brown-McLean syndrome
    Epithelial downgrowth
    Descemet's detachment
Trauma
    Blunt trauma
    Corneal laceration
    Chemical injury
    Intraocular foreign body
Angle-closure glaucoma
Infection
    Herpes simplex
        ?Iridocorneal endothelial syndrome
    Herpes zoster
    Rarer causes of disciform keratitis (e.g., mumps, acanthamoeba, fungi)
Ocular ischemia
Hypotony

Chapter 5. The causes of noninfiltrative corneal edema in adults are given in Table 18-2. Brown-McLean syndrome is characterized by peripheral corneal edema associated with golden-brown pigment on the endothelium, sparing the central cornea.[137-141] Most reported cases have occurred after intracapsular cataract extraction, but it can be seen after extracapsular cataract extraction, phacoemulsification, pars plana lensectomy, lens luxation,[138] or lens resorption.[139] It has also been observed after intermittent angle closure. The condition is usually stable, with retention of a clear central cornea. However, painful peripheral bullae and secondary infection can occur.

ENDOTHELIITIS

A linear pattern of endothelial inflammation and destruction can occur in nongrafted corneas. The appearance and the process appear to be similar to those of allogeneic corneal graft rejection. A line of keratic precipitates progresses across the cornea, destroying the endothelium and leaving stromal edema in its wake. Herpes simplex can cause such a picture unilaterally (see Chapter 12).[142-144] It can also be seen as a recurrent, bilaterally symmetric process in otherwise healthy eyes,[145,146] associated with active pars planitis,[147] or after cataract extraction.[144,148,149] The etiology is unknown, but an autoimmune process has been proposed.[144,145] Topical corticosteroids have been effective in some cases, and the combination of corticosteroids and topical and oral antiviral therapy has been successful in others.

Single or multiple inflammatory endothelial plaques are another form of endothelial inflammation seen with herpes simplex.

One pedigree has been described in which there appeared to be a dominantly inherited form of recurrent keratoendotheliitis.[150] Attacks usually began around age 10 and recurred two to three times per year, lasting days to weeks. Corneal edema, guttae, and mild anterior chamber reaction were noted during attacks, and some patients developed stromal opacities after multiple attacks.

REFERENCES

1. Krachmer JH et al: A study of 64 families with corneal endothelial dystrophy, *Arch Ophthalmol* 96:2036, 1978.
2. Adamis AP et al: Fuchs' endothelial dystrophy of the cornea, *Surv Ophthalmol* 38:149, 1993.
3. Mortelmans L: Forme familiale de la dystrophie cornéene de Fuchs, *Ophthalmologica* 123:88, 1952.
4. Cross HE, Maumenee AE, Cantolino SJ: Inheritance of Fuchs' endothelial dystrophy, *Arch Ophthalmol* 85:268, 1971.
5. Krachmer JH et al: Inheritance of endothelial dystrophy of the cornea, *Ophthalmologica* 181:301, 1980.
6. Rosenblum P et al: Hereditary Fuchs' dystrophy, *Am J Ophthalmol* 90:455, 1980.
7. Magovern M et al: Inheritance of Fuchs' combined dystrophy, *Ophthalmology* 86:1897, 1979.
8. Buxton JN et al: Tonography in cornea guttata: a preliminary study, *Arch Ophthalmol* 77:602, 1967.
9. Roberts CW et al: Endothelial guttata and facility of aqueous outflow, *Cornea* 3:5, 1984.
10. Krachmer JH et al: Corneal endothelial dystrophy, *Arch Ophthalmol* 96:2036, 1978.
11. Pitts JF, Jay JL: The association of Fuchs's corneal endothelial dystrophy with axial hypermetropia, shallow anterior chamber, and angle closure glaucoma, *Br J Ophthalmol* 74:601, 1990.
12. Loewenstein A et al: The association of Fuchs's corneal endothelial dystrophy with angle closure glaucoma, *Br J Ophthalmol* 75:501, 1991.
13. Lipman RM, Rubenstein JB, Torczynski E: Keratoconus and Fuchs' corneal endothelial dystrophy in a patient and her family, *Arch Ophthalmol* 108:993, 1990.
14. Orlin SE et al: Keratoconus associated with corneal endothelial dystrophy, *Cornea* 9:299, 1990.
15. Goar EL: Dystrophy of the corneal endothelium (cornea guttata), with a report of a histological examination, *Am J Ophthalmol* 17:215, 1934.
16. Lorenzetti DW et al: Central cornea guttata: incidence in the general population, *Am J Ophthalmol* 64:1155, 1967.
17. Zeporkes J: Glassy network in the anterior chamber: report of a case, *Arch Ophthalmol* 10:517, 1933.
18. Wolter JR, Larson BF: Pathology of cornea guttata, *Am J Ophthalmol* 48:161, 1959.
19. Forgács J: Stries hyalines rétrocornéennes post-inflammatories en toiles araignées, *Ophthalmologica* 145:301, 1963.
20. Abbott RL et al: Specular microscopic and histologic observations in non-guttate corneal endothelial degeneration, *Ophthalmology* 88:788, 1981.
21. Chi HH, Teng CC, Katzin HM: Histopathology of primary endothelial-epithelial dystrophy of the cornea, *Am J Ophthalmol* 45:518, 1958.
22. Krachmer JH, Schnitzer JI, Fratkin J: Cornea pseudoguttata: a clinical and histopathologic description of endothelial cell edema, *Arch Ophthalmol* 99:1377, 1981.
23. Irvine AR: The role of the endothelium in bullous keratopathy, *Arch Ophthalmol* 56:338, 1956.
24. Iwamoto T, DeVoe AG: Electron microscopic studies on Fuchs' combined dystrophy: I. Posterior portion of the cornea, *Invest Ophthalmol* 10:9, 1971.
25. Hogan MJ, Wood I, Fine M: Fuchs' endothelial dystrophy of the cornea, *Am J Ophthalmol* 78:363, 1974.
26. Grayson M: The nature of hereditary deep polymorphous dystrophy of the cornea: its association with iris and anterior chamber dysgenesis, *Trans Am Ophthalmol Soc* 72:516, 1974.
27. Waring GO: Posterior collagenous layer (PCL) of the cornea, *Arch Ophthalmol* 100:122, 1982.
28. Bourne WM, Johnson DH, Campbell RJ: The ultrastructure of Descemet's membrane: III. Fuchs' dystrophy, *Arch Ophthalmol* 100:1952, 1982.
29. Kenney MC et al: Characterization of the Descemet's membrane isolated from Fuchs' endothelial dystrophy corneas, *Exp Eye Res* 39:267, 1984.
30. Robinson MR, Streeten BW: Energy dispersive x-ray analysis of the cornea: application to paraffin sections of normal and diseased cornea, *Arch Ophthalmol* 102:1678, 1984.
31. Bahn CF et al: Classification of corneal endothelial disorders based on neural crest origin, *Ophthalmology* 91:558, 1984.
32. Kuwabara T, Quevedo AR, Logan DC: An experimental study of dichloroethane poisoning, *Arch Ophthalmol* 79:321, 1968.

33. Thomann U, Meier-Gibbons F, Schipper I: Phototherapeutic keratectomy for bullous keratopathy, *Br J Ophthalmol* 79:335, 1995.

34. Olson RJ et al: Visual results after penetrating keratoplasty for aphakic bullous keratopathy and Fuchs' dystrophy, *Am J Ophthalmol* 88:1000, 1979.

35. Price FW, Whitson WE, Marks RG: Graft survival in four common groups of patients undergoing penetrating keratoplasty, *Ophthalmology* 98:322, 1991.

36. Stocker FW, Irish A: Fate of successful corneal graft in Fuchs' endothelial dystrophy, *Am J Ophthalmol* 68:820, 1969.

37. Olson T, Ehlers N, Favini E: Long-term results of corneal grafting in Fuchs' endothelial dystrophy, *Acta Ophthalmol (Copenh)* 62:445, 1984.

38. Aquavella JV, Shaw EL, Rao GN: Intraocular lens implantation combined with penetrating keratoplasty, *Ophthalmic Surg* 8:113, 1977.

39. Lindstrom RL, Harris WS, Doughman DJ: Combined penetrating keratoplasty, extracapsular cataract extraction, and posterior chamber intraocular lens implantation, *Am Intraocular Implant Soc J* 7:130, 1981.

40. Binder PS: Intraocular lens powers used in the triple procedure, *Ophthalmology* 92:1561, 1985.

41. Busin M et al: Combined penetrating keratoplasty, extracapsular cataract extraction, and posterior chamber intraocular lens implantation, *Ophthalmic Surg* 18:272, 1987.

42. Arentsen JJ, Laibson PR: Penetrating keratoplasty and cataract extraction: combined vs nonsimultaneous surgery, *Arch Ophthalmol* 96:75, 1978.

43. Miller CA, Krachmer JH: *Endothelial dystrophies.* In Kaufman HE et al, editors: *The cornea,* New York, 1988, Churchill Livingstone.

44. Martin TP et al: Cataract formation and cataract extraction after penetrating keratoplasty, *Ophthalmology* 101:113, 1994.

45. Payant JA et al: Cataract formation following corneal transplantation in eyes with Fuchs' endothelial dystrophy, *Cornea* 9:286, 1990.

46. Pietruschka G: Ueber eine Familiäre Endothel-dystrophie der Hornhaut (in Kombination met Glaukom, Vitiligo, und Otosklerose), *Klin Monatsbl Augenheilkd* 136:794, 1960.

47. Maumenee AE: Congenital hereditary corneal dystrophy, *Am J Ophthalmol* 50:1114, 1960.

48. Pearce WG, Tripathi RC, Morgan G: Congenital endothelial corneal dystrophy: clinical, pathological and genetic study, *Br J Ophthalmol* 53:477, 1969.

49. Harboyan G et al: Congenital corneal hereditary dystrophy: progressive sensorineural deafness in a family, *Arch Ophthalmol* 85:27, 1971.

50. Kanai A: Further electron microscopic study of hereditary corneal edema, *Invest Ophthalmol* 10:545, 1971.

51. Kanai A et al: Electron microscopic study of hereditary corneal edema, *Invest Ophthalmol* 2:197, 1971.

52. Judisch GF, Maumenee IH: Clinical differentiation of recessive congenital hereditary endothelial dystrophy and dominant hereditary endothelial dystrophy, *Am J Ophthalmol* 85:606, 1978.

53. Waring GO, Rodrigues MM, Laibson PR: Corneal dystrophies: II. Endothelial dystrophies, *Surv Ophthalmol* 23:147, 1978.

54. Kirkness CM et al: Congenital hereditary corneal oedema of Maumenee: its clinical features, management, and pathology, *Br J Ophthalmol* 71:130, 1987.

55. Antine BE: Congenital corneal dystrophy, *Am J Ophthalmol* 70:656, 1970.

56. Antine BE: Congenital hereditary corneal dystrophy (CHCD), *South Med J* 63:946, 1970.

57. Antine BE: Histology of congenital hereditary corneal dystrophy, *Am J Ophthalmol* 69:964, 1970.

58. Twomey JM et al: Ocular enlargement following infantile corneal opacification, *Eye* 4:497, 1990.

59. Kenyon KR, Antine B: The pathogenesis of congenital hereditary endothelial dystrophy of the cornea, *Am J Ophthalmol* 72:787, 1971.

60. Kenyon KR, Maumenee AE: The histological and ultrastructural pathology of congenital hereditary corneal dystrophy: a case report, *Invest Ophthalmol* 7:475, 1968.

61. Rodrigues MM et al: Endothelial alterations in congenital corneal dystrophy, *Am J Ophthalmol* 80:678, 1975.

62. Kenyon KR, Maumenee AE: Further studies of congenital hereditary corneal dystrophy of the cornea, *Am J Ophthalmol* 76:419, 1973.

63. Stainer GA et al: Correlative microscopy and tissue culture of congenital hereditary endothelial dystrophy, *Am J Ophthalmol* 93:456, 1982.

64. Sekundo W et al: Immuno-electron labelling of matrix components in congenital hereditary endothelial dystrophy, *Graefes Arch Clin Exp Ophthalmol* 232:337, 1994.

65. Daus W, Volcker HE, Homberg A: Cytology of the corneal endothelium in endothelial dystrophy, *Fortschr Ophthalmol* 87:364, 1990.

66. Mullaney PB et al: Congenital hereditary endothelial dystrophy associated with glaucoma, *Ophthalmology* 102:186, 1995.

67. Pearce WG, Tripathi RC, Morgan G: Congenital endothelial corneal dystrophy: clinical, pathological and genetic study, *Br J Ophthalmol* 53:477, 1969.

68. Levenson JE, Chandler JW, Kaufman HE: Affected asymptomatic relatives in congenital hereditary endothelial dystrophy, *Am J Ophthalmol* 76:976, 1973.

69. Waring GO, Laibson PR: Keratoplasty in infants and children, *Trans Am Acad Ophthalmol Otolaryngol* 83:283, 1977.

70. Stulting RD et al: Penetrating keratoplasty in children, *Ophthalmology* 91:1222, 1984.

71. Dreizen NG, Stulting RD, Cavanagh HD: *Penetrating keratoplasty and cataract surgery in chil-*

dren. In Reinecke R, editor: *Ophthalmology annual: nineteen eighty-seven,* Norwalk, CT, 1987, Appleton-Century Crofts.

72. Sajjake H et al: Results of penetrating keratoplasty in CHED: congenital hereditary endothelial dystrophy, *Cornea* 14:18, 1995.

73. Cibis GW et al: The clinical spectrum of posterior polymorphous dystrophy, *Arch Ophthalmol* 95:1529, 1977.

74. Hogan MJ, Bietti G: Hereditary deep dystrophy of the cornea (polymorphous), *Am J Ophthalmol* 65:777, 1968.

75. Hansen TE: Posterior polymorphous corneal dystrophy, *Acta Ophthalmol (Copenh)* 61:454, 1983.

76. Boruchoff SA, Kuwabara T: Electron microscopy of posterior polymorphous degeneration, *Am J Ophthalmol* 72:879, 1971.

77. Snell AC Jr, Irwin ES: Hereditary deep dystrophy of the cornea, *Am J Ophthalmol* 45:636, 1958.

78. Cibis GW, Tripathi RC: The differential diagnosis of Descemet's tears and posterior polymorphous dystrophy bands, *Ophthalmology* 89:614, 1982.

79. Hirst LW, Waring GO III: Clinical specular microscopy of posterior polymorphous endothelial dystrophy, *Am J Ophthalmol* 95:143, 1983.

80. Mashima Y et al: Specular microscopy of posterior polymorphous endothelial dystrophy, *Ophthalmic Pediatr Genet* 7:101, 1986.

81. Laganowski HC, Sherrard E, Kerr Muir MG: The posterior corneal surface in posterior polymorphous dystrophy: a specular microscopical study, *Cornea* 10:224, 1991.

82. Laganowski HC et al: Distinguishing features of the iridocorneal endothelial syndrome and posterior polymorphous dystrophy: value of endothelial specular microscopy, *Br J Ophthalmol* 75:212, 1991.

83. Pratt AW, Saheb ME, Leblanc R: Posterior polymorphous corneal dystrophy in juvenile glaucoma, *Can J Ophthalmol* 11:180, 1976.

84. Rubenstein RA, Silverman JJ: Hereditary deep dystrophy of the cornea associated with glaucoma and ruptures in Descemet's membrane, *Arch Ophthalmol* 79:123, 1968.

85. Teekhasaenee C et al: Posterior polymorphous dystrophy and Alport syndrome, *Ophthalmology* 98:1207, 1991.

86. Polack FM et al: Scanning electron microscopy of posterior polymorphous corneal dystrophy, *Am J Ophthalmol* 89:575, 1980.

87. Rodrigues MM et al: Glaucoma due to endothelialization of the anterior chamber angle: a comparison of posterior polymorphous dystrophy of the cornea and Chandler's syndrome, *Arch Ophthalmol* 98:688, 1980.

88. Rodrigues MM et al: Epithelialization of the corneal endothelium in posterior polymorphous dystrophy, *Invest Ophthalmol Vis Sci* 19:832, 1980.

89. Tripathi RC, Casey TA, Wise EG: Hereditary

posterior polymorphous dystrophy: an ultrastructural and clinical report, *Trans Ophthalmol Soc UK* 94:211, 1974.

90. Chan CC et al: Similarities between posterior polymorphous and congenital hereditary endothelial dystrophies: a study of 14 buttons of 11 cases, *Cornea* 1:155, 1982.

91. Presberg SE et al: Posterior polymorphous corneal dystrophy, *Cornea* 4:239, 1985.

92. Richardson WP, Hettinger ME: Endothelial and epithelial-like cell formations in a case of posterior polymorphous dystrophy, *Arch Ophthalmol* 103:1520, 1985.

93. McCartney ACE, Kirkness CM: Comparison between posterior polymorphous dystrophy and congenital hereditary endothelial dystrophy of the cornea, *Eye* 2:63, 1988.

94. Krachmer JH: Posterior polymorphous corneal dystrophy: a disease characterized by epithelial-like endothelial cells which influence management and prognosis, *Trans Am Ophthalmol Soc* 83:413, 1985.

95. Rodrigues MM et al: Posterior polymorphous dystrophy of the cornea: cell culture studies, *Exp Eye Res* 33:535, 1981.

96. Tetsumotos K et al: Epithelial transformation of the corneal endothelium in forceps birth-injury-associated keratopathy, *Cornea* 12:65, 1993.

97. Sekundo W et al: An ultrastructural investigation of an early manifestation of the posterior polymorphous dystrophy of the cornea, *Ophthalmology* 101:1422, 1994.

98. de Felice GP et al: Posterior polymorphous dystrophy of the cornea: an ultrastructural study, *Graefes Arch Clin Exp Ophthalmol* 223:265, 1985.

99. Witschel H et al: Posterior polymorphous dystrophy of the cornea (Schlichting): an unusual clinical variant, *Graefes Arch Clin Exp Ophthalmol* 214:15, 1980.

100. Boruchoff SA, Weiner MJ, Albert DM: Recurrence of posterior polymorphous corneal dystrophy after penetrating keratoplasty, *Am J Ophthalmol* 109:323, 1990.

101. Sekundo W et al: Multirecurrence of corneal posterior polymorphous dystrophy: an ultrastructural study, *Cornea* 13:509, 1994.

102. Eagle RC et al: Proliferative endotheliopathy with iris abnormalities: the iridocorneal endothelial syndrome, *Arch Ophthalmol* 97:2104, 1979.

103. Harms C: Einseitige spontane Luckenbildung der iris durch atrophie ohne mechanische Zerrung, *Klin Monatsbl Augenheilkd* 41:522, 1903.

104. Chandler PA: Atrophy of the stroma of the iris: endothelial dystrophy, corneal edema, and glaucoma, *Am J Ophthalmol* 41:607, 1956.

105. Cogan DG, Reese AB: A syndrome of iris nodules, ectopic Descemet's membrane, and unilateral glaucoma, *Arch Ophthalmol* 93:963, 1975.

106. Shields MB, Campbell DG, Simmons RJ: The es-

sential iris atrophies, *Am J Ophthalmol* 85:749, 1978.

107. Setala K, Vannas A: Corneal endothelial cells in essential iris atrophy: a specular microscopic study, *Acta Ophthalmol* 57:1020, 1979.

108. Hirst LW et al: Specular microscopy of iridocorneal endothelial syndrome, *Am J Ophthalmol* 89:1, 1980.

109. Neubauer L, Lund O-E, Leibowitz HM: Specular microscopic appearance of the corneal endothelium in iridocorneal endothelial syndrome, *Arch Ophthalmol* 101:916, 1983.

110. Sherrard ES, Grangoulis MA, Muir MG: On the morphology of cells of posterior cornea in the iridocorneal endothelial syndrome, *Cornea* 10:233, 1991.

111. Bourne WM: Partial corneal involvement in the iridocorneal endothelial syndrome, *Ophthalmology* 94:774, 1982.

112. Bourne WM, Brubaker RF: Progression and regression of partial corneal involvement in the iridocorneal endothelial syndrome, *Trans Am Ophthalmol Soc* 90:201, 1992.

113. Kupfer C et al: The contralateral eye in the iridocorneal endothelial (ICE) syndrome, *Ophthalmology* 90:1343, 1983.

114. Hemady RK et al: Bilateral iridocorneal endothelial syndrome: case report and review of the literature, *Cornea* 13:368, 1994.

115. Campbell DG, Shields MB, Smith TR: The corneal endothelium and the spectrum of essential iris atrophy, *Am J Ophthalmol* 86:317, 1978.

116. Scheie HG, Yanoff M: Iris nevus (Cogan-Reese) syndrome: a cause of unilateral glaucoma, *Arch Ophthalmol* 93:963, 1975.

117. Shields MB et al: Iris nodules in essential iris atrophy, *Arch Ophthalmol* 94:406, 1976.

118. Daicker B, Sturrock G, Guggenheim R: Clinico-pathological correlation in Cogan-Reese syndrome, *Klin Monatsbl Augenheilkd* 180:531, 1982.

119. Shields MB et al: Corneal edema in essential iris atrophy, *Ophthalmology* 86:1533, 1979.

120. Quigley HA, Forster RF: Histopathology of cornea and iris in Chandler's syndrome, *Arch Ophthalmol* 96:1878, 1978.

121. Richardson RM: Corneal decompensation in Chandler's syndrome: a scanning and transmission electron microscopic study, *Arch Ophthalmol* 97:2112, 1979.

122. Patel A et al: Clinicopathologic features of Chandler's syndrome, *Surv Ophthalmol* 27:327, 1983.

123. Hirst LW et al: Epithelial characteristics of the endothelium in Chandler's syndrome, *Invest Ophthalmol Vis Sci* 24:603, 1983.

124. Rodrigues MM, Stulting RD, Waring GO: Clinical, electron microscopic and immunohistochemical study of the corneal endothelium and Descemet's membrane in the irido-corneal endothelial syndrome, *Am J Ophthalmol* 101:16, 1986.

125. Alvarado JG et al: Pathogenesis of Chandler's

126. syndrome, essential iris atrophy and the Cogan-Reese syndrome: I. Alterations of the corneal endothelium, *Invest Ophthalmol Vis Sci* 27:853, 1986.

126. Lee WR, Marshall GE, Kirkness CM: Corneal endothelial cell abnormalities in an early stage of the iridocorneal syndrome, *Br J Ophthalmol* 78:624, 1994.

127. Kramer TR et al: Cytokeratin expression in corneal endothelium in the iridocorneal endothelial syndrome, *Invest Ophthalmol Vis Sci* 33:3581, 1992.

128. Eagle RC et al: The iris nevus (Cogan-Reese) syndrome: light and electron microscopic observations, *Br J Ophthalmol* 64:446, 1980.

129. Radius RL, Herschler J: Histopathology in the iris-nevus (Cogan-Reese) syndrome, *Am J Ophthalmol* 89:780, 1980.

130. Bahn CF et al: Classification of corneal endothelial disorders based on neural crest origin, *Ophthalmology* 91:558, 1984.

131. Alvarado JA et al: Detection of herpes simplex viral DNA in the iridocorneal endothelial syndrome, *Arch Ophthalmol* 112:1601, 1994.

132. Shields MB: *Textbook of glaucoma*, ed 2, Baltimore, 1987, Williams & Wilkins.

133. Buxton JN, Lash RS: Results of penetrating keratoplasty in the iridocorneal endothelial syndrome, *Am J Ophthalmol* 98:297, 1984.

134. Crawford GJ et al: Penetrating keratoplasty in the management of iridocorneal endothelial syndrome, *Cornea* 8:34, 1989.

135. Chang PC et al: Prognosis for penetrating keratoplasty in iridocorneal endothelial syndrome, *Refract Corneal Surg* 9:129, 1993.

136. Debroff BM, Thoft RA: Surgical results of penetrating keratoplasty in essential iris atrophy, *J Refract Corneal Surg* 10:428, 1994.

137. Brown SI, McLean JM: Peripheral corneal edema after cataract extraction: a new clinical entity, *Trans Am Acad Ophthalmol Otolaryngol* 73:465, 1969.

138. Brown SI: Peripheral corneal edema after cataract extraction, *Am J Ophthalmol* 70:326, 1970.

139. Charlin R: Peripheral corneal edema after cataract extraction, *Am J Ophthalmol* 99:298, 1985.

140. Lim JI, Lam S, Sugar J: Brown-McLean syndrome, *Arch Ophthalmol* 109:22, 1991.

141. Reed JW et al: Clinical and pathologic findings of aphakic peripheral corneal edema: Brown-McLean syndrome, *Cornea* 11:577, 1992.

142. Vannas A, Ahonen R: Herpetic endothelial keratitis: a case report, *Acta Ophthalmol (Copenh)* 59:296, 1981.

143. Robin JB, Steigner JB, Kaufman HE: Progressive herpetic corneal endotheliitis, *Am J Ophthalmol* 100:336, 1985.

144. Olsen TW et al: Linear endotheliitis, *Am J Ophthalmol* 117:468, 1994.

145. Khodadoust AA, Attarzadeh A: Presumed autoimmune corneal endotheliopathy, *Am J Ophthalmol* 93:718, 1982.

146. Ohashi Y et al: Idiopathic corneal endotheliopathy, *Arch Ophthalmol* 103:1666, 1985.

147. Khodadoust AA et al: Pars planitis and autoimmune endotheliopathy, *Am J Ophthalmol* 102:633, 1986.

148. Sugar A, Smith T: Presumed autoimmune corneal endotheliopathy, *Am J Ophthalmol* 94:689, 1982.

149. Rice RL, Tuberville AW, Wood TO: Endothelial line associated with pseudophakic bullous keratopathy, *Cornea* 4:42, 1986.

150. Ruusuvaara P, Setäläka K: Keratoendotheliitis fugax hereditaria: a clinical and specular microscopic study of a family with dominant inflammatory corneal disease, *Acta Ophthalmol (Copenh)* 65:159, 1987.

Nineteen

Immunologic Disorders

IMMUNOLOGIC CHARACTERISTICS OF THE OCULAR SURFACE

The immunology of the eye is influenced by its unique anatomy and physiology. The surface of the eye is protected by several different mechanisms. Nonimmunologic protective mechanisms include physical protection and removal of foreign material by the lids and tears, the normal bacterial flora, mucus, tear proteins (e.g., lactoferrin and lysozyme), and the barrier function of the epithelium (see Chapter 6). Several current general reviews[1-3] of the immune system provide an overview of the basic mechanisms of immunology.

Conjunctiva

The mucosa of the gastrointestinal, respiratory, and urogenital tracts is associated with lymphoid tissues, which together are referred to as the *mucosal immune system*. These lymphoid tissues are considered a distinct immunologic entity because they exhibit several unique characteristics that distinguish them from the systemic immune system: They contain some mucosa-specific cell types, such as the mucosal mast cell, as well as specialized immunoregulatory cells. The lymphocytes of mucosal follicles are a subpopulation that remains largely confined to mucosal tissues; even after release into the circulation they home to mucosal tissues and often specifically to the organ from which they originated. In some cases the epithelium over the lymphoid tissue is composed of specialized cells that transfer antigens to the lymphocytes and can transform into class II major histocompatibility complex antigen-presenting cells.

The mast cells present in mucosa are distinct from mast cells found in other body tissues. They are important in immediate-type hypersensitivity (ITH) reactions; they contain a num-

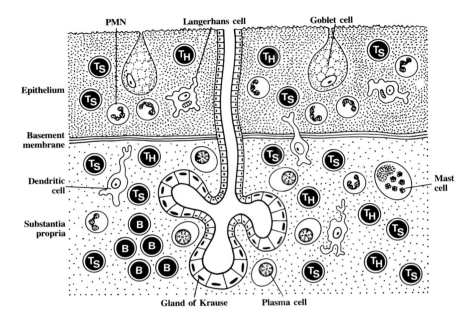

Figure 19-1
Immunologic cell population of the conjunctiva (see text). T_H, Helper T lymphocyte; T_S, suppressor T lymphocyte; B, B lymphocyte. (Modified from Sacks EH et al: *Ophthalmology* 93:1276, 1986.)

ber of inflammatory mediators, such as histamine, proteases, prostaglandins, and leukotrienes, which are released in response to activation of IgE by an allergen. One important difference between mucosal and nonmucosal mast cells is that disodium cromoglycate (cromolyn) inhibits the release of inflammatory mediators by mucosal mast cells but not by nonmucosal mast cells.

The lymphocyte population of the conjunctiva may be analogous to other mucosa-associated lymphoid tissue, such as gut-associated lymphoid tissue and bronchus-associated lymphoid tissue.[4] In one immunohistologic study, lymphocytes bearing a mucosa-specific antigen (human mucosal lymphocyte-1) were found in the conjunctiva, limbus, and lacrimal gland.[5] In another study,[6] however, lymphoid tissue with morphologic and immunophenotypic features of mucosa-associated lymphoid tissue was seen in the forniceal conjunctiva of only 31% of specimens obtained at autopsy.

Lymphocytes are interspersed in the epithelial layer and form a distinct layer within the substantia propria (Fig. 19-1). Those in the epithelium are mainly cytotoxic-suppressor T cells, and a nearly equal proportion of cytotoxic-suppressor and helper-inducer T cells is found in the substantia propria.[7] A smaller population of B cells is present in the substantia pro-

pria; these are arranged in aggregates and localized to the fornices. This distribution of T and B cells is similar to that seen in the intestinal mucosa.[8]

The lymphoid tissue of the conjunctiva is able to acquire and process antigens. After interaction of the lymphocytes with antigen the activated lymphoblasts are thought to travel to the local lymph nodes, the preauricular and submandibular nodes. From there they are probably released into the blood, and through an unknown mechanism migrate back to the ocular tissues and, to a lesser extent, to other mucosal tissue. Antibody production appears to occur first in the regional lymph nodes and then travel via the circulation to the eye.[9] Once the lymphocytes sensitized to the original antigen travel to the ocular tissue, local antibody production occurs.[10]

Mast cells are also present in the substantia propria, but they are seen in the epithelium only in disease states, such as vernal keratoconjunctivitis and giant papillary conjunctivitis. Small numbers of neutrophils may be present in the epithelium and substantia propria, but eosinophils and basophils are not found in normal conjunctiva. Langerhans' cells, which function as antigen-presenting cells, are found in large numbers in the epithelium. They are most plentiful in the bulbar and forniceal conjunctiva. Dendritic antigen-presenting cells are present in the substantia propria.

Lacrimal Tissue

The lacrimal gland and accessory lacrimal glands also belong to the mucosa-associated lymphoid tissue system. Their chief contribution appears to be the production of secretory IgA, which is released into the tears. IgA-producing plasma cells are found in the lymphoid aggregates associated with the intralobular ducts, both in the main and accessory lacrimal glands. These cells produce J-linked dimeric IgA, which is taken up by the overlying acinar cells, bound to a secretory component, and released into the gland lumen. Secretory IgA is relatively resistant to proteolysis and is a relatively poor activator of complement (possibly to decrease the inflammatory response and lessen damage to the epithelial surface). IgA appears to be important in protecting against microbial infection by promoting microbial phagocytosis, inhibiting microbial binding to surface epithelium, interfering with bacterial exotoxins, and enhancing antibody-dependent cell-mediated cytotoxicity.

Cornea

Although the cornea is normally devoid of blood vessels, lymphatics, and inflammatory cells, a number of immunologically active cells and substances are present in the cornea. Immunoglobulins and complement components are present, probably through diffusion from the limbal vessels. C3, C4, and C5 are found throughout the corneal stroma; but the larger C1q molecule is localized to the corneal periphery.[11] IgG and IgA are also present throughout the stroma, but at levels much lower than in the serum.[12] The much larger IgM is found only in the peripheral cornea. Langerhans' cells, which are antigen-presenting cells, are found in the corneal epithelium; their density is greatest at the limbus and decreases markedly toward the central cornea.[13]

The cornea enjoys a relative "immune privilege," meaning that foreign antigens, such as a corneal graft, are tolerated much more readily in the cornea than at other sites, partly because of the absence from the cornea of blood vessels and lymphatics, impairing both the afferent and efferent limbs of the immune system. It may also be related to the relative lack of antigen-presenting cells, or the development of anterior chamber–associated immune deviation (ACAID) (see next section).

In pathologic states vascularization of the cornea can occur and is accompanied by the development of lymphoid channels and an increase in the number of Langerhans' cells. Their presence diminishes the relative immune privilege of the cornea.

Anterior Chamber

The anterior chamber also appears to enjoy a relative immune privilege. When certain foreign antigens are introduced into the anterior chamber, a selective suppression of delayed-type hypersensitivity (DTH) occurs (also referred to as ACAID).[14] Systemic production of antigen-specific antibodies and cytotoxic T cells appears to be normal. Suppression of DTH is mediated by the induction of antigen-specific suppressor T cells.[15-17]

Development of ACAID may influence the ability of the immune system to respond to virus or tumor in the anterior chamber or to corneal allografts. It has been hypothesized that DTH is selectively suppressed to avoid the amount of "innocent bystander" tissue destruction that often accompanies it.

DISORDERS OF IMMUNE-MEDIATED INJURY

Mechanisms of Immune-Mediated Injury (Hypersensitivity Responses)

The immune response can cause injury to the host if it is excessive or inappropriate. Such reactions are called *hypersensitivity reactions,* and four different mechanisms have been described by Gell et al.[18] Type I, called *anaphylaxis* or *immediate hypersensitivity,* involves the reaction of antigen (allergen) with IgE (and possible IgG4) antibody bound to mast cells or circulating basophils. This reaction leads to the release of inflammatory mediators, such as histamine, serotonin, heparin, leukotrienes, prostaglandins, and proteases from the mast cells or basophils. Type II, called *cytotoxic hypersensitivity,* involves formation of antibodies directed against antigens present on cells. Once bound to the cells the antibodies can activate complement, stimulate mediator release and/or phagocytosis by macrophages and other leukocytes, or activate killer cells. Type III, called *immune complex hypersensitivity,* occurs when circulating antigen-antibody complexes become deposited in tissues, where they activate complement, cause platelet aggregation, and stimulate mediator release and/or phagocytosis by macrophages and other leukocytes. In Type IV, or *cell-mediated hypersensitivity,* antigen-specific lymphocytes are stimulated by contact with macrophage-bound antigen. The lymphocytes release lymphokines, which attract and stimulate other mononuclear cells and may play a role in direct cytotoxicity. In some cases, the T lymphocytes transform into blast cells, which can kill cells bearing the sensitizing antigen.

With the knowledge that has been acquired about the interaction between different cells in the immune system, it has become apparent that this classification is an oversimplification. In reality there is a great deal of overlap between antibody-mediated and cell-mediated mechanisms. For example, in asthma, considered a form of ITH involving reaction of allergen with IgE bound to pulmonary mast cells, T cells were found to have a strong influence on production of IgE antibodies and the inflammatory response to activated mast cells. Therefore, it is better to examine the specific defects in immune regulation that occur in each disease.

Approaches to Treatment

Although our knowledge of the processes involved in these types of reactions has become much more sophisticated, the means of treatment remain largely limited to generalized immunosuppression with corticosteroids or other immunosuppressive agents. Cyclosporine and FK-506 are the only exceptions to this practice because they act primarily on T cells and T cell–produced mediators, although they appear to have some direct B-cell activity.

Corticosteroids

Corticosteroids have both immunosuppressive and antiinflammatory effects. The mechanism of their immunosuppressive action is poorly understood, but they appear to exert direct effects on all inflammatory cells. Corticosteroids bind to intracytoplasmic receptors in target cells, leading to multiple intracellular changes. One of these is the production of lipomodulin, a protein that inhibits release of arachidonic acid, blocking both the cyclooxygenase and lipoxygenase pathways of prostaglandin formation. Corticosteroids increase the intracellular levels of cAMP, diminishing the release of inflammatory mediators from mast cells and basophils. Corticosteroids have a broad range of other effects on the immune system, including decreases in: vascular permeability; neutrophil chemotaxis; the number of circulating lymphocytes, eosinophils, and macrophages; lymphocyte proliferation; synthesis or release of prostaglandins, plasminogen activator, lymphokines,

and monokines; the movement of antigen-antibody complexes across basement membranes; and cidal activity by macrophages.

In most cases, short-acting corticosteroids, such as prednisone or prednisolone, are used for immune-mediated diseases. The initial dose is usually 1 mg/kg/day. Because the circulating half-life of these agents is less than 2 hours, maximum immunosuppression is achieved with divided-dose therapy, such as four times daily.[19] However, this regimen is also more likely to induce adverse effects. Therefore, as disease activity subsides the regimen is gradually consolidated to a single daily dose, usually over a period of less than 3 weeks. Once the patient's condition is clinically improved and stable, an attempt can be made to switch to an alternate-day regimen, because this lessens the risk of opportunistic infections. This is gradually tapered as disease activity and patient tolerance allow.

High-dose intravenous pulses of methylprednisolone can sometimes achieve greater immunosuppressive effects. These are indicated for acute graft rejection, a flare in disease activity in a patient already receiving corticosteroids, for disease exacerbation in a patient who has experienced unacceptable corticosteroid side effects, and for rapidly progressive, fulminant disease. Five hundred milligrams to 1 g of intravenous methylprednisolone is given daily for 3 days, once monthly.

Cytotoxic Agents

Cytotoxic agents interfere with the synthesis of proteins and nucleic acids, inhibiting cell replication and preferentially killing dividing cells; therefore, they kill B and T cells that are stimulated to divide. However, this is probably not the only mechanism for their action. Alkylating agents such as cyclophosphamide and chlorambucil alkylate the DNA of both resting and dividing cells, resulting in cross-linkage of double-stranded DNA and leading to cell death during mitosis. Cyclophosphamide also suppresses a variety of leukocyte functions, including antibody formation, soluble mediator production, monocyte and macrophage production, and cutaneous delayed hypersensitivity.

Cyclophosphamide is usually initiated at 2 mg/kg/day as a single oral dose. A clinical response is usually noted within 2 to 3 weeks, and the dose is adjusted according to the white blood cell count. In most conditions an optimal therapeutic response can be seen without lowering the total leukocyte count below 3000.[20] If no response is observed after 2 to 3 weeks, the daily dose is increased by 25 mg and continued for another 2 weeks. Adjustments are made until a clinical response is achieved or leukopenia or other toxicity appears. Complications include bone marrow toxicity, hemorrhagic cystitis, bladder malignancy, infertility, hepatotoxicity, leukemia, and lymphoma.

Purine analogs such as azathioprine and mercaptopurine inhibit DNA synthesis by interfering with purine metabolism. They primarily destroy proliferating rather than resting lymphocytes, making them less potent immunosuppressive agents than cyclophosphamide. Azathioprine inhibits antibody production, but less than cyclophosphamide, and has no effect on soluble mediator production or release. The therapeutic protocol for azathioprine is similar to that for cyclophosphamide. A clinical response is generally seen within 3 to 4 weeks. Bone marrow suppression, hepatitis, stomatitis, and lymphoreticular and other neoplasms can be seen.

Folic acid analogs such as methotrexate impair DNA synthesis by inhibiting the formation of folic acid, which is important in the synthesis of thymidine. Methotrexate also inhibits neutrophil 5-lipoxygenase, reducing the generation of leukotrienes. Methotrexate is the most commonly used cytotoxic drug for rheumatoid arthritis. At low doses (12.5 mg/week) it has a relatively low frequency and severity of adverse effects. It can be effective for some patients with ocular inflammatory disease who do not respond to or are intolerant to corticosteroid therapy.[21] Methotrexate has also been shown to be effective in some patients with less aggressive forms of Wegener's granulomatosis.[22] Treatment is usually begun at 5 mg weekly, increasing gradually until a dose of 10 to 20 mg per week is attained. Methotrexate toxicities include bone marrow suppression, hepatitis, stomatitis, dermatitis, nausea, vomiting, and diarrhea.

The use of these agents should be undertaken only in conjunction with someone who is familiar with them, such as an oncologist, and with careful monitoring of their systemic effects.

Cyclosporine

Cyclosporine is a potent immunosuppressive agent that relatively selectively suppresses T-cell function. It appears to act by interfering with the activation of T cells. Cyclosporine inhibits T-cell proliferation, production of cytokines, mast cell degranulation, and the proliferation, function, and interaction of various other immunocompetent cells. It appears to bind an intracellular peptide known as *cyclophilin,* which is involved in the regulation of transcriptional activation of lymphokine genes.[23] Cyclosporine also has an effect on humoral immunity via indirect and direct inhibition of B cells and inhibits monocyte production of tumor necrosis factor-α. Cyclosporine has been used primarily in organ transplantation, and some efficacy has also been reported in autoimmune disease, primarily rheumatoid arthritis. The immunosuppressive dose is 10 to 20 mg/kg/day, which produces serum levels of 100 to 400 ng/ml. Treatment is usually initiated at this dose and is gradually tapered to a maintenance dose of 4 to 8 mg/kg/day.[24] Toxic effects include nephrotoxicity, hepatotoxicity, reactivation of latent viral infections, and lymphomas.

Systemic treatment has been used in a variety of ocular inflammatory disorders, including scleritis,[25] uveitis,[26] Behçet's syndrome, and prevention of graft rejection. However, significant side effects, particularly nephrotoxicity, limit its use. Topical administration of cyclosporine (2%) has also been reported to be effective in inflammatory diseases of the anterior segment, including vernal keratoconjunctivitis,[27] ligneous conjunctivitis,[28] scleritis,[29] Mooren's ulcer,[30] rheumatoid corneal ulceration,[31-34] and high-risk keratoplasty.[35-37] In one report topical cyclosporine appeared to be most effective in cases of atopic and vernal conjunctivitis and least effective for scleritis and cicatricial pemphigoid.[37]

FK-506 is a macrolide antibiotic derived from *Streptomyces* spp. that is more potent than cyclosporine but appears to act through a similar mechanism.[38] FK-506 inhibits T-cell proliferation and suppresses cytokine production. The toxicity appears to be similar to that seen with cyclosporine. Experience with systemic immune disease has been limited. One study reported a beneficial effect in some patients with ocular inflammatory disease.[39]

Diseases of Immediate-Type Hypersensitivity

Diseases with ITH, such as allergic conjunctivitis, vernal keratoconjunctivitis, atopic dermatitis with keratoconjunctivitis, and giant papillary conjunctivitis, are discussed in Chapter 8.

Systemic Lupus Erythematosus

Systemic lupus erythematosus (SLE) is a chronic multisystem disease related to immunologic dysfunction and characterized by the production of autoantibodies. It is seen more fre-

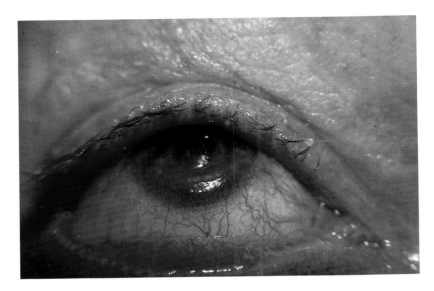

Figure 19-2
Noninfiltrative marginal melt of cornea seen in a case of lupus erythematosus. The eye is also dry, with a lusterless appearance.

quently in women, with the peak age of onset in the twenties to thirties.

Pathogenesis

Systemic lupus erythematosus appears to result from a dysfunction in immunoregulation: Impaired suppressor T-cell function allows for production of autoantibodies, such as antinuclear antibodies, anticell membrane antibodies, and antithyroid antibodies. Immune complexes are formed that become deposited in many tissues, causing local inflammation and damage (a type III hypersensitivity reaction). Double-stranded DNA autoantibodies are highly specific for SLE and correlate with disease activity. Ribosomal P, proliferating cell nuclear antigen, and Sm (to uridine-rich RNA molecules) autoantibodies are fairly specific for SLE but do not correlate with disease activity. Production of phospholipid antibodies correlates with thrombotic complications.[40]

A similar condition can develop in patients taking certain drugs, such as hydralazine, procainamide, isoniazid, methyldopa, and hydantoins, through production of autoantibodies.

Clinical Manifestations

The most common cutaneous feature of SLE is an erythematous rash, which can appear on the nose and cheeks in a "butterfly" distribution and on the neck and extremities, especially the tips and dorsa of the fingers, palms, and areas of skin above the elbows. Discoid rashes, alope-

cia, and mucosal ulcers can also be seen. Other findings include arthritis, polyarthralgia, pleuritis, pericarditis, myocarditis, lymphadenopathy, splenomegaly, nephritis, and hematologic and neurologic disease.

The most common findings in the eye involve the retina: cotton-wool spots, retinal hemorrhages, and edema of the retina and disc, all probably related to a retinal vasculitis. Lupus anticoagulants and antiphospholipid antibodies are much more frequent in patients with thrombotic disease, in the retina as well as in other tissues.[41] The lids may exhibit telangiectasia just above the lid margins. Episcleritis or scleritis can occur and can be the presenting sign of the disease.[42] Necrotizing scleritis is less common than in other systemic vasculitic diseases.[43] Chemosis can also occur as a presenting sign of the disease.[44] Anterior uveitis can also be seen, usually in association with scleritis.

Keratoconjunctivitis sicca has been reported as common in SLE,[45,46] but Sjögren's syndrome is relatively rare and usually mild.[47] Patients also exhibit punctate keratitis unrelated to dryness.[48,49] Interstitial keratitis[50,51] and quiet, relatively noninfiltrated marginal melts (Fig. 19-2) can be seen. Infiltrative lesions also occur and respond to topical steroid therapy (Fig. 19-3).

Discoid Lupus Erythematosus

Discoid lupus erythematosus (DLE) refers to the presence of characteristic skin lesions that may be seen either in isolation or in association with

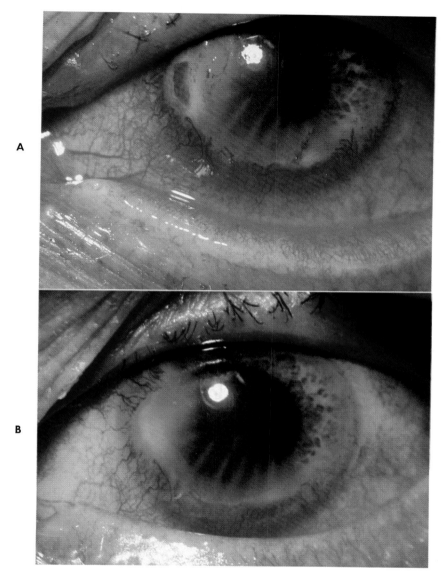

Figure 19-3
A, Infiltrative marginal melt in a case of lupus erythematosus. **B,** Its response to topical steroid medication.

SLE. The lesions are sharply demarcated, raised, erythematous, and scaly and may exhibit telangiectasia and follicular plugging. Central scarring produces depigmentation and permanent loss of appendages. The lesions can affect any part of the body but are most common in light-exposed areas, especially the face and scalp. Approximately 5% of patients with DLE progress to SLE; however, 20% of patients with SLE have DLE lesions. Immunoglobulin, complement, and a mononuclear infiltrate are present at the dermal-epidermal junction in involved areas.

Discoid lupus erythematosus skin lesions may affect the eyelid skin (Fig. 19-4).[52] The lesions can extend over the lid margins and into the conjunctival sac. Conjunctival scarring and lid margin distortion can result.[42,53] One patient presented with chronic conjunctivitis without lid involvement.[54]

Superficial punctate keratitis, recurrent epithelial erosions, neovascularization, and mar-

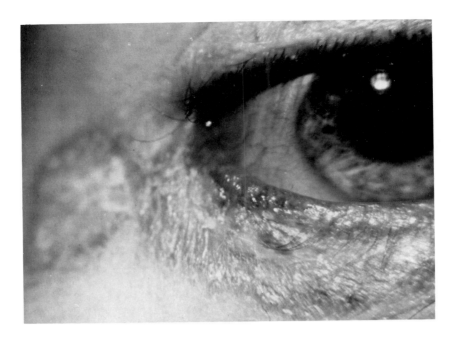

Figure 19-4
Discoid lupus. (From Grayson M, Keates RH: *Manual of diseases of the cornea,* Boston, 1969, Little, Brown & Co.)

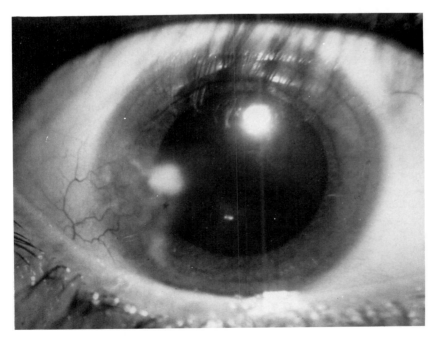

Figure 19-5
Scarring and vascularization of the cornea occur occasionally in discoid lupus. (From Grayson M, Keates RH: *Manual of diseases of the cornea,* Boston, 1969, Little, Brown & Co.)

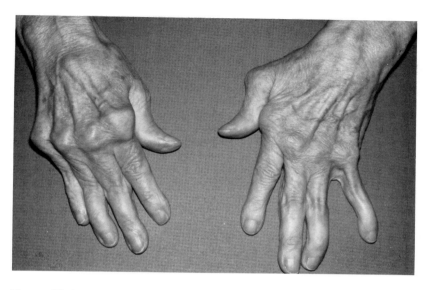

Figure 19-6
Characteristic appearance of the hands in rheumatoid arthritis.

ginal corneal infiltrates occasionally occur[54-57] (Fig. 19-5). The inferior, light-exposed portion of the cornea is more affected. In one patient the ocular lesions responded to systemic treatment with quinacrine hydrochloride.[56] Two other patients responded to topical corticosteroid therapy.[57]

Rheumatoid Arthritis

Rheumatoid arthritis is a multisystem, inflammatory autoimmune disorder that primarily affects the joints. It is found more frequently in women, with an average age of onset of 30 to 40 years. The onset of the arthritis is usually gradual, but acute, fulminant cases can occur. The small joints of the hands and feet are most commonly involved, followed by involvement of the wrists, elbows, ankles, knees, and hips. Joint inflammation is characterized by morning stiffness, pain, and swelling. With time characteristic joint deformities develop (Fig. 19-6). Many extraarticular manifestations can be seen, and their presence correlates with the chronicity and severity of the articular disease. Affected tissues include the skin, lungs, heart, lymphatic system, peripheral nervous system, and eye. A generalized vasculitis can occur, manifested by peripheral neuropathy, cutaneous lesions, and gastrointestinal ulcers.

Pathogenesis

There is a high prevalence of human leukocyte antigen–DR4 in rheumatoid arthritis, mainly subtypes Dw4 and Dw14. It is likely that every patient with rheumatoid arthritis shares a common epitope of Dr β-chains, but only a small percentage of individuals with these epitopes develop rheumatoid arthritis.[58]

Rheumatoid arthritis appears to be caused by a chronic T-lymphocyte and macrophage-dependent response to foreign antigens or autoantigens present in synovial tissue. Articular inflammation results from the production of cytokines and other inflammatory mediators by activated T lymphocytes and macrophages. Circulating cytokines may play a role in many of the extraarticular manifestations of rheumatoid arthritis. IgG and IgM antiimmunoglobulin antibodies are formed (rheumatoid factors); these react with immunoglobulins, forming immune complexes. Immune complexes are often found in serum, joints, and other tissues; and although they can contribute to the disease, they are probably not the primary cause. However, those patients with rheumatoid factors have a worse prognosis.

Diagnosis

The diagnosis of rheumatoid arthritis is primarily clinical. No tests are specific for rheumatoid arthritis. Diagnostic criteria include symptoms and signs of typical joint disease, the presence of subcutaneous nodules, demonstration of serum rheumatoid factor, characteristic histologic changes in synovium and subcutaneous nodules, and a poor mucin precipitate from synovial fluid.[59] Other inflammatory processes must be excluded. In a majority of patients the disease manifests characteristic clinical features within 1 to 2 years of onset.

Rheumatoid factors are found in more than two thirds of adults with the disease. However, they are not specific for rheumatoid arthritis; 10% to 20% of adults over 65 years of age have a positive test, and rheumatoid factor may be seen in many other inflammatory diseases, such as SLE, Sjögren's syndrome, sarcoidosis, hepatitis, syphilis, and malaria. The erythrocyte sedimentation rate is increased in nearly all patients with active rheumatoid arthritis. Radiographs of affected joints are usually not helpful in establishing the diagnosis in early disease.

Ocular Complications

The ocular complications usually occur in patients with severe disease, especially those who have other extraarticular complications.[60] The most common ophthalmic finding is keratoconjunctivitis sicca, which occurs in approximately 15% to 25% of patients.[61-63] Xerostomia is also present in some cases (see Sjögren's syndrome, Chapter 14).

Episcleritis and scleritis are commonly seen (see Chapter 20).[43,64-66] They are probably caused by an immune complex vasculitis of the conjunctival or scleral vessels.[66] The scleritis can take any of the typical forms: diffuse anterior, nodular anterior, necrotizing with inflammation, posterior scleritis, or scleromalacia perforans, but diffuse anterior scleritis is the most frequent type. Rheumatoid arthritis is the most common disease associated with scleritis and is present in nearly all cases of scleromalacia perforans.[67] The presence of necrotizing scleritis in a patient with rheumatoid arthritis indicates systemic disease activity and a poor overall prognosis; without aggressive treatment a majority of the patients die within 5 years.[64,68-71]

The most common corneal manifestations of rheumatoid arthritis are those caused by keratitis sicca (see Chapter 14).[61,62] The cornea is also affected in approximately 50% to 70% of patients with scleritis.[60,65] Corneal involvement usually occurs as a direct extension of perilimbal scleritis onto the peripheral cornea (sclerokeratitis). It is seen in 36% to 50% of patients with rheumatoid scleritis.[65,72,73] Watson has divided the corneal changes in scleritis into four types: sclerosing keratitis, acute stromal keratitis, marginal furrowing, and keratolysis; each can occur in rheumatoid arthritis.[66,67] (These types are described in more detail in Chapter 20.) Episcleritis can also be associated with peripheral corneal lesions, most commonly peripheral stromal infiltration and edema.[70]

Peripheral corneal melting can also occur in the absence of scleritis.[72,74] The cornea may show a noninfiltrative, slowly melting lesion either at the limbus or 1 to 2 mm inside the limbus (Fig. 19-7). Infiltrative peripheral corneal lesions also occur (Fig. 19-8). Occasionally the furrows or melting areas perforate (Fig. 19-9). Corneal ulceration and scleritis can occur after cataract extraction.[75,76] Central ulceration is most often related to dryness, while superior marginal ulceration and scleritis are related to vasculitis. The outcome of these cases is often poor.[77,78]

Some of the drugs used in treating rheumatoid arthritis, such as systemic corticosteroids, gold salts, and antimalarials, can produce ocular complications (see Chapter 24). Antimalarial agents, such as hydroxychloroquine sulfate, can cause a whorllike pattern of intraepithelial deposits, resembling the keratopathy of Fabry's disease (verticillate or vortex dystrophy). Lens pigmentation and peripheral corneal infiltration (Fig. 19-10) and ulceration can result from gold therapy.

Progressive Systemic Sclerosis (Scleroderma)

Progressive systemic sclerosis is a multisystem disorder characterized by inflammatory, fibrotic, degenerative, and vascular changes in the skin and in some internal organs, particularly the gastrointestinal tract, lungs, heart, and kidney.[79,80] Women are affected more often than men, with an onset typically in the third or fourth decade. The hallmark of progressive systemic sclerosis is induration of the skin (scleroderma), most commonly over the digits, resulting from collagen deposition in the dermis (Fig. 19-11). Raynaud's phenomenon (present in 90% of cases), arthritis, pulmonary fibrosis, impaired gastrointestinal motility (particularly esophageal), calcinosis, renal failure, and telangiectasia are other manifestations. The pathogenesis is unknown.

Both keratoconjunctivitis sicca[81,82] and conjunctival fornix foreshortening[83,84] occur in the majority of patients. Lid distortions can result from involvement of the skin of the lid, and lid telangiectasias can be seen. Corneal infiltration and vascularization occur rarely (Fig. 19-12).[85] It has been reported that the diagnosis can be made on conjunctival biopsy, even in early cases. Fibrosis around capillaries, in a bandlike pattern, and degranulating mast cells are present.[86]

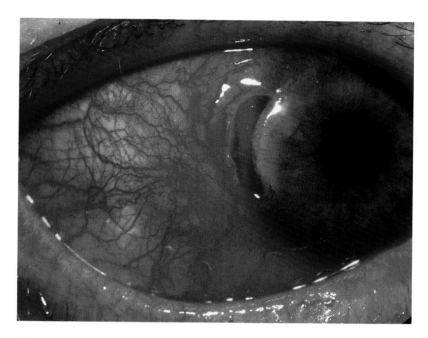

Figure 19-7
Marginal noninfiltrative melting of the limbal tissues in rheumatoid arthritis.

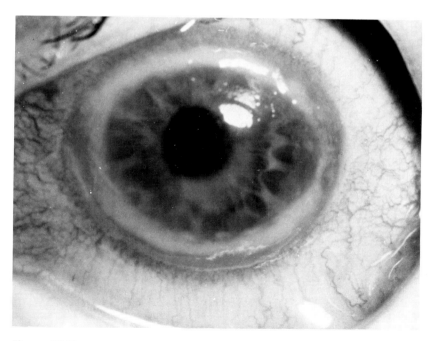

Figure 19-8
Infiltrative circumferential lesion of the cornea in a patient with rheumatoid arthritis.

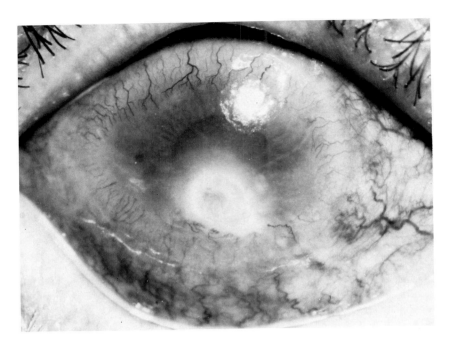

Figure 19-9
Central corneal perforation in rheumatoid arthritis.

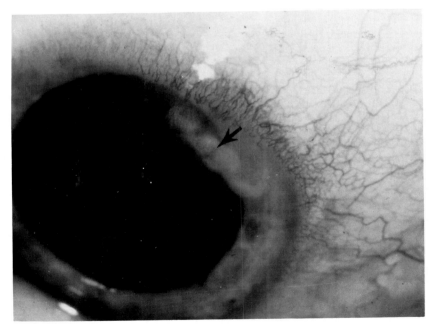

Figure 19-10
Marginal infiltration noted in a patient treated with gold for rheumatoid arthritis (*arrow*).

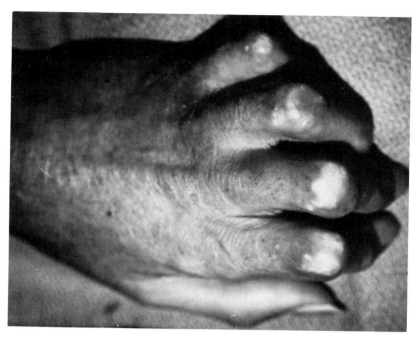

Figure 19-11
Progressive systemic sclerosis. Tightening of skin and contraction of fingers with Raynaud's phenomenon can be seen. (From Grayson M: *The cornea in systemic disease.* In Duane TD, editor: *Clinical ophthalmology,* vol 4, Hagerstown, MD, 1976, Harper & Row. Used with permission of Lippincott-Raven Publishers.)

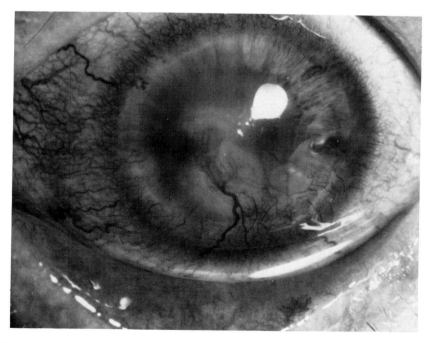

Figure 19-12
Marked injection, vascularization, and infiltration of the cornea in progressive systemic sclerosis. (From Grayson M: *The cornea in systemic disease.* In Duane TD, editor: *Clinical ophthalmology,* vol 4, Hagerstown, MD, 1976, Harper & Row. Used with permission of Lippincott-Raven Publishers.)

Relapsing Polychondritis

This disease, characterized by recurrent inflammation of cartilaginous tissues, occurs equally often in men and women, with onset usually between 40 and 60 years of age. Polychondritis can occur in patients with many connective tissue diseases or vasculitides, including rheumatoid arthritis, Sjögren's syndrome, Wegener's granulomatosis, and systemic lupus erythematosus. The pathogenesis is unknown, but both humeral and cell-mediated immunities are thought to bring about tissue damage. Anticartilage antibodies have been found in patients with polychondritis.[87]

Inflammation in the cartilage of the pinnae of the ears, nose (Fig. 19-13), larynx, trachea, and joints occurs, as does heart valve disease, vasculitis, and glomerulonephritis.[88]

Eye involvement occurs in approximately 60% of patients and includes episcleritis (40% of patients), conjunctivitis (25% of patients), scleritis, keratitis, and iritis.[43,89-91] Episcleritis or conjunctivitis may be the presenting sign of the disease. The scleritis is often not amenable to treatment with systemic steroids and dapsone, so more potent immunosuppressive agents such as azathioprine and cyclophosphamide are required.[73] Corneal involvement usually occurs as a result of adjacent scleritis, but isolated marginal keratitis also can occur.[70,79,92] Peripheral corneal infiltration and noninfiltrated marginal melts can be seen.[93] The latter can extend circumferentially to encircle the cornea and can lead to perforation.

Inflammatory Bowel Disease

Inflammatory bowel diseases are idiopathic disorders in which there is chronic gastrointestinal inflammation. The two forms of inflammatory bowel disease are ulcerative colitis and Crohn's disease. Ulcerative colitis affects only the large bowel and is characterized by ulceration and relatively superficial inflammation. Crohn's disease can affect any portion of the gastrointestinal tract but typically involves the terminal ileum and ascending colon. The inflammation involves the entire intestinal wall and contains granulomas. Extraintestinal inflammation, involving the eyes, skin, joints, liver, or vasculature, has been reported in 25% to 36% of patients.[94]

The pathogenesis of Crohn's disease is unknown. It appears to involve a tendency to mount immunologic responses to one or more antigens of the gastrointestinal mucosa.[95] In early Crohn's disease, focal accumulation of mononuclear cell is seen. Both B- and T-cell responses to mucosal antigens are increased, as are the responses to some bacterial antigens. Antibodies are synthesized that cross-react with normal bowel epithelium, but these probably do not play a major role in the disease process. The mechanism for eye involvement is also unclear. However, a unique peptide was recently identified in the colon, chondrocytes, and nonpigmented epithelial cells of the ciliary processes.[96] Theoretically, autoantibodies against this peptide could cause bowel and joint inflammation and uveitis.

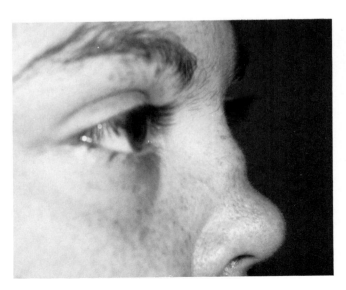

Figure 19-13
Collapse of the nose in relapsing polychondritis.

Crohn's disease may be associated with retinal edema, neuroretinitis, periorbital edema, and recurrent iridocyclitis.[97-99] Episcleritis, scleritis, sclerokeratitis, scleromalacia,[100] and subconjunctival nodules[101] have been reported.[102,103] Ocular inflammation is more likely in patients with inflammation of the colon (not limited to the small bowel), arthritis, or arthralgia.[104] There is little correlation between inflammatory bowel activity and ocular inflammation, with the possible exception of episcleritis.[104,105] Infiltrative marginal ulcerations of the cornea occur. In addition, small white nonfluorescein-staining opacities can be seen in the midperipheral superficial stroma.[103,105a]

Episcleritis and scleritis can also occur in patients with ulcerative colitis. Necrotizing infiltrative marginal corneal melting and marginal infiltrates may be present.[98,99]

Corticosteroids are often not sufficient for control of ocular inflammation. Systemic nonsteroidal antiinflammatory drugs are often helpful in the treatment of uveitis, episcleritis, and scleritis.[106] Cytotoxic immunosuppressive agents, cyclosporine, or FK-506 may be necessary in some cases.

Behçet's Syndrome

Behçet's syndrome is a rare, idiopathic, multisystem inflammatory disease associated with prominent mucocutaneous and ocular findings. The underlying pathologic condition appears to be an inflammatory obliterative vasculitis, particularly involving the venous system.

The hallmarks of Behçet's syndrome are recurrent aphthous (Fig. 19-14) and genital ulceration and uveitis. One can also find pustular skin lesions, polyarthritis, thrombophlebitis, involvement of the central nervous system, and gastrointestinal disturbances. The conjunctiva may exhibit inflammation, ulcerations (Fig. 19-15), edema, and hemorrhages.[107] These lesions may be recurrent. Corneal opacification, vascularization, ulceration, and punctate keratopathy can occur. Cyclosporine appears to be the most effective treatment.[108]

Vasculitis Syndromes

Vasculitis syndromes are a heterogeneous group of disorders characterized by inflammation of blood vessels. They are generally believed to be immune complex diseases, similar to the Arthus reaction.[24] Circulating antigen-antibody complexes formed in a state of relative antigen excess are deposited in blood vessel walls. Once deposited, antibody activates the classic complement cascade. Neutrophils invade the blood vessel wall and release lysosomal enzymes after interaction with the immune complex, resulting in tissue necrosis. The nature of the antigen is not known, but in some cases it appears to be microbial.

Antineutrophil cytoplasmic antibodies, present in many of these diseases, can activate neutrophils, leading to degranulation and stimulation of the respiratory burst, resulting in vascular endothelial injury. Cell-mediated immune mechanisms may also be involved, particularly

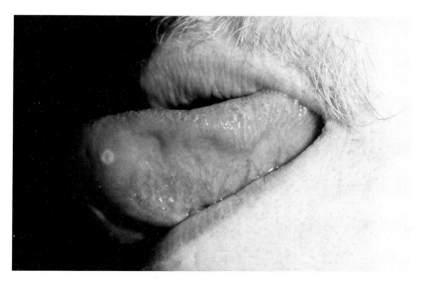

Figure 19-14
Aphthous ulcer of tongue in Behçet's syndrome.

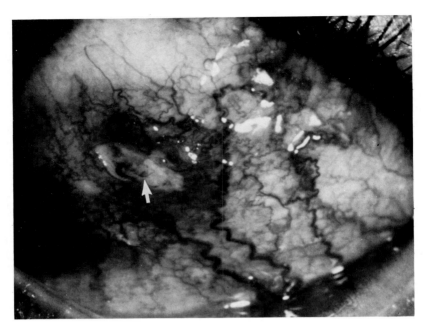

Figure 19-15
Ulceration of the conjunctiva (*arrow*) in Behçet's syndrome.

in those diseases in which granuloma formation is observed (e.g., Wegener's granulomatosis).[109] Antigen-sensitized lymphocytes can interact with circulating antigens. Endothelial cells can also participate in the inflammatory reaction: they can secrete cytokines and express class I and class II major histocompatibility complex antigens and adhesion molecules.

Cranial Arteritis

Cranial arteritis, also referred to as giant cell or temporal arteritis, is an inflammatory disorder of large- and medium-sized arteries, occurring mostly in the elderly. Multiple arteries can be affected, but it characteristically affects branches of the carotid artery, particularly the temporal artery. Ocular findings include ischemic optic neuropathy, central retinal artery occlusion, cranial nerve palsies, uveitis, and scleritis.[110] Although rare, marginal corneal ulceration has been reported in this condition. In addition, both corneal and conjunctival ulceration was seen in one patient.[111]

Polyarteritis Nodosa

Polyarteritis nodosa is a systemic necrotizing vasculitis of small- and medium-sized muscular arteries, particularly the renal and visceral arteries. Men are affected more than twice as often as women, and the average age at onset is 45 years. The cause is unknown, but there is some

evidence that polyarteritis occurs as a complication of hepatitis B infection in some patients.[24]

Because the blood vessels of any organ system of the body can be involved, the systemic manifestations are quite variable. Patients often present with nonspecific signs and symptoms, such as fever, weight loss, weakness, abdominal pain, and myalgia, either alone or in addition to complaints related to dysfunction of a specific organ.

Ophthalmic involvement occurs in approximately 20% of patients, most commonly as choroidal vasculitis.[112] Other findings include choroiditis, retinal vasculitis, optic atrophy, papilledema, exudative retinal detachment, central retinal artery occlusion, iritis, and cranial nerve palsies.[103]

The conjunctiva can be hyperemic and may contain subconjunctival hemorrhages. Pale yellow, waxy, raised, and very friable conjunctival lesions can occur[113]; these are associated with edema and necrosis and a surrounding inflammatory reaction. Nodular episcleritis and nodular, diffuse, or necrotizing scleritis can be seen (Fig. 19-16). The scleritis is nearly always painful and progresses unless control of the systemic disease is achieved.

Melting of the margins of the cornea, with or without infiltration, can be seen. It can appear similar to a Mooren's ulcer and can be the presenting sign of the disease.[114-118] However,

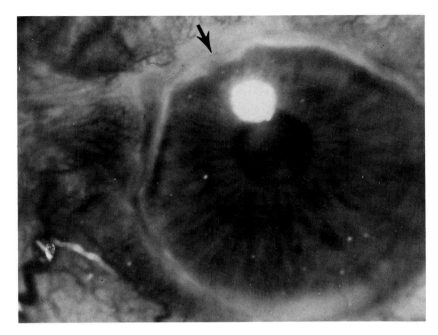

Figure 19-16
Marginal melt in periarteritis (*arrow*).

unlike Mooren's ulcer, in most cases polyarteritis nodosa is associated with an adjacent scleritis. The ulcers can spread circumferentially or centrally and can form a ring ulcer. The keratitis is associated with marked injection of the eye and severe pain. The final result may be scarring, vascularization, or perforation of the globe.

Polyarteritis nodosa is present in approximately 25% of patients with Cogan's syndrome (see below). The diagnosis must be made histopathologically. Biopsy of nodular skin lesions, symptomatic muscle, or the testes is most likely to be diagnostic. The most effective systemic treatment is with a combination of a corticosteroid and cytotoxic immunosuppressive agent.

Antiphospholipid Syndrome

Antiphospholipid antibodies can develop either in association with other autoimmune disorders or without evidence of any other systemic disease, in which case it is called *primary antiphospholipid antibody syndrome*.[119] Conjunctival telangiectases and microaneurysms, episcleritis, and limbal keratitis have been reported in patients with primary antiphospholipid antibody syndrome.[120] Posterior segment abnormalities were present in 15 of 17 patients in one series.[120] These abnormalities included venous tortuosity, optic disk edema, vitreous hemorrhages, cotton-wool spots, serous macular detachment, and vasoocclusive retinopathy. The prevalence of vasoocclusive disease in patients with lupus increases fourfold if antiphospholipid antibody syndrome is present.

Allergic Angiitis and Granulomatosis (Churg-Strauss Syndrome)

Allergic angiitis and granulomatosis is a form of necrotizing systemic vasculitis that is similar to polyarteritis nodosa. The arterial lesions resemble those of polyarteritis, except in allergic angiitis small arteries and veins and capillaries are affected. Also, unlike polyarteritis nodosa, pulmonary involvement is the dominant manifestation. Granulomas and eosinophils are found in affected tissues, and there is a strong association with severe asthma and peripheral eosinophilia. The eosinophil may be the primary mediator of tissue damage.

Ocular complications include conjunctival granulomas,[121,122] episcleritis, and marginal corneal ulceration.[123,124]

Wegener's Granulomatosis

Wegener's granulomatosis is a distinct form of vasculitis that mostly affects the upper and lower respiratory tracts and the renal glomeruli. It can be seen at any age but has a peak incidence in the third and fourth decades. Patients typically present with upper respiratory tract findings, such as recurrent epistaxis, chronic

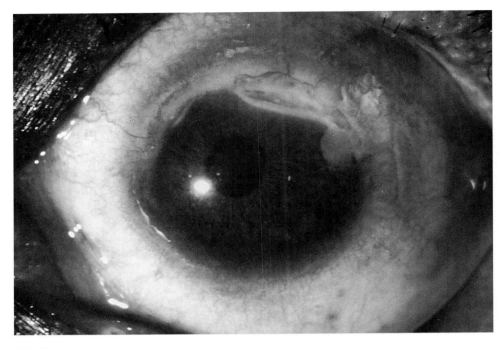

Figure 19-17
Infiltrative peripheral corneal lesion in Wegener's granulomatosis. (Courtesy of Diane Curtin, Pittsburgh, PA.)

rhinorrhea, sinus pain and drainage, or chronic otitis media. Pulmonary involvement may be manifested as chronic cough, hemoptysis, dyspnea, or asymptomatic infiltrates on chest radiography. Many other tissues can be involved, particularly the kidneys, skin, peripheral and central nervous systems, and heart. The main pathologic features are a necrotizing vasculitis of small arteries and veins with granuloma formation and focal and segmental glomerulonephritis.

The pathogenesis of Wegener's granulomatosis is unknown, but it is reasonable to suspect that it occurs as an aberrant immunologic reaction to an antigen that enters through or resides in the upper airway.[125] As in other forms of vasculitis, immune complexes appear to play a role: circulating immune complexes and immune-complex–mediated vasculitis have been observed in some patients. Antibodies to a corneal epithelial antigen have been found in patients with peripheral ulcerative keratitis associated with Wegener's granulomatosis.[126]

Ocular involvement occurs in approximately 60% of patients and is the presenting sign in 16%.[127-129] Both the complete and limited forms of Wegener's granulomatosis can affect the eye. Orbital inflammation, which often occurs as a result of extension from adjacent si-

nus disease, commonly causes proptosis and can be severe enough to cause corneal exposure, restricted motility, and papilledema. Ulcerative lesions of the palpebral conjunctiva can be seen.[130] Retinal vasculitis, uveitis, optic neuropathy, episcleritis, scleritis, and conjunctivitis can also occur.

The cornea in patients with Wegener's granulomatosis may exhibit a necrotizing infiltrative marginal ulcer (Fig. 19-17),[72,131-133] which is usually associated with adjacent nodular or necrotizing scleritis. Localized conjunctivitis or episcleritis is often the initial sign, followed by development of scleritis and adjacent keratitis.[98] Marginal corneal infiltrates occur in nearly all patients with anterior scleritis and correlate with disease activity.[134] Typically, peripheral intrastromal infiltrates form, and, with progression, the overlying epithelium breaks down, leading to formation of a crescentic ulcer. This ulcer extends both centrally and circumferentially and can have an overhanging edge, making the corneal appearance indistinguishable from that of Mooren's ulcer, although the sclera is usually not involved in Mooren's ulcer. Perforation of these ulcers can occur.[135]

Histologically, the corneoscleral lesions are characterized by necrosis and an inflammatory infiltrate with eosinophils, neutrophils, and lymphocytes.[72,114,131,133] Extracellular deposition of eosinophil major basic protein and neutrophil elastase was detected in corneoscleral specimens in one study, supporting the role of eosinophils and neutrophils in the pathogenesis of these lesions.[136] A granulomatous reaction, with plasma cells, lymphocytes, and multinucleated giant cells, is present in the adjacent sclera.

Autoantibodies against neutrophil cytoplasmic determinants (ANCA) are positive in nearly all cases with ocular disease and are specific for Wegener's granulomatosis and related forms of vasculitis.[134,137-139] The erythrocyte sedimentation rate is invariably elevated. The diagnosis of Wegener's granulomatosis is clinicopathologic. It requires demonstration of necrotizing granulomatous vasculitis in biopsy specimens of appropriate tissue in a patient with the clinical findings of upper and lower respiratory tract disease together with evidence of glomerulonephritis. Other vasculitides, particularly allergic angiitis, granulomatosis, and Goodpasture's syndrome, need to be excluded.

Systemic immunosuppression is indicated for treatment of both the ocular and the systemic disease.[116,134] Without institution of appropriate systemic treatment, Wegener's granulomatosis is fatal, usually within a few months of the onset of renal disease. Combined therapy with corticosteroids and cyclophosphamide has achieved long-term survival in over 90% of patients.[22,125,129] However, long-term follow-up has demonstrated that this treatment is associated with high incidences of cancer and disease recurrence.[22,129,140] Low-dose weekly methotrexate can be effective in patients with less aggressive disease.[22,129] Failure of ANCA levels to revert to normal during immunosuppressive therapy was reported to be associated with a greater risk of relapse in one study of patients with ocular disease,[141] but others have not found this to be the case.[24] Oral trimethoprim/sulfamethoxazole may be a safer alternative in patients with limited disease.[142]

Treatment

Systemic Evaluation. Many of the diseases just described have similar external ocular manifestations, including episcleritis, scleritis, and marginal corneal infiltration and ulceration (Table 19-1). The approach to treatment differs, depending on whether the patient has an identified immunologic disease. If a patient with no previous history of immunologic disease presents with scleritis, marginal corneal ulceration or infiltration, or severe or recurrent episcleritis, a systemic evaluation should be performed. The

ophthalmologist should obtain a review of systems. The presence of suggestive symptoms can lead to the diagnosis of latent systemic disease. Many of these symptoms and the diseases with which they are associated are provided in Table 19-2. Patients should also undergo a thorough history and physical examination, preferably by a rheumatologist. Diagnostic testing is directed by the results of this evaluation (Table 19-3). If the results of the examination are not suggestive of a systemic inflammatory disease, further evaluation is generally not informative; however, the following tests are suggested: complete blood count with differential, erythrocyte sedimentation rate, antinuclear antibody titer, rheumatoid factor assay, complete blood count, blood urea nitrogen, creatinine, chest radiography, serum uric acid, serologic test for syphilis, and possibly serum complement levels and biopsy of skin lesions.

Management of Systemic Disease

If the patient is known to have an immunologic disease, such as rheumatoid arthritis, the physician managing the systemic disease should be notified of the ocular involvement and informed that it is a sign of activity of the systemic disease, requiring systemic treatment. Treatment usually entails initiation or enhancement of immunosuppression. All patients with Wegener's granulomatosis or polyarteritis should be treated with cytotoxic immunosuppressive therapy. Foster and Sainz de la Maza[73] also recommend cytotoxic immunosuppressive therapy for patients with rheumatoid arthritis or relapsing polychondritis who develop necrotizing scleritis. Without immunosuppressive therapy these patients have a high mortality. Management of marginal corneal ulceration and infiltration is discussed in the next section. Episcleritis and scleritis are discussed in more detail in the next chapter.

Management of Marginal Corneal Infiltration or Ulceration

Local ocular therapy is usually insufficient for marginal corneal infiltration and ulceration. However, some measures can help to limit corneal damage while waiting for systemic immunosuppression to take effect. Use of topical corticosteroids can lessen corneal infiltration, but in general, they should be applied only when the epithelium is intact. Topical lubrication and bandage contact lenses can help promote epithelial healing, particularly when keratoconjunctivitis sicca is present. Topical cyclosporine 2% has been reported to be effective in a few cases.[31-34]

Table 19-1   Anterior Segment Involvement in Immune-Mediated Diseases

	Lid Disease	Kerato-conjunctivitis Sicca	Conjunctivitis	Conjunctival Scarring	Episcleritis	Scleritis	Marginal Infiltrates	Ulcerative Keratitis
Systemic lupus erythematosus	+	++			+	+	+	+
Discoid lupus erythematosus	++	?+		+			+	+
Rheumatoid arthritis		+++			++	++	+	+
Progressive systemic sclerosis	+	+++		+++			+	
Relapsing polychondritis			++		++	+	+	+
Crohn's disease					++	+	++	+
Ulcerative colitis			+(ulcers)		++	+	++	+
Behçet's syndrome					+	+	?+	+
Polyarteritis nodosa			+(granulomas)		+	+		+
Churg-Strauss syndrome					+	+		
Wegener's granulomatosis			+		+	+	+	+

Table 19-2 Review of Systems Questionnaire for Episcleritis and Scleritis

Manifestations	Associated Systemic Diseases
Skin, hair, and nails	
Rash/vesicles/ulcers	Connective tissue, vasculitic, and infectious diseases, atopy, Ros
Sunburn easily	SLE
Hyper/depigmentation	SLE, leprosy
Loss of hair	SLE, leprosy
Painfully cold fingers	RA, SLE, GCA
Scaling	Reit, PA, atopy
Nail lesions	Reit, PA, vasculitic diseases
Respiratory	
Constant coughing	RA, SLE, AS, RP, Ch-S, Weg, TB, Lyme
Coughing blood	RA, SLE, AS, Weg, TB
Shortness of breath	RA, SLE, AS, RP, Ch-S, Weg, atopy, TB
Asthma attacks	Ch-S, atopy
Pneumonia	SLE, AS, RP, Ch-S, Weg, atopy, TB
Cardiac	
Anginal chest pain	RA, SLE, PAN, GCA
Genitourinary	
Blood in urine	SLE, Reit, RP, PAN, Ch-S, Weg, TB
Urinary discharge	Reit
Pain during urination	Reit
Prostate trouble	AS, Reit, IBD, Ch-S, TB
Testicular pain	PAN, mumps, Lyme
Genital lesions	Reit, Behçet, mumps, TB, Syph
Kidney stones	Gout, IBD
Rheumatological	
Painful joints	Connective tissue and vasculitic diseases, gout, TB, Lyme
Morning stiffness	RA, SLE, AS
Muscle aches	RA, SLE, AS, PAN, GCA, Lyme
Back pain	AS, Reit, PA, IBD
Heel pain	AS, Reit, gout
Big toe pain	Gout, PA
Gastrointestinal	
Abdominal pain	SLE, Reit, IBD, PAN, Ch-S, Behçet
Nausea, vomiting	SLE, IBD, RP, PAN, Cogan
Difficult swallowing	RA, SLE
Blood in stool	IBD, PAN, Ch-S, Behçet
Diarrhea	SLE, Reit, IBD, PAN
Constipation	IBD
Anal lesions	IBD
Neurological	
Headaches	SLE, RP, GCA, mumps, Lyme
Numbness/tingling	Connective tissue, vasculitic, and infectious diseases
Paralysis	Connective tissue, vasculitic, and infectious diseases
Seizures	SLE, RP, PAN, Ch-S, mumps, Lyme
Psychiatric	SLE, Reit, Ch-S, Behçet, GCA, mumps, Lyme
Neuralgia	Leprosy, VZV
Ear	
Deafness	RP, Weg, GCA, Cogan, mumps, Syph
Swollen ear lobes	RP
Ear infections	RP, Weg
Vertigo	RP, Cogan
Noises in ears	RP, Cogan

From Foster CS, Sainz de la Maza: *The sclera,* New York, 1994, Springer-Verlag.
SLE, Systemic lupus erythematosus; RA, Rheumatoid arthritis; GCA, Giant cell arteritis; Reit, Reiter's syndrome; PA, Polyarteritis; AS, Ankylosing spondylitis; RP, Relapsing polychondritis; Ch-S, Churg-Strauss syndrome; Weg, Wegener's granulomatosis; TB, Tuberculosis; IBD, Inflammatory bowel disease; PAN, Polyarteritis nodosa; Lyme, Lyme disease; Behçet, Behçet's syndrome; Syph, Syphilis; Cogan, Cogan's syndrome; VZV, Varicella-zoster virus infection.

Table 19-3   Laboratory Tests for Suspected Systemic Disease[a]

Systemic Disease	Laboratory Test[b]
Noninfectious	
Rheumatoid arthritis	RF, ANA (anti-DNA-histone), CIC, C, Cryog, limb joint X rays, HLA typing
Systemic lupus erythematosus	ANA (anti-dsDNA, anti-Sm), CIC, IgC, C, Cryog, UA
Ankylosing spondylitis	CIC, sacroiliac X ray, HLA typing
Reiter's syndrome	CIC, sacroiliac X ray, UA, HLA typing
Psoriatic arthritis	Limb and sacroiliac X rays
Arthritis and IBD	Limb, sacroiliac, and abdominal X rays
Relapsing polychondritis	CIC, C
Polyarteritis nodosa	HBsAg, Cryog, C, CIC, angiography, UA
Churg-Strauss syndrome	WBC/eosinophil count, IgE, CIC, chest X ray
Wegener's granulomatosis	IgA, IgE, RF, ANCA, CIC, sinus and chest X ray, BUN, Creat clearance, UA
Behçet's disease	CIC, C, HLA, typing
Giant cell arteritis	ESR, CIC, IgG
Cogan's syndrome	CIC, C
Atopy	Eosinophil count, IgE, chest X ray
Gout	Uric acid, limb X ray
Infectious	Serologies

From Foster CS, Sainz de la Maza M: *The sclera*, New York, 1994, Springer-Verlag.
[a]Blood, urine, and X-ray-based tests.
[b]ESR, Erythrocyte sedimentation rate; ANA, anti-nuclear antibodies; anti-dsDNA, antibody to double-stranded DNA; anti-Sm, antibodies to small nuclear ribonucleoproteins—Sm; anti-RNP, antibodies to small nuclear ribonucleoproteins—RNP; CIC, circulating immune complex; IgG, IgA, and IgE, immunoglobulins; C, complement (C3 and C4, as tested by CH50); Cryog, cryoglobulins; RF, rheumatoid factor; HBsAg, hepatitis B surface antigen; WBC, white blood count; ANCA, anti-neutrophil cytoplasmic antibodies; immunofluorescence method; UA, urinalysis; BUN, blood urea nitrogen; Creat, creatinine.

If there is no history of systemic disease and no contraindication to systemic corticosteroids, I treat initially with prednisone (1 mg/kg/day). If the patient has been diagnosed with a systemic inflammatory disease, such as rheumatoid arthritis, the managing physician is contacted and an immediate increase in immunosuppression arranged. In general this regimen allows healing of the ulceration in 1 to 2 weeks. First the perilimbal injection and edema are reduced, and ulceration is slowed or halted; then the epithelium gradually closes over the ulcer bed.

Cytotoxic immunosuppressive agents can also be used in addition to or instead of corticosteroids in patients who require a high maintenance dose of corticosteroids or who do not respond to corticosteroids. Cyclophosphamide or methotrexate are most commonly used.[143] It can take 2 to 3 weeks before the effect of systemic immunosuppression is evident, so the disease must be controlled by other means until that time.

Sometimes this treatment is not sufficient or rapid enough and progressive ulceration occurs. In these cases, or when systemic immunosuppression is not possible, resection of adjacent conjunctiva is often helpful.[144,145] The conjunctiva may be a source of inflammatory cells and destructive enzymes, such as collagenase. Limbal conjunctivectomy is a simple procedure that can be performed in the office with the use of topical anesthetic drops and a subconjunctival injection of 1% lidocaine in the area of the limbal melt. The conjunctiva is excised for 3 to 4 mm from the limbus, extending circumferentially past the margins of the ulceration. The conjunctiva is not sutured.

Application of cyanoacrylate tissue adhesive can also retard ulceration and seal perforations. I use it if the ulceration is approaching Descemet's membrane or is progressing rapidly. After perforation, lamellar or penetrating keratoplasty is often successful in restoring integrity to the globe, but functional vision is achieved much less often.[78] Aggressive management of the disease process, such as by immunosuppression or protection of the ocular surface, is necessary to prevent recurrent corneal melting.

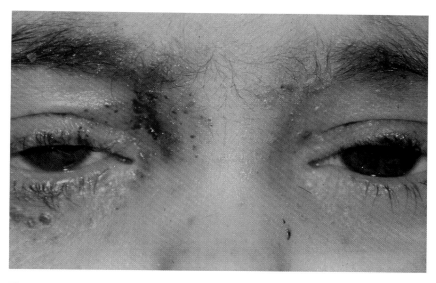

Figure 19-18
Wiskott-Aldrich syndrome with ulcerative lid lesions.

DISORDERS OF THE IMMUNE SYSTEM

Wiskott-Aldrich Syndrome

The classic findings in Wiskott-Aldrich syndrome, an X-linked recessive immune disease, are eczema, thrombocytopenia, and susceptibility to bacterial, viral, fungal, and protozoal infections. Defects in both the cellular and humoral immune systems are present. Most patients die from bleeding or infection. Autoimmune disorders also are common, and more than 20% of patients develop malignancy, most often lymphoma or leukemia.

Although the numbers of lymphocytes are normal, patients cannot mount delayed hypersensitivity responses. Serum IgM is reduced, IgA and IgE are elevated, and catabolism of all immunoglobulins is increased. Antibody production to microbial antigens is reduced, particularly to polysaccharide antigens, such as those present in the capsules of pneumococci.[146] These findings may be related to a deficiency of a cell-membrane glycoprotein normally present on T lymphocytes and platelets.[147]

Conjunctivitis, conjunctival bleeding, necrotizing lid ulcers (Fig. 19-18), blepharitis, and episcleritis can occur. In addition, ulcerative keratitis and chronic or recurrent viral infection can be seen.

Acquired Immune Deficiency Syndrome

Acquired immune deficiency syndrome is an immunodeficiency disease caused by infection with a T-cell lymphotrophic virus (HIV). The major clinical manifestations are related to deficiencies of cell-mediated immunity and include a variety of opportunistic infections and malignancies. Between 40% and 70% of patients with AIDS will develop ocular complications.[148] The most frequent ocular manifestations are retinal microvasculopathy, which is seen as cotton-wool spots, retinal hemorrhages and microaneurysms, and opportunistic infection, especially with cytomegalovirus and *Candida* and *Toxoplasma* spp. Retinal necrosis, optic neuropathy, and other neuroophthalmic disorders are also common.[149]

Anterior segment manifestations of AIDS include herpes zoster or herpes simplex infection, microsporidiosis, molluscum contagiosum, Kaposi's sarcoma, dry eye, and ulcerative keratitis. The incidence of epithelial herpes simplex does not appear to be greater than normal, but the disease is more severe and prolonged, and recurrences may be more frequent.[150] The dendrites are more likely to affect the marginal cornea, and the median healing time is longer than in immunocompetent patients (approximately 3 weeks). Herpes zoster occurs more frequently in patients with AIDS and is often a presenting manifestation.[151-153] The incidences of corneal involvement, uveitis, and postherpetic neuralgia may be higher than in immunocompetent patients.[152] The clinical course of herpes zoster can be more severe and less responsive to antiviral therapy. Prolonged intravenous acyclovir may be required.

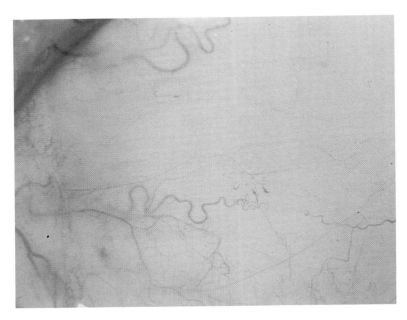

Figure 19-19
Conjunctival vessel tortuosity in multiple myeloma.

Microsporidial infection of the conjunctiva and cornea occurs almost exclusively in AIDS patients. This condition is discussed in Chapter 11. Molluscum contagiosum is common in patients with AIDS and can affect the lid, conjunctiva, and limbus.[154,155] In patients with AIDS, the number of lesions tends to be greater, and they are longer lasting and more resistant to therapy. Molluscum contagiosum is discussed in Chapter 13. Kaposi's sarcoma affects the lids or conjunctiva in 20% to 24% of patient with AIDS.[156] The lids are most commonly affected. Conjunctival lesions are seen most often in the inferior fornix. Kaposi's sarcoma is discussed in Chapter 26.

The incidence of dry eye also seems to be higher in patients with HIV infection; from 12% to 21% of patients are affected.[157] The cause of dry eye is not known. Most cases of ulcerative keratitis in HIV patients are infectious and are associated with typical risk factors, such as contact lens wear, exposure, and intravenous drug use.[158-160] Some cases, however, occur without obvious risk factors. There appears to be a tendency for the clinical course to be more complicated and the infection less responsive to standard treatment.

Drug-induced corneal lipidosis, related to acyclovir and ganciclovir, was observed in two patients with AIDS.[161] Clinically, translucent vacuoles were seen in the corneal epithelium.

Reticular deposits may be seen on the corneal endothelium of patients with cytomegalovirus retinitis.[162]

Multiple Myeloma and Dysproteinemias

Multiple myeloma is a malignant proliferation of plasma cells. It results in bone pain, anemia, bleeding, susceptibility to infection, hypercalcemia, renal failure, neurologic symptoms, amyloidosis, and serum hyperviscosity. Onset is usually between 50 and 70 years of age.

Ocular Manifestations

Lytic lesions of the orbital bones, nerve palsies, papilledema, and visual field defects occur in multiple myeloma.[163] In addition, one may find infiltration of adnexal tissue by myeloma cells, proteinaceous cysts of the nonpigmented ciliary epithelium, and hyperviscosity retinopathy.

Marked tortuosity of the conjunctival vessels, with sludging of the circulation, can result from increased blood viscosity (Fig. 19-19). Crystals can be seen in the conjunctiva, cornea (Fig. 19-20A), and retina (Fig. 19-20B).[164] Fine, punctate or needlelike, multicolored crystals occur in the corneal epithelium or anterior stroma.[32,165,166] A diffuse stromal haze may be noted (Fig. 19-20A). In some cases amorphous gray-white epithelial and subepithelial deposits are seen in the corneal periphery[167-169] that can extend like fingers from the superior cornea. In

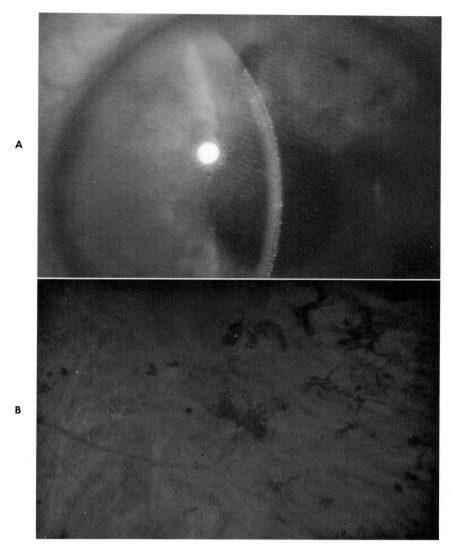

Figure 19-20
Multiple myeloma. **A,** Crystals in corneal epithelium and stromal haze. **B,** Retinal crystals.

most cases vision is only mildly reduced. Crystalline deposition in a vortex pattern was described in one case.[169a]

Histologically, corneal crystals have been found in keratocytes and epithelium.[166,169b] In some cases the deposits are intracellular, whereas in others they are extracellular. The deposits are composed of immunoglobulin-related proteins; immunoperoxidase staining has been most strongly positive for IgG and IgA κ and λ light chains.[169c]

A polychromatic, dustlike deposition of copper can occur in central Descemet's membrane, with sparing of the peripheral cornea. This dep-

osition is also seen in the anterior lens capsule. Both appear to be related to the ability of some myeloma proteins to bind copper.[169d]

Similar changes can be seen in patients with other forms of dysproteinemia, such as benign monoclonal gammopathy[169b,170] (Figs. 19-21 and 19-22) and essential cryoglobulinemia.[168] In addition, patches of myeloma cells can be deposited on the corneal endothelium, and calcific band keratopathy can result from the hypercalcemia often present in multiple myeloma. Dystrophic corneal changes have been reported in multiple myeloma, Waldenström's macroglobulinemia, and cryo-

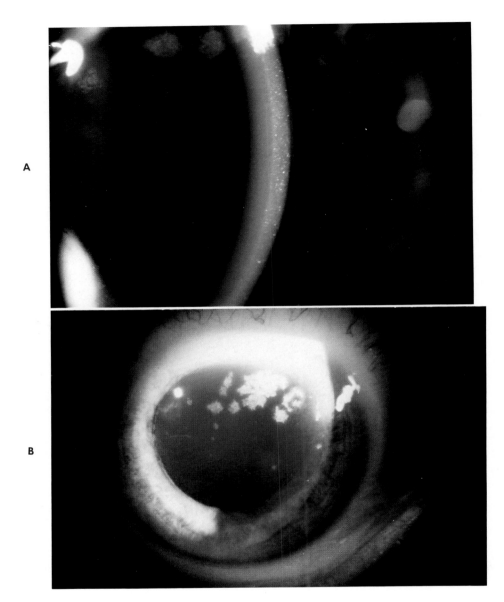

Figure 19-21
Benign monoclonal gammopathy. **A,** Subepithelial glistening deposits. **B,** Large geographic crystalline patches involving full thickness of cornea. (From Miller KH et al: *Ophthalmology* 87:944, 1980.)

globulinemia.[171,172] These dystrophic changes appear as reticulated and undulating patterns of opacification in the posterior stroma.[172]

Others

Langerhans' cell granulomatosis (eosinophilic granuloma, Hand-Schüller-Christian syndrome) is a group of diseases characterized by proliferation of Langerhans' cells. Hand-Schüller-Christian syndrome includes exophthalmos, diabetes insipidus, and destructive bone lesions and is seen in 25% of cases of multifocal eosinophilic granuloma. Large xanthelasmas of the lids can be seen. Yellow-white infiltration of the corneal limbus and peripheral stroma can occur (Fig. 19-23), possibly representing a nodular xanthoma.

Graft-versus-host disease (GVHD) is the major complication of bone marrow transplantation. T lymphocytes in the transplanted marrow recognize antigens of the host as foreign, become sensitized, and attack the host tissue. The major

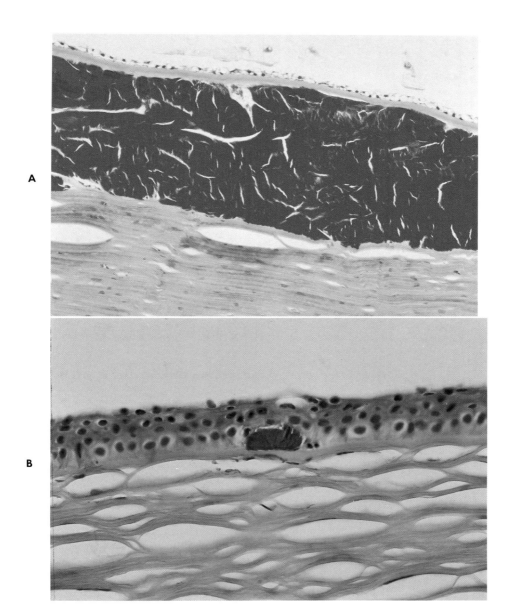

Figure 19-22
Benign monoclonal gammopathy. **A,** Large deposits in the posterior corneal stroma. Descemet's membrane and the endothelium are normal (Masson's trichrome stain, original magnification ×400). **B,** Subepithelial corneal deposit and surrounding normal epithelium, Bowman's membrane, and stroma (Van der Grift stain, original magnification ×100). (From Miller KH et al: *Ophthalmology* 87:944, 1980.)

targets are the skin, gastrointestinal tract, and liver.[173] The most frequent ocular manifestations are keratoconjunctivitis sicca, cicatricial lagophthalmos, and sterile conjunctivitis and uveitis.[174,175] Persistent epithelial defects and stromal ulceration, both sterile and infectious, can result from the dry eye and lagophthalmos. The amount of conjunctival inflammation appears to be a good indicator of the severity of GVHD and of the prognosis for survival.[176] Conjunctival histology specific for GVHD can be present in bone marrow transplant patients without evidence of systemic GVHD.[177]

A perforating corneal ulcer developed in a patient with *mycosis fungoides*.[178] T cells typical of mycosis fungoides were found in the corneal stroma.

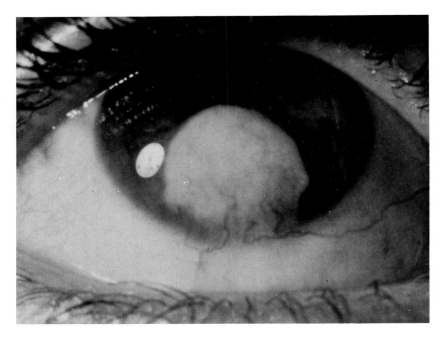

Figure 19-23
Yellow infiltrate involving all layers of the cornea in Hand-Schüller-Christian disease. (Courtesy of
L. Calkins, Kansas City, MO.)

MISCELLANEOUS IMMUNOLOGIC DISEASES OF THE CORNEA

Phlyctenulosis

Phlyctenulosis is an inflammatory disorder involving the cornea or conjunctiva that appears to be caused by cell-mediated hypersensitivity (type IV).[179-181] A phlycten, derived from the Greek word, *phlyctaena,* which means blister, is a small vesicle, blister, or pustule. In the past, sensitivity to tuberculoprotein was the most common cause of phlyctenulosis, and it was associated with poor hygiene and poor nutrition. Now phlyctenulosis is most commonly associated with staphylococcal infection. It is most often seen in the first two decades of life.

Clinical Manifestations

Phlyctenulosis usually occurs in self-limited attacks, although some cases can persist for many weeks. In purely conjunctival cases the symptoms are mild, but severe photophobia is characteristic when the cornea is involved.

The first attack usually occurs at the limbus; later attacks can occur in the cornea or on the bulbar (Fig. 19-24) or tarsal conjunctiva. The lesion can be pinpoint to several millimeters in size; in general, the older the child the larger the phlyctenule. In addition, phlyctenules tend

to be large and succulent if active tuberculosis is present. Each lesion follows a course of elevation, infiltration, ulceration, and resolution over a total period of 6 to 12 days. The phlyctenule begins as a small round or oval, hard, red, elevated lesion. Within 2 to 3 days a yellowish-white center develops and then ulcerates. When it occurs at the limbus, approximately two thirds of the phlyctenule lies on the conjunctival side and one third on the cornea. The phlyctenule usually leaves a scar only on the corneal side (Fig. 19-25). The scar is typically triangular, with its base at the limbus and its apex toward the central cornea. Although it is usually superficial, deep stromal scarring can also occur.

Later attacks also tend to occur at the limbus; they develop adjacent to the limbus or at the central edge of pannus from previous attacks. In this manner the phlyctenulosis can become confluent at the limbus or march across the cornea ("wandering" phlyctenule). More than one phlyctenule can occur simultaneously. Corneal phlyctenules are seen as an amorphous infiltrate (Fig. 19-26), which ulcerates and usually becomes vascularized. A fascicle of vessels can extend to the infiltrate (Fig. 19-27), resembling the ulcer of herpes simplex.

Corneal perforations occur more commonly

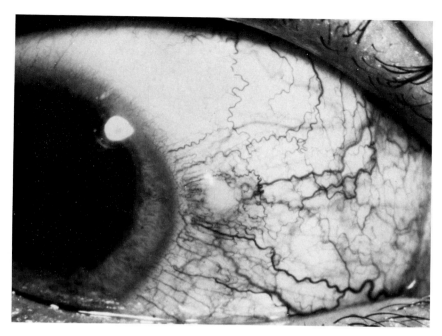

Figure 19-24
Conjunctival phlyctenule.

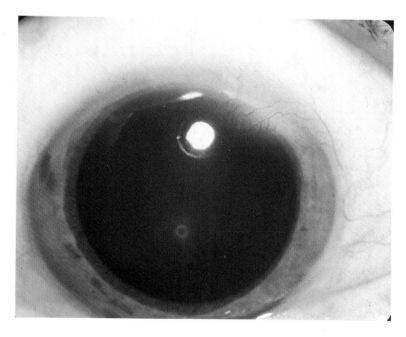

Figure 19-25
Scarring of the cornea with superficial vascularization resulting from limbal phlyctenular disease.
(Courtesy of F. Wilson II, Indianapolis, IN.)

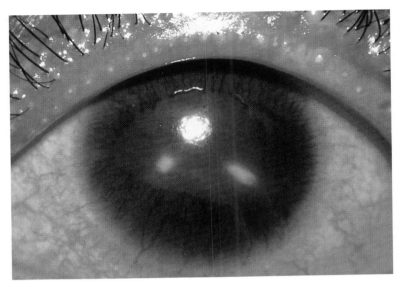

Figure 19-26
Corneal infiltrate resulting from tuberculous phlyctenular disease.

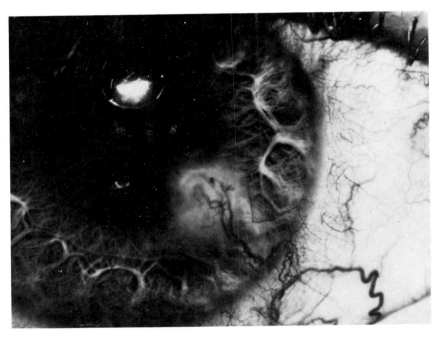

Figure 19-27
Fascicular type of phlyctenular corneal disease.

in tubercular phlyctenulosis, particularly in blacks and Eskimos, but staphylococcal disease can also lead to perforation, usually after many attacks, and with topical steroid use. Old phlyctenular disease is a cause of Salzmann's nodular corneal degeneration.

Etiology
Phlyctenulosis appears to be a cell-mediated hypersensitivity response to a topical foreign antigen. In addition to tuberculosis, phlyctenular disease is associated with staphylococci, *Coccidioides immitis*, *Candida albicans* (Fig. 19-28),

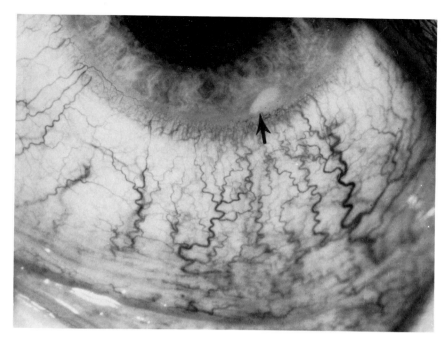

Figure 19-28
Candida albicans phlyctenulosis (*arrow*).

lymphogranuloma venereum, parasites, adenoviruses, and herpes simplex.[180,182,183] The greatest number of cases today are associated with staphylococcal blepharitis. Phlyctenulosis is also seen occasionally during convalescence from coccidioidomycosis. In coccidioidomycosis, there are no corneal stromal phlyctenules; the phlyctenules are confined to the limbal area. Therefore the visual disability that often occurs in tuberculous phlyctenulosis is not seen. The phlyctenulosis of cutaneous candidiasis is recurrent but usually not visually damaging.

Mondino et al.[184,185] were able to create both marginal infiltrates and phlyctenule-like lesions in rabbits, by immunization with *Staphylococcus aureus* followed by topical application of live staphylococci or staphylococcal cell wall antigen (ribitol teichoic acid). The phlyctenules contain plasma cells, lymphocytes, and macrophages, and polymorphonuclear leukocytes invade when necrosis occurs.[3]

Treatment

The primary treatment is removal of the inciting infection. The lid margins should be cultured and skin testing for tuberculosis performed. Staphylococcal blepharitis should be treated by lid hygiene and topical antibiotics. Tuberculous phlyctenulosis responds extremely well to topical corticosteroids. Staphylococcal phlyctenulosis does not respond as well; often the disease recurs despite apparent elimination of the organism from the lid margin.[186] However, low-dose topical corticosteroid and cycloplegia usually greatly increase comfort and lessen corneal scarring. Oral tetracycline (250 mg three times daily for 3 weeks followed by 250 mg daily for 2 months) or erythromycin (25 mg/kg/day in four divided doses) may induce more prolonged remission.[187,188] Keratoplasty may be necessary for treating perforation or central corneal scarring. Penetrating keratoplasty for visual rehabilitation has a favorable prognosis.[189]

Marginal (Catarrhal) Infiltrates and Ulcers

Catarrhal ulcers and infiltrates of the cornea are usually associated with chronic staphylococcal blepharoconjunctivitis. The experimental work in rabbits[184,185] has suggested that it is caused by an antibody response to *S. aureus* cell wall antigen, with immune complex formation in the peripheral corneal stroma. However, many of these patients have only nonaureus staphylococci on their lids.[190]

The catarrhal infiltrate or ulcer is a gray-white, painful lesion that is circumferential with the limbus. A lucid corneal interval is usu-

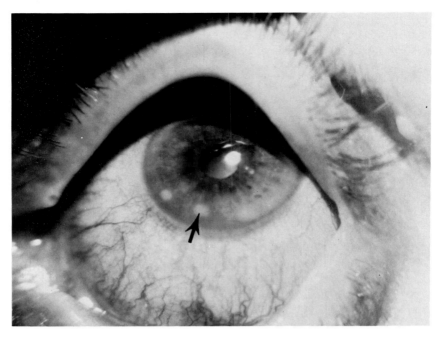

Figure 19-29
Catarrhal ulcers of staphylococcal origin (*arrow*).

ally seen between the lesion and the limbus (Fig. 19-29) or the central edge of corneal vessels. It has been hypothesized that the position of the infiltrate is related to the deposition of the immune complexes formed between the corneal staphylococcal antigen and the antibodies entering from the limbal vessels.[181]

The lesions can be single or multiple, narrow or broad; they are most often located in an area where the lid margin crosses the limbus. Without treatment they usually clear within 2 to 3 weeks. Catarrhal infiltrates can also be caused by *Haemophilus aegyptius, Moraxella lacunata,* beta-hemolytic streptococci, bacillary dysentery, food or drug allergy, lymphogranuloma, *Neisseria gonorrhoeae, Escherichia coli,* and actinomyces.[191,192]

Treatment

Clinically, these lesions cannot be definitively distinguished from peripheral corneal infection, infiltrates, and ulcers associated with rheumatoid arthritis and other collagen vascular diseases and peripheral herpes simplex infection. Therefore, it is important to consider these possibilities, particularly when taking a history; to obtain a bacterial and, in some cases, a viral culture; and to look for scleritis.

In most cases lid scrubs and antibiotic ointment (bacitracin, erythromycin, or gentamicin) are initiated and a bacterial culture is per-

formed. If the culture is negative after 48 hours, topical corticosteroid (e.g., prednisolone acetate two to four times daily) is begun. Oral tetracycline is sometimes necessary for control of meibomitis.

Sterile Corneal Infiltrates Associated with Contact Lenses

Conjunctival hyperemia and anterior stromal infiltrates can develop in contact lens wearers, especially those wearing hydrophilic lenses. The cause of these infiltrates is unclear. Delayed hypersensitivity to thimerosal may be responsible in some cases (see Fig. 9-2).[193] Most infiltrates are now unrelated to thimerosal and may be caused by a reaction to other chemicals absorbed by the lens, to microbes or their products in the lens, to protein deposits on the lens, or to foreign material trapped under the lens. As seen with infectious keratitis, the risk of sterile ulceration is greatest with extended-wear soft contact lenses, followed by daily-wear soft contact lenses and rigid gas-permeable lenses.[194,195] Differentiating these infiltrates from infectious infiltrates can be difficult (see Chapter 10).

Cogan's Syndrome

Cogan's syndrome of nonsyphilitic interstitial keratitis is bilateral and painful[196] and can occur at any age. Symptoms may include photo-

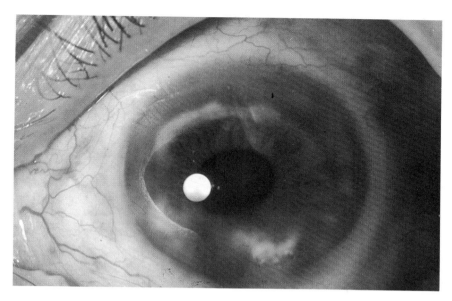

Figure 19-30
Cogan's interstitial keratitis. (From Grayson M: *The cornea in systemic disease.* In Duane TD, editor: *Clinical ophthalmology,* vol 4, Hagerstown, MD, 1976, Harper & Row.)

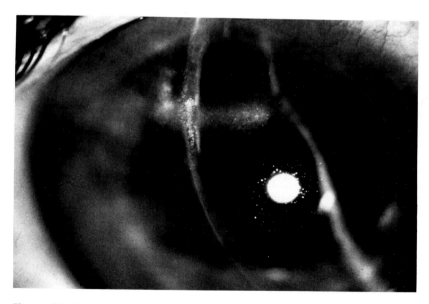

Figure 19-31
Anterior stromal infiltrates in early Cogan's interstitial keratitis.

phobia, fever, periorbital edema, and unilateral proptosis. The syndrome is associated with vestibuloauditory symptoms, which can be more severe than the ocular disease.[197] Cogan's syndrome is characterized by deep yellow nodular corneal stromal opacities (Fig. 19-30). Early in the disease, peripheral subepithelial nummular opacities are most commonly seen (Fig. 19-31)[198]; if these are treated with steroids, the clas-

sic picture may never develop. Deep corneal vascularization, mild uveitis, episcleritis, and scleritis[199] can also occur.

The vestibuloauditory symptoms can precede or follow the ocular symptoms. They are usually closely associated, but in some cases ocular disease develops as much as 2 years after the vestibuloauditory disease.[197] Typically, high-pitched unilateral tinnitus is followed rap-

Table 19-4 Clinical Features of Two Types of Mooren's Ulcer		
Feature	**Type I**	**Type II**
Prevalence	Common form	Atypical form; common in Africa
Pathogenic factors	Trauma	Trauma; ?helminthiasis
Age (years)	Usually >40	Usually 20–30
Sex	M > F	M > F
Laterality	25% Bilateral	75% Bilateral
Pain	Moderate to severe	Variable
Course	Slowly progressive	May be rapid
Response to treatment	Moderate	Poor
Perforation	Uncommon	One third of patients

Modified from Schanzlin D: *Mooren's ulceration.* In Smolin G, Thoft RA, editors: *The cornea: scientific foundations and clinical practice,* Boston, 1986, Little, Brown & Co.

idly by sensorineural deafness in the ipsilateral ear. Symptoms follow in the other ear within a few days. Balance symptoms are also present in most cases. In one study the majority of the patients ended up totally deaf with no vestibular function; in some cases, however, complete resolution occurred after early corticosteroid treatment. Nearly all other organ systems can be affected, with gastrointestinal hemorrhage and aortic insufficiency most common.[200] The etiology is unknown, but approximately 25% of patients with this syndrome have had clinical or tissue findings consistent with polyarteritis nodosa.[201] In two patients circulating antibodies to corneal antigens were identified.[202]

Cogan's interstitial keratitis responds to topical corticosteroid therapy. Systemic corticosteroids are indicated for treatment of vestibuloauditory disease or polyarteritis. It is important to consider this diagnosis, particularly when only subepithelial infiltrates are present. If the cause is assumed to be viral keratitis and no systemic treatment is given, permanent hearing loss can occur.

Mooren's Ulcer

Mooren's ulcer is a localized disease of the cornea characterized by chronic ulceration. It can develop at any age but is rare in individuals younger than 20 years of age. It is bilateral in 25% to 50% of cases. Mooren's ulcer tends to occur in two clinical types (Table 19-4).[203] A relatively benign, unilateral form usually occurs in older people (past the fourth decade) and is more responsive to therapy. The more severe, atypical, bilateral form is found in younger patients (third decade) and is much more difficult to treat. The latter form appears to be more common in black men.[204,205] Physical or chemical trauma may antedate the development of Mooren's ulcers.

Clinical Findings

Patients usually complain of severe pain, redness, and light sensitivity. The first sign is an infiltrate in the peripheral anterior stroma, most often located in the interpalpebral space. Within a few weeks, the overlying epithelium is lost and stromal thinning begins (Fig. 19-32); this thinning slowly deepens and spreads centrally and circumferentially (Fig. 19-33). The central margin often has an overhanging edge; the peripheral edge extends to the limbus and occasionally onto the sclera. Some portions of the ulcer can be quiescent, while others are active; the epithelium is absent over areas of activity. In the wake of the ulceration, the stroma is thinned by one half to three quarters and is covered by superficial vascularization.

The ulceration normally runs a course of 3 to 12 months[3]; periods of total remission are not uncommon. In severe cases the entire cornea can be involved and perforation can occur.

Histopathology

Histopathologic examination of the conjunctiva adjacent to Mooren's ulcer shows heavy infiltration with plasma cells and lymphocytes.[144,206,207] The corneal stroma shows active inflammation, particularly in the area of the overhanging edge.[206,208,209] The principal cells are neutrophils, but plasma cells, eosinophils, and lymphocytes are also present.

Etiology

Some have hypothesized that corneal injury, by surgery, infection, or trauma, alters corneal antigens and elicits an autoimmune response.[3] In many cases such an injury can be identified. In Nigeria, Mooren's ulcer is frequently associated with systemic helminth infections[205]; in these cases an immunologic reaction to helminth-related antigens in the cornea or to corneal an-

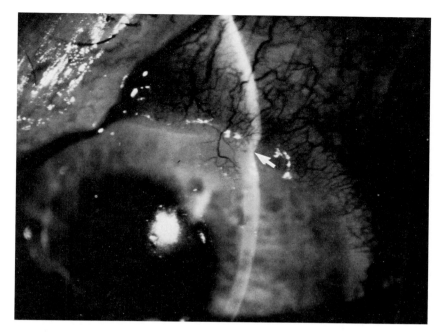

Figure 19-32
Slit-lamp microscope section of early Mooren's ulcer (*arrow*).

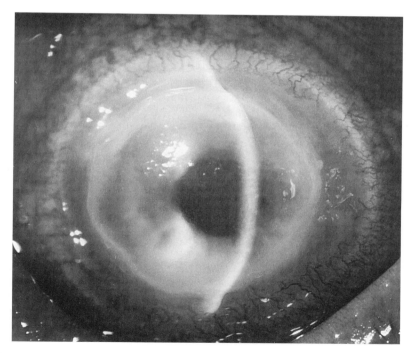

Figure 19-33
Mooren's ulcer with thinning involving the entire limbal cornea. (Courtesy of Diane Curtin, Pittsburgh, PA.)

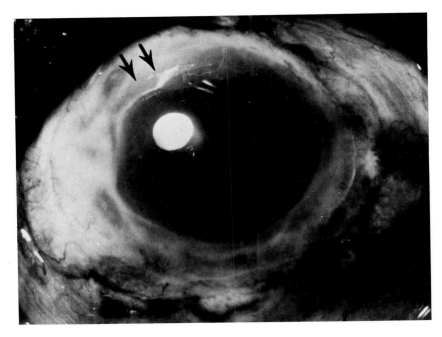

Figure 19-34
Healed Mooren's ulcer after limbal conjunctival resection (*double arrow*).

tigens altered by the infection may be responsible.[210]

Several findings suggest the role of autoimmunity: the high concentration of plasma cells in the adjacent conjunctiva, circulating autoantibodies against corneal and conjunctival tissue,[30,206,207,211,212] tissue-fixed antibodies and complement in the conjunctiva,[206] elevated circulating immune complex and IgA levels,[212] and reduced suppressor T-cell levels.[207] Cell-mediated immunity against corneal tissue has also been demonstrated in some patients.[208,213] However, these findings can be secondary to the destructive corneal inflammation.

Chronic hepatitis C virus infection was present in three patients with bilateral Mooren's ulcer.[214,215] In each case there was significant improvement in the corneal disease during treatment with interferon-α, an effective therapy for hepatitis caused by hepatitis C virus infection.

The corneal changes in Mooren's ulcer are very similar to those seen in systemic diseases with vasculitis, such as Wegener's granulomatosis and polyarteritis nodosa. Therefore, a perilimbal vasculitis may be able to produce the same manifestations.

The tissue destruction appears to be at least partially mediated by collagenase and other degradative enzymes. Metabolic products from tissue culture of the conjunctiva are able to degrade collagen and corneal proteoglycan.[206]

Diagnosis

The diagnosis of Mooren's ulcer can only be made once these collagen vascular diseases and other causes of vasculitis are excluded. A thorough history, medical examination, chest radiography, erythrocyte sedimentation rate, complete blood count, rheumatoid factor, antinuclear antibody titer, Venereal Disease Research Laboratory (VDRL) test, fluorescent-treponemal antibody absorption test (FTA-ABS), blood urea nitrogen level, and creatinine level should be obtained.

In most cases, Mooren's ulcer can be distinguished clinically from other causes of peripheral corneal ulceration. Terrien's marginal degeneration is noninflammatory and nonpainful, and the epithelium is intact (see Table 16-4). Bacterial corneal ulcers usually have more yellowish infiltrate, purulent discharge, and greater anterior chamber, conjunctival, and scleral reaction. Peripheral herpetic ulceration does not exhibit an overhanging central edge and may be associated with decreased corneal sensation. However, bacterial and viral cultures should be performed. Catarrhal ulcers can be distinguished by the presence of blepharitis, the lucid interval between the ulcer and the limbus, the lack of an overhanging central edge, and the lack of severe pain.

Treatment

There is no well established and generally successful treatment for Mooren's ulcer. Whether the ulceration can be arrested depends largely on the aggressiveness of the disease. In general, unilateral ulcers in elderly individuals tend to respond more than bilateral ulcers in young individuals.[203]

I treat initially with topical and (if possible) systemic corticosteroids: prednisolone acetate 1% (four to eight times a day) and oral prednisone (1 mg/kg/day). Cycloplegics, and sometimes a bandage contact lens, are also given to help relieve discomfort. If progression occurs despite 4 to 5 days of treatment, or if perforation is threatened, limbal conjunctival excision is performed (Fig. 19-34).[216] The effect of the excision appears to be temporary and can be repeated several times. Cryotherapy of the perilimbal conjunctiva may have a similar effect.[217]

If progression occurs despite these measures, and perforation or extensive destruction of the eye is threatened, stronger immunosuppressive agents should be considered.[143] Cyclophosphamide and methotrexate both have been successful in many cases.[218,219] These agents should be administered only after discussing the risks and benefits with the patient and coordinating the therapy with a hematologist or rheumatologist who monitors their systemic effects. Systemic administration of cyclosporine has been reported to be effective in several cases, even when cytotoxic agents were not, and may have a lower risk of systemic complications.[32,33] Topical cyclosporine has also been reported to be effective in some cases.[30,37] Very high doses of corticosteroids (1 g methylprednisolone intravenously three times during the first 7 days, followed by 1 g weekly, with gradual tapering) are another option.[220] Cyanoacrylate adhesive can be helpful in sealing small perforations or retarding progression of deep ulceration. Lamellar keratectomy of the central island of remaining stroma can quiet the process and retain some useful vision.[221,222] Keratoepithelioplasty, either alone or in combination with a lamellar graft, has been reported to heal Mooren's ulcer and reduce recurrences.[223] If perforation occurs, lamellar or penetrating keratoplasty can be performed.[224]

REFERENCES

1. Roitt I, Brostoff J, Male D, editors: *Immunology,* ed 2, New York, 1989, Mosby/Gower.
2. Barrett JT: *Textbook of clinical immunology,* ed 5, St Louis, 1988, Mosby–Year Book.
3. Smolin G, O'Connor GR: *Ocular immunology,* Philadelphia, 1981, Lea & Febiger.
4. Franklin RM, Remus LE: Conjunctival-associated lymphoid tissue: evidence for a role in the secretory immune system, *Invest Ophthalmol Vis Sci* 25:181, 1983.
5. Dua HS et al: Mucosa specific lymphocytes in the human conjunctiva, corneoscleral limbus and lacrimal gland, *Curr Eye Res* 13:87, 1994.
6. Wotherspoon AC, Hardman LS, Isaacson PG: Mucosa-associated lymphoid tissue (MALT) in the human conjunctiva, *J Pathol* 174:33, 1994.
7. Sacks EH et al: Lymphocytic subpopulations in the normal human conjunctiva: a monoclonal antibody study, *Ophthalmology* 93:1276, 1986.
8. Strober W, Brown WR: *The mucosal immune system.* In Samter M, editor: *Immunological diseases,* ed 4, Boston, 1988, Little, Brown & Co.
9. Smolin G, Hall J, Stein M: Afferent arc of the corneal immunological reaction, *Can J Ophthalmol* 7:336, 1972.
10. Shimada K, Silverstein AM: Local antibody formation within the eye, *Invest Ophthalmol* 14:573, 1975.
11. Mondino BJ, Brady KJ: Distribution of hemolytic complement in the normal cornea, *Arch Ophthalmol* 99:1430, 1981.
12. Allansmith MR, McClennan B: Immunoglobulins in the human cornea, *Am J Ophthalmol* 80:125, 1975.
13. Gillete TE, Chandler JW, Greiner JV: Langerhans cells of the ocular surface, *Ophthalmology* 89:700, 1982.
14. Streilein JW: Anterior chamber associated immune deviation: the privilege of immunity in the eye, *Surv Ophthalmol* 35:67, 1990.
15. Ferguson TA, Kaplan HJ: The immune response and the eye: I. The effects of monoclonal antibodies to T suppressor factors in anterior chamber associated immune deviation (ACAID), *J Immunol* 139:346, 1987.
16. Ferguson TA, Waldrep JC, Kaplan HJ: The immune response and the eye: II. The nature of T suppressor cell induction in anterior chamber associated immune deviation (ACAID), *J Immunol* 139:352, 1987.
17. Wilbanks GA, Streilein JW: Characterization of suppressor cells in anterior chamber-associated immune deviation (ACAID) induced by soluble antigen: evidence of two functionally and phenotypically distinct T-suppressor cell populations, *Immunology* 71:383, 1990.
18. Gell PGH, Coombs RA, Lackmann P, editors: *Clinical aspects of immunology,* ed 3, Oxford, 1974, Blackwell Scientific Publications.
19. Katz P, Fauci AS: *Drugs that regulate the immune response.* In Frank MM et al, editors: *Samter's immunologic diseases,* ed 5, New York, 1995, Little, Brown & Co.
20. Fauci AS, Haynes BF, Katz P: The spectrum of vasculitis: clinical, pathologic, immunologic, and therapeutic considerations, *Ann Intern Med* 89:660, 1978.
21. Shah SS et al: Low-dose methotrexate therapy for ocular inflammatory disease, *Ophthalmology* 99:1419, 1992.

22. Hoffman GS et al: The treatment of Wegener's granulomatosis with glucocorticoids and methotrexate, *Arthritis Rheum* 35:1322, 1992.

23. Harding MW, Handschumacher RE: Cyclophilin is a primary target molecule for cyclosporine A: structural and functional implications, *Transplantation* 46:29S, 1988.

24. Katz P, Fauci A: *Systemic vasculitis.* In Frank MM et al, editors: *Samter's immunologic diseases,* ed 5, New York, 1995, Little, Brown & Co.

25. McCarthy JM et al: Cyclosporine A for the treatment of necrotizing scleritis and corneal melting in patients with rheumatoid arthritis, *J Rheumatol* 19:1358, 1992.

26. Nussenblatt RB et al: Treatment of intraocular inflammatory disease with cyclosporin A, *Lancet* 2:235, 1983.

27. Ben Ezra D et al: Cyclosporin eyedrops for the treatment of severe vernal keratoconjunctivitis, *Am J Ophthalmol* 101:278, 1986.

28. Holland EJ et al: Immunohistologic findings and results of treatment with cyclosporin in ligneous conjunctivitis, *Am J Ophthalmol* 107:160, 1989.

29. Rosenfeld SI et al: Topical cyclosporine for treating necrotizing scleritis, *Arch Ophthalmol* 113:20, 1995.

30. Zhao J-C, Jin X-Y: Immunological analysis and treatment of Mooren's ulcer with cyclosporin A applied topically, *Cornea* 12:481, 1993.

31. Kervick GN et al: Paracentral rheumatoid corneal ulceration: clinical features and cyclosporine therapy, *Ophthalmology* 99:80, 1992.

32. Hill JC, Potter P: Treatment of Mooren's ulcer with cyclosporin A: report of three cases, *Br J Ophthalmol* 71:11, 1987.

33. Wakefield D, Robinson LP: Cyclosporin therapy in Mooren's ulcer, *Br J Ophthalmol* 71:415, 1987.

34. Zierhut M et al: Topical treatment of severe corneal ulcers with cyclosporin A, *Graefes Arch Clin Exp Ophthalmol* 227:30, 1989.

35. Belin MW et al: Topical cyclosporin in high-risk corneal transplants, *Ophthalmology* 96:1144, 1989.

36. Belin MW, Bouchard CS, Phillips TM: Update on topical cyclosporin A: background, immunology, and pharmacology, *Cornea* 9:184, 1990.

37. Holland EJ et al: Topical cyclosporin A in the treatment of anterior segment inflammatory disease, *Cornea* 12:413, 1993.

38. Starzl TEJ, Makowka L, Todo S: FK506: a potential breakthrough in immunosuppression, *Transplant Proc* 19:3, 1987.

39. Ishioka M et al: FK506 treatment of noninfectious uveitis, *Am J Ophthalmol* 118:723, 1994.

40. Frank MM et al, editors: *Samter's immunologic diseases,* ed 5, New York, 1995, Little, Brown & Co.

41. Fitzpatrick EP, Chesen N, Rahn EK: The lupus anticoagulant and retinal vaso-occlusive disease, *Am J Ophthalmol* 22:148, 1990.

42. Frith P et al: External ocular findings in lupus erythematosus: a clinical and immunopathological study, *Br J Ophthalmol* 74:163, 1990.

43. Sainz de la Maza M, Foster CS, Jabbur NS: Scleritis associated with systemic vasculitic diseases, *Ophthalmology* 102:687, 1995.

44. Leahy AB et al: Chemosis as a presenting sign of systemic lupus erythematosus, *Arch Ophthalmol* 110:609, 1992.

45. Ramos-Niembro F, Alarcon-Segovia D: Development of sicca symptoms in SLE patients with existing subclinical abnormalities, *Arthritis Rheum* 22:935, 1979.

46. Dubois EI, Tuffanelli DL: Clinical manifestations of SLE: analysis of 520 cases, *JAMA* 190:104, 1964.

47. Andonopoylos AP et al: Sjögren's syndrome in systemic lupus erythematosus, *J Rheumatol* 17:201, 1990.

48. Gold DH, Morris DA, Henkind P: Ocular findings in SLE, *Br J Ophthalmol* 56:800, 1972.

49. Spaeth GL: Corneal staining in systemic lupus erythematosus, *N Engl J Med* 276:1168, 1967.

50. Halmay O, Ludwig K: Bilateral band-shaped deep keratitis and iridocyclitis in systemic lupus erythematosus, *Br J Ophthalmol* 48:558, 1964.

51. Reeves JA: Keratopathy associated with systemic lupus erythematosus, *Arch Ophthalmol* 74:159, 1965.

52. Huey C et al: Discoid lupus erythematosus of the eyelids, *Ophthalmology* 90:1389, 1983.

53. Frith P et al: External ocular findings in lupus erythematosus: a clinical and immunopathological study, *Br J Ophthalmol* 74:163, 1990.

54. Foster RE et al: An unusual ocular manifestation of discoid lupus erythematosus, *Cleve Clin J Med* 61:232, 1994.

55. Doesschat JT: Corneal complications in lupus erythematosus discoidus, *Ophthalmologica* 132:153, 1956.

56. Foster CS: Ocular surface manifestations of neurological and systemic diseases, *Int Ophthalmol Clin* 19:207, 1979.

57. Raizman MB, Baum J: Discoid lupus keratitis, *Arch Ophthalmol* 107:545, 1989.

58. Wolfe AM: The epidemiology of rheumatoid arthritis: a review, *Bull Rheum Dis* 19:518, 1968.

59. Arnett FC: Revised criteria for the classification of rheumatoid arthritis, *Bull Rheum Dis* 38:1, 1989.

60. Jayson MIV, Easty DL: Ulceration of the cornea in rheumatoid arthritis, *Ann Rheum Dis* 36:428, 1977.

61. Thompson M, Eadie S: Keratoconjunctivitis sicca and rheumatoid arthritis, *Ann Rheum Dis* 15:21, 1956.

62. Ericson S, Syndmark E: Studies on the sicca syndrome in patients with rheumatoid arthritis, *Acta Rheum Scand* 16:60, 1970.

63. Talal N: *Sjögren's syndrome.* In Samter M, editor: *Immunological diseases,* ed 4, Boston, 1988, Little, Brown & Co.

64. Jayson MI, Jones DEP: Scleritis and rheumatoid arthritis, *Ann Rheum Dis* 30:343, 1971.

65. McGavin DDM et al: Episcleritis and scleritis: a study of their clinical manifestations and associations with rheumatoid arthritis, *Br J Ophthalmol* 60:192, 1976.

66. Watson PG, Hazelman BL: *The sclera and systemic disorders*, London, 1976, WB Saunders.

67. Watson PG: *Diseases of the sclera and episclera*. In Duane TD, Jaeger EA, editors: *Clinical ophthalmology*, vol 4, Philadelphia, 1988, Harper & Row.

68. Foster CS, Forstot SL, Wilson LA: Mortality rate in rheumatoid arthritis patients developing necrotizing scleritis or peripheral ulcerative keratitis: effects of systemic immunosuppression, *Ophthalmology* 91:1253, 1984.

69. Erhardt CC et al: Factors predicting a poor life prognosis in rheumatoid arthritis: an eight year prospective study, *Ann Rheum Dis* 48:7, 1989.

70. Watson PG, Hayreh SS: Scleritis and episcleritis, *Br J Ophthalmol* 60:163, 1976.

71. Jones P, Jayson MIV: Rheumatoid scleritis: a long-term follow up, *Proc R Soc Med* 66:1161, 1973.

72. Sevel D: Necrogranulomatous keratitis associated with Wegener's granulomatosis and rheumatoid arthritis, *Am J Ophthalmol* 63:250, 1967.

73. Foster CS, Sainz de la Maza M: *The sclera*, New York, 1994, Springer-Verlag.

74. Brown SI, Grayson M: Marginal furrows: a characteristic corneal lesion of rheumatoid arthritis, *Arch Ophthalmol* 79:563, 1968.

75. Radtke N, Meyers S, Kaufman HE: Sterile corneal ulcers after cataract surgery in keratoconjunctivitis sicca, *Arch Ophthalmol* 96:51, 1978.

76. Insler MS, Boutros G, Boulware DW: Corneal ulceration following cataract surgery in patients with rheumatoid arthritis, *Am Intraocular Implant Soc J* 11:594, 1985.

77. Maffett MJ et al: Sterile corneal ulceration after cataract extraction in patients with collagen vascular disease, *Cornea* 9:279, 1990.

78. Bernauer W et al: The management of corneal perforations associated with rheumatoid arthritis: an analysis of 32 eyes, *Ophthalmology* 102:1325, 1995.

79. Gilliland BC: *Progressive systemic sclerosis (diffuse scleroderma)*. In Braunwald E et al, editors: *Harrison's principles of internal medicine*, ed 11, New York, 1987, McGraw-Hill.

80. Silver RM: *Systemic sclerosis (scleroderma)*. In Frank MM et al, editors: *Samter's immunologic diseases*, ed 5, New York, 1995, Little, Brown & Co.

81. Alarcón-Segovia D et al: Sjögren's syndrome and progressive systemic sclerosis (scleroderma), *Am J Med* 57:78, 1974.

82. Kirkham TH: Scleroderma and Sjögren's syndrome, *Br J Ophthalmol* 53:131, 1969.

83. Horan EC: Ophthalmic manifestations of progressive systemic sclerosis, *Br J Ophthalmol* 53:388, 1969.

84. Stucci CA, Geiser JD: Manifestations oculares de la sclérodermie generalisée (points communs avec le syndrome de Sjögren), *Doc Ophthalmol* 22:72, 1967.

85. Manschot S: Über die pathologie und pathogenese von sclerodermia universalis, *Mitt Med Fakult Kaiserl Univ Tokyo* 31:55, 1924.

86. Macel E et al: Conjunctival biopsy in scleroderma and primary Sjögren's syndrome, *Am J Ophthalmol* 115:792, 1993.

87. Meyer O et al: Relapsing polychondritis: pathogenic role of anti-native collagen type II antibodies, *J Rheumatol* 8:820, 1981.

88. Herman JH: *Polychondritis*. In Kelly WN et al, editors: *Textbook of rheumatology*, Philadelphia, 1985, WB Saunders.

89. McKay DAR, Watson PG, Lyne AJ: Relapsing polychondritis and eye disease, *Br J Ophthalmol* 58:600, 1974.

90. Anderson B: Ocular lesions in relapsing polychondritis and other rheumatoid syndromes, *Trans Am Acad Ophthalmol Otolaryngol* 71:227, 1967.

91. Rucker CW, Ferguson RH: Ocular manifestations of relapsing polychondritis, *Trans Am Ophthalmol Soc* 62:167, 1979.

92. Matoba A et al: Keratitis in relapsing polychondritis, *Ann Ophthalmol* 16:367, 1984.

93. Michelson JB: Melting corneas with collapsing nose, *Surv Ophthalmol* 29:148, 1984.

94. Danzi JT: Extraintestinal manifestations of idiopathic inflammatory bowel disease, *Arch Intern Med* 148:297, 1988.

95. Brown WR, Claman HR, Strober W: *Immunologic diseases of the gastrointestinal tract*. In Frank MM et al, editors: *Samter's immunologic diseases*, ed 5, New York, 1995, Little, Brown & Co.

96. Bhaqat S, Das KM: A shared and unique peptide in the human colon, eye, and joint detected by a monoclonal antibody, *Gastroenterology* 107:103, 1994.

97. Ernst BB et al: Posterior segment manifestations of inflammatory bowel disease, *Ophthalmology* 98:1272, 1991.

98. Ellis PP, Gentry JH: Ocular complications of ulcerative colitis, *Am J Ophthalmol* 58:779, 1964.

99. Billson FA et al: Ocular complications of ulcerative colitis, *Gut* 8:102, 1967.

100. Evans JP, Eustace P: Scleromalacia perforans associated with Crohn's disease treated with sodium versenate (EDTA), *Br J Ophthalmol* 57:330, 1973.

101. Grewal RK, Rush D, Burde RM: Subconjunctival nodules: an unusual ocular complication of Crohn's disease, *Can J Ophthalmol* 29:238, 1994.

102. Hopkins DJ et al: Ocular disorders in a series of 332 patients with Crohn's disease, *Br J Ophthalmol* 58:732, 1974.

103. Macoul KL: Ocular changes in granulomatous ileocolitis, *Arch Ophthalmol* 84:95, 1970.

104. Salmon JF, Wright JP, Murray AD: Ocular inflammation in Crohn's disease, *Ophthalmology* 98:480, 1991.

105. Knox DL, Schachat AP, Mustonen EP: Primary, secondary and coincidental ocular complications of Crohn's disease, *Ophthalmology* 91:163, 1984.

105a. Schulman MF, Sugar A: Peripheral corneal infiltrates in inflammatory bowel disease, *Ann Ophthalmol* 13:109, 1981.

106. Soukiasian SH, Foster CS, Raizman MB: Treatment strategies for scleritis and uveitis associated with inflammatory bowel disease, *Am J Ophthalmology* 118:601, 1994.

107. Ouertani A, Lasram L, Mili I: Behçet's disease disclosed by ocular conjunctival aphthous ulcer: apropos of a case, *J Fr Ophtalmol* 15:131, 1992.

108. Nussenblatt RB, Palestine AG: *Uveitis: fundamentals and clinical practice*, Chicago, 1989, Mosby–Year Book.

109. Katz P, Fauci AS: *Systemic vasculitis*. In Frank MM et al, editors: *Samter's immunologic diseases*, ed 5, New York, 1995, Little, Brown & Co.

110. Gold DH: *Ocular manifestations of connective tissue (collagen) diseases*. In Duane T, editor: *Clinical ophthalmology*, vol 5, Philadelphia, 1988, Harper & Row.

111. Gerstle CS, Friedman AH: Marginal corneal ulceration (limbal guttering) as a presenting sign of temporal arteritis, *Ophthalmology* 87:1173, 1980.

112. Foster CS: *Ocular manifestations of the nonrheumatic acquired collagen vascular diseases*. In Smolin G, Thoft RA, editors: *The cornea: scientific foundations and clinical practice*, Boston, 1983, Little, Brown & Co.

113. Purcell JJ, Birkenkamp R, Tsai CC: Conjunctival lesions in periarteritis nodosa, *Arch Ophthalmol* 102:736, 1984.

114. Cogan DG: Corneoscleral lesions in periarteritis and Wegener's granulomatosis, *Trans Am Ophthalmol Soc* 53:321, 1955.

115. Moore JG, Sevel D: Corneoscleral ulceration in periarteritis nodosa, *Br J Ophthalmol* 50:651, 1966.

116. Foster CS: Systemic immunosuppressive therapy for progressive bilateral Mooren's ulcer, *Ophthalmology* 92:1436, 1985.

117. Harbart F, McPherson SD: Scleral necrosis in periarteritis nodosa, *Am J Ophthalmol* 30:727, 1947.

118. Wise GN: Ocular periarteritis nodosa, *Arch Ophthalmol* 48:1, 1952.

119. Asherson RA et al: The "primary" antiphospholipid syndrome: major clinical and serological features, *Medicine* 68:366, 1989.

120. Castañón C, Amigo M-C, Bañãles JL et al: Ocular vaso-occlusive disease in primary antiphospholipid syndrome, *Ophthalmology* 102:256, 1995.

121. Meisler DM et al: Conjunctival inflammation and amyloidosis in allergic granulomatosis and angiitis (Churg-Strauss syndrome), *Am J Ophthalmol* 91:216, 1981.

122. Shields CL, Shields JA, Rozanski TI: Conjunctival involvement in Churg-Strauss syndrome, *Am J Ophthalmol* 102:601, 1986.

123. Chumbley LC, Harrison EG, DeRemee RA: Allergic granulomatosis and angiitis (Churg-Strauss syndrome): report and analysis of 30 cases, *Mayo Clin Proc* 52:477, 1977.

124. Robin JB et al: Ocular involvement in the respiratory vasculitides, *Surv Ophthalmol* 30:127, 1985.

125. Fauci AS: *The vasculitis syndromes*. In Braunwald E et al, editors: *Harrison's principles of internal medicine*, ed 11, New York, 1987, McGraw-Hill.

126. John SL et al: Corneal autoimmunity in patients with peripheral ulcerative keratitis (PUK) in association with rheumatoid arthritis and Wegener's granulomatosis, *Eye* 6:630, 1992.

127. Bullen CL et al: Ocular complications of Wegener's granulomatosis, *Ophthalmology* 90:270, 1983.

128. Haynes BF et al: The ocular manifestations of Wegener's granulomatosis: fifteen years experience and review of the literature, *Am J Med* 63:131, 1977.

129. Hoffman GS et al: Wegener's granulomatosis: an analysis of 158 patients, *Ann Intern Med* 116:488, 1992.

130. Jordan DR, Addison DJ: Wegener's granulomatosis. Eyelid and conjunctival manifestations as the presenting feature in two individuals, *Ophthalmology* 101:602, 1994.

131. Austin P et al: Peripheral corneal degeneration and occlusive vasculitis in Wegener's granulomatosis, *Am J Ophthalmol* 85:311, 1978.

132. Brady HR, Israel MR, Lewin WH: Wegener's granulomatosis and corneoscleral ulcer, *JAMA* 193:148, 1965.

133. Ferry AP, Leopold IH: Marginal (ring) corneal ulcer as a presenting manifestation of Wegener's granuloma: a clinicopathologic study, *Trans Am Acad Ophthalmol Otolaryngol* 74:1276, 1970.

134. Charles SJ, Meyer PA, Watson PG: Diagnosis and management of systemic Wegener's granulomatosis presenting with anterior ocular inflammatory disease, *Br J Ophthalmol* 75:201, 1991.

135. Biglan AW et al: Corneal perforation in Wegener's granulomatosis treated with corneal transplantation, *Ann Ophthalmol* 9:799, 1979.

136. Trocme SD et al: Eosinophil and neutrophil degranulation in ophthalmic lesions of Wegener's granulomatosis, *Arch Ophthalmol* 109:1585, 1991.

137. Nolle B, Coners H, Duncker G: ANCA in ocular inflammatory disorders, *Adv Exp Med Biol* 336:305, 1993.

138. Pulido JS et al: Ocular manifestations of patients with circulating antineutrophil cytoplasmic antibodies, *Arch Ophthalmol* 108:845, 1990.

139. Cohen-Tervaert JW et al: Association between

active Wegener's granulomatosis and anticytoplasmic antibodies, *Arch Intern Med* 149:2461, 1989.

140. McCune WJ, Friedman AW: Immunosuppressive drug therapy for rheumatic disease, *Curr Opin Rheumatol* 5:282, 1993.

141. Power WJ et al: Disease relapse in patients with ocular manifestations of Wegener's granulomatosis, *Ophthalmology* 102:154, 1995.

142. Soukiasian SH et al: Trimethoprim-sulfamethoxazole for scleritis associated with limited Wegener's granulomatosis: use of histopathology and anti-neutrophil cytoplasmic antibody (ANCA) test, *Cornea* 12:174, 1993.

143. Tauber J et al: An analysis of therapeutic decision making regarding immunosuppressive chemotherapy for peripheral ulcerative keratitis, *Cornea* 9:66, 1990.

144. Wilson FM, Grayson M, Ellis FD: Treatment of peripheral corneal ulcers by limbal conjunctivectomy, *Br J Ophthalmol* 60:713, 1976.

145. Feder RS, Krachmer JH: Conjunctival resection for the treatment of the rheumatoid corneal ulceration, *Ophthalmology* 91:111, 1984.

146. Waldmann TA: *Immunodeficiency diseases: primary and acquired.* In Samter M, editor: *Immunological diseases,* ed 4, Boston, 1988, Little, Brown & Co.

147. Remold-O'Donnell E et al: Characterization of a human lymphocyte surface sialoglycoprotein that is defective in Wiskott-Aldrich syndrome, *J Exp Med* 159:1705, 1984.

148. Jabs DA et al: Ocular manifestations of acquired immune deficiency syndrome, *Ophthalmology* 96:1092, 1989.

149. Stenson SM, Friedberg DN: *AIDS and the eye,* New Orleans, 1995, Contact Lens Association of Ophthalmologists.

150. Young TI et al: Herpes simplex keratitis in patients with acquired immunodeficiency syndrome, *Ophthalmology* 96:1476, 1989.

151. Cole IL et al: Herpes zoster ophthalmicus and the acquired immune deficiency syndrome, *Ophthalmology* 102:1027, 1984.

152. Kestelyn P et al: Severe herpes zoster ophthalmicus in young African adults: a marker for HTLV-III seropositivity, *Br J Ophthalmol* 71:806, 1987.

153. Sandor EV et al: Herpes zoster ophthalmicus in patients at risk for the acquired immune deficiency syndrome (AIDS), *Am J Ophthalmol* 101:153, 1986.

154. Kohn SR: Molluscum contagiosum in patients with acquired immunodeficiency syndrome, *Arch Ophthalmol* 105:458, 1987.

155. Robinson MR et al: Molluscum contagiosum of the eyelids in patients with acquired immune deficiency syndrome, *Ophthalmology* 99:1745, 1992.

156. Shuler JD et al: Kaposi's sarcoma of the conjunctiva and eyelids associated with the acquired immunodeficiency syndrome, *Arch Ophthalmol* 107:859, 1988.

157. Lucca JA et al: Keratoconjunctivitis sicca in male patients infected with human immunodeficiency virus type I, *Ophthalmology* 97:1008, 1990.

158. Shuler JD, Engstrom RE, Holland GN: External ocular disease and anterior segment disorders associated with AIDS, *Int Ophthalmol Clin* 29:98, 1989.

159. Aristimuno B et al: Spontaneous ulcerative keratitis in immunocompromised patients, *Am J Ophthalmol* 115:202, 1993.

160. Hemady RK: Microbial keratitis in patients infected with the human immunodeficiency virus, *Ophthalmology* 102:1026, 1995.

161. Wilhelmus KR et al: Corneal lipidosis in patients with the acquired immunodeficiency syndrome, *Am J Ophthalmol* 119:14, 1995.

162. Mitchell SM, Barton K, Lightman S: Corneal endothelial changes in cytomegalovirus retinitis, *Eye* 8:41, 1994.

163. Orellana J, Friedman AH: Ocular manifestations of multiple myeloma, Waldenström's macroglobulinemia and benign monoclonal gammopathy, *Surv Ophthalmol* 26:3, 1981.

164. Pinkerton RMH, Robertson DM: Corneal and conjunctival changes in dysproteinemia, *Invest Ophthalmol* 8:357, 1969.

165. Aronson SB, Shaw R: Corneal crystals in multiple myeloma, *Arch Ophthalmol* 61:541, 1959.

166. Perry HD, Donnenfeld ED, Font RL: Intraepithelial corneal immunoglobulin crystals in IgG-kappa multiple myeloma, *Cornea* 12:448, 1993.

167. Beebe WE, Webster RG, Spencer WB: Atypical corneal manifestations of multiple myeloma: a clinical histopathologic, and immunohistochemical report, *Cornea* 8:274, 1989.

168. Kremer I et al: Corneal subepithelial monoclonal kappa IgG deposits in essential cryoglobulinaemia, *Br J Ophthalmol* 73:669, 1989.

169. Hill JC, Mulligan GP: Subepithelial corneal deposits in IgG lambda myeloma, *Br J Ophthalmol* 73:552, 1989.

169a. Auran JD, Donn A, Hyman GA: Multiple myeloma presenting as vortex crystalline keratopathy and complicated by endocapsular hematoma, *Cornea* 11:584, 1992.

169b. Barr CC, Gelender H, Font R: Corneal crystalline deposits associated with dysproteinemia: report of two cases and review of literature, *Arch Ophthalmol* 98:884, 1980.

169c. Miller KH et al: Immunoprotein deposition in the cornea, *Ophthalmology* 87:944, 1980.

169d. Lewis RA, Falls HF, Troyer DO: Ocular manifestations of hypercupremia associated with multiple myeloma, *Arch Ophthalmol* 93:1050, 1975.

170. Steuhl KP et al: Paraproteinemic corneal deposits in plasma cell myeloma, *Am J Ophthalmol* 111:312, 1991.

171. Gloor B: Diffuse corneal degeneration in a case of Waldenström's macroglobulinemia, *Ophthalmologica* 155:449, 1968.

172. Oglesby RB: Corneal opacities in a patient with

cryoglobulinemia and reticulohistiocytosis, *Arch Ophthalmol* 65:63, 1961.

173. Thomas ED et al: Bone-marrow transplantation, *N Engl J Med* 292:832, 1975.

174. Jack M et al: Ocular manifestations of graft-vs-host disease, *Arch Ophthalmol* 101:1080, 1983.

175. Franklin R et al: Ocular manifestations of graft-vs-host disease, *Ophthalmology* 90:4, 1983.

176. Jabs DA et al: The eye in bone marrow transplantation: III. Conjunctival graft vs host disease, *Arch Ophthalmol* 107:1343, 1989.

177. West RH, Szer J, Pedersen JS: Ocular surface and lacrimal disturbances in chronic graft-versus-host disease: the role of conjunctival biopsy, *Aust N Z J Ophthalmol* 19:187, 1991.

178. McCaa CS et al: Corneal ulcer with perforation and T-cell lymphocyte corneal infiltration in mycosis fungoides, paper presented at the Ocular Microbiology and Immunology Group, October 29, 1994, San Francisco.

179. Thygeson P: The etiology and treatment of phlyctenular keratoconjunctivitis, *Am J Ophthalmol* 34:1217, 1951.

180. Thygeson P: Observations on nontuberculous phlyctenular keratoconjunctivitis, *Trans Am Acad Ophthalmol Otolaryngol* 58:128, 1954.

181. Smolin G, Okumoto M: Staphylococcal blepharitis, *Arch Ophthalmol* 95:812, 1977.

182. Jeffrey MP: Ocular diseases caused by nematodes, *Am J Ophthalmol* 40:41, 1953.

183. Al-Hussaini MK et al: Phlyctenular eye disease in association with *Hymenolepsis nana* in Egypt, *Br J Ophthalmol* 63:627, 1979.

184. Mondino BJ, Dethlefs B: Occurrence of phlyctenules after immunization with ribitol teichoic acid of *Staphylococcus aureus*, *Arch Ophthalmol* 102:461, 1984.

185. Mondino BJ, Laheji AK, Adamu SA: Ocular immunity to *Staphylococcus aureus*, *Invest Ophthalmol Vis Sci* 28:560, 1987.

186. Thygeson P, Fritz MH: Cortisone in the treatment of phlyctenular keratoconjunctivitis, *Am J Ophthalmol* 34:357, 1951.

187. Culbertson WW et al: Effective treatment of phlyctenular keratoconjunctivitis with oral tetracycline, *Ophthalmology* 100:1358, 1993.

188. Zaidman GW, Brown SI: Orally administered tetracycline for phlyctenular keratoconjunctivitis, *Am J Ophthalmol* 92:173, 1981.

189. Smith RE, Dippe DW, Miller SD: Phlyctenular keratoconjunctivitis: results of penetrating keratoplasty in Alaskan natives, *Ophthalmic Surg* 6:62, 1975.

190. Bowers R et al: Non-aureus staphylococcus in corneal disease, *Invest Ophthalmol Vis Sci* 30(suppl):380, 1989.

191. Thygeson P: Marginal corneal infiltrates and ulcers, *Trans Am Acad Ophthalmol Otolaryngol* 51:198, 1946.

192. Duke-Elder S, Leigh AG: *System of ophthalmology*, vol VIII, *Diseases of the outer eye*, St Louis, 1965, Mosby–Year Book.

193. Mondino BJ, Groden LR: Conjunctival hyper-

194. Stapleton F, Dart J, Minassian D: Nonulcerative complications of contact lens wear: relative risks for different lens types, *Arch Ophthalmol* 110:1601, 1992.

195. Stapleton F, Dart JK, Minassian D: Risk factors with contact lens related suppurative keratitis, *CLAO J* 19:204, 1993.

196. Cogan DG: Syndrome of nonsyphilitic interstitial keratitis and vestibuloauditory symptoms, *Arch Ophthalmol* 33:144, 1945.

197. McDonald TJ, Vollertsen RS, Younge BR: Cogan's syndrome: audiovestibular involvement and prognosis in 18 patients, *Laryngoscope* 95:650, 1985.

198. Cobo LM, Haynes BF: Early corneal findings in Cogan's syndrome, *Ophthalmology* 91:903, 1984.

199. Shah P et al: Posterior scleritis: an unusual manifestation of Cogan's syndrome, *Br J Rheumatol* 33:774, 1994.

200. Vollertsen RS: Vasculitis and Cogan's syndrome, *Rheum Dis Clin North Am* 16:433, 1990.

201. Cheson BD, Bluming AZ, Alroy J: Cogan's syndrome: a systemic vasculitis, *Am J Ophthalmol* 60:549, 1976.

202. Majoor MH et al: Corneal autoimmunity in Cogan's syndrome? Report of two cases, *Ann Otol Rhinol Laryngol* 101:679, 1992.

203. Wood TO, Kaufman HE: Mooren's ulcer, *Am J Ophthalmol* 71:417, 1971.

204. Kietzman B: Mooren's ulcer in Nigeria, *Am J Ophthalmol* 65:679, 1968.

205. Majekodunmi AA: Ecology of Mooren's ulcer in Nigeria, *Doc Ophthalmol* 49:211, 1980.

206. Brown SI: Mooren's ulcer: histopathology and proteolytic enzymes of adjacent conjunctiva, *Br J Ophthalmol* 59:670, 1975.

207. Murray PE, Rahi AHS: Pathogenesis of Mooren's ulcer: some new concepts, *Br J Ophthalmol* 68:182, 1984.

208. Foster CS et al: The immunopathology of Mooren's ulcer, *Am J Ophthalmol* 88:149, 1979.

209. Young RG, Watson PG: Light and electron microscopy of corneal melting syndrome (Mooren's ulcer), *Br J Ophthalmol* 66:341, 1982.

210. Ban der Gaag R et al: Circulating antibodies against corneal epithelium and hookworm in patients with Mooren's ulcer from Sierra Leone, *Br J Ophthalmol* 67:623, 1983.

211. Brown SI, Mondino BJ, Rabin BS: Autoimmune phenomenon in Mooren's ulcer, *Am J Ophthalmol* 82:835, 1976.

212. Berkowitz PT et al: Presence of circulatory immune complexes in patients with peripheral corneal diseases, *Arch Ophthalmol* 101:242, 1983.

213. Mondino BJ, Brown SI, Rabin BS: Cellular immunity in Mooren's ulcer, *Am J Ophthalmol* 85:788, 1978.

214. Wilson SE et al: Mooren-type hepatitis C virus-

associated corneal ulceration, *Ophthalmology* 101:736, 1994.

215. Moazami G et al: Interferon treatment of Mooren's ulcers associated with hepatitis C, *Am J Ophthalmol* 119:365, 1995.

216. Brown SI: Mooren's ulcer: treatment by conjunctival excision, *Br J Ophthalmol* 59:675, 1975.

217. Aviel E: Combined cryoapplications and peritomy in Mooren's ulcer, *Br J Ophthalmol* 56:48, 1972.

218. Foster CS: Systemic immunosuppressive therapy for progressive bilateral Mooren's ulcer, *Ophthalmology* 92:1436, 1985.

219. Brown SI, Mondino BJ: Therapy of Mooren's ulcer, *Am J Ophthalmol* 98:1, 1984.

220. Wakefield D, McCluskey P, Penny R: Intrave- nous pulse methylprednisolone therapy in severe inflammatory eye disease, *Arch Ophthalmol* 104:847, 1986.

221. Brown SI, Mondino BJ: Penetrating keratoplasty in Mooren's ulcer, *Am J Ophthalmol* 89:255, 1980.

222. Martin NF, Stark WJ, Maumenee AE: Treatment of Mooren's-like ulcer by lamellar keratectomy: report of six eyes and literature review, *Ophthalmic Surg* 18:564, 1987.

223. Kinoshita S et al: Long-term results of keratoepithelioplasty in Mooren's ulcer, *Ophthalmology* 98:438, 1991.

224. Bessant DA, Dart JK: Lamellar keratoplasty in the management of inflammatory corneal ulceration and perforation, *Eye* 8:22, 1994.

Twenty

Episcleritis and Anterior Scleritis

Scleral inflammation can be divided into two clinically important categories—episcleritis and scleritis. Episcleritis is a benign disease that is usually not associated with systemic disease, whereas scleritis can be painful and destructive and is often associated with serious systemic disease. In most cases episcleritis and scleritis can be clinically differentiated.

IMMUNOLOGY

The sclera contains immunoglobulins and the components of the classic and alternative complement pathways.[1,2] Scleral fibroblasts produce C1 and can be induced to produce collagenase, elastase, and other matrix-degrading enzymes.[3] They normally express class I human leukocyte antigens (HLA) but can be induced to express class II HLA antigens by exposure to an inflammatory stimulus.[4,5] Macrophages, neutrophils, lymphocytes, and Langerhans' cells are absent or present in very low numbers.

Scleritis associated with autoimmune disease is thought to be related to immune-complex vasculitis.[5] Vessel thrombosis and inflammatory infiltration of the vessels walls is seen. The complexes may be deposited from the circulation or formed in the sclera itself. Deposition of the complexes results in activation of complement, which stimulates neutrophil chemotaxis and enzyme release. Chronic inflammation can lead to a granulomatous response, with macrophages, epithelioid cells, multinucleated giant cells, and lymphocytes.

EPISCLERITIS

Clinical Manifestations
Episcleritis occurs most often in adults in the fourth decade of life but can develop at any age.[3,6] More common in women than in men, episcleritis is characterized by injection of the episcleral vessels (Table 20-1). The injection can be localized or diffuse and is occasionally bilateral. It can be associated with mild tenderness; a feeling of heat, pin-pricking, or irritation; or

Table 20-1 Features of Conjunctivitis, Episcleritis, and Scleritis

	Conjunctivitis	Episcleritis	Scleritis
Symptoms	Discharge, gritty sensation, itching	Usually none, may have mild discomfort, pricking	Deep, boring pain; may have tearing, photophobia
Injection			
Location	Diffuse, forniceal	Usually sectoral but can be diffuse, nodular	Diffuse or nodular
Hue	Red	Red	Purplish
Tenderness	None	Mild or none	Usually
Blanching with phenylephrine 10%	Yes	Moderate	No
Other findings	Follicles, chemosis, superficial punctate keratopathy, focal keratitis	Rarely fine peripheral corneal scarring	Scleral edema, scleral thinning, scleral necrosis, iritis, keratitis, serous elevations of choroid

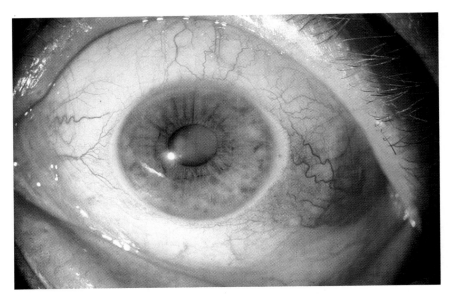

Figure 20-1
Most common appearance of episcleritis, with sectoral interpalpebral injection. (Courtesy of Diane Curtin, Pittsburgh, PA.)

tearing or mild photophobia. The episcleritis develops rapidly. When examined in daylight the redness does not have a bluish hue (Fig. 20-1). Episcleral (but not scleral) edema can be present. The vessels constrict after application of 10% phenylephrine (Fig. 20-2). Mild peripheral corneal infiltrates or opacities and a mild iritis can occasionally be seen. Most attacks of episcleritis are self-limited, resolving in 5 to 10 days[7]; however, some can last for months or years. Recurrences in the same or opposite eye are seen in approximately 60% of cases.[6] Most commonly, patients experience recurrences for 3 to 6 years, with a gradual decrease in frequency.

In some cases a nodule develops within a lo-

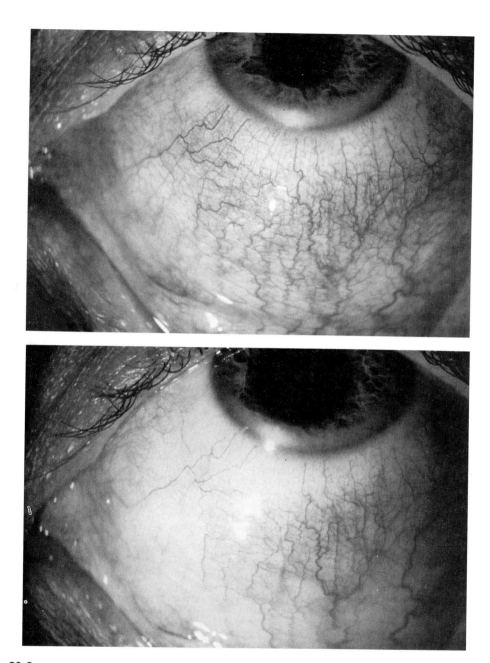

Figure 20-2
Diffuse episcleritis before (*top*) and after (*bottom*) application of 10% phenylephrine. (From Wiley L, Arffa R, Fireman P: *Allergic and immunologic diseases of the eye.* In Fireman P, Slavin R, editors: *Atlas of allergies,* New York, 1991, Gower.)

calized area of inflammation (Fig. 20-3). The nodule is red, round, or oval and 2 to 6 mm in diameter. The conjunctiva can be moved over the nodule, but the nodule is fixed to the sclera. The nodule is translucent, and slit-beam microscopy will demonstrate that the sclera is flat. More than one nodule may be present. This condition is called *nodular episcleritis,* and the course differs from that seen in simple episcleritis. It usually arises over 2 to 3 days and resolves over 4 to 6 weeks. The nodule gradually becomes paler and flatter, and the area heals without scarring or scleral thinning.

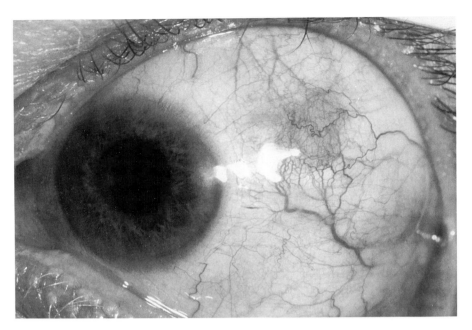

Figure 20-3
Nodular episcleritis. (Courtesy of Diane Curtin, Pittsburgh, PA.)

Associated Diseases

The diseases associated with episcleritis are listed in Table 20-2. Approximately 30% of patients have an associated disease.[3,6,8-10] In those cases associated with viral infection or systemic inflammatory disease, the systemic disease is usually well established when episcleritis develops. Evaluation of patients for systemic disease is discussed in the section on scleritis.

Episcleritis in herpes zoster ophthalmicus can occur during the acute disease or several weeks later. It can be related to direct viral invasion or an immune response to the virus. Herpes simplex episcleritis is uncommon and usually results from direct viral invasion. Yellowish conjunctival infiltrates and corneal or conjunctival dendrites may be present.[10] The episcleritis usually resolves in a few weeks without sequelae.

Treatment

In most cases episcleritis can be managed with observation. Because episcleritis does not cause injury to the eye, treatment is given for symptoms or cosmesis. Cold compresses, cool artificial tears, and topical vasoconstrictors (e.g., naphazoline) can provide some symptomatic relief. If this is not sufficient to relieve discomfort, or if the patient demands treatment for social or professional reasons, topical cortico-steroids or oral nonsteroidal antiinflammatory drugs (NSAIDs) can be used (Table 20-3). A topical corticosteroid with relatively low ocular penetration, such as fluoromethalone, is preferable. The minimum dose necessary to provide the desired effect should be used. In most cases the drops can be tapered and discontinued in 2 weeks. NSAIDs are particularly useful in patients with chronic simple or nodular episcleritis and those with associated systemic inflammatory disease. Specific treatment may be required for an associated disease: Patients with acne rosacea should be treated with an oral tetracycline; patients with gout are usually treated with allopurinol.

SCLERITIS

Clinical Manifestations

The eye can be likened to a ball-and-socket joint, and many of the conditions that affect the joints can also affect the sclera.[9] Scleritis occurs most often during the fourth to sixth decades of life and is more common in women.[9,11] It is bilateral in approximately one third of patients.[10]

Clinically, scleritis is typically accompanied by pain, lacrimation, and photophobia. The pain can be severe and can radiate from the eye

Table 20-2	Diseases Associated with Episcleritis and Scleritis
Episcleritis	**Scleritis**
SYSTEMIC INFLAMMATORY DISEASES	
Rheumatoid arthritis	Rheumatoid arthritis
Relapsing polychondritis	Ankylosing spondylitis
Rheumatic heart disease	Psoriatic arthritis
Inflammatory bowel disease	Systemic lupus erythematosus
Systemic lupus erythematosus	Polyarteritis nodosa
Psoriatic arthritis	Wegener's granulomatosis
Behçet's syndrome	Relapsing polychondritis
Cogan's syndrome	Rheumatic heart disease
	Inflammatory bowel disease
	Behçet's syndrome
	Cranial arteritis
	Cogan's syndrome
	Reiter's syndrome
INFECTIOUS DISEASES	
Tuberculosis	Tuberculosis
Syphilis	Syphilis
Herpes simplex	Herpes simplex
Herpes zoster	Herpes zoster
	Bacteria, especially *Pseudomonas* and *Acanthamoeba*
	Fungi
METABOLIC DISORDERS	
Gout	Gout
	Thyrotoxicosis
SKIN DISEASES	
Erythema nodosum	Erythema nodosum
Erythema multiforme	Acne rosacea
Acne rosacea	

Table 20-3	Dosages of Nonsteroidal Anti-inflammatory Agents in Episcleritis and Scleritis	
Agent	**Dosage (mg)**	
Diclofenac (Voltaren)	75 delayed release bid	
Diflunisal (Dolobid)	500 bid	
Fenoprofen (Nalfon)	600 tid	
Flurbiprofen (Ansaid)	100 tid	
Ibuprofen (Motrin)	800 tid	
Indomethacin (Indocin)	75 sustained release bid	
Ketoprofen (Orudis)	100 tid	
Naproxen (Naprosyn)	500 bid	
Piroxicam (Feldene)	20 qd	
Tolmetin (Tolectin)	400–600 tid	

to the jaw, forehead, or sinuses. Vision can be decreased. There is dilation of the deep episcleral vessels, giving the eye a bluish-red hue, which is best appreciated in daylight (Table 20-1). The vessels do not blanch after application of topical phenylephrine (10%). The sclera can be either edematous or necrotic and devoid of overlying vessels. Scleral edema is best appreciated with slit-beam microscopy, where it is seen as anterior displacement of the deep edge of the beam. Scleral thinning (seen as increased visibility of the darker choroid), chemosis, iritis

and corneal ulceration, vascularization, and opacification can be seen.

Anterior scleritis can be divided into the following four types:[9]

1. *Diffuse*—Broad area(s) of scleral inflammation, with minimal or diffuse scleral edema and no necrosis (Fig. 20-4)
2. *Nodular*—One or more localized areas of scleral inflammation, with nodular scleral edema and no necrosis (Fig. 20-5); the nodule is opaque, immobile, and firm to the touch
3. *Necrotizing with inflammation*—One or more avascular patches of necrotic sclera, surrounded by scleral inflammation and pain (Figs. 20-6 and 20-7)
4. *Necrotizing without inflammation* (scleromalacia perforans)—Scleral necrosis without surrounding inflammation or pain; longstanding rheumatoid arthritis in most cases (Fig. 20-8)

It can be difficult to distinguish diffuse anterior scleritis from simple episcleritis, and nodular scleritis from nodular episcleritis. The presence of deep pain, lack of constriction of vessels with phenylephrine, and a bluish hue to the injection suggest the diagnosis of scleritis. It is also important to differentiate scleromalacia perforans from degenerative scleral thinning. Degenerative scleral thinning is usually seen in individuals over 60 years of age. It is typically 1 to 2 mm in width and 2 to 6 mm in length.[12-15] It is most often seen between the insertion of the medial and lateral recti and the limbus. The lesions are bilateral and symmetric. It is caused

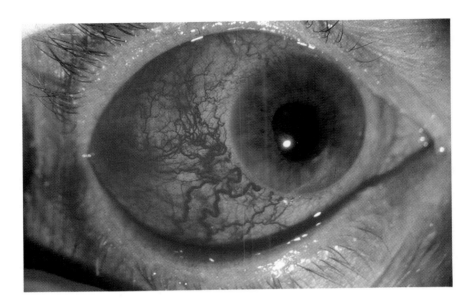

Figure 20-4
Diffuse scleritis. (Courtesy of Diane Curtin, Pittsburgh, PA.)

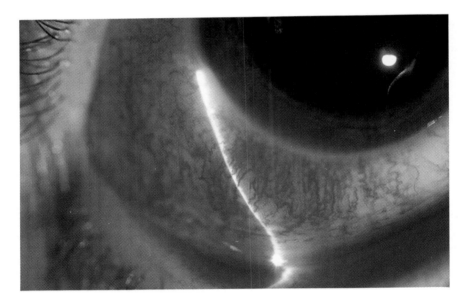

Figure 20-5
Nodular scleritis. Note bending of slit beam by the swollen sclera. (Courtesy of Diane Curtin, Pittsburgh, PA.)

by hyaline degeneration and calcification of the sclera.

The majority of patients with scleritis experience recurrences. Patients can advance from one form to another. Scleritis can occasionally complicate cataract extraction. It is almost invariably necrotizing, and in most cases a systemic vasculitic disease can be identified.

The percentages of patients with associated disease and visual loss vary according to the type of scleritis present (Table 20-4).[16]

Associated Diseases
The most common systemic disease associated with scleritis is rheumatoid arthritis, but a wide variety of other inflammatory diseases can also

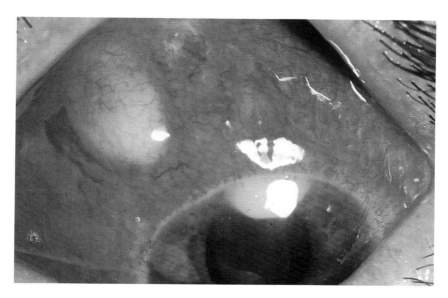

Figure 20-6
Severe sclerouveitis with large necrotizing granulomas. One lesion extends into the anterior chamber.

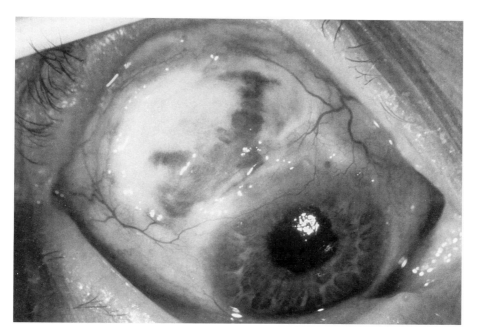

Figure 20-7
Large area of necrotizing scleritis with scleral thinning. (Courtesy of Diane Curtin, Pittsburgh, PA.)

be seen[8,10-17] (Table 20-2). In the most recent series from the Massachusetts Eye and Ear Infirmary,[3] an associated systemic disease was identified in 98 of 172 patients (57%). Forty-eight percent of patients had connective tissue or vasculitic disease and 7% had infectious disease. Of 100 patients whose only presenting complaint was scleritis, connective tissue disease or vasculitic disease was diagnosed in 26. Fifteen of these 26 patients had necrotizing scleritis with inflammation. The most common diagnosis was Wegener's granulomatosis, followed by relapsing polychondritis. However, because this is a referral center, the patient pop-

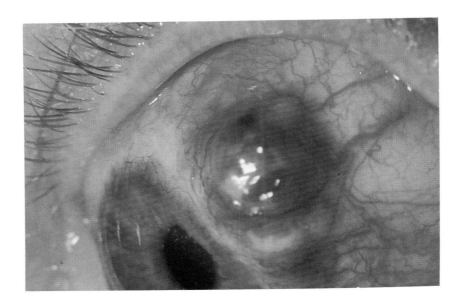

Figure 20-8
Large area of scleral melting without much inflammatory reaction (scleromalacia perforans) in a case of rheumatoid arthritis.

Table 20-4	Risk of Associated Disease and Visual Loss According to Type of Scleritis	
Disease	**Risk of Associated Disease***	**Risk of Loss of Visual Acuity†**
Episcleritis	30	0
Diffuse anterior scleritis	13–45	10–26
Nodular anterior scleritis	28–50	13–26
Necrotizing; with inflammation	50–95	74–82
Necrotizing; without inflammation	90–100	33

*References 3, 9.
†References 9, 67.

ulation may have been biased. In support of this, the mean duration of symptoms prior to diagnosis was 3 years. In my experience a systemic disease is diagnosed in only a small percentage of patients who do not have an identified associated disease on presentation.

Diagnostic Evaluation

Anterior segment fluorescein angiography can be helpful in differentiating scleritis from episcleritis, in identifying early necrotizing scleritis, in monitoring the effect of therapy, and in guiding tectonic surgery.[18-20] A low intravenous dose of fluorescein is used (0.6 ml of 20% sodium fluorescein) because fluorescein rapidly leaks from the episcleral and conjunctival vessels.[21,22] Use of fluorescein-labeled isothiocya-

nate-dextran conjugates—larger molecules that do not leak from anterior segment vessels—may be superior but is not approved for human use at this time.

Biopsy of the involved sclera is most useful in identifying infectious agents. Bacteria, fungi, parasites, and viruses can be isolated from conjunctiva, episclera, or sclera. In noninfectious cases biopsy can demonstrate vascular inflammation. Because nearly all patients with necrotizing scleritis have evidence of vascular inflammation, biopsy is not necessary to demonstrate this. However, vascular inflammation is present in approximately 60% of biopsies in nonnecrotizing scleritis, and granulomatous inflammation is present in only 23%.[3] The presence of vascular inflammation is not diagnostic

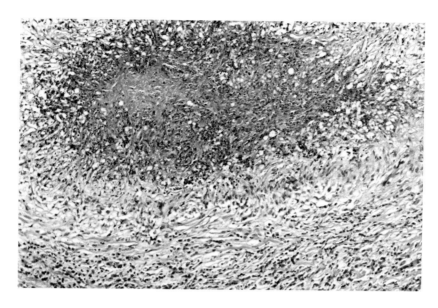

Figure 20-9
Granulomatous inflammation of sclera in rheumatoid arthritis. Fibrinoid necrosis is surrounded by a zone of palisading epithelioid cells and lymphocytes (hematoxylin-eosin stain, ×200). (Courtesy of Bruce L. Johnson, Pittsburgh, PA.)

of systemic vasculitic disease, but together with compatible systemic findings it can be highly suggestive of a specific vasculitic disease. The presence of granulomas in association with typical clinical features can confirm the diagnosis of Wegener's granulomatosis, even in the absence of positive anti-neutrophil cytoplasmic antibodies testing.

Histopathology
Histologically, necrotizing scleritis is seen as a granulomatous reaction (Fig. 20-9). Fibrinoid necrosis is seen in the center of the reaction, surrounded by epithelioid cells, multinucleated giant cells, plasma cells, lymphocytes, and less often, neutrophils. In areas of necrosis there is perivascular cuffing with neutrophils, lymphocytes, and medial necrosis, leading to vascular thrombosis, occlusion, or aneurysm formation.[3,23-27] A granulomatous reaction was seen in 23% of biopsies from patients with diffuse and nodular scleritis.[3] In these patients, lymphocytes, macrophages, and plasma cells are most plentiful, but neutrophils, mast cells, and eosinophils can also be present.

Immunopathologic examination indicated that the numbers of macrophages and T lymphocytes, particularly helper lymphocytes, were increased over normal sclera.[23] Neutrophil and lymphocyte infiltration in and around the vessel walls is accompanied by deposition of antibody and complement in the vessel wall. Because the episcleral and perforating scleral vessels are capillary and postcapillary venules and do not have a tunica media, the classical histologic diagnosis of vasculitis cannot be applied to them. Foster et al.[23] have used the term *inflammatory microangiopathy.* Inflammatory microangiopathy is nearly always present in necrotizing scleritis. It is present in approximately 60% of patients with nonnecrotizing scleritis, both those with and without systemic vasculitic disease.

Complications
Corneal Changes
Watson[9] reported that corneal involvement occurred in 37% of patients with scleritis. He divided corneal involvement into four types: acute stromal keratitis, sclerosing keratitis, limbal guttering, and keratolysis.

Acute Stromal Keratitis. Acute stromal keratitis can accompany diffuse or nodular nonnecrotizing scleritis. Superficial and midstromal opacities are most commonly seen near the limbus adjacent to areas of scleral inflammation (Figs. 20-10 through 20-12) but can also involve the central cornea. The peripheral and central corneal stroma can become diffusely edematous and cloudy. Vascularization and permanent scarring can develop with time.

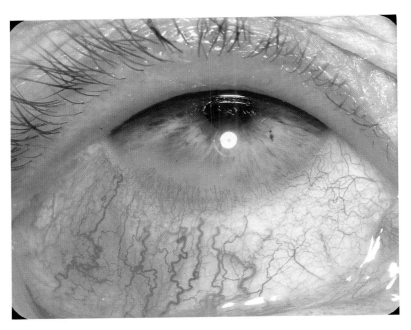

Figure 20-10
Nodular sclerokeratitis in a patient with rheumatoid arthritis.

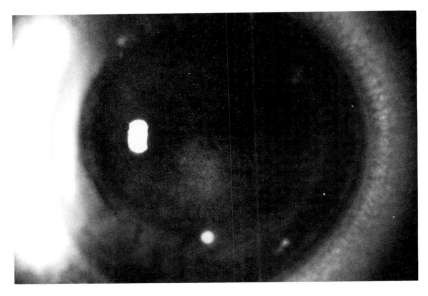

Figure 20-11
Acute stromal keratitis in scleritis, with central and peripheral stromal infiltration.

Sclerosing Keratitis. Sclerosing keratitis is the most common form of corneal involvement and can occur in any form of scleritis. The perilimbal cornea becomes thickened and gray; with time the opacification advances toward the central cornea. Crystalline opacities caused by lipid deposition can be seen behind the leading edge. Nodular corneal opacities, ring infiltrates, vascularization, and lipid deposition can develop (Fig. 20-13).

Limbal Guttering. Peripheral corneal thinning can occur with or without ulceration. Nonulcerative thinning is most commonly seen in middle-aged or elderly individuals with rheumatoid arthritis and develops over a period of

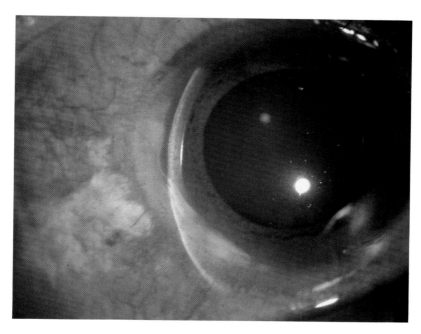

Figure 20-12
Midstromal peripheral corneal infiltration adjacent to an area of scleritis. (Courtesy of Diane Curtin, Pittsburgh, PA.)

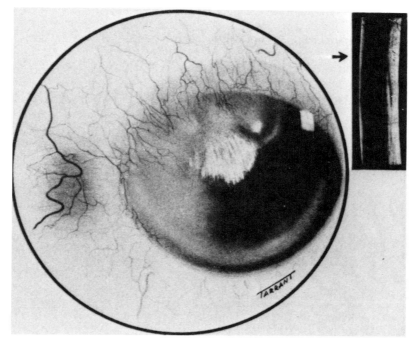

Figure 20-13
Sclerokeratitis. A diffuse peripheral change affects the whole corneal stroma at the site of the scleritis. Behind the advancing edge the corneal lamellae take on a crystalline appearance like floss candy. A "precipitin ring" has formed around one opacity. (From Watson PG: *Diseases of the sclera and episclera.* In Duane TD, Jaeger EA, editors: *Clinical ophthalmology,* vol 4, Philadelphia, 1988, Harper & Row. Used with permission of Lippincott-Raven Publishers.)

years. The thinning usually does not extend more than 2 mm from the limbus. It can be accompanied by vascularization and lipid deposition. Vision is rarely affected. In some cases the thinning can be severe enough to cause ectasia, resulting in an appearance similar to that of Terrien's degeneration. Rarely, perforation can occur. Limbal corneal thinning can also occur without scleritis in patients with longstanding rheumatoid arthritis (see Chapter 19).[28,29]

Peripheral Ulcerative Keratitis. Peripheral ulcerative keratitis (keratolysis) most often occurs in severe cases of necrotizing scleritis, with or without inflammation. Most of these patients have systemic inflammatory disease. The process is similar to the peripheral ulcerative keratitis seen in the absence of scleritis, including Mooren's ulcer (see Chapter 19). It is a destructive and dangerous process, frequently associated with loss of vision. Adjacent to an area of scleritis, the peripheral cornea becomes swollen and infiltrated. An epithelial defect develops and the stroma melts away. The process extends circumferentially and sometimes centrally and can lead to a descemetocele or rupture.

Others

Anterior uveitis frequently occurs in patients with scleritis, especially those with necrotizing scleritis with inflammation. Approximately 65% of patients enucleated for scleritis have evidence of anterior uveitis.[30,31] The presence of uveitis increases the risk of damage to the intraocular structures and loss of vision. Aggressive therapy is indicated to control the scleritis and uveitis.

Glaucoma occurs in 12% to 22% of patients with scleritis.[3,10,16,32] Angle-closure glaucoma can be precipitated by swelling of the angle structures, particularly if the patient has narrow angles. Inflammatory and steroid-induced glaucomas can occur. Cataract formation can result from intraocular inflammation and local or systemic steroid treatment. Cataract surgery should be attempted only in the absence of scleral inflammation.

Systemic Evaluation

The evaluation of patients for systemic inflammatory disease is discussed in Chapter 19. Patients should undergo a thorough history and examination, preferably by a rheumatologist. Diagnostic testing is directed by the results of this evaluation. If the results are not suggestive of a systemic inflammatory disease, further evaluation is generally not informative; however, the following tests are suggested: complete blood count with differential, erythrocyte sedimentation rate, serum uric acid, serologic test for syphilis, tuberculous skin testing, chest radiography, and radiography of the sacroiliac joints.

Infectious Scleritis

All classes of microbial organisms can cause scleral infection. Most bacterial, fungal, and amoebal cases occur as extension of a corneal infection. Primary scleral infection most commonly occurs after surgical or nonsurgical trauma. Immune compromise of the eye or host frequently plays a role. Endogenous spread of systemic infection to the sclera occurs in some conditions, such as tuberculosis, syphilis, and leprosy.

The clinical presentation of infectious scleritis is usually indistinguishable from that of noninfectious scleritis. Therefore, it is important to evaluate the risk factors for scleral infection in any patient with scleritis and to obtain cultures or perform a biopsy in suspicious cases. The following conditions increase the risk of scleral infection: trauma, surgical procedures, radiation, contact lens wear, chronic topical corticosteroid administration, recurrent herpes simplex, herpes zoster, and systemic immune compromise (e.g., diabetes, AIDS). The most common surgical procedures associated with scleral infection are pterygium excision, particularly if followed by beta-irradiation, topical thiotepa or mitomycin, retinal detachment repair with scleral buckling, and strabismus surgery.

Bacterial Scleritis

Bacterial scleritis usually occurs as scleral extension of a bacterial keratitis (see Fig. 10-8).[33-35] *Pseudomonas* is the most commonly encountered organism, but many other bacteria, including *Streptococcus pneumoniae, Staphylococcus aureus, Staphylococcus epidermidis, Proteus,* and *Nocardia asteroides,* as well as atypical mycobacteria have been reported.[33,36-40] The scleritis is necrotizing and usually suppurative (Fig. 20-14). The prognosis is poor, particularly in eyes with sclerokeratitis. Early diagnosis and aggressive and prolonged treatment can preserve vision in some eyes.

Tuberculous scleritis is usually acquired by hematogenous spread of pulmonary tuberculosis[41,42] but can also occur by extension of lesions in the cornea, conjunctiva, or iris or by direct injury.[43-45] Scleritis can also occur as an immune response to tubercular antigens. Tuberculous scleritis typically presents as nodular scleritis that, if left untreated, can progress to necrotiz-

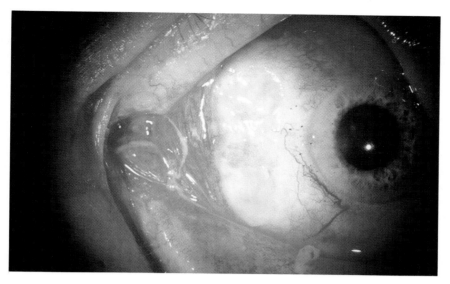

Figure 20-14
Scleral infection with *Pseudomonas aeruginosa* 20 years after beta-irradiation for a pterygium.

ing scleritis. Mucopurulent discharge may be present. Infiltrates and neovascularization can affect the adjacent cornea. Immune-mediated scleritis is usually seen in association with interstitial keratitis or phlyctenulosis.

Both episcleritis and scleritis can occur in leprosy and can be the initial manifestation. They can be a result of direct *Mycobacterium leprae* invasion or can be immune-mediated. The scleritis is usually bilateral and nodular and can progress to necrotizing. It is usually recurrent over many years, with exacerbations lasting 3 to 4 weeks. Peripheral corneal opacification and interstitial keratitis can occur (see Chapter 11).

Scleritis can occur during the course of congenital, secondary, or tertiary syphilis. Episcleritis can occur during primary syphilis, usually associated with an overlying conjunctival chancre. Scleritis in congenital syphilis is late in onset. It tends to be diffuse, prolonged, of mild severity, and resistant to treatment.[6] In secondary syphilis, scleritis and episcleritis appear at the same time as or after the onset of the skin rash. Conjunctivitis is often present, and the inflammation often involves the limbus. Primary scleritis must be differentiated from extension of a ciliary body gumma.[46] The scleritis in tertiary syphilis is indistinguishable from immune-mediated scleritis. The scleritis can be of any type and is often recurrent.[6] It may respond to systemic penicillin treatment, but some cases are unresponsive to both this regimen and oral antiinflammatory therapy.[47]

Episcleritis and scleritis have been reported in Lyme disease,[3,48,49] and *Nocardia* scleritis has also been reported.[50,51]

Fungal Scleritis

Fungal infections of the sclera nearly always affect compromised eyes or hosts. They frequently follow trauma (especially with organic matter) or surgery and may be associated with a fungal keratitis or endophthalmitis.[3,52,53] Hematogenous spread of a systemic fungal infection can also occur.[54] Fungal scleritis typically occurs as a slowly progressive necrotizing scleritis with suppuration. Smears and cultures from scrapings may be diagnostic, but in some cases biopsy is necessary.

Viral Scleritis

The most common viral cause of scleritis is herpes zoster. Although scleritis can occur during the acute episode, it more commonly occurs months or years later. Therefore, it may involve either direct viral invasion or an immune response to the viral infection. The incidence of scleritis in herpes zoster ophthalmicus is 1% to 8%.[6,10,55] The scleritis can be diffuse, nodular, or necrotizing. It can take months to resolve and often results in marked scleral thinning. Staphyloma formation can occur, and scleral homografting may be necessary.[56] Recurrences are frequent.

Herpes simplex can also cause scleritis both through direct tissue invasion and through an immune response.[10] Active infectious scleritis is usually diffuse or nodular, whereas immune-mediated scleritis is most often necrotizing. Scleritis and episcleritis can also occur with mumps.[57,58] They usually resolve spontaneously.

Parasitic Scleritis

Acanthamoebic scleritis is usually the result of extension of corneal disease (see Chapter 11). The scleritis is usually diffuse or nodular (see Fig. 11-16) but progression to necrotizing can occur.[59] Scleritis and episcleritis can also occur in toxoplasmosis,[60] usually as an extension of chorioretinitis.

Treatment
Immune-Mediated Scleritis

If a systemic inflammatory disease is present, it should be treated primarily, in conjunction with an internist or rheumatologist. Immunosuppressive therapy is often indicated for these patients.

Scleritis almost never responds to topical treatment alone; systemic treatment with an NSAID, corticosteroid, or other immunosuppressive agents is required. In patients with nonsevere, nonnecrotizing scleritis and no evidence of systemic disease, an NSAID (e.g., indomethacin, 75 mg sustained release twice daily, or ibuprofen, 800 mg three times daily) is usu-

Table 20-5   Treatment Summary for Patients with Collagen Vascular Disease and Scleritis

| Disease | Scleritis | | |
	Diffuse	Nodular	Necrotizing
Rheumatoid arthritis	Oral NSAID* Topical steroids Topical cyclosporine (?) Systemic corticosteroids	Oral NSAID Topical cyclosporine (?) Systemic corticosteroids Low-dose (once a week) methotrexate	Methotrexate Azathioprine Cyclophosphamide Systemic cyclosporine Systemic corticosteroids
Systemic lupus erythematosus	Oral NSAID Hydroxychloroquine sulfate (Plaquenil) Systemic corticosteroids	Oral NSAID Hydroxychloroquine sulfate (Plaquenil) Systemic corticosteroids Low-dose (once a week) methotrexate	Oral corticosteroids Intravenous pulse corticosteroids Azathioprine Cyclophosphamide, oral, or intravenous pulse
Polyarteritis nodosa	Cyclophosphamide and prednisone	Cyclophosphamide and prednisone	Cyclophosphamide and prednisone Azathioprine, methotrexate, cyclosporine alternatives
Wegener's granulomatosis	Cyclophosphamide and prednisone	Cyclophosphamide and prednisone	Cyclophosphamide and prednisone Azathioprine, methotrexate, cyclosporine alternatives
Relapsing polychondritis	Oral NSAID Dapsone Systemic corticosteroids Low-dose (once a week) methotrexate Azathioprine	Oral NSAID Dapsone Systemic corticosteroids Low-dose (once a week) methotrexate Azathioprine	Cyclophosphamide and prednisone Azathioprine and prednisone
Behçet's disease	Oral NSAID Colchicine	Oral NSAID Colchicine Systemic corticosteroids	Prednisone and chlorambucil Prednisone and cyclophosphamide Prednisone and cyclosporine

From Foster CS, Sainz de la Maza M: *The sclera,* New York, 1994, Springer-Verlag.
*Nonsteroidal antiinflammatory drug.

ally tried first (Table 20-3). Generally the first response to therapy is relief from pain. Some reduction in injection, tenderness, or corneal disease should be noted within 2 weeks. Once the eye is quiet the dose can be tapered gradually. If one agent is not effective another should be tried. Effective treatment can usually be achieved.

If the scleritis is severe, necrotizing, or unresponsive to NSAIDs, systemic corticosteroids are indicated. The initial dose of prednisone is approximately 1 mg/kg. Once the inflammation is controlled the dose can be reduced relatively quickly (over about 2 weeks) to 20 to 40 mg/day; thereafter the dose is slowly tapered (see Chapter 19). If this regimen is not effective, high-dose intravenous pulse therapy can be considered (1 g methylprednisolone intravenously three times during the first 7 days, followed by 1 g weekly, with gradual tapering).[61] Concomitant prophylactic therapy for gastrointestinal mucosal irritation or ulceration is probably worthwhile. Oral antacids and/or carafate (sucralfate) can be used.

Immunosuppressive therapy is used primarily in patients with a known systemic inflammatory disease. All patients with Wegener's granulomatosis or polyarteritis should be treated with cytotoxic immunosuppressive therapy. Foster and Sainz de la Maza[3] also recommend cytotoxic immunosuppressive ther-

apy for patients with rheumatoid arthritis or relapsing polychondritis who develop necrotizing scleritis. Without immunosuppressive therapy these patients have a high mortality rate. Treatment of these and other systemic inflammatory diseases should be coordinated with an internist or rheumatologist. The guidelines given by Foster and Sainz de la Maza[3] are summarized in Table 20-5.

Cytotoxic immunosuppressive agents can also be used in addition to or instead of corticosteroids in patients who require a high maintenance dose of corticosteroids or in those who do not respond to corticosteroids. They are frequently necessary for treatment of patients with necrotizing scleritis. Cyclophosphamide appears to be the most effective agent. Topical or systemic cyclosporine has been used successfully in a few patients.[62-64]

In severe cases large areas of scleral thinning can develop, with protrusion of the choroid (Fig. 20-15). It is sometimes necessary to surgically reinforce areas of thinning or perforation. The disease process should be controlled or the patch will melt quickly. Cornea, sclera, or periosteum can be used, depending on the size and location of the defect (Fig. 20-16). Hyperbaric oxygen therapy appeared to stimulate revascularization in one patient with scleral necrosis after beta-radiation.[62]

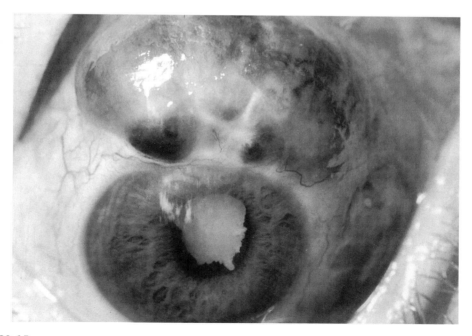

Figure 20-15
Extensive scleromalacia perforans, with bulging of choroid. (Courtesy of Diane Curtin, Pittsburgh, PA.)

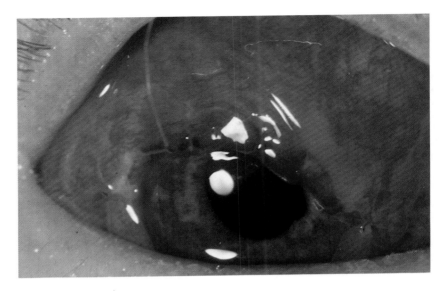

Figure 20-16
Autogenous tibial periosteum used to reinforce the sclera in the case seen in Figure 20-15.

Infectious Scleritis

Treatment of bacterial scleritis is fortified topical and systemic antibiotic therapy, guided by the suspected pathogen (see Chapter 10). This therapy may be modified once definitive culture and sensitivity results are obtained. If the infection is around a foreign body, such as a scleral buckle, the foreign body should be removed and cultured. If the scleritis does not respond to treatment after several days of therapy, surgical therapy should be considered. Debridement of infected sclera, cryotherapy,[33,65] and periosteal grafting may be beneficial.

Syphilis scleritis is treated using the neurosyphilis regimen: 24 million U of aqueous penicillin G intravenously daily for 10 days, followed by intramuscular penicillin, 2.4 million U of penicillin G benzathione intramuscularly once a week for 3 weeks.[66] In penicillin-allergic patients, tetracycline or erythromycin is used.

Fungal scleritis is treated with topical subconjunctival and systemic antifungal agents, according to the type of fungus involved (see Chapter 10). Surgical debridement and tectonic grafts may be necessary. Prolonged medical therapy is required.

Herpes simplex episcleritis and scleritis can be treated with topical antiviral agents, such as trifluridine. Oral acyclovir, 400 mg five times daily, may also be useful.

REFERENCES

1. Brawman-Mintzer O, Mondino BJ, Mayer FJ: The complement system in sclera, *Invest Ophthalmol Vis Sci* 29:1756, 1988.
2. Brawman-Mintzer O, Mondino BJ, Mayer FJ: Distribution of complement in the sclera, *Invest Ophthalmol Vis Sci* 30:2240, 1989.
3. Foster CS, Sainz de la Maza M: *The sclera,* New York, 1994, Springer-Verlag.
4. Harrison SA, Mondino BJ, Mayer FJ: Scleral fibroblasts, *Invest Ophthalmol Vis Sci* 31:2412, 1990.
5. Fong LP et al: Immunopathology of scleritis, *Ophthalmology* 98:472, 1991.
6. Watson PG, Hazelman BL: *The sclera and systemic disorders,* London, 1976, WB Saunders.
7. Watson PG et al: Treatment of episcleritis: a double blind trial comparing betamethasone 0.1%, oxyphenbutazone 10% and placebo eye ointments, *Br J Ophthalmol* 57:866, 1973.
8. Lyne AJ, Pitkeathley DA: Episcleritis and scleritis: association with connective tissue disease, *Arch Ophthalmol* 80:171, 1968.
9. Watson PG: *Diseases of the sclera and episclera.* In Duane TD, Jaeger EA, editors: *Clinical ophthalmology,* vol 4, Philadelphia, 1988, Harper & Row.
10. Watson PG, Hayreh SS: Scleritis and episcleritis, *Br J Ophthalmol* 60:163, 1976.
11. McGavin DDM et al: Episcleritis and scleritis: a study of their clinical manifestations and associations with rheumatoid arthritis, *Br J Ophthalmol* 60:192, 1976.
12. Sorensen TB: Paralimbal scleromalacia, *Acta Ophthalmol* 53:901, 1975.
13. Roper KL: Senile hyaline scleral plaques, *Arch Ophthalmol* 34:283, 1945.

14. Katz D: A localized area of calcareous degeneration in the sclera, *Arch Ophthalmol* 2:30, 1929.
15. Duke-Elder S, Leigh AG: *Diseases of the outer eye: cornea and sclera*. In Duke-Elder S, editor: *System of ophthalmology*, vol 8, part 2, St Louis, 1965, Mosby–Year Book.
16. Sainz de la Maza M, Jabbur NS, Foster CS: Severity of scleritis and episcleritis, *Ophthalmology* 101:389, 1994.
17. Sevel D: Necrogranulomatous keratitis associated with Wegener's granulomatosis and rheumatoid arthritis, *Am J Ophthalmol* 63:250, 1967.
18. Watson PG, Bovey E: Anterior segment fluorescein angiography in the diagnosis of scleral inflammation, *Ophthalmology* 92:1, 1985.
19. Bron AJ, Easty DL: Fluorescein angiography of the globe and anterior segment, *Trans Ophthalmol Soc UK* 90:339, 1970.
20. Watson PG: Anterior segment fluorescein angiography in the surgery of immunologically induced corneal and scleral destructive disorders, *Ophthalmology* 94:1452, 1987.
21. Meyer PA, Watson PG: Low dose fluorescein angiography of the conjunctiva and episclera, *Br J Ophthalmol* 71:2, 1987.
22. Meyer PA: Pattern of blood flow in episcleral vessels studied by low-dose fluorescein videoangiography, *Eye* 2:533, 1988.
23. Fong LP et al: Immunopathology of scleritis, *Ophthalmology* 98:472, 1991.
24. Ferry AP: Histopathology of rheumatoid episcleral nodules: an extra-articular manifestation of rheumatoid arthritis, *Arch Ophthalmol* 82:77, 1969.
25. Watson PG: The nature and treatment of scleral inflammation (Doyne Memorial Lecture), *Trans Ophthalmol Soc UK* 102:257, 1982.
26. Fraunfelder FT, Watson PG: Evaluation of eyes enucleated for scleritis, *Br J Ophthalmol* 60:227, 1976.
27. Rao NA, Marak GE, Hidayat AA: Necrotizing scleritis: a clinico-pathologic study of 41 cases, *Ophthalmology* 92:1542, 1985.
28. Brown SI, Grayson M: Marginal furrows: a characteristic corneal lesion of rheumatoid arthritis, *Arch Ophthalmol* 79:563, 1968.
29. Jayson MIV, Easty DL: Ulceration of the cornea in rheumatoid arthritis, *Ann Rheum Dis* 36:428, 1977.
30. Fraunfelder FT, Watson PG: Evaluation of eyes enucleated for scleritis, *Br J Ophthalmol* 60:227, 1976.
31. Wilhelmus KR, Watson PG, Vasavada AR: Uveitis associated with scleritis, *Trans Ophthalmol Soc UK* 101:351, 1981.
32. Wilhelmus KR, Grierson I, Watson PG: Histopathologic and clinical associations of scleritis and glaucoma, *Am J Ophthalmol* 91:697, 1981.
33. Reynolds MG, Alfonso E: Infectious scleritis and keratoscleritis: management and outcome, *Am J Ophthalmol* 112:543, 1991.
34. Alfonso E et al: *Pseudomonas* corneoscleritis, *Am J Ophthalmol* 103:90, 1987.
35. Raber IM et al: *Pseudomonas* corneoscleral ulcers, *Am J Ophthalmol* 92:353, 1981.
36. Altman AJ et al: Scleritis and *Streptococcus pneumoniae*, *Cornea* 10:341, 1991.
37. Sainz de la Maza M, Foster CS: Necrotizing scleritis after ocular surgery, *Ophthalmology* 98:1720, 1991.
38. Basti S, Gopinathan U, Gupta S: Nocardial necrotizing scleritis after trauma: successful outcome using cefazolin, *Cornea* 13:274, 1994.
39. Brooks JG, Mills RAD, Coster DJ: Nocardial scleritis, *Am J Ophthalmol* 114:371, 1992.
40. Kattan HM, Pflugfelder SC: *Nocardia* scleritis, *Am J Ophthalmol* 110:446, 1990.
41. Bloomfield SE, Mondino B, Gray GF: Scleral tuberculosis, *Arch Ophthalmol* 94:954, 1976.
42. Donahue HC: Ophthalmologic experience in a tuberculosis sanatorium, *Am J Ophthalmol* 64:742, 1967.
43. Swan KC: Some contemporary concepts of scleral disease, *Arch Ophthalmol* 45:630, 1951.
44. Nanda M, Pflugfelder SC, Holland S: *Mycobacterium tuberculosis* scleritis, *Am J Ophthalmol* 108:736, 1989.
45. Duke-Elder S: *System of ophthalmology*, vol 8, *Diseases of the outer eye: conjunctiva*, St Louis, 1965, Mosby–Year Book.
46. Duke-Elder S: *System of ophthalmology*, vol 8, *Diseases of the outer eye: conjunctiva*, St Louis, 1965, Mosby–Year Book.
47. Wilhelmus KR, Yokoyama CM: Syphilitic episcleritis and scleritis, *Am J Ophthalmol* 104:595, 1987.
48. Flach AJ, Lavoie PE: Episcleritis, conjunctivitis, and keratitis as ocular manifestations of Lyme disease, *Ophthalmology* 97:973, 1990.
49. Zaidman GW: Episcleritis and symblepharon associated with Lyme disease, *Am J Ophthalmol* 109:487, 1990.
50. Kattan HM, Pflugfelder SC: *Nocardia* scleritis, *Am J Ophthalmol* 110:446, 1990.
51. Brooks JG, Mills RAD, Coster DJ: Nocardial scleritis, *Am J Ophthalmol* 114:371, 1992.
52. Margo CE, Polack FM, Mood CI: *Aspergillus* panophthalmitis complicating treatment of pterygium, *Cornea* 7:285, 1988.
53. Milauskas AT, Duke JR: Mycotic scleral abscess: report of a case following a scleral buckling operation for retinal detachment, *Am J Ophthalmol* 63:951, 1967.
54. Stenson S, Brookner A, Rosenthal S: Bilateral endogenous necrotizing scleritis due to *Aspergillus oryzae*, *Ann Ophthalmol* 14:67, 1982.
55. Womack LW, Liesegang TJ: Complications of herpes zoster ophthalmicus, *Arch Ophthalmol* 101:42, 1983.
56. Arducci G, Capelli I: Scleral staphyloma after scleritis caused by herpes zoster, *Ann Ottalmologia* 94:187, 1968.
57. Swan KC, Penn RF: Scleritis following mumps: report of a case, *Am J Ophthalmol* 53:366, 1962.
58. North DP: Ocular complications of mumps, *Br J Ophthalmol* 37:99, 1953.
59. Lindquist TD, Fritsche TR, Grutzmacher RD:

Scleral ectasia secondary to *Acanthamoeba* keratitis, *Cornea* 9:74, 1990.

60. Zimmerman LE: Ocular pathology of toxoplasmosis, *Surv Ophthalmol* 6:832, 1961.
61. Wakefield D, McCluskey P, Penny R: Intravenous pulse methylprednisolone therapy in severe inflammatory eye disease, *Arch Ophthalmol* 104:847, 1986.
62. Hoffman F, Wiederholt M: Local treatment of necrotizing scleritis with cyclosporin A, *Cornea* 4:3, 1985.
63. Holland EJ et al: Topical cyclosporin A in the treatment of anterior segment inflammatory disease, *Cornea* 12:413, 1993.
64. Rosenfeld SI et al: Topical cyclosporine for treating necrotizing scleritis, *Arch Ophthalmol* 113:20, 1995.
65. Eiferman RA: Cryotherapy of *Pseudomonas* keratitis and scleritis, *Arch Ophthalmol* 97:1637, 1979.
66. Spoor TC et al: Ocular syphilis: acute and chronic, *J Clin Neuroophthalmol* 3:197, 1983.

Twenty-One

Metabolic Diseases

ENDOCRINE DISORDERS

Hyperthyroidism (Graves' Disease)

Hyperthyroidism most commonly occurs as part of a syndrome that may include goiter, exophthalmos, and pretibial myxedema. The eye changes seem to be independent of thyroid activity; they can be seen in the hyperthyroid state, or they may appear after a euthyroid or hypothyroid state has been reached. In some patients typical eye changes are present but no clinical history of thyroid dysfunction can be elicited. Graves' disease appears to be an autoimmune condition, but the mechanism of the ocular changes is unclear.

Ophthalmic involvement occurs in approximately 50% of patients. Patients may complain of a sandy feeling in the eyes, lacrimation, photophobia, decreased vision, or double vision. The most common signs are lid retraction, lid lag, conjunctival injection with chemosis, and proptosis. There is often a fullness and edema of the lids (Fig. 21-1). The conjunctival vessels are most dilated over the muscle insertions, and marked hyperemia and chemosis can occur (Fig. 21-2). The lids occasionally show increased pigmentation (Fig. 21-3).

Corneal involvement is related to exposure from proptosis and lid retraction. The earliest change is punctate staining of the cornea and conjunctiva in the interpalpebral zone. With more severe drying, chemosis, epithelial defects, ulceration, and even perforation can result. Hyperthyroidism may also be associated with superior limbal keratoconjunctivitis (see Chapter 8).

Mild exposure can be treated with lubricants and nocturnal taping of the lids or moisture barriers. In more advanced cases, lid surgery, such as lateral tarsorrhaphy or lid relaxation procedures, may be helpful. Exophthalmos can be reduced with oral corticosteroids, radiation, or surgical decompression.

Hypothyroidism

Superficial punctate keratopathy can occasionally be seen in hypothyroidism. Some have also suggested that hypothyroidism can cause an increase in tear production.

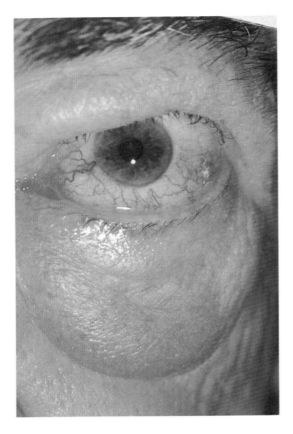

Figure 21-1
Edema of the lids, proptosis, conjunctival injection, and exposure keratitis of the lower one fourth of the cornea in thyroid orbitopathy.

Multiple Endocrine Neoplasia

Multiple endocrine neoplasia (MEN) is a rare hereditary condition in which neoplasias arise in multiple endocrine glands. The cell type involved in the neoplastic process is usually one that produces a polypeptide or biogenic amine. Three major disease patterns are seen, although overlap syndromes do exist. MEN type I and MEN type II arise from different genetic lesions. MEN types IIa and IIb are probably related to more than one genetic abnormality, at least one of which involves chromosome 10. MEN type I includes the following:

1. Autosomal dominant inheritance
2. Parathyroid adenoma or hyperplasia (nearly all)
3. Pancreatic islet cell tumors (80%)
4. Pituitary adenomas (>50%)
5. Thyroid adenomas
6. Subcutaneous lipomas
7. Adrenocortical adenomas
8. Carcinoid tumors

MEN type IIa (Sipple's syndrome) includes the following:

1. Autosomal dominant inheritance
2. Medullary carcinoma of the thyroid
3. Pheochromocytomas (50%)
4. Parathyroid adenoma or hyperplasia (10% to 20%)

MEN type IIb (Froboese's syndrome)[1] includes the findings in type IIa plus:

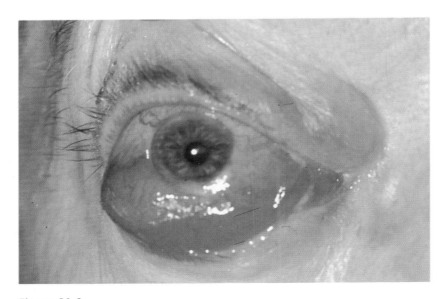

Figure 21-2
Marked chemosis of the lower conjunctiva in Graves' disease.

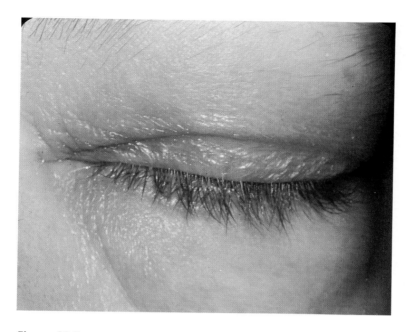

Figure 21-3
Pigmentation of the lids (Jellinek's sign) in a patient with hyperthyroidism.

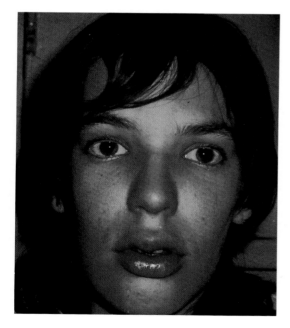

Figure 21-4
Marfanoid habitus and facies in multiple endocrine neoplasia.

1. Multiple mucosal neuromas involving the tongue, lips, gastrointestinal tract, and subconjunctival areas
2. Abnormal facies, including thick lips and soft tissue prognathism (Fig. 21-4)

3. Marfanoid habitus
4. Enlarged corneal nerves

The only ocular involvement in MEN type I is visual field defects caused by pituitary adenomas. Prominent corneal nerves are rarely present in type IIa. Ophthalmic signs are relatively common in type IIb.[2,3] Thickened nerves are seen in the cornea (Fig. 21-5), iris, and conjunctiva. The nerve fibers form an irregular lattice pattern across the entire cornea. They are seen as large white trunks entering the stroma, with smaller branches into the anterior and posterior stroma. Enlarged nerves can also be seen in the bulbar or tarsal conjunctiva. The nerves frequently appear as flat, poorly circumscribed bundles. They can also be smooth, yellow, and elevated and can resemble pingueculae. Multiple white cords may be seen radiating from the cornea. Paralimbal nerve bundles may be associated with dilated conjunctival vessels.

Less commonly seen is thickening of the lids or irregular prominences along the free margins (Fig. 21-6) that are caused by neuromas. Nasal displacement of the puncta, everted eyelids, decreased tear formation, and poor pupillary dilation can also be seen.

The nerves in the cornea do not appear to be myelinated; they contain numerous closely packed axons and Schwann cells. The latter have abundant basal lamina material but do not ensheathe the axons with myelin. The nod-

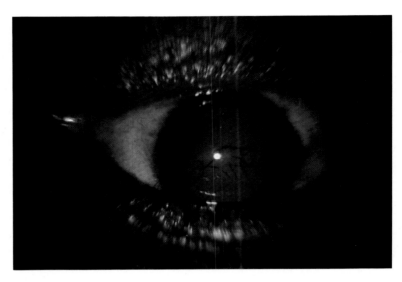

Figure 21-5
Increased visibility of the corneal nerves in multiple endocrine neoplasia.

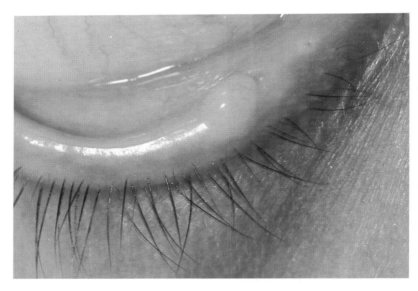

Figure 21-6
Neuromas of conjunctival lid margin in multiple endocrine neoplasia. (From Grayson M: *The cornea in systemic disease.* In Duane TD, editor: *Clinical ophthalmology,* vol 4, Hagerstown, MD, 1976, Harper & Row. Used with permission of Lippincott-Raven Publishers.)

ules of the conjunctiva and lid are composed of coiled myelinated nerves, with thickened perineurium and sometimes ganglion cells.

The ophthalmologist may have the opportunity to make the diagnosis of MEN by recognizing the prominent corneal nerves and other ocular findings. The differential diagnosis of increased visibility of the corneal nerves is discussed in Chapter 9. Investigation for MEN and

medullary carcinoma of the thyroid is very important. Serum concentration of calcitonin is elevated in medullary carcinoma of the thyroid and is a useful diagnostic test.

Multiple endocrine neoplasia type IIb and neurofibromatosis have many similarities in their clinical picture, and most likely they have been confused in the past. It is questionable whether neurofibromatosis is associated with

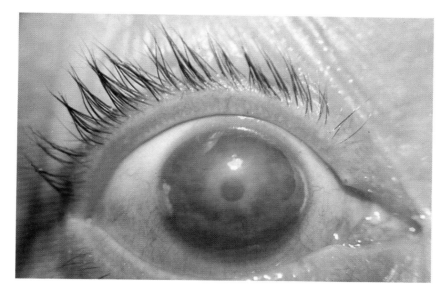

Figure 21-7
Hyperparathyroidism with calcium deposition in the anterior cornea.

prominent corneal nerves; such cases may have been unrecognized MEN type IIb.

Disorders of Calcium Metabolism

Hypercalcemia of any cause can be associated with calcium deposition in the cornea and conjunctiva. Corneal calcium deposition occurs most often in an interpalpebral band pattern but can be more diffuse[4] or appear as a circumferential limbal pattern. The cornea calcification associated with disorders of calcium metabolism cannot be clinically differentiated from idiopathic calcium deposition or deposition associated with intraocular inflammation. Band keratopathy usually begins in the peripheral interpalpebral cornea and extends centrally (see Chapter 15). A lucid interval is present between the calcific band and the limbus. Small holes are seen within the calcific opacity. Initially, the deposits are grayish and flat, but with progression they become white and elevated.

Hypercalcemia is often associated with conjunctival calcification. This gives the conjunctiva a granular appearance, which can be associated with injection and irritation, although most patients are asymptomatic. In band keratopathy associated with ocular inflammation the calcium is deposited extracellularly, whereas in systemic disease the deposits are often intracellular.

Hyperparathyroidism

In hyperparathyroidism, calcium can be deposited as hydroxyapatite crystals in the corneal (Fig. 21-7) and conjunctival epithelium, corneal endothelium, and anterior sclera.[5,6] The calcium is seen intracellularly in the nucleus and cytoplasm, in contrast to the extracellular deposition seen from most other causes.

Chronic Kidney Failure

Patients with renal failure often develop hypercalcemia or hyperphosphatemia, and calcium phosphate can be deposited in the cornea and conjunctiva.[7-9] The corneal deposits are seen as either band keratopathy or a more diffuse limbal opacification (Fig. 21-8). Conjunctival calcium deposition gives the limbal deposits a granular appearance. Mild calcification is very common and usually asymptomatic, but it can be associated with redness and irritation.[7] The calcium is deposited extracellularly.[7] Interestingly, a kidney transplant will result in resolution of conjunctival and corneal calcification, but hemodialysis does not.[8]

Idiopathic Hypercalcemia of Infancy

Idiopathic hypercalcemia of infancy is a rare cause of hypercalcemia that begins between 3 and 9 months of age.[10] The manifestations may include failure to thrive, apathy, polyuria, muscular weakness, hypertension, mental retardation, osteosclerosis, aortic stenosis, dwarfed habitus, and peculiar "elfin" facies. There appears to be abnormal sensitivity to vitamin D and increased calcium absorption from the intestines.[11] In addition to corneal calcium deposition, papilledema, strabismus, nystagmus, pu-

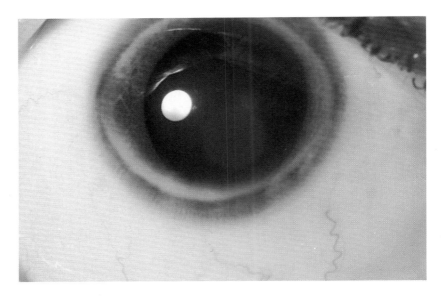

Figure 21-8
Calcific deposits of calcium in the cornea in a patient with renal failure.

pillary changes, and lenticular opacities have been described. Ultrastructurally, the corneal calcium deposition is usually intracellular, often confined to the nucleus. Extracellular deposits have also been seen.[12]

Hypophosphatasia

Hypophosphatasia is a rare familial disease characterized by multiple skeletal abnormalities and malformations, increased intracranial pressure, failure to thrive, and often early death from nephrocalcinosis.[13,14] It appears to result from an autosomal recessive deficiency of the tissue nonspecific alkaline phosphatase isoenzyme. Patients with infantile hypophosphatasia are homozygous for the abnormal trait, while childhood and adult patients are compound heterozygotes. Serum calcium is normal or elevated, serum phosphorus is normal, and alkaline phosphatase is low. Urine calcium is high, and all patients excrete excessive amounts of phosphoryl ethanolamine in the urine. Defective skeletal mineralization leads to rickets in children and osteomalacia in adults. There is no established treatment.

Band keratopathy and conjunctival calcification have been noted and may be accompanied by blue sclera, a malformation of the orbits (harlequin orbits), cataracts, optic atrophy, and pathologic lid retraction.[13,14]

Hypoparathyroidism

Acquired hypoparathyroidism is usually related to mechanical injury to or surgical removal of the parathyroid glands. The clinical manifestations are the result of hypocalcemia and include tetany, seizures, mental abnormalities, intestinal upset, and ectodermal abnormalities. A variety of ocular problems can occur, including lenticular abnormalities, blepharospasm, strabismus, nystagmus, papilledema, ptosis, and photophobia. Corneal vascularization and keratopathy are less commonly seen.

Hypoparathyroidism also occurs idiopathically, possibly on a hereditary basis, and can be associated with deficiencies of other organs, such as the adrenals, ovaries, and thymus. In the candidiasis-endocrinopathy syndrome, hypoparathyroidism, Addison's disease, pernicious anemia, ovarian failure, and mucocutaneous candidiasis appear in childhood. An autoimmune pathogenesis has been suggested, but the evidence is minimal. Ulcerating vascularization and opacification of the cornea can occur, possibly as a phlyctenular response to candidiasis.

DISORDERS OF LIPID METABOLISM

Sphingolipidoses

Sphingolipids are lipids that contain a long chain base, such as ceramides, cerebrosides, gangliosides, and sphingomyelins. The *sphingolipidoses* are disorders of sphingolipid catabolism; enzymatic defects result in intracellular accumulation of the lipid enzyme substrates. Depending on the specific enzymatic defect,

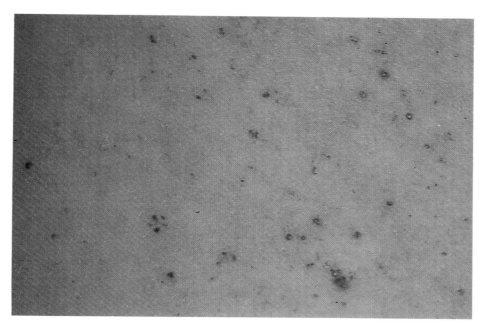

Figure 21-9
Skin lesions in Fabry's disease.

nervous tissue, reticuloendothelial cells, viscera, or vascular tissue can be affected.

Fabry's Disease

Fabry's disease, also known as angiokeratoma corporis diffusum, results from deficiency of α-galactosidase A.[15] It is transmitted as an X-linked recessive trait. The substrates are neutral glycosphingolipids with terminal α-galactosyl moieties, primarily globotriosylceramide. These accumulate in vascular endothelium, smooth muscle, heart muscle, renal glomeruli, sweat glands, central nervous system (CNS), spleen, liver, lymph nodes, and bone marrow. Fabry's disease is characterized clinically by telangiectatic skin lesions, hypohidrosis, febrile episodes, peripheral neuropathy, renal failure, cardiovascular disease, gastrointestinal symptoms, and CNS disturbances. The skin eruptions appear in childhood or around puberty and consist of small (pinpoint to several millimeters), round, red to blue-black spots (Fig. 21-9), some of which become hyperkeratotic (Fig. 21-10). They are noted particularly on the breasts, glutea, hips, thighs, and upper extremities.

Ocular findings occur in the majority of patients.[16-18] The most common finding is corneal opacity, which is present in nearly all affected males as well as in 90% of female carriers.[19] The opacity consists of fine, superficial, white, yellow, or brown dots, distributed in a vortex pattern (Fig. 21-11). The opacities can be seen only with the aid of a slit-lamp microscope and do not affect vision. They appear to result from accumulation of sphingolipid in the epithelium. Histologically, intracytoplasmic lamellar inclusions are noted, especially in the basal epithelial cells.[20,21] Similar inclusions can also be present in stromal keratocytes, Bowman's layer, endothelium, and conjunctival epithelium.[22,23]

Other causes of opacities in a vortex distribution (cornea verticillata) are deposition of chloroquine, amiodarone, and other drugs; Tangier disease; striate melanokeratosis; and Melkersson-Rosenthal syndrome (see Chapter 9).

Dilation and tortuosity of the conjunctival vessels, sometimes with aneurysm formation, occurs in approximately 60% of patients (Fig. 21-12). Posterior spokelike sutural cataracts, consisting of 9 to 12 spokes (Fig. 21-13), occur in about 50% of patients. Sphingolipid is probably deposited in the lens suture line. Cream-colored anterior capsular deposits, sometimes in a propeller-like pattern, may also be noted. Vision is not affected. Other ocular manifestations include periorbital edema (25% of cases), papilledema, retinal edema, optic atrophy, and dilation and tortuosity of the retinal vessels.

Gaucher's Disease

Gaucher's disease is an inherited deficiency of β-glucosidase, the enzyme that divides gluco-

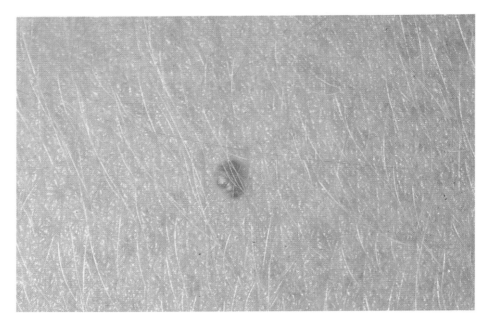

Figure 21-10
Skin lesions in Fabry's disease may become hyperkeratotic.

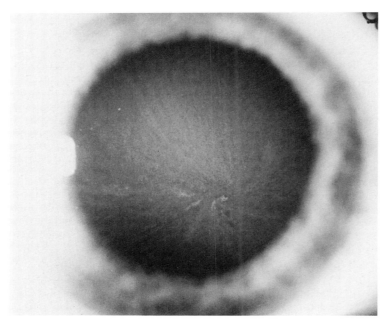

Figure 21-11
Whorllike opacification of the epithelium in Fabry's disease. (Courtesy of Diane Curtin, Pittsburgh, PA.)

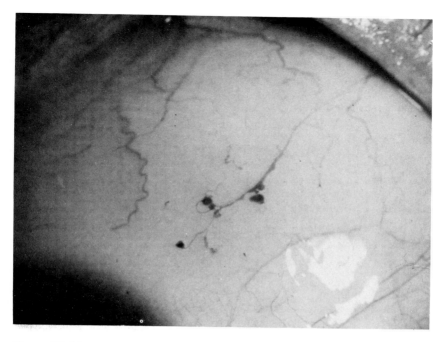

Figure 21-12
Conjunctival aneurysms in Fabry's disease.

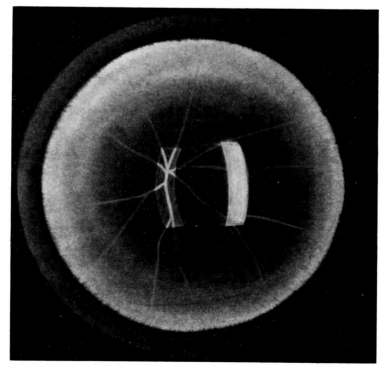

Figure 21-13
Spokelike cataract in Fabry's disease.

sylceramide into ceramide and glucose, resulting in an accumulation of glucosylceramide in reticuloendothelial cells throughout the body, particularly the liver and spleen. A variety of genetic mutations, all affecting chromosome 1, can produce this disease. Three clinical forms are recognized: (1) an adult form with liver and spleen enlargement, bone lesions, and skin pigmentation, but no primary CNS involvement; (2) an infantile form, with severe CNS disease and usually death by 3 years of age; and (3) a juvenile form, combining the features of the adult form with milder, slowly progressive neurologic impairment. All are inherited as an autosomal recessive trait.

The adult form of the disease may exhibit prominent, dark yellow pingueculae,[24] which are noted nasally and occur in approximately 25% of cases. Histologically, they contain foamy epithelioid cells (Gaucher's cells) instead of the elastosis seen in the usual pinguéculum. White deposits were observed in the peripheral corneal endothelium, chamber angle, and pupillary margin in one patient.[25] Occasionally, a cherry-red spot can be seen in the macula. Perimacular degeneration and ring granular opacities around the fovea occasionally occur. Retinal hemorrhages, edema, and nystagmus are seen in juveniles.

Metachromatic Leukodystrophy
Metachromatic leukodystrophy is a disorder of myelin metabolism with progressive neurologic deterioration, affecting both the CNS and peripheral nervous system.[26] It occurs in several forms, including congenital, late infantile, juvenile, and adult, and all appear to be related to abnormalities of arylsulfatase A (cerebroside sulfatase). Galactosyl sulfatide (cerebroside sulfate) accumulates in the white matter of the CNS, kidney, gallbladder, and other visceral organs. In the congenital and infantile forms, corneal clouding can occur,[27] as well as optic atrophy, abnormal extraocular movements, pupillary abnormalities, and graying of the macula.[26, 28]

GM₁ Gangliosidosis
GM_1 gangliosidosis is a rare autosomal recessive disease that occurs in congenital, juvenile, and adult forms, all caused by a deficiency of β-galactosidase.[29] The mucopolysaccharidosis Morquio type B is caused by a deficiency of the same enzyme. The infantile form is characterized by coarse facies, hepatosplenomegaly, a macular cherry-red spot (50% of cases), developmental delay, and skeletal changes resembling those of the mucopolysaccharidoses. The infant is affected at birth or shortly thereafter and survives only 1 to 2 years. Mild diffuse corneal clouding and conjunctival microvascular abnormalities are present in some patients.[30-32] In the adult form, corneal clouding can occur, as well as spondyloepiphyseal dysplasia, similar to that seen in mucopolysaccharidosis IV, spasticity, and ataxia, but intelligence is normal.[33] No ocular abnormalities have been reported in patients with the juvenile form.

Other Diseases
Niemann-Pick disease may rarely be associated with clouding of the corneas.[34] In the Niemann-Pick group of diseases a deficiency of acid sphingomyelinase leads to accumulation of sphingomyelin and other lipids. Lamellar and membranous cytoplasmic inclusions are found in epithelium, keratocytes, and endothelium.[34-37] In one case of Sandhoff disease (GM_2 gangliosidosis) corneal clouding was present.[38] In other cases the corneas are clear, but on pathologic examination single membrane-bound vacuoles are seen in keratocytes.[39] Table 21-1 summarizes the enzymatic defects and ocular signs in the sphingolipidoses that affect the anterior segment.

Hyperlipoproteinemias
Hyperlipoproteinemia is commonly associated with earlier onset of corneal arcus, xanthelasma (Fig. 21-14), and occasionally xanthomas and other external ocular disease. Lipoproteins are divided into prebeta or very low-density lipoproteins (VLDLs), beta- or low-density lipoproteins (LDLs), alpha- or high-density lipoproteins (HDLs), and chylomicrons. Six patterns of serum lipoprotein elevation were distinguished by Freidrickson et al. in 1967 (Table 21-2).[40]

More recently it has become apparent that most of the lipoprotein patterns are not specific to a single disease, but rather can be caused by several different genetic diseases as well as by other metabolic diseases. In addition, some specific genetic diseases can produce more than one lipoprotein type. However, past descriptions of ocular complications have referred only to Freidrickson types and have not distinguished between the different causes, so the ophthalmic findings are discussed here in terms of Freidrickson types. In general, premature arcus and xanthelasma (raised yellow plaques near the inner canthus of the eyelids [Fig. 21-14]) occur in types with hypercholesterolemia, and eruptive xanthomas occur in types with hypertriglyceridemia (Table 21-2).

Table 21-1 Sphingolipidoses with Anterior Segment Findings*

Disease	Fabry's Disease	Gaucher's Disease	Metachromatic Leukodystrophy†	GM_1 Gangliosidosis	Niemann-Pick Disease
Heredity	Sex-linked recessive	Autosomal recessive	Autosomal recessive	Autosomal recessive	Autosomal recessive
Enzyme defect	α-galactosidase A	β-glucosidase	Arylsulfatase A	β-galactosidase	Acid sphingomyelinase
Tissue storage	Glycosphingolipids	Glucosylceramide	Galactosylsulfatide (cerebroside sulfate)	GM_1 ganglioside; glycoproteins; keratan sulfate	Sphingomyelin and cholesterol
Corneal clouding	+ (Epithelial)	−			
Macular grayness or cherry-red spots	−	±	+	±	+ (Rare)
Optic atrophy	−	−	+	+	+ (Neuropathic forms)
Conjunctiva	Vascular dilation and tortuosity	Dark-yellow pingueculae (25%)	−	−	−

*Corneal clouding has also been reported in one case of Sandhoff disease (GM_2 gangliosidosis II).
†Congenital and infantile forms.

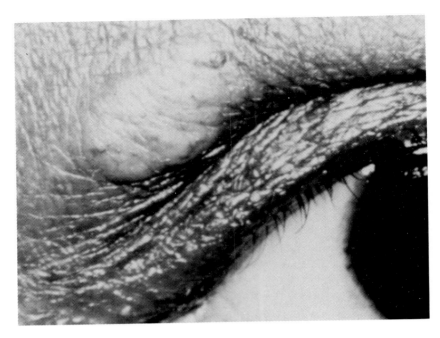

Figure 21-14
Xanthelasma of lid.

Type I (Hyperchylomicronemia, or Buerger-Grütz Disease)

Hyperlipoproteinemia type I is rare and can be caused by either of two autosomal recessive disorders: familial lipoprotein lipase deficiency and familial apoprotein CII deficiency. The serum is creamy-white because of an accumulation of chylomicrons containing mainly triglycerides; this can be seen as lipemia retinalis when plasma levels exceed 2000 mg/ml. In familial lipoprotein lipase deficiency, eruptive xanthomata, which are small, yellow-orange papules surrounded by an erythematous halo, can develop when the lipemia is severe. They are most commonly seen on the face, buttocks, and limbs and can involve the lids. Hepatomegaly, splenomegaly, and foam cell infiltration of the bone marrow also develop. In familial apoprotein CII deficiency, VLDL level is also elevated, and a type V lipoprotein pattern can be present. Eruptive xanthomata are rare. Rarely, lipid keratopathy occurs in type I lipoproteinemia, but premature corneal arcus usually does not.[41]

Type IIa (Hyperbetalipoproteinemia, Hypercholesterolemia)

Most individuals with this lipid profile have polygenic hypercholesterolemia as a result of an interaction between multiple genetic and environmental factors, such as diet and obesity. Type IIa can be related to single gene mutations, as in familial hypercholesterolemia and multiple lipoprotein-type hyperlipidemia, common autosomal dominant disorders, or secondary to a variety of systemic conditions, including Cushing's syndrome, hypothyroidism, Werner's syndrome, acute intermittent porphyria, and nephrotic syndrome. Type IIa is characterized by increased LDLs of normal composition. In familial hypercholesterolemia, heterozygous individuals have a higher than normal incidence of premature coronary disease and peripheral atherosclerotic occlusive disease. Xanthomatous lesions develop in the tendons, particularly the Achilles, plantar, patellar, and digital extensors of the hands. In individuals homozygous for familial hypercholesterolemia, the disease is much more severe, and death from myocardial infarction usually occurs before age 20.[42,43] Patients with multiple lipoprotein–type hyperlipidemia tend to have mild and variable elevations of plasma lipids. Premature atherosclerosis and coronary artery disease are more common than normal, but xanthomata do not occur. In familial cases corneal arcus develops at an earlier age: It is present in 50% of heterozygotes over 30 years of age and in 75% over age 40[44]; in homozygotes it usually appears in the first decade. In familial hyper-

Table 21-2 Major Hyperlipoproteinemias

Type	Primary Disorders	Major Elevation in Plasma		Premature Corneal Arcus	Lid/Conjunctiva	Lipemia Retinalis
		Lipoprotein	Lipid			
I	Familial lipoprotein lipase deficiency Familial apoprotein CII deficiency	Chylomicrons	Triglycerides	–	Eruptive xanthomata in lids	+
IIa	Familial hypercholesterolemia Multiple lipoprotein-type hyperlipidemia Polygenic/exogenous hypercholesterolemia	LDL*	Cholesterol	+	Xanthelasma Lid and conjunctival xanthomata	–
IIb	Multiple lipoprotein-type hyperlipidemia Familial hypercholesterolemia	LDL and VLDL†	Cholesterol and triglycerides	+	– (Xanthomata)	–
III	Familial dysbetalipoproteinemia	VLDL remnants	Triglycerides and cholesterol	+	Xanthelasma (lid xanthomata)	+
IV	Familial hypertriglyceridemia (mild form) Multiple lipoprotein-type hyperlipidemia Sporadic hypertriglyceridemia Tangier disease	VLDL	Triglycerides	–	(Lid xanthomata)	+
V	Familial hypertriglyceridemia (severe form) Familial apoprotein CII deficiency Multiple lipoprotein-type hyperlipidemia	VLDL and chylomicrons	Triglycerides and cholesterol	–	Eruptive xanthomata (rare)	+

*Low-density lipoprotein.
†Very low-density lipoprotein.

cholesterolemia xanthelasmas occur frequently, and conjunctival xanthomata and lipid keratopathy can also occur.

Type IIb

Type IIb is characterized by elevated VLDL and LDL levels. Both total serum cholesterol and serum triglyceride levels are elevated. It may be hereditary, most commonly caused by multiple lipoprotein–type hyperlipidemia and rarely by familial hypercholesterolemia. This pattern can also be seen in Cushing's syndrome and the nephrotic syndrome. Corneal arcus is more common, and xanthomata can be seen in familial hypercholesterolemia cases.

Type III (Dysbetalipoproteinemia)

Type III is rare and is usually inherited as an autosomal recessive trait. Serum triglyceride and cholesterol levels are elevated as a result of accumulation of abnormal beta-lipoproteins derived from partial catabolism of VLDL (VLDL remnants or intermediary density lipoprotein). Two types of xanthomata are seen: xanthoma striata palmaris, orange or yellow discolorations of the palmar and digital creases; and tuberous xanthomata, nodular elevations most often seen on the elbows and knees. Premature coronary vascular disease and peripheral vascular disease are common. Obesity, diabetes mellitus, and hypothyroidism are often present. Premature corneal arcus, xanthelasma, and lipemia retinalis can be seen.

Type IV (Hyperprebetalipoproteinemia)

Type IV can be inherited, due to familial hypertriglyceridemia, a common autosomal dominant disorder; idiopathic; or related to one of many systemic conditions, including diabetes mellitus, oral contraceptive use, alcoholism, uremia, emotional stress, acromegaly, and von Gierke's disease. Typically, patients with familial and sporadic hypertriglyceridemia exhibit obesity, hyperglycemia, and hyperinsulinemia. Serum VLDL and triglyceride levels are usually mildly to moderately elevated; but severe exacerbations occur with excessive alcohol consumption, use of oral contraceptives, hypothyroidism, poorly controlled diabetes, or other precipitating factors. During such exacerbations chylomicrons are also elevated (type V pattern), and eruptive xanthomata and pancreatitis can occur. Lipemia retinalis can be seen.

Type V (Hyperprebetalipoproteinemia, Hyperchylomicronemia)

Type V is a rare type in which VLDLs and chylomicrons accumulate in the blood in individuals on a normal diet. The serum is creamy, and the triglyceride level is high. It typically results from familial apoprotein CII deficiency and rarely occurs in individuals with familial hypertriglyceridemia (as described previously) or multiple lipoprotein–type hyperlipidemia. Homozygous individuals with familial apoprotein CII deficiency present in adolescence or early adult life with recurrent attacks of pancreatitis. Eruptive xanthomata rarely occur. Heterozygotes do not develop pancreatitis. Patients with familial hypertriglyceridemia who develop a type V pattern can develop pancreatitis and eruptive xanthomata. Lipemia retinalis is common, but corneal arcus is not.

A number of other, relatively rare disorders of lipid metabolism can affect the cornea,[45] and these are discussed in the rest of this chapter and summarized in Table 21-3.

Apolipoprotein A-1 Deficiency

Apolipoprotein A-1 is a protein that serves as the principle structural component of HDL. Only six patients with a deficiency of apolipoprotein A-1 have been described, and these deficiencies have been caused by a variety of mutations.[46,47] Diffuse corneal clouding was present in four of six cases. HDL levels are very low. Early coronary artery disease, planar xanthomata, and hepatosplenomegaly were present in some cases.

Familial Lecithin-Cholesterol Acyltransferase Deficiency

Lecithin-cholesterol acyltransferase (LCAT) is an enzyme that circulates in the plasma and catalyzes the formation of plasma lipoprotein cholesteryl esters. Familial LCAT deficiency is a rare autosomally inherited disorder in which there is absence or near absence of LCAT activity in plasma. Serum-unesterified cholesterol and VLDL levels are increased, and esterified cholesterol and lysolecithin are reduced. The structures of all lipoproteins are abnormal. Anemia, uremia, and proteinuria are frequently present, but the risk of myocardial infarction is not increased. Both familial LCAT deficiency and fish-eye disease involve mutations in the LCAT gene on chromosome 16.

Corneal opacities consisting of many small gray dots can be seen throughout the stroma, beginning in early childhood (Fig. 21-15).[47-53] The opacities can become dense in the periphery, resembling a corneal arcus. There is usually a lucid interval at the limbus, but occasionally crystals (presumably cholesterol) are seen near Descemet's membrane. Visual acuity is not affected. Membranous deposits are present in keratocyte vacuoles and extracellularly. The presence of unesterified cholesterol was documented in one cornea.[54]

Fish-Eye Disease

Fish-eye disease is a rare hereditary disease in which LCAT activity toward HDL is absent, but LCAT activity toward LDL is present.[55] Marked corneal clouding is the most prominent finding. The eyes are said to resemble those of boiled fish. The HDL abnormalities are comparable with those seen in familial LCAT deficiency. LDL, triglyceride, and VLDL levels can be elevated.[49,56,57] Corneal clouding begins late in the second decade of life and can become sufficiently dense as to require keratoplasty. Gray-white-yellow dots are seen throughout the stroma and are densest in the periphery. Corneal thickness is increased. On histopathologic examination, numerous extracellular vacuoles made of a cholesterol-containing lipid are seen throughout the stroma.[56] One pedigree

with a similar clinical presentation but different serum lipid profile has been described.[58]

Tangier Disease

Tangier disease (familial HDL deficiency) is transmitted as an autosomal recessive trait. The exact biochemical defect is unknown. In homozygotes, a complete absence of plasma HDL is noted; in its place an abnormal HDL is found. There may be an abnormally low level of LDL and cholesterol. Chylomicron and VLDL levels are highly abnormal. Triglycerides are normal or increased. Cholesteryl esters are diffusely deposited in reticuloendothelial cells. One sees a yellowish-orange tinge of the tonsils, tonsil beds, rectal mucosa, and conjunctiva. There is enlargement of the liver, spleen, and lymph nodes and relapsing peripheral neuropathy. There is a minimally increased risk of coronary artery disease.

The cornea shows stromal clouding, presum-

Table 21-3	Other Disorders of Lipid Metabolism			
Disease	**Primary Abnormality**	**Serum**	**Cornea**	**Lid/Conjunctiva**
Apolipoprotein A-1 deficiency	Apolipoprotein A-1	Absent HDL*	Diffuse clouding; mild to marked	
Familial LCAT† deficiency	LCAT	High VLDL‡, unesterified cholesterol	Diffuse dotlike opacities; arcuslike	
Tangier disease	?	Absent HDL	Stromal clouding, vision normal	Yellowish-orange conjunctival tinge
Fish-eye disease	LCAT	Low HDL, ± increased LDL§, triglyceride, VLDL	White-yellow dotlike opacities; increased thickness	
Refsum disease	β-oxidation of β-methylated fatty acids	Increased phytanic acid	Thickened epithelium; pannus; increased visibility of nerves; guttae; edema	
Cerebrotendinous xanthomatosis	Hepatic mitochondrial 27-hydroxylase	Increased cholesterol		Xanthelasma
Phytosterolemia	Unknown	Increased phytosterols	Premature arcus	Xanthelasma
Farber disease	Lysosomal acid ceramidase	Increased tissue ceramide	Clouding	Conjunctival granulomas (type I)

*High-density lipoprotein.
†Lecithin-cholesterol acyltransferase.
‡Very low-density lipoprotein.
§Low-density lipoprotein.

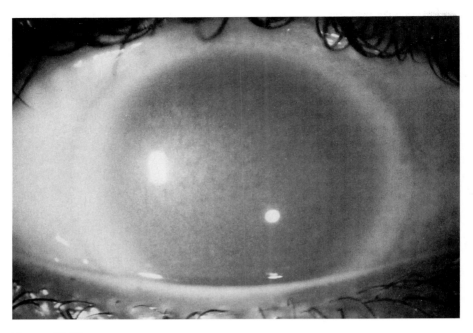

Figure 21-15
Diffuse opacification of the corneal stroma in lecithin-cholesterol acyltransferase deficiency. (Courtesy of Robert D. Deitch Jr., Indianapolis, IN.)

ably caused by the deposition of cholesteryl esters.[59,60] Many small dots are seen throughout the stroma, sometimes in a whorllike fashion, densest posteriorly and in the horizontal meridian. A lipid arcus is not present, and vision is usually not affected.

Refsum Disease

Refsum disease is an autosomal recessive disease of lipid metabolism that results in accumulation of phytanic acid, a C_{20} branched-chain fatty acid. The enzymatic defect is in the alpha-oxidation of beta-methylated fatty acids. It is an important disease to recognize because dietary restriction of phytols and plasmapheresis therapy can significantly improve the outcome. Phytanic acid accumulation also occurs in Zellweger syndrome and some other peroxisomal disorders.

The major manifestations are neurologic (caused by demyelination) and retinal. Common findings include peripheral neuropathy, cerebellar ataxia, nerve deafness, anosmia, pupillary abnormalities, retinal pigmentary degeneration, ichthyosis, and skeletal abnormalities. Irregular, thick, hazy corneal epithelium; fibrovascular pannus; and increased visibility of the corneal nerves can be present.[61] Corneal guttae, stromal edema, and cataracts can also occur.

Cerebrotendinous Xanthomatosis

Cerebrotendinous xanthomatosis is a rare familial disorder of sterol metabolism caused by a deficiency of hepatic mitochondrial 27-hydroxylase, which is involved in the synthesis of bile acids. Cholesterol and cholestanol are stored in most tissues, particularly in xanthomata, bile, and brain.[62] The manifestations include dementia, cerebellar ataxia, tuberous and tendon xanthomata, spinal cord paresis, and early atherosclerosis. Patients have a high incidence of xanthelasmas and cataracts and should be treated with chenodeoxycholic acid.

Phytosterolemia

Phytosterolemia is another rare, inherited sterol storage disease. It is inherited as an autosomal recessive trait and is characterized by tendon and tuberous xanthomata and premature coronary artery disease.[62] Increased amounts of phytosterols (plant sterols) are found in serum and erythrocytes and in some tissues. Premature corneal arcus and xanthelasmas are seen. Patients are treated with diets low in plant and shellfish sterols and with cholestyramine.

Farber Disease

Farber disease is a genetic disorder of lipid metabolism that is associated with a deficiency of lysosomal acid ceramidase and tissue accumulation of ceramide. The manifestations include painful and progressively deformed joints; subcutaneous nodules; hoarseness; nervous system dysfunction; lung, heart, and lymph node involvement; and usually death within a few years. Corneal opacities have been noted in these patients;[63] granulomatous, xanthoma-like conjunctival lesions occur in type I.[64] Macular cherry-red spots are also found in some patients. Histologically, granulomas and accumulation of lipid-laden macrophages are noted in affected tissues. Round inclusions, surrounded by a bilaminar membrane, are seen in conjunctival and corneal epithelium and in keratocytes.[65]

DISORDERS OF CARBOHYDRATE METABOLISM

Systemic Mucopolysaccharidoses

The extracellular matrix plays a vital role in the maintenance and regulation of cellular function as well as in intercellular support. It is composed primarily of proteoglycans, which are a type of glycoprotein composed of noncollagenous protein chains with covalently bound oligosaccharides and glycosaminoglycan (GAG) side chains. GAGs, previously known as mucopolysaccharides, are composed of repeating disaccharide units, typically a hexosamine plus a uronic acid. In the past, the GAG portions of the proteoglycans were much better characterized than the core proteins, so many proteoglycans were named according to the type(s) of GAG side chain (e.g., chondroitin sulfate proteoglycan). More information is now available about the structure of the core protein, and the nomenclature is changing. More often the proteoglycan is given a single simple name that reflects the properties of the core protein (e.g., aggrecan).

Keratan sulfate and dermatan/chondroitin sulfate are the primary GAGs of the stroma, in approximately a 3:1 ratio.[66] The core protein that contains the chondroitin/dermatan sulfate chains is decorin,[67] which has also been found in other body tissues. The core protein of the proteoglycan containing keratan sulfate is similar to decorin, and has been named *lumican*.[68] Lumican is also found in the aorta and intestines. Heparan sulfate, another major mucopolysaccharide, is not present in the cornea but is found in the retina, CNS, and aorta.

The mucopolysaccharidoses are recessively inherited deficiencies of enzymes that degrade GAGs (mucopolysaccharides).[69] Degradation of GAGs involves four glycosidases, five sulfatases, and one nonhydrolytic transferase, all present in lysosomes.[69] The absence or abnormal structure of one of these enzymes leads to accumulation of its substrates intracellularly. The specific enzyme defect determines which GAGs accumulate and which tissues are affected. There are 10 known enzyme deficiencies that give rise to six distinct mucopolysaccharidoses. Deficiencies in enzymes that normally degrade dermatan sulfate or keratan sulfate lead to accumulation of these substances in the cornea, resulting in corneal clouding. Accumulation of heparan sulfate can cause retinopathy and optic atrophy. In both cases the stored mucopolysaccharides apparently also spill out of the cells into the blood, from which they can be deposited in reticuloendothelial cells, blood vessels, and heart valves, or be excreted in the urine.

The clinical characteristics of the mucopolysaccharidoses are summarized in Table 21-4, and the heredity and enzymatic defects in Table 21-5.

Hurler Syndrome

Hurler syndrome (mucopolysaccharidosis IH) is characterized by gargoyle-like facies, marked skeletal abnormalities (dysostosis multiplex), and progressive mental retardation. Skeletal abnormalities include dorsal and lumbar kyphosis with gibbus, short stature (Fig. 21-16), flaring of the lower ribs, and broad hands with stubby fingers (Fig. 21-17). Hepatosplenomegaly, deafness, and cardiac problems are common. Those affected can appear normal at birth, but the disease becomes evident during the first 1 to 2 years of life. Death usually occurs during the teenage years as a result of cardiorespiratory complications. There is a deficiency of α-L-iduronidase resulting in accumulation of heparan sulfate and dermatan sulfate.

The cornea can be clear at birth, but soon afterward becomes characterized by an avascular noninflammatory clouding (Fig. 21-18). Fine, gray, punctate opacities are first seen in the anterior stroma, then in the posterior stroma and endothelium, resulting in a diffuse, ground-glass haze. Corneal thickness may be increased. Pigmentary retinopathy and optic atrophy also commonly occur.[70] Glaucoma caused by trabecular involvement has been reported.[71] Short-term success of corneal transplantation in Hurler syndrome has also been reported.[72]

Scheie's Syndrome

Scheie's syndrome (mucopolysaccharidosis IS) is caused by a different defect in the same enzyme affected in Hurler syndrome, α-L-iduronidase. Hurler and Scheie syndromes are caused by al-

Table 21-4 Ocular and Systemic Features of Mucopolysaccharidoses

	Syndrome	Corneal Opacification	Retinal Pigmentary Degeneration	Optic Atrophy	Mental Retardation	Cardio-vascular	Skeletal Dysplasia
Mucopolysaccharidosis IH	Hurler syndrome	+	+	+	+	+	+
Mucopolysaccharidosis IS	Scheie's syndrome	+	+	+	−	+	+
Mucopolysaccharidosis IH/S	Hurler-Scheie compound	+	+	+	±	+	+
Mucopolysaccharidosis IIA	Hunter's syndrome, severe	−*	+	+	+	+	+
Mucopolysaccharidosis IIB	Hunter's syndrome, mild†	+	+	+	±	+	+
Mucopolysaccharidosis III	Sanfilippo's syndrome A–D	−	+	+	+	−	+
Mucopolysaccharidosis IV	Morquio syndrome	+‡	−	+	−	+	+
Mucopolysaccharidosis VI	Maroteaux-Lamy syndrome, severe§	+	−	+	−	+	+
Mucopolysaccharidosis VI	Maroteaux-Lamy syndrome, mild	+	−	−	−	−	−
Mucopolysaccharidosis VII	Sly syndrome	+§	?	?	+	?	+

*Ciliary body involved. Subclinical corneal clouding is demonstrable histochemically.
†Sclera involved.
‡Corneal clouding may not be grossly evident after age 10, extent variable.
§Corneal clouding present in infantile and in some cases of adult form.

	Syndrome	Enzymatic Defect	Excessive Urinary Mucopolysaccharide	Inheritance
Mucopolysaccharidosis IH	Hurler	α-L-iduronidase	Dermatan sulfate* Heparan sulfate	Recessive
Mucopolysaccharidosis IS	Scheie's	α-L-iduronidase	Dermatan sulfate Heparan sulfate	Recessive
Mucopolysaccharidosis II	Hunter's A–B	Sulfoiduronate sulfatase	Dermatan sulfate Heparan sulfate	X-linked recessive
Mucopolysaccharidosis IIIA	Sanfilippo's A	Heparan sulfate sulfatase	Heparan sulfate	Recessive
Mucopolysaccharidosis IIIB	Sanfilippo's B	N-Acetyl-α-D-glucosa-minidase	Heparan sulfate	Recessive
Mucopolysaccharidosis IIIC	Sanfilippo's C	Acetyl-CoA: gluco-saminide N-acetyltransferase	Heparan sulfate	Recessive
Mucopolysaccharidosis IIID	Sanfilippo's D	N-acetylglucosamine 6-sulfate sulfatase	Heparan sulfate	Recessive
Mucopolysaccharidosis IV	Morquio	N-acetylgalactosamine 6-sulfate sulfatase	Keratan sulfate	Recessive
Mucopolysaccharidosis VI	Maroteaux-Lamy	Arylsulfatase B	Dermatan sulfate	Recessive
Mucopolysaccharidosis VII	Sly	β-Glucuronidase	Dermatan sulfate (?) Heparan sulfate	Recessive

*Dermatan sulfate was previously called chondroitin sulfate B.

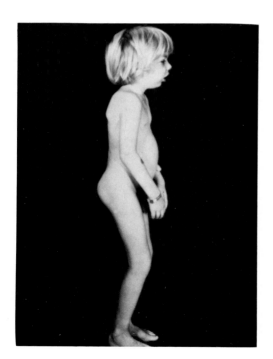

Figure 21-16
Physical stature in Hurler disease. (From Grayson M, Keates RH: *Manual of diseases of the cornea*, Boston, 1969, Little, Brown & Co.)

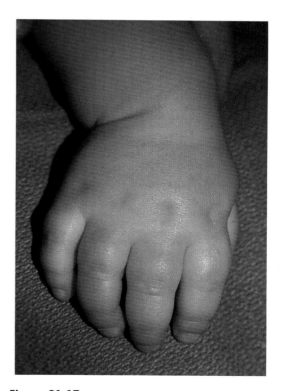

Figure 21-17
Deformity of hands in Hurler disease. (From Grayson M, Keates RH: *Manual of diseases of the cornea*, Boston, 1969, Little, Brown & Co.)

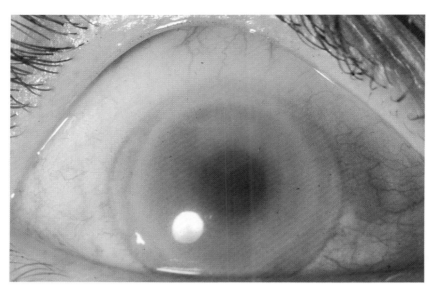

Figure 21-18
Cloudy cornea in Hurler disease.

lelic mutations of the same gene; the disease is demonstrated when patients are homozygous for the abnormal allele. Systemically, Scheie syndrome is less severe; growth and intelligence are usually near normal. Claw hand, coarse facial features, joint stiffness, hepatomegaly, and aortic regurgitation can be present.

Progressive corneal clouding occurs, and is more marked in the periphery.[73,74] It may be present at birth or develop early in life. Clouding can become severe later in life. Pigmentary retinopathy, optic atrophy, and glaucoma also occur. Acute narrow-angle glaucoma has been seen as a result of limbal corneal thickening from mucopolysaccharide deposition.[75]

Penetrating keratoplasty can remove the corneal opacity, but vision may be limited by retinal or optic nerve disease.[73,76-78]

Hurler-Scheie Compound

Rarely, a patient has one Hurler allele and one Scheie allele. This Hurler-Scheie compound (mucopolysaccharidosis IH/S) results in a phenotype halfway between the two diseases. Corneal clouding, abnormal facies, skeletal deformities, moderate mental retardation, and aortic valve disease occur.[79,80]

Hunter's Syndrome

Hunter's syndrome (mucopolysaccharidosis II) is the only mucopolysaccharidosis transmitted as an X-linked recessive trait. It is caused by a deficiency of iduronate sulfate sulfatase, resulting in accumulation of heparan sulfate and dermatan sulfate. Severe and mild forms occur, and both are similar to Hurler syndrome, with skeletal dysplasia (dysostosis multiplex), mental retardation, deafness, and cardiovascular changes. The severe form is still milder than Hurler syndrome, but death usually occurs before 15 years of age. Patients with the mild form have fair intelligence and live 30 to 50 years. Gross corneal clouding is not seen; however, in patients with the mild form, a corneal opacity can occur later in life. Mucopolysaccharide deposits have been seen in pathologic specimens (see below). Retinal pigmentary changes and optic atrophy occur, and involvement of the sclera and cilia may be present.[81]

It has been stated that the lack of early corneal clouding can be used to discriminate clinically between Hunter's and Hurler syndromes,[82] but this may not always be true; patients with Hurler syndrome up to 14 years of age with clear corneas have been reported.[83]

Sanfilippo's Syndrome

Sanfilippo's syndrome (mucopolysaccharidosis III) can be caused by any of four different enzymatic defects, with the same phenotype (but not all involving the same gene). All of the enzymes are involved in the degradation of heparan sulfate (Table 21-5). These patients have progressive severe mental retardation but less severe hepatosplenomegaly and skeletal and facial abnormalities (Fig. 21-19). They usually live only into the teens. The corneas are grossly clear, but some opacity may be evident on slit-

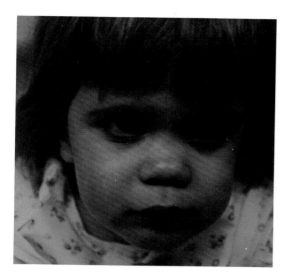

Figure 21-19
Characteristic facial appearance in a patient with Sanfilippo's syndrome. (From Grayson M, Keates RH: *Manual of diseases of the cornea*, Boston, 1969, Little, Brown & Co.)

lamp microscope examination.[66,84] Pigmentary retinal degeneration and optic atrophy occur.

Morquio Syndrome

Morquio syndrome (mucopolysaccharidosis IV) occurs in severe and mild types (types A and B, respectively), with different enzymatic defects (Table 21-5). Both defects result in accumulation of keratan sulfate. Characteristic facies, marked dwarfism, and skeletal dysplasia occur, but mental retardation is not present. Spinal cord or medullary compression can develop from vertebral dysplasia, and deafness, hepatosplenomegaly, and cardiac disease may occur. Corneal clouding commonly develops but is variable. It may not be grossly evident until after the patient is 10 years of age; it can exhibit only a mild diffuse stomal haze; or it can be severe at any age.[85] Optic atrophy is common, but retinopathy is not.

Maroteaux-Lamy Syndrome

Maroteaux-Lamy syndrome (mucopolysaccharidosis VI) exhibits many of the skeletal anomalies seen in Hurler syndrome, but intelligence is normal and aortic disease is absent. Arylsulfatase B deficiency leads to accumulation of dermatan sulfate. Corneal opacities are present in all cases, although a slit-lamp microscope is sometimes needed to see them.[86] Optic atrophy and hydrocephalus may be seen, but there is no retinal degeneration. Successful corneal trans-

plantation has been reported in some cases,[87,88] but in another case recurrence of deposition clouded the graft in less than 1 year.[89]

Sly Syndrome

Individuals with Sly syndrome, also known as β-glucuronidase deficiency and mucopolysaccharidosis VII, exhibit mental retardation, skeletal dysplasia, and hepatosplenomegaly. Corneal clouding is present in the infantile type, appearing between 7 months and 8 years of age.[90,91] Corneal clouding also can be present in the milder adult form.

Histopathology

The corneal findings in all of the mucopolysaccharidoses are similar.[92-95] Vacuolization of the cytoplasm affects conjunctival and corneal epithelium, endothelium, and keratocytes (Fig. 21-20). Ultrastructurally, the vacuoles are either single membrane–bound structures containing fibrillogranular material or membranous lamellar inclusions (Fig. 21-21). Extracellular mucopolysaccharide deposition can also be found in the stroma or subepithelially.[81] The changes are noted in all cases with clinically cloudy corneas. Less marked changes are also found in patients with mucopolysaccharidosis II and mucopolysaccharidosis III and clear corneas.[96,97]

Treatment

As mentioned earlier, corneal transplantation has resulted in at least short-term clear corneas, but vision may still be limited by optic nerve or retinal disease. Bone marrow transplantation can correct the enzymatic deficiency by providing cells with normal enzyme activity.[98] Early results suggest that corneal clouding and retinal function can stabilize or even improve;[99] however, there is no improvement in CNS function.

Other approaches have been attempted in animal models. In one study in mice with mucopolysaccharidosis VII, partial correction of the disease was achieved by retrovirus-mediated transfer of a β-glucuronidase gene into mutant hematopoietic stem cells. Intravenous infusion of the deficient enzyme (α-L-iduronidase) significantly decreased tissue storage of GAG in a canine model of Hurler disease.

Local Corneal Mucopolysaccharidoses
Macular Corneal Dystrophy

Macular dystrophy is a hereditary disorder of keratan sulfate synthesis (see Chapter 17). Mucopolysaccharide accumulates in stromal keratocytes and endothelial cells and is deposited between the stromal lamellae, resulting in corneal clouding. The accumulated mucopolysaccha-

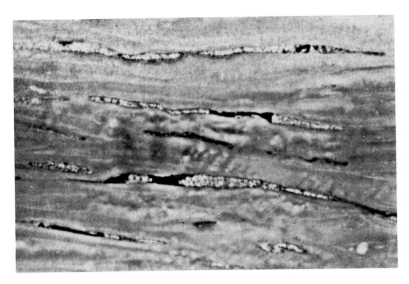

Figure 21-20
Vacuolization of keratocyte cytoplasm in a patient with Maroteaux-Lamy syndrome. (From Kenyon KR et al: *Am J Ophthalmol* 73:718, 1972.)

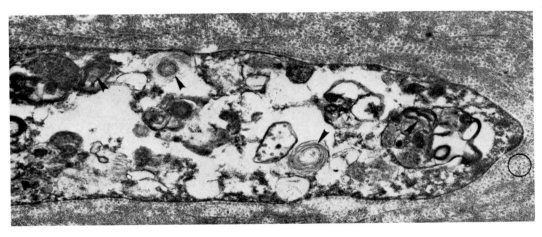

Figure 21-21
Higher magnification of a keratocyte, showing membranous lamellar inclusions and fibrillogranular material. (From Kenyon KR et al: *Am J Ophthalmol* 73:718, 1972.)

ride appears to be related to keratan sulfate, and in some patients normal keratan sulfate is absent from the serum and cartilage; however, no systemic manifestations have been observed.

Mucopolysaccharidoses of Bowman's Layer
Several cases of isolated conjunctival and corneal clouding caused by acid mucopolysaccharide deposition have been described in infants and in a 20-year-old patient. The corneal deposits were limited to Bowman's layer. Systemic mucopolysaccharidosis was not evident, but in one case cardiovascular anomalies and telangi-

ectasias involving multiple organ systems were present. In addition, peripheral edema, cyanosis, and inguinal hernia have been seen.

Diabetes Mellitus
Patients with diabetes mellitus can have decreased corneal sensation and decreased epithelial adhesion. The sensation is usually only mildly reduced,[100-102] but neurotrophic ulcers can occur.[103] Decreased adhesion of the corneal epithelium and delayed epithelial wound healing are often noted in diabetics.[104,105] Thickening of the epithelial basement membrane

and reduced penetration of anchoring fibrils into Bowman's layer may be responsible.[106] More rapid epithelial clouding during intraocular surgery, decreased epithelial barrier function,[107] decreased tear production,[108] and intraepithelial fructose and sorbitol (normally not present)[109] have been noted in diabetic patients. Morphologic endothelial abnormalities, such as a decreased percentage of hexagonal endothelial cells and a higher coefficient of variation of cell size, have been reported.[110,111] Impaired endothelial cell regulation of stromal hydration, as documented by fluorophotometry and recovery from cataract surgery, has been observed in patients with retinopathy[112-115] and in diabetic rabbits.[116] Reversal of abnormal corneal epithelial cell morphology and decreased sensation[117] as well as abnormal endothelial cell morphology[118] were observed after topical treatment with an aldose reductase inhibitor.

Glycogen Storage Disease
Type 1A (Von Gierke's Disease)

Von Gierke's disease, also known as glucose-6-phosphatase deficiency, is an autosomal recessive disorder marked by hypoglycemia, hepatomegaly, bleeding diathesis, hyperlipidemia, and short stature. A faint brown peripheral corneal clouding maybe noted. Lipemia retinalis and eruptive xanthomas can occur with hyperlipidemia, and multiple yellowish, discrete paramacular lesions can be seen. The disease is treated by nocturnal nasogastric infusion of glucose or oral administration of uncooked cornstarch.

Type II (Pompe's Disease)

Pompe's disease is a relatively common deficiency of lysosomal acid α-glucosidase. It has no ocular manifestations, but distinctive pathologic findings were present in a conjunctival specimen.[119] Glycogen-engorged fibroblasts were seen in the substantia propria. In addition, membrane-bound inclusions containing glycogen particles were found in the corneal epithelium and endothelium.

DISORDERS OF COMBINED CARBOHYDRATE AND LIPID METABOLISM

Mucolipidoses

Mucolipidoses are lysosomal storage diseases involving some combination of mucopolysaccharide, glycoprotein, glycolipid, and oligosaccharide metabolism (Table 21-6). Some forms exhibit features of both mucopolysaccharidoses and sphingolipidoses. Corneal clouding is seen in several of the disorders.

Mucolipidosis I

Most of the patients previously categorized as having mucolipidosis I actually have a specific glycoprotein storage disease, so it has been recommended that this term be abandoned.[120] Some of these patients have sialidosis or mannosidosis.

Mucolipidosis II (I-Cell Disease)

Mucolipidosis II shows many of the clinical and radiographic features of Hurler syndrome but presents earlier and does not show mucopolysacchariduria. It is characterized by gargoyle-like facies, severe growth and psychomotor retardation, thickened skin, and mucopolysacchariosis-like skeletal dysplasia (dysostosis multiplex). Mild hepatomegaly, progressive corneal clouding, glaucoma, and megalocornea can occur as well.[121,122] Cherry-red spots are not seen.

Striking granular inclusions are seen in fibroblast and keratocytes (I-cells), and this can be demonstrated in conjunctival biopsy specimens.[122,123] The disease is caused by a defect in the posttranslational processing of lysosomal enzymes. Both types II and III are deficiencies of the same enzyme, UDP-N-acetylglucosamine (GlcNAc):lysosomal enzyme glycoprotein GlcNAc 1-phosphotransferase, which is involved in posttranslational synthesis of the oligosaccharide portion of many lysosomal enzymes. Targeting of lysosomal enzymes to lysosomes is mediated by receptors that bind mannose 6-phosphate recognition markers on the enzymes. The recognition marker is synthesized in the golgi complex using the enzyme that is abnormal in this disease. In the absence of this marker the lysosomal enzymes are not bound by the lysosomes, resulting in their secretion into the extracellular space.[124]

Mucolipidosis III (Pseudo-Hurler Polydystrophy)

Mucolipidosis III is a milder disorder than type II, but patients also exhibit many of the manifestations of the mucopolysaccharidoses, particularly dysostosis multiplex. During the first decade of life, restricted joint mobility, small stature, claw-hand deformity, hip dysplasia, and scoliosis develop. Mild mental retardation and cardiac valve disease are also present. Corneal clouding is consistently present by age 10.[125,126] Fine, discrete opacities are seen initially in the anterior or posterior stroma and progress to involve the entire stroma. The inclusions in fibroblasts, including conjunctival fibroblasts, are similar to those in mucolipidosis type II but are less marked.[127]

Table 21-6 Disorders of Combined Carbohydrate and Lipid Metabolism

	Enzyme Defect	Stored	Heredity	Corneal Clouding	Retinopathy	Retardation	Skeletal Dysplasia
MUCOLIPIDOSES							
II (I cell disease)	UDP-N-acetylglucosamine (GlcNAc):glycoprotein GlcNAc 1-photo-transferase	Mucopolysac-charides; lipids	AR*	Common	−+†	+	+
III (pseudo-Hurler polydystrophy)	UDP-N-acetylglucosamine (GlcNAc):glycoprotein GlcNAc 1-photo-transferase	Mucopolysac-charides; lipids	AR	+ (Mild)	+	+ (Mild)	+
IV (Berman's syndrome)	Unknown	Gangliosides; phospholipids; acid mucopoly-saccharidosis	AR	+	−	+	−
GLYCOPROTEIN STORAGE DISORDERS							
Goldberg-Cotlier syndrome (a sialidosis)	Glycoprotein neuraminidase + β-galactosidase	Sialoglycopeptides + N-glycosidically linked oligosaccharides	AR	+	Cherry-red spot	−	±†
Mannosidosis	β-D-mannosidase	N-glycosidically linked oligosaccharides	AR	+ Superficial	−	+	+
Fucosidosis	β-L-fucosidase	Oligosaccharides and glycoasparagines	AR	+ Superficial	+	+	+

*Autosomal recessive.
†One case described.

Mucolipidosis IV (Berman's Syndrome)

Berman's syndrome is manifested by mental retardation, retinal degeneration, and corneal clouding without other somatic features.[128] It has been reported mainly in Ashkenazi Jews. The exact enzyme deficiency is not known. Bilateral diffuse corneal haze is usually evident at birth or by 6 weeks of age.[129-132] A milder variant with corneal clouding and no psychomotor retardation has been described in teenagers.[133] Multiple dotlike opacities are present in all layers of the stroma, homogeneously from the center of the periphery. On histologic examination, characteristic inclusions are found in the epithelium of the cornea and conjunctiva and, to a much lesser extent, in keratocytes and conjunctival substantia propria.[134-136] Two types of single membrane–bound vesicles are seen: Some contain whorled membranous inclusions, thought to represent phospholipids, and others contain granular material, consistent with mucopolysaccharides (Fig. 21-22).

Because the corneal clouding is largely caused by epithelial disease, conjunctival transplantation (with donor conjunctiva from an unaffected sibling) was performed in one patient.[137] The central cornea remained clear at 1 year, but extensive peripheral vascularization occurred.

Glycoprotein Storage Disorders

These are rare autosomal recessive disorders involving enzymes that hydrolyze polysaccharide linkages. All are characterized by mental retardation, coarse facies, and skeletal dysplasia.

Sialidosis

Sialidosis is an autosomal recessive disorder caused by a deficiency of glycoprotein neuraminidase, sometimes in association with β-galactosidase deficiency. Patients have a cherry-red spot in the macula, spokelike lens opacities, mental retardation, myoclonus, hepatosplenomegaly, and mucopolysaccharidosis-like skeletal dysplasia. Progressive stromal and epithelial corneal clouding occurs in some patients.[138] On histopathologic examination, single membrane–bound inclusions are found in corneal epithelial cells and keratocytes, as in the mucopolysaccharidoses, and rare lamellar bodies, as seen in the sphingolipidoses, are also present.

Goldberg-Cotlier syndrome is a sialidosis with a combined deficiency of neuraminidase and β-galactosidase. The characteristics are the same

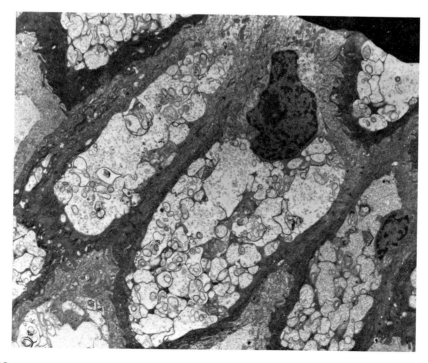

Figure 21-22

Electron micrograph of mucolipidosis type IV, showing membrane-bound vesicles containing whorled membranous inclusions and granular material. (Courtesy of Bruce L. Johnson, Pittsburgh, PA.)

as in neuraminidase deficiency alone, and corneal clouding is present.[139,140] Inclusions, mostly membrane bound, are seen in conjunctival fibroblasts and epithelium.[141]

Alpha-Mannosidosis

Individuals with mannosidosis demonstrate coarse facies, cardiac dysfunction, hepatosplenomegaly, gingival hyperplasia, and skeletal dysplasia. It is most often lethal in childhood. Due to a deficiency of α-mannosidase, glycoprotein-derived, mannose-containing oligosaccharides accumulate in tissues and are excreted in the urine. Spokelike posterior cortical cataracts are commonly seen.[142] They consist of numerous punctate vacuoles arranged in a cartwheel-like or spokelike configuration. Superficial corneal opacities have been reported in a few cases. Similar clinical changes have been observed in cats with mannosidosis. In these animals a low activity of acid α-mannosidase has been detected in keratocytes, and accumulation of partially degraded oligosaccharides occurs in keratocytes, lens, and vitreous.

Fucosidosis

Fucosidosis is an autosomal recessive disorder with a range of severities. Patients with fucosidosis differ from those with mannosidosis by the presence of abnormal sweat electrolytes and cutaneous angiokeratomas. Deficiency of α-fucosidase leads to tissue accumulation of oligosaccharides, glycolipids, and glycopeptides. Dilated, tortuous conjunctival vessels and central anterior corneal opacification have been reported.[143,144] Cytoplasmic, membrane-bound inclusions, containing fibrillogranular and multilaminated material, are found in corneal, conjunctival, and vascular endothelium.[145,146]

OTHER DISORDERS OF METABOLISM

Disorders of Amino Acid Metabolism

Anterior segment involvement in disorders of amino acid metabolism is summarized in Table 21-7.

Alkaptonuria

One of the prominent clinical features of this autosomal recessive metabolic disorder is a characteristic bluish gray or black pigmentation of connective tissue, known as *ochronosis*.[147] It is caused by a deficiency of homogentisic acid oxidase, an enzyme normally present in the liver and kidneys. Homogentisic acid is an intermediate in the metabolism of tyrosine and phenylalanine, and homogentisic acid oxidase normally converts it to maleylacetoacetic acid. The enzyme deficiency leads to excessive amounts of homogentisic acid, most of which is excreted in the urine; however, the acid and its oxidized, pigmented polymers (alkapton) can also bind collagen, leading to their accumulation in connective tissue. In addition, for unknown reasons, degenerative changes occur, particularly in cartilage and intervertebral discs.

The earliest signs are usually pigmentation of the sclerae and ears (Fig. 21-23), which becomes manifest between 20 and 40 years of age. Pigmentation of the nasal and internal cartilage and ligaments can also be seen. Degenerative arthropathy, involving mainly the large joints and the spine, develops in the majority of patients. The urine darkens on standing as a result of the oxidation of homogentisic acid; however, in the presence of reducing agents or if the urine has an acid pH, darkening does not occur.

Ocular Manifestations. Ocular pigmentation occurs in the interpalpebral fissure. The conjunctiva, episclera, sclera, and the tendons of the horizontal recti can become pigmented with this material[148-150] (Fig. 21-24). In addition, the cornea immediately inside the limbus may exhibit areas of pigmentation. The pigment is usually brownish black, appears like "oil droplets," and is located in the area of Bowman's layer and deep epithelium. Their appearance is similar to the droplets of spheroidal degeneration. Pigmentation of the tarsal plates and lids can also be seen.

Histopathology. The pigment is seen with light microscopy as amber-(ochre) colored globules or fiberlike structures in the peripheral cornea, conjunctiva, and sclera. Ultrastructurally, the pigment is extracellular, attached to collagen fibers and fibrocytes.[151]

Cystinosis

Cystinosis is an autosomal recessive disorder characterized by intralysosomal accumulation of free cystine in body tissues, particularly in the reticuloendothelial cells of the bone marrow, liver, spleen, and lymphatic system. Deposition can also occur in the kidneys, leading to generalized proximal tubular dysfunction (Fanconi's syndrome), and in ocular tissues, including the cornea, conjunctiva, and retina. The defect appears to involve impaired efflux of cystine from lysosomes rather than a defect in catabolism. Cystine and cysteine levels in plasma and urine are not elevated, but increased concentrations can be detected in leukocytes or cultured fibroblasts or in biopsies of rectal mucosa.[152]

Table 21-7 Disorders of Amino Acid Metabolism with Corneal Findings

Disorder	Enzyme Deficiency	Accumulated Material	Heredity	Corneal Findings	Other Findings
Alkaptonuria	Homogentisic acid oxidase	Homogentisic acid	AR*	Ochre-colored deposits in limbal area	Interpalpebral pigmentation of conjunctiva, episclera, sclera, and rectus tendons
Cystinosis	Impaired transport of cystine across lysosomal membranes	Cystine	AR	Diffuse stromal crystals; recurrent erosions (late)	Peripheral retinopathy; crystals in conjunctiva, sclera, and uvea
Tyrosinemia II (Richner-Hanhart syndrome)	Cytoplasmic tyrosine aminotransferase	Tyrosine	AR	Epithelial deposits, dendritic or sunburst pattern; vascularization	Conjunctival plaques

*Autosomal recessive.

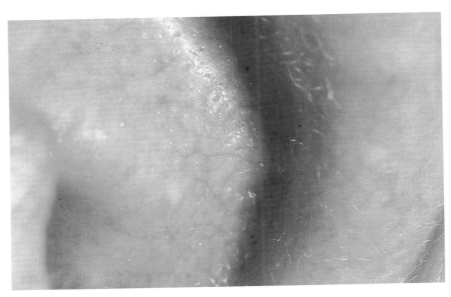

Figure 21-23
Pigmentation of the ear cartilage in alkaptonuria. (From Grayson M: *The cornea in systemic disease.* In Duane TD, editor: *Clinical ophthalmology,* vol 4, Hagerstown, MD, 1976, Harper & Row. Used with permission of Lippincott-Raven Publishers.)

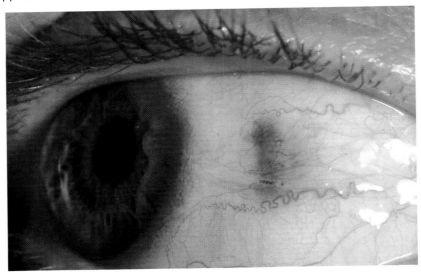

Figure 21-24
Pigmentation of the lateral rectus tendon in alkaptonuria. (From Grayson M: *The cornea in systemic disease.* In Duane TD, editor: *Clinical ophthalmology,* vol 4, Hagerstown, MD, 1976, Harper & Row. Used with permission of Lippincott-Raven Publishers.)

Clinical Manifestations. Cystinosis occurs in three forms: infantile, adolescent, and adult. The infantile form usually becomes apparent by 4 to 6 months of age. Growth retardation, vitamin D–resistant rickets, hypopigmentation of the skin and hair, and progressive renal failure occur, with death occurring usually before 10 years of age. The adolescent form exhibits less

severe renal impairment, which usually becomes apparent in the second decade.[153,154] In the adult form the patients are in good health; they are usually free of symptoms, except perhaps for photophobia.[155] The only manifestations are corneal; renal function is normal and retinopathy is absent.

Corneal and conjunctival involvement oc-

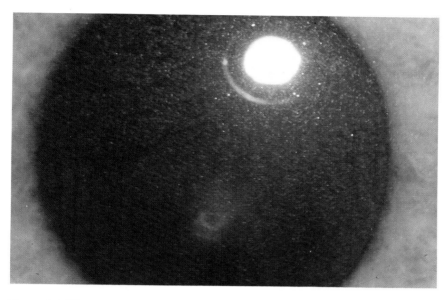

Figure 21-25
Corneal crystals in cystinosis.

curs in all three forms of cystinosis, and the appearance is similar. In the cornea, glistening, polychromatic, needlelike to rectangular crystals are seen (Fig. 21-25). They first appear anteriorly and gradually spread posteriorly, always more peripherally than centrally.[156] In the infantile form they first appear from 6 to 15 months of age and involve the entire stroma by age 7 years. In the adult form they may become evident in the teen years or as late as 50 years of age.

The crystals become denser with age.[157,158] They may cause a rather intense photophobia but do not decrease acuity. In advanced cases corneal erosions can occur as often as several times each month, and the cornea can become thickened. Band keratopathy is a frequent complication. Crystal deposition can also be seen on the anterior lens surface and can thicken the iris stroma.[158]

Crystal deposits are also evident in the conjunctiva, particularly in the bulbar and forniceal areas, where they create a ground-glass appearance.[159] Peripheral retinopathy is consistently present only in the infantile form. There is extensive depigmentation in the periphery, with irregular clumps of pigment (Fig. 21-26). The retinal pigmentary changes may precede the corneal and conjunctival changes by many months and rarely may be seen as early as the fifth week of life.

Histopathology. With electron microscopy the corneal crystals are seen to be intracellular,

within epithelium and keratocytes, and membrane bound.[152,160,161] Crystal deposition results in thinning and focal breaks in Bowman's membrane that may be related to the photophobia.[161] Crystals are also present in subepithelial conjunctiva, sclera, iris, ciliary body, choroid, extraocular muscles, and retinal pigment epithelium.[152,160-164] The crystals in the conjunctiva and uvea have been identified as L-cystine by x-ray diffraction.

A conjunctival biopsy specimen can confirm the diagnosis and may be taken fairly easily. It should be fixed in absolute ethanol and examined with polarized light for detection of typical crystals (Fig. 21-27). However, the diagnosis can also be made by leukocyte cystine assay, which is less invasive.

Differential Diagnosis. A number of other conditions are associated with crystals in the cornea (see Chapter 9). In most cases corneal appearance, patient age, and systemic findings can differentiate the disorders. However, multiple myeloma and other dysproteinemias can be difficult to distinguish from adult cystinosis. The corneal changes are very similar, and systemic manifestations are often absent. Examination of a conjunctival biopsy specimen or leukocyte cystine assay can indicate the proper diagnosis.

Treatment.   Cysteamine (β-mercaptoethylamine) can be used to reduce corneal crystal content. The cysteamine reacts with intracellu-

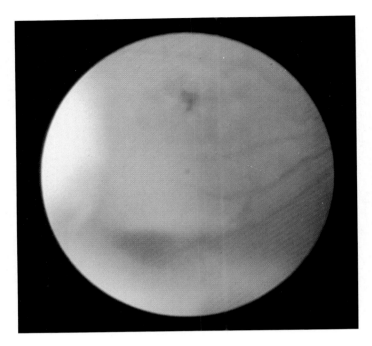

Figure 21-26
Peripheral retinal depigmentation with irregular clumps of pigment in cystinosis. (From Grayson M: *The cornea in systemic disease.* In Duane TD, editor: *Clinical ophthalmology,* vol 4, Hagerstown, MD, 1976, Harper & Row. Used with permission of Lippincott-Raven Publishers.)

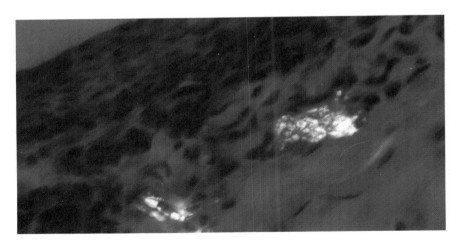

Figure 21-27
Typical crystals of cystinosis seen with polarized light in a biopsy of the conjunctiva.

lar cystine, forming a cysteine-cysteamine disulfide, which resembles lysine and is transported out of the lysosome by the normal lysine transport system. The cysteamine is given as a 0.2% to 0.5% drop four to six times daily.[165-167] A corneal transplant was clear after 2 years in one case,[168] but in another case crystal deposition recurred in less than 6 weeks.[169]

Tyrosinemia II (Richner-Hanhart Syndrome)

Two major disorders are associated with hypertyrosinemia—tyrosinemia types I and II. *Tyrosinemia type I* (also known as hepatorenal tyrosinemia) is a rare autosomal recessive disease characterized by cirrhosis of the liver and renal tubular dysfunction, but there are no ocular

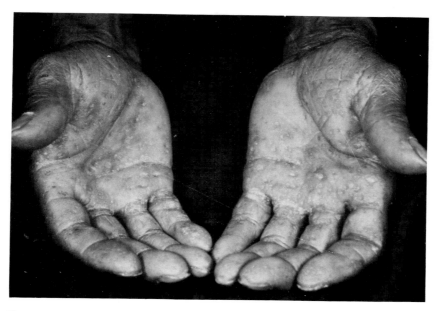

Figure 21-28
Painful hyperkeratotic lesions on the hands in tyrosinemia.

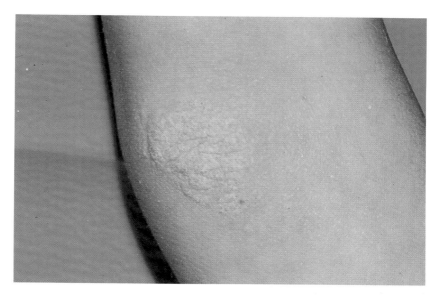

Figure 21-29
Hyperkeratotic skin lesion in tyrosinemia.

manifestations. Patients with *tyrosinemia type II* (also known as oculocutaneous tyrosinemia or Richner-Hanhart syndrome) exhibit skin lesions and corneal opacities, and 50% have mental retardation.[170] Autosomal recessively transmitted, it appears to be caused by a deficiency of cytoplasmic tyrosine aminotransferase, resulting in high levels of tyrosine in the blood and urine.[171]

In most cells, the excess tyrosine is removed by mitochondrial aspartate transaminase (converting it to pHPPA), but this enzyme is not present in cells of ectodermal origin. The palms and soles are affected by hyperhidrosis, blisters, and painful erosions that become crusted and hyperkeratotic (Fig. 21-28). Hyperkeratotic plaques can also be found on the knees and elbows (Fig. 21-29).

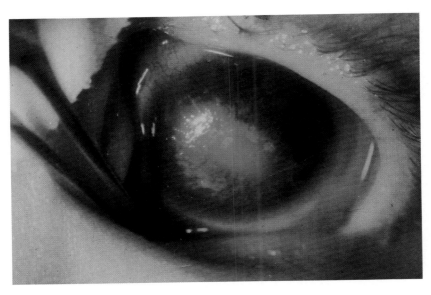

Figure 21-30
Tyrosine in the cornea. (Courtesy of Robert Burns, Columbia, MO.)

Ocular Manifestations. Corneal involvement occurs in most cases and usually precedes the skin lesions. In one case, however, ocular involvement developed 17 years after the skin lesions.[172] The patient can develop photophobia, tearing, redness, and pain anywhere from 2 weeks to 8 years of age. Intraepithelial and subepithelial opacification occurs, sometimes with erosions or ulcerations.[171,173-176]

Grayson[177] described a case in which the corneal lesions consisted of dustlike opacities randomly distributed in the lower aspect of the cornea. The lesions did not stain with fluorescein; there was neither vascularization nor decreased sensation. The only complaint was that of photophobia. Similar findings were observed in a premature infant with temporary hypertyrosinemia. Multiple subepithelial punctate crystalline deposits developed and disappeared after 5 days in patients on a low-tyrosine diet.[178]

The corneal lesions may have a dendritic or sunburst configuration (Fig. 21-30), with surrounding ground-glass haze.[179] The dendritic lesions have often been confused with herpetic dendrites, but there are distinguishing features: The lesions in tyrosinemia type II are thick and plaquelike; they do not exhibit the fine, delicate club-shaped edges of herpes simplex dendrites; they are bilateral, which is rare in herpes simplex; they do not stain with fluorescein; they are usually not associated with vascularization; and the sensation is intact. Subcapsular lens opacities, conjunctival thickening, and an extensive papillary hypertrophy of the tarsal conjunctiva have also been observed.

Histopathology. In one case the cornea was examined with light microscopy and demonstrated hyperplastic stratified epithelium with intracellular edema.[180] In Grayson's case, histologic examination revealed thickening of the basement membrane with tiny fingerlike projections extending into the basal layer of the epithelium[177] (Fig. 21-31). Examination of a conjunctival plaque revealed membrane-bound inclusions in superficial epithelial cells and blood vessel endothelium.[171]

Rats fed a diet high in tyrosine develop snowflakelike corneal opacities and paw erythema.[181] Intracytoplasmic crystals are found in the corneal epithelium.[182] The crystals probably disrupt the epithelial cells and lysosomes, eliciting an inflammatory response.

Treatment. Institution of a diet low in tyrosine and phenylalanine can lead to resolution of the eye and skin lesions. In two cases the corneal lesion recurred after a penetrating graft.[183,184] In one of these cases the recurrence appeared to be related to systemic corticosteroid treatment.[184]

Phenylketonuria

Phenylketonuria is a group of disorders characterized by reduced activity of phenylalanine hydroxylase. The most common is classic phenylketonuria, which is inherited as an autosomal recessive trait and results in mental retardation, seizures, hypopigmentation, and eczema. In most cases phenylketonuria is diagnosed shortly after birth because of routine

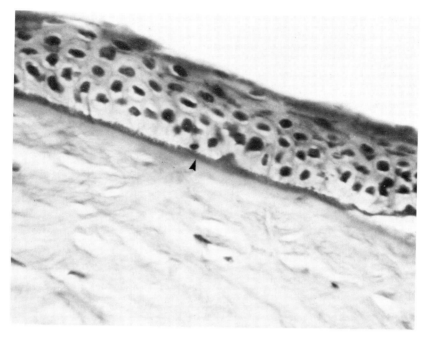

Figure 21-31
Thickening of the basement membrane with tiny fingerlike projections extending into the basal layer of the epithelium.

testing, and early institution of dietary therapy can prevent complications.

Cataracts, partial albinism, and photophobia can be seen. Small corneal opacities were reported in one patient, but the etiology was unclear.

Amyloidosis

Amyloidosis is a disorder of protein metabolism in which there is tissue deposition of a characteristic extracellular protein material. Amyloid deposits can be localized (e.g., corneal amyloid degeneration and lattice dystrophy) or systemic, and primary or secondary. Amyloidosis has been classified in many ways, but the following appears to be most useful clinically: (1) association with immunocyte dyscrasia, with or without frank malignancy, such as multiple myeloma, in which the amyloid fibrils are derived from immunoglobulin light chains (AL type); (2) association with chronic inflammatory or infectious disease (AA type); (3) heredofamilial amyloidosis, the type associated with familial Mediterranean fever (AA type) and a variety of neuropathic, nephropathic, cardiomyopathic, and other forms, in which the amyloid fibrils are most commonly derived from transthyretin, also known as plasma prealbumin (AF prealbumin type); (4) a common nonhereditary pathologic finding in elderly individuals (AS type); and (5) localized amyloidosis,

without evidence of systemic disease. The eye can be affected by primary and secondary localized amyloidosis and in AL and familial types of systemic amyloidosis.

Primary Localized Amyloidosis

Primary localized amyloidosis can affect the bulbar or palpebral conjunctiva, Tenon's capsule, tarsus, limbus, lacrimal gland, or orbit.[184-187] In the lid and conjunctiva the amyloid appears as a soft, yellow nodule. The conjunctival deposit is usually subepithelial. Types I and III lattice corneal dystrophy and gelatinous droplike dystrophy can also be classified as types of primary localized amyloidosis of the cornea (see Chapter 17).

Secondary Localized Amyloidosis

Secondary localized amyloidosis of the cornea can occur after trauma or can be associated with a chronic ocular inflammatory disorder (see Amyloid Degeneration, Chapter 16). The amyloid may appear as a small, salmon pink to yellow-white, fleshy, waxy, sometimes nodular mass or masses on the cornea or conjunctiva; as grayish perivascular deposits; as lamellar deposits; or as a subepithelial pannus. Such amyloid deposits are nearly always clinically insignificant and are most often found only on histologic examination.

Primary Systemic Amyloidosis

Nonfamilial primary systemic amyloidosis is almost always related to an immunocyte disorder, even if one is not clinically apparent.[188] Purpuric and papillary lesions of the eyelids and conjunctiva can be seen (Fig. 21-32).[189,190] In one patient lattice dystrophy was present.[52] Nonamyloid corneal immunoglobulin deposits occur in multiple myeloma and benign monoclonal gammopathy (see Chapter 19). Neurologic involvement can lead to ptosis, ophthalmoplegia, neuroparalytic keratitis, and pupillary abnormalities. In familial forms the findings are similar, but veillike vitreous opacities, retinal periphlebitis, conjunctival vascular abnormalities,[191] and glaucoma can occur. Scalloped pupils can occur and appear to be diagnostic.[192] Subclinical conjunctival amyloid deposition is present in most patients, and a conjunctival biopsy can be used for diagnosis of the disease.[191,193]

A rare form of dominantly inherited primary systemic amyloidosis, familial amyloid polyneuropathy type IV or Meretoja's syndrome, is associated with lattice dystrophy of the cornea. The latticelike corneal changes usually become manifest between 20 and 35 years of age; in later decades one sees involvement of the skin, peripheral nerves, and cranial nerves (see Chapter 17). The exact nature of the amyloid protein has not been determined, but abnormal apolipoprotein A-1, or gelsolin, an action-severing protein, is found in some kindreds.

Variant gelsolin molecules have been identified, always at nucleotide 654 in the gelsolin gene, which is on chromosome 9q.[194-198] Antibodies to the mutated gelsolin protein and to protein AP bind to amyloid deposits in the cornea and conjunctiva, the perineurium of ciliary nerves, the walls of ciliary vessels, the optic nerve sheaths, the stroma of the ciliary body, and the choriocapillaris.[199]

Wilson's Disease

Wilson's disease is characterized by progressive neurologic impairment and liver dysfunction. Copper is deposited in almost all body tissues, especially in the liver, brain, kidneys, and cornea. The exact metabolic defect has not been identified, but the rate of copper excretion into bile is reduced, with accumulation of copper in the liver that eventually spills over into the blood, leading to extrahepatic deposition. It is transmitted as an autosomal recessive trait.

Approximately one half of patients present with hepatic involvement: acute hepatitis, cirrhosis, or asymptomatic hepatosplenomegaly. Neurologic or psychiatric disturbances, such as tremors, spasticity, chorea, rigidity, and psychoses, are the first clinical signs in most other patients. Occasionally amenorrhea or spontaneous abortions can be the only manifestations.

Ocular Manifestations

In Wilson's disease copper deposition can be seen in the cornea, as the Kayser-Fleischer ring,

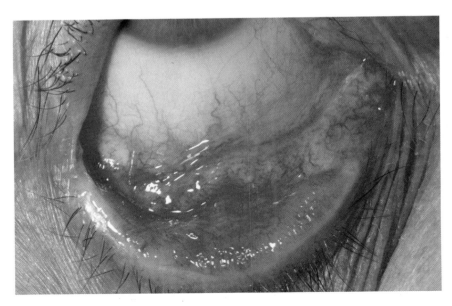

Figure 21-32
Amyloid deposition in the lid and conjunctiva in primary systemic amyloidosis. (Courtesy of Diane Curtin, Pittsburgh, PA.)

and in the lens, as "sunflower cataracts"[200] (Table 21-8). The Kayser-Fleischer copper ring is a peripheral band, 1 to 3 mm wide, at the level of Descemet's membrane and extending to the limbus without a lucid interval (Fig. 21-33). It is usually yellow-brown but may appear gold, red, blue, green, or any mixture of these colors.[201-203] The color can change depending on

Table 21-8 Other Metabolic Disorders with Anterior Segment Findings		
Disorder	**Corneal Findings**	**Other Ocular Findings**
Familial amyloid polyneuropathy IV	Lattice dystrophy	Cranial neuropathy
Wilson's disease	Kayser-Fleischer ring	Sunflower cataract
Hyperuricemia (Gout)	Urate crystal deposition	Conjunctivitis; episcleritis; scleritis
Porphyria cutanea tarda	Blistering and scarring crystals*	Cicatricial ectropion; punctal stenosis; conjunctival vesicles and scarring; scleral thinning
Congenital erythropoietic porphyria	Scarring	Cicatricial ectropion; keratoconjunctivitis; scleral thinning; optic atrophy; retinal hemorrhages
Hemochromatosis	—	Rusty-brown pigmentation of perilimbal conjunctiva
Zellweger syndrome	Clouding	Cataracts; glaucoma; retinal pigmentary abnormalities; optic disc pallor
Biotinidase deficiency	—	Conjunctivitis; optic neuropathy; motility disturbances; retinal pigmentary abnormalities

*One case.

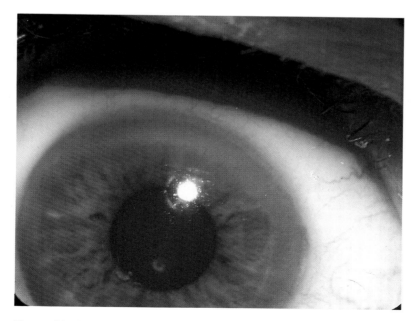

Figure 21-33
Kayser-Fleischer ring.

the angle of illumination. On occasion a double ring can be seen, with an outer ruby-red ring and a green inner ring. The deposition is first noted as a thin crescent superiorly, then inferiorly, and eventually circumferentially. If posterior embryotoxon is present, a clear space separates the ring from the limbus, because Descemet's membrane ends anteriorly. Gonioscopic examination is sometimes required to detect an early Kayser-Fleischer ring because deposition occurs most peripherally first, and the ring may be obscured by an arcus or wide limbus.

A Kayser-Fleischer ring is seen in approximately 95% of patients with Wilson's disease.[204,205] It is present in all patients who have neurologic involvement and in 70% to 90% of hepatic patients; however, it is absent in over 30% of children presenting with acute liver disease and may be absent in those without neurologic or hepatic symptoms.

A characteristic "sunflower" cataract is also present in 15% to 20% of patients. It is seen as a green or brown pigmentation of the central anterior and posterior lens capsule, in a central and petaloid distribution.[203-206]

The corneal pigmentation is caused by granular copper deposition in peripheral Descemet's membrane.[203,207-209] Using more sensitive means of detection, copper deposition has also been demonstrated centrally, and it appears to be bound to sulfur.[210]

Differential Diagnosis
The diagnosis of Wilson's disease can be made by demonstration of a serum ceruloplasmin level less than 20 mg/dl and either Kayser-Fleischer rings or increased concentration of copper in a liver biopsy. However, approximately 5% of patients with the disease have higher ceruloplasmin levels, and some patients with other liver diseases have both elevated liver copper and pigmented corneal rings. These rings are clinically identical to Kayser-Fleischer rings and have been reported in primary biliary cirrhosis, progressive intrahepatic cholestasis of childhood, chronic active hepatitis with cirrhosis, other cholestatic syndromes, and exogenous chalcosis.[211-213] Patients with Wilson's disease can be differentiated from those with these disorders by their inability to incorporate radioactive copper into ceruloplasmin.[214]

Other conditions that cause pigmentation of the posterior corneal surface and can be mistaken for Wilson's disease are multiple myeloma, extensive copper treatment for trachoma (corneal and lenticular changes), copper intraocular foreign bodies, and carotenemia. In multiple myeloma, copper is deposited cen-

trally in Descemet's membrane, Bowman's layer, and the anterior and posterior lens capsules. In carotenemia, golden yellow rings are present at the site of a corneal arcus; in addition, night blindness can be present.

Treatment
The most effective treatment of Wilson's disease is removal of tissue deposits with D-penicillamine, which prevents as well as reverses the clinical manifestations. The Kayser-Fleischer rings regress with penicillamine treatment and are a good indicator of the effectiveness of therapy. The most dramatic response is in the neurologic symptoms, but some patients show improvement in their liver disease. The most symptomatic patients may show the most remarkable improvement.[215,216] Lifetime therapy is required. Regression of Kayser-Fleischer rings has also been observed after liver transplantation.[217]

Hyperuricemia
Elevation of serum uric acid occurs in a wide variety of disorders. *Gout* is the combination of hyperuricemia with any of the following: characteristic arthritis, urate deposition in joints (tophi), interstitial renal disease, or uric acid nephrolithiasis. It primarily occurs in men, with a peak incidence in the fifth decade. It represents a heterogeneous group of disorders, often caused by a combination of genetic and environmental influences.

Ocular Manifestations
Monosodium urate can be deposited in the cornea, conjunctiva, and sclera: An acute conjunctival inflammation can occur, with marked hyperemia and a scanty foamy discharge (Fig. 21-34). The patient complains of photophobia, burning, and pain.[218,219] Conjunctival tophi can also occur. Conjunctival inflammation can be associated with acute attacks of gouty arthritis. Scleritis, episcleritis, and iritis can also be seen.[218]

Fine, punctate or needlelike, refractile crystals can appear in the anterior corneal stroma and epithelium and are most dense in the palpebral fissure.[220] This deposition can occur in cases of hyperuricemia with or without gouty symptoms. The corneal appearance can be similar to band keratopathy, but it is brownish rather than the whitish gray seen with calcium deposition (Fig. 21-35). Urate crystals can be demonstrated in the nuclei of the epithelial cells and in the superficial stroma.[220]

Identical uric acid crystal deposition can also occur without hyperuricemia or gout, in which case it is called *urate keratopathy*. Urate keratop-

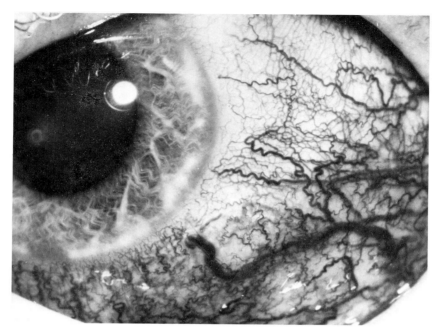

Figure 21-34
Severe hyperemia of the conjunctiva and episclera as seen in gout.

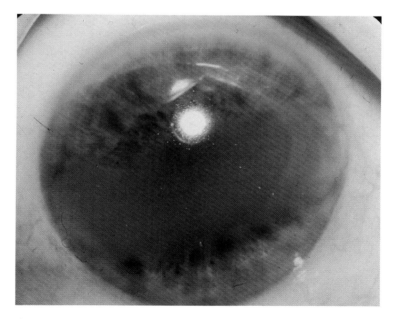

Figure 21-35
Urate band keratopathy.

athy appears to be caused by local disturbance of uric acid metabolism.

Treatment

Acute gouty arthritis is treated with anti-inflammatory agents, typically colchicine or indomethacin and occasionally corticosteroids. Presumably, acute conjunctivitis, episcleritis, and scleritis could be treated similarly. Antihyperuricemic agents (e.g., allopurinol, probenecid, or sulfinpyrazone) are given to prevent further complications. Corneal epithelial deposits can be removed by scraping or superficial keratectomy.[221]

Porphyria

The porphyrias are a group of disorders of heme biosynthesis. Heme functions as a prosthetic, oxygen-carrying group for many proteins in the body, including hemoglobin, cytochromes, and catalase. It is essential for life and is present in all aerobic cells. The two major sites of heme synthesis are the liver and red blood cells, and depending on the specific form of porphyria, the erythropoietic or hepatic site can be predominantly affected, or both can be equally affected. The main clinical symptoms are intermittent attacks of nervous system dysfunction, sensitivity of the skin to light, or both.

Porphyria Cutanea Tarda

Porphyria cutanea tarda (PCT), also known as symptomatic porphyria, is the most common form of porphyria. It can be inherited as an autosomal dominant trait or can be sporadic. There is a deficiency of hepatic uroporphyrinogen decarboxylase. Abnormal porphyrins accumulate in skin from local synthesis and distribution from the liver. Irradiation of the deposits leads to activation of the complement system. Alcohol, estrogen, and iron overload (hepatic siderosis) are aggravating factors. Twenty-five percent to 100% of patients have a history of heavy alcohol intake, but a small percentage of patients with alcoholism develop PCT. PCT is characterized by photosensitive cutaneous lesions, liver disease, and urinary excretion of porphyrins; neurologic symptoms do not occur. It usually becomes manifest between 40 and 60 years of age. Skin abnormalities include increased facial pigmentation, increased fragility to trauma, erythema, scleroderma-like changes, and vesicular and ulcerative lesions.

Recurrent vesication of the lid skin can lead to scarring, with cicatricial ectropion and punctal stenosis.[222-224] The conjunctiva can be hyperemic and chemotic and vesicles can form, leading to necrosis, scarring, and symblepharon

formation.[222,223,225,226] The interpalpebral conjunctiva is most affected. In one study the incidences of pingueculae and pterygia were higher than expected.[227] Scarring of the cornea can result from blistering or can be complication of cicatricial ectropion. In one case, white-tan nonrefractile crystals were present in the peripheral anterior stroma.[200] Scleritis, chiefly interpalpebral scleromalacia, has been described,[228] but histologic examination of one such case indicated scleral dehydration and elastotic degeneration, not inflammation or thinning.[223] In one report the scleral lesions showed pink fluorescence with ultraviolet light.[200]

Congenital Erythropoietic Porphyria

This rare, recessively inherited form of porphyria affects only erythropoiesis. It involves a deficiency of uroporphyrinogen III cosynthase, which leads to overproduction and excretion of uroporphyrinogen I. Abnormal porphyrins are distributed throughout the body. Congenital erythropoietic porphyria becomes manifest at or shortly after birth and is recognized by the excretion of pink or red urine. Later, affected individuals develop hemolytic anemia, splenomegaly, and cutaneous photosensitivity, causing bullous eruptions of the skin. Neurologic dysfunction does not occur.

Optic nerve atrophy and retinal hemorrhages may be found on fundus examination. Scarring and depigmentation of the eyelids, ectropion, keratoconjunctivitis, conjunctival necrosis, scleromalacia, and corneal melting and scarring can occur.[222,229]

Other Forms of Porphyria

Photosensitivity is also a feature of variegate porphyria and erythrohepatic porphyria, and it is likely that similar ocular lesions can occur in these patients. The most extensive report of ocular involvement in the porphyrias was published in 1952,[222] and our understanding and classification of porphyrias was limited at that time. However, conjunctival blistering and scarring were noted in many of these patients with skin involvement.

Hemochromatosis

Hemochromatosis is an iron storage disorder in which increased absorption of iron from the intestine results in tissue deposition. It can occur on a genetic basis, with autosomal recessive inheritance, or secondary to other disease, particularly chronic disorders of erythropoiesis such as thalassemia or sideroblastic anemia. The liver, pancreas, and heart are most affected. A rusty brown pigmentation of the perilimbal bulbar conjunctiva, greater inferiorly than superiorly, has been described.[230,231]

Zellweger Syndrome

Zellweger syndrome is a rare hereditary abnormality of peroxisomes. Peroxisomes are membrane-bound organelles that lack DNA and are found in all cells. They catalyze beta-oxidation of fatty acids and related substrates and are the principle site of peroxide metabolism. In Zellweger syndrome there is a failure to import newly synthesized peroxisomal proteins into peroxisomes. The proteins remain in the cytosol where they are rapidly degraded.

Zellweger syndrome is characterized by severe hypotonia, high forehead, large anterior fontanelle, midface hypoplasia, and hepatomegaly. Affected infants usually die within a few months of birth. Cloudy corneas and cataracts are present in the majority of cases, and glaucoma, Brushfield spots, persistent pupillary membrane, epicanthus, rapidly progressive retinal dystrophy, and optic disc pallor can also be present.[232]

Biotinidase Deficiency

Biotin is a B vitamin that serves as a prosthetic group in carboxylase enzymes involved in gluconeogenesis, fatty acid synthesis, and amino acid catabolism. *Biotinidase deficiency* is a rare disorder of the recycling of endogenous biotin. It occurs in two forms, neonatal and juvenile. The neonatal form presents in the first few days of life with lactic acidosis, organic acidemia, and hyperammonemia. Children with the juvenile form have seizures, hypotonia, ataxia, breathing problems, developmental delay, skin rash, alopecia, hearing loss, and optic atrophy. Affected individuals present at 3 weeks to several years of age, usually with metabolic ketolactic acidosis. The treatment is 5 to 20 mg of oral biotin daily.

Conjunctivitis, which is present in one half of patients with biotinidase deficiency, is one of the initial findings in about 10% of patients.[233,234] In one series of 78 patients, ophthalmologic abnormalities were found in 51%: keratoconjunctivitis (30%), optic neuropathy (13%), motility disturbances (13%), retinal pigment changes (4%), and pupillary findings (1%).[235] Corneal ulcers occur rarely.

REFERENCES

1. Norton JA et al: Multiple endocrine neoplasia type IIb: the most aggressive form of medullary thyroid carcinoma, *Surg Clin North Am* 59:109, 1979.
2. Robertson DM, Sizemore GW, Gordon H: Thickened corneal nerves as a manifestation of multiple endocrine neoplasia, *Trans Am Acad Ophthalmol Otolaryngol* 79:772, 1975.
3. Spector B, Klintworth GK, Wells SA: Histologic study of the ocular lesions in multiple endocrine neoplasia syndrome type IIb, *Am J Ophthalmol* 91:204, 1981.
4. Cogan DG, Henneman PH: Diffuse calcification of the cornea in hypercalcemia, *N Engl J Med* 257:451, 1957.
5. Berkow JW, Fine SB, Zimmerman LE: Unusual ocular calcification in hyperparathyroidism, *Am J Ophthalmol* 66:812, 1968.
6. Jensen OA: Ocular calcification in primary hyperparathyroidism, *Acta Ophthalmol* 53:173, 1971.
7. Berlyne GM: Microcrystalline conjunctival calcification in renal failure, *Lancet* 2:366, 1968.
8. Harris LS et al: Conjunctival and corneal calcific deposits in uremic patients, *Am J Ophthalmol* 72:130, 1971.
9. Porte R, Crombie AL: Corneal and conjunctival calcification in chronic renal failure, *Br J Ophthalmol* 57:339, 1973.
10. Fraser D et al: A new look at infantile hypercalcemia, *Pediatr Clin North Am* 13:503, 1966.
11. Garabédian M et al: Elevated plasma 1,25-$(OH_2)D$ concentrations in infants with hypercalcemia and elfin facies, *N Engl J Med* 312:948, 1985.
12. Harley RD et al: Idiopathic hypercalcemia of infancy: optic atrophy and other ocular changes, *Trans Am Acad Ophthalmol Otolaryngol* 69:977, 1965.
13. Brenner RL et al: Eye signs of hypophosphatasia, *Arch Ophthalmol* 81:614, 1969.
14. Fraser D: Hypophosphatasia, *Am J Ophthalmol* 22:730, 1957.
15. Hashimoto K, Lieberman P, Lamkin N: Angiokeratoma corporis diffusum (Fabry disease), *Arch Dermatol* 112:1416, 1976.
16. Grace EV: Diffuse angiokeratosis (Fabry's disease), *Am J Ophthalmol* 62:139, 1966.
17. Sher NA, Letson RD, Desnick RJ: The ocular manifestations in Fabry's disease, *Arch Ophthalmol* 97:671, 1979.
18. Spaeth GL, Frost P: Fabry's disease: its ocular manifestations, *Arch Ophthalmol* 74:760, 1965.
19. Weingeist TA, Blodi FC: Fabry's disease: ocular findings in a female carrier, *Arch Ophthalmol* 85:169, 1971.
20. Font RL, Fine BS: Ocular pathology in Fabry's disease, *Am J Ophthalmol* 73:419, 1973.
21. Francois J, Hanssens M, Teuchy H: Corneal ultrastructural changes in Fabry's disease, *Ophthalmologica* 176:313, 1978.
22. Frost P, Tamala Y, Spaeth GL: Fabry's disease-glycolipid lipidosis: histochemical and electron microscopic studies of two cases, *Am J Med* 40:618, 1966.
23. Riegel EM et al: Ocular pathology of Fabry's disease in a hemizygous male following renal transplantation, *Surv Ophthalmol* 26:247, 1982.

24. Petrohelos M et al: Ocular manifestations of Gaucher's disease, *Am J Ophthalmol* 80:1006, 1975.

25. Sasaki T, Tsukahara S: New ocular findings in Gaucher's disease: a report of two brothers, *Ophthalmologica* 191:206, 1985.

26. Kolodny EH: *Metachromatic leukodystrophy and multiple sulfatase deficiency: sulfatide lipidosis.* In Scriver CR et al, editors: *The metabolic basis of inherited disease,* ed 6, New York, 1989, McGraw-Hill.

27. Quigley HA, Green RW: Clinical and ultrastructural ocular histopathologic studies of adult onset metachromatic leukodystrophy, *Am J Ophthalmol* 82:471, 1976.

28. Libert J et al: Ocular findings in metachromatic leukodystrophy, *Arch Ophthalmol* 97:1495, 1979.

29. O'Brien J: Generalized gangliosidosis, *J Pediatr* 75:167, 1969.

30. Emery JM et al: GM1 gangliosidosis: ocular and pathological manifestations, *Arch Ophthalmol* 85:177, 1971.

31. Weiss MJ et al: GM1 gangliosidosis type I, *Am J Ophthalmol* 76:999, 1973.

32. Sorcinelli R, Sitzia A, Loi M: Cherry-red spot, optic atrophy and corneal cloudings in a patient suffering from GM1 gangliosidosis type I, *Metab Pediatr Syst Ophthalmol* 10:62, 1987.

33. Beaudet AL: *Lysosomal storage diseases.* In Braunwald E et al, editors: *Harrison's principles of internal medicine,* ed 11, New York, 1987, McGraw-Hill.

34. Robb RM, Kuwabara T: The ocular pathology of type A Niemann-Pick disease: a light and electron microscopic study, *Invest Ophthalmol* 12:366, 1973.

35. Howes EL et al: Ocular pathology of infantile Niemann-Pick disease: study of fetus of 23 weeks' gestation, *Arch Ophthalmol* 93:494, 1975.

36. Libert J, Toussaint D, Guiselings R: Ocular findings in Niemann-Pick disease, *Am J Ophthalmol* 80:991, 1975.

37. Walton DS, Robb RM, Crocker AC: Ocular manifestations of group A Niemann-Pick disease, *Am J Ophthalmol* 84:174, 1978.

38. Tremblay M, Szots F: GM$_2$ Type 2-gangliosidosis (Sandhoff's disease): ocular and pathological manifestations, *Can J Ophthalmol* 9:338, 1974.

39. Brownstein S et al: Sandhoff's disease (GM$_2$ gangliosidosis type 2): histopathology and ultrastructure of the eye, *Arch Ophthalmol* 98:1089, 1980.

40. Freidrickson DS, Levy RI, Lees RS: Fat transport in lipoproteins: an integrated approach to mechanisms and disorders, *N Engl J Med* 276:34, 1967.

41. Vinger PF, Sacks BA: Ocular manifestations of hyperlipoproteinemia, *Am J Ophthalmol* 70:563, 1970.

42. Brown MS, Goldstein JL: *The hyperlipoproteinemias and other disorders of lipid metabolism.* In

Braunwald E et al, editors: *Harrison's principles of internal medicine,* ed 11, New York, 1987, McGraw-Hill.

43. Spaeth GL: Ocular manifestations of lipoprotein disease, *JCE Ophthalmol* 41:11, 1979.

44. Jaeger W, Eisenhauer GG: Der diagnostische wert des arcus cornae als hinsweis auf lipoidstoff-wechselstorungen, *Klin Monatsbl Augenheilkd* 171:321, 1977.

45. Barchiesi BJ et al: The cornea and disorders of lipid metabolism, *Surv Ophthalmol* 36:1, 1991.

46. Funke H et al: A frameshift mutation in the human apolipoprotein A-1 gene causes high density lipoprotein deficiency, partial lecithicin: cholesterol acyltransferase deficiency and corneal opacification, *J Clin Invest* 87:375, 1991.

47. Breslow JL: *Familial disorders of high density lipoprotein metabolism.* In Scriver CR et al, editors: *The metabolic and molecular basis of inherited disease,* ed 7, New York, 1995, McGraw-Hill.

48. Horven I, Egge K, Gjone E: Corneal and fundus changes in familial LCAT deficiency, *Acta Ophthalmol (Copenh)* 52:201, 1974.

49. Bron AJ: Corneal changes in the dyslipoproteinemias, *Cornea* 8:135, 1989.

50. Bron AJ et al: Primary LCAT deficiency disease, *Lancet* 1:929, 1975.

51. Bethell W, McCullocoh C, Ghosh M: Lethicin cholesterol acyltransferase deficiency: light and electron microscopic finding from 2 corneas, *Can J Ophthalmol* 10:494, 1975.

52. Vrabec MP et al: Ophthalmic observations in lecithin cholesterol acyltransferase deficiency, *Arch Ophthalmol* 106:225, 1988.

53. Langmann A et al: Ophthalmological findings in three patients with cholesterol acyltransferase deficiency syndrome before and after kidney transplantation, *Graefes Arch Clin Exp Ophthalmol* 231:607, 1993.

54. Cogan DG et al: Corneal opacity in LCAT disease, *Cornea* 11:595, 1992.

55. Funke H et al: A molecular defect causing fish eye disease: an amino acid exchange in lecithin-cholesterol acyltransferase (LCAT) leads to the selective loss of alpha-LCAT activity, *Proc Natl Acad Sci USA* 88:4855, 1991.

56. Philipson BT: Fish eye disease, *Birth Defects* 18:441, 1982.

57. Carlson LA: Fish eye disease: a new familial condition with massive corneal opacities and dyslipoproteinemia. Clinical and laboratory studies in two affected families, *Eur J Clin Invest* 12:41, 1982.

58. Koster H et al: A fish-eye disease-like familial condition with massive corneal clouding and dyslipoproteinemia: report of clinical, histologic, electron microscopic, and biochemical features, *Cornea* 11:452, 1992.

59. Chu FC et al: Ocular manifestations of familial high-density lipoprotein deficiency (Tangier disease), *Arch Ophthalmol* 97:1926, 1979.

60. Pressly TA et al: Ocular complications of Tangier disease, *Am J Med* 83:991, 1987.

61. Baum JL, Tannenbaum M, Kolodny EH: Refsum's syndrome with corneal involvement, *Am J Ophthalmol* 60:699, 1965.
62. Björkhem I, Bober KM: *Inborn errors in bile acid biosynthesis and storage of sterols other than cholesterol.* In Scriver CR et al, editors: *The metabolic and molecular basis of inherited disease,* ed 7, New York, 1995, McGraw-Hill.
63. Ozaki H et al: Farber's disease (disseminated lipogranulomatosis): the first case reported in Japan, *Acta Med Okayama* 32:69, 1978.
64. Zetterstrom R: Disseminated lipogranulomatosis (Farber's disease), *Acta Paediatr* 47:501, 1958.
65. Zarbin MA et al: Farber's disease: light and electron microscopic study of the eye, *Arch Ophthalmol* 103:73, 1985.
66. Sanfilippo SJ et al: Mental retardation associated with acid mucopolysacchariduria (heparitin sulfate type), *J Pediatr* 63:837, 1963.
67. Li W et al: cDNA clone to chick corneal chondroitin/dermatan sulfate proteoglycan reveals identity to decorin, *Arch Biochem Biophys* 296:190, 1992.
68. Blochberger TC et al: cDNA to chick lumican (corneal keratan sulfate proteoglycan) reveals homology to the small interstitial proteoglycan gene family and expression muscle and intestine, *J Biol Chem* 267:347, 1992.
69. Neufeld EF, Muenzer J: *The mucopolysaccharidoses.* In Scriver CR et al, editors: *The metabolic and molecular basis of inherited disease,* ed 7, New York, 1995, McGraw-Hill.
70. Gills PF et al: Electroretinography and fundus oculi findings in Hurler's disease and allied mucopolysaccharidoses, *Arch Ophthalmol* 74:596, 1965.
71. Spellacy E et al: Glaucoma in a case of Hurler disease, *Br J Ophthalmol* 64:773, 1980.
72. Rosen DA et al: Keratoplasty and electron microscopy of the cornea in systemic mucopolysaccharidosis (Hurler's disease), *Can J Ophthalmol* 3:218, 1968.
73. Scheie HG, Hambrick GW, Barnes LA: A newly recognized form of Hurler's disease (gargoylism), *Am J Ophthalmol* 53:753, 1962.
74. Summers CG et al: Dense peripheral corneal clouding in Scheie syndrome, *Cornea* 13:277, 1994.
75. Quigley HA, Maumenee AE, Stark WJ: Systemic mucopolysaccharidosis, *Am J Ophthalmol* 80:1, 1975.
76. Canstantopoulas B, Dekaban AS, Scheie HG: Heterogeneity of disorders in patients with corneal clouding, normal intellect, and mucopolysaccharidosis, *Am J Ophthalmol* 72:1106, 1971.
77. Quigley HA, Goldberg MF: Scheie syndrome and macular corneal dystrophy: an ultrastructural comparison of conjunctiva and skin, *Arch Ophthalmol* 85:553, 1971.
78. Sugar J: Corneal manifestations of the systemic mucopolysaccharidoses, *Ann Ophthalmol* 11:531, 1979.
79. Chijiiwa T et al: Ocular manifestations of Hurler/Scheie phenotype in two sibs, *Jpn J Ophthalmol* 27:54, 1983.
80. Kajii T et al: Hurler/Scheie genetic compounds (mucopolysaccharidosis IH/IS) in Japanese brothers, *Clin Genet* 6:394, 1974.
81. Goldberg MF, Duke JR: Ocular histopathology in Hunter's syndrome: systemic mucopolysaccharidosis, type II, *Arch Ophthalmol* 77:503, 1967.
82. DiFerrante H et al: Mucopolysaccharide storage diseases: corrective activity of normal human serum and lymphocyte extracts, *Birth Defects* 9:31, 1973.
83. Gardner RJM, Hay JR: Hurler's syndrome with clear corneas, *Lancet* 2:845, 1974.
84. Bartsocas C et al: San Filippo type C disease: clinical findings in four patients with a new variant of mucopolysaccharidosis III, *Eur J Pediatr* 130:251, 1979.
85. Van Noorden GK, Zellweger H, Ponseti I: Ocular findings in Morquio-Ullrich's disease, *Arch Ophthalmol* 64:585, 1960.
86. Goldberg MF, Scott CI, McKusick VA: Hydrocephalus and papilledema in Maroteaux-Lamy syndrome (mucopolysaccharidosis type VI), *Am J Ophthalmol* 69:969, 1970.
87. Suveges I: Histological and ultrastructural studies of the cornea in Maroteaux-Lamy syndrome, *Graefes Arch Clin Exp Ophthalmol* 212:29, 1979.
88. Naumann GO, Rummelt V: Clearing of the para-transplant host cornea after perforating keratoplasty in Maroteaux-Lamy syndrome (type VI A mucopolysaccharidosis), *Klin Monatsbl Augenheilkd* 203:351, 1993.
89. Schwartz MF, Werblin TP, Green WR: Occurrence of mucopolysaccharide in corneal grafts in the Maroteaux-Lamy syndrome, *Cornea* 4:58, 1985.
90. Hoyme HE et al: Presentation of mucopolysaccharidosis VII (β-glucuronidase deficiency) in infancy, *J Med Genet* 18:237, 1981.
91. Beaudet AL et al: Variation in the phenotypic expression of beta glucuronidase deficiency, *J Pediatr* 86:388, 1975.
92. Kenyon KR et al: The systemic mucopolysaccharidoses: ultrastructural and histological studies of conjunctiva and skin, *Am J Ophthalmol* 73:811, 1972.
93. Kenyon KR et al: Ocular pathology of the Maroteaux-Lamy syndrome (systemic mucopolysaccharidosis type VI): histologic and ultrastructural report of two cases, *Am J Ophthalmol* 73:718, 1972.
94. McDonnell JM, Green WR, Maumenee IH: Ocular histopathology of systemic mucopolysaccharidosis, type II-A (Hunter syndrome, severe), *Ophthalmology* 92:1772, 1985.
95. Rummelt V, Meyer HJ, Naumann GO: Light and electron microscopy of the cornea in systemic mucopolysaccharidosis type I-S (Scheie's syndrome), *Cornea* 11:86, 1992.
96. DelMonte MA et al: Histopathology of Sanfil-

ippo's syndrome, *Arch Ophthalmol* 101:1255, 1983.

97. Lavery MA et al: Ocular histopathology and ultrastructure of Sanfilippo's syndrome, type III-B, *Arch Ophthalmol* 101:1263, 1983.

98. Birkenmeier EH et al: Increased life span and correction of metabolic defects in murine mucopolysaccharidosis type VII after syngeneic bone marrow transplantation, *Blood* 78:3081, 1991.

99. Summers CG et al: Ocular changes in the mucopolysaccharidoses after bone marrow transplantation: a preliminary report, *Ophthalmology* 96:977, 1989.

100. Schwartz DE: Corneal sensitivity in diabetics, *Arch Ophthalmol* 91:174, 1974.

101. Schultz RO et al: Diabetic keratopathy as a manifestation of peripheral neuropathy, *Am J Ophthalmol* 96:368, 1983.

102. Ruben ST: Corneal sensation in insulin dependent and non-insulin dependent diabetics with proliferative retinopathy, *Acta Ophthalmol (Copenh)* 72:576, 1994.

103. Hyndiuk R et al: Neurotrophic corneal ulcers in diabetes mellitus, *Arch Ophthalmol* 95:2193, 1977.

104. Perry HD et al: Corneal complications after closed vitrectomy through the pars plana, *Arch Ophthalmol* 96:401, 1978.

105. Foulks GN et al: Factors related to corneal epithelial complications after closed vitrectomy in diabetics, *Arch Ophthalmol* 97:1076, 1979.

106. Kenyon KR: Recurrent corneal erosion: pathogenesis and therapy, *Int Ophthalmol Clin* 19:169, 1979.

107. Göbbels M, Spitznas M, Oldendoerp J: Impairment of corneal epithelial barrier function in diabetics, *Graefes Arch Clin Exp Ophthalmol* 227:142, 1989.

108. Seifart H, Strempel I: The dry eye and diabetes mellitus I, *Ophthalmology* 91:235, 1994.

109. Schultz RO et al: Diabetic keratopathy, *Trans Am Ophthalmol Soc* 79:180, 1981.

110. Schultz RO et al: Corneal endothelial changes in type I and type II diabetes mellitus, *Am J Ophthalmol* 98:401, 1984.

111. Itoi M et al: Specular microscopic studies of the corneal endothelium of Japanese diabetics, *Cornea* 8:2, 1989.

112. Ravalico G et al: Corneal endothelial function in diabetes: a fluorophotometric study, *Ophthalmologica* 208:179, 1994.

113. Pierro L et al: Correlation of corneal thickness with blood glucose control in diabetes mellitus, *Acta Ophthalmol (Copenh)* 71:169, 1993.

114. Lass JH et al: A morphologic and fluorophotometric analysis of the corneal endothelium in type I diabetes mellitus and cystic fibrosis, *Am J Ophthalmol* 100:783, 1985.

115. Göbbels M, Spitznas M: Endothelial barrier function after phacoemulsification: a comparison between diabetic and nondiabetic patients, *Graefes Arch Clin Exp Ophthalmol* 229:254, 1991.

116. Herse PR: Corneal hydration control in normal and alloxan-induced diabetic rabbits, *Invest Ophthalmol Vis Sci* 31:2205, 1990.

117. Hosotani H et al: Reversal of abnormal corneal epithelial cell morphologic characteristics and reduced corneal sensitivity in diabetic patients by aldose reductase inhibitor, CT-112, *Am J Ophthalmol* 119:228, 1995.

118. Datiles MR et al: The effects of sorbinil, an aldose reductase inhibitor, on the corneal endothelium in galactosemic dogs, *Invest Ophthalmol Vis Sci* 31:2201, 1990.

119. Libert J et al: Ocular ultrastructural study in a fetus with type II glycogenosis, *Br J Ophthalmol* 61:476, 1977.

120. Beaudet AL: *Lysosomal storage diseases.* In Braunwald E et al, editors: *Harrison's principles of internal medicine,* ed 11, New York, 1987, McGraw-Hill.

121. Borit A, Sugarman GI, Spencer WH: Ocular involvement in I-cell disease (mucolipidosis II) light and electron-microscopic findings, *Graefes Arch Clin Ophthalmol* 198:25, 1976.

122. Libert J et al: Ocular findings in I-cell disease (mucolipidosis type II), *Am J Ophthalmol* 83:617, 1977.

123. Kenyon KR, Sensenbrenner JA: Mucolipidosis II (I-cell disease): ultrastructural observations of conjunctiva and sclera, *Invest Ophthalmol* 10:555, 1971.

124. Komfeld S, Sly WS: *I-cell disease and pseudo-Hurler polydystrophy: disorders of lysosomal enzyme phosphorylation and localization.* In Scriver CR et al, editors: *The metabolic and molecular basis of inherited disease,* ed 7, New York, 1995, McGraw-Hill.

125. Kelly TE et al: Mucolipidosis III (pseudo-Hurler polydystrophy): clinical and laboratory studies in a series of 12 patients, *Johns Hopkins Med J* 137:156, 1975.

126. Traboulsi EI, Maumenee IH: Ophthalmic findings in mucolipidosis III (pseudo-Hurler polydystrophy), *Am J Ophthalmol* 102:592, 1986.

127. Quigley HA, Goldberg MF: Conjunctival ultrastructure in mucolipidosis 3 (pseudo Hurler polydystrophy), *Invest Ophthalmol* 10:568, 1971.

128. Newell FW, Matalon R, Meyer S: A new mucolipidosis with psychomotor retardation, corneal clouding and retinal degeneration, *Am J Ophthalmol* 80:440, 1975.

129. Berman ER et al: Congenital corneal clouding with abnormal systemic storage bodies: a new variant of mucolipidosis, *J Pediatr* 84:519, 1974.

130. Merin S et al: Mucolipidosis IV: ocular systemic and ultrastructural findings, *Invest Ophthalmol Vis Sci* 14:437, 1975.

131. Amir N, Zlotogora J, Bach G: Mucolipidosis type IV: clinical spectrum and natural history, *Pediatrics* 79:953, 1987.

132. Newman NJ et al: Corneal surface irregularities and episodic pain in a patient with mucolipidosis IV, *Arch Ophthalmol* 108:251, 1990.

133. Casteels I et al: Mucolipidosis type IV: presentation of a mild variant, *Ophthalmic Paediatr Genet* 13:205, 1992.

134. Kenyon KR et al: Mucolipidosis IV: histopathology of conjunctiva, cornea and skin, *Arch Ophthalmol* 97:1106, 1979.

135. Zwann J, Kenyon KR: Two brothers with presumed mucolipidosis IV, *Birth Defects* 18:381, 1982.

136. Riedel KG et al: Ocular abnormalities in mucolipidosis IV, *Am J Ophthalmol* 99:125, 1985.

137. Dangel ME, Bremer DL, Rogers GL: Treatment of corneal opacification in mucolipidosis IV with conjunctival transplantation, *Am J Ophthalmol* 99:137, 1985.

138. Cibis GW et al: Mucolipidosis I, *Arch Ophthalmol* 101:933, 1983.

139. Emery JM et al: Gm₁-gangliosidosis: ocular and pathological manifestations, *Arch Ophthalmol* 85:177, 1971.

140. Goldberg MF et al: Macular cherry-red spot, corneal clouding, and beta-galactosidase deficiency: clinical, biochemical, and electron microscopic study of a new autosomal recessive storage disease, *Arch Intern Med* 128:387, 1971.

141. Usui T et al: Conjunctival biopsy in adult form galactosialidosis, *Br J Ophthalmol* 77:165, 1993.

142. Arbisser AI et al: Ocular findings in mannosidosis, *Am J Ophthalmol* 82:465, 1976.

143. Borrone C et al: Fucosidosis: clinical, biochemical, immunologic, and genetic studies in two new cases, *J Pediatr* 84:727, 1974.

144. Snyder RO et al: Ocular findings in fucosidosis, *Birth Defects* 12:241, 1976.

145. Libert J, Van Hoof F, Tonduer M: Fucosidosis: ultrastructural study of conjunctiva and skin and enzyme analysis of tears, *Invest Ophthalmol* 15:626, 1976.

146. Hoshino M et al: Fucosidosis: ultrastructural study of the eye in an adult, *Graefes Arch Clin Exp Ophthalmol* 227:162, 1989.

147. La Du BN: Alcaptonuria. In Scriver CR et al, editors: *The metabolic basis of inherited disease*, ed 6, New York, 1989, McGraw-Hill.

148. Smith JW: Ochronosis of the sclera and cornea complicating alkaptonuria: review of the literature and report of four cases, *JAMA* 120:1282, 1942.

149. Garrett EE: Ocular ochronosis with alkaptonuria, *Am J Ophthalmol* 55:617, 1963.

150. Wirtschafter JD: The eye in alkaptonuria, *Birth Defects* 12:279, 1976.

151. Kampik A, Sani JN, Green WR: Ocular ochronosis: clinicopathological, histochemical and ultrastructural studies, *Arch Ophthalmol* 98:1441, 1980.

152. Kenyon KR, Sensenbrenner JA: Electron microscopy of cornea and conjunctiva in childhood cystinosis, *Am J Ophthalmol* 78:68, 1974.

153. Goldman H et al: Adolescent cystinosis: comparison with infantile and adult forms, *Pediatrics* 47:979, 1971.

154. Zimmerman TJ, Hood CI, Gasset AR: "Adolescent" cystinosis: a case presentation and re-

view of the recent literature, *Arch Ophthalmol* 92:265, 1974.

155. Richler M et al: Ocular manifestations of nephropathic cystinosis: the French-Canadian experience in a genetically homogeneous population, *Arch Ophthalmol* 109:359, 1991.

156. Melles RB et al: Spatial and temporal sequence of corneal crystal deposition in nephropathic cystinosis, *Am J Ophthalmol* 104:598, 1987.

157. Yamamoto GK et al: Long-term ocular changes in cystinosis: observation in renal transplant recipients, *J Pediatr Ophthalmol Strabismus* 16:21, 1979.

158. Kaiser-Kupfer MI et al: Long-term ocular manifestations in nephropathic cystinosis, *Arch Ophthalmol* 104:706, 1986.

159. Wong VG: Ocular manifestations in cystinosis, *Birth Defects* 12:181, 1976.

160. Sanderson PO et al: Cystinosis: a clinical, histopathologic, and ultrastructural study, *Arch Ophthalmol* 91:270, 1974.

161. Kaiser-Kupfer MI et al: Nephropathic cystinosis: immunohistochemical and histopathologic studies of cornea, conjunctiva and iris, *Curr Eye Res* 6:617, 1987.

162. Cogan DG, Kuwabara T: Ocular pathology of cystinosis, *Arch Ophthalmol* 63:51, 1960.

163. Wong VG, Schulman JD, Seegmiller JE: Conjunctival biopsy for the biochemical diagnosis of cystinosis, *Am J Ophthalmol* 70:278, 1970.

164. Francois J et al: Cystinosis: a clinical and histopathologic study, *Am J Ophthalmol* 73:643, 1972.

165. Bradbury JA et al: A randomised placebo-controlled trial of topical cysteamine therapy in patients with nephropathic cystinosis, *Eye* 5:755, 1991.

166. Jones NP, Postlethwaite RJ, Noble JL: Clearance of corneal crystals in nephropathic cystinosis by topical cysteamine 0.5%, *Br J Ophthalmol* 75:311, 1991.

167. Kaiser-Kupfer MI et al: A randomized placebo-controlled trial of cysteamine eye drops in nephropathic cystinosis, *Arch Ophthalmol* 108:689, 1990.

168. Kaiser-Kupfer MI, Datiles MB, Gahl WA: Clear graft two years after keratoplasty in nephropathic cystinosis, *Am J Ophthalmol* 105:318, 1988.

169. Katz B, Melles RB, Schneider JA: Recurrent crystal deposition after keratoplasty in nephropathic cystinosis, *Am J Ophthalmol* 104:190, 1987.

170. Goldsmith LA, Laberge C: *Tyrosinemia and related disorders*. In Scriver CR et al, editors: *The metabolic basis of inherited disease*, ed 6, New York, 1989, McGraw-Hill.

171. Bienfang DC, Kuwabara T, Pueschel SM: The Richner-Hanhart syndrome: report of a case with associated tyrosinemia, *Arch Ophthalmol* 94:1133, 1976.

172. Colditz PB et al; Tyrosinaemia II, *Med J Aust* 141:244, 1984.

173. Burns RP: Soluble tyrosine aminotransferase de-

ficiency: an unusual cause of corneal ulcers, *Am J Ophthalmol* 73:400, 1972.

174. Sandberg HO: Bilateral keratopathy in tyrosinosis, *Acta Ophthalmol* 53:760, 1975.

175. Jaeger W et al: Herpetiform bilateral epithelial corneal dystrophy caused by tyrosinemia (Richner-Hanhart syndrome), *Klin Monatsbl Augenheilkd* 173:506, 1978.

176. Rabinowitz LG et al: Painful keratoderma and photophobia: hallmarks of tyrosinemia type II, *J Pediatr* 126:266, 1995.

177. Grayson M: Corneal manifestations of keratosis plantaris and palmaris, *Am J Ophthalmol* 59:483, 1965.

178. Driscoll DJ et al: Corneal tyrosine crystals in transient neonatal tyrosinemia, *J Pediatr* 113:91, 1988.

179. Charlton KH et al: Pseudodendritic keratitis and systemic tyrosinemia, *Ophthalmology* 88:355, 1981.

180. Zaleski WA, Hill A, Murray RG: Corneal erosions in tyrosinosis, *Can J Ophthalmol* 8:556, 1973.

181. Rich LF, Beard ME, Burns RP: Excess dietary tyrosine and corneal lesions, *Exp Eye Res* 17:87, 1973.

182. Gipson IK, Burns RP, Wolfe-Lande JD: Crystals in corneal epithelial lesions of tyrosine-fed rats, *Invest Ophthalmol* 14:937, 1975.

183. Larregue M et al: Syndrome du Richner-Hanhart ou tyrosinose oculo-cutanee, *Ann Dermatol Venereol* 106:53, 1979.

184. Sayar RB et al: Clinical picture and problems of keratoplasty in Richner-Hanhart syndrome, *Ophthalmologica* 197:1, 1988.

185. Knowles DM II et al: Amyloidosis of the orbit and adnexae, *Surv Ophthalmol* 19:367, 1975.

186. Smith ME, Zimmerman LE: Amyloidosis of the eyelid and conjunctiva, *Arch Ophthalmol* 75:42, 1966.

187. Blodi FC, Apple DJ: Localized conjunctival amyloidosis, *Am J Ophthalmol* 88:346, 1979.

188. Pepys MB: *Amyloidosis*. In Samter M, editor: *Immunological diseases*, ed 4, Boston, 1988, Little, Brown & Co.

189. Lijima S: Primary systemic amyloidosis: a unique case complaining of diffuse eyelid swelling and conjunctival involvement, *J Dermatol* 19:113, 1992.

190. Patrinely JR, Koch DD: Surgical management of advanced ocular adnexal amyloidosis, *Arch Ophthalmol* 110:882, 1992.

191. Ando E et al: Ocular microangiopathy in familial amyloidotic polyneuropathy, type I, *Graefes Arch Clin Exp Ophthalmol* 230:1, 1992.

192. Lessell S et al: Scalloped pupils in familial amyloidosis, *N Engl J Med* 293:914, 1975.

193. Sandgren O, Hofer PA: Conjunctival involvement in familial amyloidotic polyneuropathy, *Acta Ophthalmol (Copenh)* 68:292, 1990.

194. Gorevic PD et al: Amyloidosis due to a mutation of the gelsolin gene in an American family with lattice corneal dystrophy type II, *N Engl J Med* 325:1780, 1991.

195. Haltia M et al: Gelsolin gene mutation at codon 187-in familial amyloidosis, Finnish: DNA diagnostic assay, *Am J Med Genet* 42:357, 1992.

196. de la Chapelle A et al: Gelsolin-derived familial amyloidosis caused by asparagine or tyrosine substitution for aspartic acid at residue 197, *Nature Genet* 2:157, 1992.

197. Sunada Y et al: Inherited amyloid polyneuropathy type IV (gelsolin variant) in a Japanese family, *Ann Neurol* 33:57, 1993.

198. Maury CP: Gelsolin-related amyloidosis: identification of the amyloid protein in Finnish hereditary amyloidosis as a fragment of variant gelsolin, *J Clin Invest* 87:1195, 1991.

199. Kivela T et al: Ocular amyloid deposition in familial amyloidosis, Finnish: an analysis of native and variant gelsolin in Meretoja's syndrome, *Invest Ophthalmol Vis Sci* 35:3759, 1994.

200. Chumbley LC: Scleral involvement in symptomatic porphyria, *Am J Ophthalmol* 84:729, 1977.

201. Manschot WA: Ring of Kayser and Fleischer, *Ophthalmologica* 132:164, 1956.

202. Slovis TL et al: The varied manifestations of Wilson's disease, *J Pediatr* 78:578, 1971.

203. Tso MOM, Fine BS, Thorpe HE: Kayser-Fleischer ring and associated cataract in Wilson's disease, *Am J Ophthalmol* 79:479, 1975.

204. Wiebers DO, Hollenhorst RW, Goldstein NP: The ophthalmological manifestations of Wilson's disease, *Mayo Clin Proc* 52:409, 1977.

205. Dobyns WB, Goldstein NP, Gordon H: Clinical spectrum of Wilson's disease (hepatolenticular degeneration), *Mayo Clin Proc* 54:35, 1979.

206. Cairns JE, Williams HP, Walshe JM: Sunflower cataract in Wilson's disease, *Br Med J* 3:95, 1969.

207. Uzman LL, Jakus MA: The Kayser-Fleischer ring: a histochemical and electron microscope study, *Neurology* 7:341, 1957.

208. Ellis PP: Ocular deposition of copper in hypercupremia, *Am J Ophthalmol* 68:423, 1969.

209. Johnson BL: Ultrastructure of the Kaiser-Fleischer ring, *Am J Ophthalmol* 76:455, 1973.

210. Johnson RE, Campbell RJ: Wilson's disease: electron microscopic, x-ray energy spectroscopic, and atomic absorption spectroscopic studies of cornea copper deposition and distribution, *Lab Invest* 46:564, 1982.

211. Fleming CR et al: Pigmented rings in non-Wilsonian liver disease, *Ann Intern Med* 86:285, 1977.

212. Frommer D et al: Kayser-Fleischer-like rings in patients without Wilson's disease, *Gastroenterology* 72:1331, 1977.

213. Tauber J, Steinert RF: Pseudo-Kayser-Fleischer ring of the cornea associated with non-Wilsonian liver disease: a case report and literature review, *Cornea* 12:74, 1993.

214. Scheinberg IH: *Wilson's disease*. In Braunwald E et al, editors: *Harrison's principles of internal medicine*, ed 11, New York, 1987, McGraw-Hill.

215. Mitchell AM, Heller GL: Changes in Kayser-Fleischer ring during treatment of hepatolentic-

ular degeneration, *Arch Ophthalmol* 80:622, 1968.

216. Sussman W, Scheinberg IH: Disappearance of Kayser-Fleischer rings: effects of penicillamine, *Arch Ophthalmol* 82:738, 1969.

217. Schoenberger M, Ellis PP: Disappearance of Kayser-Fleischer rings after liver transplantation, *Arch Ophthalmol* 97:1914, 1979.

218. McWilliams JR: Ocular findings in gout, *Am J Ophthalmol* 35:1778, 1952.

219. Ferry AP, Safir A, Melikan HE: Ocular abnormalities in patients with gout, *Ann Ophthalmol* 17:632, 1985.

220. Slansky HH, Kuwabara T: Intranuclear urate crystals in corneal epithelium, *Arch Ophthalmol* 80:338, 1968.

221. Fishman RS, Sunderman FW: Band keratopathy in gout, *Arch Ophthalmol* 75:367, 1967.

222. Barnes HD, Boshoff PH: Ocular lesions in patients with porphyria, *Arch Ophthalmol* 48:567, 1952.

223. Sevel D, Burger D: Ocular involvement in cutaneous porphyria: a clinical and histological report, *Arch Ophthalmol* 85:580, 1970.

224. Sober AJ, Grove AS Jr, Muhlbauer JE: Cicatricial ectropion and lacrimal obstruction associated with sclerodermoid variant of porphyria cutanea tarda, *Am J Ophthalmol* 91:400, 1981.

225. Duke-Elder S, Leigh AG: *System of ophthalmology,* vol VIII, *Diseases of the outer eye,* St Louis, 1965, Mosby–Year Book.

226. Stokes WH: Ocular manifestations in hydroa vacciniforme, *Arch Ophthalmol* 23:1131, 1940.

227. Hammer H, Korom I: Photodamage of the conjunctiva in patients with porphyria cutanea tarda, *Br J Ophthalmol* 76:592, 1992.

228. Salmon JF et al: Acute scleritis in porphyria cutanea tarda, *Am J Ophthalmol* 109:400, 1990.

229. Mohan M et al: Corneoscleral ulceration in congenital erythropoietic porphyria (a case report), *Jpn J Ophthalmol* 32:21, 1988.

230. Cibis PA, Brown EB, Hong WM: Ocular aspects of systemic siderosis, *Am J Ophthalmol* 44:158, 1957.

231. Davies G et al: Deposition of melanin and iron in ocular structures in haemochromatosis, *Br J Ophthalmol* 56:338, 1972.

232. Cohen SMZ et al: Ocular histopathologic and biochemical studies of the cerebrohepatorenal syndrome (Zellweger's syndrome) and its relationship to neonatal adrenoleukodystrophy, *Am J Ophthalmol* 96:488, 1984.

233. Campana G et al: Ocular aspects in biotinidase deficiency: clinical and genetic original studies, *Ophthalmic Paediatr Genet* 8:125, 1987.

234. Wolf B, Heard GS: *Disorders of biotin metabolism.* In Scriver CR et al, editors: *The metabolic basis of inherited disease,* ed 6, New York, 1989, McGraw-Hill.

235. Salbert BA, Astruc J, Wolf B: Ophthalmologic findings in biotinidase deficiency, *Ophthalmologica* 206:177, 1993.

Twenty-Two

Diseases of the Skin

BULLOUS OCULOCUTANEOUS DISEASES

The conjunctiva or cornea can be involved in a wide variety of blistering skin diseases (Table 22-1). Most of these diseases cause conjunctival inflammation, and secondary conjunctival and corneal scarring is the main complication.

Pemphigoid skin diseases are a group of disorders characterized by subepidermal bulla formation and deposition of immunoglobulins within the lamina lucida of the epithelial basement membrane in skin and mucous membrane. These diseases include cicatricial pemphigoid (CP), bullous pemphigoid, herpes gestationis, and localized scarring pemphigoid. Only CP and bullous pemphigoid affect the eye.

Cicatricial Pemphigoid
Cicatricial pemphigoid is a cicatricial disease of the conjunctiva and, to a lesser extent, other mucous membranes and skin, which is presumed to be of autoimmune origin. It has also been called benign mucous membrane pemphigoid, ocular pemphigoid, and essential shrinkage of the conjunctiva. It is generally believed to result from formation of autoantibodies against a component of the epithelial basement membrane (type-II hypersensitivity reaction).

Table 22-1 Bullous Skin Diseases

	Age (Most Common)	Skin Lesions	Course	Site of Blister Formation	Immunopathology Immunoglobulin Deposition	Immunopathology Localization	Conjunctival Involvement Frequency	Scarring	Other
Cicatricial pemphigoid	>60 yr; F > M	Vesiculo-bullous 25%	Chronic	SE*	Linear IgG	Lamina lucida	70%–90%	+	
Stevens-Johnson syndrome (erythema multiforme)	10–30 yrs	Multiform: target lesions, macules, papules, bullae	4–6 wk (rarely recurrent)	SE	C3 protein ± IgM	Superficial micro-vessels; ± dermo-epidermal junction	Frequent	+	Entropion, trichiasis, dry eye, secondary corneal disease
Toxic epidermal necrolysis	10–30 yr	Flaccid, necrotic sheets	4–6 wk (rarely recurrent)	IE† (basal)			Common	+	
Bullous pemphigoid	40–60 yr	Large, tense bullae	Usually self-limited	SE	Linear IgG	Lamina lucida	Infrequent	–	
Pemphigus vulgaris	30–50 yr	Bullae, Nikolsky's sign	Chronic	IE	Linear IgG	Intercellular spaces	16%	–	Palpebral conjunctiva

Paraneoplastic pemphigus	Elderly	Polymorphous	Acute	IE			?Common	+	Associated neoplasm
Dermatitis herpetiformis	20–40 yr; M > F	Pruritic, vesicles, papules, bullae	Chronic	SE	Granular IgA	Tips of dermal papillae	Rare	+	Gluten-sensitive enteropathy
Linear IgA disease	30–50 yr	Tense bullae	?Usually self-limited	SE	Linear IgA	Lamina lucida	Common	+	
Epidermolysis bullosa‡	Varies with type	Blisters after trauma	Chronic	IE or SE	Varies	Varies	Frequent	+	Blepharitis, corneal erosion, vesicles, ulcers
Chronic bullous disease of childhood	<5 yr	Large, tense bullae	<10 yr	SE	Linear IgA	Lamina lucida	?Common	+	

*SE, Subepidermal.
†IE, Intraepidermal.
‡See Table 25-2.

Clinical Manifestations

Cicatricial pemphigoid primarily affects older people, and it is more common in women. It seldom develops before 50 years of age but cases in children have been reported.[1] Oral mucosal lesions (Fig. 22-1) occur in 50% to 90% of patients,[2-4] and lesions of the nose, larynx, anus, esophagus, and vagina can also be seen.[5] The oral lesions include a chronic desquamative gingivitis and short-lived vesicles and bullae. Skin lesions (Fig. 22-2) occur in approximately one third of patients.[3,4,6] Skin involvement generally appears in one of two forms: (1) scattered tense vesicles or bullae, sometimes on an erythematous or urticarial base, that heal without residual scarring and are usually limited in extent and few in number; and (2) blisters that occur repeatedly on one or several erythematous areas,[7] often around the head and neck, leading to scarring.

Ocular involvement occurs in the majority of cases and can be the only manifestation of the disease. The most serious complications of CP result from the ocular involvement, except for rare cases of death due to esophageal strictures.

The onset is usually insidious with recurrent attacks of mild and clinically nonspecific conjunctival inflammation. Mucopurulent discharge occurs occasionally, and erroneous diagnoses of bacterial conjunctivitis are not uncommon. During these early episodes conjunctival hyperemia, edema, ulceration, and vesicles can be present. In the absence of coexisting vesiculobullous inflammation of the skin or other mucosa, the first clinical clue to the true nature of the problem is usually slight foreshortening of the inferior conjunctival fornices (Fig. 22-3). Gossamer subepithelial scarring of the conjunctiva may also be found. These subtle conjunctival signs should be sought in any older patient with chronic or recurrent eye redness of unknown origin.

Cicatricial pemphigoid occasionally presents with severe acute inflammation. The patient suddenly develops lid swelling, intense conjunctival hyperemia and edema, and infiltration with rapid scarring of the subepithelial conjunctiva. Bullae are encountered only rarely.

The disease is nearly always bilateral, although it may be very asymmetric. CP is a chronic disease, with exacerbations and remissions. Conjunctival surgery can be associated with marked exacerbation of the disease. Progressive conjunctival scarring occurs and can lead to symblepharon formation (Fig. 22-4), misdirected lashes (Fig. 22-5), entropion, and keratoconjunctivitis sicca. The extent of symblepharon formation is best determined by pulling the lower lid down and having the patient look up, and then pulling the upper lid up and having the patient look down. Scarring usually affects the inferior forniceal conjunctiva first, then the medial and/or nasal bulbar conjunctiva.

Tear deficiency occurs as a result of closure of the tear ductules, and loss of goblet cells leads to mucus deficiency. The lids can become

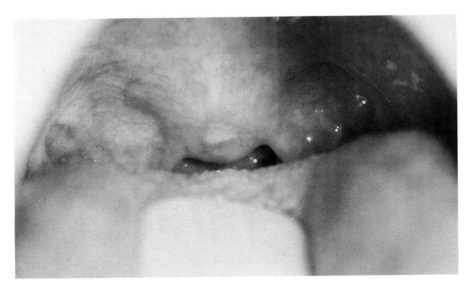

Figure 22-1
Ulcer of the oral mucous membrane (*arrow*) in cicatricial pemphigoid. (Courtesy of Diane Curtin, Pittsburgh, PA.)

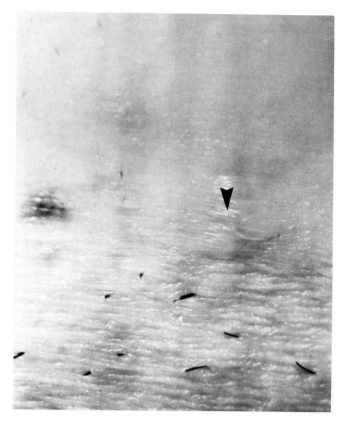

Figure 22-2
Skin bulla (*arrow*) in pemphigoid.

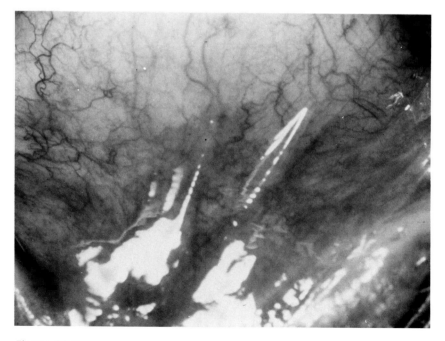

Figure 22-3
Early symblepharon of the lower cul-de-sac in cicatricial pemphigoid.

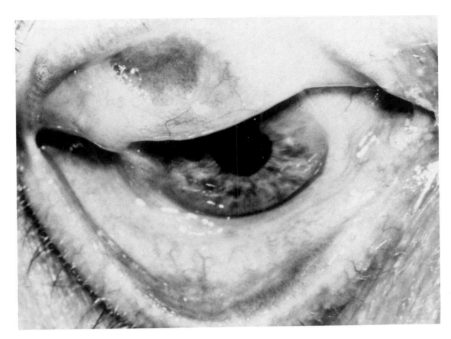

Figure 22-4
Extensive scarring of the upper tarsal conjunctiva in cicatricial pemphigoid.

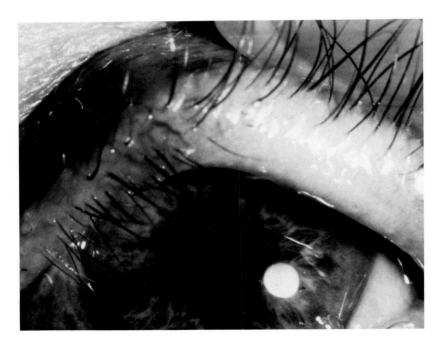

Figure 22-5
Secondary distichiasis in cicatricial pemphigoid.

fixed to the globe, with constant exposure of the cornea and conjunctiva, called *ankyloblepharon* (Fig. 22-6). The cornea is remarkably spared except in the late stages, when it may be seriously compromised by the secondary effects of cicatrization, drying, and trichiasis. The compromised cornea is then subject to superficial scarring and vascularization, persistent epithelial defects, sterile ulceration, and bacterial infection (Fig. 22-7).

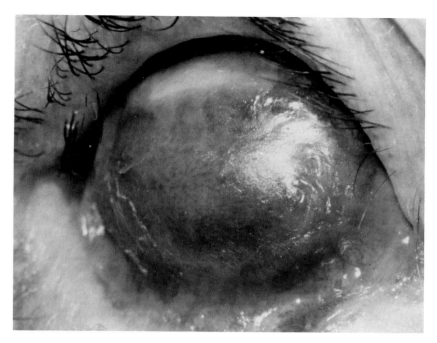

Figure 22-6
Advanced ocular disease in cicatricial pemphigoid, with ankyloblepharon, drying, and keratinization of the corneal and conjunctival epithelium.

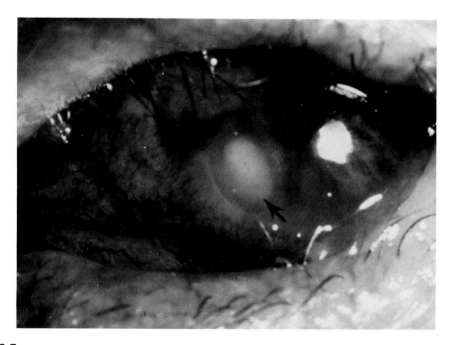

Figure 22-7
The cornea in cicatricial pemphigoid is prone to bacterial invasion. In this case, *Staphylococcus aureus* infection is present (*arrow*).

It is essential to document the extent of conjunctival scarring at each visit, to determine the disease stage, and to detect progression. Foster et al.[8] have divided CP into four stages:

Stage 1—Conjunctival inflammation, mucoid discharge, rose bengal staining of the conjunctiva, and subtle subepithelial fibrosis (fine striae)

Stage 2—Conjunctival shrinkage, with foreshortening of the inferior fornix

Stage 3—Presence of symblepharon formation

Stage 4—End-stage disease, with ankyloblepharon, severe dry eye, and ocular surface keratinization

As noted by the same group,[9] this staging classification is not sufficient to detect progression. It is best to determine the severity of conjunctival shrinkage by measuring the distance from the inferior fornix to the lid margin and to the inferior limbus. Symblepharon formation is described according to the number of symblephara present and the percentage of the width of the horizontal fissure involved. I find it most useful to make measurements and draw symblephera and forniceal depth at each visit, rather than using an alphanumeric classification system.

Histopathology

During active disease subepithelial bullae may be seen. There is inflammation in the epithelium and substantia propria of the conjunctiva, with lymphocytes, plasma cells, macrophages, polymorphonuclear leukocytes, and eosinophils.[10,11] Later, subepithelial fibrosis, loss of goblet cells,[12,13] and keratinization of the epithelium occur.[10,14] Increased numbers of desmosomes and tonofilaments have been observed in the conjunctival epithelium,[15] and this reverted to normal with immunosuppression.[16]

Pathogenesis

The formation of the bullae appears to be caused by autoimmune response against components of the basement membrane. During active disease, immunoglobulins (IgG and sometimes IgA and IgM) and complement components can often be found along the epithelial basement membrane of the conjunctiva[8,17-20] (Fig. 22-8). However, the presence of circulating anti–basement membrane antibodies is uncommon[18,20,21] (in contrast to bullous pemphigoid, in which circulating anti–basement membrane antibodies are present in most cases). The exact antigen against which these antibodies are directed has not been identified, but the bulla forms in the lamina lucida.[22]

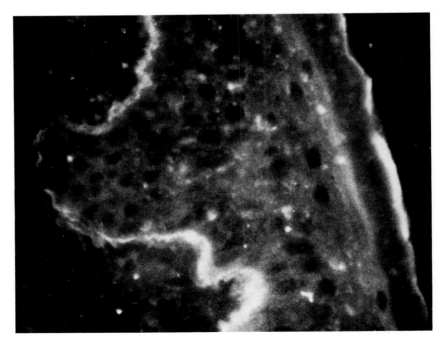

Figure 22-8
Deposition of immunoglobulin in the epithelial basement membrane in a patient with cicatricial pemphigoid. (Courtesy of S.F. Bean, Houston, TX.)

Several other immunologic abnormalities have been observed. In some cases immunoglobulins have also been found to be bound to the conjunctival epithelium,[23,24] and circulating antibodies that bind to the conjunctival and corneal epithelia were present.[23] Also, approximately half of the patients with CP have elevated serum levels of IgA,[23,25] and antinuclear antibodies are often present.[26] Serum levels of interleukin-6 were depressed and levels of tumor necrosis factor-α were increased in CP patients.[27] In one study there was a high frequency of human leukocyte antigen (HLA)–DQB1*0301 in patients with CP.[28] HLA-B12 has been found more frequently in these patients—in 45% compared with 20% of controls.[29]

Diagnosis

The diagnosis of CP is usually clinical, based on progressive bilateral conjunctival scarring. Further support for the diagnosis can often be obtained by finding a few eosinophils in a conjunctival scraping. Eosinophils are more likely to be found during acute inflammatory exacerbations of the disease.

Immunopathologic examination of a conjunctival biopsy may demonstrate antibodies at the level of the basement membrane. However, biopsy must be obtained from an area of active disease, and the absence of antibodies does not rule out the diagnosis. The biopsy can also exacerbate the disease; scarring is probably less if the biopsy is taken from the bulbar conjunctiva, away from the fornix. Foster et al.[30] recommend performing immunopathologic studies on fresh, snap-frozen specimens embedded in a cryostat embedding compound and sectioned on a cryostat microtome. Cryosections are stained with fluorescein-conjugated antisera directed against human immunoglobulins IgG, IgM, IgA, and IgD as well as C3 and C4 complement components. The sensitivity of this technique was 52%.[30] When this immunofluorescence analysis was negative or inconclusive, an immunoperoxidase technique was performed on additional sections, increasing the sensitivity to 83%.

Chronic cicatrization of the conjunctiva can also occur from other causes, and these should be considered particularly in any patient with unilateral disease (see Chapter 6). Prolonged topical administration of echothiophate iodide, pilocarpine, epinephrine, or idoxuridine can cause conjunctival scarring. Drug-induced pemphigoid is clinically identical to cicatricial pemphigoid, except that it is often unilateral, and there are no systemic signs. Cicatrization can cease when medication is stopped, or it can continue to progress. Systemic administration of practolol and D-penicillamine can lead to conjunctival scarring. Other causes include chemical burns, radiation, Stevens-Johnson syndrome, sarcoidosis,[31] infectious conjunctivitis, masquerade syndrome (Fig. 22-9), and trauma.

The other bullous skin diseases, discussed later, should also be considered in the differential diagnosis. The conjunctiva is infrequently involved in bullous pemphigoid. Conjunctival lesions occur in the majority of patients with pemphigus vulgaris, but they produce transient symptoms and rarely cause permanent scarring. Conjunctival involvement can also occur in dermatitis herpetiformis and epidermolysis bullosa.

Treatment

The treatment of CP is disappointing. At this time the most effective means of inhibiting the progression of disease is by immunosuppressive therapy. In general, dapsone appears to be as effective as cyclophosphamide and azathioprine in halting progression of disease and is better tolerated. Dapsone is probably the best initial immunosuppressive therapy for patients with mild to moderate inflammation and slowly progressive scarring, and cyclophosphamide is best for patients with severe, rapidly progressive disease.[32-34] Prednisone is useful in quieting active inflammation but is less effective in preventing cicatrization. Therefore, it is given in addition to other immunosuppressive agents when marked conjunctival inflammation is present.[8,32,35] Topical cyclosporine does not appear to be effective.[36] Immunosuppression is indicated only for patients with active inflammation or progressive scarring.

The initial dose of dapsone is 50 mg daily for 1 to 2 weeks, then 50 mg twice daily. Maintenance doses range from 50 to 150 mg daily. Dapsone should not be given to patients with a history of sulfone allergy or glucose-6-phosphate dehydrogenase deficiency. Complications include hemolysis (dose-dependent), bone marrow suppression, gastrointestinal complaints, and renal and liver dysfunction. A clinical response is seen in 1 to 4 weeks. If progression occurs despite dapsone therapy, or adverse reactions limit its use, another immunosuppressive agent (e.g., cyclophosphamide) should be given.

The initial doses of cyclophosphamide and prednisone are 100 to 150 and 80 to 120 mg/day, respectively (both 1 to 2 mg/kg/day). The use of these agents is discussed in Chapter 19. Prednisone is tapered relatively rapidly, achiev-

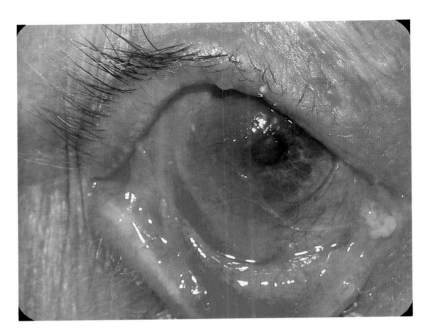

Figure 22-9
Conjunctival pathologic condition resembling cicatricial pemphigoid. In this case, however, conjunctival carcinoma is present.

ing alternate day therapy within 1 month and discontinuing therapy in about 2 months. If significant disease activity is still present after 1 month of treatment, the dose of cyclophosphamide can be increased by 25 mg/day. The dose can be increased monthly, as tolerated. Patients who do not respond to cyclophosphamide may respond to dapsone or azathioprine.[32]

Once remission is achieved, the dose of cyclophosphamide is gradually tapered. The rate should be guided by the patient's clinical response and the occurrence of side effects. As with any immunosuppressive therapy, the patient should also be followed up for adverse effects by someone familiar with the use of these agents. Prolonged therapy is required. It is probably best to continue immunosuppressive therapy for 1 year before attempting to discontinue it. The majority of patients will relapse, but prolonged periods of remission can be obtained, and control of the disease can be regained readily upon reinstitution of therapy.[33,37]

Complications of conjunctival scarring must also be addressed. Topical artificial tear solutions are used to alleviate drying and exposure. Punctal occlusion can be performed if the puncta are not already scarred by the disease. A bandage contact lens can be used to manage drying, trichiasis, and epithelial defects, but there must be adequate space for the lens, and the risk of infection is increased. These patients are prone to infectious blepharitis, conjunctivitis, and keratitis. Prompt diagnosis and treatment of infections are essential. Electrolysis, cryotherapy, and lid surgery may be necessary to treat trichiasis. Recurrence is common and repeated treatments are often necessary. External lid rotation procedures are usually performed if electrolysis and cryotherapy are not successful. Buccal mucous membrane grafting to the inferior lid margin and fornix can treat resistant cases of entropion and trichiasis; however, patients must be carefully selected, and the complication rate is high.[38]

Lid, conjunctival, and intraocular procedures should be undertaken with caution, because they can exacerbate the disease. Many eyes have progressed to atrophy bulbi after otherwise uncomplicated cataract extraction. The presence of severe dry eye significantly increases the risk of corneal complications. Trichiasis and entropion should be repaired before intraocular surgery is attempted.

If surgery is performed, the patient should be immunosuppressed and quiescent before the procedure and probably for at least 2 months after surgery.[39] The addition of oral prednisone (1 mg/kg) for 2 days before surgery and 10 days afterward is probably worthwhile.[38] Penetrating keratoplasty is nearly always unsuccessful.[40] A keratoprosthesis can be placed as a last resort.

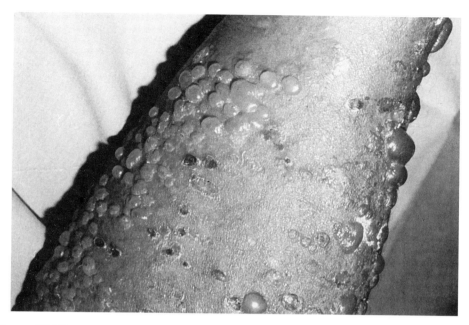

Figure 22-10
Typical large, tense blisters in bullous pemphigoid. (Courtesy of Judy Small, Pittsburgh, PA.)

Bullous Pemphigoid

Bullous pemphigoid is another member of the pemphigoid group of diseases. It is characterized by the presence of large, tense, nongrouped blisters occurring mainly on the sides of the neck and axillary and inguinal regions, and these resolve without scarring (Fig. 22-10). Bullous pemphigoid most commonly arises in the seventh and eighth decades of life, although it can occur at any age. It is generally a benign, self-limited disease. The oral mucosa is involved in approximately one third of patients, and the eye is affected only rarely.[41]

Bullous pemphigoid appears to be an autoimmune disease, with autoantibodies directed against an antigen (bullous pemphigoid antigen) in the lamina lucida of basement membranes. Linear deposition of IgG, and occasionally IgA, IgM, or IgE, is seen at the lamina lucida of the epithelial basement membrane.[42] Circulating antibodies directed against this same antigen are found in the majority of patients.[42,43]

Erythema Multiforme Major (Stevens-Johnson Syndrome)

Erythema multiforme is an episodic, self-limited, mucocutaneous inflammatory disorder. Clinically, the disease manifests as a spectrum from mild to severe; the severe form is called *erythema multiforme major*, or Stevens-Johnson syndrome. It is more commonly precipitated by herpes simplex infection or drugs, but it can be associated with other infectious agents or carcinoma, and often no precipitating factor can be identified. The pathogenesis of the mucocutaneous lesions is thought to be related to immune complexes, cell-mediated immunity, or both.[44]

Erythema multiforme major most often affects children and young adults and is seldom encountered in the elderly. A prodrome of fever, malaise, sore throat, and arthralgia may precede the skin eruptions by 1 to 14 days. The skin lesions can take many forms but are predominantly either "bull's eye" (Fig. 22-11) or bullous formations. The dorsal hands and feet and extensor surfaces of the forearms and legs are most frequently involved, often with a strikingly symmetric distribution (Fig. 22-12). The mucous membranes, especially of the eyes and mouth, are frequently affected by bullous and erosive lesions. Individual skin lesions tend to have life cycles of about 2 weeks. Recurrent cycles of lesions can occur, with most appearing by 6 weeks after onset. Recurrences develop in approximately one third of patients.

Ocular Manifestations

Conjunctival inflammation occurs in a large proportion of cases and correlates with systemic severity. The conjunctivitis is diffuse and bilateral (Fig. 22-13) and can be catarrhal, mucopurulent, hemorrhagic, or membranous and ultimately cicatrizing.[45,46] Conjunctival bullae

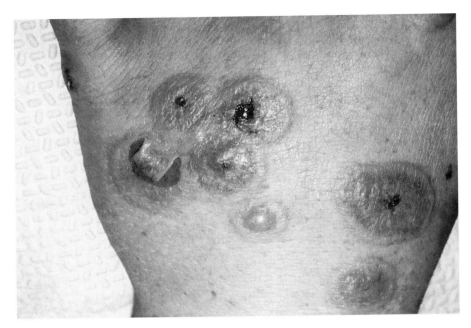

Figure 22-11
Target skin lesions in erythema multiforme. (Courtesy of Judy Small, Pittsburgh, PA.)

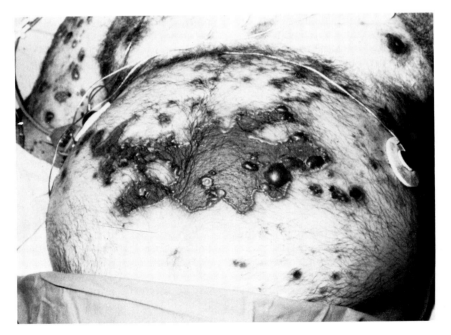

Figure 22-12
Hemorrhagic bullae in Stevens-Johnson syndrome.

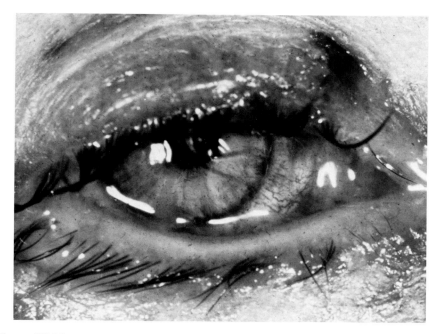

Figure 22-13
Diffuse mucopurulent and membranous conjunctivitis in Stevens-Johnson syndrome.

and ulcerative lesions can also occur. There is a tendency for relative sparing of the cornea until the late complications of conjunctival scarring ensue. However, corneal ulceration, drying, and peripheral vascularization can be seen during the acute phase of the disease. Unlike CP, the corneal and conjunctival inflammation does not progress indefinitely. Once the systemic disease has resolved, the ocular inflammation quiets. Recurrences of erythema multiforme usually do not involve the conjunctiva. Rarely, however, recurrent conjunctival inflammation is observed for many years after the initial episode.[47]

The final result can vary from no visible sequelae to severe scarring, keratoconjunctivitis sicca, corneal vascularization (Fig. 22-14), keratinization of the lid margins (Fig. 22-15), symblepharon (Fig. 22-16), and lid distortions with trichiasis and entropion.[48,49] Iridocyclitis and even panophthalmitis can occur. The subsequent effects of these complications can be disabling and can lead to blindness.

Treatment

Treatment of the systemic disease is primarily supportive. Suspected etiologic factors are eliminated, fluid balance is maintained, and antipruritics and analgesics are administered. Systemic corticosteroids are recommended by some, but their efficacy for the systemic disease

is unclear,[50] and they appear to have no effect on the ocular disease.

In the presence of conjunctivitis, topical steroids and antibiotic ointment are given, but their effect is questionable. If there is evidence of conjunctival ulceration or synechiae, I take measures to decrease symblepharon formation, although the benefits of this procedure are questionable. Daily lysis of synechiae can be performed, but preventing contact between the bulbar and palpebral conjunctivae appears to be more effective. This can be accomplished with a symblepharon ring, or a plastic wrap can be sutured around the lid; both usually require use of a bandage lens.

Management of the complications of Stevens-Johnson syndrome is similar to that described for CP. If lid function and tear production are not very impaired, surgical measures can be successful. Mucous membrane grafts can be used to treat cicatricial entropion and trichiasis.[51,52] Lamellar dissection or keratoepithelioplasty can be performed to remove superficial corneal scarring and improve vision.

Toxic Epidermal Necrolysis

Toxic epidermal necrolysis (TEN) appears to be a severe form of erythema multiforme.[50] It is characterized by broad areas of skin necrosis and sloughing, resembling a thermal burn. Intraepithelial cleavage occurs at the basal layer

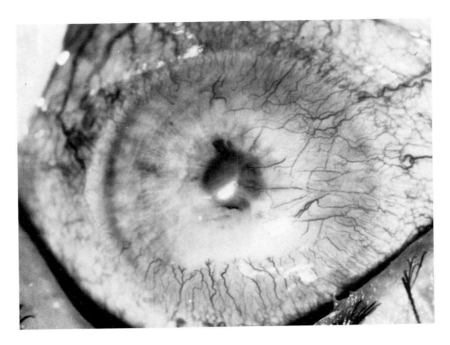

Figure 22-14
Perforation of the cornea after treatment of vascularized and dry cornea of Stevens-Johnson syndrome
with frequent topical steroids.

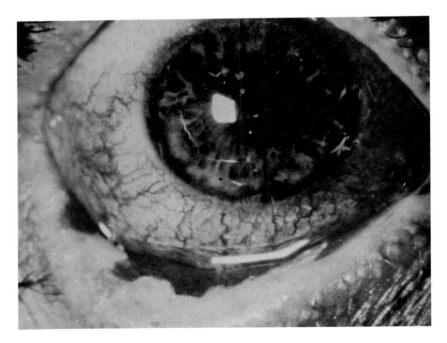

Figure 22-15
Keratinization of the lid margin after Stevens-Johnson syndrome.

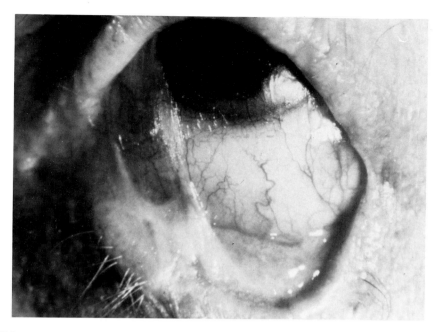

Figure 22-16
Corneal keratinization, symblepharon formation, dry eye, and corneal vascularization resulting from Stevens-Johnson syndrome.

of the epidermis. TEN should be distinguished from staphylococcal scalded skin syndrome, an unrelated disorder with a similar clinical appearance. Scalded skin syndrome usually affects children and is related to infection with staphylococci that produce exfoliation or epidermolytic toxins, usually *Staphylococcus aureus* bacteriophage group 2.[50] Mucous membranes are not affected in this condition.

Toxic epidermal necrolysis begins with a prodrome like that of erythema multiforme. A few days later erythema and bullae of the skin and mucous membranes appear. The bullae become flaccid, and large areas of epidermis fall away, leaving an appearance of scalded skin (Figs. 22-17 and 22-18). Remaining areas of skin are often wrinkled and can be made to slide away like a "slipped rug" when pressure is applied (Nikolsky's sign). Mucous membranes of the mouth, genitalia, and rectum are frequently affected. Necrolysis can be generalized within 24 hours but usually spreads gradually from a Stevens-Johnson syndrome–like initial appearance.[53] The mortality rate is about 20%.[54]

The ocular findings are the same as those of erythema multiforme, except that they tend to be milder in TEN.[53-55] Conjunctival involvement is common; mucopurulent conjunctivitis is most frequent, but ulcerative and membranous conjunctivitis with subsequent scarring can also occur.[56,57] The conjunctival scarring can lead to the same complications as were described for erythema multiforme, including trichiasis, lid distortion, dry eye, and corneal vascularization and opacification.[58,59] Sjögren's syndrome, with xerostomia and lymphocytic infiltration of the salivary glands, can also occur after TEN.[60]

Epidermolysis Bullosa

Epidermolysis bullosa is a group of rare diseases characterized by the formation of bullous lesions after minor mechanical trauma (Figs. 22-19 through 22-21). Dystrophic nail problems also occur. Most of these diseases are hereditary. Their pathogenesis is not well understood, but they appear to be disorders of the epithelial cell attachment complex—hemidesmosomes, basement membrane, or anchoring fibrils. The exact layer of separation between the epidermis and dermis differs in the various forms of the disease, and this is related to different defects in the components of the epithelial attachment complex.[61-64] There are many clinical variants, which are divided into four major hereditary types and an acquired type (Table 22-2).

Ocular involvement has been reported in most types of epidermolysis bullosa and appears to be most common in the autosomal re-

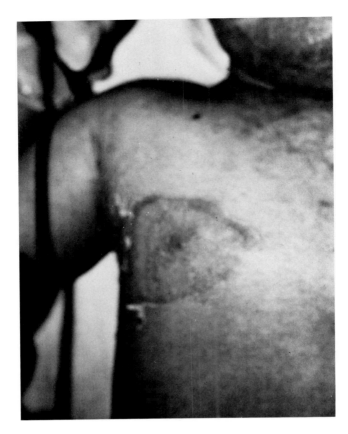

Figure 22-17
Toxic epidermal necrolysis. The skin bullae become flaccid, and large areas of epidermis fall away, leaving "scalded skin."

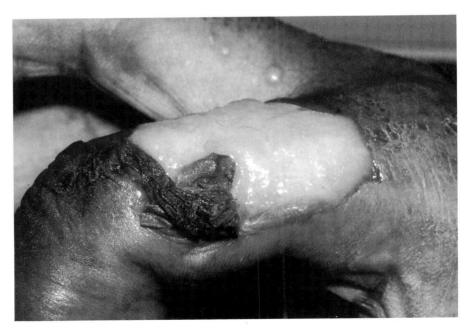

Figure 22-18
Toxic epidermal necrolysis. The blister on the finger has fallen away, with exposure of denuded skin. (Courtesy of Judy Small, Pittsburgh, PA.)

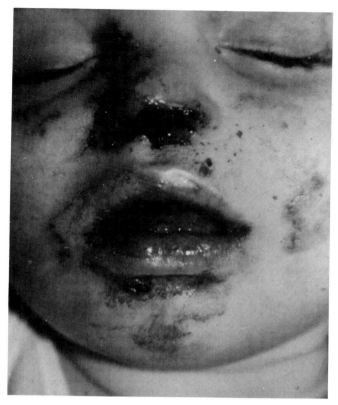

Figure 22-19
Epidermolysis bullosa with hemorrhagic lesions of the mucous membranes.

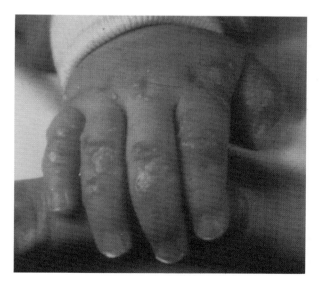

Figure 22-20
Typical bullous lesions of the hand in epidermolysis bullosa.

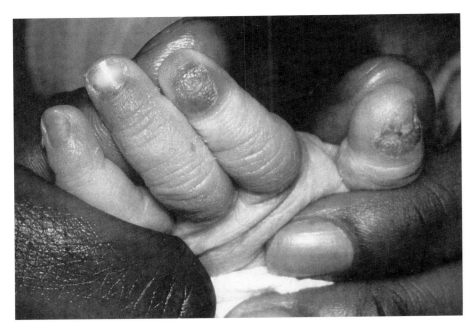

Figure 22-21
Dystrophic nails in epidermolysis bullosa. (Courtesy of Judy Small, Pittsburgh, PA.)

cessive dermolytic (dystrophic) type.[65,66] Eyelid blisters, conjunctival vesicles, and corneal erosions can occur.[2,67-70] Corneal erosions appear to be the most common ocular complication, occurring in all types, and their frequency is proportional to the frequency of blistering of the skin.[65] Conjunctival involvement can lead to ulceration, pseudomembrane formation, and symblepharon. These changes appear to be localized and slowly progressive. Corneal pannus, ulceration, and scarring can result from the conjunctival changes or from erosions (Fig. 22-22); even perforation can occur.[71] Eyelid scarring can develop after blistering in the junctional and dermolytic types and can lead to ectropion.

Blepharitis is treated with lid hygiene. Antibiotic ointment and bandage contact lenses can be given for corneal erosions, but patching should be avoided because the skin frequently blisters beneath the tape. Bandage contact lenses can also be used to decrease recurrences. Symblepharon can be reduced by lysis, with resuturing of the cut ends to avoid contact of deepithelialized limbal and palpebral surfaces. Lubricants, moisture chambers, or skin grafts may be necessary for treatment of cicatricial ectropion.

Dermatitis Herpetiformis

Dermatitis herpetiformis is a chronic inflammatory dermatosis with erythematous, papular,

vesicular, or pustular lesions occurring in groups, with a symmetric distribution and accompanied by intense itching.[72] The skin lesions usually heal without scarring. Granular and occasionally linear deposits of IgA are seen along the dermal-epidermal junction at the tips of dermal papillae (Fig. 22-23) both in lesional and in clinically uninvolved areas of skin.[72a] The majority of patients also have gluten-sensitive enteropathy, but the relationship between the two conditions is unclear. The disease may lessen after long-term adherence to a gluten-free diet. Eye involvement is not very common and usually occurs only in severe cases. Shrinkage of the conjunctiva and conjunctival eosinophilia can occur.[73]

Linear IgA Disease

Linear IgA disease (linear IgA bullous dermatosis) is a recently recognized form of bullous dermatosis that is closely related to dermatitis herpetiformis, bullous pemphigoid, and chronic bullous disease of childhood.[74,75] Linear deposition of IgA is seen along the epithelial basement membrane.[76] The disease occurs in both adults and children; it is designated adult linear IgA disease in the former and chronic bullous disease of childhood in the latter. It is characterized by tense blisters of varying size. The majority of cases have mucosal involvement.

Conjunctival inflammation occurs in many patients and can lead to scarring and sym-

Table 22-2 Epidermolysis Bullosa

Type	Inheritance	Site of Blister Formation	Defect	Severity	Scarring	Conjunctival Involvement	Corneal Involvement
Epidermolytic (simplex)	Autosomal dominant	Within basal epithelial cells	?Mutant protein involved in intercellular adhesion	Mild	–	Rare	Uncommon
Junctional (letalis)	Autosomal recessive	Superficial lamina lucida of basement membrane	Decreased + abnormal hemidesmosomes	Severe (survive <2 years)	– (Atrophy)	Uncommon	Common
Dystrophic (dermolytic) Dominant (hyperplastic, others)	Autosomal dominant	Lamina densa of basement membrane and anchoring fibrils	Decreased + abnormal anchoring fibrils	Moderate	+	Uncommon	Common
Recessive (polydysplastic, others)	Autosomal recessive	Lamina densa of basement membrane and anchoring fibrils	Decreased + abnormal anchoring fibrils ?Excess collagenase activity	Moderate to severe	+	Majority	Common
Epidermolysis bullosa acquisita	– Autoimmune	Linear IgG and C3 along basement membrane	Antibody against type VII collagen	Variable	+	Occasionally	?

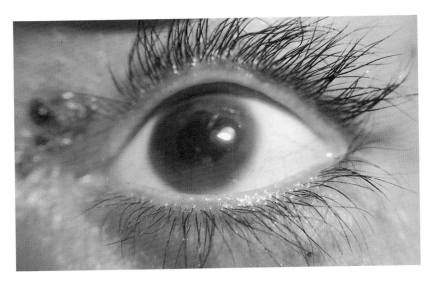

Figure 22-22
Corneal involvement in epidermolysis bullosa.

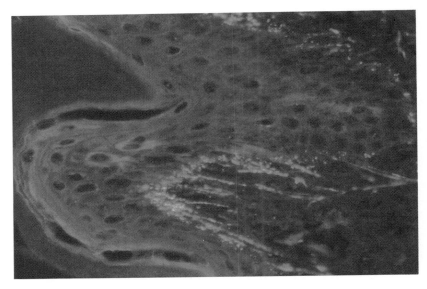

Figure 22-23
Immunopathology of dermatitis herpetiformis. Fluorescence indicates the detection of deposits of IgA along the dermal-epidermal junction at the tips of the dermal papillae. (From IFTesting Service, Buffalo, NY.)

blepharon (Fig. 22-24).[74,77,78] In one review of 25 cases, conjunctival inflammation occurred in 72% of patients and scarring in 40%.[74]

Chronic Bullous Disease of Childhood

Chronic bullous disease of childhood is an uncommon blistering disease that affects young children. Large, tense bullae affect the abdomen, lower extremities, perioral region, neck, axillae, groin, and other areas (Fig. 22-25). Annular lesions, such as those seen in erythema multiforme, can also be present. Chronic bullous disease of childhood runs a course of exacerbations and remissions, with gradually decreasing severity and resolution before the teens or adulthood.

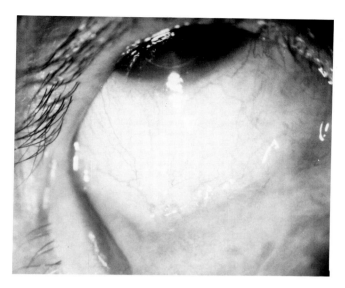

Figure 22-24
Conjunctival scarring in linear IgA disease. (Courtesy of Eric Donnenfeld, Rockville Center, NY.)

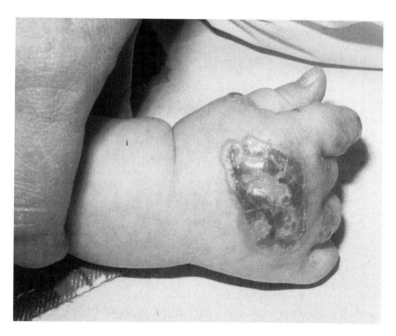

Figure 22-25
Chronic bullous disease of childhood, with large, tense blisters on the back of the hand. (Courtesy of Judy Small, Pittsburgh, PA.)

Linear IgA deposits are seen in the epithelial basement membrane, and most patients have low circulating titers of anti–basement membrane IgA as well.[79] In one recent study, ocular symptoms of pain, redness, grittiness, or discharge were present in 40% of children, and conjunctival scarring was seen in two of seven patients examined by an ophthalmologist.[74]

Pemphigus

Pemphigus is a group of blistering skin diseases characterized by intraepithelial bulla formation. Autoantibodies are directed against an antigen that is part of desmosomal and adherens junctions in both epidermal and mucosal squamous epithelium.[80-82] IgG and complement components can be demonstrated in the intercellular spaces of early acantholytic lesions in nearly all cases (Fig. 22-26).[83]

The most common type of pemphigus encountered in the United States is pemphigus vulgaris. A chronic disease, it most commonly occurs in the fourth and fifth decades of life but can develop at any age. The skin lesions are flaccid, weeping bullae that erode, leaving large denuded areas (Fig. 22-27). The mucous membranes are commonly involved, particularly the oral mucosa, and can be the site of onset. Because the bullae form within the epithelium and the substantia propria and dermis are not involved, scarring does not occur.

Ocular lesions occur in approximately 16% of patients[84] (Fig. 22-28). Intraepithelial conjunctival bullae are seen, mainly on the palpebral conjunctiva and commonly near the inner canthus. The bullae rupture and nearly always heal without scarring. Conjunctival inflammation without bullae can also occur and may be more common.[85] The cornea is not affected.

A recently described variant of pemphigus, paraneoplastic pemphigus, is an autoimmune disease associated with an underlying neoplasm. It is characterized by painful mucosal erosions and polymorphous skin eruptions. Conjunctivitis, sloughing of conjunctival epi-

thelium, and conjunctival scarring have been observed.[82,86,87]

Hydroa Vacciniforme

Patients with hydroa vacciniforme exhibit a congenitally abnormal sensitivity to sunlight. *Hydroa* refers to the vesicular nature of the eruption, and *vacciniforme* refers to the tendency for the lesions to heal without scarring. The sun-exposed areas, particularly the face and eyelids, are primarily involved (Fig. 22-29).

A hypertrophic conjunctivitis can occur. Conjunctival epithelial thickening and cyst formation are seen. The conjunctiva can be hyperemic, and vesicles, ulceration, and scarring can be present. Scarring and vascularization of the cornea can also occur.[88]

EXFOLIATIVE ERYTHRODERMA (EXFOLIATIVE DERMATITIS)

Exfoliative erythroderma refers to a group of papulosquamous eruptions that produce a diffuse erythroderma with desquamation (exfoliation). There are multiple causes; it often represents a generalized extension of a preexisting dermatosis, such as psoriasis, atopic dermatitis, pityriasis rubra pilaris, or ichthyosis. It can be associated with leukemia, lymphoma, or drug reaction, or it can be idiopathic. The prognosis is variable, depending on the underlying etiology; overall, approximately 60% of patients re-

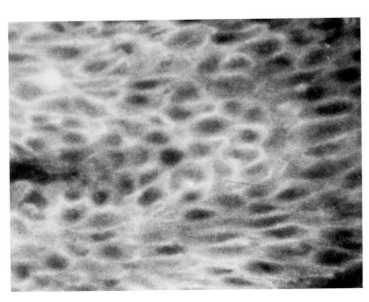

Figure 22-26
Deposition of immunoglobulin in the intercellular spaces in pemphigus vulgaris. (Courtesy of S.F. Bean, Houston, TX.)

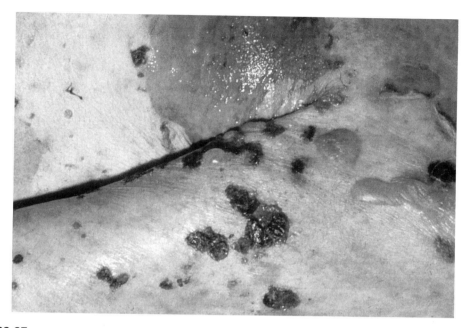

Figure 22-27
Skin lesions in pemphigus vulgaris: flaccid weeping bullae that erode, leaving large denuded areas. (From the American Academy of Dermatology, 1978.)

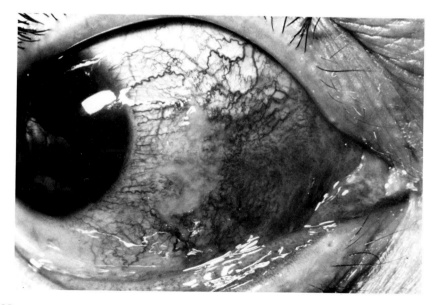

Figure 22-28
Conjunctival lesion in pemphigus vulgaris. (From Roat MI, Thoft RA: *Pemphigus.* In Gold DH, Weingeist TA, editors: *The eye in systemic disease,* Philadelphia, 1990, JB Lippincott.)

cover within 8 to 10 months, and 30% of patients die. Multiple recurrences can be seen in idiopathic cases.

Nonspecific conjunctival irritation can be caused by desquamation of scales from adjacent skin into the conjunctival sac. Chronic inflammation of the lid skin can produce cicatricial ectropion (Fig. 22-30). Some shrinkage of the lower conjunctival fornix can be seen. The cornea is not affected, except secondarily from ectropion or scaling.

ROSACEA

Rosacea is a dermatosis in which significant ocular morbidity can occur with relatively mild skin disease. Rosacea is a chronic disorder that affects women more than men, and its onset is usually between 25 and 50 years of age. However, ocular involvement has been seen in patients as young as 4 years of age.[89] It involves the skin primarily in the area of the forehead, nose, cheeks, and chin. It has a vascular compo-

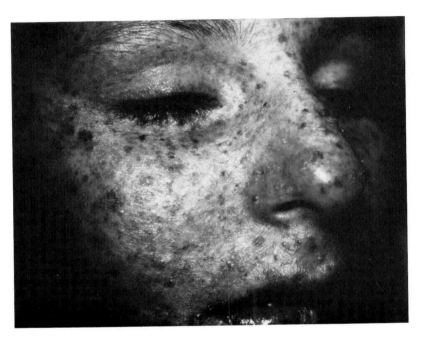

Figure 22-29
Hydroa vacciniforme with papulovesicular lesions on exposed skin.

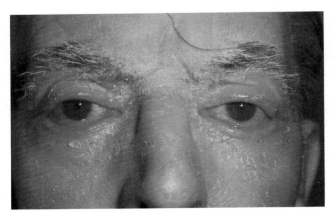

Figure 22-30
Exfoliative dermatitis resulting in cicatricial ectropion.

nent (erythema and telangiectasia) with or without an acneiform component (papules, pustules, and nodules) (Fig. 22-31). No comedones are seen.

Rhinophyma is an advanced form of the nasal disease in which there is hypertrophy of the nose with hyperplasia of sebaceous glands, fibrosis, and increased vascularity (Fig. 22-32). The skin condition is often overlooked, and certainly this disease is more common than realized.

Ocular Manifestations

The most commonly associated eye findings are meibomitis and blepharitis. The lid margins are red and slightly thickened, and telangiectasia can be present. Inspissation of meibomian gland secretions, inflammation around the gland orifices, and foaming of the lid margins may also be present. Chalazia are frequently observed, as are staphylococcal infections of the lids.

The blood vessels of the conjunctiva can be dilated in a manner similar to the vessels of the skin of the eyelids, nose, and face. The dilated vessels are seen most often in the interpalpebral areas of the bulbar conjunctiva. A nodular conjunctivitis, similar to a phlyctenule, can also be seen. These are small, gray, highly vascularized elevations of the bulbar conjunctiva, most of-

ten located near the limbus in the interpalpebral area. They can be sufficiently elevated to cause dellen formation.

The cornea can become extensively involved with scarring and vascularization. Rosacea keratitis is accompanied by pain, photophobia, and foreign body sensation. Superficial punctate keratopathy, involving the lower two thirds of the cornea, often accompanies the blepharitis or meibomitis.[90] Frequently, a leash of superficial vessels grows onto the cornea, most commonly in the inferior interpalpebral area, and can be associated with fluorescein staining and sometimes superficial infiltrates at the central edge (Fig. 22-33).

Progression usually occurs with a series of intermittent attacks. Ophthalmic remissions and exacerbations can occur independently of the course of the skin disease. Broad areas of pannus can form, and even the entire circumference of the limbus can be affected; but the disease usually remains worse inferiorly. Dense white scars can form, with heavy vascularization. Marginal or, less commonly, central corneal melting can develop (Fig. 22-34). Progressive thinning can occur during a single episode or with repeated bouts of inflammation. Perforation can occur, especially if topical corticosteroids have been used injudiciously. Nodular

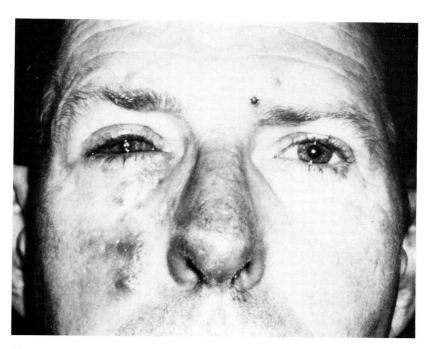

Figure 22-31
Erythema and telangiectasia of the facial skin in acne rosacea.

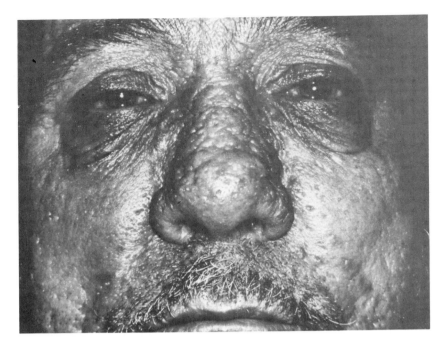

Figure 22-32
Rhinophyma caused by acne rosacea.

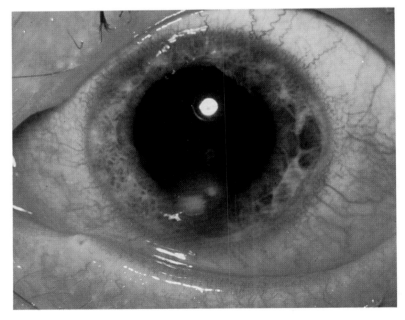

Figure 22-33
Keratitis, with dense white opacities and vascularization in rosacea.

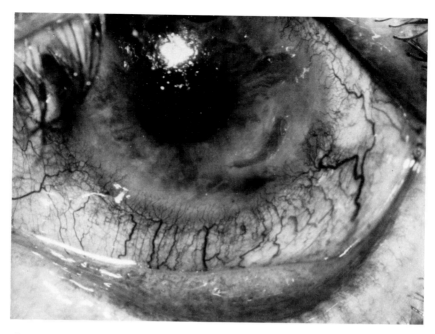

Figure 22-34
Marginal corneal ulceration in rosacea.

episcleritis, scleritis, and conjunctival granuloma formation occur rarely.[91,92]

Pathogenesis

The cause of rosacea and the relationship between the skin disease and the eye disease are not known. Conjunctival biopsy specimens demonstrated infiltration of the epithelium by inflammatory cells, mainly helper/inducer T cells, phagocytic cells, and antigen-presenting cells.[93] Large subepithelial infiltrates of chronic inflammatory cells were present, and frank granuloma formation was seen in some cases. The authors felt this appearance was most consistent with a type-IV hypersensitivity reaction.

The associated blepharitis and meibomitis do not appear to be solely responsible for the eye complications. Attempts at relating the disease to staphylococcal infection have not been very successful.

Treatment

The patient with severe rosacea should be under the joint care of a dermatologist and ophthalmologist. The most effective treatment is systemic tetracycline, 250 mg four times a day.[94,95] The reason that rosacea responds to tetracycline is not really known. Doxycycline or minocycline (both 50 mg twice daily) appears to be as effective, with a simpler regimen.[96] Ampicillin and erythromycin (both 250 mg four times a day) can also be used, but they seem to be less effective. Lid hygiene should also be instituted, and any staphylococcal infection of the lid margins should be eliminated.

The tetracycline is continued four times a day for 1 month and is then decreased by 250 mg/day each month. Many patients require 250 to 500 mg of tetracycline or 50 mg of doxycycline daily to prevent exacerbation of disease.

Topical corticosteroid therapy can reduce ocular inflammation, vascular invasion, and infiltration. However, it is essential to ensure that infiltrates are not infectious before initiating treatment. In addition, attention must be paid to the length of treatment and the dose given, because this is a chronic disease, prone to superinfection, thinning, and perforation.

It may be necessary to perform a corneal graft if the cornea becomes extensively scarred, but the long-term results are not satisfactory.

SEBORRHEIC DERMATITIS

Seborrheic dermatitis is an oily skin eruption, seen as greasy scales on an erythematous patch of skin. The scalp, eyebrows, eyelids, nasolabial folds, retroauricular skin, chest, and back can be involved. Sebaceous gland dysfunction, with excess sebum production, is thought to be responsible for the skin findings. Nearly all pa-

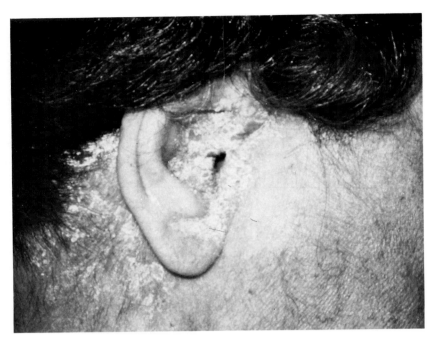

Figure 22-35
Involvement of the ear in psoriasis. The skin typically exhibits erythematous patches covered with silvery white scales.

tients with seborrheic blepharitis, and approximately one third of patients with meibomian gland dysfunction, have evidence of seborrheic dermatitis, but it is usually mild and easily overlooked.[97]

PSORIASIS

Psoriasis is a chronic skin disorder characterized by excessive proliferation of the epidermis. This is most often seen as geographic, demarcated, erythematous patches of skin covered with silvery white scales (Fig. 22-35). Psoriasis typically affects the scalp, nails, extensor surfaces of the extremities, and sacral region. Auspitz sign is present; when hyperkeratotic scales are removed by scratching, small blood droplets appear within a few seconds.

It is a common disease that can be seen in any age group, but it typically arises in the third decade. It usually lasts for life, but many patients experience remissions, which can last for years. It is more common in whites and in women.

The primary defect in psoriasis is not known.[98] Many patients have relatives with psoriasis, so heredity may be a factor. The psoriatic patient exhibits a tendency toward acceler-

ated epidermopoiesis in response to external and internal stimuli. The nature of the stimuli is controversial, although it has been shown that the condition improves when the patient is in a warmer climate. Trauma, infection, and stress may also be trigger factors. There is some evidence to support participation of the immune system in the disease process.

Ocular Manifestations

Ocular signs of psoriasis occur in approximately 10% of cases. The eyelids are frequently involved (Fig. 22-36) and can become swollen, red, and scaly. Scaling may also be seen at the base of the lashes. Trichiasis and madarosis occur in severe cases. A nonspecific conjunctivitis is common, and yellow plaquelike lesions can occur. Phlyctenule-like lesions can be seen at the limbus.

The cornea can be affected by superficial and deep opacities, vascularization, peripheral infiltration, and melting[99-101] (Fig. 22-37). Corneal involvement usually occurs when there is active disease in the skin of the lids.

Treatment of psoriasis with psoralens and long ultraviolet light can cause superficial punctate keratitis.[102] Uveitis can occur, usually in patients with psoriatic arthritis.

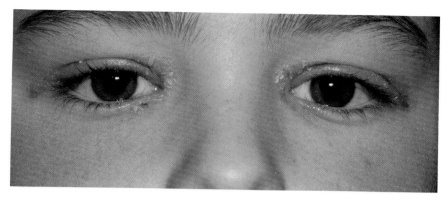

Figure 22-36
Involvement of the lids in psoriasis.

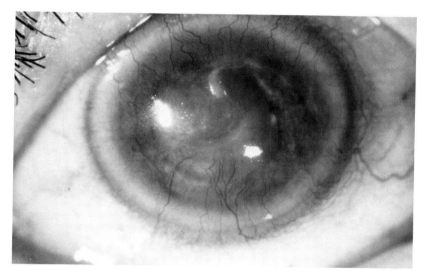

Figure 22-37
Corneal ulceration and vascularization in psoriasis.

Treatment

Treatment of the systemic and dermatologic problems should be undertaken by an internist and dermatologist, respectively. Topical therapy includes anthralin, tar, and corticosteroids. Systemic therapy with methotrexate, oral vitamin A (etretinate), and psoralens and long ultraviolet light can be used in more severe cases.

Corneal melting is treated with lubrication, bandage contact lenses, tarsorrhaphy, and treatment of the systemic disease.

ICHTHYOSIS

Ichthyosis is a large group of disorders characterized by thickening (hyperkeratosis), fissuring, and scaling of the skin (Fig. 22-38). It can be hereditary or acquired. Acquired disease is usually associated with lymphoma. All of these disorders involve retardation of desquamation or hyperproliferation of the epidermal cells. Four main hereditary groups exist (Table 22-3): (1) ichthyosis vulgaris (autosomal dominant); (2) recessive X-linked ichthyosis (steroid sulfatase deficiency); (3) lamellar ichthyosis, which includes both classic lamellar ichthyosis and congenital ichthyosiform erythroderma (autosomal recessive); and (4) epidermolytic hyperkeratosis (autosomal dominant). Heterozygous females with the X-linked form (carriers) do not develop the full-blown dermatosis but manifest some of the clinical features. Ichthyosis is also seen as part of the keratitis, ichthyosis, and deafness syndrome, which is discussed later.

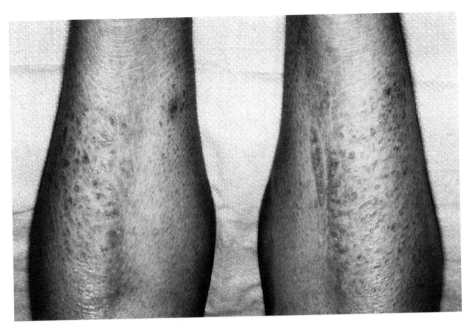

Figure 22-38
Scaling of the skin in ichthyosis. (Courtesy of Judy Small, Pittsburgh, PA.)

Table 22-3	Major Forms of Ichthyosis			
Features	**Ichthyosis Vulgaris**	**X-linked Ichthyosis**	**Lamellar Ichthyosis***	**Epidermolytic Hyperkeratosis**
Onset	>1 year	>1 year	Birth	Birth
Inheritance	Autosomal dominant	X-linked recessive	Autosomal recessive (Autosomal dominant)	Autosomal dominant
Scales on skin	Fine, extensor surfaces	Brownish, extensor surfaces of extremities	White → brown, fine → large, over most of body;	Often dark, warty; generalized
Palmoplantar hyperkeratosis	Mild	—	Moderate	Mild to severe
Associated disease	Atopy	Cryptorchidism; arylsulfatase C + steroid sulfatase deficiency	Prematurity, sepsis, heat intolerance	Sepsis
Eye findings	None	Pre-Descemet opacities; band keratopathy; superficial nodular lesions; increased corneal nerve visibility	Ectropion; conjunctivitis (CIE); keratitis (CIE)	None

*There are at least two different forms: classic lamellar ichthyosis and congenital ichthyosiform erythroderma (CIE).

Ocular Manifestations

Lid ectropion can be seen in lamellar ichthyosis.[103] In the X-linked form, diffuse dotlike or striate opacities can be seen on Descemet's membrane or immediately anterior to it (Fig. 22-39).[104-106] These opacities usually are not present until adulthood in affected males. In one series corneal opacities were present in approximately 24% of affected males and were present in the same percentage of carrier mothers.[107] Larger white or gray deep stromal opacities[108]; small refractile bodies in the epithelium, superficial stroma, and endothelium; granular subepithelial opacities[109]; prominent corneal nerves; and band keratopathy have also been reported.[110,111] Superficial nodular corneal degeneration and ulceration are rarely part of the clinical picture (Fig. 22-40).

Conjunctivitis and keratitis can be present in the congenital ichthyosiform erythroderma form of lamellar ichthyosis (Fig. 22-41),[112] and superficial punctate keratopathy can be present in all forms.

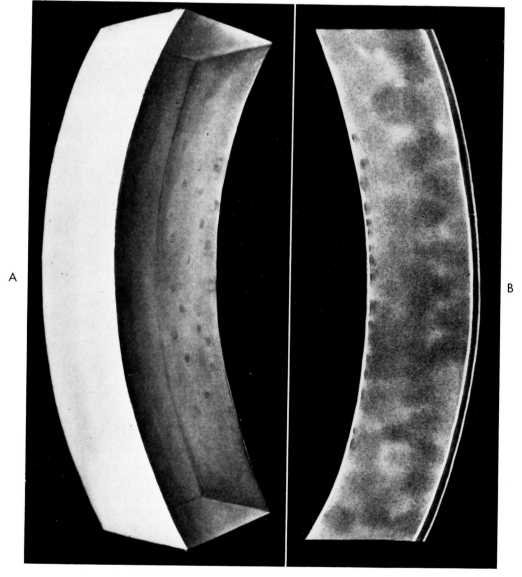

A

B

Figure 22-39
Punctate or striate opacities on or anterior to Descemet's membrane in X-linked ichthyosis.
A, Parallel-piped section. **B,** Optical section.

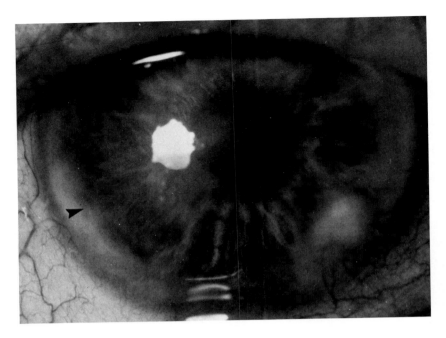

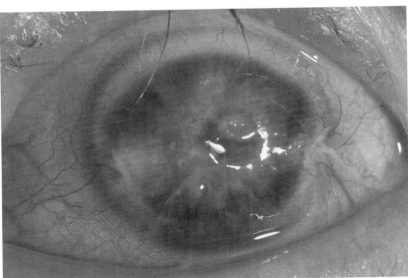

Figure 22-40
Superficial nodular corneal degeneration and ulceration in ichthyosis.

KERATITIS, ICHTHYOSIS, AND DEAFNESS SYNDROME

Keratitis, ichthyosis, and deafness syndrome is a rare congenital syndrome.[113,114] Some cases exhibit autosomal dominant transmission,[115,116] whereas others are sporadic. The ichthyosis is usually present at an early age. Hyperkeratosis of the palms and soles with a characteristic dotted and waxy pattern in bas-relief is noted (Fig. 22-42). A reticulated pattern of hyperkeratosis on the face, perioral furrowing, heavy grain–leatherlike keratoderma, leukoplakia of the buccal mucosa, deep lingual fissuring along the dorsal midline of the tongue, and rugae of the buccal mucosa can be seen. Follicular plugging and scant or absent hair, eyebrows, and eyelashes are noted (Fig. 22-43). The nails can be thick and dystrophic (Fig. 22-44). Many patients have decreased sweating caused by hyperkeratosis and plugging of the eccrine glands.

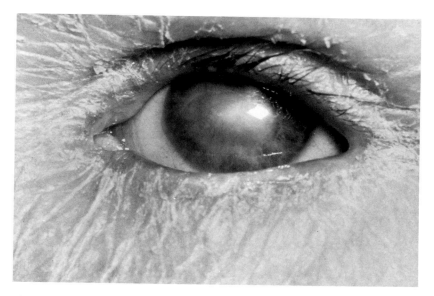

Figure 22-41
Congenital ichthyosiform erythroderma with scaling of the skin and corneal opacification.

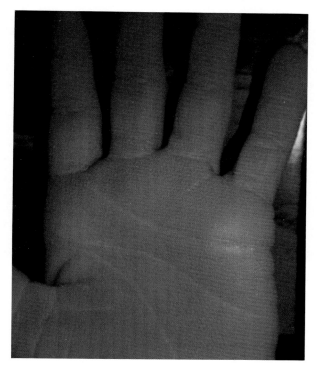

Figure 22-42
Palmar hyperkeratosis in keratitis, ichthyosis, and deafness syndrome.

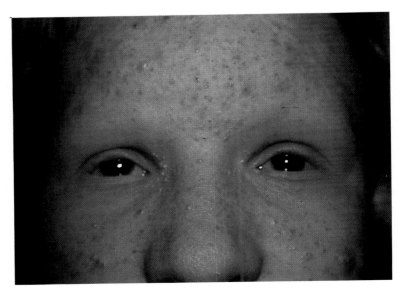

Figure 22-43
Facial sebaceous dysfunction in keratitis, ichthyosis, and deafness syndrome.

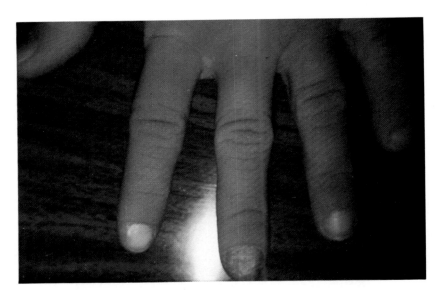

Figure 22-44
Fingernail malformation in keratitis, ichthyosis, and deafness syndrome.

Deafness is severe and of the neurosensory type; it is either present at birth or develops in the first 2 years of life. These patients also appear to be prone to recurrent bacterial, fungal, or viral infections of the skin and squamous cell carcinoma. Hypoplasia of the cerebellum has been noted in some patients.[117]

Punctate epithelial keratopathy and vascularizing keratitis (Fig. 22-45) are prominent features. The pannus is superficial and can extend 360°. It can be accompanied by numerous intraepithelial cysts. Corneal thinning and stromal opacification also occur.

JUVENILE XANTHOGRANULOMA

Juvenile xanthogranulomas are firm skin nodules that are reddish at first and then turn yellow-orange (Fig. 22-46). They usually appear before the end of the first year of life (80%) and resolve within 3 to 6 years. Histology of early

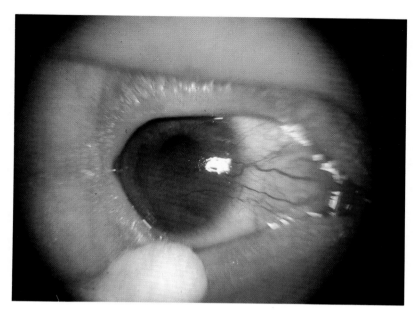

Figure 22-45
Superficial vascularization, thinning, and opacification of the cornea in keratitis, ichthyosis, and deafness syndrome.

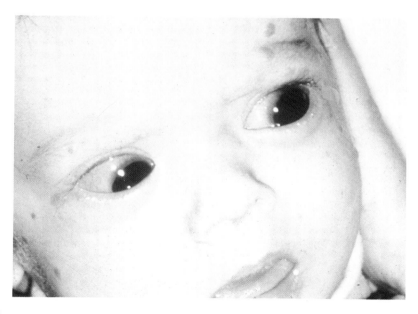

Figure 22-46
Yellow-red papular lesions of the skin in juvenile xanthogranuloma. These lesions can occur as epibulbar lesions that may extend onto the cornea.

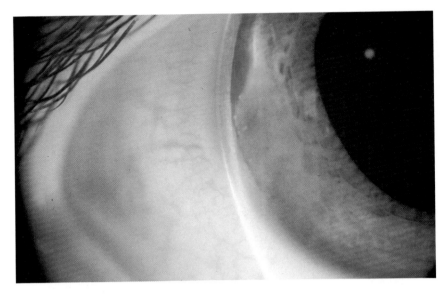

Figure 22-47
Iris lesion in juvenile xanthogranuloma. (Courtesy of Diane Curtin, Pittsburgh, PA.)

lesions reveals a monomorphous non–lipid-containing histiocytic infiltrate. In mature lesions a granulomatous infiltrate is present, containing lipid-laden macrophages (foamy cells), lymphocytes, eosinophils, neutrophils, foreign body giant cells, and Touton giant cells.

Xanthogranulomas can involve the iris and ciliary body (Fig. 22-47). The iris lesions can cause spontaneous anterior chamber hemorrhages, and secondary glaucoma can ensue.[118] Phlyctenule-like epibulbar lesions occasionally occur and can extend onto the cornea.[119,120] They are yellow-white to pink and can resemble the salmon-pink nodules seen in lymphoma. Corneal blood staining can result from hyphema, and corneal edema and enlargement can result from glaucoma.

KERATOSIS FOLLICULARIS SPINULOSA DECALVANS

The hallmarks of *keratosis follicularis spinulosa decalvans* (keratosis pilaris decalvans, follicular ichthyosis, Sieman's disease) are hyperkeratotic, conical, horny plugs at the hair follicle openings that give the skin a coarse texture. Sites of predilection are the face, scalp, eyebrows, neck, arms, and fingers. In addition, some loss of hair occurs at the lateral portion of the eyebrow and occiput. Skeletal hypoplasia, failure to thrive, deafness, and recurrent infections have been reported.[121]

Ocular Manifestations

Keratosis follicularis spinulosa decalvans affects the cornea only rarely. Corneal abnormalities result most commonly from mechanical trauma from keratotic spines on the eyelids or hardened secretions of the meibomian glands. A circumferential pannus with diffuse, superficial, farinaceous opacities has been reported[122] (Fig. 22-48). Female carriers may show recurrent erosions, epithelial or subepithelial opacities, and prominent corneal nerves. The epithelium can be thick and irregular and can contain irregularly shaped nuclei, vacuoles, and keratotic spines (Fig. 22-48).

KYRLE'S DISEASE

Kyrle's disease is a very rare disorder of keratinization characterized by multiple hyperpigmented keratotic papules that have a central plug. They can be located on any part of the body, with relative sparing of the palms, soles, and face. The cause is unknown; it can be associated with chronic renal failure or diabetes mellitus.

Ocular Manifestations

The corneal lesions of Kyrle's disease have a unique appearance. They consist of minute, yellow-brown, subepithelial opacities (Fig. 22-49). Their greatest density and deepest penetration occur at the limbus, the least at the cor-

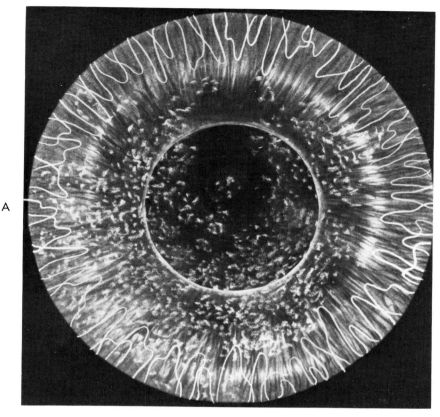

A

Figure 22-48
In Sieman's disease, circumferential pannus with diffuse superficial farinaceous opacities may be seen.
A, Diagrammatic representation of corneal findings.
Continued

neal center.[123] Posterior subcapsular cataracts can also be found.

KERATOSIS FOLLICULARIS (DARIER'S DISEASE)

In *keratosis follicularis,* small, brown scaly papules affect mainly the scalp, face, and upper trunk (Fig. 22-50). The nails and oral mucosa are frequently affected. Histologic findings are diagnostic: focal acantholysis and abnormal cornification with dyskeratotic cells. Keratosis follicularis is inherited as an autosomal dominant trait.

Ocular Manifestations
Corneal involvement in keratosis follicularis is varied, but peripheral opacities and central epithelial irregularity in a radiating cobweb pattern are most often seen[124,125] (Fig. 22-51). In addition, a dense yellow peripheral pannus and a central stromal opacity can be noted. The eyelids may exhibit keratotic plaques, and sometimes staphylococcal blepharitis and trichiasis

are seen. In one eye examined histologically, focal keratinization of the limbal conjunctiva and diffuse thickening of the basement membrane of the corneal epithelium were present.[126] The skin lesions improve with oral retinoid therapy, but the corneal lesions do not.

WERNER SYNDROME

Werner syndrome is a rare autosomal recessive disorder marked by progeroid features. A cessation of growth occurs during the second decade of life, and graying of the hair, balding, atrophy of skin and muscles, high-pitched voice, trophic ulcers of the legs, painful hyperkeratotic skin lesions, metastatic calcification, osteoporosis, and hypogonadism are among the other features.

Bilateral posterior stellate cataracts usually appear between the ages of 20 and 35 years. Bullous keratopathy has followed cataract extraction in many cases.[127,128] Metastatic corneal calcification has been observed after both cata-

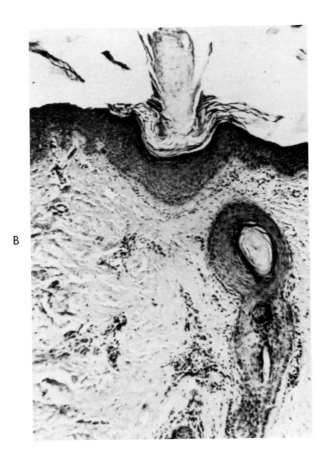

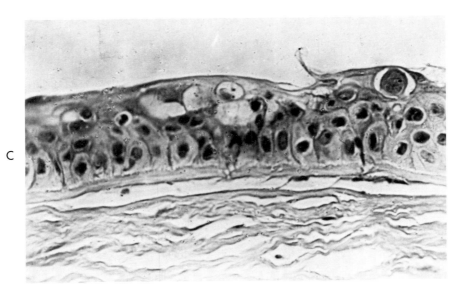

Figure 22-48, cont'd
B, Skin with thickened epithelium and keratotic spine. **C,** Erosion of the superficial epithelium. (Courtesy of A. Franceschetti, Geneva, Switzerland.)

ract extraction and penetrating keratoplasty.[129] Blue sclera,[123] iris telangiectasia, and retinitis pigmentosa have been reported.[130,131]

ACRODERMATITIS ENTEROPATHICA

This rare familial disease usually appears in early infancy and follows a characteristic clini-

cal course. A rash is symmetrically distributed over the face and bony prominences (Fig. 22-52). The rash first goes through a vesiculobullous stage, then assumes a more erythematous, squamous, psoriasiform appearance. Dystrophy of the nails and alopecia, with loss of eyelashes and eyebrows, are also seen. The infant is withdrawn and irritable and has diarrhea.

This disease appears to result from faulty absorption of zinc. The synthesis of keratins is affected by the zinc deficiency. Systemic administration of zinc sulfate often results in rapid improvement. Zinc treatment must be maintained for life.

Ocular Manifestations

Blepharitis, photophobia, and conjunctivitis can be seen. Bilateral superficial punctate lesions and nebulous subepithelial opacities of the cornea, located mainly in the upper paralimbal region, are also seen.[132,133] These are radiating, linear, white to light-brown, slightly whorllike opacities passing from the limbus about two thirds of the distance to the corneal center (Fig. 22-53). In some cases a corneal opacity occurs at the tips of these radiating lines, and in one case anterior corneal vascularization occurred.[134] Histologic examination of this case indicated thinning and loss of polarity of the epithelium and absence of Bowman's layer.[134]

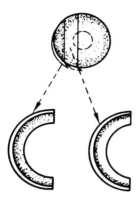

Figure 22-49
In Kyrle's disease, minute, yellow-brown opacities can be seen subepithelially and in the anterior stroma. (From Tessler HH, Apple DJ, Goldberg M: *Arch Ophthalmol* 90:278, 1973.)

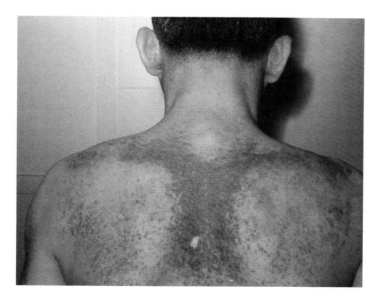

Figure 22-50
Darier's disease, showing thick vegetative plaques and papulomatous growths covered with greasy crusts. (From Grayson M, Keates RH: *Manual of diseases of the cornea,* Boston, 1969, Little, Brown & Co.)

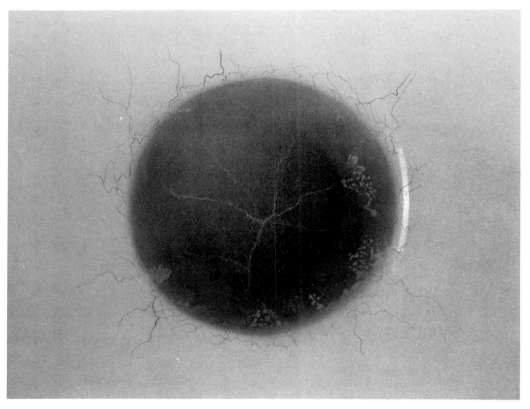

Figure 22-51
Schematic illustration of peripheral opacities and central radiating lines in the corneal epithelium of a 43-year-old woman with Darier's disease. (From Blackman HJ, Rodrigues MM, Peck GL: *Ophthalmology* 87:931, 1980.)

MALIGNANT ATROPHIC PAPULOSIS (DEGOS' DISEASE)

Malignant atrophic papulosis is a rare systemic disease with skin, gastrointestinal, and central nervous system manifestations. The underlying process is a lymphocyte-mediated vasculitis, the etiology of which is unknown; it has been hypothesized that a transmissible agent (e.g., a slow virus) is responsible.[135] The skin lesions may be the first sign of the disease and are pathognomonic. The lesions are firm, pink or pale red, smooth, dome-shaped papules 2 to 5 mm in diameter that can develop central necrosis, resulting in a porcelain white color (Fig. 22-54). Thin white scales can overlie the lesion, which can demonstrate pink, telangiectatic borders.

Gastrointestinal involvement occurs in the majority of patients; it is usually manifested as cramps, pain, vomiting, or bleeding. Infarcts and vascular thromboses can affect the central nervous system and other organs. Approximately 50% of patients die within 3 years.

Ocular involvement occurs in about one third of patients. Conjunctival lesions are seen as avascular patches, sometimes accompanied by telangiectasias and microaneurysms.[136-138] They can be mistaken for a Bitot's spot. Avascular areas can also involve the sclera, retina, choroid, and optic nerve. Ptosis, neuritis, diplopia, papilledema, and visual field abnormalities can result from neurologic involvement.

XERODERMA PIGMENTOSUM

Xeroderma pigmentosum is an autosomal recessive disorder characterized by intolerance to sunlight. It is caused by a defect in the repair of ultraviolet light–induced DNA damage. Prolonged erythema and edema occur even with minimal sun exposure. With time, the sun-exposed skin develops macules and atrophies, with hypopigmented plaques, telangiectasias, dryness, and scaling (Fig. 22-55). Beginning as early as the first decade, these children develop

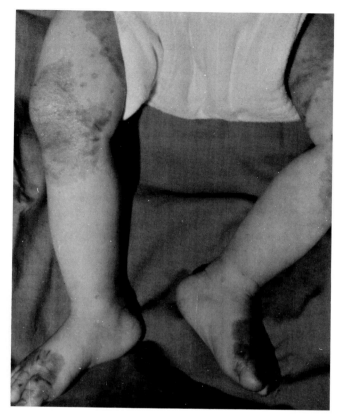

Figure 22-52
Acrodermatitis with lesions distributed on the buttocks, legs, and feet.

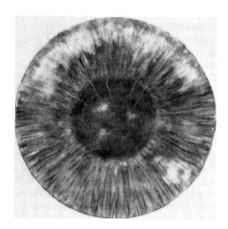

Figure 22-53
The corneal lesions seen in some cases of acrodermatitis enteropathica are radiating, linear, white-brown, slightly whorllike opacities passing from the limbus about two thirds of the distance to the corneal center. (From Matta CS, Felker GV, Ide CH: *Arch Ophthalmol* 93:140, 1975.)

numerous malignant cutaneous tumors, particularly basal cell carcinomas and squamous cell carcinomas. There is a predilection for the circumoral and circumorbital areas.

Ocular Manifestations

Most patients with xeroderma pigmentosum have photophobia, and many have conjunctivitis.[139,140] The conjunctivae are dry and hyperemic. Telangiectasias, pigmented lesions, and tumors occur on the bulbar conjunctiva. There can be recurrent inflammation, sometimes with membrane formation, and symblepharon can result. Loss of cilia, ectropion, and entropion are common and can result in conjunctival or corneal exposure. The cornea can become vascularized, ulcerated, and scarred (Fig. 22-56), and limbal tumors, particularly squamous cell carcinoma, are frequently encountered.[141] Endothelial cell density is less than normal for cell age, and the coefficient of variation of cell size is increased, suggesting an increased rate of endothelial injury and loss due to ultraviolet exposure.[142]

The major treatment is avoidance of ultravi-
Text continued on p. 638.

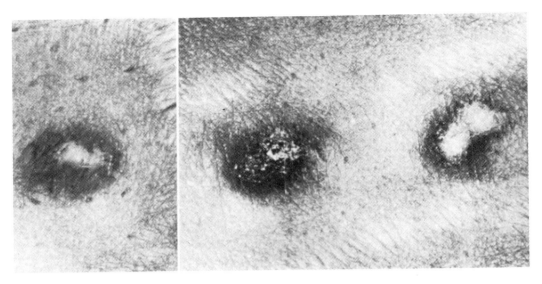

Figure 22-54
Skin lesions with atrophic porcelain white centers are characteristic of malignant atrophic papulosis. (From Howsden SM et al: *Arch Dermatol* 112:1582, 1976.)

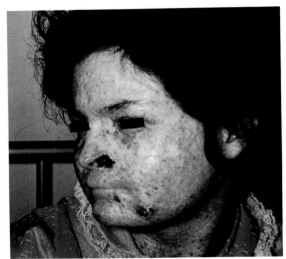

Figure 22-55
Skin changes in xeroderma pigmentosum, including squamous and basal cell carcinomas of the skin.

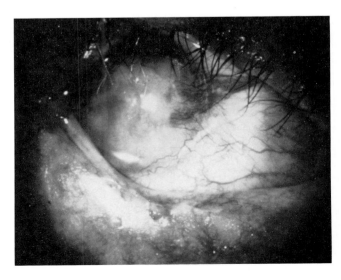

Figure 22-56
Corneal scarring resulting from exposure and trichiasis in xeroderma pigmentosum. (From Sugar J: *Metabolic disorders of the cornea.* In Kaufman HE et al: *The cornea,* New York, 1989, Churchill Livingstone.)

Table 22-4 Other Skin Diseases with Corneal or Conjunctival Findings			
Disorder	**Inheritance**	**Major Findings**	**Anterior Segment Findings**
Hereditary benign intraepithelial dyskeratosis[1,2]	Autosomal dominant	Oral dyskeratoses (white spongy folds and plaques of thickened mucosa)	Conjunctival hyperemia; foamy gelatinous perilimbal plaques; corneal vascularization
Hereditary mucoepithelial dysplasia	Autosomal dominant	Mucosal dyskeratoses; follicular keratoses; alopecia; lung disease	Photophobia; tearing; conjunctival dyskeratoses; corneal vascularization; keratitis; cataracts
Dyskeratosis congenita	?X-linked recessive	Reticulated hyperpigmentation; nail dystrophy; mucosal leukoplakia	Punctal stenosis; blepharitis; ectropion; madarosis; bullous conjunctivitis[145]
Epidermal nevus syndrome	?	Linear epidermal or sebaceous nevi; central nervous system and skeletal abnormalities	Nevus involving ocular surface; lid coloboma; limbal lipodermoids; corneal opacities[146]
Pili torti	Autosomal dominant	Twisted hairs	Corneal opacities[147]
Progressive facial hemiatrophy (Parry-Romberg syndrome)	—	Atrophy of the soft tissues of half the face (Fig. 22-57); seizures; trigeminal neuralgia	Ectropion; corneal exposure; iritis; band keratopathy (Fig. 22-58); bullous keratopathy; pupil and extraocular muscle abnormalities
Sjögren-Larson syndrome	Autosomal recessive	Ichthyosis; mental retardation; spasticity	"Corneal dystrophy"[148]
Incontinentia pigmenti	X-linked dominant	Vesicular lesions leave linear, whorled hyperpigmentation (Fig. 22-59)	Conjunctival pigmentation; corneal opacity; interstitial keratitis[149]
Papillon-LeFèvre syndrome (diffuse keratoderma with periodontopathy)	Autosomal recessive	Hyperkeratosis of palms and soles; periodontitis; calcification of falx cerebri	Peripheral corneal vascularization; corneal epithelial hypertrophy
Pachyonychia congenita (Jackson-Lawler type)	Autosomal dominant	Nail thickening (pachyonychia); palmoplantar hyperkeratoses; follicular keratosis	Corneal dyskeratoses
Pityriasis rubra pilaris	Sporadic or autosomal dominant	Follicular squamous papules; palmar plantar keratoderma (Fig. 22-60)	Conjunctival and corneal keratinization; fibrovascular pannus; interstitial scarring; corneal epithelial erosions; corneal vascularization
Rothmund-Thomson syndrome	Autosomal recessive	Poikiloderma; atrophy; hypo- or	

Continued

Table 22-4   Other Skin Diseases with Corneal or Conjunctival Findings—cont'd

Disorder	Inheritance	Major Findings	Anterior Segment Findings
		hyperpigmentation; telangiectasia; hyperkeratosis; skeletal anomalies; hypogonadism	Cataracts; band keratopathy; keratoconus
Anhidrotic ectodermal dysplasia	X-linked recessive; autosomal recessive	Hypohidrosis; hypotrichosis; defective dentition; absence of sebaceous glands	Keratoconjunctivitis sicca; peripheral pannus; tiny intraepithelial cysts; punctal atresia
Ectrodactyly-ectodermal dysplasia-cleft lip/palate syndrome	Autosomal dominant	Lobster-claw deformity of hands; anomalies of the central face; sparse hair; hypohidrosis; deafness	Abnormal or absent meibomian glands; lacrimal drainage system abnormalities; conjunctival scarring; entropion; secondary corneal disease[3–6]
Hidradenitis suppurativa	—	Chronic suppurative and cicatricial disease of apocrine gland–bearing skin; bacterial infection of involved skin	Interstitial keratitis[7]; peripheral corneal infiltrates; peripheral ulcerative keratitis[8]
Cutis verticis gyrata (Rosenthal-Kloepfer syndrome)		Convoluted folds and furrows in skin, especially the scalp; acromegaloid habitus; mental retardation; epilepsy	Corneal leukomas[150]
Lichen planus		Grayish-white papules that coalesce, often forming a reticular pattern; affects skin and mucosa of genitalia and mouth	Cicatrizing conjunctivitis[9] (rare)

[1]Von Sallmann L, Paton D: Hereditary benign intraepithelial dyskeratosis: I. Ocular manifestations, *Arch Ophthalmol* 63:421, 1960.

[2]Witkop CJ Jr et al: Hereditary benign intraepithelial dyskeratosis: II. Oral manifestations and hereditary transmission, *Arch Path* 70:696, 1960.

[3]Wilson FM II, Grayson M, Pieroni D: Corneal changes in ectodermal dysplasia, *Am J Ophthalmol* 75:11, 1973.

[4]Baum JL, Bull MJ: Ocular manifestations of the ectrodactyly, ectodermal dysplasia, cleft lip-palate syndrome, *Am J Ophthalmol* 78:211, 1976.

[5]McKnab AA, Potts MJ, Welham RAN: The EEC syndrome and its ocular manifestations, *Br J Ophthalmol* 73:261, 1989.

[6]Mader TH, Stulting RD: Penetrating keratoplasty in ectodermal dysplasia, *Am J Ophthalmol* 110:319, 1990.

[7]Bergeron JR, Stone OJ: Interstitial keratitis associated with hidradenitis suppurativa, *Arch Dermatol* 95:473, 1965.

[8]Mahmood MA, Pillai S, Limaye SR: Peripheral ulcerative keratitis associated with hidradenitis suppurativa, *Cornea* 10:75, 1991.

[9]Neumann R, Dutt CJ, Foster CS: Immunohistopathologic features and therapy of conjunctival lichen planus, *Am J Ophthalmol* 115:494, 1993.

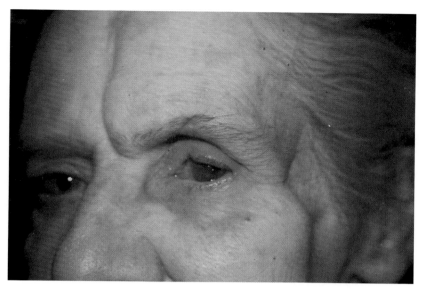

Figure 22-57
Parry-Romberg syndrome of progressive hemifacial atrophy showing severe depression of the zygomatic and temporal areas. (From Grayson M, Pieroni D: *Am J Ophthalmol* 70:42, 1970.)

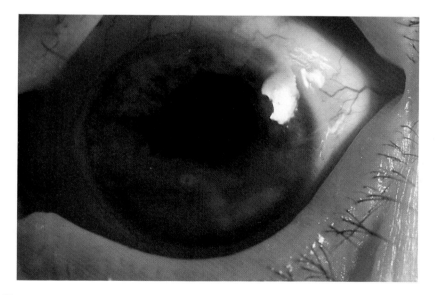

Figure 22-58
Early corneal edema and band keratopathy in Parry-Romberg syndrome. (From Grayson M, Pieroni D: *Am J Ophthalmol* 70:42, 1970.)

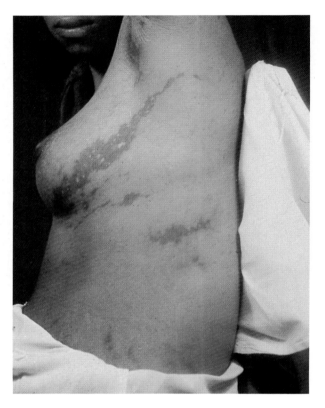

Figure 22-59
Pigmented, whorllike striae and hypertrophic skin changes are typical of incontinentia pigmenti.

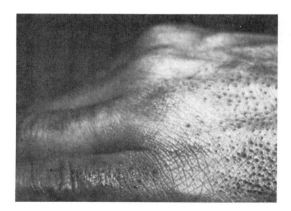

Figure 22-60
Pityriasis rubra pilaris lesions exhibit spiny, keratotic, scaly, acuminate follicular papules on an erythematous base. (From Grayson M, Keates RH: *Manual of diseases of the cornea,* Boston, 1969, Little, Brown & Co.)

olet radiation. Close monitoring for the development of tumors and early excision are essential. Lid deformities should be corrected surgically to prevent corneal complications. Penetrating keratoplasty can be successful in some patients.[143,144]

ACANTHOSIS NIGRICANS

Acanthosis nigricans refers to a complex of skin findings observed in a number of conditions. In the elderly it is often associated with malignancy, most often adenocarcinoma. A pigmented, velvety, rugated hypertrophy of the skin affects the face, neck, groin, axillae, and periumbilical area. Soft papillomas can also be seen in affected areas. Histologically, the primary abnormality is papillomatosis of the epidermis with hyperkeratosis. The skin condition may result from peptide production by the tumor.

The lid skin can be involved, resulting in thickening and pigmentation.[145] Palpebral conjunctival epithelial hypertrophy, with hyperkeratosis, has been observed in some cases.[146-149] A diffuse papillary conjunctivitis, giant papillae, or papillomatous growths may be seen. The affected conjunctiva may or may not be pigmented. In one child with the benign form of acanthosis nigricans, infiltration and vascularization of the cornea occurred, possibly secondary to eyelid involvement.[145]

DERMOCHONDROCORNEAL DYSTROPHY OF FRANÇOIS

This condition is transmitted as an autosomal recessive trait. Deformities of the hands and feet occur in the first 5 years of life. Xanthomalike nodules appear in the skin of the nose, ears, and extensor aspects of the elbows and joints of the fingers.

By the end of the first decade of life, white or brownish, irregular subepithelial opacities appear.[150] The corneal periphery is clear, and the stroma and endothelium are normal. Vision is somewhat decreased, but the corneal changes do not advance.

OTHER SKIN DISEASES

A number of other skin disease that can affect the cornea or conjunctiva are described in Table 22-4.[128,151,152]

REFERENCES

1. Iglesias LS et al: Ocular cicatricial pemphigoid in a twelve-year-old boy, *Cornea* 11:365, 1992.
2. Wright PG: Cicatrizing conjunctivitis, *Trans Ophthalmol Soc UK* 105:1, 1986.
3. Foster CS: Cicatricial pemphigoid, *Trans Am Ophthalmol Soc* 84:527, 1986.
4. Mondino BJ: Cicatricial pemphigoid and erythema multiforme, *Ophthalmology* 97:939, 1990.
5. Hanson RD, Olsen KD, Rogers RS: Upper aerodigestive tract manifestations of cicatricial pemphigoid, *Ann Otol Rhinol Laryngol* 97:493, 1988.
6. Mondino BJ, Brown SI: Ocular cicatricial pemphigoid, *Ophthalmology* 88:95, 1981.
7. Stanly JR: *Bullous pemphigoid, cicatricial pemphigoid and chronic bullous disease of childhood.* In Fitzpatrick TB et al, editors: *Dermatology in general medicine,* ed 4, New York, 1993, McGraw-Hill.
8. Foster CS, Wilson LA, Ekins MB: Immunosuppressive therapy for progressive ocular cicatricial pemphigoid, *Ophthalmology* 89:340, 1982.
9. Tauber J, Jabbur N, Foster CS: Improved detection of disease progression in ocular cicatricial pemphigoid, *Cornea* 11:446, 1992.
10. Person JR, Rogers RS: Bullous and cicatricial pemphigoid: clinical, histopathologic, and immunopathologic correlations, *Mayo Clin Proc* 52:54, 1977.
11. Bernauer W et al: The conjunctiva in acute and chronic mucous membrane pemphigoid: an immunohistochemical analysis, *Ophthalmology* 100:339, 1993.
12. Ralph RA: Conjunctival goblet cell density in normal subjects and in dry eye syndromes, *Invest Ophthalmol* 14:299, 1975.
13. Nelson JD, Wright JC: Conjunctival goblet cell densities in ocular surface disease, *Arch Ophthalmol* 102:1049, 1984.
14. Anderson SR et al: Benign mucous membrane pemphigoid: III. Biopsy, *Acta Ophthalmol (Copenh)* 52:455, 1974.
15. Carroll JM, Kuwabara T: Ocular pemphigus: an electron microscopic study of conjunctival and corneal epithelium, *Arch Ophthalmol* 80:683, 1968.
16. Galbavy EJ, Foster CS: Ultrastructural characteristics of conjunctiva in cicatricial pemphigoid, *Cornea* 4:127, 1985.
17. Furney N et al: Immunofluorescent studies of ocular cicatricial pemphigoid, *Am J Ophthalmol* 80:825, 1975.
18. Griffith MR et al: Immunofluorescent studies in mucous membrane pemphigoid, *Arch Dermatol* 109:195, 1974.
19. Proia AD, Foulks GN, Sanfilippo FP: Ocular cicatricial pemphigoid with granular IgA and complement deposition, *Arch Ophthalmol* 103:1669, 1985.
20. Leonard J et al: Immunofluorescent studies in ocular cicatricial pemphigoid, *Br J Dermatol* 118:209, 1988.
21. Waltman SR, Yarran D: Circulating autoantibodies in ocular pemphigoid, *Am J Ophthalmol* 77:891, 1974.
22. Meyer JR et al: Localization of basement membrane components in mucous membrane pemphigoid, *J Invest Dermatol* 84:105, 1985.
23. Mondino BJ et al: Autoimmune phenomena in ocular cicatricial pemphigoid, *Am J Ophthalmol* 83:443, 1977.
24. Rice BA, Foster CS: Immunopathology of cicatricial pemphigoid affecting the conjunctiva, *Ophthalmology* 97:1476, 1990.
25. Bean SF et al: Ocular cicatricial pemphigoid, *Trans Am Acad Ophthalmol Otolaryngol* 81:806, 1976.
26. Waltman SR, Yarian D: Circulating autoantibodies in ocular pemphigoid, *Am J Ophthalmol* 77:891, 1974.
27. Lee SJ et al: Serum levels of tumor necrosis factor-alpha and interleukin-6 in ocular cicatricial pemphigoid, *Invest Ophthalmol Vis Sci* 34:3522, 1993.
28. Chan LS et al: High frequency of HLA-DQB1*0301 allele in patients with pure ocular

cicatricial pemphigoid, *Dermatology* 189(suppl):99, 1994.

29. Mondino BJ, Brown SI, Rabin BS: HLA antigens in ocular cicatricial pemphigoid, *Br J Ophthalmol* 62:265, 1978.

30. Power WJ et al: Increasing the diagnostic yield of conjunctival biopsy in patients with suspected ocular cicatricial pemphigoid, *Ophthalmology* 102:1158, 1995.

31. Flach A: Symblepharon in sarcoidosis, *Am J Ophthalmol* 85:210, 1978.

32. Tauber J, Sainz de la Maza M, Foster CS: Systemic chemotherapy for ocular cicatricial pemphigoid, *Cornea* 10:185, 1991.

33. Fern AI et al: Dapsone therapy for the acute inflammatory phase of ocular pemphigoid, *Br J Ophthalmol* 76:332, 1992.

34. Elder MJ, Lightman S, Dart JK: Role of cyclophosphamide and high dose steroid in ocular cicatricial pemphigoid, *Br J Ophthalmol* 79:264, 1995.

35. Mondino BJ, Brown SI: Immunosuppressive therapy in ocular cicatricial pemphigoid, *Arch Ophthalmol* 96:453, 1983.

36. Holland EJ et al: Topical cyclosporin A in the treatment of anterior segment inflammatory disease, *Cornea* 12:413, 1993.

37. Foster CS, Neumann R, Tauber J: Long term results of systemic chemotherapy for ocular cicatricial pemphigoid, *Doc Ophthalmol* 82:223, 1992.

38. Heiligenhaus A et al: Long-term results of mucous membrane grafting in ocular cicatricial pemphigoid: implications for patient selection and surgical considerations, *Ophthalmology* 100:1283, 1993.

39. Sainz de la Maza M, Tauber J, Foster CS: Cataract surgery in ocular cicatricial pemphigoid, *Ophthalmology* 95:481, 1988.

40. Tugal-Tutkun I, Akova YA, Foster CS: Penetrating keratoplasty in cicatrizing conjunctival diseases, *Ophthalmology* 102:576, 1995.

41. Venning B et al: Mucosal involvement in bullous and cicatricial pemphigoid, *Br J Dermatol* 118:7, 1988.

42. Jordan RE, Triftshauser CT, Schroeter AL: Direct immunofluorescent studies of pemphigus and bullous pemphigoid, *Arch Dermatol* 103:486, 1971.

43. Ahmed AR, Maize J, Provost TT: Bullous pemphigoid: clinical and immunologic follow-up after successful therapy, *Arch Dermatol* 113:1043, 1977.

44. Soter NA, Wuepper KD: *Erythema multiforme and Stevens-Johnson syndrome*. In Samter M, editor: *Immunological diseases*, ed 4, Boston, 1988, Little, Brown & Co.

45. Mondino BJ: Cicatricial pemphigoid and erythema multiforme, *Ophthalmology* 97:939, 1990.

46. Power WJ et al: Analysis of the acute ophthalmic manifestations of the erythema multiforme/Stevens-Johnson syndrome/toxic epidermal necrolysis disease spectrum, *Ophthalmology* 102:1669, 1995.

47. Chan LS et al: Ocular cicatricial pemphigoid occurring as a sequela of Stevens-Johnson syndrome, *JAMA* 266:1543, 1991.

48. Arstikoitis MJ: Ocular aftermath of Stevens-Johnson syndrome, *Arch Ophthalmol* 90:376, 1973.

49. Dohlman CH, Doughman DJ: The Stevens-Johnson syndrome, *Trans New Orleans Acad Ophthalmol* 24:236, 1972.

50. Fritsch PO, Elias PM: *Erythema multiforme and toxic epidermal necrolysis*. In Fitzpatrick TB et al, editors: *Dermatology in general medicine*, ed 4, New York, 1993, McGraw-Hill.

51. McCord CD, Shen WP: Tarsal polishing and mucous membrane grafting for cicatricial entropion, trichiasis and epidermalization, *Ophthalmic Surg* 14:1021, 1983.

52. Mannor GE et al: Hard-palate mucosa graft in Stevens-Johnson syndrome, *Am J Ophthalmol* 118:786, 1994.

53. Revuz J et al: Toxic epidermal necrolysis: clinical findings and prognosis factors in 87 patients, *Arch Dermatol* 123:1160, 1987.

54. Lyell A: A review of toxic epidermal necrolysis in Britain, *Br J Dermatol* 79:662, 1967.

55. Revuz J et al: Treatment of toxic epidermal necrolysis: Créteil's experience, *Arch Dermatol* 123:1156, 1987.

56. Bjornberg A, Bjornberg K, Gisslen H: Toxic epidermal necrolysis with ophthalmic complications, *Acta Ophthalmol* 42:1084, 1964.

57. Belfort R et al: Ocular complications of Stevens-Johnson syndrome and toxic epidermal necrolysis in patients with AIDS, *Cornea* 10:536, 1991.

58. Binaghi M et al: Ocular complications of Lyell's syndrome, *J Fr Ophthalmol* 8:239, 1985.

59. de Felice GP, Caroli R, Autelitano A: Long-term complications of toxic epidermal necrolysis (Lyell's disease): clinical and histopathological study, *Ophthalmologica* 195:1, 1987.

60. Roujeau J-C et al: Sjögren-like syndrome after toxic epidermal necrolysis, *Lancet* 2:609, 1985.

61. Hintner H et al: Immunofluorescence mapping of antigenic determinants within the dermal-epidermal junction in mechanobullous diseases, *J Invest Dermatol* 76:113, 1981.

62. Bauer EA, Briggaman RA: *Hereditary epidermolysis bullosa*. In Fitzpatrick TB et al, editors: *Dermatology in general medicine*, ed 4, New York, 1993, McGraw-Hill.

63. Iwamoto M et al: The ultrastructural defect in conjunctiva from a case of recessive dystrophic epidermolysis bullosa, *Arch Ophthalmol* 109:1382, 1991.

64. Shimizu H et al: Epidermolysis bullosa acquisita antigen and the carboxyl terminus of type VII collagen have a common immunolocalization to anchoring fibrils and lamina densa of basement membrane, *Br J Dermatol* 122:577, 1990.

65. Gans LA: Eye lesions of epidermolysis bullosa: clinical features, management, and prognosis, *Arch Dermatol* 124:762, 1988.

66. Lin AN et al: Review of ophthalmic findings in 204 patients with epidermolysis bullosa, *Am J Ophthalmol* 118:384, 1994.

67. Aurora A, Madhaven M, Rao S: Ocular changes in epidermolysis bullosis letalis, *Am J Ophthalmol* 79:464, 1975.

68. Zierhut M et al: Ocular involvement in epidermolysis bullosa acquisita, *Arch Ophthalmol* 107:398, 1989.

69. McDonnell PJ et al: Eye involvement in junctional epidermolysis bullosa, *Arch Ophthalmol* 107:1635, 1989.

70. Granek H, Howard B: Corneal involvement in epidermolysis bullosa simplex, *Arch Ophthalmol* 98:469, 1980.

71. Adamis AP, Schein OD, Kenyon KR: Anterior corneal disease of epidermolysis bullosa simplex, *Arch Ophthalmol* 111:499, 1993.

72. Katz SI: *Dermatitis herpetiformis*. In Fitzpatrick TB et al, editors: *Dermatology in general medicine*, ed 4, New York, 1993, McGraw-Hill.

72a. Huff JC: The immunopathogenesis of dermatitis herpetiformis, *J Invest Dermatol* 84:237, 1985.

73. Duke-Elder S, Leigh AG: *System of ophthalmology,* vol VIII, Diseases of the outer eye, St Louis, 1965, Mosby–Year Book.

74. Wojnarowska F et al: Chronic bullous disease of childhood, childhood cicatricial pemphigoid, and linear IgA disease of adults: a comparative study demonstrating clinical and immunopathologic overlap, *J Am Acad Dermatol* 19:792, 1988.

75. Wilson BD et al: Linear IgA bullous dermatosis: an immunologically defined disease, *Int J Dermatol* 24:569, 1985.

76. Leonard JN et al: Linear IgA disease in adults, *Br J Dermatol* 107:301, 1982.

77. Kelly SE et al: A clinicopathological study of mucosal involvement in linear IgA disease, *Br J Dermatol* 119:161, 1988.

78. Aultbrinker EA, Starr MB, Donnenfeld ED: Linear IgA disease: the ocular manifestations, *Ophthalmology* 95:340, 1988.

79. Drabonski J, Chorzelski TP, Jablonska S: The ultrastructural localization of IgA deposits in chronic bullous disease of childhood (CBDC), *J Invest Dermatol* 72:291, 1979.

80. Ahmed AR et al: Pemphigus: current concepts, *Ann Intern Med* 92:396, 1980.

81. Woo TT et al: Specificity and inhibition of the epidermal cell detachment induced by pemphigus IgG in vitro, *J Invest Dermatol* 81:115, 1983.

82. Anhalt GJ et al: Paraneoplastic pemphigus, *N Engl J Med* 323:1729, 1990.

83. Jordan RE, Triftshauser CT, Schroeter AL: Direct immunofluorescent studies of pemphigus and bullous pemphigoid, *Arch Dermatol* 103:486, 1971.

84. Bean SF, Holubar K, Gillet RB: Pemphigus involving the eyes, *Arch Dermatol* 111:1484, 1975.

85. Hodak E et al: Conjunctival involvement in pemphigus vulgaris: a clinical histopathological and immunofluorescence study, *Br J Dermatol* 123:615, 1990.

86. Meyers SJ et al: Conjunctival involvement in paraneoplastic pemphigus, *Am J Ophthalmol* 114:621, 1992.

87. Lam S et al: Paraneoplastic pemphigus, cicatricial conjunctivitis, and acanthosis nigricans with pachydermatoglyphy in a patient with bronchogenic squamous cell carcinoma, *Ophthalmology* 99:108, 1992.

88. Bennion SD, Johnson C, Weston WL: Hydroa vacciniforme with inflammatory keratitis and secondary anterior uveitis, *Pediatr Dermatol* 4:320, 1987.

89. Erzurum SA, Feder RS, Greenwald MJ: Acne rosacea with keratitis in childhood, *Arch Ophthalmol* 111:228, 1993.

90. Jenkins MS et al: Ocular rosacea, *Am J Ophthalmol* 88:618, 1979.

91. Watson PG, Hayreh SS: Scleritis and episcleritis, *Br J Ophthalmol* 60:163, 1976.

92. Albert DL, Brownstein S, Jackson WB: Conjunctival granulomas in rosacea, *Am J Ophthalmol* 113:108, 1992.

93. Hoang-Xuan T et al: Ocular rosacea: a histologic and immunopathologic study, *Ophthalmology* 97:1468, 1990.

94. Brown SI, Shahinian L: Diagnosis and treatment of ocular rosacea, *Trans Am Acad Ophthalmol* 85:779, 1978.

95. Knight AG, Vickers CFH: A follow-up of tetracycline-treated rosacea, *Br J Dermatol* 93:577, 1975.

96. Frucht-Perry J et al: Efficacy of doxycycline and tetracycline in ocular rosacea, *Am J Ophthalmol* 116:88, 1993.

97. McCulley JP, Dougherty JM: Blepharitis associated with acne rosacea and seborrheic dermatitis, *Int Ophthalmol Clin* 25:159, 1985.

98. Christophers E, Sterry W: *Psoriasis.* In Fitzpatrick TB et al, editors: *Dermatology in general medicine*, ed 4, New York, 1993, McGraw-Hill.

99. Boss JM et al: Peripheral corneal melting syndrome in association with psoriasis, *Br Med J* 282:609, 1981.

100. Cram DL: Corneal melting in psoriasis, *J Am Acad Dermatol* 5:617, 1981.

101. Catsarou-Catsari A et al: Ophthalmological manifestations in patients with psoriasis, *Acta Derm Venereol (Stockh)* 64:557, 1984.

102. Backman HA: The effects of PUVA on the eye, *Am J Optom Physiol Opt* 59:86, 1982.

103. Shindle R, Leone C: Cicatricial entropion associated with lamellar ichthyosis, *Arch Ophthalmol* 89:62, 1973.

104. Franceschetti A, Maeder G: Dystrophie profonde de la cornée dans un cas d'ichtyose congénitale, *Bull Mem Soc Fr Ophthalmol* 67:146, 1954.

105. Sever RJ, Frost P, Weinstein G: Eye changes in ichthyosis, *JAMA* 206:2283, 1968.

106. Piccirillo A et al: Ocular findings and skin histology in a group of patients with X-linked ichthyosis, *Br J Dermatol* 119:185, 1988.

107. Costagliola C et al: Ocular findings in X-linked ichthyosis: a survey on 38 cases, *Ophthalmologica* 202:152, 1991.

108. Friedman B: Corneal findings in ichthyosis, *Am J Ophthalmol* 39:575, 1955.

109. Macsai MS, Doshi H: Clinical pathologic correlation of superficial corneal opacities in X-linked ichthyosis, *Am J Ophthalmol* 118:477, 1994.

110. Franceschetti A, Schlaeppe V: Dégénérescence en bandelette et dystrophie, prédescemétique de la cornée dans un d'ichtyose congénitale, *Dermatologica* 115:217, 1957.

111. Jay B, Black RK, Wells RS: Ocular manifestations of ichthyosis, *Br J Ophthalmol* 52:217, 1968.

112. Van Everdingen JJ, Rampen FH, Van der Schaar WW: Normal tearing and tear production in congenital ichthyosiform erythroderma with deafness and keratitis, *Acta Dermatol Venereol (Stoch)* 62:76, 1982.

113. Skinner BA, Greist MC, Norins AL: The keratitis, ichthyosis, and deafness (KID) syndrome, *Arch Dermatol* 117:285, 1981.

114. Baden HP, Alper JC: Ichthyosiform dermatosis, keratitis, deafness, *Arch Dermatol* 113:1701, 1977.

115. Tuppurainen K et al: The KID-syndrome in Finland: a report of four cases, *Acta Ophthalmol (Copenh)* 66:692, 1988.

116. Grob JJ et al: Keratitis, ichthyosis, and deafness (KID) syndrome: vertical transmission and death from multiple squamous cell carcinomas, *Arch Dermatol* 123:777, 1987.

117. Hsu HC, Lin GS, Li WM: Keratitis, ichthyosis, and deafness (KID) syndrome with cerebellar hypoplasia, *Int J Dermatol* 27:695, 1988.

118. Zimmerman LE: Ocular lesions of juvenile xanthogranuloma, *Am J Ophthalmol* 60:1011, 1965.

119. Cogan DG, Kuwabara T, Parke D: Epibulbar nevo-xantho-endothelioma, *Arch Ophthalmol* 59:717, 1958.

120. Yanoff M, Perry H: Juvenile xanthogranuloma of the corneoscleral limbus, *Arch Ophthalmol* 113:915, 1995.

121. Britton H et al: Keratosis follicularis spinulosa decalvans: an infant with failure to thrive, deafness and recurrent infections, *Arch Dermatol* 114:761, 1978.

122. Forgács J, Franceschetti A: Histologic aspect of corneal changes due to hereditary metabolic and cutaneous affections, *Am J Ophthalmol* 47:191, 1959.

123. Tessler HH, Apple DJ, Goldberg MF: Ocular findings in a kindred with Kyrle disease: hyperkeratosis follicularis et parafollicularis in cutem penetrans, *Arch Ophthalmol* 90:278, 1973.

124. Blackman HJ, Rodrigues MM, Peck GL: Corneal epithelial lesions in keratosis follicularis (Darier's disease), *Ophthalmology* 87:941, 1980.

125. Wright JC: Darier's disease, *Am J Ophthalmol* 55:134, 1963.

126. Daicker B: Ocular involvement in keratosis follicularis associated with retinitis pigmentosa: clinicopathological case report, *Ophthalmologica* 209:47, 1995.

127. Rud E: Werner's syndrome in 3 siblings, *Acta Ophthalmol* 34:255, 1956.

128. Petrohelos MA: Werner's syndrome: a survey of 3 cases with review of the literature, *Am J Ophthalmol* 56:941, 1956.

129. Kremer I, Ingber A, Ben-Sira I: Corneal metastatic calcification in Werner's syndrome, *Am J Ophthalmol* 106:221, 1988.

130. Kleeberg J: Werner's syndrome, *Acta Med Orient* 8:146, 1949.

131. Valero A, Gellei B: Retinitis pigmentosa, hypertension and uremia in Werner's syndrome, *Br J Med* 2:351, 1960.

132. Matta CS, Felker GV, Ide CH: Eye manifestations in acrodermatitis enteropathica, *Arch Ophthalmol* 93:140, 1975.

133. Warshawsky RS et al: Acrodermatitis enteropathica: corneal involvement with histochemical and electron micrographic studies, *Arch Ophthalmol* 93:194, 1975.

134. Cameron JD, McClain CJ: Ocular histopathology of acrodermatitis enteropathica, *Br J Ophthalmol* 70:662, 1986.

135. Soter NA, Livingston DL, Mihm MC: *Malignant atrophic papulosis*. In Fitzpatrick TB et al, editors: *Dermatology in general medicine*, ed 3, New York, 1987, McGraw-Hill.

136. Henkind P, Clark DE: Ocular pathology in malignant atrophic papulosis: Dego's disease, *Am J Ophthalmol* 65:164, 1968.

137. Howard RO, Nishida S: A case of Degos' disease with electron microscope findings, *Trans Am Acad Ophthalmol Otolaryngol* 73:1097, 1969.

138. Sibillat M et al: Papulose atrophiante maligne (maladie de Degos): revue clinique, *J Fr Ophthalmol* 9:299, 1986.

139. Goyal JL et al: Oculocutaneous manifestations in xeroderma pigmentosa, *Br J Ophthalmol* 78:295, 1994.

140. Kraemer KH et al: Xeroderma pigmentosum: cutaneous, ocular and neurologic abnormalities in 830 published cases, *Arch Dermatol* 123:241, 1987.

141. Gaasterland D, Rodrigues M, Mashell A: Ocular involvement in xeroderma pigmentosum, *Ophthalmology* 89:980, 1982.

142. Okubo K et al: The corneal endothelium in xeroderma pigmentosum, *Ophthalmologica* 195:178, 1987.

143. Jalali S et al: Penetrating keratoplasty in xeroderma pigmentosum: case reports and review of the literature, *Cornea* 13:527, 1994.

144. Calonge M et al: Management of corneal com-

plications in xeroderma pigmentosum, *Cornea* 11:173, 1992.

145. Lamba P, Lal S: Ocular changes in benign acanthosis nigricans, *Dermatologica* 1140:356, 1970.

146. Newman G, Carsten M: Acanthosis nigricans: conjunctival and lid lesions, *Arch Ophthalmol* 90:259, 1973.

147. Tabandeh H et al: Conjunctival involvement in malignancy-associated acanthosis nigricans, *Eye* 7:648, 1993.

148. Groos EB et al: Eyelid involvement in acanthosis nigricans, *Am J Ophthalmol* 115:42, 1993.

149. Wedge CCI et al: Malignant acanthosis nigricans: a case report, *Ophthalmology* 100:1590, 1993.

150. François J: Heredo-familial corneal dystrophies, *Trans Ophthalmol Soc UK* 86:367, 1966.

151. Steir W, Van Voolen A, Selmanowitz V: Dyskeratosis congenita: relationship to Fanconi's anemia, *Blood* 39:510, 1972.

152. McCray J, Smith JL: Conjunctival and retinal incontinentia pigmenti, *Arch Ophthalmol* 79:417, 1968.

Twenty-Three

Other Systemic Disorders

NUTRITIONAL DISORDERS

Vitamin A Deficiency

Vitamin A deficiency is relatively rare in the United States, but it is common in some developing countries. The leading cause of childhood blindness throughout the world,[1] vitamin A deficiency primarily occurs in preschool-aged children and is usually seen in association with other nutritional deficits, such as multiple vitamin deficiency and protein-calorie malnutrition (marasmus). In the well-fed populations of developed countries, vitamin A deficiency is rarely seen but can result from systemic disease (e.g., malabsorption, cystic fibrosis, liver disease) or dietary indiscretion.[2-6]

Clinical Manifestations

The classification scheme of ocular findings in xerophthalmia that has been developed by the World Health Organization is illustrated in the box on p. 646. The earliest symptom of vitamin A deficiency is usually night blindness, followed by conjunctival xerosis and keratinization, blepharitis, and meibomitis. Nonocular findings can include hyperkeratosis of the skin, lengthening of the eyelashes, enhanced keratinization and xerosis of other mucosal surfaces, increased intracranial pressure, and mental retardation.

In conjunctival xerosis the conjunctiva can be lusterless, wrinkled, red, and opaque.[7,8] The signs are first noted in the temporal quadrant, appearing as an unwettable portion of the conjunctiva. Later, all portions of the conjunctiva can be involved, but the bulbar conjunctiva tends to be more affected than the palpebral conjunctiva. A *Bitot's spot* (Fig. 23-1) is a small white-gray irregular plaque with a foamy surface. It is seen on the bulbar conjunctiva, usually temporal to the limbus, and is often bilateral.

Non–vitamin A–responsive Bitot's spots can also be seen in patients who have had previous vitamin A deficiency.[1,8] In addition, not all cases of vitamin A deficiency manifest a Bitot's spot.

Corneal xerosis is usually seen in individuals

with conjunctival xerosis (Fig. 23-2). The earliest sign is a superficial punctate keratopathy, which usually begins inferiorly.[9] When the punctate keratopathy becomes confluent, the cornea develops a peau d'orange or ground-glass appearance. Keratinization, stromal edema, and rapid tear break-up can also be noted. These findings are often present despite normal aqueous tear production.

The preceding changes are readily reversible with vitamin A treatment.[9,10] However, these

eyes are prone to corneal ulceration, often with severe visual consequences[7,11,12] (Fig. 23-3). Minor trauma or conjunctival infection (e.g., measles) often leads to marked stromal loss and scarring.[13]

The earliest and most common form of corneal ulceration is small, sharply punched-out lesions, most often affecting the peripheral nasal cornea.[9] These may begin as localized, sharply demarcated areas of swollen, opaque, grayish-yellow stroma that sloughs, leaving a descemetocele. Larger and more irregularly shaped ulcers can also occur.

Keratomalacia is an extreme form of corneal ulceration in vitamin A deficiency. It is particularly common in children with advanced starvation and those with systemic disease, such as diarrhea, parasitic infection, or measles in addition to malnutrition. Keratomalacia can develop suddenly. There is generalized softening of the stroma, which turns yellow-white and sloughs, leaving a descemetocele or perforation. The cause is not known: Both clinically and histologically it appears that an inflammatory response does not play a significant role.

Histologically, the main feature of vitamin A deficiency is squamous metaplasia of the conjunctival and corneal epithelium[14-16] (Fig. 23-4). There is acanthotic thickening of the epithelium, with keratinization of the surface. Goblet cells are greatly reduced in number, resulting in

World Health Organization Classification of Findings in Vitamin A Deficiency	
Classification	**Finding**
XN	Night blindness
X1A	Conjunctival xerosis
X1B	Bitot's spots
X2	Corneal xerosis
X3A	Corneal ulceration or keratomalacia involving < one third of corneal surface
X3B	Corneal ulceration or keratomalacia involving ≥ one third of corneal surface
XS	Corneal scarring
XF	Xerophthalmic fundus

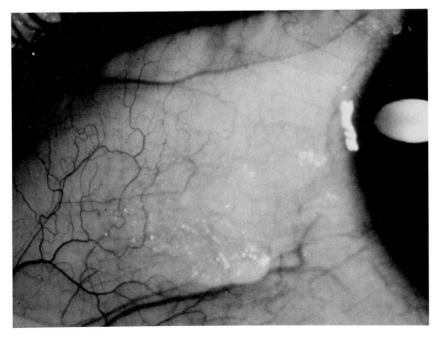

Figure 23-1
Bitot's spot.

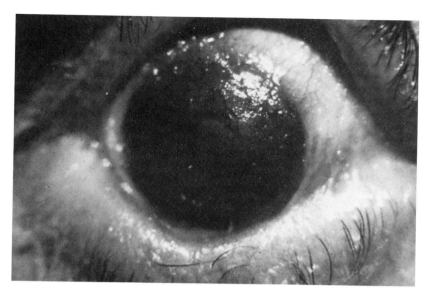

Figure 23-2
Lusterless and dry conjunctiva and cornea with epidermization in a patient with vitamin A deficiency.

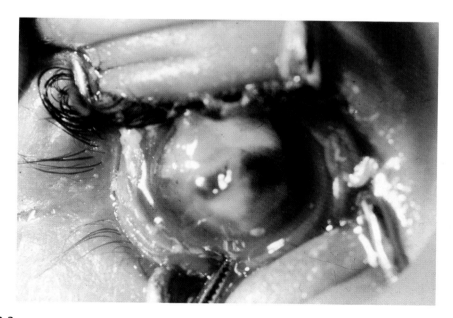

Figure 23-3
Keratomalacia in a patient with vitamin A deficiency. (Courtesy of D. Paton, Houston, TX.)

a lack of mucin. A chronic inflammatory infiltrate is often present in the substantia propria. Bitot's spots are areas of marked keratinization.[16] The foamy appearance is caused by mucus and xerosis bacilli (*Corynebacterium xerosis*).[17]

The normal function of vitamin A in the conjunctiva and cornea and the mechanism by which its deficiency causes disease are unclear. Conjunctival and corneal xerosis occur in vitamin A–deficient animals, but Bitot's spots are not seen.[14,18,19] In vitamin A–deficient animals

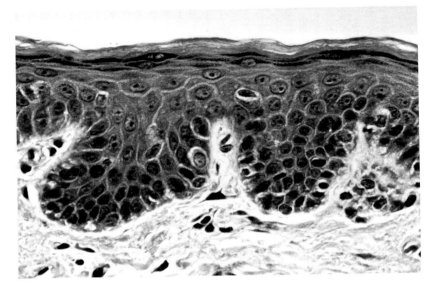

Figure 23-4
Bitot's spot. Note epidermalization of the conjunctival epithelium with a stratified squamous configuration, rete peg formation, absence of goblet cells, and keratinization of surface. (Hematoxylin-eosin stain; × 800.) (Courtesy of Bruce L. Johnson, Pittsburgh, PA.)

there is decreased adhesion of the corneal epithelium to its basement membrane; this appears to be related to decreased hemidesmosomes and other abnormalities of the adhesion complex.[20] Vitamin A stimulates the conversion of limbal stem cells to transient amplifying cells but inhibits the amplification of corneal and limbal transient amplifying cells.[21]

In vitamin A–deficient rats spontaneous corneal stromal ulceration is rare, but ulceration after thermal burns[13] or stromal incisions[22] is increased. These corneas produce much higher levels of interleukin-1 and chemotactic activity after injury than normal corneas.[23]

Treatment
Vitamin A can be administered either orally or parentally, if necessary. The recommended dose for children over 1 year of age is 200,000 IU on each of 2 consecutive days, followed by another dose 1 to 2 weeks later.[24] Adjunctive topical vitamin A administration also appears to be beneficial.[25-27] Improvement is seen in 1 to 4 days, with complete resolution usually within 1 week.

Riboflavin Deficiency
Riboflavin is the precursor of flavin coenzymes involved in the transfer of electrons in oxidation-reduction reactions. Riboflavin defi-

ciency causes *cheilosis,* which is fissuring and ulceration of the oral mucous membranes, particularly at the corners of the mouth. Facial seborrhea and glossitis also occur. The tongue has a purplish hue, and the filiform papillae are flattened out.

The patient complains of photophobia, irritation, and twitching and burning of the eyes. The lid margins and conjunctivae are injected. Increased prominence of the limbal vessels occurs early, and these vessels can later extend onto the cornea. A superficial epithelial keratitis, corneal opacification, mydriasis, and increased iris pigmentation can be seen.[28]

NEUROLOGIC DISORDERS

Familial Dysautonomia (Riley-Day Syndrome)
Familial dysautonomia is an autosomal recessive disease that seems to be confined to Ashkenazi Jews (Table 23-1). The abnormal gene has been localized to chromosome 9.[29] There is a deficiency of plasma dopamine β-hydroxylase, the enzyme that catalyzes the conversion of dopamine to norepinephrine. This results in a deficiency of norepinephrine and epinephrine and elevation of serum and urine homovanillic acid, the breakdown product of dopamine.

Table 23-1 Neurologic Disorders with Corneal Manifestations				
Disorder	**Inheritance**	**Pathogenesis**	**Major Systemic Findings**	**Ocular Findings**
Familial dysautonomia (Riley-Day syndrome)	AR*	Dopamine-beta-hydrox-ylase deficiency	Autonomic instability; emotional lability; dysphagia	Tear deficiency; corneal anesthesia; retinal vascular tortuosity
Shy-Drager syndrome	—	Degeneration of central autonomic nervous system	Progressive autonomic instability in elderly; orthostatic hypotension; urinary incontinence; impotence; hypohidrosis	Dry eye; iris atrophy; convergence insufficiency; anisocoria; Horner's syndrome
Neurofibromatosis (von Recklinghausen's disease)	AD†	Unknown	Neurofibromas; other neural tumors; pigmented skin lesions	Corneal hypesthesia; plexiform neuroma of the upper lid; iris nodules; glaucoma
Myotonic dystrophy	AD	Unknown	Progressive muscle weakness; myotonia	Corneal exposure; cataracts; hypotony; ophthalmoplegia; ptosis; enophthalmos
Wilson's disease (see Chapter 24)	AR	Impaired liver excretion of copper	Progressive neurologic impairment; liver dysfunction	Kayser-Fleischer ring; sunflower cataract
Ataxia-telangiectasia	AR	Unknown	Cerebellar ataxia; cutaneous telangiectasia; immunodeficiency	Conjunctival telangiectasias

*Autosomal recessive.
†Autosomal dominant.

Patients with familial dysautonomia usually have a history of feeding difficulty from birth and show an extreme emotional lability. Autonomic instability is demonstrated by abnormal sweating, labile hypertension, and postural hypotension. Other findings include decreased lacrimation, corneal hypesthesia, absence of the fungiform papillae of the tongue (Fig. 23-5), diminished pain and temperature sensation, hyporeflexia, motor incoordination, episodic fever, and episodic vomiting. Few patients reach adulthood because of recurrent pulmonary infections caused by aspiration and renal failure secondary to hypertension.

Corneal complications result from tear deficiency and corneal anesthesia. There is a wide variation in the severity of corneal disease; some cases may be free of disease, whereas others experience ulceration (Fig. 23-6), scarring, vascularization, or perforation.[30-33] Retinal vascular tortuosity, ptosis, anisocoria, and exotropia have been observed.[34] Prompt pupillary constriction occurs after instillation of a dilute miotic (e.g., 2.5% methacholine).[35]

Early diagnosis of Riley-Day syndrome will permit routine protective care of the patient's cornea so that complications are minimized. Therapy includes artificial tear solutions, punctal occlusion, and tarsorrhaphy. (Treatment of dry eyes and neurotrophic keratitis is discussed in Chapters 14 and 15, respectively.) Parenteral administration of pilocarpine or neostigmine will increase tear production;[35] however, side effects prevent the therapeutic use of these drugs. General anesthesia is risky in these patients; they are intolerant to thiopental sodium, and they are prone to severe hypotension and cardiac arrest.

Shy-Drager Syndrome

Shy-Drager syndrome is a progressive degenerative disorder of the autonomic nervous system, with onset usually in the sixth or seventh decade of life. Findings include orthostatic hypotension, urinary incontinence, impotence, and decreased sweating. The cornea and conjunctiva may become affected by keratoconjunctivitis sicca. Other eye findings are iris atrophy, convergence insufficiency, anisocoria, and Horner's syndrome.

Other Neurologic Disorders

Neurofibromatosis (von Recklinghausen's disease) is an autosomal dominant disease characterized by multiple neurofibromas, hyperpigmented skin lesions (Fig. 23-7), and other tumors of the central and peripheral nervous systems. Plexiform neuromas can occur in the upper lid, simulating a "bag of worms" (Figs. 23-8 and 23-9). Decreased corneal sensation, sometimes leading to neurotrophic keratitis, can also be seen.

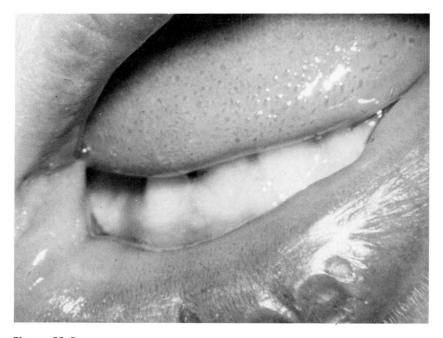

Figure 23-5
Absence of fungiform papillae of the tongue in Riley-Day syndrome.

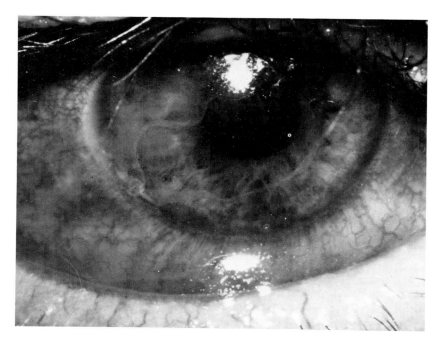

Figure 23-6
Corneal ulcer in a patient with Riley-Day syndrome with severe hypolacrima.

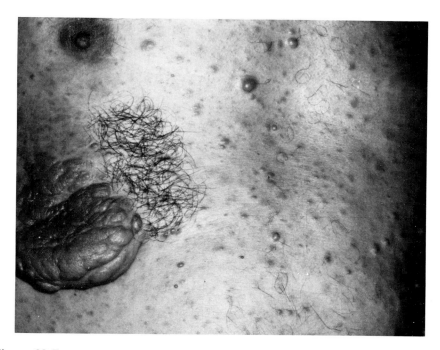

Figure 23-7
Subcutaneous tumors are firm, nodular, and attached to a nerve in neurofibromatosis.

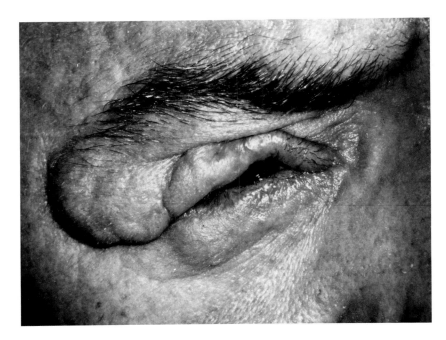

Figure 23-8
Plexiform neuroma of the upper lid in neurofibromatosis.

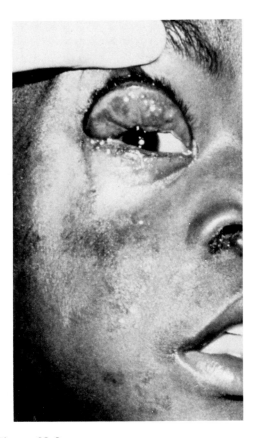

Figure 23-9
Lid involvement in neurofibromatosis.

Myotonic muscular dystrophy is another autosomal dominant disease in which there is slowly progressive muscle weakness. Exposure keratitis can be noted in the inferior cornea. Orbicularis muscle weakness and a poor Bell's phenomenon contribute to the corneal exposure. Multicolored granular cortical opacities can be seen in the lens. Other ocular findings include hypotony, ophthalmoplegia, ptosis, and enophthalmos.

HEREDITARY DISORDERS AFFECTING MULTIPLE ORGAN SYSTEMS

Ehlers-Danlos Syndrome

This syndrome is produced by a group of hereditary disorders and is characterized by hypermobile joints and hyperextensibility of the skin. Ehlers-Danlos type VI, known as the ocular form, is inherited as an autosomal recessive trait and appears to be caused by a deficiency of lysyl hydroxylase, the enzyme responsible for hydroxylation of lysine residues in collagen types I and III. In its absence, cross-linkage of the collagen molecules does not occur. Patients exhibit joint hypermobility, skin hyperextensibility, scoliosis, marfanoid habitus, and aortic rupture. Ocular signs include microcornea, recurrent intraocular bleeding, corneal curvature abnormalities, acute hydrops, sclerocornea, and susceptibility to rupture of the globe.[36] Some patients with similar clinical findings, including keratoglobus, blue sclera, ocular fragility, and mild joint hypermobility, have normal lysyl hydroxylase levels (see Chapter 17).[37-40]

Alport's Syndrome

Alport's syndrome is a hereditary disorder consisting of nephritis and sensorineural deafness. It can be inherited as an autosomal dominant or X-linked trait. Progressive anterior and posterior lenticonus and spherophakia are seen. Subcapsular cataract, macular changes, albipunctate fundus, and optic nerve drusen can also occur.

In one study, 11 of 17 Thai patients with Alport's syndrome had endothelial changes consistent with posterior polymorphous dystrophy.[41] Arcus juvenilis,[42] keratoconus, and pigment dispersion[43] have been noted in some cases. Several corneal ulcers resistant to treatment have also been observed.

Alport's syndrome appears to be related to a mutation of the genes for the α chains of type IV collagen, most commonly α-5. This protein is normally present in basement membranes of the kidney, skin, lung, and eye, including Descemet's membrane, the lens capsule, and the epithelial basement membrane of the ciliary processes.[44] Absence of the α-3, α-4, and α-5 chains has been observed in the anterior lens capsules of patients with Alport's syndrome.[45]

Lowe Oculocerebrorenal Syndrome

Lowe syndrome includes congenital bilateral cataracts, nystagmus, glaucoma, Fanconi's syndrome (aminoaciduria, renal tubular acidosis, hypercalciuria, glucosuria, hypouricemia), mental and psychomotor retardation, oculodigital sign of Franceschetti (ocular manipulation with the hands), hypotonia, and areflexia. The disease is often, but not always, transmitted as a sex-linked recessive trait. Most patients with Lowe syndrome have been fair-haired boys; however, the disease has also been described in females and in a black individual.

Cataracts are found in all patients with Lowe syndrome. The female carrier can have white, punctate, anterior and posterior lens opacities. Congenital glaucoma is present in approximately 60% of patients. A mild haze can occur in the cornea, involving the peripheral stroma.[46] Buphthalmos, stromal vascularization, and scarring can also occur, and exuberant corneal scarring (corneal keloid formation) has been described.[47,48] The cause of the corneal scarring is unclear, but it may be related to oculodigital manipulation or surgical procedures

for glaucoma and cataracts. Iris and retinal abnormalities can also be found.[49]

Rubella can cause both cataracts and glaucoma, but usually not together in the same patient. It would be wise to check the mother of a boy with cataracts and glaucoma.

REFERENCES

1. Tielsch JM, Sommer A: The epidemiology of vitamin A deficiency and xerophthalmia, *Annu Rev Nutr* 4:183, 1984.
2. Fells P, Bors F: Ocular complications of self-induced vitamin A deficiency, *Trans Ophthalmol Soc UK* 89:221, 1969.
3. Olver J: Keratomalacia on a "healthy" diet, *Br J Ophthalmol* 70:357, 1986.
4. Matsuo T et al: Keratomalacia in a child with familial hypo-retinol-binding proteinemia, *Jpn J Ophthalmol* 32:249, 1988.
5. Susan EP et al: Corneal perforation in patients with vitamin A deficiency in the United States, *Arch Ophthalmol* 108:350, 1990.
6. Brooks HL, Driebe WT, Schemmer GG: Xerophthalmia and cystic fibrosis, *Arch Ophthalmol* 108:354, 1990.
7. Paton D: Keratomalacia: a review of its relationship to xerophthalmia and its response to treatment, *Eye Ear Nose Throat Mon* 46:186, 1967.
8. Paton D, McLaren DS: Bitot spots, *Am J Ophthalmol* 50:568, 1960.
9. Sommer A, Sugana T: Corneal xerophthalmia and keratomalacia, *Arch Ophthalmol* 100:404, 1982.
10. Sommer A: *Nutritional blindness: xerophthalmia and keratomalacia*, New York, 1982, Oxford University Press.
11. Smith RS, Farrell T, Bailey T: Keratomalacia, *Surv Ophthalmol* 20:213, 1975.
12. Venkataswamy G: Ocular manifestations of vitamin A deficiency, *Br J Ophthalmol* 51:854, 1967.
13. Sent WL et al: The effect of thermal burns on the release of collagenase from corneas of vitamin A–deficient rats, *Invest Ophthalmol Vis Sci* 19:1461, 1980.
14. Pirie A: Xerophthalmia, *Invest Ophthalmol* 15:417, 1976.
15. Sullivan WR, McCulley JP, Dohlman CH: Return of goblet cells after vitamin A therapy in xerosis of the conjunctiva, *Am J Ophthalmol* 75:720, 1973.
16. Sommer A, Green R, Kenyon KR: Clinical histopathologic correlations of vitamin A responsive and nonresponsive Bitot's spots, *Arch Ophthalmol* 99:2014, 1981.
17. Ganley JP, Payne CM: Clinical and electron microscopic observations of the conjunctiva of adult patients with Bitot's spots, *Invest Ophthalmol Vis Sci* 20:632, 1981.
18. Pfister RR, Renner ME: The corneal and conjunctival surface in vitamin A deficiency: a scanning electron microscope study, *Invest Ophthalmol Vis Sci* 17:874, 1978.

19. Van Horn DL et al: Xerophthalmia in vitamin A deficient rabbits: clinical and ultrastructural alterations in the cornea, *Invest Ophthalmol Vis Sci* 9:1067, 1980.

20. Shams NB et al: Effect of vitamin A deficiency on the adhesion of rat corneal epithelium and the basement membrane complex, *Invest Ophthalmol Vis Sci* 34:2646, 1993.

21. Kruse FE, Tseng SC: Retinoic acid regulates clonal growth and differentiation of cultured limbal and peripheral corneal epithelium, *Invest Ophthalmol Vis Sci* 35:2405, 1994.

22. Hayashi K et al: Stromal degradation in vitamin A–deficient rat cornea: comparison of epithelial abrasion and stromal incision, *Cornea* 9:254, 1990.

23. Shams NB et al: Increased interleukin-1 activity in the injured vitamin A–deficient cornea, *Cornea* 13:156, 1994.

24. Sovani I et al: Response of Bitot's spots to a single oral 100,000- or 200,000-IU dose of vitamin A, *Am J Ophthalmol* 118:792, 1994.

25. Sommer A, Emran N: Topical retinoic acid in the treatment of corneal xerophthalmia, *Am J Ophthalmol* 86:615, 1978.

26. Van Horn DL et al: Topical retinoic acid in the treatment of experimental xerophthalmia in the rabbit, *Arch Ophthalmol* 99:317, 1981.

27. Ubels JL et al: The efficacy of retinoic acid ointment for treatment of xerophthalmia and corneal epithelial wounds, *Curr Eye Res* 4:1049, 1985.

28. Syndenstricker VP et al: The ocular manifestations of ariboflavinosis, *JAMA* 114:2437, 1940.

29. Blumenfeld A et al: Localization of the gene for familial dysautonomia on chromosome 9 and definition of DNA markers for genetic diagnosis, *Nat Genet* 4:160, 1993.

30. Liebman SD: Ocular manifestations of Riley-Day syndrome, *Arch Ophthalmol* 56:719, 1956.

31. Boruchoff SA, Dohlman CH: The Riley-Day syndrome: ocular manifestations in a 35-year-old patient, *Am J Ophthalmol* 63:523, 1967.

32. Dunnington JH: Congenital alacrima in familial autonomic dysfunction, *Arch Ophthalmol* 52:925, 1954.

33. Liebman SD: Riley-Day syndrome, *Arch Ophthalmol* 58:188, 1957.

34. Goldberg MF, Payne JW, Brunt PW: Ophthalmologic studies of familial dysautonomia, *Arch Ophthalmol* 80:732, 1968.

35. Smith AA, Dancis J, Breinin G: Ocular responses to autonomic drugs in familial dysautonomia, *Invest Ophthalmol* 4:358,1965.

36. Cameron J: Corneal abnormalities in Ehlers-Danlos syndrome type VI, *Cornea* 12:54, 1993.

37. Biglan AW, Brown SI, Johnson BC: Keratoglobus and blue sclera, *Am J Ophthalmol* 83:225, 1977.

38. Stein R, Lazar M, Adam A: Brittle cornea: a familial trait associated with blue sclera, *Am J Ophthalmol* 66:67, 1968.

39. Judisch F, Wariri M, Krachmer J: Ocular Ehlers-Danlos syndrome with normal lysyl hydrolase activity, *Arch Ophthalmol* 94:1489, 1976.

40. Royce PM et al: Brittle cornea syndrome: an heritable connective tissue disorder distinct from Ehlers-Danlos syndrome type VI and fragilitas oculi, with spontaneous perforations of the eye, blue sclerae, red hair, and normal collagen lysyl hydroxylation, *Eur J Pediatr* 149:465, 1990.

41. Teekhasainee C et al: Posterior polymorphous dystrophy and Alport syndrome, *Ophthalmology* 98:1207, 1991.

42. Chavis RM, Groshong T: Corneal arcus in Alport's syndrome, *Am J Ophthalmol* 75:793, 1973.

43. Davies PD: Pigment dispersion in a case of Alport's syndrome, *Br J Ophthalmol* 54:557, 1970.

44. Yoshioka K et al: Type IV collagen alpha 5 chain: normal distribution and abnormalities in X-linked Alport syndrome revealed by monoclonal antibody, *Am J Pathol* 144:986, 1994.

45. Cheong HI et al: Immunohistologic studies of type IV collagen in anterior lens capsules of patients with Alport syndrome, *Lab Invest* 70:553, 1994.

46. Wilson WA, Richards W, Donnell GR: Oculocerebral-renal syndrome of Lowe, *Arch Ophthalmol* 70:5, 1963.

47. Cibis GW et al: Corneal keloid in Lowe's syndrome, *Arch Ophthalmol* 100:1795, 1982.

48. Sugar J: *Metabolic disorders of the cornea*. In Kaufman HE et al, editors: *The cornea*, New York, 1988, Churchill Livingstone.

49. Ginsberg J, Bore KE, Fogelson MH: Pathological features of the eye in the oculocerebrorenal (Lowe) syndrome, *J Pediatr Ophthalmol Strabismus* 18:16, 1981.

Twenty-Four

Drugs and Metals

This chapter deals first with the deposition of metals in the conjunctiva and the cornea. Metal-containing therapeutic agents can cause lesions that may aggravate the initial disease. The effect of systemic drugs on the conjunctiva and cornea is also discussed. The adverse effects of topical drugs are reviewed in Chapter 25.

METALS

Gold

Gold can accumulate in the cornea after systemic administration of gold compounds, typically for rheumatoid arthritis.[1-5]* Both oral (e.g., auranofin) and intramuscular (e.g., gold sodium thiomalate or thiosulfate) preparations are used; their mechanism of action is not known.

Gold deposition in the cornea is known as *corneal chrysiasis*. The presence of corneal deposits is related to the total dose of gold, the duration of treatment, and the intensity of gold therapy (total dose/duration of therapy).[3] The density of the deposits is correlated with the duration of treatment but not with the total dose.[3,4] In general, corneal changes are not seen until the total dose exceeds 1 g; the majority of patients receiving a total of more than 1.5 g or more than 25 mg/wk for 6 months will exhibit corneal deposits.[3,4,6] These deposits usually clear within 3 to 5 months after gold therapy is discontinued.

Stromal involvement appears to be most common. Slit-lamp microscopy reveals fine, dustlike, yellow-brown to purple-violet granules that affect mainly the posterior stroma and are denser inferiorly. On transillumination, the cornea can appear purple. Deposition can also occur in the corneal epithelium (Fig. 24-1A). In one large study[4] of patients relatively early in the course of therapy, deposits were seen only in the epithelium. The deposits are usually diffuse and can have a vortex pattern, as in Fabry's disease. In other cases they can be peripheral, or only central, like a Hudson-Stähli line.

Some fine gold granules may also be seen in the conjunctiva.[2] Histologically, the conjuncti-

*The article by Roberts and Wolter[5] contains an excellent illustration of stromal deposits.

val gold deposits are both intracellular and extracellular, found in the epithelium and superficial substantia propria.

Inflammatory corneal reactions can also occur. Marginal ulcerative keratitis (Fig. 24-1) and iritis can be seen, most likely caused by a hypersensitivity reaction to the gold deposits.[7] The keratitis is seen as a white, crescent-shaped ulcer bordering the limbus and associated with conjunctival hyperemia and pain. Infiltration without ulceration can also be seen. This infiltration may start as a flat, distinct, superficial white opacity at one side of the cornea, with no line of normal cornea between the opacity and the sclera. The ulceration and infiltration tend to remain in the anterior layers of the cornea, but they spread from the periphery centrally and along the limbus.

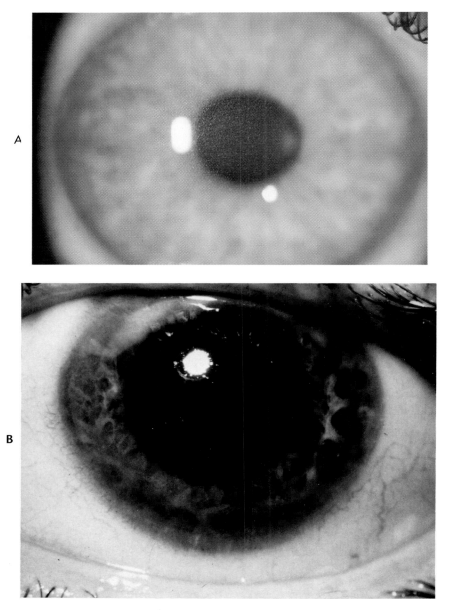

Figure 24-1
A, Corneal chrysiasis. Note the fine gold deposits in the superficial cornea. (Courtesy of Robert D. Deitch Jr, Indianapolis, IN.) **B,** Ulcerative and infiltrative corneal lesion seen in gold therapy for rheumatoid arthritis.

Lens deposition (lenticular chrysiasis) occurs later than corneal deposition, usually after more than 3 years of therapy.[3,8,9] Several patterns of deposition can be seen: fine, diffuse, granular deposits without a purplish hue, on or within the central anterior lens capsule; fine deposits within the anterior embryonic suture lines; flakelike deposits within the central cortex; and diffuse, anterior subcapsular deposits, with or without posterior subcapsular deposits.

The gold deposits in the cornea, conjunctiva, and lens do not interfere with vision and are not an indication to discontinue gold therapy. If keratitis occurs, however, therapy should be stopped. The keratitis heals, but a vascularized scar can remain. Penicillamine therapy also appears to be effective.

Mercury

Chronic exposure to mercury can result in changes in the lens and cornea.[10,11] Exposure can occur through occupational exposure to mercury vapor and mercurial compounds or from chronic topical application of ophthalmic medications containing organomercurial compounds. These compounds serve as antiseptics or preservatives; examples are thimerosal, mercuric oxide, and phenylmercuric nitrate.

Bluish-gray mercurial deposits can be seen around conjunctival blood vessels and in peripheral Descemet's membrane. In rare cases fine, glistening, particulate opacities have been seen in the central corneal stroma. Follicular conjunctivitis, punctate keratitis, subepithelial infiltrates, edema, and vascularization have been reported.[12] Calcific band keratopathy can also develop[13] (Fig. 24-2) (see Chapter 16). Chelation with ethylenediaminetetraacetic acid is effective in removing the mercury deposits.

Mercurialentis consists of a rose-brown or pinkish homogeneous opacity that can involve the whole anterior surface of the lens but sometimes is limited to an anterior subcapsular disk.[14] Phenylmercuric nitrate and acetate penetrate the eye readily and can bind persistently to sulfhydryl groups in the lens. This reaction occurs more readily than with other mercurial antimicrobial preservatives, such as thimerosal. Mercurialentis has not been seen with thimerosal at the normal concentration used in ophthalmic solutions (0.005%).

Thimerosal in contact lens solutions can elicit a delayed hypersensitivity reaction in some patients.[15] Sterile corneal infiltrates (see Chapters 9 and 19), papillary conjunctivitis, and contact lens–induced keratoconjunctivitis may be related to thimerosal hypersensitivity.

Copper

Chalcosis is the term used to describe deposition of copper in tissues. Deposition in the eye most

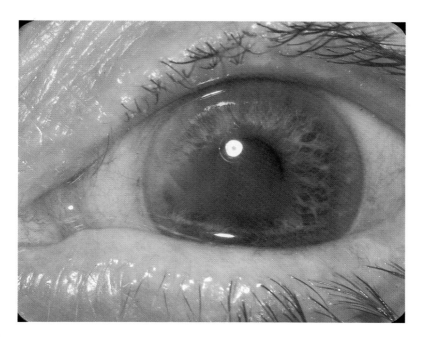

Figure 24-2
Band keratopathy caused by mercurial toxicity (topical use of medication containing phenylmercuric nitrate as a preservative).

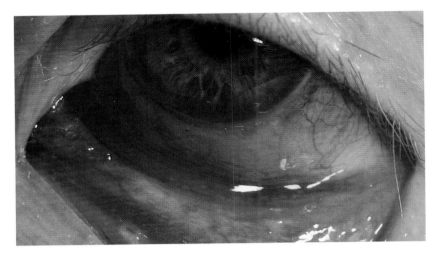

Figure 24-3
Silver pigmentation of the conjunctiva in argyrosis.

commonly results from copper-containing intraocular foreign bodies. Pure copper tends to cause a violent purulent reaction that usually leads to panophthalmitis and loss of the eye. Alloy metals composed of less than 85% copper tend to cause chalcosis.[16]

Copper has an affinity for basement membranes, such as Descemet's membrane and the lens capsule, but deposition can occur in any tissue.[17] Corneal deposition is seen as yellow-brown, red, blue, or green coloration of peripheral Descemet's membrane. The iris can be slightly greenish, the vitreous a yellowish green-blue. Iridescent, multicolored particles are seen beneath the anterior lens capsule and can take on the form of a sunflower.[18]

The deposition of copper in the cornea and lens in systemic diseases, such as Wilson's disease, is described in Chapter 21.

Silver

Argyrosis is the deposition of silver in mucous membranes and skin, usually after long-term use of silver-containing medications. Colloidal silver, silver protein, and silver nitrate are topical antibacterial agents that are used rarely in the United States today but are relatively common in other countries. A silver nitrate compound, Argyrol, was used extensively early in this century. Today ocular argyrosis is usually a result of industrial exposure to organic salts of silver.[19,20]

Similar manifestations occur after both topical and systemic administration. Silver deposition can result in a slate gray discoloration of the conjunctiva (Fig. 24-3), lids, and nasolacri-

mal apparatus.[21-23] The nasal conjunctiva tends to be most affected because of pooling of tears. The cornea can also be affected: Fine blue, gray, green, or gold opacities are found in the deep stroma and Descemet's membrane.[24-26] Iridescent anterior subcapsular lens opacities can also occur.[22]

Histologically, the silver is deposited intracellularly in the substantia propria of the conjunctiva, in the basement membrane of the conjunctival epithelium (Fig. 24-4), in conjunctival vascular endothelium, and in Descemet's membrane[25,27,28] (Fig. 24-5).

The silver deposition rarely interferes with vision and gradually fades after cessation of exposure. If the appearance is unacceptable, the following treatment can reduce the discoloration: A sterile solution containing 6% sodium thiosulfate and 0.25% potassium ferricyanide, prepared within 30 minutes of use, is injected into the skin or subconjunctival tissue.

Iron

Iron deposition, or *siderosis,* can occur either as a result of the presence of an iron-containing foreign body, systemic hemochromatosis, or systemic iron administration, or as a degenerative change in the epithelium (Table 24-1). When iron is released from particles inside the eye, the surrounding tissues develop a rust-brown discoloration, and their function can be impaired. In general, iron-containing particles in the anterior chamber or cornea are better tolerated than those in the posterior segment. In the anterior chamber, iron compounds are slowly released and carried away by the flow of

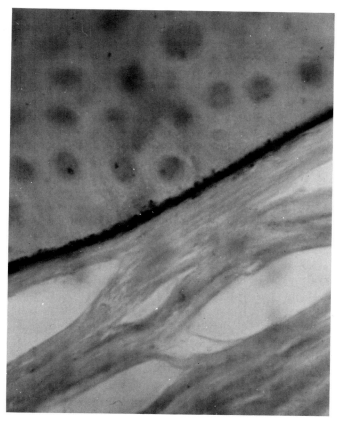

Figure 24-4
Silver impregnation of the epithelial basement membrane in argyrosis.

aqueous, so the deposits affect only the tissues adjacent to the foreign body.

The cornea is seldom discolored by intraocular iron, but it can display a rust-brown color as a result of fine deposits in the deepest layers. These deposits impart a gray and dirty appearance, but on oblique illumination the cornea can appear greenish blue or golden. Histopathologic examination of one case demonstrated iron deposits only within keratocytes, and there was no relationship between siderosome accumulation and cell degeneration.

An iron-containing foreign body buried in the conjunctiva or cornea can lead to localized brownish-red pigmentation of the adjacent tissues (Fig. 24-6). If allowed to remain long enough and if large enough, it can cause more diffuse pigmentation of the cornea by spreading through the epithelium, stroma, and endothelium.[29]

Coats' white ring is a small ring of iron deposition that remains after removal of a superficial corneal metallic foreign body (see Chapter 16).[30,31] It is made up of discrete white dots and

is most common in the interpalpebral area.

After persistent hemorrhage in the anterior chamber, iron deposition can be seen in the posterior stroma (Fig. 24-7). The development of such "corneal blood staining" appears to be related to both the elevation of intraocular pressure and the duration of the hyphema. In a rabbit model the corneal blood staining was uniformly accompanied by endothelial cell injury.[32] After resolution of the hemorrhage, the corneal deposits gradually fade; however, penetrating keratoplasty may be necessary.

Systemic hemochromatosis usually does not involve the cornea.[33,34] Scleral iron deposition can occur and is usually only evident histologically. However, rusty discoloration anterior to the horizontal recti has been noted. Such deposition can rarely occur after numerous blood transfusions or markedly prolonged iron therapy.[35] A bilateral circular pigmented line of the corneal epithelium can be seen in hereditary spherocytosis (Dalgleisch lines).[36]

Iron deposition in the corneal epithelium occurs with aging and with conditions that dis-

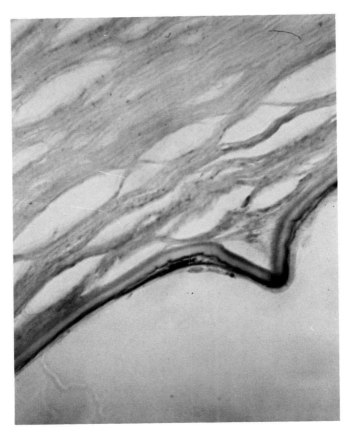

Figure 24-5
Deposition of silver in Descemet's membrane.

Table 24-1	Corneal Iron Deposition		
Condition	**Color**	**Location**	**Pattern**
Hereditary spherocytosis (Dalgleisch line)	Brown	Epithelium	Horizontally oval
Coats' white ring	White	Epithelium, anterior stroma	Small interpalpebral circle
Hudson-Stähli line	Brown	Epithelium	Linear, junction of inferior and middle thirds
Fleischer ring	Brown	Epithelium	Base of cone in keratoconus
Stocker line	Brown	Epithelium	Linear, central to pterygium
Ferry line	Brown	Epithelium	Linear, central to filtering bleb
Blood staining	Yellow-brown-red	Deep stroma	Diffuse, central
Intraocular foreign body	Yellow-brown-red	Deep stroma	Diffuse, central

turb the normal pattern of epithelial migration over the cornea. The typical form of iron deposition is the *Hudson-Stähli line*, which occurs in the majority of patients over 50 years of age.[37] It is seen as a brown, green, yellow, or white irregular horizontal line in the central deep epithelium, at the juncture of the lower and middle thirds of the cornea. Histologically, iron is present in the basal corneal epithelial cells.[38] Such iron deposits can be found in nearly all corneas of any age,[37,38] suggesting that this is a normal, progressive process related to epithelial turnover.

Epithelial iron lines also occur adjacent to

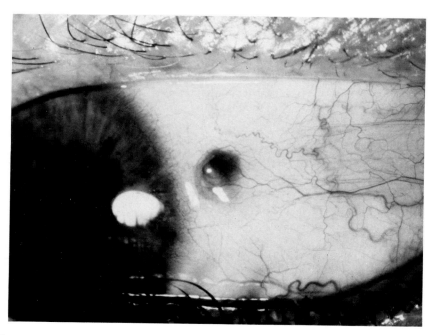

Figure 24-6
Pigmented spot near the limbus caused by a retained subconjunctival metallic (ferrous) foreign body.

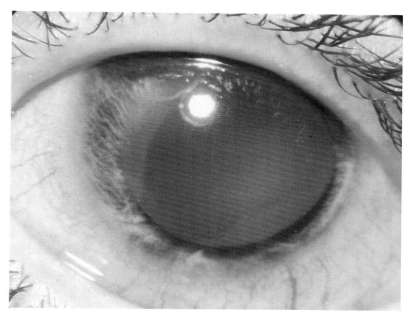

Figure 24-7
Blood staining of cornea.

acute elevations of the corneal surface: central to filtering blebs (Ferry)[39] or pterygia (Stocker),[40] at the base of the cone in keratoconus (Fleischer),[41] around Salzmann's nodules,[42] inside the rim of corneal grafts,[43] and around radial keratotomy incisions and other refractive procedures.[44,45]

SYSTEMIC DRUGS

A wide variety of medications can affect the conjunctiva or cornea when administered systemically. Some of the more common ones are discussed here; others are listed in Table 24-2. Some, such as amiodarone and tilorone, cause

Table 24-2	Systemic Medications that Affect the Cornea and Conjunctiva	
Drug	**Uses**	**Effects**
Adriamycin (doxorubicin)	Malignancy	Nonspecific conjunctivitis, lacrimation, keratitis[20]
Alkylating agents (busulfan, chlorambucil, cyclophosphamide, melphalan)	Malignancy, systemic inflammatory diseases	Blepharoconjunctivitis, dry eye, hyperpigmentation, corneal opacities and edema (nitrosourea)[46]
Aminoquinolones (amodiaquine, chloroquine, hydroxychloroquine)	Malaria, rheumatoid arthritis	Vortex keratopathy, yellow discoloration of the conjunctiva
Amiodarone	Cardiac arrhythmias	Vortex keratopathy, halos, blurred vision
Antacids	Dyspepsia	Band keratopathy (hypercalcemia), bluish discoloration of conjunctiva, corneal deposits[47]
Clofazimine	Leprosy	Reddish pigmentation of the skin and conjunctiva, vortex keratopathy
Cytarabine (Ara-C, cytosine arabinoside)	Malignancy, herpes simplex	Corneal epithelial microcysts, conjunctivitis
Diethylcarbamazine	Filariasis	Punctate keratitis, corneal opacities (related to dead organisms), conjunctivitis
Digoxin	Arrhythmias, heart failure	Corneal edema at very high serum levels[45]
Fluorouracil	Malignancy	Blepharitis, lacrimation, punctal stenosis, cicatricial ectropion, conjunctivitis
Gold-containing compounds	Rheumatoid arthritis	Corneal and lens deposits, keratitis, ulceration
Indomethacin	Antiinflammatory	Conjunctivitis, photosensitivity, edema, vortex keratopathy, superficial punctate keratitis, crystalline deposits
Iron dextran	Iron deficiency	Conjunctival erythema, edema, scleral pigmentation
Methotrexate	Malignancy, systemic inflammatory diseases, psoriasis	Blepharoconjunctivitis, hypopigmentation, hyperpigmentation, lacrimation, dry eye
Naproxen	Antiinflammatory	Vortex keratopathy, ? corneal ulcers
Perhexilene	Arrhythmias	Vortex keratopathy,[48] dry eye
Phenothiazines	Psychosis	Deposits, first on anterior lens surface, then near Descemet's membrane, and only in extreme cases in the epithelium
Phenylbutazone	Antiinflammatory	Peripheral vascularization, corneal opacities, keratitis, scarring, ulceration (?due to lupoid reaction to drug)[12]

Table 24-2 Systemic Medications that Affect the Cornea and Conjunctiva—cont'd

Drug	Uses	Effects
Practolol	Angina, hypertension	Conjunctival inflammation,[49] scarring, keratinization, dry eye,[50] dense yellow or white stromal opacities, ulceration
Quinacrine (Atabrine)	Antimalarial, antihelminthic	Yellow, white, brown, blue, or gray deposits in conjunctiva and cornea
Retinoids (etretinate, isotretinoin)	Psoriasis, acne	Blepharoconjunctivitis, dry eye, fine subepithelial opacities[51]
Suramin	Onchocerciasis, trypanosomiasis	Vortex keratopathy, keratitis
Tamoxifen	Breast carcinoma	Vortex keratopathy
Thioxanthene derivatives (chlorprothixene, thiothixene)	Antipsychotics	Fine particulate corneal deposits, keratitis[12]
Tilorone	Immunoadjuvant, malignancy, graft-versus-host disease	Vortex keratopathy[52]
Vitamin D		Calcium deposits in cornea and conjunctiva

Modified from Curran CCF, Luce JK: *Am J Ophthalmol* 108:709, 1989 and Madrepaerla SA, Johnson M, O'Brien TP: *Am J Ophthalmol* 113:211, 1992.

vortex dystrophy, which is discussed in Chapter 9.

Phenothiazines

Phenothiazines are a group of medications used primarily in the treatment of psychoses. Their action is believed to be related to blockage of dopamine receptors in the central nervous system. The incidence of ocular side effects, which are dose- and drug-dependent, is low. Chlorpromazine is the drug most commonly associated with pigmentary deposits in the eye. The deposits are first seen in the lens as anterior, subcapsular yellow-brown-white dots in the pupillary aperture[53] (Fig. 24-8). In more advanced cases similar deposits can be seen near Descemet's membrane (Fig. 24-9). They tend to involve the interpalpebral cornea and are accompanied by similar granules in the interpalpebral conjunctiva. In extreme cases pigmented streaks or lines can be seen in the interpalpebral corneal epithelium.[54] The distribution of the deposits suggests that exposure to light contributes to their formation.

The deposits in the lens, cornea, and conjunctiva have no adverse effects. They tend to subside slowly with cessation of drug administration.[55]

Aminoquinolones

Chloroquine and hydroxychloroquine are aminoquinolones used as antimalarial agents and in treating rheumatoid arthritis, systemic lupus erythematosus, and other systemic inflammatory diseases. Their major ocular side effect is retinopathy, which can result in permanent visual loss. Ocular toxicity is most common with cloroquine, but it can also occur with hydroxychloroquine. Chronic administration of chloroquine can also produce deposits in the cornea that are visible with the biomicroscope. They are seen as many fine yellowish or white dots in the epithelium.[56-59] At first they may appear as a Hudson-Stähli line or as an increase in an existing iron line, but the most common appearance is as an epithelial vortex. These deposits usually do not disturb the surface of the epithelium. They can also be seen in individuals who work in the manufacturing of chloroquine.

The corneal deposits do no harm and disappear after the medication is discontinued or if the dose is reduced. They are not a contraindication to continued use of the drug, and there appears to be no correlation between corneal deposition and retinopathy.

Similar deposits can be seen with administration of quinacrine, indomethacin,[60] amio-

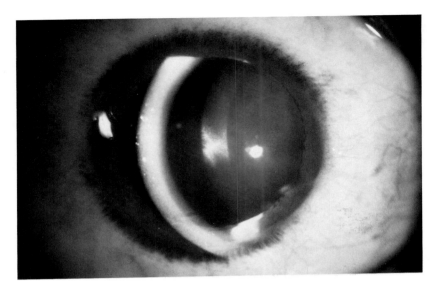

Figure 24-8
Lens deposits resulting from thorazine administration.

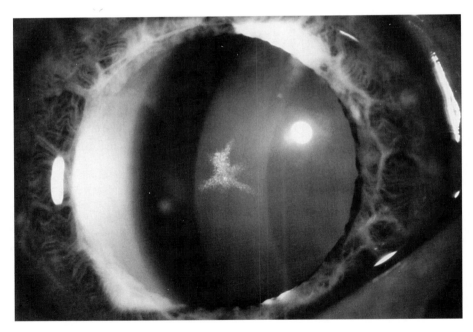

Figure 24-9
Corneal deposits resulting from chlorpromazine administration. (Courtesy of Diane Curtin, Pittsburgh, PA.)

darone (Fig. 24-10),[61,62] naproxen,[63] suramin,[64] tamoxifen, clofazimine,[65] and other medications. Many of the drugs associated with this picture exhibit cationic amphiphilia, and it has been hypothesized that these drugs form complexes with polar intracellular lipids that cannot be metabolized by lysosomal phospholipases.[66,67] The complexes accumulate in the epi-

thelial cells, resulting in a condition similar to Fabry's disease.

Cytarabine

Cytarabine (Ara-C, cytosine arabinoside) is an antimetabolite used in the treatment of leukemias and other malignancies as well as systemic herpes simplex infection. Ocular complications

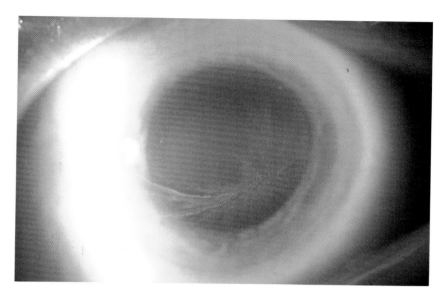

Figure 24-10
Corneal epithelial pigmentation resulting from amiodarone administration.

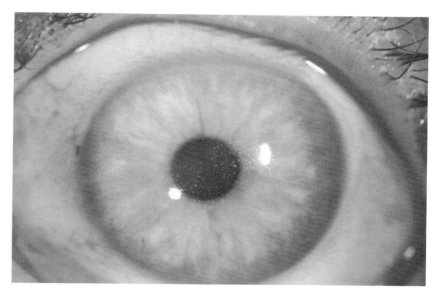

Figure 24-11
Corneal epithelial cysts related to cytarabine therapy.

are common in patients receiving high-dose (> 3 g/m²) chemotherapy. Conjunctivitis and ocular irritation are most common, but corneal epithelial cysts can also occur[68] (Fig. 24-11). These cysts can produce marked photophobia, tearing, and reduced vision. Symptoms usually develop 5 to 7 days after initiation of therapy and reverse 1 to 2 weeks after cessation. The incidence and severity appear to be reduced by

prophylactic use of corticosteroids.[69] In one study 2-deoxycytidine was found to be equally effective, with a theoretically lower risk of complications.[70]

Fluorouracil

Fluorouracil (5-FU) is another antimetabolite used systemically in the treatment of malignancies, particularly carcinoma of the colon, rectum, breast, stomach, and pancreas. It has also been injected subconjunctivally to reduce scar formation after filtering surgery.[71] Systemic administration is associated with excess tearing, conjunctival irritation, occlusion of the lacrimal puncta (Fig. 24-12), and blepharitis.[72,73] In addition, limbal conjunctivitis can occur (Fig. 24-13). Cicatricial ectropion can result from topical administration to the facial skin.[74]

Subconjunctival 5-FU is used to reduce scarring after filtering surgery. It can lead to persistent epithelial defects, subepithelial scarring,

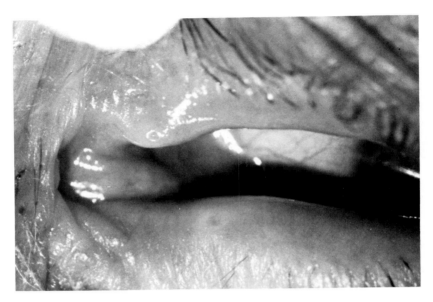

Figure 24-12
Punctal stenosis resulting from systemic administration of 5-fluorouracil.

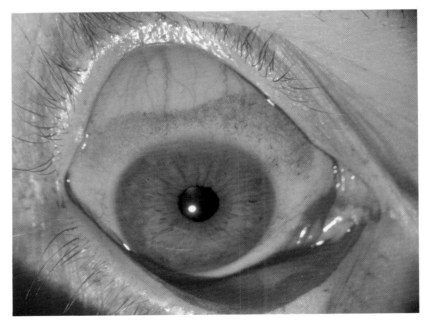

Figure 24-13
Superior limbal staining with rose bengal related to systemic administration of 5-fluorouracil.

and corneal ulceration.[75-77] Experimentally, 5-FU inhibits epithelial wound healing.[78]

Retinoids

Etretinate and isotretinoin are vitamin A–related compounds that are used in the treatment of psoriasis, cystic acne, and other skin disorders. They are commonly associated with blepharoconjunctivitis, dry eyes, and transient blurred vision.[79,80] Fine, round subepithelial opacities have also been observed in the central and peripheral corneas of patients taking these medications.[51] The opacities usually do not interfere with vision.

REFERENCES

1. Hashimoto A et al: Corneal chrysiasis: a clinical study in rheumatoid arthritis receiving gold therapy, *Arthritis Rheum* 15:309, 1972.
2. Kincaid MC et al: Ocular chrysiasis, *Arch Ophthalmol* 100:1791, 1982.
3. McCormick SA et al: Ocular chrysiasis, *Ophthalmology* 92:1432, 1985.
4. Bron AJ, McLendon BF, Camp AV: Epithelial deposition of gold in the cornea in patients receiving systemic therapy, *Am J Ophthalmol* 88:354, 1979.
5. Roberts WH, Wolter JR: Ocular chrysiasis, *Arch Ophthalmol* 56:48, 1956.
6. Hashimoto A et al: Corneal chrysiasis: a clinical study in rheumatoid arthritis patients receiving gold therapy, *Arthritis Rheum* 15:309, 1972.
7. Rodenhäuser JH, von Behrend T: Type 2 incidence of eye involvement after parenteral gold therapy, *Dtsch Med Wochenschr* 94:2389, 1969.
8. Gottlieb NL, Major JC: Ocular chrysiasis correlated with gold concentrations in the crystalline lens during chrysotherapy, *Arthritis Rheum* 21:704, 1978.
9. Weidle EG: Lenticular chrysiasis in oral chrysotherapy, *Am J Ophthalmol* 103:240, 1987.
10. Gourlay JS: Mercurialentis, *Trans Ophthalmol Soc* 74:441, 1954.
11. Locket Z, Nazroo IA: Eye changes following exposure to metallic mercury, *Lancet* 1:528, 1952.
12. Fraunfelder FT: *Drug-induced ocular side effects and drug interactions,* ed 3, Philadelphia, 1989, Lea & Febiger.
13. Kennedy RE, Roca PD, Platt DS: Further observations on atypical band keratopathy in glaucomatous patients, *Trans Am Ophthalmol Soc* 72:107, 1974.
14. Burn RA: Mercurialentis, *Proc R Soc Med* 55:322, 1962.
15. Wilson LA, McNatt J, Reitschel R: Delayed hypersensitivity to thimerosal in soft contact lens wearers, *Ophthalmology* 88:804, 1981.
16. Rao NA, Tso MOM, Rosenthal AR: Chalcosis in the human eye, *Arch Ophthalmol* 94:1379, 1976.
17. Rosenthal AR, Appleton B, Hopkins JL: Intraocular copper foreign bodies, *Am J Ophthalmol* 78:671, 1974.
18. Rao NA, Tso MOM, Rosenthal R: Chalcosis in the human eye, *Arch Ophthalmol* 94:1379, 1976.
19. Moss AP et al: The ocular manifestations and functional effect of occupational argyrosis, *Arch Ophthalmol* 97:906, 1979.
20. Scroggs MW, Lewis JS, Proia AD: Corneal argyrosis associated with silver soldering, *Cornea* 11:264, 1992.
21. Yanoff M, Scheie HG: Argyrosis of the conjunctiva and lacrimal sac, *Arch Ophthalmol* 72:57, 1964.
22. Bartlett RE: Generalized argyrosis with lens involvement, *Am J Ophthalmol* 38:402, 1954.
23. Spencer WH et al: Endogenous and exogenous ocular and systemic silver deposition, *Trans Ophthalmol Soc UK* 100:171, 1980.
24. Weiler HH et al: Argyria of the cornea due to self-administration of eyelash dye, *Ann Ophthalmol* 14:822, 1982.
25. Hanna C, Fraunfelder FT, Sanchez J: Ultrastructural study of argyrosis of the cornea and conjunctiva, *Arch Ophthalmol* 92:18, 1974.
26. Gutman FA, Crosswell HH: Argyrosis of the cornea without clinical conjunctival involvement, *Am J Ophthalmol* 65:183, 1968.
27. Spencer WH et al: Endogenous and exogenous ocular and systemic silver deposition, *Trans Ophthalmol Soc UK* 100:171, 1980.
28. Karcioglu ZA, Caldwell DR: Corneal argyrosis: histologic, ultrastructural and microanalytic study, *Can J Ophthalmol* 20:257, 1985.
29. Zuckerman BD, Lieberman TW: Corneal rust ring, *Arch Ophthalmol* 63:254, 1960.
30. Coats G: Small superficial opaque white rings in the cornea, *Trans Ophthalmol Soc UK* 32:53, 1912.
31. Nevins RC, Davis WH, Elliott JH: Coats' white ring of the cornea: unsettled metal fettle, *Arch Ophthalmol* 80:145, 1968.
32. Gottsch FD et al: Corneal blood staining: an animal model, *Ophthalmology* 93:797, 1986.
33. Cibis PA, Brown EB, Hong SM: Ocular aspects of systemic siderosis, *Am J Ophthalmol* 44:158, 1957.
34. Davies G et al: Deposition of melanin and iron in ocular structures in haemochromatosis, *Br J Ophthalmol* 56:338, 1972.
35. Salminen L, Paasio P, Ekfors T: Epibulbar siderosis induced by iron tablets, *Am J Ophthalmol* 93:660, 1982.
36. Dalgleisch R: Ring-like corneal deposits in a case of congenital spherocytosis, *Br J Ophthalmol* 49:40, 1965.
37. Gass JD: The iron lines of the superficial cornea, *Arch Ophthalmol* 71:348, 1964.
38. Barraquer-Somers E, Chan CC, Green WR: Corneal epithelial iron deposition, *Ophthalmology* 90:729, 1983.
39. Ferry AP: A new iron line of the superficial cornea, *Arch Ophthalmol* 79:142, 1968.

40. Stocker FW: Eine pigmentierte hornhautline bei pterygium, *Schweiz Med Wochenschr* 20:19, 1939.

41. Fleischer B: Über keratoconus und eigenartige figuren bildung in der cornea, *Munchen Med Wochenschr* 53:625, 1906.

42. Reinach NW, Baum J: A corneal pigmented line associated with Salzmann's nodular degeneration, *Am J Ophthalmol* 91:677, 1981.

43. Mannis MJ: Iron deposition in the corneal graft, *Arch Ophthalmol* 101:1858, 1983.

44. Koenig SB et al: Corneal lines after refractive keratoplasty, *Arch Ophthalmol* 101:1862, 1983.

45. Seiler T, Holschbach A: Central corneal iron deposit after photorefractive keratectomy, *Ger J Ophthalmol* 2:143, 1993.

46. Kapp JP et al: Limitations of high dose intra-arterial 1,3- bis(2-chloroethyl)-1 nitrosourea (BCNU) chemotherapy for malignant gliomas, *Neurosurgery* 10:715, 1982.

47. Fischer FP: Bismuthiase secondaire de la cornee, *Ann Oculist (Paris)* 183:615, 1950.

48. Gibson JM et al: Severe ocular side effects of perhexilene maleate: case report, *Br J Ophthalmol* 68:553, 1984.

49. Garner A, Rahi AHS: Practolol and ocular toxicity: antibodies in serum and tears, *Br J Ophthalmol* 60:684, 1976.

50. Wright P: Untoward effects associated with practolol administration: oculomucocutaneous syndrome, *Br Med J* 1:595, 1975.

51. Fraunfelder FT, LaBraico JM, Meyer SM: Adverse ocular reactions possibly associated with isotretinoin, *Am J Ophthalmol* 100:534, 1985.

52. Weiss JN, Weinberg RS, Regelson W: Keratopathy after oral administration of tilorone hydrochloride, *Am J Ophthalmol* 89:46, 1980.

53. McClanahan WS et al: Ocular manifestations of chronic phenothiazine derivative administration, *Arch Ophthalmol* 75:319, 1966.

54. Johnson AW, Buffaloe WJ: Chlorpromazine epithelial keratopathy, *Arch Ophthalmol* 76:664, 1966.

55. Lal S et al: Replacement of chlorpromazine with other neuroleptics: effect on abnormal skin pigmentation and ocular changes, *J Psychiatr Neurosci* 18:173, 1993.

56. Bernstein HN: Chloroquine ocular toxicity, *Surv Ophthalmol* 12:415, 1967.

57. Carr RE et al: Ocular toxicity of antimalarial drugs, *Am J Ophthalmol* 66:738, 1968.

58. Lawwill T, Appleton B, Alstatt L: Chloroquine accumulation in human eyes, *Am J Ophthalmol* 65:530, 1968.

59. Jeddi A et al: The cornea and synthetic antimalarials, *J Fr Ophtalmol* 17:36, 1994.

60. Burns DA: Indomethacin, reduced retinal sensitivity, and corneal deposits, *Am J Ophthalmol* 66:825, 1968.

61. Kaplan LJ, Cappaert WE: Amiodarone keratopathy, *Arch Ophthalmol* 100:601, 1982.

62. Wilson FM, Schmitt TE, Grayson M: Amiodarone-induced cornea verticillata, *Ann Ophthalmol* 12:657, 1980.

63. Szmyd L, Perry HD: Keratopathy associated with the use of naproxen, *Am J Ophthalmol* 99:598, 1985.

64. Teich SA et al: Toxic keratopathy associated with suramin therapy, *N Engl J Med* 314:1455, 1986.

65. Walinder PE, Gip L, Stempa M: Corneal changes in patients treated with clofazimine, *Br J Ophthalmol* 60:526, 1976.

66. Lullman H, Lullmann-Rauch R, Wassermann O: Lipidosis induced by amphiphilic cationic drugs, *Biochem Pharmacol* 27:1103, 1978.

67. D'Amico DJ, Kenyon KR: Drug-induced lipidoses of the cornea and conjunctiva, *Int Ophthalmol* 4:67, 1981.

68. Hopen G et al: Corneal toxicity with systemic cytarabine, *Am J Ophthalmol* 91:500, 1981.

69. Lass J et al: Topical corticosteroid therapy for corneal toxicity from systemically administered cytarabine, *Am J Ophthalmol* 94:617, 1982.

70. Lazarus HM et al: Comparison of the prophylactic effects of 2-deoxycytidine and prednisolone for high-dose intravenous cytarabine-induced keratitis, *Am J Ophthalmol* 104:476, 1987.

71. Heuer DK et al: 5-Fluorouracil and glaucoma filtering surgery: III. Intermediate follow-up of a pilot study, *Ophthalmology* 93:1537, 1986.

72. Caravella LP, Burns JA, Zangmeister M: Punctal-canalicular stenosis related to systemic fluorouracil therapy, *Arch Ophthalmol* 99:284, 1981.

73. Imperia PS, Lazarus HM, Lass JH: Ocular complications of systemic cancer chemotherapy, *Surv Ophthalmol* 34:209, 1989.

74. Galentine P et al: Bilateral cicatricial ectropion following topical administration of 5-fluorouracil, *Ann Ophthalmol* 13:575, 1981.

75. Knapp A et al: Serious corneal complications of glaucoma filtering surgery with postoperative 5-fluorouracil, *Am J Ophthalmol* 103:183, 1987.

76. Shapiro MS et al: 5-Fluorouracil toxicity to the ocular surface epithelium, *Invest Ophthalmol Vis Sci* 26:580, 1985.

77. Capone A et al: In vivo effects of 5-FU on ocular surface epithelium following corneal wounding, *Invest Ophthalmol Vis Sci* 28:1661, 1987.

78. Ando H et al: Inhibition of corneal epithelial wound healing: a comparative study of mitomycin C and 5-fluorouracil, *Ophthalmology* 99:1809, 1992.

79. Mathers WD et al: Meibomian gland morphology and tear osmolarity: changes with Accutane therapy, *Cornea* 10:286, 1991.

80. Lerman S: Ocular side effects of Accutane therapy, *Lens Eye Toxic Res* 9:428, 1992.

Twenty-Five

Toxic and Allergic Reactions to Topical Ophthalmic Medications

*Fred M. Wilson II, MD**

TOXIC REACTIONS
Toxic Papillary Keratoconjunctivitis
Toxic Papillary Keratoconjunctivitis with
    Scarring (Pseudopemphigoid)
Toxic Follicular Conjunctivitis
Toxic Follicular Conjunctivitis with
    Scarring (Pseudotrachoma)
Anesthetic Toxicity
Toxic Calcific Band-Shaped Keratopathy

ALLERGIC REACTIONS
Allergic Contact Dermatoconjunctivitis
Anaphylactoid Blepharoconjunctivitis

MISCELLANEOUS REACTIONS

RECOVERY FROM DRUG REACTIONS

PREVENTION OF DRUG REACTIONS

*Professor of Ophthalmology, Director, Cornea and External Ocular Disease Service, Indiana University School of Medicine, Department of Ophthalmology, 702 Rotary Circle, Indianapolis, IN 46202.

Toxic and allergic reactions to topical ophthalmic medications are common and troublesome. They are second in frequency only to keratoconjunctivitis sicca among all external ocular diseases.[1]

Toxicity is the result of direct chemical irritation of tissues by drugs or preservatives. *Allergy* requires sensitization to and induction of ocular inflammation by the patient's immune system. Contrary to widespread belief, toxic reactions are much more common than allergic ones, the former accounting for about 90% of all reactions (Table 25-1).

TOXIC REACTIONS

Toxic Papillary Keratoconjunctivitis
Toxic papillary keratoconjunctivitis is the most common of all adverse reactions to topical medications (Table 25-1). It results from the ability of certain medications to be irritating simply by being applied repeatedly to the ocular surface. The toxic effects usually take at least 2 weeks to develop.

Punctate staining, more prominent with rose bengal red than with fluorescein, is the most common finding. The staining is usually most pronounced on the inferonasal conjunctiva and cornea (Fig. 25-1), where medications gravitate on their way to the lacrimal outflow system. Worsening of preexisting corneal staining can occur, even before the typical inferonasal staining, if corneal surface disease precedes development of the drug reaction (Fig. 25-2). Rarely, ointments are trapped beneath the upper eyelid, producing staining along the upper limbus. Medications toxic to the epithelium can also cause, or inhibit the healing of, chronic epithelial defects of the cornea, sometimes producing pseudodendrites or pseudo-geographic ulcers, which can be mistaken for herpes simplex keratitis[1,2] (Fig. 25-3).

Other signs include hyperemia, nonspecific papillary conjunctivitis, and scant mucoid or mucopurulent discharge. Itching is absent, and eosinophils are not seen in conjunctival scrapings.

The main causes of toxic papillary reactions

Table 25-1	Relative Frequencies of Various Types of Adverse Reactions to Topical Ophthalmic Medications[1]	
Type of Reaction		**Relative Frequency (%)**
TOXIC REACTIONS		90
Toxic papillary reactions		76
Toxic follicular reactions		9
Toxic calcific band keratopathy		2
Pseudopemphigoid		2
Pseudotrachoma		1
ALLERGIC REACTIONS		10
Allergic contact reactions		10
Anaphylactoid reactions		Very rare

(see box on p. 672) are aminoglycoside antibiotics, antiviral agents, and the preservative benzalkonium chloride. Benzalkonium is an especially common offender because it is one of the most frequently used preservatives (in concentrations from 0.004% to 0.02%) and because it is a surfactant with detergent-like properties. Damage to corneal epithelium occurs even at the lower concentrations.[1-3]

The factors that predispose to toxic papillary reactions include keratoconjunctivitis sicca, other ocular surface problems, prolonged use of medications, and the use of multiple preparations. The dry eye is especially susceptible, so even relatively nontoxic preservatives, such as chlorobutanol, can cause toxicity. The major problem is that benzalkonium is still present in several artificial-tear preparations, and dry eyes in patients who use such tears often are made worse by them sooner or later. These difficulties have led to the advent of an artificial tear solution (Tear Naturale II, Alcon Laboratories, Fort Worth, TX) with a preservative that is presumably nontoxic to epithelial cells; artificial tears and contact lens solutions that are preserved with sorbic acid or sorbate (also thought to be nontoxic); preservative-free tears such as Refresh (Allergan, Irvine, CA), Refresh Plus (Cellufresh) (Allergan, Irvine, CA), Celluvisc (Allergan, Irvine, CA), Hypotears PF (CIBA Vision Ophthalmics, Duluth, GA), Tears Naturale Free

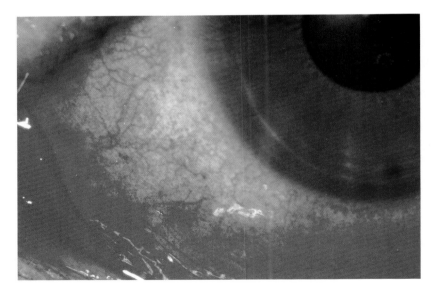

Figure 25-1
Characteristic punctate staining, with rose bengal red, of the inferonasal bulbar conjunctiva in a patient with toxic papillary keratoconjunctivitis secondary to neomycin. Such staining occurs in association with toxic reactions to many other drugs and preservatives and several other types of medication-induced toxicities and allergies. Similar but usually less impressive staining can be seen with fluorescein.

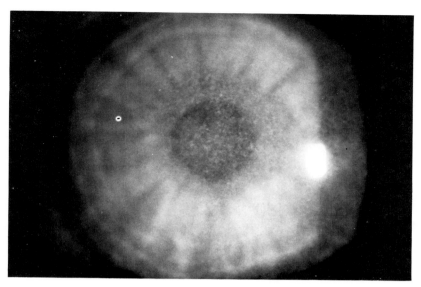

Figure 25-2
Toxic keratitis secondary to neomycin. Extensive punctate staining of the cornea, in this case with fluorescein, can precede or develop in conjunction with the typical inferonasal staining of toxic papillary keratoconjunctivitis (and other medication-induced reactions) when preexisting ocular surface disease, such as keratoconjunctivitis sicca, is present. Such corneal staining develops eventually, even in the absence of predisposing surface disease.

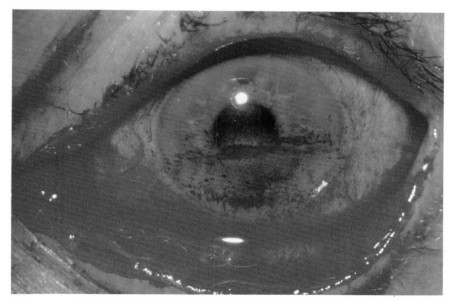

Figure 25-3
Chronic epithelial defect of the cornea secondary to neomycin toxicity (rose bengal red stain). Such toxic epithelial defects are often mistaken for herpes simplex dendrites or geographic ulcers. The toxic lesions have relatively smooth and rolled-under edges and change very little with time, whereas herpetic defects have finely irregular edges and change their shapes fairly rapidly. Note also the drug-induced staining of the inferonasal bulbar conjunctiva.

(Alcon Laboratories, Fort Worth, TX), and Bion Tears (Alcon Laboratories, Fort Worth, TX), which are dispensed in small, sterile, "unit dose" containers; and preservative-free lubricating ointments (Hypotears, CIBA Vision Ophthalmics, Duluth, GA, and Refresh PM, Allergan, Irvine, CA).

The mainstay of treatment of toxic papillary reactions, and virtually all other reactions, is the withdrawal of offending medications and preservatives. Preservative-free artificial tears or

---

Main Causes of Toxic Papillary Reactions

AMINOGLYCOSIDE ANTIBIOTICS
  Neomycin
  Gentamicin
  Tobramycin
NEARLY ALL "CONCENTRATED" OR "FORTIFIED" ANTIBIOTICS AND ANTIFUNGAL AGENTS
ANTIVIRAL AGENTS
  Idoxuridine
  Vidarabine
  Trifluorothymidine*
TOPICAL ANESTHETIC AGENTS
  Proparacaine
  Tetracaine
PRESERVATIVES†
  Benzalkonium

---

*Trifluorothymidine is the least toxic of the three antiviral agents.
†Chlorobutanol is occasionally toxic to the dry eye.

---

lubricants may be prescribed if necessary. Topical corticosteroids are of no value (and are usually preserved with benzalkonium). Patching or therapeutic soft contact lenses are sometimes helpful for treating chronic epithelial defects or keratopathy.

Toxic Papillary Keratoconjunctivitis with Scarring (Pseudopemphigoid)

Prolonged and severe toxic papillary reactions can lead to conjunctival scarring or keratinization, worse below inferior conjunctivitis, producing a clinical picture that mimics cicatricial pemphigoid (Fig. 25-4). Corneal pannus can also develop. This kind of reaction is probably most often the result of longstanding and severe toxic papillary keratoconjunctivitis, although evidence exists that type-III (antigen-antibody-mediated) hypersensitivity might play a role in some cases.[4,5] Progression ceases when the causative medications are discontinued.

Pseudopemphigoid is usually caused by the long-term use of glaucoma medications, perhaps because of the chronicity of their use (see box on p. 673).

Toxic Follicular Conjunctivitis

Although the exact mechanism by which toxic follicular conjunctivitis develops is uncertain, it is presumed to be toxic rather than allergic.[1] Itching, eczematoid dermatitis, eosinophils in conjunctival scrapings, and positive cutaneous patch tests are all absent unless the patient also

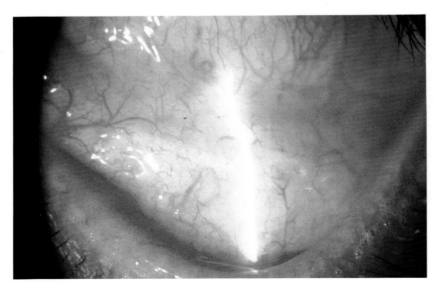

Figure 25-4
Pseudopemphigoid from the chronic use of dipivalyl epinephrine. Note conjunctival scarring and cicatricial foreshortening of the inferior conjunctival fornix.

happens to react allergically to the causative drug. Even ocular hyperemia and punctate staining are often, but not invariably, lacking or unimpressive: these findings, too, if present, can indicate superimposed toxic papillary or allergic reactions. The toxic follicular response itself probably results from the ability of certain drugs to act as nonantigenic mitogens (as do, for example, phytohemagglutinin and pokeweed mitogen) to induce mitoses and lymphoblastic transformations of lymphocytes by nonimmunologic means.

Toxic follicular reactions come about slowly, usually requiring at least several weeks, and sometimes years, to develop. Follicular conjunctivitis is the main finding (Fig. 25-5). This represents a proliferation of subepithelial conjunctival lymphocytes. True lymphoid follicles, with germinal centers containing lymphoblasts, are present[1] (Fig. 25-6). The folli-

cles are most prominent in the lower fornix and the inferior palpebral conjunctiva but can occur at the limbus, in the superior palpebral conjunctiva, and in the semilunar fold. As mentioned previously, hyperemia and punctate staining are usually mild, if present at all. The same is true of mucoid or mucopurulent discharge. The exudate seldom shows any purulence clinically, although a few neutrophils sometimes can be found in conjunctival scrapings.

The causes of toxic follicular conjunctivitis are shown in the box below. No preservatives

---

Antiglaucoma Agents: Main Causes of Drug-Induced Pseudopemphigoid*

Echothiophate
Epinephrine
Dipivalyl epinephrine
Pilocarpine

Some of these reactions, especially those caused by epinephrine or dipivalyl epinephrine, may have associated type-III hypersensitivity and so may not be purely toxic.

Causes of Drug-Induced Toxic Follicular Conjunctivitis*

ANTIVIRAL AGENTS
Idoxuridine
Vidarabine
Trifluorothymidine
ANTIGLAUCOMA AGENTS
Pilocarpine
Echothiophate
Epinephrine
Dipivalyl epinephrine
Carbachol
CYCLOPLEGIC AGENTS
Atropine
Homatropine

With prolonged use, these drugs can cause conjunctival scarring, producing a pseudotrachoma syndrome.

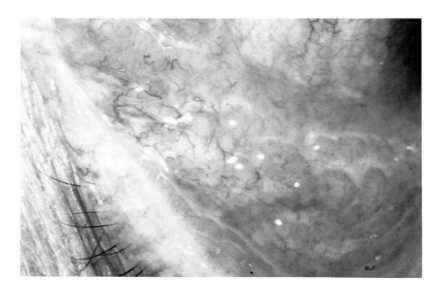

Figure 25-5
Toxic follicular conjunctivitis caused by topical dipivalyl epinephrine. Similar reactions can be produced by epinephrine itself, antiviral agents, miotic drugs, and certain cycloplegic agents (atropine and homatropine).

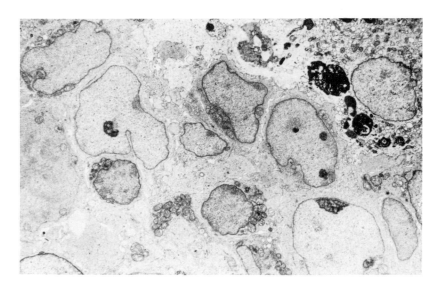

Figure 25-6
Electron microscopy of the germinal center of the dipivalyl epinephrine-induced follicle from the patient shown in Figure 25-5. That this is a true lymphoid follicle is indicated by the presence of the large, pale lymphoblasts with prominent nuclei (and often nucleoli) and the dark, irregular "tingible bodies" (*upper right*). *Tingible bodies* are macrophages that have engulfed nuclear material and are evidence of follicular maturity. As is also characteristic of lymphoid follicles, masses of lymphocytes (produced by the metabolically active lymphoblasts) were found more peripherally (not shown here). (Original magnification, ×3000.) (From Wilson FM II: *Trans Am Ophthalmol Soc* 81:854, 1983.)

are known to produce follicular reactions, and only a few specific drugs do so. Although various drugs and preservatives cause toxic papillary reactions in susceptible individuals, only the drugs listed in the box are known to induce follicles.

The factors that predispose to toxic follicular conjunctivitis are prolonged use of one of the causative drugs and individual susceptibility. Some evidence suggests that the use of old or outdated medications that have undergone deterioration might also predispose to the problem.[6]

The best treatment is withdrawal of the drug that is causing the reaction. Occasionally, substitution of a new and fresh preparation of the same drug can be helpful. Topical corticosteroid slows but does not prevent the development of the follicular hypertrophy and would hardly ever be useful as treatment except, perhaps, as a temporizing measure. Of course, simple observation, with continuation of the offending drug, is permissible if the drug is needed and the symptoms are not severe.

Toxic Follicular Conjunctivitis with Scarring (Pseudotrachoma)
Longstanding toxic follicular conjunctivitis can lead to conjunctival scarring and corneal pan-

nus, producing (with the follicles) a *pseudotrachoma* syndrome (Fig. 25-7). Even preauricular lymphadenopathy can be present, representing lymphocytic hypertrophy in the regional lymph node. Punctal occlusion can occur in the absence of other evidence of conjunctival scarring. Molluscum contagiosum of the eyelid margin is another cause of pseudotrachoma.

Anesthetic Toxicity
Toxic keratoconjunctivitis secondary to the abuse of topical anesthetic agents is an uncommon but potentially severe problem. It is primarily a particularly severe form of toxic papillary keratoconjunctivitis, although it has some features of its own that warrant consideration as a separate entity.

Chronic use of a topical anesthetic is extremely toxic to epithelial microvilli, organelles, and desmosomes (intercellular bridges), and to cellular metabolism, mitosis, and migration.[2] The loss of microvilli causes instability of the tear film, adding to the drying and neurotrophic keratopathy that result from the loss of corneal sensation. Some of the inflammation might be secondary to a superimposed antibody-mediated reaction.

Anesthetic toxicity develops within a few days to weeks. The ability of the drug to relieve

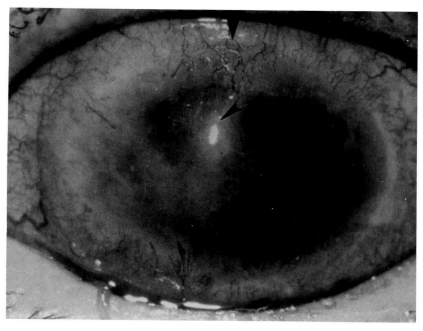

Figure 25-7
Pseudotrachoma secondary to idoxuridine. Note the corneal pannus (*large arrow*) and corneal infiltrate (*small arrow*). Although the infiltrate is probably of herpetic origin, it is often uncertain whether corneal vascularization is secondary to drug toxicity or to underlying disease. Associated conjunctival follicles and scarring, which were clearly drug induced, combined to create a trachoma-like picture.

pain is short-lived, so the patient soon begins to use it more frequently (often every few minutes), with progressively less relief or response and more rebound pain as the effect of the drop wears off. Patients who abuse topical anesthetics sometimes have psychologic or psychiatric problems and continually gain access to the drug on their own, although physicians are occasionally at fault for providing the medication.

Clinical manifestations can include severe ocular pain, lid swelling, hyperemia, mucopurulent discharge, extensive punctate staining, chronic epithelial defects of the cornea, Wessely-immune ringlike or disciform stromal infiltrates, corneal edema, superficial or deep corneal vascularization, and iridocyclitis with keratic precipitates (Fig. 25-8). The corneal stroma does not show ulceration or necrosis as often occurs with bacterial, fungal, or acanthamoebic corneal ulcers, and corneal cultures are negative or noncontributory. Hypopyon and hyphema have also developed secondary to anesthetic toxicity.

Treatment of anesthetic abuse requires stopping the drug and substituting other means for relieving pain and encouraging healing, such as cycloplegia, patching, therapeutic soft contact lenses, or systemic analgesic agents. Topical corticosteroids can reduce pain and inflammation to some extent. Hospitalization and psychiatric consultation are occasionally advisable.

Toxic Calcific Band-Shaped Keratopathy

Medications preserved with phenylmercuric nitrate, such as sulfisoxazole diolamine and, in the past, certain preparations of pilocarpine, can cause deposition of calcium in the cornea (Fig. 25-9) and mercury in the lens.[2,7,8] The preservative is believed to damage protein in the superficial corneal stroma, so the calcium is then deposited as a degenerative change.[9] The mercury itself accumulates in the anterior lens capsule (mercurialentis).[10] A closely related preservative, phenylmercuric acetate, can also cause mercurialentis but not band keratopathy.[10] These deposits appear only after months or years of exposure to the mercurial preservatives.[2]

Unlike other forms of calcific band keratopathy, the preservative-induced form sometimes begins centrally rather than peripherally. Eventually, the calcium extends as a horizontal band across the interpalpebral zone of the cornea. The deposits lie superficially in Bowman's layer. Mercurialentis appears as a circular, pink to

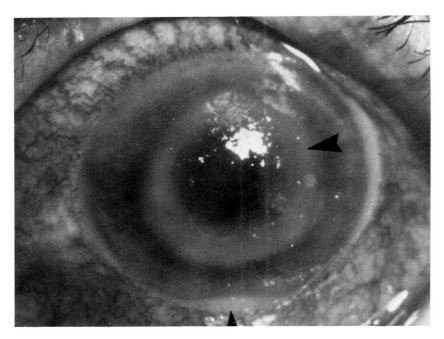

Figure 25-8
Keratitis caused by abuse of topical proparacaine. Hyperemia, chronic epithelial defect, stromal edema surrounded by a Wessely-immune ringlike infiltrate (*large arrow*), and small hypopyon (*small arrow*) without stromal ulceration or necrosis can be seen. (Courtesy of Merrill Grayson, Indianapolis, IN.)

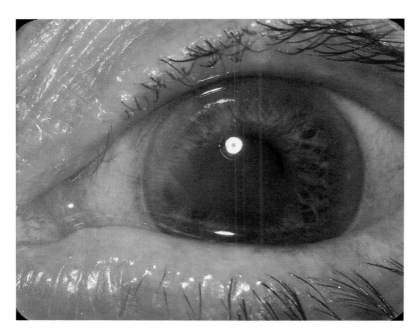

Figure 25-9
Toxic calcific band-shaped keratopathy induced by a phenylmercuric nitrate preservative in pilocarpine eye drops.

rose-brown dusting of the central anterior lens capsule.

The band keratopathy can be removed by debridement and chelation therapy as is used for other forms of calcific band keratopathy. Obviously, use of the medication containing the phenylmercuric preservative should be discontinued.

ALLERGIC REACTIONS

Allergic Contact Dermatoconjunctivitis

Allergic contact dermatoconjunctivitis is the second most common type of drug reaction (see Table 25-1).[1] Allergic contact reactions occur after sensitization of thymus-derived lymphocytes (T cells) in the regional lymph nodes and represent type-IV (delayed) hypersensitivity. Topical medications act as haptens (partial antigens) and must combine with tissue proteins to form complete antigens that can sensitize lymphocytes in nearby lymph nodes. The lymphocytes then return to the site of application and accumulation of the medication, combine with the drug-protein antigen, and produce inflammation by releasing various lymphokines.

These reactions usually take weeks to years to develop, depending on the amount of hapten applied, the degree of its penetrability, and the extent to which it is a sensitizer.[2] However, allergic contact reactions can appear in as little as 48 hours if the patient has been sensitized previously to the drug involved.

The only important predisposing factor, other than individual susceptibility and the prolonged use of medication, is the presence of preexisting cutaneous disease of the eyelids, which permits enhanced penetration of the hapten. It should be remembered that cross-sensitization to similar haptens is to be expected. For example, a patient who is allergic to one aminoglycoside antibiotic will probably react to any of the other ones.

The hallmark of this kind of reaction is eczematoid blepharitis and periocular dermatitis (Fig. 25-10). If the cause is an eye drop, the eczema begins at the nasal aspect of the lower eyelid (where drugs first spill onto the skin [Fig. 25-11]). The dermatitis is preceded by generalized hyperemia of the conjunctiva and the same findings as occur with toxic papillary reactions and can finally spread extensively to affect the upper eyelid, the temporal and malar regions, and the cheek. If the cause is an ointment or a nonophthalmic substance such as a cosmetic, the eczema appears first wherever the

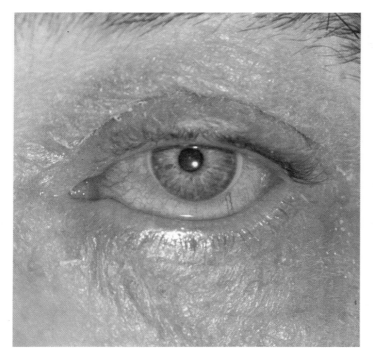

Figure 25-10
Periocular cutaneous eczema of allergic contact dermatoconjunctivitis secondary to idoxuridine.

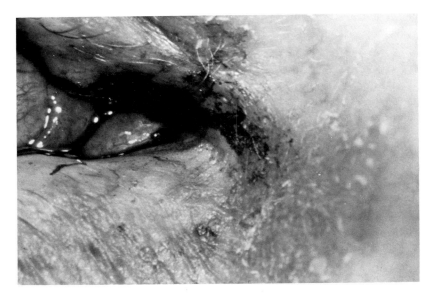

Figure 25-11
Early allergic contact dermatoconjunctivitis affects the skin of the medial canthal area and the inferonasal eyelid. This example was caused by dipivalyl epinephrine. Rose bengal red stain has been instilled (appears black).

hapten has been applied (e.g., the upper eyelid), and the eye itself can be uninflamed. Itching is prominent, and eosinophils are present in conjunctival scrapings in about 25% of cases because the sensitized lymphocytes can produce an eosinophil chemotactic factor.[1,2] Rarely, contact allergy can be associated with marginal corneal infiltration and ulceration.[2,11,12]

The most common causes of allergic contact dermatoconjunctivitis are shown in the box at the right. Thimerosal use (in contact lens care solutions) is often associated with and may be at least partially responsible for a specific clinical syndrome (*contact lens–induced keratoconjunctivitis,* see Chapter 8) seen in people who wear contact lenses. Severe inflammation of the conjunctiva and cornea can occur, but there is seldom any dermatitis, probably because insufficient amounts of the preservative are present in and on the contact lens to result in any significant spillover to the skin. Nevertheless, a type-IV allergic contact reaction may be responsible.

Secondary infection of eczematoid dermatitis, usually by *Staphylococcus* or *Streptococcus* and less often by *Candida,* is not uncommon.[2,13] Any of these organisms alone can cause spreading eczema, with or without a preexisting drug allergy. Such infectious eczematoid dermatitis should be suspected whenever cutaneous ulcerations are present in the affected skin; when rel-

Main Causes of Drug-Induced Allergic Contact Reactions

AMINOGLYCOSIDE ANTIBIOTICS
  Neomycin
  Gentamicin
  Tobramycin
ANTIVIRAL AGENTS
  Idoxuridine
  Vidarabine
  Trifluorothymidine (rarely)
CYCLOPLEGIC AGENTS
  Atropine
  Homatropine
GLAUCOMA AGENTS
  Apraclonidine
  Dorzolamide
PRESERVATIVES OR OTHER ADDITIVES
  Thimerosal*
  Chlorhexidine*
  Edetate (EDTA)

*Thimerosal and (very rarely) chlorhexidine cause contact allergy almost exclusively in people who wear contact lenses.

atively remote areas such as the nose, forehead, lower face, or neck are involved; or when the eczema fails to clear after the supposedly causative drug is withdrawn. Patients with atopic eczema are highly susceptible to both drug-induced and infectious eczematoid reactions.

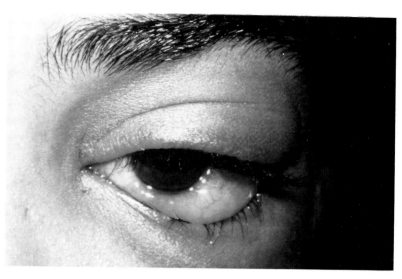

Figure 25-12
Anaphylactoid blepharoconjunctivitis. Note erythema and angioedema of the eyelids, as well as conjunctival edema (chemosis).

Once the skin is broken down, even poorly sensitizing drugs can induce contact allergy; this type of reaction should be treated by stopping all topical medications whenever possible. Cool compresses may be used for relief of discomfort. Contact allergy does respond well to topical corticosteroids, but I prefer not to prescribe them because secondary infection may develop, and some of the ingredients (or even the steroid itself[14-16]) could possibly lead to further contact reactions. If infection is unlikely, I sometimes apply a topical steroid ointment once to the affected skin, in the office only; this approach can achieve considerable and rapid relief while avoiding the risks of ongoing treatment. Any suspicion of infection is a reason to take cultures (or at least scrapings) and perhaps to prescribe appropriate oral antibiotic therapy.

Anaphylactoid Blepharoconjunctivitis

Anaphylactoid reactions to topical ophthalmic medications are rare. I have seen only six cases in the past 27 years.

These reactions are mediated by previously formed IgE humoral antibodies (type I, immediate hypersensitivity). Patients who have had prior sensitization to a drug and already have circulating IgE antibodies to it can upon reexposure react within seconds or minutes by manifesting urticaria (in the epidermis) or angioedema (in the dermis) of the eyelids, as well as chemosis and itching (Fig. 25-12). The eye is mildly to moderately hyperemic and has only a watery or slightly mucoid discharge. Itching

is intense. Although eosinophils are present in the conjunctival stroma, few if any are detected in scrapings because they do not quickly reach the conjunctival surface. Systemic anaphylactoid symptoms, and even true anaphylaxis, are possible but fortunately are extremely rare.[17,18]

The causes of anaphylactoid reactions are few and include some medications (bacitracin and sulfacetamide) that otherwise seldom cause either allergic or toxic reactions (see box on p. 680).

Therapy of anaphylactoid blepharoconjunctivitis should include immediate instillation of a vasoconstricting agent and topical corticosteroid and the application of a cold compress. An oral antihistamine should be given if the problem persists for more than a few minutes, and one should be prepared to treat systemic anaphylaxis if necessary. The offending drug should never be used again.

MISCELLANEOUS REACTIONS

Several other kinds of adverse effects of topical ophthalmic medications are possible,[2] many of which are seldom encountered, including phototoxic and photoallergic reactions (requiring interaction between drugs and light and, in the case of photoallergy, participation of the patient's immune system); cutaneous changes secondary to the application of fluorinated corticosteroids; drug-induced alterations of melanin (producing hyperpigmentation or hypopig-

Main Causes of Anaphylactoid Reactions to Topical Ophthalmic Medications

ANTIMICROBIAL AGENTS
  Penicillin
  Bacitracin
  Sulfacetamide
ANESTHETIC AGENTS
  Proparacaine
  Benoxinate
  Tetracaine

Benign (Relatively Nontoxic and Nonallergic) Topical Ophthalmic Medications

ANTIMICROBIAL AGENTS
  Sulfacetamide
  Erythromycin
  Bacitracin
  Polymyxin B
OCULAR LUBRICANTS
  Preservative-free artificial tears and ointments
  Preserved artificial tears and ointments without
    benzalkonium or thimerosal

mentation); and cumulative depositions of drugs (e.g., pigmentation secondary to mercury or silver, the deposition of silver being referred to as *argyria* in the skin and *argyrosis* in the conjunctiva).

A more common cumulative deposition is the so-called *adrenochrome deposit,* which is an accumulation of oxidized and polymerized epinephrine in preexisting conjunctival cysts. These deposits appear as discrete, dark brown to black, round spots, one to several millimeters in diameter, in the subepithelial conjunctiva of patients who have been treated chronically with epinephrine or dipivalyl epinephrine eyedrops for glaucoma (Fig. 25-13). The deposits are harmless and should not be mistaken for melanomas.

Antibiotics and steroids can alter the normal microbial flora of the eyelids and conjunctiva, sometimes predisposing to the development of opportunistic infections. Steroids can also inhibit wound healing, exert biotropism (drug-induced reactivations of latent infections by dermatophytes, *Candida,* and possibly herpes simplex), and enhance the activity of the enzyme collagenase (leading to corneal "melting" and perforation).

RECOVERY FROM DRUG REACTIONS

Except for anaphylactoid reactions, drug reactions often resolve slowly after the causative medications are stopped. Some reactions improve or clear within a few days to a week or two, but many require at least 2 or 3 weeks even to show improvement, and 6 to 8 weeks to clear completely; this is especially true of many toxic papillary and follicular reactions. If a topical steroid is discontinued abruptly along with other medications, the patient actually can appear worse for several days as a result of "rebound inflammation," which can occur when a steroid is suddenly withdrawn.

PREVENTION OF DRUG REACTIONS

An effort to make an accurate diagnosis is probably the single most important measure that can be taken to prevent drug-induced diseases.[19] Lack of diagnosis tends to lead to excessive and prolonged treatment—excessive treatment because the practitioner hopes to cover all possibilities ("shotgun therapy") and prolonged treatment because it is impossible to know the prognosis and natural history of the disease without first knowing the diagnosis. This approach can cause the *overtreatment syndrome,* in which harmful therapy is continued past the time when the underlying disease has improved or resolved because the adverse effects of treatment are misinterpreted as a failure or insufficiency of therapy; more medications are then prescribed, producing a relentless cycle that is interrupted only when treatment is greatly reduced or stopped.

The second most important factor in prevention is knowledge of and respect for the potential toxicities and allergenicities of specific drugs and preservatives (Table 25-2).[1,2]

The third most common problem is the mistaken belief on the part of both patients and practitioners that adverse drug reactions should clear quickly after medications are stopped. As discussed earlier, many reactions resolve slowly. Even when a drug reaction is correctly suspected, reducing treatment will be of little benefit if more drugs are prescribed a week or two later because the patient has not improved.

Finally, prevention requires dispelling the idea that most drug reactions are allergies and not toxicities. This misconception leads one to expect that almost any change in therapy should solve the problem (because the patient is thought simply to be "allergic" to a particular medication); but no improvement can occur if the patient is actually suffering from toxicity

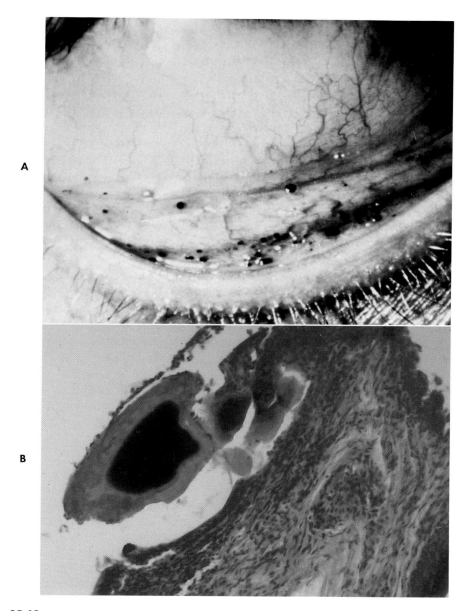

Figure 25-13
A, Adrenochrome deposits of oxidized and polymerized epinephrine in the lower palpebral conjunctiva. **B,** Histopathologic appearance of a conjunctival adrenochrome deposit. The deposit lies within a conjunctival cyst and consists of a dark central area of fully oxidized and polymerized drug, surrounded by a lighter peripheral zone of incomplete polymerization. (Hematoxylin-eosin stain, ×100.) (From Wilson FM II: *Surv Ophthalmol* 24:57, 1979.)

and the new medications are as toxic as the previous ones.

Adverse reactions to topical ophthalmic medications usually result from diagnostic uncertainty, leading to the prescribing of inappropriately numerous or potent medications for unnecessarily prolonged periods. Problems can

occur, but they are much less frequent when medications are prescribed prudently and wisely. When possible, and especially when the diagnosis is in doubt, it is usually best to prescribe relatively "bland" medications that are unlikely to cause irritation or allergy, as discussed in the box on p. 680 (e.g., erythromycin,

Table 25-2   Potential Toxicities and Allergenicities of Preservatives and Other Additives in Topical Ophthalmic Medications

Preservative or Additive	Toxicity	Allergenicity
Benzalkonium	++++	0
Boric acid	+	0
Chlorhexidine	+	+*
Chlorobutanol	+	0
Edetate (EDTA)	0	+
Parabens	0	+
Phenol	+	0
Phenylethyl alcohol	+	0
Phenylmercuric acetate	++†	0
Phenylmercuric nitrate	++†	0
Polyquaternium-1	0	+
Sodium bisulfate or thiosulfate	+	0
Sorbic acid or sorbate	0	+
Thimerosal	0	+++*

*Thimerosal and (very rarely) chlorhexidine cause contact allergy almost only in people who wear contact lenses (contact lens–induced keratoconjunctivitis); these patients nearly always have contact allergy only on the eye itself and do not manifest cutaneous eczema.

†Phenylmercuric nitrate causes toxic calcific band-shaped keratopathy and mercurialentis, whereas phenylmercuric acetate causes only mercurialentis.

bacitracin, sulfacetamide, polymyxin B, or artificial tears and lubricating ointments without benzalkonium, especially for patients who have dry eyes).

Although generally benign, such medications can be very useful. Potency, "newness," and popularity are not necessarily indicative of efficacy, although these features too often influence the selection of drugs. Medications should be prescribed for specific purposes and with specific goals in mind. If the goals are not attained within 2 or 3 weeks, the treatment probably should be changed or stopped and reevaluated. It is usually pointless to treat for several months with an antibiotic-steroid preparation, an antiviral agent, and an aminoglycoside antibiotic. Any conditions that might respond to such a regimen (and there are very few) should do so within a few days; continuing the treatment too long almost always makes the patient worse.

Admittedly, rapid and accurate diagnosis of the red or irritated eye is not always easy or possible. When the diagnosis is in doubt, it is generally better to prescribe relatively harmless drugs, or even placebo therapy, unless the eye is imminently and seriously threatened. Intensive therapy and polypharmacy are neither necessary nor efficacious for most external ocular diseases. Such treatment is apt to obscure spontaneous or therapy-induced improvement and to make diagnosis more difficult.

ACKNOWLEDGMENTS

This work was supported in part by grants from the Indiana Lions Eye Bank, Inc., Indianapolis, IN, and Research to Prevent Blindness, Inc., New York.

This material was presented in part in a thesis (1983) written for partial fulfillment of membership requirements of the American Ophthalmological Society.[1]

DISCLAIMER

The author has no proprietary interest in any of the medications discussed.

REFERENCES

1. Wilson FM II: Adverse external ocular effects of topical ophthalmic therapy: an epidemiologic, laboratory, and clinical study, *Trans Am Ophthalmol Soc* 81:854, 1983.
2. Wilson FM II: Adverse external ocular effects of topical ophthalmic medications, *Surv Ophthalmol* 24:57, 1979.
3. Gardner SK: *Ocular drug penetration and pharmacokinetic principles.* In Lamberts W, Potter DE, editors: *Clinical ophthalmic pharmacology,* Boston, 1987, Little, Brown & Co.
4. Pattern JT, Cavanagh HD, Allansmith MR: Induced ocular pseudopemphigoid, *Am J Ophthalmol* 82:272, 1986.
5. Ostler HB et al: *Drug-induced cicatrization of the*

conjunctiva. In O'Connor GR, editor: *Immunologic diseases of the mucous membranes: pathology, diagnosis, and treatment,* New York, 1980, Masson Publishing.

6. Theodore FH, Schlossman A: *Ocular allergy,* Baltimore, 1958, Williams & Wilkins.
7. Kennedy RE, Roca PD, Landers PH: Atypical band keratopathy in glaucomatous patients, *Am J Ophthalmol* 72:917, 1971.
8. Kennedy RE, Roca PD, Platt DS: Further observations on atypical band keratopathy in glaucoma patients, *Trans Am Ophthalmol Soc* 72:107, 1974.
9. Galin MA, Ostbaum SA: Band keratopathy in mercury exposure, *Ann Ophthalmol* 6:1257, 1974.
10. Garron LK et al: A clinical pathologic study of mercurialentis medicamentosus, *Trans Am Ophthalmol Soc* 74:295, 1966.
11. Theodore FH, Schlossman A: *Ocular allergy,* Baltimore, 1958, Williams & Wilkins.
12. Thygeson P: Marginal corneal infiltrates and ulcers, *Trans Am Acad Ophthalmol Otolaryngol* 51:198, 1947.
13. Thygeson P: Etiology and treatment of blepharitis, *Arch Ophthalmol* 36:445, 1946.
14. Fisher AA: *Contact dermatitis,* ed 2, Philadelphia, 1973, Lea & Febiger.
15. Smolin G: Medrysone hypersensitivity: report of a case, *Arch Ophthalmol* 85:478, 1971.
16. Theodore FH, Schlossman A: *Ocular allergy,* Baltimore, 1958, Williams & Wilkins.
17. Carter ES Jr, Cope CB: Anaphylaxis due to topical penicillin, *J Allergy* 25:270, 1954.
18. McCuiston CF: Penicillin-sensitivity test, *N Engl J Med* 25:1114, 1957.
19. Wilson FM II: *Prevention of iatrogenic drug-induced external ocular disease.* In Frielaender MH, editor: *Prevention of eye disease,* New York, 1988, Mary Ann Liebert, Inc.

Twenty-Six

Corneal Trauma

RADIATION INJURY

Ultraviolet radiation injury usually occurs after exposure to a welder's arc or sunlamp without adequate protection. Pain, photophobia, and irritation develop 6 to 12 hours after exposure. Pain results from epithelial cell and epithelial nerve axon loss, but the subepithelial nerve plexuses are spared.[1] Cycloplegia and a nonsteroidal antiinflammatory drug (NSAID) can be administered until the epithelium recovers (usually a few days). Antibiotic prophylaxis may be given.

Therapeutic ionizing radiation can cause injury to the lacrimal system, cornea, and sclera. This most commonly complicates radiation treatment of skin, orbital, and sinus neoplasms.

Keratoconjunctivitis sicca can result from radiation injury to the lacrimal glands. Ocular radiation can cause progressive superficial corneal vascularization and opacification, which can be complicated by ulceration and perforation (Fig. 26-1). The effects of radiation may not become manifest for several years. No treatment is clearly beneficial. Application of cyanoacrylate adhesive or keratoplasty may be necessary for perforation.

Corneal and scleral ulceration can also occur after beta-irradiation for pterygia.[2-5] In one study, 4.5% of patients had severe scleromalacia after an average dose of 22 Gy.[3] The risk of complications does not appear to be directly related to the total dose of radiation,[2] and the effects are delayed for several years. In a review of infectious complications, the mean latency before infection was over 14 years.[4] The affected sclera is avascular, heals poorly, and is prone to infection.

The diagnosis is made by the history of radiation of the eye and the exclusion of other causes of noninfiltrative ulceration, such as vasculitic scleritis and peripheral ulcerative keratitis. Treatment is supportive. Perforations can be repaired with cyanoacrylate adhesive or lamellar patch grafts, although the grafted tissue often ulcerates as well. Periosteal grafts may be more resistant to ulceration.

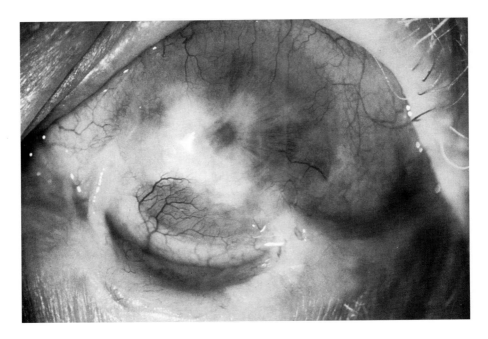

Figure 26-1
Corneal vascularization and scarring after radiation. (Courtesy of Diane Curtin, Pittsburgh, PA.)

BLUNT TRAUMA

Blunt trauma to the cornea can cause endothelial injury and rupture of Descemet's membrane. Stromal edema, Descemet's folds, and an anterior chamber reaction can be seen. Breaks in Descemet's membrane appear as linear or fusiform openings in the posterior layer, sometimes with curling of the edges into the anterior chamber. There is usually marked overlying stromal and epithelial edema. The area of stroma that is affected depends on the type of injury; a direct, focal blow, such as from a BB pellet, causes a ring of corneal edema (Fig. 26-2). Corneal rupture is rare and nearly always occurs in the setting of previous corneal surgery, such as penetrating keratoplasty or radial keratotomy, or a corneal thinning disorder, such as Terrien's marginal degeneration or keratoglobus. With healing, Descemet's ruptures can resemble fine-branching striae, broad bands of increased relucency with blurred margins (called Haab's striae in eyes with congenital glaucoma), or broad bands projecting posteriorly from the endothelial surface (Fig. 26-3).

The endothelial injury appears to result from mechanical deformation. Healing of the endothelium occurs by recovery of injured cells or their replacement by the sliding of adjacent endothelial cells.[6] Healthy endothelium slides over breaks in Descemet's membrane and restores normal endothelial pump function. Translucent ridges remain as permanent markers of the injury, but they do not affect vision. Recovery usually occurs within 3 months. Treatment is only indicated to provide comfort and can include hypertonic drops or ointment, bandage contact lens application, cycloplegia, and an NSAID.

LACERATIONS

Lacerations of the conjunctiva usually do not require repair. However, it is important to determine whether a foreign body is present or if ocular penetration has occurred. The risk can be determined by evaluating the history of the injury, the extent of subconjunctival hemorrhage (ability to visualize the sclera), and the presence or absence of intraocular hemorrhage and retinal injury. If the presence of a foreign body or ocular penetration cannot be excluded, exploration of the wound should be performed. Whether this requires use of the operating room and general anesthesia depends on the extent of injury and the cooperation of the patient. In the absence of perforating injury, conjunctival lacerations less than 1 cm in length do not require suturing. Larger lacerations are

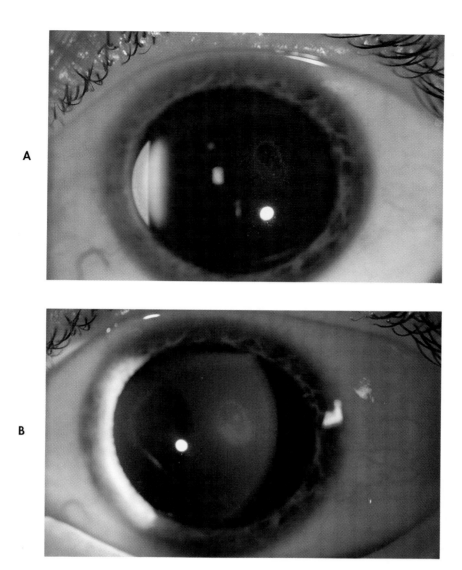

Figure 26-2
Endothelial injury after blunt trauma. A ring of endothelial opacification (Vossius' ring) can be seen by retroillumination (**A**) and direct illumination (**B**). (Courtesy of Diane Curtin, Pittsburgh, PA.)

usually closed with absorbable (collagen or polyglactin 910) sutures.

The management of corneal lacerations depends on their extent, the risk of infection, and whether or not perforation has occurred. Occult perforation can be detected by assessment of anterior chamber depth and intraocular pressure, careful slit-microscopic examination of the cornea, and Seidel's testing (after application of 2% fluorescein, gentle pressure is applied to the globe, and aqueous leakage is seen as dilution of the dye with a change in color to yellow or green).

Nonperforating corneal lacerations do not require suturing if the edges of the wound are well opposed, without overriding (Fig. 26-4). Small, self-sealing perforating lacerations, without iris, lens, or vitreous incarceration (Fig. 26-5), do not require suturing either. A bandage contact lens can be used to increase comfort and provide support to the wound. Cultures should be obtained and antibiotic treatment given. In most cases a broad-spectrum single agent, such as a fluoroquinolone, is given four to eight times daily. Nonpenetrating lacerations with wound gape, override, or loose avulsed flaps should be sutured.

Non–self-sealing lacerations (Fig. 26-6) re-

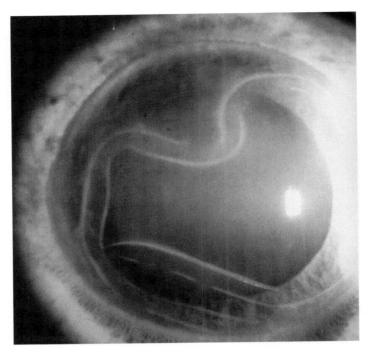

Figure 26-3
Broad bands protruding from endothelial surface after Descemet's rupture. (Courtesy of Diane Curtin, Pittsburgh, PA.)

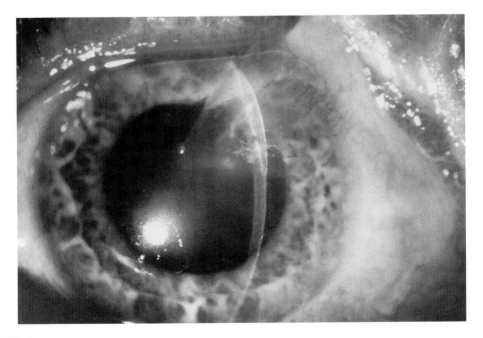

Figure 26-4
Lamellar corneal laceration, producing a flap of loose anterior stroma. (Courtesy of Diane Curtin, Pittsburgh, PA.)

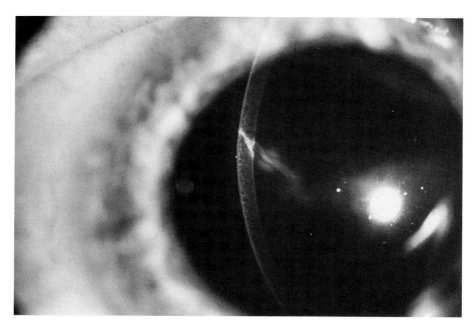

Figure 26-5
Self-sealing full-thickness corneal laceration. (Courtesy of Diane Curtin, Pittsburgh, PA.)

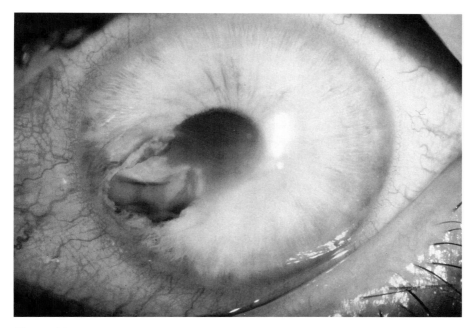

Figure 26-6
Full-thickness corneal laceration with uveal prolapse.

quire surgical closure. Tissue adhesive alone can be used for some small lacerations, but most require suturing. Lamellar or penetrating keratoplasty may be necessary if there is tissue loss.

If perforation is present there is a risk of endophthalmitis and intraocular foreign body. The overall risk of endophthalmitis in penetrating injury has been reported to be 3.2% to 7.4%, with increased incidence seen with delay in primary wound closure, retained intraocular foreign body, rural injury site, and rupture of the crystalline lens.[7-9] Gram-positive organisms are responsible in approximately 95% of cases, with *Bacillus* spp. accounting for 24% to 46%, most commonly in rural injury.[10]

Cultures should be obtained in all cases. Antibiotic treatment is controversial. Some authors recommend intravenous, periocular, and topical antibiotics in all cases of penetrating ocular trauma.[11] Others have recommended intraocular injection of antibiotics in all cases.[12] In a recent multicenter, controlled study of the treatment of endophthalmitis, systemic antibiotics had no significant effect on outcome.[13]

If surgical repair is warranted, subconjunctival injection of vancomycin, 25 mg, and ceftazidime, 100 mg (or cefazolin, 100 mg, and gentamicin, 20 mg) should be performed. Intravitreal antibiotic injection (e.g., amikacin, 0.4 mg, and vancomycin, 1.0 mg) can be performed in cases with rupture of the lens, retained intraocular foreign body, or posterior penetration. Depending on the nature of the injury, topical treatment can range from ofloxacin every 2 hours to combined vancomycin and gentamicin or amikacin every hour. In cases in which contamination with vegetable matter has occurred, *Bacillus* spp. infection is more likely, and clindamycin or vancomycin should be administered.

THERMAL BURNS

Thermal burns most often result from flames, but explosions or splashing of hot materials can also cause this injury.[14-16] Thermal burns cause immediate, local injury that is readily apparent. Usually the lids are affected most, and the cornea and conjunctiva are relatively protected. In my experience, isolated corneal burns occur most often during ocular surgery or as a result of contact with hot hair curlers. Whitening and contraction of tissues is seen. Astigmatism can result from contraction at the burn site. Most of these minor corneal injuries heal spontaneously without sequelae. However, vascularization and scarring can result in most severe cases (Fig. 26-7). More often the corneas are affected by exposure due to contracture and deformity of the burned lids. Frequent lubrication, moisture chambers, tarsorrhaphy, skin grafting, and other surgical procedures may be necessary to preserve corneal integrity.

CHEMICAL INJURIES

A wide variety of chemicals can cause ocular surface injury. In most cases the injury is relatively mild and recovery is rapid; however, some chemicals cause severe ocular damage and even permanent blindness. Burns of the external eye from strong acids or alkalies are the most common serious chemical injuries. The severe effects of these agents result mainly from an alteration of the local concentration of hydrogen and hydroxide ions. If ionization in solution is weak, the agent will be relatively harmless, as demonstrated by the potentially acidic substance carbon dioxide, which is lipid soluble and penetrates the epithelial layer of the cornea well. The carbolic acid is not harmful because ionization is weak. The amount of damage also depends on the amount and concentration of the chemical, the time that the eye is exposed to the chemical, and the ability of the chemical to penetrate the eye. Many chemicals also have specific toxic effects, such as acting as organic solvents, binding to proteins, inactivating enzymes, or impairing other metabolic processes.

Any chemical injury should be treated as an acute ophthalmic emergency. This is the only situation, outside of the operating room, in which literally seconds can affect the outcome. Regardless of the nature of the specific chemical, prompt irrigation with any benign fluid, such as water, can lessen or prevent blinding sequelae. Irrigation must be performed at the time of injury; by the time the patient arrives at the emergency room or the ophthalmologist's office, most of the damage has already been done. Nevertheless, irrigation is repeated by the clinician to ensure elimination of the chemical from the ocular surface. Of course, any solid material should be located and removed. The chemical(s), their concentrations, and the duration of exposure should also be determined. The patient should be asked to bring the chemical container or its label, particularly if the agent is uncommon or has a mixture of ingredients. Toxicology books, such as Grant's *Toxicology of the Eye*,[17] poison control centers, package inserts, and manufacturers can also provide valuable information.

Alkali Burns
Alkaline Chemicals
The most caustic alkalies are ammonium hydroxide (NH_4OH), sodium hydroxide (NaOH), calcium hydroxide ($Ca[OH]_2$), potassium hydroxide (KOH), and magnesium hydroxide ($Mg[OH]_2$). As evident from their names, each is a combination of a cation and hydroxide and readily dissociates in solution, releasing large amounts of the toxic hydroxide.

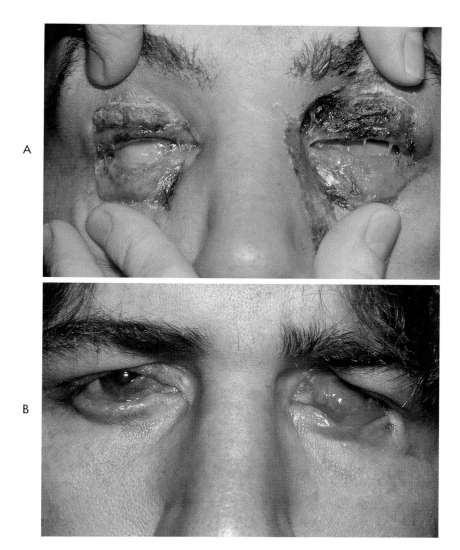

Figure 26-7
Thermal burns caused by molten iron. **A,** Early effects of injury on the lids and conjunctiva. **B,** Late scarring of the lids, producing exposure and scarring and vascularization of corneas. (Courtesy of Diane Curtin, Pittsburgh, PA.)

Ammonia. Ammonia (NH_3), a common cleaning agent, is found in fertilizers and refrigerants and is used in the manufacturing of other chemicals. NH_3 can dissolve in water (including tears), and forms ammonium hydroxide, which is very caustic. The ammonia penetrates ocular tissues readily because it is both lipid- and water-soluble; it can reach the anterior chamber in less than a minute.[18] Thus it can cause extensive internal ocular injury and is not readily removed by topical irrigation.

Sodium Hydroxide. Sodium hydroxide is commonly referred to as lye or caustic soda and is used as a cleanser and in manufacturing. Injuries probably occur most commonly during its use in the unclogging of household drains. In these cases a combination of crystals and solution explode out of the drain into the eyes. Lye also appears to be a common choice in deliberate attempts at blinding. Sodium hydroxide penetrates the eye quickly, but not as quickly as ammonia; peak anterior chamber alkalinity occurs 3 to 5 minutes after exposure.[18] Severe injuries are common.

Calcium Hydroxide. Lime, plaster, cement, mortar, and whitewash contain calcium hydroxide and are common sources of ocular injury. The solids usually fall or are splashed into the eye and can become trapped in the fornices, resulting in prolonged ocular exposure. Calcium hydroxide penetrates relatively poorly; it reacts with the epithelial cell membrane to form calcium soaps, which precipitate and hinder further penetration. Therefore, it tends to cause more superficial injury but early opacification. This often suggests a worse outcome than is actually observed.

Others. Potassium hydroxide, also known as caustic potash, is commonly used both as a cleanser and in manufacturing. Its penetration and severity are similar to those of sodium hydroxide. Magnesium hydroxide is a component of flares and fireworks and is therefore seen in the context of thermal and sometimes concussive injuries. By itself, magnesium hydroxide causes minor epithelial injury.

Pathogenesis
Strongly alkaline chemicals result in disruption of cells because the high pH causes saponification and dissociation of fatty acids in the cell membranes. A local pH of 11.5 or greater appears to be associated with permanent injury. In the stroma, the hydroxyl ions cause swelling of collagen fibers, which results in their thickening and shortening. They also lead to hydrolyzation of interfibrillar glycosaminoglycans.[19] The severity of stromal injury is also related to the nature of the cation, which influences penetration and itself can bind collagen and glycosaminoglycans.[20]

Injury to conjunctiva, corneal nerves, keratocytes, endothelium, and limbal blood vessels can also occur by the same mechanisms. Corneal anesthesia, obliteration of keratocytes, diffuse endothelial cell loss, and ischemia can result. Stimulation of the free nerve endings in the corneal and conjunctival epithelium is responsible for the intense pain associated with alkali injury.[21] Intraocular structures, including the iris, lens, trabecular meshwork, and ciliary body can also be affected depending on the aqueous pH. Aqueous pH can remain alkaline for up to 3 hours after injury, regardless of external irrigation.[18,22] Aqueous glucose and ascorbate levels are decreased and can remain so for prolonged periods.[23-25]

Epithelial healing involves migration and proliferation of the remaining epithelial cells. The rate of healing of a corneal epithelial defect is influenced by the source of the epithelium. If limbal epithelium remains, healing is much more rapid than if conjunctival epithelium

must be the sole source.[26] The healing rate is proportional to the percentage of the limbal circumference that is healthy. Epithelial healing is also delayed by inflammation and damage to the basement membrane.[27,28] If the cornea is covered with epithelium derived entirely from the conjunctiva, the epithelium may retain its conjunctival morphology, and vascularization, opacification, and thickening can occur. The effect of alkali injury on the goblet cell population is unclear; some have found decreased goblet cell density, as in cicatricial pemphigoid and other scarring diseases.[29] Others, surprisingly, have found goblet cell density to be increased significantly.[30]

Neutrophils infiltrate the peripheral stroma within 12 to 24 hours after an alkali injury. In severe injuries, and if the epithelial defect persists, progressive leukocytic infiltration occurs. Mononuclear cell infiltration begins 14 to 21 days after injury.[31] Keratocytes migrate into the stroma to replace keratocytes destroyed by the alkali injury. Keratocytes are necessary for repair of the stroma, secreting collagen and the mucopolysaccharide ground substance. Collagen synthesis requires ascorbate, which can be deficient in these corneas (see below).

Stromal ulceration commonly occurs in alkali-burned corneas. Several factors contribute to stromal ulceration, including persistent epithelial defects, tear deficiency, inflammation, release of proteolytic enzymes,[32,33] antioxidant deficiency,[34,35] anesthesia, and impairment of collagen synthesis. One type of proteolytic enzyme, collagenase, appears to play a significant role and has been the subject of a great deal of investigation. Epithelium, fibroblasts, and polymorphonuclear leukocytes (PMNs) are capable of releasing collagenase, and collagenase activity has been detected in ulcerating corneas after alkali burns.[18,36,37] Collagenase appears within 9 hours after the burn and reaches a peak level at 14 to 21 days.

Production of plasmin by epithelial cells, PMNs, and keratocytes may also play a role in stromal ulceration (see Chapter 15). It has also been proposed that the host's immunologic response contributes to ulceration,[38,39] as suggested by the following findings: In rabbits, if a second eye is burned 2 to 4 weeks after the first, the rate of ulceration in the second eye is much higher than in the first. In addition, administration of convalescent serum from burned rabbits increases the rate of ulceration.

Localized corneal ascorbate deficiency has been observed after alkali burns and may play a role in corneal ulceration.[25,40,41] Aqueous levels of ascorbate are normally 20 times higher than in plasma, presumably because of active transport by the ciliary body. Damage to the ciliary body can impair or eliminate this function and lead to a relative ascorbate deficiency. Ascorbate is required for collagen synthesis, the conversion of monocytes to fibroblasts, and the formation of normal rough endoplasmic reticulum and plays a role in the synthesis of glycosaminoglycans.

Clinical Manifestations

Acute. Within minutes after a severe alkali injury, extensive injury can occur in all cell types in the cornea, including epithelium, keratocytes, nerves, vessels, and endothelium. Damage to cellular and vascular components of the conjunctiva, iris, and ciliary body and to the lens epithelium can also occur in the first few hours. The conjunctiva is injected and can exhibit areas of necrosis, which appear white and devoid of blood vessels (Figs. 26-8 through 26-11). Large epithelial defects can be present, involving the entire cornea and extending into the fornices. The corneal stroma is often cloudy and edematous; in severe injuries it can be opaque. The anterior chamber may be shallow and exhibit fibrin formation.

The intraocular pressure can rise rapidly.[42,43] This early increase appears to be caused by the shrinkage of collagen in the cornea and trabecular meshwork, with compression of the anterior chamber and trabecular outflow channels. Within a few hours other mechanisms can come into play: increased episcleral venous

pressure, blockage of the trabecular meshwork with inflammatory debris, and possibly prostaglandin release from damaged intraocular structures. Although these mechanisms can contribute to a pressure rise, ciliary body injury can also occur, leading to decreased aqueous production. Over the first few days the balance between these factors is precarious, and the eye can fluctuate between hypotony and marked pressure elevation.

The severity of injury and the prognosis for healing of the eye can be estimated based on initial examination. A useful classification scheme developed by Hughes[44,45] and modified by Roper-Hall[46] divides the injuries into four groups (Table 26-1). A more detailed classification scheme has been devised by Ralph,[47] as shown in Table 26-2. These schemes are helpful, particularly for those unaccustomed to caring for patients with chemical injuries. They can be used as an indication of the likelihood of complications and the long-term prognosis. Clearly the most important prognostic signs are the degree of limbal necrosis (ischemia) and the cloudiness of the corneal stroma. Signs of anterior chamber injury, such as a fixed, dilated pupil, iridocyclitis, and a sustained increase in intraocular pressure also indicate more severe injury. These signs are considered only in Ralph's scheme.

Early Reparative Phase. Typically the epithelium begins to grow in from the periphery of the defect within a few days. Depending on the

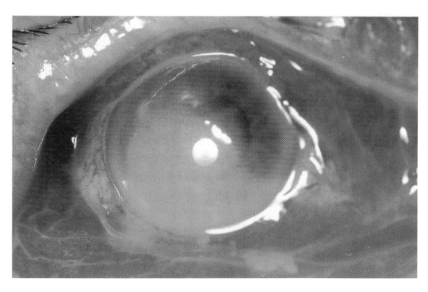

Figure 26-8
Alkali burn with injection and chemosis of the conjunctiva and increased relucency of the cornea.

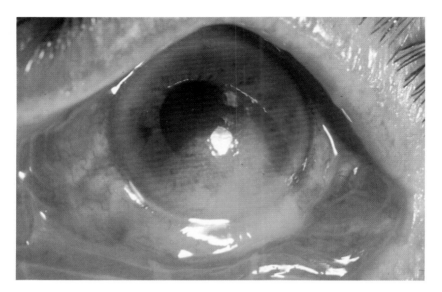

Figure 26-9
Small area of limbal ischemia.

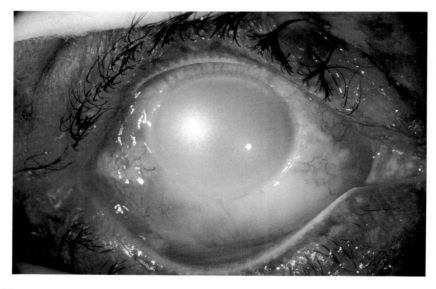

Figure 26-10
Alkali burn with total loss of corneal epithelium, stromal haze, and ischemia of approximately one third of the limbus.

extent of injury, however, it can take 1 to 2 weeks to reach the cornea. In the meantime, symblepharon can develop as a result of fusion of the denuded palpebral and bulbar conjunctival surfaces. Its progression across the cornea can be agonizingly slow, taking many weeks, especially in cases with marked stromal injury. The epithelial healing rate depends on the extent of limbal involvement, the amount of tis-

sue necrosis, adequacy of lid function, tear production, and patient age. Peripheral vascularization and inflammatory cell infiltration often accompany the epithelium.

With time the stroma gradually clears, and anterior chamber inflammation subsides. However, fibrotic membranes can form on the iris, endothelium, or lens, and the lens can become swollen and cloudy. The intraocular pressure

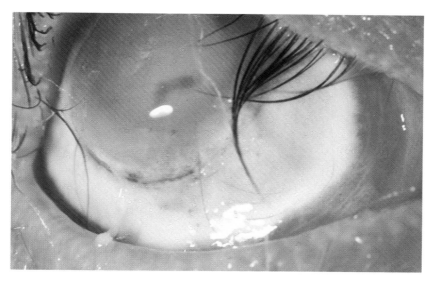

Figure 26-11
Marbleization of the cornea and severe limbal ischemia.

Table 26-1	Hughes–Roper-Hall Classification of Chemical Burns	
Grade	**Clincal Findings**	**Prognosis**
Grade I	Corneal epithelial damage; no limbal ischemia (Fig. 26-8)	Good
Grade II	Cornea hazy but iris detail seen; ischemia at less than one third of limbus (Fig. 26-9)	Good
Grade III	Total loss of corneal epithelium; stromal haze blurring iris details; ischemia at one third to one half of limbus (Fig. 26-10)	Guarded
Grade IV	Cornea opaque, obscuring view of iris or pupil; ischemia at more than one half of limbus (Fig. 26-11)	Poor

can range from hypotony to a glaucoma that is difficult to control, but it is usually not as labile as in the acute phase.

Stromal ulceration can occur anytime after the first 7 to 10 days, but it most typically begins 2 to 3 weeks after injury. It occurs only in areas in which epithelium and superficial vessels are not present. In most cases the epithelium covers the cornea before there is significant thinning, and vessels are seen peripherally or not at all; however, the longer an epithelial defect is present the greater the likelihood of ulceration. In severe cases epithelial healing can take months, and progressive stromal ulceration can occur before the epithelium reaches the central cornea (Fig. 26-12). Stromal ulceration stops with reepithelialization or neovascularization of the stroma. If perforation can be avoided, healing will eventually be realized, albeit often with severe vascularization and scarring.

Late Reparative Phase. If initial epithelial healing is achieved without marked vascularization and scarring, the eye can look fairly good at this stage, even after severe burns. A closer inspection, however, can often indicate obstacles yet to be dealt with. Conjunctival scarring can progress for weeks after injury and can lead to closure of the lacrimal gland ductules, entropion, trichiasis, and impaired lid closure (Fig. 26-13). In addition to aqueous tear deficiency, the lipid component of tears can be reduced by scarring of the meibomian gland orifices, mucin deficiency can result from goblet cell loss, and sometimes tear surfacing is also impaired. Corneal sensation is often reduced because of nerve injury. Although it is not readily evident, there may also be extensive endothelial and keratocyte injury.

All of these problems can take their toll with time. In the more severe cases corneal scarring and vascularization progress for 6 to 12 months

Table 26-2   Classification of Chemical Burns

Total Score	Prognosis
CONJUNCTIVA	
Perilimbal hyperemia	0
Chemosis	1
LIMBUS	
No ischemia	0
Spotty limbal ischemia	1
Ischemia < one third of circumference	2
Ischemia one third to one half of circumference	3
Ischemia > one half of circumference	4
CORNEAL EPITHELIUM	
Clouded epithelium	1
Epithelial loss ≤ 50%	2
Epithelial loss > 50%	3
CORNEAL STROMA	
Mild stromal haze; iris details visible	2
Moderate stromal haze; iris details barely visible	3
Severe stromal haze; no iris details visible	4
INTRAOCULAR STRUCTURES	
Oval, fixed pupil or aqueous cells	2
Sustained increase of intraocular pressure during first 24 hr	3

Total Score	Prognosis
0–3	Insignificant injury; rapid recovery without sequelae
4–6	Mild injury with rapid replacement of damaged epithelium and clearing of any stromal haze; return of visual acuity to baseline usually occurs within 1 to 2 wk
7–9	Moderately severe injury, usually with a delay of 1 to 3 wk in complete reepithelialization; some reduction in visual acuity may result from persistent stromal haze; peripheral pannus is common
10–12	Severe burn, with sluggish regrowth of the epithelium and frequent development of pannus; stromal loss is common and perforation can occur; visual acuity usually

Table 26-2   Classification of Chemical Burns—cont'd

Total Score	Prognosis
	permanently reduced by pannus and stromal haze
13–17	Most severe burns with worst prognosis; prolonged epithelial recovery, with dense pannus formation and stromal loss; perforation is common; cataract is expected; end result, after many months or years, is dense corneal scarring and vascularization, phthisis, or loss of the globe

Adapted from Ralph RA: *Chemical burns of the eye.* In Duane T, editor: *Clinical ophthalmology,* vol 4, Hagerstown, MD, 1988, Harper & Row. Used with permission of Lippincott-Raven Publishers.

after injury. Damage to the endothelium can lead to retrocorneal fibrous membrane formation. The trabecular meshwork, iris, and ciliary body also can be affected by fibrous proliferation. Pupillary membranes and cataracts are often present and must be removed before visual rehabilitation. Intraocular pressure can remain elevated, or the eye can become hypotonous and subsequently phthisical.

Treatment

Immediate. The chemically injured eye must be copiously irrigated as soon as possible (Table 26-3).[48] In most cases the fate of the eye is determined in the first few minutes after injury; therefore, irrigation is best performed at the site of injury with any nontoxic liquid. After the patient arrives at the emergency room or doctor's office, irrigation should be repeated. It is useful to determine the pH in the inferior cul-de-sac before irrigation, using litmus paper, but not if it delays irrigation. Theoretically, an isotonic, neutral pH, buffered solution would be the ideal irrigation fluid, but these do not appear to be superior to water, Ringer's lactate, normal saline, or similar solutions.[49] Balanced Saline Solution Plus (BSS Plus, Alcon Laboratories, Fort Worth, TX) was found to be more comfortable than normal saline or Ringer's lactate.

Irrigation is usually accomplished by running the solution through intravenous tubing, retracting the lids, and manually holding the tubing so that the fluid drips into the eye. Irri-

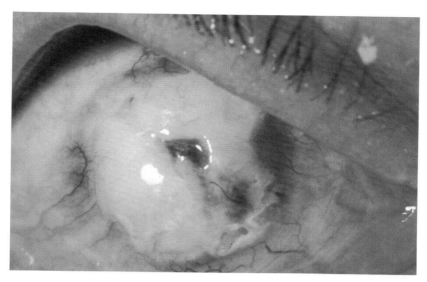

Figure 26-12
Perforation of the cornea after an alkali burn.

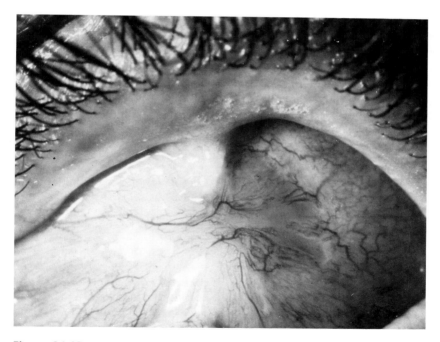

Figure 26-13
Cicatrization of the conjunctiva and symblepharon formation after an alkali burn.

gation tubes attached to polymethylmethacry-late scleral contact lenses (Medi-Flow therapeu-tic lens, Mor-Tan, Inc., Torrington, WY) and a perforated silicone tube shaped to lie in the conjunctival fornix (Oklahoma eye irrigating tube, Edward Weck and Co., Inc., Long Island City, NY) are commercial products designed to facilitate this process.[50] Irrigation is continued for a minimum of 30 minutes or until the pH becomes neutral. Topical anesthetic agents or lid block may be required for this initial treatment.

Removal of solid material is essential and may require double eversion of the lid to prop-erly ensure that this area is free of chemical. The sticky paste or powder of calcium hydrox-

Table 26-3　Initial Treatment of Alkali Injury
1. Irrigate at the site of injury with water or other nontoxic liquid.
2. Irrigate on presentation with water or intravenous solution for at least 30 minutes or until pH is neutral.
3. Remove any solid material. This may be facilitated by 0.01% ethylenediaminetetraacetic acid solution on swab or irrigation.
4. Use cycloplegia to decrease pain: atropine 1% twice a day, or scopolamine 0.25% two to four times a day.
5. Use prophylactic antibiotics (e.g., sulfacetamide, gentamicin, or erythromycin four times a day) to reduce the incidence of infection.
6. Control intraocular pressure, primarily with drugs that reduce aqueous inflow (e.g., timolol and acetazolamide).
7. Use topical corticosteroids (e.g., prednisolone acetate 1% four times a day) for 7 to 10 days to decrease pain and inflammation.
8. If opposing conjunctival surfaces are denuded of epithelium, consider physical separation with a scleral shell or plastic wrap (combined with bandage contact lens).

ide can be particularly difficult to remove. Irrigation with a 0.01- to 0.05-M solution of ethylenediaminetetraacetic acid (EDTA) and cotton swabs soaked in the same solution can help loosen it.[20]

Paracentesis with removal of aqueous or irrigation has been recommended,[21,51,52] but its benefit has not been established,[53] and there are significant risks. Therefore, I do not recommend this procedure.

A cycloplegic drop is usually instilled for comfort, and a prophylactic antibiotic is administered. If the injury is relatively mild (e.g., grade I), the eye can be patched and the patient reexamined the next day. With more severe burns, particularly with bilateral injury, the patient should be admitted to the hospital.

Early (1 to 2 Weeks). The role of the ophthalmologist in the early period of treatment is to ease discomfort, control intraocular pressure, and promote epithelial healing. A cycloplegic, such as scopolamine or atropine, is used to increase comfort, and a relatively nontoxic antibiotic is applied two to four times a day to lessen the risk of infection. Intraocular pressure elevation is treated primarily with drugs that decrease inflow, such as timolol and carbonic anhydrase inhibitors.

If conjunctival epithelial injury is extensive,

affecting both the palpebral and bulbar conjunctiva, or synechiae begin to form, measures can be taken to physically separate the two conjunctival surfaces. Whether these affect the final result is unclear. They certainly do not prevent subepithelial scarring, but they may reduce forniceal shortening. In most cases, I prefer to use a symblepharon ring, in combination with a bandage contact lens (Fig. 26-14). Alternatively, the palpebral surface can be lined with a thin plastic material, such as plastic food wrap, or adhesions can be lysed daily with a glass rod.

Epithelial healing can be promoted by lubrication, patching, bandage contact lenses, or tarsorrhaphy. Bandage contact lenses are helpful when epithelial healing is prolonged or there is recurrent epithelial loss. The lens is left in place until adequate adhesion is achieved, which may require as long as 3 months. Incomplete lid closure, entropion, ectropion, or trichiasis may develop and should be corrected as much as possible. Bandage contact lenses are also helpful in ameliorating the effects of these conditions.

Several medications have been advocated to promote epithelial healing and reduce corneal ulceration. These are discussed more thoroughly in Chapter 15. Both fibronectin[54,55] and epidermal growth factor (EGF)[56-59] promote epithelial healing after alkali injury in rabbits. However, epithelial defects recur, even with continued fibronectin or EGF treatment. The incidence of secondary epithelial breakdown was reduced by the combined use of EGF and fibronectin or by the addition of topical steroid treatment to EGF or fibronectin treatment.[60] A controlled, multicenter clinical trial of fibronectin for persistent epithelial defects failed to demonstrate efficacy of the medication.[61] In one placebo-controlled study of patients undergoing penetrating keratoplasty, EGF did not promote epithelial healing,[62] but in another controlled study of traumatic corneal epithelial defects EGF significantly enhanced healing.[63] Oral doxycycline promoted epithelialization in a rabbit alkali-burn model.[64]

The use of topical corticosteroids is controversial. The steroids reduce inflammation and provide some comfort, but they have the potential to promote stromal ulceration.[65,66] Because the risk of stromal ulceration is low in the first 10 days after injury,[66] I use 1% prednisolone acetate four times a day during the first 7 to 10 days. After this point topical corticosteroids are applied only if the epithelium is intact. In cases with marked inflammation and progressive scarring and vascularization, I grad-

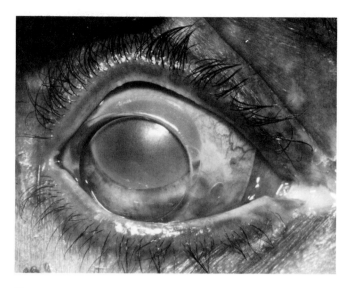

Figure 26-14
Symblepharon ring and bandage contact lens.

ually taper the steroid dose until the eye is stable, but whether this regimen affects the final outcome is debatable.

As mentioned earlier, aqueous and stromal levels of ascorbate are decreased after alkali burns. In experimental animals, administration of ascorbate prevented alkali-related corneal ulceration if treatment was begun before the onset of ulceration.[24,67] When ascorbate was compared with a control group receiving citrate, however, the incidence of ulceration and perforation was much less in the citrate group.[68] Unlike ascorbate, citrate was also effective if begun after the onset of stromal ulceration.[69] Citrate has been found to decrease PMN activity, including mediator release, and phagocytosis.[33,70] Citrate may exert its effect by binding extracellular calcium, decreasing its availability as an intraocular second messenger in PMNs. Combined use of citrate and ascorbate was significantly better in reducing ulceration than citrate alone in alkali-injured rabbits.[71] Neither ascorbate nor citrate has been demonstrated to be of benefit in a controlled human trial.

Intermediate (2 Weeks to 6 Months). The major complication in the intermediate period is stromal ulceration. The main goal is to promote epithelial healing, as described earlier, because this will prevent further ulceration. Cultures should be obtained regularly because of the possible role of microbial infection. A variety of substances have been suggested to reduce the progression of ulceration, including collagenase inhibitors (such as EDTA, cysteine, penicillamine, and acetylcysteine,[72-74]) heparin,[75] citrate, aprotinin,[76] and medroxyprogesterone[77,78]; however, no agent has been clearly demonstrated to be clinically beneficial. In a rabbit alkali burn model, placement of collagen shields exacerbated corneal ulceration.[79]

If medical treatment is not successful, a conjunctival flap can often halt ulceration. Ipsilateral conjunctiva is preferred, but if it is necrotic or scarred, contralateral conjunctiva or oral mucosa can be used.[80] Tissue adhesive can also be used to impede ulceration or to seal a small perforation. Larger perforations can be repaired by lamellar or penetrating keratoplasty, but the grafts usually succumb to ulceration as well. Covering the grafts with conjunctiva or mucosa may increase their resistance.

Long-term (Longer than 6 Months). If there is severe scarring of the cornea or conjunctival sac, keratoplasty or reconstructive plastic surgery is an option. Although results of penetrating keratoplasty have been encouraging in some instances, the overall prognosis for the marbleized corneas from alkali burns is still guarded. The odds of success are primarily determined by the severity of the injury; however, results can be improved by paying special attention to the ocular environment in which the graft is placed. Lid scarring and distortion, trichiasis, symblepharon, inflammation, and tear and mucus deficiency can threaten the graft.

Penetrating keratoplasty should be delayed until the eye is healed completely and inflammation has resolved—a process that usually requires at least 1 year and often 1.5 to 2 years.[81] Lid position abnormalities and trichiasis should be corrected first, and glaucoma should be controlled. Fresh donor tissue with healthy epithelium is important to lessen the risk of early epithelial defects. The graft epithelium should be protected during and after surgery; bandage contact lens wear, continuous patching, or suture tarsorrhaphy are used for at least 4 to 6 weeks after surgery. While the eye is open it must be kept well lubricated with artificial tears and ointments. Ocular inflammation should be minimized with topical or systemic corticosteroids.

The risk of rejection is relatively high because of the presence of corneal vessels.[82] Systemic treatment with immunosuppressives, such as cyclosporine and FK506, may increase the rate of graft survival.

In addition, the grafts often opacify because of poor epithelial healing. If epithelial defects occur they are slow to heal, and stromal ulceration or wound separation can develop. If there has been extensive limbal injury, the host epithelium is abnormal with less capacity for healing and maintenance of corneal clarity. Eventually the abnormal epithelium grows over the graft and can become affected by recurrent defects, superficial opacification, and vascularization.

Conjunctival transplantation was designed to provide healthy epithelium for resurfacing of corneas damaged by chemical and thermal burns[83-85] to prevent recurrent epithelial breakdown and reduce central corneal scarring and vascularization (see Chapter 15). A superficial lamellar keratectomy is performed first. In the traditional form, four circular areas of perilimbal conjunctiva are taken from the fellow eye and sutured at the limbus (Fig. 26-15). Alternatively, a crescentic lamellar graft containing several clock hours of limbus can be transplanted.[86,87] In bilateral injury donor limbal epithelium can be used, and the procedure is called *keratoepithelioplasty*.[88] The rate of graft rejection has been high in keratoepithelioplasty cases, but systemic cyclosporine treatment and use of human leukocyte antigen–matched donor tissue can increase the success rate.[89-91]

The surgery can be performed early for persistent epithelial defects to facilitate reepithelialization and reduce the risk of ulceration. In some patients removal of superficial scarring and vascularization, combined with conjunctival transplantation, is sufficient to restore vision. Such surgery should be delayed until at least 1 year after injury. However, epithelial

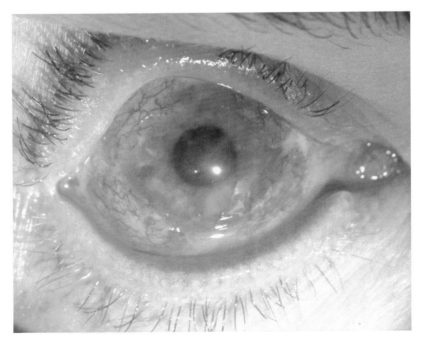

Figure 26-15
Conjunctival transplant. Note four conjunctival grafts at the limbus. (Courtesy of Richard A. Thoft, Pittsburgh, PA.)

transplantation clearly cannot remove deep corneal scarring or replace damaged endothelium. In such cases the pannus and opacified anterior stroma are removed before placement of the conjunctival grafts. The surface environment should be optimized, as with keratoplasty. Conjunctival transplantation can also be performed prior to keratoplasty in patients with ocular surface disease, which is characterized by epithelial thickening, opacification, and vascularization and recurrent erosions, to provide a more stable surface prior to penetrating keratoplasty.

Keratoprosthesis. In patients with severe bilateral injury and multiple failed keratoplasties,

keratoprostheses can be used as a last resort to obtain useful vision[92,93] (Fig. 26-16). These devices are fraught with complications and are successful for only a few years at best, but they can provide good visual acuity, albeit with a very narrow field.

Acid Burns

Exposure of the eye to weak acids tends to result in less severe injury than exposure to weak alkalies, but strong acids can cause devastating injury (Fig. 26-17). In general, the clinical manifestations and treatment of acid burns are similar to those of alkali burns, so emphasis will be placed on those features that are unique.

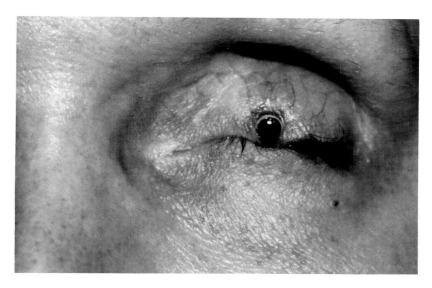

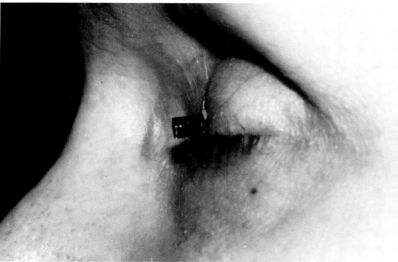

Figure 26-16
Keratoprosthesis, front and side views. (Courtesy of Massimo Busin, Bonn, Germany.)

Acidic Chemicals

Sulfuric acid (H_2SO_4) is probably the most commonly encountered acid in ocular burns. Although it is widely used in industry, most burns result from battery explosions. Lead-acid batteries contain a 20% to 25% solution of sulfuric acid. When it is exposed to an electric current, hydrogen and oxygen gasses are released, producing an explosive mixture.[94] This mixture is ignited when a match or lighter is used to illuminate the engine compartment, or jumper cables are connected improperly, resulting in sparks. The ocular injury is a combination of acid burn and contusion or laceration resulting from the explosion.

Sulfurous acid (H_2SO_3) is formed when sulfur dioxide gas combines with the water in tears or the cornea. Sulfurous acid is highly soluble in both lipid and water and therefore penetrates rapidly. It also damages the corneal nerves, resulting in anesthesia.

Hydrofluoric (HF) acid is widely used in industry and tends to cause severe injury.[95] Although it is a weak acid, the fluoride ion is a strong solvent and can dissolve cellular membranes.[96] This characteristic, plus its low molecular weight and small size, enables hydrofluoric acid to penetrate tissues easily.

Hydrochloric (HCl) acid solutions release hydrogen chloride gas, which is irritating to the eye but usually not damaging; however, concentrated solutions can cause severe damage. Exposure to small amounts of chromic acid (Cr_2O_3), used in the chrome-plating industry and in washing laboratory glassware, can cause chronic conjunctivitis and a brownish discoloration of the conjunctival epithelium.

Nitric acid (HNO_3) burns are unusual in that the epithelial opacities are yellowish rather than white. High concentrations of silver nitrate ($AgNO_3$) can result in opacification of the cornea that may be permanent.[97] Some injuries have occurred as a result of inadvertent neonatal prophylaxis, with a solution much more concentrated than the usual 1%. The use of solid silver nitrate sticks to cauterize lesions on the lids or conjunctiva has resulted in severe corneal injury as well as cataract formation. Thermal injury, acid burn, and silver deposition occur.

Pathogenesis

When exposed to an acidic environment, proteins coagulate and precipitate. In the cornea acids coagulate the epithelial cells, shrink stromal collagen, and precipitate glycosaminoglycans.[98] Fortunately, this process occurs on the surface and tends to inhibit further penetration of the chemical. Deeper injury can occur, however, especially where the anion penetrates well or the anion itself is toxic, as exemplified by hydrofluoric acid, in which the fluoride both penetrates well and dissolves membranes.

Collagen shrinkage can lead to increased intraocular pressure, as occurs in alkali injury.[99] Intraocular damage can occur; lowering of

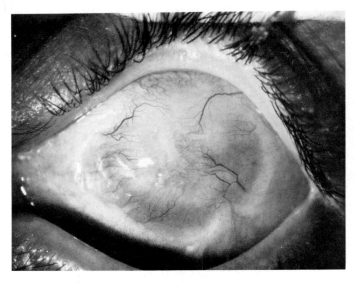

Figure 26-17
Corneal scarring resulting from a severe acid burn.

aqueous pH and increased aqueous protein and prostaglandin levels have been observed after experimental hydrochloric acid injury.[99] Ciliary body damage can result in decreased aqueous and stromal levels of ascorbate, as occurs in severe alkali burns.[41]

Clinical Manifestations

Although no classification scheme has been designed specifically for acid burns, both the Hughes–Roper-Hall (see Table 26-1) and Ralph (see Table 26-2) schemes for alkali burns are applicable. The most important prognostic indicators are limbal ischemia and evidence of intraocular injury. Corneal opacification is an indication of severity but is less significant in acid injuries because epithelial and anterior stromal coagulation can occur without extensive deep stromal or anterior chamber injury. The epithelium of the cornea and conjunctiva can turn white and opaque or, with nitric or chromic acid burns, yellow-brown. This necrotic epithelium sloughs off within a few days, sometimes revealing a clear stroma.

As in alkali burns, corneal anesthesia, conjunctival scarring, stromal ulceration, iritis, glaucoma, and lens opacification can occur. Any acid can cause these complications if it is sufficiently concentrated and the exposure is long enough. Certain acids, however, such as sulfurous acid and hydrofluoric acid, are more likely to produce severe burns because they penetrate the corneal stroma more readily or the anions are more toxic.

Treatment

The treatment of acid burns is the same as for alkali burns of the same severity. The primary emergency treatment is irrigation. Although less time is generally required for neutralization of the tears, a minimum of 20 to 30 minutes of irrigation is still recommended. Specific neutralizing chemicals have been suggested for hydrofluoric acid burns, including benzalkonium chloride, calcium chloride, and calcium gluconate, but these are toxic themselves and should be avoided.[96,100]

Other Chemicals
Tear Gas

Tear gasses disarm their targets by causing ocular stinging, smarting, and tearing through selective stimulation of sensory nerve endings in the cornea. A variety of active ingredients, or lacrimators, may be used, the most common of which is chloroacetophenone. The mechanism of effect is not understood, but the active agents in tear gasses are toxic to sulfhydryl- or thiol-containing enzymes.[17] At the concentrations encountered in normal use, no ocular injury occurs; however, at high concentrations severe damage can result.

Tear gas weapons come in explosive and solvent spray types. The explosive type includes

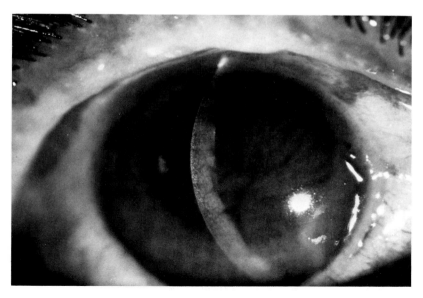

Figure 26-18
Stromal swelling after a tear gas injury.

cartridges for pistols, grenades, and canisters, all of which contain concentrated lacrimator and explosives or combustibles. Direct blasts from these weapons at close range expose the eye to mechanical damage, flying debris, and sometimes thermal injury, as well as concentrated lacrimator. The solvent spray type, such as mace, can also cause damage if the chemical is sprayed directly into the eye at close range.

Corneal epithelial loss, stromal edema, and stromal scarring can occur (Fig. 26-18). The lacrimator appears to be able to penetrate the cornea and appears to be toxic to the endothelium.[101,102]

Others

Most organic solvents are not acidic or alkaline and do not exhibit much chemical reactivity with tissues. Epithelial injury can occur, but deeper involvement is unusual. The chemicals are readily eliminated by a few minutes of irrigation.

A few chemicals cause an epithelial injury in which the symptoms are delayed until several hours after exposure, similar to what is seen in ultraviolet keratitis. Superficial punctate keratopathy is the most common finding, but diffuse epithelial loss, stromal edema, and, rarely, stromal scarring and vascularization can occur. Such chemicals include Diving Mask Defogger, formaldehyde, hydrogen sulfide, mustard gas, osmic acid, and poison ivy.[17]

Mustard gas or dichloroethyl sulfide has been used as a chemical weapon, most recently in the Iran-Iraq War. It is a highly lipid-soluble vapor that exerts its toxicity through alkylation of DNA. Exposure to mustard gas causes erythema, blistering, and ulceration of the lids, severe conjunctivitis, chemosis, and local thrombosis of conjunctival blood vessels, leading to ischemia. Corneal epithelial edema, superficial punctate keratitis, and stromal edema also occur. In most cases the corneal changes resolve within several days, but corneal ulceration, vascularization, opacification, and perforation can occur.[103] Treatment is palliative.

REFERENCES

1. Bargamanson JP: Corneal damage in photokeratitis: why is it so painful?, *Optom Vis Sci* 67:407, 1990.
2. Dusenbery KE et al: Beta irradiation of recurrent pterygia: results and complications, *Int J Radiat Oncol Biol Phys* 24:315, 1992.
3. Mackenzie FD et al: Recurrence rate and complications after beta irradiation for pterygia, *Ophthalmology* 98:1776, 1991.
4. Moriarty AP et al: Fungal corneoscleritis complicating beta-irradiation-induced scleral necrosis following pterygium excision, *Eye* 7:525, 1993.
5. Moriarty AP et al: Severe corneoscleral infection: a complication of beta irradiation scleral necrosis following pterygium excision, *Arch Ophthalmol* 111:947, 1993.
6. Slingsby JG, Forstot SL: Effect of blunt trauma on the corneal endothelium, *Arch Ophthalmol* 99:1041, 1981.
7. Barr CC: Prognostic factors in corneoscleral lacerations, *Arch Ophthalmol* 101:919, 1983.
8. Boldt HC et al: Rural endophthalmitis, *Ophthalmology* 96:1722, 1989.
9. Brinton GS et al: Posttraumatic endophthalmitis, *Arch Ophthalmol* 102:547, 1984.
10. Thompson WS et al: Endophthalmitis following penetrating ocular trauma, *Ophthalmology* 102:1696, 1995.
11. Levin MR, D'Amico DJ: *Traumatic endophthalmitis*. In Shingleton BJ, Hersh PS, Kenyon KR, editors: *Eye trauma*, St Louis, 1991, Mosby–Year Book.
12. Peyman GA, Carroll CP, Raichand M: Prevention and management of traumatic endophthalmitis, *Ophthalmology* 87:320, 1980.
13. The Endophthalmitis Study Group: Results of the endophthalmitis vitrectomy study: a randomized trial of immediate vitrectomy and of intravenous antibiotics for the treatment of postoperative bacterial endophthalmitis, *Arch Ophthalmol* 113:1479, 1995.
14. Asch MJ et al: Ocular complications associated with burns: review of a five-year experience including 104 patients, *J Trauma* 11:857, 1971.
15. Burns CL, Chylack LT: Thermal burns: the management of thermal burns of the lids and globes, *Ann Ophthalmol* 11:1358, 1971.
16. Guy RH et al: Three-years' experience in a regional burn center with burns of the eyes and eyelids, *Ophthalmic Surg* 13:383, 1982.
17. Grant WM: *Toxicology of the eye*, ed 3, Springfield, IL, 1983, Charles C Thomas.
18. Pfister RR et al: Collagenase activity of intact corneal epithelium in peripheral alkaline burns, *Arch Ophthalmol* 86:308, 1971.
19. Cejkova J et al: Alkali burns of the rabbit cornea: II. A histochemical study of glycosaminoglycans, *Histochemistry* 45:71, 1975.
20. Grant WM, Kern HLL: Action of alkalies on the corneal stroma, *Arch Ophthalmol* 54:931, 1955.
21. Pfister RR: Chemical injuries of the eye, *Ophthalmology* 90:1246, 1983.
22. Paterson CA, Pfister RR, Levinson RA: Aqueous humor pH changes after experimental alkali burns, *Am J Ophthalmol* 79:414, 1975.
23. Pfister RR, Friend J, Dohlman CH: The anterior segments of rabbits after alkali burns, *Arch Ophthalmol* 86:189, 1971.
24. Levinson RA, Paterson CA, Pfister RR: Ascorbic acid prevents corneal ulceration and perforation following experimental alkali burns, *Invest Ophthalmol* 15:986, 1976.

25. Pfister RR, Paterson CA: Ascorbic acid in the treatment of alkali burns of the eye, *Ophthalmology* 87:1050, 1980.
26. Shapiro MS, Friend J, Thoft RA: Corneal reepithelialization from the conjunctiva, *Invest Ophthalmol Vis Sci* 21:135, 1981.
27. Pfister RR: The alkali-burned cornea: I. Epithelial and stromal repair, *Exp Eye Res* 23:519, 1976.
28. Wagoner MD et al: Polymorphonuclear neutrophils delay corneal epithelial wound healing in vitro, *Invest Ophthalmol Vis Sci* 25:1217, 1984.
29. Nelson JD, Wright JC: Conjunctival goblet cell densities in ocular surface disease, *Arch Ophthalmol* 102:1049, 1984.
30. Ohji M et al: Goblet cell density in thermal and chemical injuries, *Arch Ophthalmol* 105:1686, 1987.
31. Paterson CA, Williams RN, Parker RV: Characteristics of polymorphonuclear leukocyte infiltration into the alkali burned eye and the influence of sodium citrate, *Exp Eye Res* 39:701, 1984.
32. Kehrer T et al: Enzyme activities in different types of severe alkali burns, *Ophthalmic Res* 16:207, 1984.
33. Reim M et al: Investigation of enzyme activities in severe burns of the anterior eye segment, *Graefes Arch Clin Exp Ophthalmol* 231:308, 1993.
34. Nirankari VS et al: Superoxide radical scavenging agents in treatment of alkali burns, *Arch Ophthalmol* 99:886, 1981.
35. Wright P: The chemically injured eye, *Trans Ophthalmol Soc UK* 102:85, 1982.
36. Berman MB et al: Characterization of collagenolytic activity in the ulcerating cornea, *Exp Eye Res* 11:255, 1971.
37. Gnädinger MC et al: The role of collagenase in the alkali burned cornea, *Am J Ophthalmol* 68:478, 1969.
38. Ben-Hanan I et al: Further evidence for the involvement of immunoregulatory processes in corneal alkali burns: effects of immunosuppression and convalescent serum, *Ophthalmic Res* 18:288, 1986.
39. Ben-Hanan Y et al: Indications for the role of the immune system in the pathogenesis of corneal alkali burns, *Br J Ophthalmol* 67:635, 1983.
40. Levinson RA, Paterson CA, Pfister RR: Ascorbic acid prevents corneal ulceration and perforation following experimental alkali burns, *Invest Ophthalmol* 15:986, 1976.
41. Pfister RR, Paterson CA: Additional clinical and morphological observations on the favorable effect of ascorbate in experimental ocular alkali burns, *Invest Ophthalmol Vis Sci* 16:478, 1977.
42. Paterson CA, Pfister RR: Intraocular pressure changes after alkali burns, *Arch Ophthalmol* 91:211, 1974.
43. Stein MR, Naidoff MA, Dawson CR: Intraocular pressure response to experimental alkali burns, *Am J Ophthalmol* 75:99, 1973.
44. Hughes WF: Alkali burns of the eye: I. Review of the literature and summary of present knowledge, *Arch Ophthalmol* 35:423, 1946.
45. Hughes WF: Alkali burns of the eye: II. Clinical and pathologic course, *Arch Ophthalmol* 36:189, 1946.
46. Roper-Hall MJ: Thermal and chemical burns, *Trans Ophthalmol Soc UK* 85:631, 1965.
47. Ralph RA: *Chemical burns of the eye.* In Duane T, editor: *Clinical ophthalmology,* vol 4, Hagerstown, MD, 1988, Harper & Row.
48. Brown SI, Tregakis MP, Pearce DB: Treatment of the alkali burned cornea, *Am J Ophthalmol* 74:361, 1972.
49. Herr RD et al: Clinical comparison of ocular irrigation fluids following chemical injury, *Am J Emerg Med* 9:228, 1991.
50. Morgan LB: A new drug delivery system for the eye, *Ind Med* 40:11, 1971.
51. Bennett TO, Payman GA, Rutgard J: Intracameral phosphate buffer in alkali burns, *Can J Ophthalmol* 13:93, 1978.
52. Paterson CA, Pfister RR, Levinson RA: Aqueous humor pH changes after experimental alkali burns, *Am J Ophthalmol* 79:414, 1975.
53. Grant WM: Experimental investigation of paracentesis in the treatment of ocular ammonia burns, *Arch Ophthalmol* 44:399, 1950.
54. Caron LA et al: Topical fibronectin in a rabbit alkali burn model of corneal ulceration, *Invest Ophthalmol Vis Sci* 26(suppl):176, 1985.
55. Tenn PF et al: Fibronectin in alkali-burned rabbit cornea: enhancement of epithelial wound healing, *Invest Ophthalmol Vis Sci* 26(suppl):92, 1985.
56. Watanabe K, Nakagawa S, Nishida T: Stimulatory effects of fibronectin and EGF on migration of corneal epithelial cells, *Invest Ophthalmol Vis Sci* 28:205, 1987.
57. Singh G, Foster CS: Epidermal growth factor in alkali-burned corneal epithelial wound healing, *Am J Ophthalmol* 103:802, 1987.
58. Chung JH, Fagerholm P: Treatment of rabbit corneal alkali wounds with human epidermal growth factor, *Cornea* 8:122, 1989.
59. Reim M et al: Effect of epidermal growth factor in severe experimental alkali burns, *Ophthalmic Res* 20:327, 1988.
60. Singh G, Foster CS: Growth factors in treatment of nonhealing corneal ulcers and recurrent erosions, *Cornea* 8:45, 1989.
61. Gordon JF et al: Topical fibronectin ophthalmic solution in the treatment of persistent defects of the corneal epithelium, *Am J Ophthalmol* 119:281, 1995.
62. Kandarakis AS, Page CS, Kaufman HE: The effect of epidermal growth factor on epithelial healing after penetrating keratoplasty in human eyes, *Am J Ophthalmol* 98:411, 1984.
63. Pastor JC, Calonge M: Epidermal growth factor and corneal wound healing: a multicenter study, *Cornea* 11:311, 1992.
64. Perry HD et al: Effect of doxycycline hyclate on corneal epithelial wound healing in the rab-

bit alkali-burn model: preliminary observations, *Cornea* 12:379, 1993.

65. Brown SI, Weller CA, Vidrich AM: Effect of corticosteroids on corneal collagenase of rabbits, *Am J Ophthalmol* 70:744, 1970.

66. Donshik PC et al: Effect of topical corticosteroids on ulceration in alkali-burned corneas, *Arch Ophthalmol* 96:2117, 1978.

67. Pfister RR, Paterson CA, Hayes SA: Effects of topical 10% ascorbate solution on established corneal ulcers after severe alkali burns, *Invest Ophthalmol Vis Sci* 22:382, 1982.

68. Pfister RR, Nicolaro ML, Paterson CA: Sodium citrate reduces the incidence of corneal ulcerations and perforations in extreme alkali-burned eyes: acetylcysteine and ascorbate have no favorable effect, *Invest Ophthalmol Vis Sci* 21:486, 1981.

69. Pfister RR, Haddox JL, Lank KM: Citrate or ascorbate/citrate treatment of established corneal ulcers in the alkali-injured rabbit eye, *Invest Ophthalmol Vis Sci* 29:1110, 1988.

70. Pfister RR: The effects of chemical injury on the ocular surface, *Ophthalmology* 90:601, 1983.

71. Pfister RR, Haddox JL, Yuille-Barr D: The combined effect of citrate/ascorbate treatment in alkali-injured rabbit eyes, *Cornea* 10:100, 1991.

72. Brown SI, Weller CA: Collagenase inhibitors in prevention of ulcers of alkali-burned cornea, *Arch Ophthalmol* 83:352, 1970.

73. Slansky HH, Dohlman CH, Berman MB: Prevention of corneal ulcers, *Trans Am Acad Ophthalmol Otolaryngol* 75:1208, 1971.

74. Slansky HH et al: Cysteine and acetylcysteine in the prevention of corneal ulcerations, *Ann Ophthalmol* 2:488, 1970.

75. Aronson SB et al: Pathogenetic approach to therapy of peripheral corneal inflammatory disease, *Am J Ophthalmol* 70:65, 1970.

76. Cejkova J et al: Histochemical study of alkali-burned rabbit anterior segment in which severe lesions were prevented by aprotinin treatment, *Histochemistry* 92:441, 1989.

77. Newsome DA, Gross J: Prevention by medroxyprogesterone of perforation in the alkali-burned rabbit cornea: inhibition of collagenolytic activity, *Invest Ophthalmol Vis Sci* 16:21, 1977.

78. Lass JH et al: Medroxyprogesterone in corneal ulceration: its effects after alkali burns in rabbits, *Arch Ophthalmol* 99:673, 1981.

79. Wentworth JS et al: Collagen shields exacerbate ulceration of alkali-burned rabbit corneas, *Arch Ophthalmol* 111:389, 1993.

80. Ballen PH: Mucous membrane grafts in chemical (lye) burns, *Am J Ophthalmol* 55:302, 1963.

81. Kramer SG: Late numerical grading of alkali burns to determine keratoplasty prognosis, *Trans Am Ophthalmol Soc* 81:97, 1983.

82. Abel R et al: The results of penetrating kera-

toplasty after chemical burns, *Trans Am Acad Ophthalmol Otolaryngol* 79:584, 1975.

83. Thoft RA: Conjunctival transplantation, *Arch Ophthalmol* 95:1425, 1977.

84. Thoft RA: Conjunctival transplantation as an alternative to keratoplasty, *Ophthalmology* 86:1084, 1979.

85. Thoft RA: Indications for conjunctival transplantation, *Ophthalmology* 89:335, 1982.

86. Kenyon KR, Tseng SCG: Limbal autograft transplantation for ocular surface disorders, *Ophthalmology* 96:709, 1989.

87. Tsai RJ-F, Sun T-T, Tseng SCG: Comparison of limbal and conjunctival autograft transplantation in corneal surface reconstruction in rabbits, *Ophthalmology* 97:446, 1990.

88. Thoft RA: Keratoepithelioplasty, *Am J Ophthalmol* 97:1, 1983.

89. Tsai RJ-F, Tseng SCG: Human allograft limbal transplantation for corneal surface reconstruction, *Cornea* 13:389, 1994.

90. Kwitko S et al: Allograft conjunctival transplantation for bilateral ocular surface disorders, *Ophthalmology* 102:1020, 1995.

91. Tsubota K et al: Reconstruction of the corneal epithelium by limbal allograft transplantation for severe ocular surface disorders, *Ophthalmology* 102:1486, 1995.

92. Aquavella JV et al: Keratoprosthesis: results, complications, and management, *Ophthalmology* 89:655, 1982.

93. Cardonna H: Prosthokeratoplasty, *Cornea* 2:179, 1983.

94. Holekamp TLR, Becker B: Ocular injuries from automobile batteries, *Trans Am Acad Ophthalmol Otolaryngol* 83:805, 1977.

95. Rubinfeld RS et al: Ocular hydrofluoric acid burns, *Am J Ophthalmol* 114:420, 1992.

96. McCulley JP et al: *Ocular hydrofluoric acid burns.* In Henkind P et al, editors: *Acta XXIV International Congress Ophthalmology,* New York, 1982, JB Lippincott.

97. Grayson M, Peroni D: Severe silver nitrate injury to the eye, *Am J Ophthalmol* 70:227, 1970.

98. Friedenwald JS, Hughes WF, Herrmann H: Acid burns of the eye, *Arch Ophthalmol* 35:98, 1946.

99. Paterson CA et al: The ocular hypertensive response following experimental acid burns in the rabbit eye, *Invest Ophthalmol Vis Sci* 18:67, 1979.

100. McCulley JP: *Chemical injuries.* In Smolin G, Thoft RA, editors: *The cornea: scientific foundations and clinical practice,* Boston, 1983, Little, Brown & Co.

101. Oaks LW, Dorman JE, Petty RW: Tear gas burns of the eye, *Arch Ophthalmol* 63:689, 1960.

102. Laibson PR, Oconor J: Explosive tear gas burns of the eye, *Trans Am Acad Ophthalmol Otolaryngol* 74:811, 1970.

103. Lashkari MH: Mustard gas keratoconjunctivitis, *Ophthalmology* 97(suppl):138, 1990.

Twenty-Seven

Conjunctival and Corneal Tumors

Many types of tumors can affect the cornea and conjunctiva: inflammatory, traumatic, congenital, degenerative, metabolic, and neoplastic (Tables 27-1 and 27-2). This chapter is concerned primarily with neoplastic tumors, but some other conditions that simulate neoplasms, such as traumatic and inflammatory tumors, are discussed as well. Some neoplasms primarily involve nonlimbal conjunctiva but can also affect the limbus and cornea; these are also discussed. Strictly corneal tumors are rare; most tumors involving the cornea arise near the limbus. The most common true neoplasms arise from the squamous epithelial cells or the melanocytes within the epithelium. Congenital lesions are discussed in Chapter 5.

OBTAINING SPECIMENS

It is often not possible to distinguish tumors clinically; histopathologic examination is required. Cytology is a simple procedure that can aid in the diagnosis of external lesions. It is used mainly to identify diffuse neoplastic processes causing conjunctivitis; a cytology specimen containing neoplastic cells points to the correct diagnosis and the need for biopsy. After topical anesthesia the surface of the mass is scraped with a stainless steel blade. The material is spread on a slide and immediately fixed with either a spray cytologic fixative or alcohol.

In nearly all cases a biopsy is preferable; more cells are obtained, the architecture is preserved, and the diagnosis is more likely to be accurate. The lesion can often be completely removed without an extensive procedure. In other cases, such as primary acquired melanosis or suspected pagetoid spread of sebaceous cell carcinoma, multiple small biopsies are taken. Topical or infiltrative local anesthesia is sufficient, and no suturing is necessary. Handling of the specimen with forceps should be minimized to prevent crushing.

It is important to make a drawing of the lesion and the site(s) of biopsy. Each specimen should be marked and preserved separately. It is best to place them flat on a carrier, such as a

Table 27-1   Conjunctival and Limbal Lesions

EPITHELIAL TUMORS
  Papillomata
  Benign hereditary dyskeratosis
  Keratoacanthoma[1]
  Pseudoepitheliomatous hyperplasia[2,3]
  Actinic keratosis
  Squamous dysplasia and carcinoma in situ
    (CIN)
  Invasive squamous cell carcinoma
  Mucoepidermoid carcinoma
  Spindle cell carcinoma
  Basal cell carcinoma[4,5]

SUBEPITHELIAL TUMORS
  Lymphoid tumors
    Lymphoid hyperplasia
    Lymphoma
  Leukemic infiltrate[6,7]
  Fibrous histiocytoma
  Myxoma
  Neurofibroma
  Schwannoma
  Oncocytoma
  Plasmacytoma
  Sarcoma
    Leiomyosarcoma[8]
  Vascular tumors
    Kaposi's sarcoma
    Lymphangioma
  Metastatic carcinoma

SEBACEOUS CELL CARCINOMA

MELANOCYTIC LESIONS
  Nevi
  Primary acquired melanosis
  Malignant melanoma

SYSTEMIC DISEASE
  Juvenile xanthogranuloma (see Chapter 22)
  Gaucher's disease (pigmented pseudopin-
    gueculae)
  Multiple endocrine neoplasia (type IIB)
  Neurofibromatosis (neurofibroma,
    schwannoma)
  Ochronosis (alkaptonuria)

INFLAMMATORY TUMORS
  Follicles
  Infectious
    Leprosy
    Mycobacterium
    Cat-scratch disease
    Syphilis
    Tularemia
    Epstein-Barr virus
    Sporotrichosis
    Nematodes
    Many others (see Parinaud's oculoglandu-
      lar syndrome, Chapter 7)
  Sarcoid
  Pyogenic granuloma
  Foreign body granuloma

Table 27-1   Conjunctival and Limbal Lesions—cont'd

INFLAMMATORY TUMORS—cont'd
  Phlyctenule
  ?Nodular fasciitis

CONGENITAL
  Choristomas
    Dermoids and lipodermoids
    Ectopic lacrimal gland
    Osseous choristomas
  Vascular hamartomas

DEGENERATIVE
  Pterygium
  Pingueculae
  Amyloid

POSTTRAUMATIC
  Pyogenic granuloma
  Corneal or conjunctival inclusion cyst
    (Fig. 27-1)
  Filtering bleb (Fig. 27-2)
  Uveal prolapse (Fig. 27-3)
  Intrastromal air (Fig. 27-4)
  Foreign body granuloma
  Keloid (Fig. 27-5)

tongue blade or flat porous paper (e.g., surgical glove wrapping paper), and indicate their orientation.

INFLAMMATORY AND POSTTRAUMATIC LESIONS

Pyogenic Granuloma

Pyogenic granulomas are exuberant growths of granulation tissue after injury, usually caused by trauma or infection. They occur most commonly after conjunctival surgery (e.g., for strabismus or pterygia) (Fig. 27-6) but can occur without an identifiable cause. Rarely, they can arise on the cornea, usually in an area with fibrovascular pannus after surgery or trauma.[9-14] They grow acutely, are intense red due to the high vascular content, and can have a narrower base, giving a pedunculated appearance (Fig. 27-7). The lesion is composed of loose vascular stroma with an infiltrate of acute and chronic inflammatory cells. Simple excision is usually sufficient; however, they can recur. Because Kaposi's sarcoma can have a similar appearance, it should be considered in the differential diagnosis.

Nodular Fasciitis

Nodular fasciitis is a rare acute reactive (nonneoplastic) proliferation of immature connec-

Table 27-2 Characteristics of Limbal Lesions

RAPIDLY GROWING
Pseudoepitheliomatous hyperplasia
Nodular fasciitis
Pyogenic granuloma
Mucoepidermoid carcinoma

NO HISTORY OF GROWTH
Dermoid
Ectopic lacrimal gland
Other choristomas
(?)Juvenile xanthogranuloma
Nevi

PAPILLARY
Benign noninfectious papilloma
Infectious (papillomavirus) papilloma
Intraepithelial neoplasia
Squamous cell carcinoma

HYPERKERATOTIC
Benign hereditary dyskeratosis
Intraepithelial neoplasia (rare)
Squamous cell carcinoma
Actinic keratosis
Pseudoepitheliomatous hyperplasia

CYSTIC
Choristomas (congenital)
Epithelial inclusion cysts
Lymphangiectasis
Filtering blebs

CHILDREN (FIRST DECADE)
Benign hereditary dyskeratosis
Dermoid
Ectopic lacrimal gland
Juvenile xanthogranuloma
Nevi

BILATERAL
Benign hereditary dyskeratosis
Dermoid
Infectious papilloma

EXTEND OVER CORNEA (> 1 mm)
Intraepithelial neoplasia
Invasive squamous cell carcinoma
Mucoepidermoid carcinoma
Dermoid
Ectopic lacrimal gland
Juvenile xanthogranuloma
Malignant melanoma
Primary corneal epithelial dysplasia

PIGMENTED
Nevi
Malignant melanoma
Primary acquired melanosis
Congenital melanosis
Kaposi's sarcoma (reddish)

METASTASIZE
Mucoepidermoid carcinoma
Malignant melanoma

Table 27-2 Characterizations of Limbal Lesions—cont'd

METASTASIZE—cont'd
Invasive squamous cell carcinoma (rare)
Lymphoma
Fibrous histiocytoma

CORNEAL STROMA EXTENSION
Dermoid
Ectopic lacrimal gland
Juvenile xanthogranuloma
Invasive squamous cell carcinoma (rare)
Malignant melanoma
(?)Mucoepidermoid carcinoma

ASSOCIATED WITH INFLAMMATION
Pyogenic granuloma
Benign hereditary dyskeratosis
Primary acquired melanosis
Nevi

HEREDITARY
Benign hereditary dyskeratosis

tive tissue. Histologically, these tumors are composed of highly cellular, generally nonencapsulated proliferations of immature fibroblasts, vascular endothelial cells, pools of mucinous material, and chronic inflammatory cells, and they can be mistaken for sarcomas (Fig. 27-8).[15,16] They often occur near rectus insertions and usually can be removed by simple excision.

Intrastromal Cysts

After trauma, epithelial cysts can form within the corneal stroma. Epithelial cells are implanted in the stroma during penetrating or perforating injury and proliferate, forming an interlamellar cyst. This cyst can be clear or become translucent as it fills with desquamated epithelium.[17]

Intraepithelial or intrastromal hemorrhage can also occur in vascularized corneas. Rarely these can lead to ulceration of the overlying stroma, presumably because of impairment of the passage of nutrients from the aqueous.[18]

Corneal Keloids

Keloids are exuberant growths of fibrous tissue that occur in response to injury.[19,20] They occur most frequently in the first two decades of life[21] after traumatic injuries or keratitis, such as corneal ulceration, measles, and ophthalmia neonatorum.[22,23] Bilateral corneal keloids seem to be common in Lowe syndrome.[24] Corneal keloids can appear as localized solitary nodules that tend to progress slowly or can diffusely involve the entire stroma.

Text continued on p. 714.

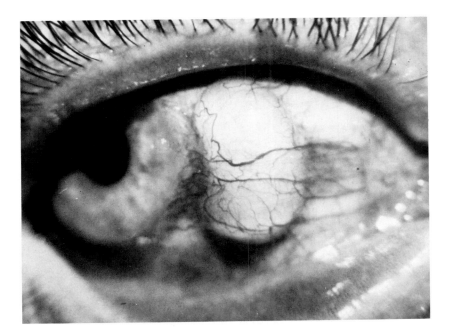

Figure 27-1
Epithelial inclusion cyst at the limbus.

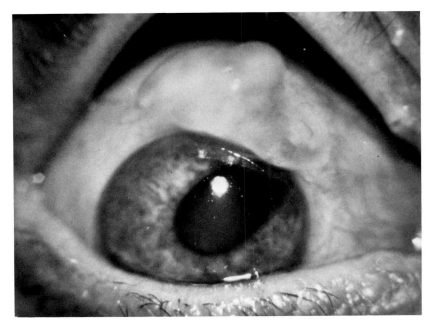

Figure 27-2
Large cystic bleb after glaucoma filtering surgery.

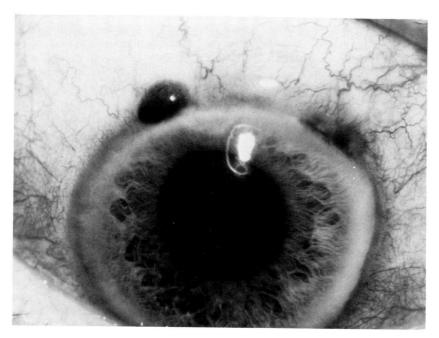

Figure 27-3
Perforation of the cornea with uveal prolapse in Terrien's marginal degeneration (see Chapter 16).

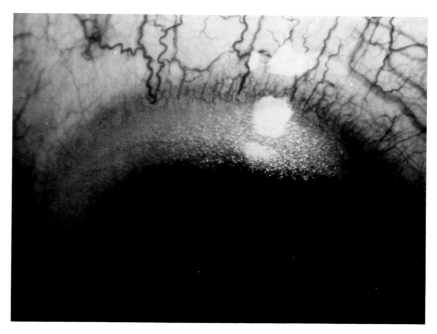

Figure 27-4
Accidental air injection into the periphery of the cornea resembling crystalline change.

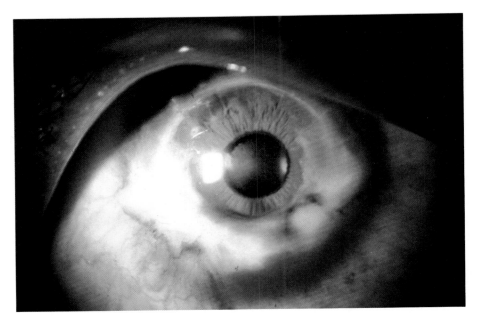

Figure 27-5
Corneal keloid that arose from the surgical wound after penetrating keratoplasty for a corneal leukoma.
(Courtesy of Massimo Busin, Bonn, Germany.)

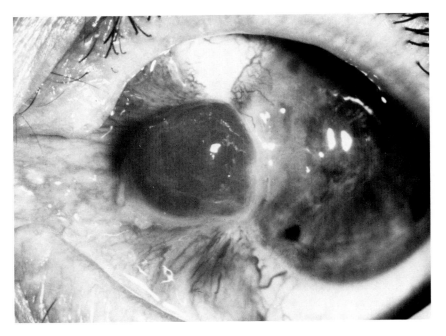

Figure 27-6
Pyogenic granuloma after pterygium surgery.

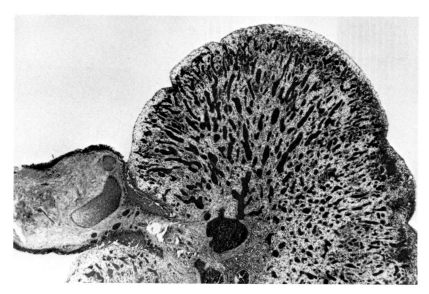

Figure 27-7
Pyogenic granuloma of the conjunctiva. This is a smooth-surfaced mass composed of vascularized granulation tissue with acute and chronic inflammatory cells. The pedunculated base is seen on the left. (Hematoxylin-eosin stain, ×50.) (Courtesy of Bruce L. Johnson, Pittsburgh, PA.)

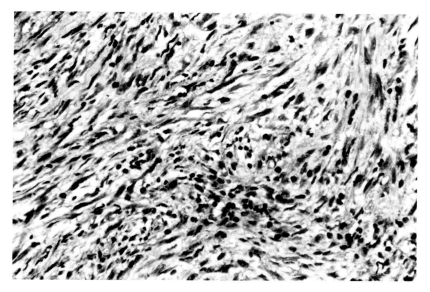

Figure 27-8
Nodular fasciitis. Loosely coherent spindle-shaped fibroblasts, intercellular myxoid material, and chronic inflammatory cells can be seen. (Hematoxylin-eosin stain, ×500.) (Courtesy of Bruce L. Johnson, Pittsburgh, PA.)

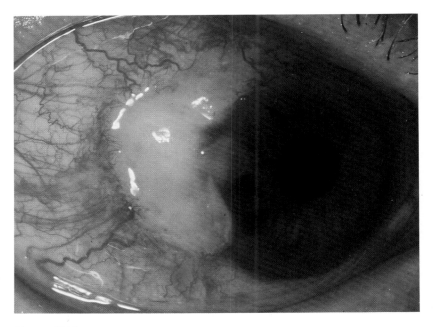

Figure 27-9
Fibrous histiocytoma.

FIBROUS HISTIOCYTOMA

Fibrous histiocytomas are solitary confined lesions composed of a mixture of fibroblasts and lipid-filled macrophages (histiocytes) that are most often found in the dermis or subcutaneous fibrous tissue. They are the most common mesenchymal orbital tumors in adults and can rarely arise from the conjunctiva, episclera, or sclera.[25-30] They can grow at the limbus and extend over the peripheral cornea. They are yellow-white and can appear as nodules at the limbus (Fig. 27-9) or as infiltrative lesions extending into the corneal stroma from the limbus. It is not clear whether the pathologic process in these external lesions is reactive or neoplastic. Excision is usually curative.

LYMPHOID TUMORS

The conjunctiva is part of the mucosal immune system and normally contains abundant lymphoid tissue. This tissue can be affected by both benign and malignant localized or systemic lymphoid proliferations. The tumors appear as single or multiple elevated masses that generally assume the contour of the globe. They are invariably salmon colored, exhibit sharply demarcated borders, lack gross blood vessels, are not tender or ulcerated, and have smooth overlying conjunctiva (Fig. 27-10). Ap-

proximately 15% to 20% of cases are bilateral. In the great majority of cases there is no history or evidence of systemic disease.

Histologic and immunologic classification of conjunctival lymphoid tumors continues to evolve. There appears to be a spectrum of lesions, ranging from polyclonal T-cell–rich tumors, in which there is a heterogeneous mix of lymphocytes, plasma cells, and histiocytes, called *reactive lymphoid hyperplasia,* to poorly differentiated monoclonal B-cell proliferations. The risk of developing systemic lymphoma, and in turn the related mortality, varies along the spectrum, but even the most benign-appearing lesions are associated with a risk of systemic disease. This may be because lesions can evolve along the spectrum, from benign to malignant.

Generally, conjunctival lymphoid tumors are divided into polyclonal T-cell–rich pseudolymphomas and monoclonal B-cell lymphomas.[31-35] The monoclonal B-cell tumors can then be subdivided into well-differentiated, intermediate, and poorly differentiated lymphomas. Polyclonal tumors and well- and intermediately differentiated B-cell tumors have a very good prognosis; the risk of extraocular manifestations appears to be low.[36,37] However, the risk of systemic disease is much higher for poorly differentiated B-cell lymphomas. Further immunohistochemical differentiation, such as T- and B-cell subsets, has not proved clinically

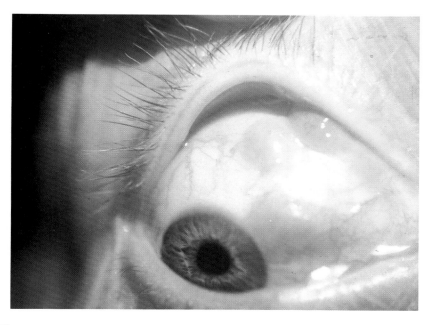

Figure 27-10
Malignant lymphoma in the bulbar conjunctiva appears as a smooth, raised, salmon pink tumor.

useful.[35,36] The course of conjunctival lymphoid tumors seems to be better than that of orbital lymphoid tumors, possibly because the conjunctiva normally contains lymphoid tissue, but the orbit does not.[31] Even when spread occurs, the course is often slow, and survival is prolonged.

Many conjunctival lymphoid tumors may be mucosal-associated lymphoid tissue (MALT) lymphomas. MALT is a distinct form of lymphoid tissue found in the bowel, stomach, respiratory mucosa, salivary glands, and other tissues. The conjunctiva-associated lymphoid tissue is probably a form of MALT (see Chapter 19). MALT tissue may develop neoplastic proliferations that are distinct from other lymphomas in histologic appearance and in behavior. MALT lymphomas are less aggressive than other forms of B-cell lymphoma and tend to remain localized to mucosal surfaces. Conjunctival lymphomas with the MALT phenotype have been described[36,38-41] and may be more frequent than previously realized.

The treatment recommended by Jakobiec et al.[26] for conjunctival lymphomas is as follows:

1. All patients should be evaluated for evidence of systemic disease, including chest radiography, whole-body computed tomography, complete peripheral blood count, Coombs' test, antinuclear antibodies, latex fixation, serum protein immuno- electrophoresis, bone marrow biopsy, bone scan, and liver-spleen scan.
2. If nonocular disease is not detected, patients receive 15 to 20 Gy of radiotherapy to the involved area, with shielding of the eyeball. This treatment is necessary because of the possibility of dedifferentiation and spread.
3. Systemic noninvasive evaluations are repeated every 6 months for 5 years.

Cryotherapy may be as effective for conjunctival lymphoid tumors as radiation, with fewer complications.[42] Multiple treatments are often necessary.

EPITHELIAL TUMORS

Tumors of the epithelium can be classified as benign, dysplastic, precancerous, or malignant. Benign tumors include cysts, papillomata, and keratoses. Dysplastic growths include squamous dysplasia and carcinoma in situ, which are referred to as *conjunctival intraepithelial neoplasia* and *actinic keratoses*. Invasive squamous cell carcinoma and mucoepidermoid carcinoma are malignant neoplasms.

The following terms are often used to describe epithelial growths and should be understood:

- *Squamous metaplasia*—Transformation of columnar or glandular epithelium into stratified squamous epithelium, sometimes with keratinization
- *Acanthosis*—Thickening of the prickle (malpighian) cell layer
- *Hyperkeratosis*—Increased keratin in the granular cell layer
- *Dyskeratosis*—Keratinization of individual cells at an abnormally deep level
- *Parakeratosis*—Nuclei present in the keratin layer
- *Dysplasia*—Cells showing atypical size and shape, increased nuclear:cytoplasmic ratio, and mitotic figures; maturation and polarity are disturbed
- *Neoplasia*—New growth, tumor formation; a mass of abnormal cells
- *Pseudoepitheliomatous hyperplasia*—A benign reactive epithelial proliferation

Papillomata

A *papilloma* is a circumscribed, elevated epithelial tumor. It consists of villous or arborescent fibrovascular outgrowths covered by neoplastic epithelium. Clinically the epithelium is translucent, and through it the capillaries in the connective tissue core can be seen. The tumor can arise from a thin central stalk (pedunculated type) or broad base (sessile type).

Conjunctival papillomatous lesions can be seen in both young and old patients. They can be viral papillomas, other benign lesions, or malignant growths, and it can be difficult or impossible to distinguish among them clinically. Table 27-3 lists some differentiating features.

The lesions seen in the younger age group (and possibly those seen in adults as well) are most often caused by viral infection with human papilloma virus (HPV).[43-46] Different serotypes of this virus are thought to be responsible for verrucae of the face, hands, and feet and genital and anal warts. HPV 6 and the closely related HPV 11, which cause most of the benign warts (condyloma acuminatum) of the genitals, appear to be most commonly associated with conjunctival papillomas.[43,46,47]

Viral papillomata can affect any portion of the conjunctiva, including the limbus. The papillomata are frequently multiple and bilateral. A fine epithelial keratitis can be seen. Viral papillomata can be observed for up to 2 years, because many of the papillomata resolve spontaneously in that time.[48] If they persist, simple excision should be combined with cryotherapy of the base and surrounding epithelium. Removal with the carbon dioxide laser also appears to be safe and effective.[49,50] These lesions can contain live virus, and if incompletely removed, can become alarmingly widespread (Fig. 27-11).[48]

The papillomata in older persons are commonly dysplastic or malignant. Some may be

Table 27-3 Clinical Characteristics of Conjunctival Papillomata	
Infectious (Viral)	**Noninfectious (Unknown Cause)**
Usually in children or young adults	Usually in older adults
May be bilateral	Nearly always unilateral
May be multiple	Nearly always single
Usually on palpebral conjunctiva, fornix, or caruncle, especially below; less commonly at limbus	Usually on bulbar conjunctiva or at limbus
Pedunculated	Sessile or diffuse
Smooth surface	More surface irregularity and thickening
May occur with verrucae on eyelid or elsewhere	No such association
Multiple lesions may appear after excision of single lesion	Each recurrence usually single
Transmissible	Not transmissible
Usually little or no conjunctivitis; rarely moderate conjunctivitis	Occasionally marked conjunctivitis ("masquerade syndrome")
Occasionally fine ("toxic") epithelial keratitis	Cornea involved only by direct extension or mechanical factors
Rarely, if ever, malignant	Benign, dysplastic, or malignant
Spontaneous resolution common	Spontaneous resolution uncommon

From Wilson FM II, Oster HB: *Am J Ophthalmol* 77:103, 1974.

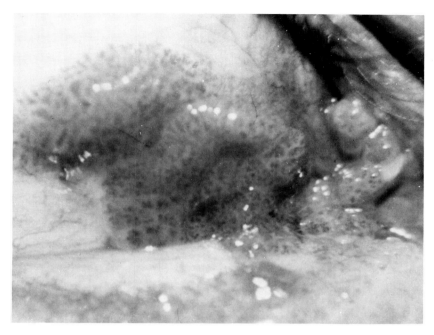

Figure 27-11
Viral papilloma extending from the limbal bulbar conjunctiva to the caruncle.

related to infection with papillomavirus.[45] They tend to be sessile and affect the limbus or bulbar conjunctiva (Fig. 27-12). The tumor can drape over the cornea or extend into the corneal epithelium or stroma. Papillary lesions in adults should be excised, particularly if they arise at the limbus, extend onto the cornea, or exhibit continued growth. Simple excision with cryotherapy of the base and surrounding epithelium is usually curative. The tumor can usually be scraped from the corneal surface, without dissection into the stroma, and cryotherapy is performed at the limbus.

Benign Hereditary Dyskeratosis

Benign hereditary dyskeratosis is a rare condition transmitted in a dominant fashion.[51,52] It affects descendants of a kindred of individuals from Halifax and Warren counties in North Carolina who have Halowar Indian, black, and white heritage and a high rate of consanguineous marriages. Cases have been seen in other parts of the country in individuals who have relocated from this area.[53,54]

Benign hyperkeratotic lesions affect the bulbar conjunctiva, typically at the limbus. The conjunctival lesions are raised, granular, semitransparent, and horseshoe-shaped (Fig. 27-13). They are usually bilateral, can be both nasal and temporal, and are located primarily in the interpalpebral fissure. They commonly appear during the first year of life and gradually progress. The lesions do not extend over the cornea or threaten vision, but corneal opacities can occur rarely and are usually deep and associated with vascularization. These lesions can be associated with conjunctival injection, foreign body sensation, papillary hypertrophy of the tarsal conjunctiva, iritis, and rubeosis iridis. Oral lesions, such as white spongy lesions on the buccal and labial mucosa and the ventral aspect of the tongue, can also be seen.

Histologically, the lesions are composed of hyperplastic epithelium, with acanthosis and dyskeratosis, but no other signs of atypia. Increased vascularization and a moderate inflammatory reaction in the conjunctival connective tissue may occur. These lesions do not evolve into truly dysplastic or carcinomatous tumors. There is no treatment; even after complete excision the lesions commonly recur.

Squamous Dysplasia and Carcinoma in Situ

Dysplasia and intraepithelial neoplasia of the conjunctival epithelium (carcinoma in situ) are uncommon tumors that are seen most often in older, fair-skinned people. The incidence of conjunctival dysplasia or carcinoma in Brisbane, Australia was estimated to be 1.9 per 100,000 per year.[55] The risk is related to the history of ultraviolet light exposure.[56] There is evi-

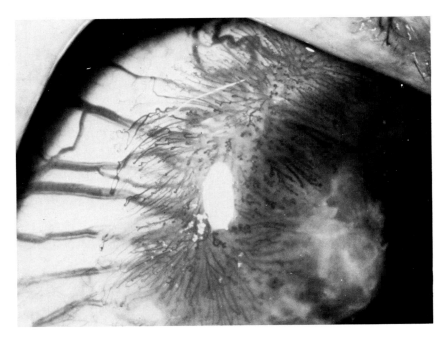

Figure 27-12
Neoplastic papilloma.

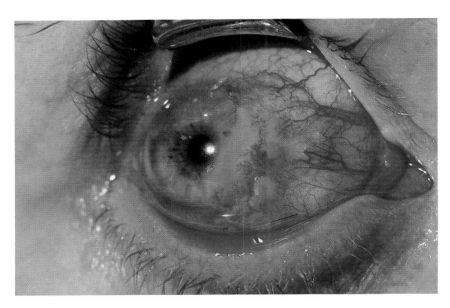

Figure 27-13
Hereditary benign intraepithelial dyskeratosis: leukoplakic limbal lesions with large conjunctival feeder vessels and corneal pannus adjacent to the lesions. (From McLean IW et al: *Ophthalmology* 88:164, 1981.)

dence that at least a portion of conjunctival epithelial neoplasms are associated with HPV. DNA from HPV types 16 and 18 has been demonstrated in neoplasms by polymerase chain reaction.[57-59] In a review of tissue samples from 38 patients, HPV 16 DNA was identified in 33 (87%).[60] HPV 16 and 18 have been implicated in the development of carcinomas in the cervix, anogenital region, upper respiratory tract, and skin.[61] The mode of transmission of the virus to the eye is not known, but in one study HPV 16 was identified in limbal conjunctival swabs from 76% of women with HPV-related cervical dysplasia.[62]

The tumors grow slowly and are usually asymptomatic. They nearly always arise at the limbus and are more common in the interpalpebral area, although lesions can arise from the bulbar or palpebral conjunctiva. The lesions appear as raised, somewhat gelatinous masses, which may be gray and slightly red, depending on the vascularity[63] (Fig. 27-14). Some dysplastic lesions have a papillary appearance, and rarely they can be hyperkeratotic and appear white (leukoplakic). In many cases the abnormal epithelium extends onto the peripheral cornea, where it can appear translucent, frosted, or white and can be associated with underlying vessels. If neglected for prolonged periods, extensive corneal involvement can develop (Fig. 27-15).

The main histopathologic feature of both dysplasia and carcinoma in situ is anaplasia of the epithelial cells. There is a high nuclear:cytoplasmic ratio; the normal polarity of the epithelium is lost; mitotic figures are more frequent; and there is dysmaturation with dyskeratosis. The process is called "dysplastic" if only a partial thickness of the epithelial layer is replaced by atypical cells (Fig. 27-16) and "carcinoma in situ" if there is total replacement of the epithelial layer (Fig. 27-17); in both cases the basement membrane is intact. The usefulness of distinguishing between dysplasia and carcinoma in situ is controversial, and some prefer just to use the term *conjunctival intraepithelial neoplasia* for both. If invasion into the subepithelial connective tissue occurs, the diagnosis of invasive squamous cell carcinoma is made.

Actinic keratoses are similar to solar keratoses, which arise on the skin and can be considered a type of dysplastic lesion. Histologically, they are differentiated from other dysplastic lesions by their surface keratinization and elastotic degeneration of the collagen in the substantia propria. However, they should be considered a form of carcinoma in situ, because their prognosis and natural history are similar.

The treatment is excision, down to bare sclera, incorporating a margin of apparently normal conjunctiva that is 2 to 3 mm wide. The extent of the tumor is best visualized by the application of rose bengal red (Fig. 27-18); areas with tumor exhibit punctate staining.[64] Portions extending over the cornea can be scraped off with a Kimura spatula or scalpel blade (e.g., Bard-Parker #64). Occasionally an adherent fibrovascular pannus is present and must be removed with sharp dissection. The limbus is carefully cleaned and scraped and can be

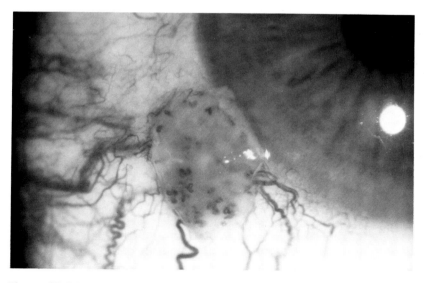

Figure 27-14
Dysplastic lesion arising at the limbus.

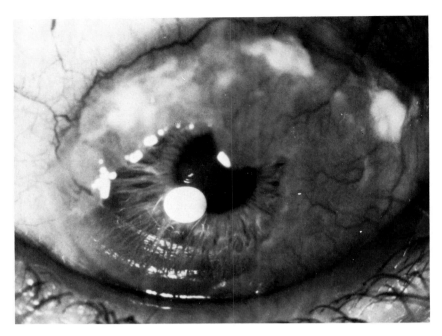

Figure 27-15
Carcinoma in situ involving the corneal epithelium.

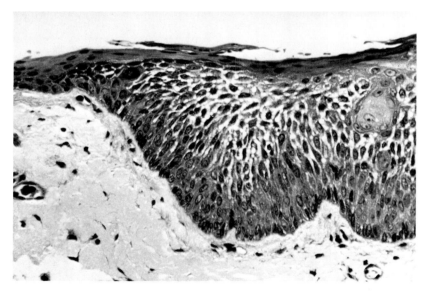

Figure 27-16
Moderately severe dysplasia of the conjunctival epithelium. Note thickening (acanthosis) of the epithelial layer with moderate atypia and loss of cellular polarity, not involving the full thickness of the epithelium. (Hematoxylin-eosin stain, ×500.) (Courtesy of Bruce L. Johnson, Pittsburgh, PA.)

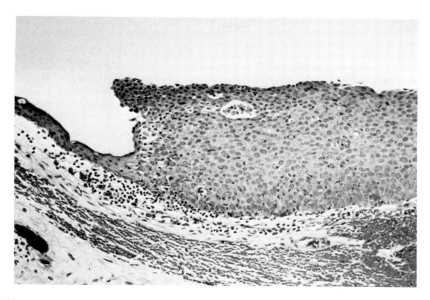

Figure 27-17
Carcinoma in situ. Note loss of cellular polarity and acanthosis involving the full thickness of the epithelial layer. (Hematoxylin-eosin stain, ×200.) (Courtesy of Bruce L. Johnson, Pittsburgh, PA.)

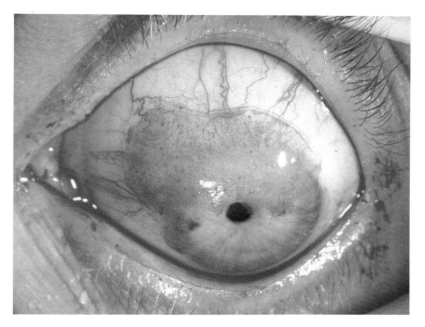

Figure 27-18
Limbal squamous tumor stained with rose bengal.

scrubbed with absolute alcohol. The limbus, base, and conjunctival margin are then frozen with a retinal cryoprobe in a rapid double freeze-thaw manner.[65] Extensive deep freezing must be carefully avoided because in a few cases ciliary body damage has led to phthisis.

Microscopically controlled excision, using an adaptation of the Mohs' micrographic technique for cutaneous tumors, may better ensure complete excision of the tumor. In a review of 19 patients, there was no evidence of recurrence in 6 to 60 months of follow-up.[66] Topical 5-fluorouracil has been used after excision or alone as treatment for noninvasive epithelial dysplasia or carcinoma in situ.[67,68] Extensive epithelial sloughing occurred, but resolution of disease without recurrence was seen in some cases.

A significant proportion of these lesions recur, even with the treatment described previously. Therefore, these patients must be followed up regularly, with rose bengal staining and reexcision of any suspicious areas. Excision of lesions that involve over 50% of the limbus can result in corneal surface disease and poor vision. In two such cases limbal autografts were successful in restoring vision.[69]

Primary Corneal Epithelial Dysplasia

Primary corneal epithelial dysplasia is a rare condition that mainly affects the corneal epithelium, without a limbal mass. It probably arises at the limbus and, for unknown reasons, spreads in a relatively flat manner over the cornea rather than accumulating at the limbus or extending into the conjunctiva.[70-72] The abnormal epithelium appears frosted or opalescent, is usually not vascularized, and has smooth or fringelike (fimbriated) edges. The lesions can be multiple, extend from the limbus or lie free in the cornea, and can be unilateral or bilateral. They progress slowly, waxing and waning in their extent. The treatment is simple removal (scraping), although the lesions can recur.

Squamous cell carcinoma of the cornea, without an associated limbal lesion, has been reported.[73] Invasion of the corneal stroma was observed. In these cases superficial keratectomy or penetrating keratoplasty was used to excise the tumor.

Invasive Squamous Cell Carcinoma

Invasive squamous cell carcinoma can arise from preexisting epithelial dysplasia or carcinoma in situ. The anaplastic cells pass through the basement membrane and invade the subepithelial tissues of the conjunctiva or cornea (Fig. 27-19). If left undetected, the invasion can extend into the deeper layers of the cornea, the sclera, or even into the eye. Only very rarely will the cells metastasize.[74]

Excision is the recommended treatment. Wide local excision, including lamellar sclerectomy if necessary, is combined with cryotherapy of the base and margins.[65] If intraocular invasion has occurred, enucleation is usually per-

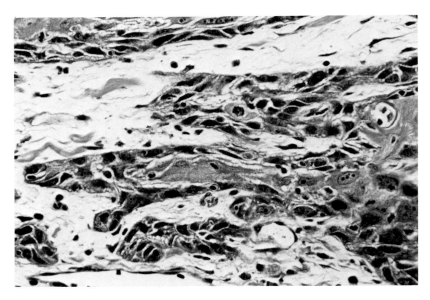

Figure 27-19
Invasive squamous cell carcinoma. The atypical epithelial cells have invaded the conjunctival stroma. (Hematoxylin-eosin stain, ×600.) (Courtesy of Bruce L. Johnson, Pittsburgh, PA.)

formed. Excision with retention of vision and no evidence of recurrence for 3.5 years was reported in one case,[75] but in another case intraocular tumor was observed 1 year after excision.[76] Exenteration is required for treatment of orbital extension.

Mucoepidermoid Carcinoma

Mucoepidermoid carcinoma is a more aggressive form of epithelial carcinoma in which there is proliferation of both squamous cells and mucin-producing goblet cells.[77-80] It cannot be clinically differentiated from typical squamous cell carcinoma. Mucoepidermoid carcinoma is usually seen in the elderly and most commonly arises at the limbus, although it can be found elsewhere in the conjunctiva. It is more likely than squamous cell carcinoma to invade the substantia propria, invade the globe, or metastasize to the regional lymph nodes. For this reason it is important to make the distinction histologically (Fig. 27-20). Mucin production can be present in only a small portion of the tumor, and in some cases it was noted in only the intraocular portion.[78,81] Wide local excision with cryotherapy is the primary treat-

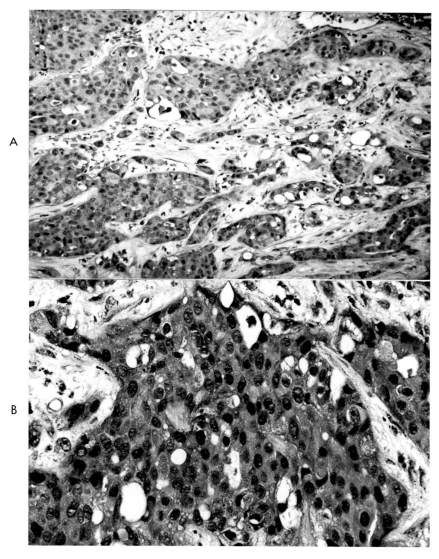

Figure 27-20
Mucoepidermoid carcinoma. **A,** Nests of abnormal cells invading the stroma. (Hematoxylin-eosin stain, ×200.) **B,** Multiple mucus-filled spaces are present within squamous cells. (Hematoxylin-eosin stain, ×500.) (Courtesy of Bruce L. Johnson, Pittsburgh, PA.)

ment. However, recurrence often leads to enucleation or exenteration. One case of recurrent mucoepidermoid carcinoma was treated successfully with excision and epibulbar iodine-125 plaque radiotherapy.[82]

Spindle Cell Carcinoma

Spindle cell carcinoma is another variant of squamous cell carcinoma in which the cells are spindle-shaped, appearing similar to fibroblasts[83,84] (Fig. 27-21). Their epithelial origin, however, has been supported by electron microscopy and immunohistochemistry.[85-87] These tumors are also relatively aggressive and are capable of intraocular extension.

SEBACEOUS CELL CARCINOMA

Although it is not a primary tumor of the conjunctiva or cornea, sebaceous cell carcinoma is important to mention because of its tendency to spread in a pagetoid fashion into the conjunctiva and cornea. Tumors of the sebaceous glands in the lids (e.g., meibomian or Zeis glands) or caruncle can spread up the gland ducts onto the epithelial surface, sometimes without a noticeable primary nodule (Fig. 27-22). These patients can present with chronic unilateral conjunctivitis, blepharoconjunctivitis, or keratoconjunctivitis (masquerade syndrome)[88-90] (Fig. 27-23). Clues to the correct diagnosis are eyelid thickening and deformity, lash loss, marked mucoid discharge, unilaterality, and an abnormal, thick papillary conjunctival appearance (see Chapter 8). In some cases sebaceous neoplasia is limited to the conjunctiva, without invasion of the basement membrane.[91] Whenever pagetoid spread of sebaceous cell carcinoma is suspected, multiple conjunctival biopsies should be taken. If the lid is thickened or a nodule is present, a wedge biopsy should be performed.

KAPOSI'S SARCOMA

This previously rare tumor has become more common because it occurs in approximately 30% of patients with AIDS.[92-96] The lesions are nodular or diffuse, blue-red or deep brown, and elevated and are usually found in the inferior forniceal conjunctiva[97] (Fig. 27-24) or eyelid. Kaposi's sarcoma usually develops in patients with an established history of the disease, but it can be a presenting manifestation. It is also more common in patients with lymphoma and leukemia. Most lesions are slowly progressive and rarely invasive.[95] Complications are usually related to the bulk of the tumor: entropion, discomfort, and obstruction of vision.

Histopathologically, the tumor is composed

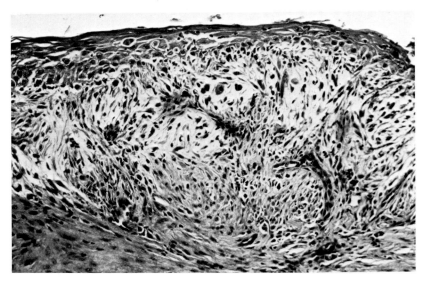

Figure 27-21
Spindle-cell variant of squamous cell carcinoma. Pleomorphic and hyperchromatic spindle-shaped cells extend from the surface epithelium and infiltrate the stroma. (Hematoxylin-eosin stain, ×250.) (Courtesy of Bruce L. Johnson, Pittsburgh, PA.)

of spindle-shaped cells with elongated oval nuclei, capillaries, and vascular slits without an apparent endothelial lining. It probably arises from vascular cells, endothelial cells, or pericytes.[97]

These tumors can be treated with simple excision,[98] cryotherapy,[98] radiation,[99,100] subconjunctival interferon-α_{2a},[101] or chemotherapy, but recurrence appears to be frequent with all forms of treatment. Fluorescein angiography may be useful prior to resection to indicate the extent of the tumor.[98] No comparative studies have been performed to determine the optimum treatment.

PIGMENTED LESIONS

The melanocytes in the conjunctiva are analogous to those in the epidermis.[102] They nor-

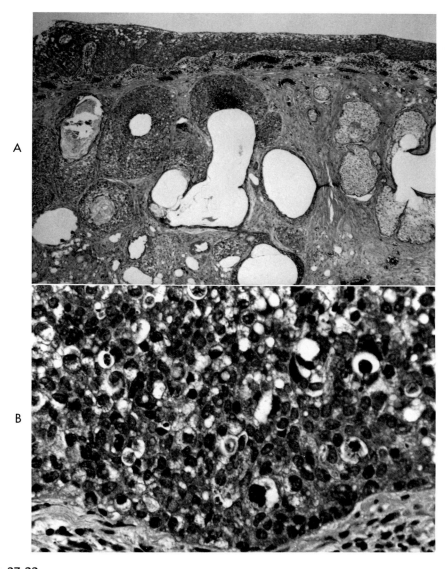

Figure 27-22
A, Sebaceous cell carcinoma arising from the meibomian glands of the tarsus. Note normal gland tissue on the right and the spread of abnormal cells superficially (pagetoid growth) on the left. (Hematoxylin-eosin stain, ×4.) **B,** Higher magnification of anaplastic superficial cells, with vacuolated cytoplasm, large nuclear forms, and abnormal mitotic figures. (Hematoxylin-eosin stain, ×500.) (Courtesy of Bruce L. Johnson, Pittsburgh, PA.)

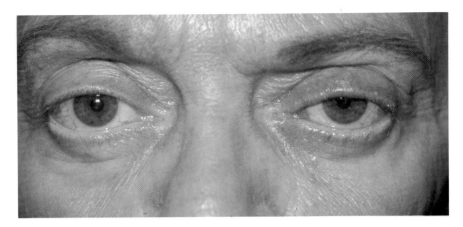

Figure 27-23
Sebaceous cell carcinoma of the left eye, producing conjunctivitis, thickening and erythema of upper lid, and loss of lashes. (Courtesy of Richard A. Thoft, Pittsburgh, PA.)

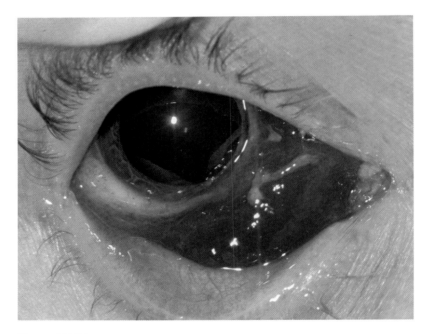

Figure 27-24
Kaposi's sarcoma.

mally are located within the basal layer of the epithelium and have delicate branching dendritic processes that contain little or no pigment. When stimulated to produce excess amounts of melanin, the melanocytes typically secrete the pigment into the adjacent epithelial or underlying stromal cells. Blacks tend to develop pigmentation of nonmelanocytic lesions, such as papillomas, through this mechanism.

The conjunctival melanocyte is most likely derived from the neural crest cells. In histologic sections stained with hematoxylin and eosin, conjunctival melanocytes are solitary dendritic cells with clear cytoplasm. The cells vary in size, number, and melanin content.

Pigmentation of the cornea and conjunctiva can also result from an increased number of melanocytes, deposition of melanin, or deposition of other pigments, such as mascara or alkapton. Conditions that can cause brownish

Table 27-4	Conditions Associated with Pigmentation of the Cornea and Conjunctiva

Benign epithelial melanosis
Congenital subepithelial melanosis
   Melanosis oculi
   Oculodermal melanocytosis (nevus of Ota)
Primary acquired melanosis
Conjunctival nevi
   Intraepithelial (junctional)
   Subepithelial
   Compound
Blue nevi
Secondary pigmentation
   Chronic conjunctival disorders
      Trachoma
      Vernal conjunctivitis
      Vitamin A deficiency
      Epithelial tumors[105]
   Skin diseases
      Xeroderma pigmentosum
      Acanthosis nigricans
   Chemicals
      Arsenic
      Phenothiazines
      Epinephrine products
      Gold
      Quinacrine
   Systemic disorders
      Addison's disease
      Folic acid deficiency anemias[106]
      Pregnancy
      Thyroid disease
      Alkaptonuria
      Alport's syndrome
   Miscellaneous
      Striate melanokeratosis
      Mascara particle inclusions
      Uveal tissue
      Hematogenous pigmentation

Some of these conditions are discussed in the following sections.

pigmentation of the cornea, limbus, or neighboring conjunctiva are given in Table 27-4.[103,104]

Benign Epithelial Melanosis

Discrete pigmented lesions can appear at birth or in early childhood, representing melanin in the basal layers of the conjunctival epithelium. These benign lesions are seen more frequently in more deeply pigmented races. They do not exhibit any malignant potential; they are always stationary. The pigmentation most often affects the perilimbal and interpalpebral areas and can extend into the peripheral corneal epithelium. It is bilateral, fairly symmetric, flat, and uninflamed.

Pigmentation can also be seen around an Axenfeld's loop, an intrascleral nerve loop approximately 4 mm from the limbus (Fig. 27-25), and around the anterior ciliary vessels. These spots occur regularly in blacks and less frequently in whites, especially those with lightly pigmented irides.

Congenital Subepithelial Melanosis

Congenital subepithelial melanosis is a group of abnormal melanin-containing cells found in the episclera and sclera, creating a slate bluegray coloration (Fig. 27-26). This condition is thought to result from incomplete migration of melanocytes destined for the surface epithelium. An increase in the number and size of melanocytes may be observed in the uvea, sclera, episclera, dermis of the eyelid, optic nerve meninges, and orbital soft tissues. These cases are more common in whites and are usually unilateral, congenital, and stationary.

The condition is called *melanosis oculi* if it is restricted to the globe, and *congenital oculodermal melanocytosis* (*nevus of Ota*) if it involves both the globe and the periorbital skin. It is usually unilateral and occurs mainly in Asians and blacks (Fig. 27-27). Malignant melanoma can occur, but the incidence does not appear to be higher than normal.

Melanocytoma

Melanocytoma is a congenital, jet-black, slowly progressive pigmented tumor composed of large polyhedral cells that are loaded with melanin. These cells are found in the deep substantia propria and episclera; therefore, the lesion often does not move with the conjunctiva. It can occur rarely in the limbal area and can be mistaken for a malignant melanoma.[107,108]

Conjunctival Nevi

Nevi are common conjunctival lesions and are similar to those of the skin. They are noted occasionally at birth, but more commonly appear during the first two decades of life. They consist of clusters of rounded, benign-appearing melanocytes and are classified according to the following layer(s) in which they are found:

1. Intraepithelial (junctional)
2. Subepithelial
3. Compound (intraepithelial plus subepithelial)

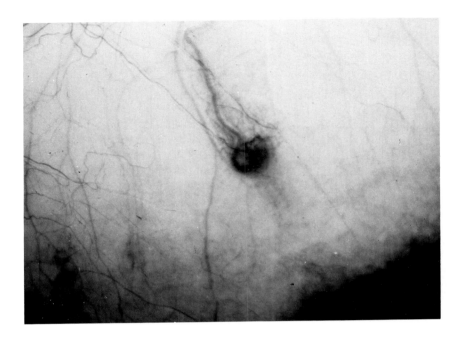

Figure 27-25
Axenfeld's loop.

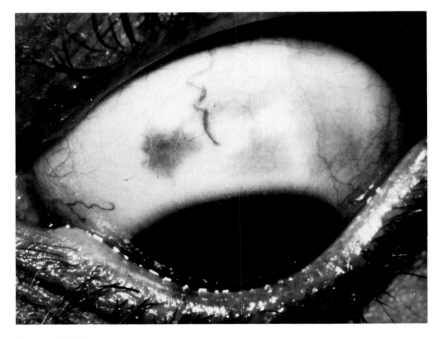

Figure 27-26
Melanosis oculi.

The nevi are initially located between the basal epithelium and the epithelial basement membrane (junctional) and gradually extend into the substantia propria in the ensuing decades, becoming compound and then subepithelial. Therefore, most conjunctival nevi are compound or subepithelial; junctional nevi are found only during the first two decades.

Conjunctival nevi occur most commonly at the limbus, in the bulbar conjunctiva, plica, caruncle, or lid margin; palpebral conjunctival or forniceal nevi are relatively rare. They may

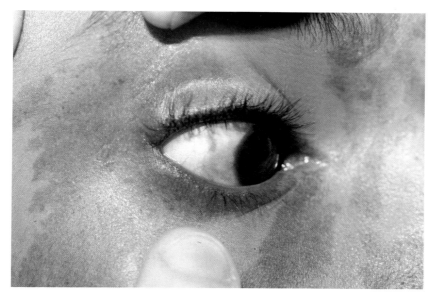

Figure 27-27
Nevus of Ota. (Courtesy of Kenneth Cheng, Pittsburgh, PA.)

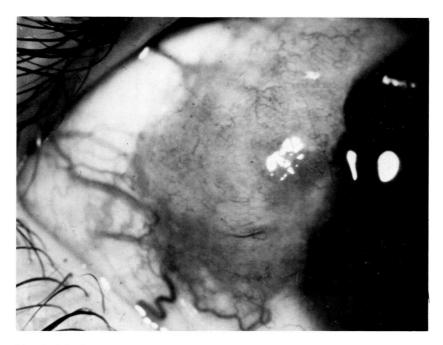

Figure 27-28
Pigmented nevus overlapping the peripheral cornea.

be focal or diffuse but are usually not multifocal. Subepithelial and compound nevi typically elevate the conjunctival surface, a process that often increases with time. All nevi are freely movable over the globe. Approximately 20% to 30% of nevi are nonpigmented. Limbal nevi can slightly overlap the peripheral cornea (Fig. 27-28), but they do not extend into the corneal stroma. (The lesion can be lifted off the cornea, revealing that the base ends at the limbus.) They can grow, especially in childhood, become more pigmented, develop clear cysts, or be associated with inflammation. Rarely do they progress to melanoma, but approximately 25% of conjunctival melanomas arise from pre-existing nevi.[109,110]

Pigmented lesions of the tarsal or forniceal conjunctiva should be excised because of the relatively greater likelihood that these lesions are malignant. Other lesions that are growing, increasing in vascularity, fixed to the underlying sclera, or associated with inflammation should be biopsied or excised, although most will be benign. Nevi can recur after excision.

Blue Nevi

Blue nevi and cellular blue nevi arise from congenital nests of melanocytes in the dermis of the skin or substantia propria of the conjunctiva.[111] They are hamartomas, resulting from incomplete migration of neural crest cells destined for the surface epithelium. When they occur in the skin they are blue, but in the conjunctiva they appear brown or black. They lack cysts, are clearly subepithelial, and move freely with the conjunctiva. They can exhibit slow growth.[112]

Primary Acquired Melanosis

Bilateral acquired racial melanosis, seen commonly in blacks, is a brown lesion located at the limbus.[113,114] There is no malignant potential, and no treatment is necessary.

Primary acquired melanosis is a unilateral idiopathic pigmentation of the conjunctival epithelium that most often occurs in whites. The pigmentation is caused by proliferation of intraepithelial melanocytes. It is patchy or diffuse and usually appears tan, black, or golden brown (Figs. 27-29 and 27-30), but it can lack pigmentation.[115,116] The onset is usually during the fourth decade of life or later, but it can arise in children. Patients with the atypical mode syndrome (dysplastic nevus syndrome) may be at a higher risk.[117,118] Any portion of the conjunctiva can be involved, and the lesions can extend onto the lid margin or the cornea. It begins as flat lesions that can wax and wane and

change location, but it generally progresses slowly. Increased activity can be associated with signs of inflammation, including hyperemia and subepithelial infiltrates. Cysts may be present. Ultraviolet light (Wood's lamp) is useful in detecting the full extent of the melanosis.[119]

Their most significant feature is their tendency for development of nodules of invasive malignant melanoma. The risk is significant enough that some have recommended changing the name of the condition to "melanoma in situ."[120] The span between onset and malignant change is variable, but probably averages 5 to 10 years. The risk of development of malignancy can be estimated by determining the histology of the lesion in multiple locations.[113,114,121-124] Multiple biopsies are taken from the different areas of pigmentation and evaluated microscopically.

The pathologist will determine the following: (1) whether or not the lesion is primary acquired melanosis; (2) if cytologic atypia is present; (3) if atypia is identified, whether cytologic features associated with high risk of progression to malignant melanoma are present; and (4) whether malignant melanoma is present. Patients having primary acquired melanosis without atypia have a low risk of developing malignant melanoma. Patients having primary acquired melanosis with atypia have a nearly 50% risk of developing malignant melanoma in the future, and if high-risk histologic features are present the risk can increase to 75% to 90%.

The high-risk features are related to the pattern of epithelial involvement and the presence of epithelioid cells.[114] When atypical melanocytes are arranged in nests or exhibit pagetoid epithelial spread the risk of melanoma approaches 90%. In addition, lesions with conspicuous epithelioid cell content are more likely to progress to melanoma.

Treatment

If the lesion is small an excisional biopsy should be performed. If the lesion is diffuse or multiple lesions are present, multiple biopsies should be taken from the portions of pigmented conjunctiva. Any area that is elevated should be biopsied.

If no atypia is present observation is indicated. If atypia is present the entire lesion should be excised, if possible. If the lesion is too extensive to excise entirely, areas with atypia should be excised if possible. Portions can be removed with histologic control unit free surgical margins are obtained (analogous to Mohs' technique for skin lesions). If large areas of the conjunctiva are affected by atypia, cryotherapy can be performed instead.[110,125,126]

These patients should be examined every 3 to 6 months for several years; if the lesion is stable, the follow-up interval can be extended to every 6 to 12 months. Photography is often helpful, and a Wood's lamp can assist in detecting the presence of early pigmentation. Repeat biopsies should be performed if there is any change in the size, elevation, or pigmentation of the lesion. The treatment of malignant melanoma is discussed later.

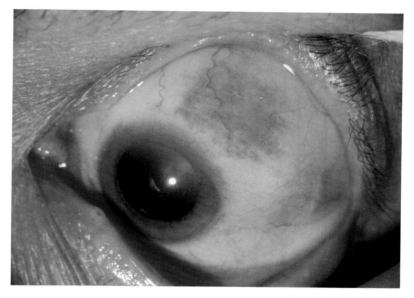

Figure 27-29
Acquired melanosis.

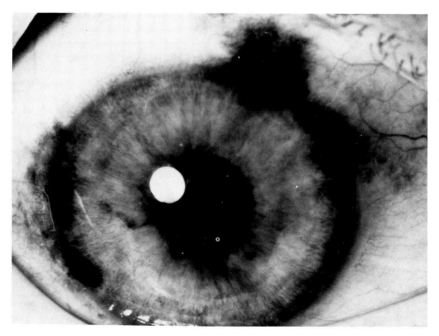

Figure 27-30
Acquired melanosis of the limbal area.

Other Causes of Melanosis
Differential Diagnosis

Complexion-associated or "racial" melanosis of the conjunctiva occurs in dark-skinned individuals, is bilateral, and tends to fade toward the fornices. Conjunctival melanoma is very rarely seen in blacks. Bilateral conjunctival pigmentation can also be seen in systemic conditions, such as Addison's disease (Fig. 27-31), pregnancy, and alkaptonuria. In alkaptonuria the pigmentation is brownish-black, interpalpebral, and can involve the episclera, sclera, and tendons of the horizontal recti. Melanosis can occur after radiation, as a result of drug deposition (e.g., epinephrine, arsenic, thorazine), and in chronic conjunctival disorders such as trachoma, vernal conjunctivitis, and vitamin A deficiency.

Striate melanokeratosis consists of lines of pigment extending out from the normal limbal pigmentation centrally across the cornea. This is seen mainly in blacks but can occur after severe inflammation and injury in other races.

Malignant Melanoma

Malignant melanoma can arise in clear conjunctiva (10% to 20%), from a preexisting nevus (20% to 30%), or from primary acquired melanosis (60%).[122,127,128] It can develop at any age but is rare before the third decade.[129] The annual incidence in Sweden was 0.024 per 100,000.[130] Clinically, the lesions can be pigmented or nonpigmented, are elevated, and can affect any portion of the conjunctiva (Figs. 27-32 and 27-33). Because nevi rarely affect the tarsal or forniceal conjunctiva, when pigmented epithelial lesions are present in these areas malignant melanoma should be suspected. Malignant melanomas can be fungating, plaquoid, or ulcerative. They can extend onto the peripheral cornea, but only rarely are they localized to the cornea.

The overall prognosis is approximately 70% survival at 10 years.[114,128,130,131] Conjunctival melanomas are closer in behavior to melanomas of the skin than to melanomas of the uvea, in that they tend to invade the lymphatics and spread first to regional lymph nodes. Further spread can be prevented in many cases by surgical excision or radiation of involved nodes. The total thickness of the tumor is important in prognosis: Lesions 1.0 mm or less in thickness are much less likely to metastasize than are thicker tumors, but even lesions less than 0.8 mm thick can be lethal.[122,131-133] Metastases are also more likely if the tumor involves the fornix, palpebral conjunctiva, plica, caruncle, or lid margin; invades the sclera or orbit; infiltrates the epithelium in a pagetoid pattern; or recurs.[128,131,133] Histologically, tumors with

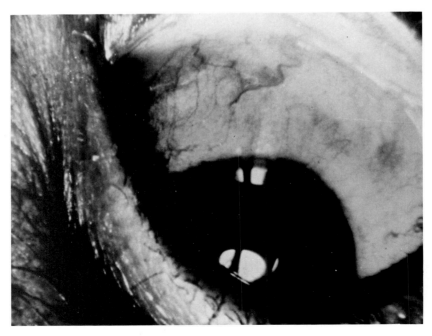

Figure 27-31
Pigmentation of the conjunctiva caused by Addison's disease.

mixed cell type and evidence of lymphatic invasion are associated with increased mortality.[130,131]

Melanomas should be treated by wide local excision, including lamellar sclerectomy or keratectomy if the tumor is fixed to the globe, followed by cryotherapy or beta-irradiation.[128,131,133] If the melanoma arose from primary acquired melanosis, the remaining melanotic areas should also be treated. Patients should be evaluated for the presence of metastasis, and must be followed up regularly for signs of local recurrence as well as distant metastasis. The average time between excision and recurrence is approximately 3.5 years.[128]

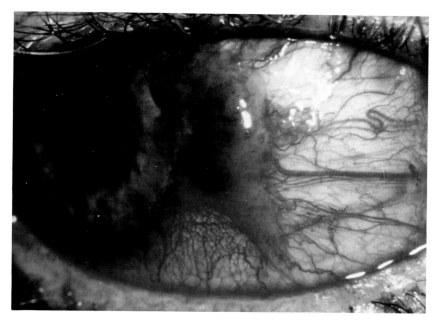

Figure 27-32
Limbal melanoma with extensive vascularization.

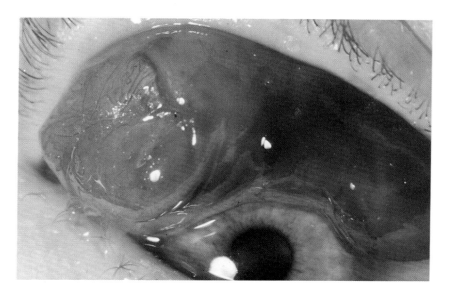

Figure 27-33
Larger limbal malignant melanoma.

REFERENCES

1. Grossniklaus HE, Martin DF, Solomon AR: Invasive conjunctival tumor with keratoacanthoma features, *Am J Ophthalmol* 109:737, 1990.
2. Kincaid MC et al: Iododerma of the conjunctiva and skin, *Ophthalmology* 88:1216, 1981.
3. Ferry AP: Granular cell tumor (myoblastoma) of the palpebral conjunctiva causing pseudoepitheliomatous hyperplasia, *Am J Ophthalmol* 91:234, 1990.
4. Husain SE et al: Primary basal cell carcinoma of the limbal conjunctiva, *Ophthalmology* 100:1720, 1993.
5. Quillen DA et al: Basal cell carcinoma of the conjunctiva, *Am J Ophthalmol* 116:244, 1993.
6. Tsumura T et al: A case of acute myelomonocytic leukemia with subconjunctival tumor, *Jpn J Ophthalmol* 35:226, 1991.
7. Kincaid MC, Green WR: Ocular and orbital involvement in leukemia, *Surv Ophthalmol* 27:211, 1983.
8. White VA et al: Leiomyosarcoma of the conjunctiva, *Ophthalmology* 98:1560, 1991.
9. Ferry AP, Zimmerman LE: Granuloma pyogenicum of limbus simulating recurrent squamous cell carcinoma, *Arch Ophthalmol* 74:229, 1965.
10. Boockvar W, Wessely Z, Ballen P: Recurrent granuloma pyogenicum of limbus, *Arch Ophthalmol* 91:42, 1974.
11. Googe JM et al: Pyogenic granulomas of the cornea, *Surv Ophthalmol* 29:188, 1984.
12. Minckler D: Pyogenic granuloma of the cornea simulating squamous cell carcinoma, *Arch Ophthalmol* 97:516, 1979.
13. De Potter P et al: Pyogenic granuloma of the cornea after penetrating keratoplasty, *Cornea* 11:589, 1992.
14. Ferry AP: Pyogenic granulomas of the eye and ocular adnexa, *Trans Am Ophthalmol Soc* 87:327, 1989.
15. Font RL, Zimmerman LE: Nodular fasciitis of the eye and adnexa: a report of 10 cases, *Arch Ophthalmol* 75:475, 1966.
16. Holds JB, Mamalis N, Anderson RL: Nodular fasciitis presenting as a rapidly enlarging episcleral mass in a 3 year old, *J Pediatr Ophthalmol Strabismus* 27:157, 1990.
17. Bloomfield SE, Jakobiec FA, Iwamoto T: Traumatic intrastromal corneal cyst, *Ophthalmology* 87:951, 1980.
18. Searl SS et al: Corneal hematoma, *Arch Ophthalmol* 102:1647, 1984.
19. O'Grady RB, Kirk HQ: Corneal keloids, *Am J Ophthalmol* 73:206, 1972.
20. Fenton RH, Tredici TJ: Hypertrophic corneal scars (keloids), *Surv Ophthalmol* 9:561, 1964.
21. Holbach LM et al: Bilateral keloid-like myofibroblastic proliferations of the cornea in children, *Ophthalmology* 97:1188, 1990.
22. Smith HC: Keloid of the cornea, *Trans Am Ophthalmol Soc* 38:519, 1940.
23. Frederique G, Howard RO, Boniuk V: Corneal ulcers in rubeola, *Am J Ophthalmol* 68:996, 1969.
24. Cibis GW et al: Corneal keloid in Lowe's syndrome, *Arch Ophthalmol* 100:1795, 1982.
25. Grayson M, Pieroni D: Solitary xanthoma of the limbus, *Br J Ophthalmol* 54:562, 1970.
26. Jakobiec FA: Fibrous histiocytoma of the corneo-scleral limbus, *Am J Ophthalmol* 78:700, 1974.
27. Iwamoto R, Jakobiec FA, Darrell RW: Fibrous histiocytoma of the corneoscleral limbus: the ultrastructure of a distinctive inclusion, *Ophthalmology* 88:1260, 1981.
28. Faludi JE, Kenyon KR, Green WR: Fibrous histiocytoma of the corneoscleral limbus, *Am J Ophthalmol* 80:619, 1975.
29. Pe'er J et al: Malignant fibrous histiocytoma of the conjunctiva, *Br J Ophthalmol* 74:624, 1990.
30. Margo CE, Horton MB: Malignant fibrous histiocytoma of the conjunctiva with metastasis, *Am J Ophthalmol* 104:433, 1989.
31. Knowles DM, Jakobiec FA: Ocular adnexal lymphoid neoplasms: clinical histopathologic, electron microscopic, and immunologic characteristics, *Hum Pathol* 13:148, 1982.
32. Knowles DM, Jakobiec FA: Immunologic characterization of ocular adnexal lymphoid neoplasms, *Am J Ophthalmol* 87:603, 1979.
33. Jakobiec FA, Iwamoto T, Knowles DM: Ocular adnexal lymphoid tumors: correlative ultrastructural and immunologic marker studies, *Arch Ophthalmol* 100:84, 1982.
34. Ellis JH et al: Lymphoid tumors of the ocular adnexa: clinical correlation with the working formulation classification and immunoperoxidase staining of paraffin sections, *Ophthalmology* 92:1311, 1985.
35. Sigelman J, Jakobiec FA: Lymphoid lesions of the conjunctiva: relation of histopathology to clinical outcome, *Ophthalmology* 85:818, 1978.
36. Jakobiec FA et al: Ocular adnexal monoclonal lymphoid tumors with a favorable prognosis, *Ophthalmology* 93:1547, 1986.
37. McNally L, Jakobiec FA, Knowles DM: Clinical morphologic, immunophenotypic, and molecular genetic analysis of bilateral ocular adnexal lymphoid neoplasms in 17 patients, *Am J Ophthalmol* 103:555, 1987.
38. Hardman-Lea S et al: Mucosal-associated lymphoid tissue lymphoma of the conjunctiva, *Arch Ophthalmol* 112:1207, 1994.
39. Petrella T et al: Report of a primary lymphoma of the conjunctiva: a lymphoma of MALT origin?, *Pathol Res Pract* 187:78, 1984.
40. Medeiros LJ, Harris NL: Lymphoid infiltrates of the orbit and conjunctiva, *Am J Surg Pathol* 13:459, 1989.
41. Sundeen JT, Longo DL, Jaffe ES: CD5 expression in B-cell small lymphocytic malignancies: correlations with clinical presentation and sites of disease, *Am J Surg Pathol* 16:130, 1992.
42. Eichler MD, Fraunfelder FT: Cryotherapy for conjunctival lymphoid tumors, *Am J Ophthalmol* 118:463, 1991.

43. Lass JH et al: Detection of human papillomavirus DNA sequences in conjunctival papilloma, *Am J Ophthalmol* 96:670, 1983.

44. Volcker HE, Holbach L: Pedicled papilloma of the conjunctiva with papilloma virus: immunohistochemical detection of species specific papilloma-virus antigens, *Klin Monatsbl Augenheilkd* 187:212, 1985.

45. McDonnell J et al: Demonstration of papillomavirus capsid antigen in human conjunctival neoplasia, *Arch Ophthalmol* 104:1801, 1986.

46. McDonnell PJ et al: Detection of human papillomavirus type 6/11 DNA in conjunctival papillomas by in situ hybridization with radioactive probes, *Hum Pathol* 18:1115, 1987.

47. Naghashfar Z et al: Genital tract papillomavirus type 6 in recurrent conjunctival papilloma, *Arch Ophthalmol* 104:1814, 1986.

48. Wilson FM II, Ostler HB: Conjunctival papillomas in siblings, *Am J Ophthalmol* 77:103, 1977.

49. Bosniak SL, Novick NL, Sachs ME: Treatment of recurrent squamous papillomata of the conjunctiva of carbon dioxide laser vaporization, *Ophthalmology* 93:1078, 1986.

50. Jackson WM, Beraja R, Codere F: Laser therapy of conjunctival papillomas, *Can J Ophthalmol* 22:45, 1987.

51. Yanoff M: Hereditary benign intraepithelial dyskeratosis, *Arch Ophthalmol* 79:291, 1968.

52. Yanoff M, Fine BS: *Ocular pathology,* New York, 1975, Harper & Row.

53. McLean IW et al: Hereditary benign intraepithelial dyskeratosis, *Ophthalmology* 88:164, 1981.

54. Reed JW, Cashwell LF, Klintworth GK: Corneal manifestations of hereditary benign intraepithelial dyskeratosis, *Arch Ophthalmol* 97:297, 1979.

55. Lee GA, Hirst LW: Incidence of ocular surface epithelial dysplasia in metropolitan Brisbane: a 10-year survey, *Arch Ophthalmol* 110:525, 1992.

56. Lee GA et al: Risk factors in the development of ocular surface epithelial dysplasia, *Ophthalmology* 100:360, 1994.

57. McDonnell JM, Mayr AJ, Martin WJ: DNA of human papillomavirus type 16 in dysplastic and malignant lesions of the conjunctiva and cornea, *N Engl J Med* 320:1442, 1989.

58. Lauer SA, Malter JS, Meier JR: Human papillomavirus type 18 in conjunctival intraepithelial neoplasia, *Am J Ophthalmol* 110:23, 1990.

59. McDonnell JM et al: Human papillomavirus DNA in a recurrent squamous carcinoma of the eyelid, *Arch Ophthalmol* 107:131, 1989.

60. McDonnell JM, McDonnell PJ, Sun YY: Human papillomavirus DNA in tissues and ocular surface swabs of patients with conjunctival epithelial neoplasia, *Invest Ophthalmol Vis Sci* 33:184, 1992.

61. Arends MJ, Wyllie AH, Bird CC: Papillomaviruses and human cancer, *Hum Pathol* 21:686, 1990.

62. McDonnell JM et al: Human papillomavirus type 16 DNA in ocular and cervical swabs of women with genital tract condylomata, *Am J Ophthalmol* 112:61, 1991.

63. Blodi FC: Squamous cell carcinoma of the conjunctiva, *Doc Ophthalmol* 34:93, 1973.

64. Wilson FM II: Rose bengal staining of epibulbar squamous neoplasms, *Ann Ophthalmol* 7:21, 1976.

65. Fraunfelder FT, Wingfield D: Management of intraepithelial conjunctival tumors and squamous cell carcinomas, *Am J Ophthalmol* 95:359, 1983.

66. Buuns DR, Tse DT, Folberg R: Microscopically controlled excision of the conjunctival squamous cell carcinoma, *Am J Ophthalmol* 117:97, 1994.

67. de Keizer RJW, de Wolff-Rouendaal D, van Delft JL: Topical application of 5-fluorouracil in premalignant lesions of cornea, conjunctiva and eyelid, *Doc Ophthalmol* 64:31, 1986.

68. Yeatts RP et al: Topical 5-fluorouracil in treating epithelial neoplasia of the conjunctiva and cornea, *Ophthalmology* 102:1338, 1995.

69. Copeland RA Jr, Char DH: Limbal autograft reconstruction after conjunctival squamous cell carcinoma, *Am J Ophthalmol* 110:412, 1990.

70. Waring GO, Ross Am, Ekins MB: Clinical and pathologic description of 17 cases of corneal intraepithelial neoplasia, *Am J Ophthalmol* 97:547, 1984.

71. Campbell RJ, Bourne WM: Unilateral central corneal epithelial dysplasia, *Ophthalmology* 88:1231, 1981.

72. Brown HH et al: Keratinizing corneal intraepithelial neoplasia, *Cornea* 8:220, 1989.

73. Cameron JA, Hidayat AA: Squamous cell carcinoma of the cornea, *Am J Ophthalmol* 111:571, 1991.

74. Zimmerman LE: The cancerous, precancerous, and pseudocancerous lesions of the cornea and conjunctiva. Proceedings of the Second Annual International Corneoplastic Conference, London, 1969, Pergamon Press.

75. Char DH et al: Resection of intraocular squamous cell carcinoma, *Br J Ophthalmol* 76:123, 1992.

76. Glasson WJ et al: Invasive squamous cell carcinoma of the conjunctiva, *Arch Ophthalmol* 112:1342, 1994.

77. Rao NA, Font RL: Mucoepidermoid carcinoma of the conjunctiva: a clinicopathologic study of five cases, *Cancer* 38:1699, 1976.

78. Brownstein S: Mucoepidermoid carcinoma of the conjunctiva with intraocular invasion, *Ophthalmology* 88:1226, 1981.

79. Gamel JW, Eiferman RA, Guibor P: Mucoepidermoid carcinoma of the conjunctiva, *Arch Ophthalmol* 102:730, 1984.

80. Carrau RL, Stillman E, Canaan RE: Mucoepidermoid carcinoma of the conjunctiva, *Ophthal Plast Reconstr Surg* 10:163, 1994.

81. Searl SS et al: Invasive squamous cell carcinoma with intraocular mucoepidermoid features: conjunctival carcinoma with intraocular

invasion and diphasic morphology, *Arch Ophthalmol* 100:109, 1982.

82. Ullman S, Augsburger JJ, Brady LW: Fractionated epibulbar I-125 plaque radiotherapy for recurrent mucoepidermoid carcinoma of the bulbar conjunctiva, *Am J Ophthalmol* 119:102, 1995.

83. Cohen BH et al: Spindle cell carcinoma of the conjunctiva, *Arch Ophthalmol* 98:1809, 1980.

84. Wise AC: A limbal spindle cell carcinoma, *Surv Ophthalmol* 12:244, 1967.

85. Battifora H: Spindle cell carcinoma: ultrastructural evidence of squamous origin and collagen production by tumor cells, *Cancer* 37:2275, 1976.

86. Huntington AC, Langloss JM, Hidayat AA: Spindle cell carcinoma of the conjunctiva: an immunohistochemical and ultrastructural study of six cases, *Ophthalmology* 97:711, 1990.

87. Ni C, Guo BK: Histological types of spindle cell carcinoma of the cornea and conjunctiva: a clinicopathologic report of 8 patients with ultrastructural and immunohistochemical findings in three tumors, *Chin Med J Engl* 103:915, 1990.

88. Foster CS, Allansmith MR: Chronic unilateral blepharoconjunctivitis caused by sebaceous carcinoma, *Am J Ophthalmol* 86:218, 1978.

89. Wolfe JT et al: Sebaceous carcinoma of the eyelid: errors in clinical and pathologic diagnosis, *Am J Surg Pathol* 8:597, 1984.

90. Margo CE, Lessner A, Stern BA: Intraepithelial sebaceous carcinoma of the conjunctiva and skin of the eyelid, *Ophthalmology* 99:227, 1992.

91. Margo CE, Grossniklaus HE: Intraepithelial sebaceous neoplasia without underlying invasive carcinoma, *Surv Ophthalmol* 39:293, 1995.

92. Curran JW, the Centers for Disease Control Task Force on Kaposi's Sarcoma and Opportunistic Infections: Epidemiologic aspects of the current outbreak of Kaposi's sarcoma and opportunistic infections, *N Engl J Med* 306:248, 1982.

93. Holland GN et al: Ocular disorders associated with a new severe acquired cellular immunodeficiency syndrome, *Am J Ophthalmol* 93:393, 1982.

94. Macher A et al: Multicentric Kaposi's sarcoma of the conjunctiva in a male homosexual with acquired immunodeficiency syndrome, *Ophthalmology* 90:879, 1983.

95. Shuler JD et al: Kaposi sarcoma of the conjunctiva and eyelids associated with the acquired immunodeficiency syndrome, *Arch Ophthalmol* 107:858, 1989.

96. Centers for Disease Control: Update: acquired immunodeficiency syndrome, *MMWR* 35:7, 1986.

97. Weiter JJ, Jakobiec FA, Iwamoto T: The clinical and morphologic characteristics of Kaposi's sarcoma of the conjunctiva, *Am J Ophthalmol* 89:546, 1980.

98. Dugel PU et al: Treatment of ocular adnexal Kaposi's sarcoma in acquired immune deficiency syndrome, *Ophthalmology* 99:1127, 1992.

99. Piedbois P et al: Radiotherapy in the management of epidemic Kaposi's sarcoma, *Int J Radiat Oncol Biol Phys* 30:1207, 1994.

100. Ghabrial R et al: Radiation therapy of acquired immunodeficiency syndrome-related Kaposi's sarcoma of the eyelids and conjunctiva, *Arch Ophthalmol* 110:1423, 1992.

101. Hummer J, Gass DJ, Huang AJW: Conjunctival Kaposi's sarcoma treated with interferon alpha-2a, *Am J Ophthalmol* 116:502, 1993.

102. Zimmerman LE: Melanocytes, melanocytic nevi and melanocytomas, *Invest Ophthalmol* 4:11, 1965.

103. Folberg R et al: Benign conjunctival melanocytic lesions: clinicopathologic features, *Ophthalmology* 96:436, 1989.

104. Jakobiec FA, Folberg R, Iwamoto T: Clinicopathologic characteristics of premalignant and malignant melanocytic lesions of the conjunctiva, *Ophthalmology* 96:147, 1989.

105. Kremer I et al: Pigmented epithelial tumors of the conjunctiva, *Br J Ophthalmol* 76:294, 1992.

106. Gilliam JN, Cox AJ: Epidermal changes in vitamin B_{12} deficiency, *Arch Dermatol* 107:231, 1973.

107. Verdaguer J, Valenzuela H, Strozzi L: Melanocytoma of the conjunctiva, *Arch Ophthalmol* 91:363, 1974.

108. Lee JS, Smith RE, Minckler DS: Scleral melanocytoma, *Ophthalmology* 89:178, 1982.

109. Folberg R, McLean IW, Zimmerman LE: Malignant melanoma of the conjunctiva, *Hum Pathol* 16:136, 1985.

110. Jakobiec FA et al: Cryotherapy for conjunctival primary acquired melanosis and malignant melanoma: experience with 62 cases, *Ophthalmology* 95:1058, 1988.

111. Gonzalez-Campora R et al: Blue nevus: classical types and new related entities. A differential diagnostic review, *Pathol Res Pract* 190:627, 1994.

112. Blicker JA, Rootman J, White VA: Cellular blue nevus of the conjunctiva, *Ophthalmology* 99:1714, 1992.

113. Folberg R, McLean IW, Zimmerman LE: Primary acquired melanosis of the conjunctiva, *Hum Pathol* 16:129, 1985.

114. Folberg R, McLean IW, Zimmerman LE: Conjunctival melanosis and melanoma, *Ophthalmology* 91:673, 1984.

115. Griffith WR, Green WR, Weinstein GW: Conjunctival malignant melanoma originating in acquired melanosis sine pigmento, *Am J Ophthalmol* 72:595, 1971.

116. Paridaens AD, McCartney AC, Hungerford JL: Multifocal amelanotic conjunctival melanoma and acquired melanosis sine pigmento, *Br J Ophthalmol* 76:163, 1992.

117. Bataille V et al: Three cases of primary ac-

quired melanosis of the conjunctiva as a manifestation of the atypical mole syndrome, *Br J Dermatol* 128:86, 1993.

118. McCarthy JM et al: Conjunctival and uveal melanoma in the dysplastic nevus syndrome, *Surv Ophthalmol* 37:377, 1993.

119. Reese AB: *Tumors of the eye,* Hagerstown, MD, 1976, Harper & Row.

120. Ackerman AB, Sood R, Koenig M: Primary acquired melanosis of the conjunctiva is melanoma in situ, *Mod Pathol* 4:253, 1991.

121. Jakobiec FA: The ultrastructure of conjunctival melanocytic tumors, *Trans Am Ophthalmol Soc* 82:599, 1984.

122. Spencer WH, Zimmerman LE: *Conjunctiva.* In Spencer WH, editor: *Ophthalmic pathology: an atlas and textbook,* ed 3, vol I, Philadelphia, 1985, WB Saunders.

123. Jakobiec FA, Folberg R, Iwamoto T: Clinicopathologic characteristics of premalignant and malignant melanocytic lesions of the conjunctiva, *Ophthalmology* 96:147, 1989.

124. Folberg R, McLean IW: Primary acquired melanosis and melanoma of the conjunctiva: terminology, classification, and biologic behavior, *Hum Pathol* 15:652, 1986.

125. Jakobiec FA et al: The role of cryotherapy in the management of conjunctival melanoma, *Ophthalmology* 89:502, 1982.

126. Brownstein S et al: Cryotherapy for precancerous melanosis (atypical melanocytic hyperplasia) of the conjunctiva, *Arch Ophthalmol* 99:1224, 1981.

127. De Potter P et al: Clinical predictive factors for development of recurrence and metastasis in conjunctival melanoma: a review of 68 cases, *Br J Ophthalmol* 77:624, 1993.

128. Lommatzsch PK et al: Therapeutic outcome of patients suffering from malignant melanomas of the conjunctiva, *Br J Ophthalmol* 74:615, 1990.

129. McDonnell JM et al: Conjunctival melanocytic lesions in children, *Ophthalmology* 96:986, 1989.

130. Seregard S, Kick E: Conjunctival malignant melanoma in Sweden 1969-91, *Acta Ophthalmol (Copenh)* 70:289, 1992.

131. Paridaens AD et al: Prognostic factors in primary malignant melanoma of the conjunctiva: a clinicopathological study of 256 cases, *Br J Ophthalmol* 78:151, 1994.

132. Silvers D et al: *Melanoma of the conjunctiva: a clinicopathologic study.* In Jakobiec FA, editor: *Ocular and adnexal tumors,* Birmingham, AL, 1978, Aesculapius Publishing Co.

133. Paridaens AD et al: Orbital exenteration in 95 cases of primary conjunctival malignant melanoma, *Br J Ophthalmol* 78:520, 1994.

Index

A

Abdominal pain, 500
Acanthamoeba
  epithelial lesions, 44
  scleritis and, 533
Acanthamoeba keratitis, 36, 269–275
  clinical manifestations of, 270–272
  contact lens wear and care and, 36
  diagnosis of, 272–273
  prevention of, 275
  treatment of, 273–275
Acanthosis nigricans, 638–639
Acetylcholinesterase, 17
Acetylcysteine, 165
Acid burns, 701–703
Acne rosacea, 37, 346
  episcleritis and, 533
  scleritis and, 533
Acquired immune deficiency syndrome, 507–508
  complications associated with, 507
  microsporidial infection, 508
  Molluscum and, 349–351
Acridine orange stain, 65
Acrodermatitis enteropathica, 631
Actinomyces israelii, 43
Acyclovir
  herpes zoster and, 315
  herpetic keratitis and, 301
Acyltransferase deficiency, familial lecithin-cholesterol, 560–561
Adenine arabinoside, herpetic keratitis and, 301
Adenoclone test, 79
Adenovirus, 317–321
  epidemic keratoconjunctivitis and, 317–318
  epidemiology of, 317
  PCR and, 80
  pharyngoconjunctival fever and, 318–321
β-adrenergic receptor blockers, 376
β-adrenergic receptors, 17
Adverse reactions to medications; *see* Toxic and allergic reactions to medications
Aerobic pathways, 23
Aging
  cornea farinata and, 387
  corneal morphological changes, 383
  corneal nerve visibility, 390
  corneal nerve visualization and, 50
  corneal nerves and, 48
  degenerations and, 383
  dellen and, 408
  pinguecula and, 384
AIDS; *see* Acquired immune deficiency syndrome
Airborne allergens, 36
Akylosing spondylitis, scleritis and, 533
Alagille syndrome, 87
Albumin fixative, 78
Alkali burns, 690–701
  pathogenesis of, 692–693
  treatment of, 696–701

Alkaptonuria, 572
Allergic reactions; *see* Toxic and allergic reactions to medications
Allograft, limbal, 378
Alpha-mannosidosis, 572
Alpha-toxin, 342
Alport's syndrome, 653
Amaurosis, Leber's congenital, 454
Amikacin, bacterial ulcerative keratitis and, 231
Amino acid metabolism disorders, 572–579
  alkaptonuria, 572
  amyloidosis, 579–580
  biotinidase deficiency, 585
  cystinosis, 572
  hemochromatosis, 584–585
  hyperuricemia, 582–584
  phenylketonuria, 578–579
  porphyria, 584
  Richner-Hanhart syndrome, 576–578
  tyrosinemia II, 576–578
  Wilson's disease, 580–582
  Zellweger syndrome, 585
Amino acids, epithelium and, 23
Aminoglycosides, 231
Aminoquinolones, 663–664
Amoebae, confocal microscopy detection of, 53
Amphotericin B, 264–265
Ampicillin, 225
Amyloid degenerations, 394–395
Amyloid deposition, 374
Amyloidosis, 394–395, 579–580
  primary, 395
    corneal nerve visualization and, 50
  systemic, lattice dystrophy and, 434
Anaerobic pathways, 23
Anaphylactic reaction, conjunctivitis and, 157
Anaphylactoid blepharoconjunctivitis, 679
Anaphylaxis, 487
Anatomy, 1–22
Anemia, hemolytic, 364
Anesthetics
  abuse of, decreased corneal sensation and, 372
  isolated congenital trigeminal, decreased corneal sensation and, 372
  topical, during cytology, 63–64
  toxicity and, 674–675
Angiitis, allergic, 501
Angioid streaks, fleck dystrophy and, 440
Aniridia, 90, 98
  cornea plana and, 88
  limbal deficiency and, 377
  microcornea and, 87
  Peters' anomaly and, 94
Ankles, hyperextensibility of, 454
Ankyloblepharon, 86
Anterior chamber
  associated immune deviation and, 487
  immunologic characteristics of, 487

Disease
  Buerger-Grütz, 558
  cat-scratch, 132–133
  Crohn's, 498
  Degos', 632
  epithelial; *see* Epithelial disease
  Fabry's, 494, 553
  Farber, 562–563
  fish-eye, 408, 561
  Gaucher's, 553–556
  graft-*versus*-host, 510–511
  Graves', 547
  I-cell, 569
  infectious, 79–80
  inflammatory bowel, 498–499
  Kawasaki, 178
  Kyrle's, 628–629
  linear IgA, 610
  Lyme, 250
  morphological record of, 13
  Newcastle, 38, 112, 322
  Niemann-Pick, 556
  Norrie's, 397
  ocular inflammatory, 395
  Paget's, 397
  peripheral inflammatory, 392
  phlyctenular, 394
  Pompe's, 569
  Refsum, 562
  rheumatic heart, 533
  Sandhoff, 556
  Siemen's, 50
  Tangier, 50, 408, 561–562
  Urbach-Wiethe, 394
  von Gierke's, 569
  von Recklinghausen's, 650–652
  Wilson's, 13, 580–582
Disorders, peripheral inflammatory, 377
DLE; *see* Discoid lupus erythematosus
Donnan's equilibrium, 26
Dots, 417
Down's syndrome, 101, 449
Doxycycline, 347
Drugs; *see also* specific types
  corneal penetration of, 28
  history of, 36–37
  physiology of penetration of, 28
  reactions to; *see* Toxic and allergic reactions
    to medications
  systemic; *see* Systemic drugs
  topical therapy history, 36–37
Dryness of eyes, 31, 358
  radiation treatment and, 37
DTH; *see* Hypersensitivity, delayed-type
Dysautonomia, familial, 648–650
Dysbetalipoproteinemia, 560
Dysgenesis, 85–86
  anterior segment; *see* Anterior segment Dys-
    genesis
  mesodermal, 88
Dyskeratosis
  benign hereditary, 717
  benign intraepithelial, 635
  congenita, 635

Dysplasia
  corneal epithelial, 722
  ectodermal, 356
  mucoepithelial, 635
  squamous, 717–722
Dyspnea, 502
Dysproteinemia, 508–510
Dysproteinemias, 50
Dystrophy, 383
  Avellino corneal, 424, 437
  basement membrane; *see* Epithelium and base-
    ment membrane dystrophy
  Bietti's marginal crystalline, 50, 441–442
  bleblike, 413, 417
  Bowman's layer; *see* Bowman's layer dystrophy
  Cogan's map-dot-fingerprint, 413
  Cogan's microcystic epithelial, 416–421
    clinical manifestations of, 417–419
  congenital hereditary endothelial, 88, 96, 471
  congenital hereditary stromal, 88, 96
  corneal
    decreased corneal sensation and, 372
    recurrent erosions and, 373
  crystalline, 440–441
  dermochondral corneal, 423–424
  dermochondrocorneal of François, 639
  Descemet's, 387
  differentiation from degenerations, 384
  ectatic; *see* Ectatic dystrophies
  endothelial; *see* Endothelial dystrophies
  epithelial basement membrane, 416–421
    recurrent erosions and, 373
  epithelium; *see* Epithelium and basement
    membrane dystrophy
  Filiform, 50
  fleck, 439–440
  François' central cloudy, 442
  François dermochondral, 423–424
  Fuchs', 50, 384
  Fuchs' endothelial; *see* Fuchs' endothelial dystrophy
  gelatinous droplike, 395, 435–437
  granular, 424
  Grayson-Wilbrandt anterior membrane, 423
  honeycomb dystrophy of Thiel and Behnke, 423
  juvenile epithelial corneal, 413
  lattice, 374, 395, 426–429
    forms of, 429
    histopathology of, 429–433
    pathogenesis of, 434–435
    treatment of, 435
  macular, 437–439
    clinical findings, 437
    pathology of, 437–439
    treatment of, 439
  macular corneal, 567–568
  map-dot-fingerprint, 373, 413, 416–421
    clinical manifestations of, 417–419
    histopathology of, 419
    treatment of, 419
  Meesmann's, 413, 415–416
  mouchetée, 439
  Pillat's parenchymatous, 442
  polymorphic stromal, 395
  polymorphous, 50